ATLAS OF
CONTEMPORARY OPHTHALMIC SURGERY

ATLAS OF
CONTEMPORARY OPHTHALMIC SURGERY

Edited by

Henry M. Clayman, M.D.

Clinical Associate Professor of Ophthalmology
Bascom Palmer Eye Institute
University of Miami School of Medicine
Chairman
Department of Ophthalmology
St. Francis Hospital
Miami, Florida

with

Bruce A. Barron, M.D.
Steve T. Charles, M.D.
Robert C. Della Rocca, M.D.
Raymond Harrison, M.D.
Eugene M. Helveston, M.D.
Maurice H. Luntz, M.D.
Marguerite B. McDonald, M.D.
Jesse L. Sigelman, M.D.
Richard R. Tenzel, M.D.

with 1539 tone drawings by
Virginia Hoyt Cantarella
and
Monika Bittman

The C. V. Mosby Company

ST. LOUIS • BALTIMORE • PHILADELPHIA • TORONTO 1990

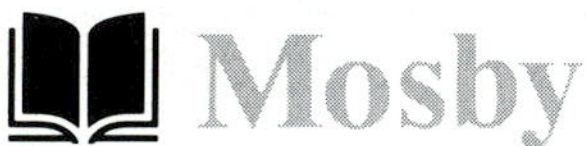

Editor: Eugenia A. Klein
Developmental Editor: Elaine Steinborn
Assistant Editor: Jo Salway
Project Editor: Kathleen L. Teal
Design: Rey Umali
Manuscript Editor: Carl Masthay
Production: Ginny Douglas, Teresa Breckwoldt

Printed in the United States of America

The C. V. Mosby Company
11830 Westline Industrial Drive, St. Louis, Missouri 63146

Library of Congress Cataloging in Publication Data

Atlas of contemporary ophthalmic surgery/edited by Henry M. Clayman, with Bruce A. Barron . . . [et al.]; with 1539 tone drawings by Virginia Hoyt Cantarella and Monika Bittman.
p. cm.
Includes bibliographical references.
ISBN 0-8016-1136-9
1. Eye—Surgery—Atlases. I. Clayman, Henry M. II. Barron, Bruce A.
[DNLM: 1. Eye—surgery—atlases. WW 17 A8803]
RE80.A85 1990
617.7'1—dc20
DNLM/DLC
for Library of Congress 89-13313
CIP

GW/MV/MV 9 8 7 6 5 4 3 2 1

CONTRIBUTORS

Bryan Arthurs, M.D., F.R.C.S.C.
Ophthalmologist
Department of Ophthalmology
Ocular Plastic Surgery
Montreal General Hospital
Sir Mortimer B. Davis—Jewish General Hospital
Lecturer
McGill University
Montreal, Quebec, Canada

Bruce A. Barron, M.D.
Assistant Professor
Department of Ophthalmology
LSU Eye Center
Louisiana State University Medical Center School of Medicine
New Orleans, Louisiana

Patricia E. Bath, M.D.
Associate Professor of Ophthalmology
Principal Investigator, Keratoprosthesis Project
Jules Stein Eye Institute
UCLA Center for Health Sciences
Los Angeles, California

Edward H. Bedrossian, Jr., M.D.
Assistant Surgeon
Department of Ophthalmic Plastic Surgery
Wills Eye Hospital
Thomas Jefferson University
Philadelphia, Pennsylvania

Steve T. Charles, M.D.
Chief, Vitreoretinal Surgery
Department of Ophthalmology
University of Tennessee School of Medicine
Adjunct Faculty Member
Biomedical Engineering Department
Memphis State University
Memphis, Tennessee

Henry M. Clayman, M.D.
Clinical Associate Professor of Ophthalmology
Bascom Palmer Eye Institute
University of Miami School of Medicine
Chairman
Department of Ophthalmology
St. Francis Hospital
Miami, Florida

Robert C. Della Rocca, M.D., F.A.C.S.
Surgeon Director
Oculoplastic and Orbital Service
The New York Eye and Ear Infirmary
New York
Associate Clinical Professor
Department of Ophthalmology
Albert Einstein–Montefiore Medical Center
Bronx
Director, Ophthalmic, Plastic, and Reconstructive Surgery
Department of Ophthalmology,
St. Luke's–Roosevelt Hospital Medical Center
New York, New York

Perry Garber, M.D.
Assistant Clinical Professor of Ophthalmology
Cornell University Medical College
Long Island Jewish Medical Center
North Shore University Hospital
New York Eye and Ear Infirmary
New York, New York

Raymond Harrison, M.D.
Chief, Glaucoma Service
Surgeon Director
Manhattan Eye Ear and Throat Hospital
Consultant Ophthalmologist
New York Eye and Ear Infirmary
New York, New York

Eugene M. Helveston, M.D.
Professor of Ophthalmology
Director, Section of Pediatric Ophthalmology
Indiana University School of Medicine
Indianapolis, Indiana

Kenneth J. Hyde, M.D.
Assistant Clinical Professor
Department of Ophthalmology
University of Texas, Health Science Center—Houston
Houston, Texas

Maurice H. Luntz, M.D.
Clinical Professor
Department of Ophthalmology
Mount Sinai School of Medicine
Consultant Ophthalmologist
Manhattan Eye Ear and Throat Hospital
New York, New York

Marguerite B. McDonald, M.D.
Professor
Department of Ophthalmology
Director, Cornea Service
LSU Eye Center
Louisiana State University Medical Center School of Medicine
New Orleans, Louisiana

Arthur Millman, M.D.
Assistant Professor of Ophthalmology
New York Medical College
Associate Adjunct
New York Eye and Ear Infirmary
New York, New York

Daniel Schaefer, M.D.
Assistant Clinical Professor
Department of Ophthalmology
Assistant Clinical Professor
Department of Otolaryngology
School of Medicine
State University of New York at Buffalo
Buffalo, New York

Jesse L. Sigelman, M.D.
Director, Retinal Vascular Service
New York Hospital–Cornell University Medical College
Director, Diabetic Eye Service
Manhattan Eye Ear and Throat Hospital
New York, New York

Philip Silverstone, M.D.
Attending Physician
Department of Ophthalmology
Hospital of St. Raphael's New Haven
Milford Hospital
Staff Physician
Yale New Haven Hospital
Milford, Connecticut

Richard R. Tenzel, M.D.
Clinical Professor
Department of Ophthalmology
University of Miami Medical School
Miami, Florida

PREFACE

When medical progress is considered, how long is an "era"? For example compare medical developments and their impact on mankind from 1350 to 1750, some 400 years, to the 50 years from 1900 to 1950. In fact there is no comparison because the roots of current medical practice such as asepsis, antibiosis, diagnostics, therapeutics, and surgical techniques are within contemporary memory. I therefore submit to you that an "era" defies temporal dimensions and is defined by the events that it encompasses.

If you accept my thesis, the last 20 years in ophthalmology are certainly an "era" and perhaps the more recent years are a "subera." The profession has seen intraocular lens (IOL) surgery move from a deprecated and vilified procedure to the customary standard of care for cataract patients. Vitreous, the nemesis of cataract surgeons, has become a subspeciality! What was formerly shunned or at the best manipulated with sable brushes, sponges, and scissors is now trimmed, tailored, and removed with a variety of mechanized instruments supported by endoilluminators and lasers. Retinas, formerly buckled externally (itself a great advance), are now amenable, in selected cases, to internal buckling with space-occupying gases and fluids. Retinopathies, heretofore considered hopeless, are often cured or at least attenuated with laser modalities, augmented by vitreous surgery as indicated.

Corneal surgery has been refined and redesigned. Its goals are not only restoration of vision, such as a successful corneal transplant, but also modification of refractive errors, a subspeciality of cornea that will continue to evolve. In glaucoma in the past 20 years we have seen trephine and punch procedures replaced by trabeculotomy and trabeculectomy, which in turn have declined in usage with the introduction of laser trabeculoplasty. Who would have thought that an advance in strabismus surgery was possible, but adjustable sutures have been invaluable in achieving better results. Both strabismus and ocular plastic surgery have benefited by the availability of botulinum toxin A, the paradoxical transformation of a human scourge to ally, and patient awareness to look better and be better has given new impetus to innovation.

This contemporary spurt of progress in ophthalmology has necessitated a new atlas, a need perceived by The C.V. Mosby Company, who asked me to edit this work. I have tried to produce a comprehensive work without miring the reader in every variation of technique. Moreover it will be noted that where subspecialities overlap the contributors do not always agree on technique and management for a given condition. This discordance is in reality a search for a "better way." It is this quest that has propelled medicine and ophthalmology to its current level of care, a level that undoubtedly will attain new heights as we move into the next "era."

The publisher and I are most grateful to the contributors for their outstanding efforts in the completion of this atlas.

Henry M. Clayman, M.D.

CONTENTS

PART ONE

CORNEAL SURGERY

Bruce A. Barron
Marguerite B. McDonald

CHAPTER 1

Essentials of Corneal Surgery

Successful corneal surgery depends on knowledge of corneal function and anatomy, a summary of which is given below. Included in this summary are descriptions of various examination techniques and the instrumentation used to clinically evaluate the cornea. The diagnosis and medical management of every corneal disorder and an exhaustive review of the indications for surgical intervention are beyond the scope of this atlas. However, concepts that are helpful in deciding when surgery is indicated are provided, and general principles of corneal surgery are outlined. Descriptions and illustrations of specific corneal surgical procedures follow in Chapters 2 to 6.

CORNEAL FUNCTIONS

There are three functions of the cornea: (1) maintenance of the integrity of the eye, (2) provision of a clear window through which light can pass to the posterior segment, and (3) refraction. Corneal surgery is directed toward preserving, restoring, or improving at least one of these functions (Table 1-1).

The most rudimentary function of the cornea is to maintain the integrity of the eye. Although this function is directly addressed with corneal trauma and thinning disorders, it should also be addressed with any corneal disorder. The importance of the epithelium in maintaining the integrity of the eye cannot be overemphasized. Trauma to the epithelium (such as exposure, dry eyes, trichiasis) that causes a chronic epithelial defect and subsequent thinning of the cornea is a frequently unrecognized condition that complicates corneal surgery.

Corneal transparency depends on the geometric arrangement of collagen fibrils and the state of relative dehydration of the stroma, in which the endothelial cells play a vital role. To provide a clear window, the cornea is avascular and must therefore meet its metabolic requirements from sources other than blood. Oxygen is obtained from the atmosphere through the anterior surface; other nutrients are obtained from the aqueous humor through the posterior surface.

The cornea is responsible for approximately two thirds of the refractive power of the eye. Actually, most of this refraction takes place at the air–tear film interface. For simplicity, however, the cornea will be considered responsible for this refraction, since the curvature of the tear film approximates the curvature of the anterior corneal surface and the refractive indices of the tear film and the

TABLE 1-1
Goals of Corneal Surgical Procedures

Goals	Surgical procedures
Corneal integrity	Penetrating keratoplasty Inlay lamellar keratoplasty Onlay lamellar keratoplasty Conjunctival flap*
Corneal transparency	Penetrating keratoplasty Lamellar keratectomy Excision of pterygium
Corneal refractive power	Penetrating keratoplasty Inlay lamellar keratoplasty Onlay lamellar keratoplasty Excision of pterygium Keratophakia Keratomileusis Intracorneal lens implantation Epikeratophakia Radial keratotomy Compression sutures Wedge resection Arcuate relaxing incisions Trapezoidal keratotomy Transverse incisions

*A conjunctival flap should not be used as the sole treatment for a corneal perforation.

cornea are similar. The refractive power of a spherical surface is dependent on the curvature of the surface and the refractive indices of the media on either side of the surface, as indicated by the following equation:

$$D = (n_2 - n_1)/r$$

where n_2 is the index of refraction of the second medium, n_1 is the index of refraction of the first medium, r is the radius of curvature of the surface in meters, and D is the refractive power of a spherical surface in diopters. The index of refraction is 1.000 for air, 1.376 for cornea, and 1.336 for aqueous humor. For an average cornea the refractive power of the anterior surface is +48.8 diopters [(1.376 − 1.000)/0.0077 meter], the refractive power of the posterior surface is −5.8 diopters [(1.336 − 1.376)/0.0069 m], and the total refractive power is +43 diopters (48.8 − 5.8). The refractive power of the cornea can be changed by alteration of the anterior curvature, the posterior curvature, or the index of refraction of the cornea. The difference between the indices of refraction of air and cornea (1.000 versus 1.376) is greater than the difference between the indices of refraction of cornea and aqueous humor (1.376 versus 1.336). Therefore a change in the anterior curvature affects the refractive power more than a change in the posterior curvature. This principle is used in virtually all refractive procedures, such as radial keratotomy, keratomileusis, keratophakia, epikeratophakia, and astigmatic keratectomy or keratotomy. The one exception is intrastromal implantation of a material with a high index of refraction, such as polysulfone—a procedure that is not clinically successful at the present time.

PATIENT EVALUATION AND PREPARATION

There are three questions to ask when one is evaluating a cornea for surgery. These questions are based on the three functions of the cornea described above.

First, is the cornea intact? If the cornea is perforated, it must be repaired. A perforation without tissue loss, as can occur from trauma, can usually be repaired with sutures. A perforation with tissue loss, which can occur from trauma, dry eyes, a chronic epithelial defect, an infection, or an immunologic disorder (such as rheumatoid arthritis), can be repaired with cyanoacrylate adhesive or tissue. The decision whether to use cyanoacrylate adhesive or tissue is discussed further in Chapter 3. If tissue replacement is indicated, corneal tissue is usually preferred and can be used as a lamellar or penetrating graft, depending on the location and cause of the perforation. A central perforation is usually best repaired with a penetrating graft; a peripheral perforation is usually best repaired with a lamellar graft. A lamellar graft is contraindicated in an active infection because of the risk of postoperative spread of the infection in the graft/host interface. An area of corneal thinning that has not perforated but is threatening the integrity of the eye, such as a descemetocele, must also be repaired. Corneal tissue is usually preferred, but periosteum is useful for peripheral thinning caused by an immunologic disorder. An important principle in the surgical management of any corneal thinning or perforation is to treat the underlying disorder. Otherwise, thinning will recur. Mild to moderate corneal thinning by itself is not an indication for surgical intervention. If the disorder responsible for the thinning is stable, the integrity of the eye is not threatened, and the thinning is not causing decreased visual acuity (such as Terrien's marginal degeneration causing astigmatism that can be corrected with glasses or a contact lens), the thinning should be left alone.

Corneal thinning is best assessed and followed by slitlamp examination. Pachymetry may also be useful. If corneal thinning is causing astigmatism, it can be followed by refraction, keratometry, and keratoscopy. The Seidel test is invaluable in allowing assessment of a possible corneal perforation. Sterile concentrated fluorescein is applied to the surface of the cornea, and the cornea is examined at the slitlamp with cobalt blue light. Leakage of aqueous humor appears as a stream of apple-green fluid. If the leakage is intermittent or the eye is hypotonus, the Seidel test may be falsely negative unless gentle pressure is applied to the eye. It may also be falsely negative if the perforation is plugged with iris.

Second, is the cornea clear enough for light to pass unimpeded to the posterior segment? The density and location of a corneal opacity and the age of the patient are important in determining whether surgery is indicated. A dense central opacity decreases visual acuity and should be removed. If the opacity is superficial, it may be removed by lamellar keratectomy. An inlay lamellar graft can be placed if the cornea underlying the opacity is thin. The bed of a lamellar keratectomy is usually irregular, however, which may limit postoperative visual acuity, and penetrating keratoplasty may be preferred in these cases. If the opacity is deep, penetrating keratoplasty is indicated.

The effect of less dense opacities on visual acuity is frequently difficult to assess. The appearance of the opacity can be deceptive. For example, opacities caused by granular dystrophy are conspicuous on slitlamp examination, but visual acuity is usually not affected because there are small intervening areas of clear cornea. A scar caused by interstitial keratitis often appears worse than the effect it has on visual acuity. Laser interferometry may be helpful in assessment of the effect corneal opacities have on visual acuity. If a corneal opacity does not permit visualization of the posterior segment, ancillary tests, such as ultrasound or electrophysiologic tests, must be used to assess the posterior segment. An opacity in a child is more visually significant than one in an adult because of the risk of deprivation amblyopia. For example, corneal blood staining that might be left to resolve in an adult would be an indication for penetrating keratoplasty in a child because of the amblyopia that would develop during the time it would take for the blood to clear.

Third, how is the cornea affecting the refractive power of the eye? The refractive power of the cornea is assessed by objective and subjective refraction (with and without a hard contact lens), keratometry, and keratoscopy. A diagnostic hard contact lens is invaluable in the determination of best corrected visual acuity in an eye with an abnormal cornea because of the smooth anterior surface it provides. Keratometry and keratoscopy are done before any type of refractive surgery is considered. The type of refractive surgery depends on the type of refractive error and whether the cornea is otherwise normal. For keratoconus, penetrating keratoplasty or onlay lamellar keratoplasty are considered. Options for aphakia include secondary intraocular lens implantation, keratophakia, keratomileusis, and epikeratophakia. Keratomileusis, epikeratophakia, and radial keratotomy are possibilities for myopia. For peripheral thinning disorders that cause astigmatism, such as Terrien's marginal degeneration, a crescentic or doughnut-shaped inlay lamellar graft or a 12 mm onlay lamellar graft may be used. There are many surgical procedures for astigmatism, which are described in detail in Chapter 5. The most important concept in the preoperative evaluation of any patient considering refractive surgery is to determine that the patient is indeed spectacle and contact lens intolerant.

SURGICAL ANATOMY

Gross anatomy

The cornea forms the outer coat of the anterior sixth of the eye. The posterior surface of the cornea is circular and measures 12 mm in diameter; the anterior surface is oval and measures 12 mm horizontally and 11 mm vertically. The oval shape of the anterior surface is the result of a more prominent limbus superiorly and inferiorly than medially and laterally.

The thickness of the cornea varies from 0.5 mm centrally to 1 mm peripherally because of the variation in the curvature of the anterior corneal surface. Corneal thickness is measured clinically with an optical or ultrasonic pachymeter. Either type of pachymeter can be used during a routine examination; only an ultrasonic pachymeter, however, can be used intraoperatively. The thickness of the central cornea is usually measured for assessment of the general health of the corneal endothelial cells. Thicknesses in other areas are measured for evaluation of corneal swelling or thinning in those areas, or as part of certain surgical procedures, such as radial keratotomy, for determination of the depth to make incisions.

There are many ways to describe the cornea topographically. The "center" of the cornea is a nonspecific term because it can refer to the geometric center, the visual center (the point where the visual axis or the line of sight intersects the cornea), or the apical center (the apex of the cornea). Geographically the cornea can be divided into "central," "paracentral," and "peripheral" areas. Although these terms may be useful in gross descriptions of the cornea, the boundaries of the areas are vague and artificially drawn. The cornea can also be mapped in terms of "axes" or "meridians," which are lines passing through the geometric center of the cornea. An axis is a straight line, whereas a meridian is a curved line that follows the anterior corneal surface. These terms are essential in understanding corneal astigmatism. Although clock hours can be used for orientation (with the superior cornea at 12 o'clock and the inferior cornea at 6 o'clock), the axis or meridian expressed in degrees (with the superior cornea at 90 degrees and the inferior cornea at 270 degrees) is more precise. Other terms used to describe the location of corneal astigmatism are "with the rule" and "against the rule." "With the rule" refers to a steep vertical meridian; "against the rule" refers to a steep horizontal meridian.

The curvatures of the anterior and posterior corneal surfaces can be expressed in millimeters or diopters (D). The curvature in millimeters can be converted to diopters by the equation

$$D = (n_2 - n_1)/r$$

where n_2 is the index of refraction of the second medium, n_1 is the index of refraction of the first medium, and r is the radius of curvature of the surface in meters. The radius of curvature of the posterior corneal surface is uniform and is 6.9 mm. The radius of curvature of the anterior corneal surface varies; it is 7.7 mm centrally and increases as the cornea flattens peripherally.

Corneal curvature can be evaluated by keratometry and keratoscopy. Keratometry evaluates a limited area of the cornea (3 mm); keratoscopy evaluates a much larger area and is therefore more useful. There are various types of keratometers, some of which can be used intraoperatively, such as the Terry keratometer. There are also various types of keratoscopes. Placido's disc is the forerunner of modern keratoscopes. The principle behind all keratoscopes involves (1) reflection of a circular object from the anterior corneal surface and

(2) examination of that reflection. The circular object can be as simple as the end of a safety pin, but it usually consists of one or more concentric rings of light. One can evaluate the reflection directly by visual inspection or indirectly by taking a photograph, which can be analyzed qualitatively or quantitatively. Quantitative computer analysis can produce a color-coded contour map of the anterior corneal surface, which is easier to interpret than the original photograph. Intraoperative keratoscopes, such as the Troutman keratoscope, are available. At present, these keratoscopes provide only qualitative information, but this information is useful at the time of certain refractive procedures.

Microscopic anatomy

Histologically the cornea is composed of six layers: (1) epithelium, (2) basement membrane of the epithelium, (3) Bowman's layer, (4) stroma, (5) Descemet's membrane (basement membrane of the endothelium), and (6) endothelium. More simply, the cornea can be thought of as stroma sandwiched between two cell layers with their basement membranes.

The corneal epithelium is nonkeratinized stratified squamous epithelium four to six cells thick. It contains a basal cell layer, a wing cell layer, and a superficial cell layer. The basal cell layer is the germinative layer. As the cells mature, they move anteriorly, become wing cells and then superficial cells, and desquamate. This anterior migration takes approximately 7 days. An epithelial defect heals by sliding of adjacent epithelial cells to cover the defect, followed by proliferation of these cells to form an epithelium of normal thickness. Corneal epithelial cells are attached to one another by desmosomes. Basal cells are secured to the basement membrane and underlying cornea by hemidesmosomes. The superficial cells have tight junctions, which form an important barrier that prevents certain substances in the tear film from moving into the cornea. This barrier is also the reason that fluid can collect underneath the epithelium to form bullae.

The basement membrane of the epithelium is secreted by the basal epithelial cells and, with the hemidesmosomes, is responsible for adherence of the epithelium to the underlying cornea. Diseases that are associated with abnormal basement membrane, such as diabetes mellitus, are frequently associated with recurrent or chronic epithelial defects.

Bowman's layer can be considered a modification of the anterior stroma. It is composed of randomly oriented collagen fibrils that have a smaller diameter than the collagen fibrils of the rest of the stroma. Bowman's layer develops during fetal life and does not regenerate if injured. Therefore diseases or surgical procedures that damage Bowman's layer result in scarring. Prevention of this scarring has become an important goal in the development of photoablative keratectomy procedures. Bowman's layer contributes to the rigidity of the anterior corneal surface, which must be taken into consideration in refractive surgery.

The corneal stroma is composed of collagen fibrils that are grouped in lamellae that extend from limbus to limbus. The lamellae are parallel to one another, which aids in lamellar dissection of the cornea. The collagen fibrils are surrounded by ground substance, which consists primarily of keratin sulfate and chondroitin sulfate. The stroma also contains keratocytes, which produce the collagen fibrils and ground substance. Normally keratocytes have a low metabolic rate, but with injury to the cornea, they can become fibroblastic. Stromal wounds heal slowly because of the avascularity of the cornea.

Descemet's membrane is the basement membrane of the corneal endothelium. It is composed of an anterior banded portion, which is secreted during fetal life, and a posterior nonbanded portion, which continues to be secreted after birth. The nonbanded portion therefore increases in thickness with age. Descemet's membrane is a relatively resilient structure. It frequently remains intact, forming a descemetocele, when the rest of the cornea has melted. When Descemet's membrane is severed, the cut ends curl toward the stroma. Adjacent endothelial cells slide over the wound and secrete a new Descemet's membrane composed only of nonbanded material.

The corneal endothelium is one cell layer thick and is vital in regulating corneal hydration. Endothelial cells have limited, if any, regenerative capacity in humans. When endothelial cells are injured, the remaining endothelial cells enlarge and spread out to cover the area of injury. When there are too few endothelial cells to cover the cornea contiguously, or they are unable to adequately regulate corneal hydration, corneal edema ensues. The number of endothelial cells is usually expressed in terms of cell density (cells/mm^2). The density is measured clinically with a specular photomicroscope. Normal cell density is approximately 4000 cells/mm^2 at birth and decreases with age. Other parameters used to describe endothelial cells are variation in shape (pleomorphism) and size (polymegathism). Although endothelial cell density indicates the number of endothelial cells, it does not assess their function. An indirect measure of endothelial cell function is corneal thickness.

GENERAL PRINCIPLES OF CORNEAL SURGERY

The general principles of corneal surgery are similar to those of other anterior segment surgery. Preoperative preparation may include a mydriatic or miotic agent, depending on whether the corneal surgery is to be intraocular or extraocular and on what concomitant intraocular surgery is planned. An osmotic agent, such as intravenous mannitol, may be given if intraocular surgery is planned and posterior pressure is unwanted. Whereas a soft eye is desirable for many intraocular procedures, it is undesirable for certain extraocular corneal procedures, such as procedures that involve lamellar keratectomy, and virtually all the refractive surgical procedures.

Anesthesia for most corneal procedures is similar to that required for cataract extraction, that is, peribulbar or retrobulbar anesthesia, and in some cases general anesthesia. Some procedures, including limited lamellar keratectomies (such as corneal biopsy) and keratotomies (such as radial keratotomy), are most safely done with a topical anesthetic, such as 1% proparacaine hydrochloride. Topical 4% cocaine solution is a valuable adjunct for obtaining limbal anesthesia, which is necessary for stabilization of the eye with forceps. One best applies cocaine solution by saturating a cotton-tipped applicator or cellulose sponge with the solution and holding it at the limbus. Cocaine is toxic to the corneal epithelium, and care is taken to keep it from touching the epithelium. (In onlay lamellar keratoplasty the toxicity of cocaine to the corneal epithelium is used as an advantage to remove the epithelium.)

There are two important differences between corneal surgery and other ocular surgery: the techniques for making incisions and the techniques for closing them. Incisions required for most corneal procedures should be perpendicular to the anterior corneal surface. The notable exception is lamellar keratectomy without placement of a lamellar graft, where the incisions should be angled so that epithelium can heal over the lamellar bed more easily. These perpendicular incisions are in contradistinction to angled cataract incisions, and a conscious effort is required to make them.

Full-thickness corneal wounds are closed with sutures placed deeply and tied with more tension than that required for limbal wounds. Partial-thickness corneal wounds are closed with sutures placed more superficially and tied more loosely. The most common suture for corneal surgery is 10-0 nylon. Thicker suture (9-0 nylon) is used in some procedures, such as penetrating keratoplasty combined with posterior segment surgery. Thinner suture (11-0 nylon) is used as an ancillary suture in penetrating keratoplasty; it is not strong enough to secure wound closure alone, however. Mersilene (polyethylene terephthalate polyester fiber) and Prolene (polypropylene) may also be used. Larger sutures and sutures that incite inflammation are undesirable. Because of the slow healing rate of the stroma, corneal sutures must be left in place much longer than sutures used in other areas of the eye.

The various corneal procedures, with emphasis on surgical principles, are described and illustrated in the following chapters in this section.

CHAPTER 2

Penetrating Keratoplasty

There are five primary indications for penetrating keratoplasty: (1) maintenance of the integrity of the eye (as in repair of a corneal perforation), (2) restoration of corneal clarity (as in removal of a corneal scar), (3) restoration of a normal anterior corneal surface (as in penetrating keratoplasty for keratoconus), (4) restoration of normal corneal physiology (as in treatment of bullous keratopathy), and (5) elimination of a central corneal infection (as in surgical management of central infectious keratitis that is unresponsive to medical therapy and is spreading toward the periphery). Elimination of pain, may be a secondary indication for penetrating keratoplasty but is not an indication by itself. Frequently there is a combination of the above indications in many of the corneal disorders for which penetrating keratoplasty is done.

The surgical techniques of penetrating keratoplasty have improved dramatically since 1906, when Zirm reported a successful penetrating keratoplasty in a patient with a chemical burn. Advances have been made in eye banking and donor corneal preservation, microsurgical instruments, needles and suture material, and medications.

With current techniques the success rate for penetrating keratoplasty is greater than 95% in good prognosis cases, such as keratoconus. In poor prognosis cases, such as severe dry eyes, chemical burns, pemphigoid, or Stevens-Johnson syndrome, the success rate is much lower and approaches zero percent. Nevertheless, penetrating keratoplasty should be done initially in patients in whom there is some chance for success because the only alternative is prosthokeratoplasty, which has a high incidence of long-term complications (see Chapter 6).

There are many techniques for penetrating keratoplasty. The techniques described in this chapter are those that, in our experience, produce the best results.

PREOPERATIVE MEDICATIONS

Three types of preoperative medications are considered in penetrating keratoplasty: miotic or mydriatic agents, hypotensive agents, and corticosteroids. A topical miotic agent, such as pilocarpine hydrochloride, is given to a phakic eye with a clear lens, to an eye with an intraocular lens that will not be removed, and to an aphakic eye with an intact vitreous face that is posterior to the pupil.

A topical mydriatic agent is given to an eye with a cataract that will be extracted and to an eye with a posterior chamber intraocular lens that will be removed. A miotic or mydriatic agent is not given to an aphakic eye if a vitrectomy is anticipated. A soft eye is usually desirable in penetrating keratoplasty and is achieved by preoperative intermittent external pressure. In addition, a systemic hypotensive agent, such as intravenous mannitol, may be given if there are no contraindications. Systemic corticosteroids are given for several days preoperatively to a patient with ocular inflammation (including patients with a history of keratitis), a previous corneal graft rejection, or an increased risk for corneal graft rejection.

POSTOPERATIVE MEDICATIONS

At the end of penetrating keratoplasty, methylprednisolone acetate is injected subconjunctivally except in an eye with an active infection, a history of herpes simplex keratitis, or corticosteroid-induced glaucoma. A topical corticosteroid, antibotic, cycloplegic agent,and, if appropriate, hypotensive agent are applied, and an eye pad and shield are placed.

Postoperatively, a topical antibiotic, cycloplegic agent, and corticosteroid are started. The antibiotic is usually only necessary until the corneal epithelium has healed; prolonged use may be toxic to the epithelium. The choice of cycloplegic agent depends on the corneal disorder for which penetrating keratoplasty is done and concomitant intraocular procedures. A mild cycloplegic agent, such as cyclopentolate hydrochloride, is used in keratoconus because of reports of permanent pupillary dilatation after the use of stronger cycloplegic agents. If a posterior chamber intraocular lens has been implanted, it may be wise to use a mild cycloplegic agent, such as cyclopentolate, instead of a stronger cycloplegic agent, which can cause the iris to capture the edge of the intraocular lens. A strong cycloplegic agent, such as scopolamine hydrobromide or atropine sulfate, is indicated in a phakic or aphakic eye with inflammation. The frequency and duration of topical corticosteroids depend on the corneal disorder for which penetrating keratoplasty is done, the amount of postoperative inflammation, and the phakic status of the eye. If penetrating keratoplasty is done for a failed graft from a prior graft rejection, or if there is pronounced postoperative inflammation, systemic and topical corticosteroids are given. Topical corticosteroids are not used as long in a phakic eye as in an aphakic or pseudophakic eye because of the risk of corticosteroid-induced cataract. We usually use once-a-day or once-every-other-day topical corticosteroids indefinitely in an aphakic or pseudophakic eye if there are no contraindications, such as corticosteroid-induced glaucoma. In an eye with a history of herpes simplex keratitis, topical trifluridine is given with a frequency equal to that of the topical corticosteroids.

Providing Scleral Support

The shape of a normal phakic eye is maintained by the cornea, sclera, lens-iris diaphragm, vitreous, and aqueous humor (intraocular pressure). In every penetrating keratoplasty at least two of these factors are eliminated: corneal integrity and intraocular pressure. Removal of the lens eliminates another support, and removal of the vitreous leaves only the sclera to support the eye. The sclera alone is infrequently rigid enough to maintain the shape of the eye, especially in a young patient. Therefore, a ring is sutured to the superficial sclera so that the eye will not collapse. Although a ring may not be necessary in some older patients in whom the lens and vitreous are not removed, we routinely use a ring in all patients because once an eye starts to collapse it is difficult to suture a ring to the sclera without the risk of prolapsing the intraocular contents.

There are a variety of rings for supporting the sclera. We prefer the McNeill-Goldman ring, which is a combined scleral support ring and blepharostat (Fig. 2-1). It consists of a small anterior ring connected to a larger posterior ring by four radial struts. Two blepharostats are attached to the anterior ring. The anterior ring is sutured to the superficial sclera with four interrupted 5-0 Dacron sutures. To prevent rotation of the eye, at least one of the sutures is wrapped around one of the struts. The McNeill-Goldman ring thus provides scleral support, blepharostasis, and stabilization of the eye. It does not permit much intraoperative movement of the eye, however. Therefore, in a patient in whom intraoperative movement of the eye is desirable (as in one undergoing combined penetrating keratoplasty and posterior segment surgery), we use Jaffe lid specula, a Flieringa ring, and sutures through the superior and inferior rectus muscles instead of the McNeill-Goldman ring. We also use this method if it becomes apparent that the posterior ring of the McNeill-Goldman ring is applying pressure on the eye as the anterior ring is sutured to the sclera.

Improper suturing of any scleral support ring can distort the cornea and lead to postoperative astigmatism. A misplaced or tight suture distorts the cornea, which may cause noticeable corneal striae, or may not become apparent until after the recipient corneal button has been removed and the edge of the corneal opening is pulled toward the tight suture (Fig. 2-2). It is therefore important that the scleral sutures be placed immediately beneath the ring in a radial fashion and that they be tied just tight enough to support the sclera.

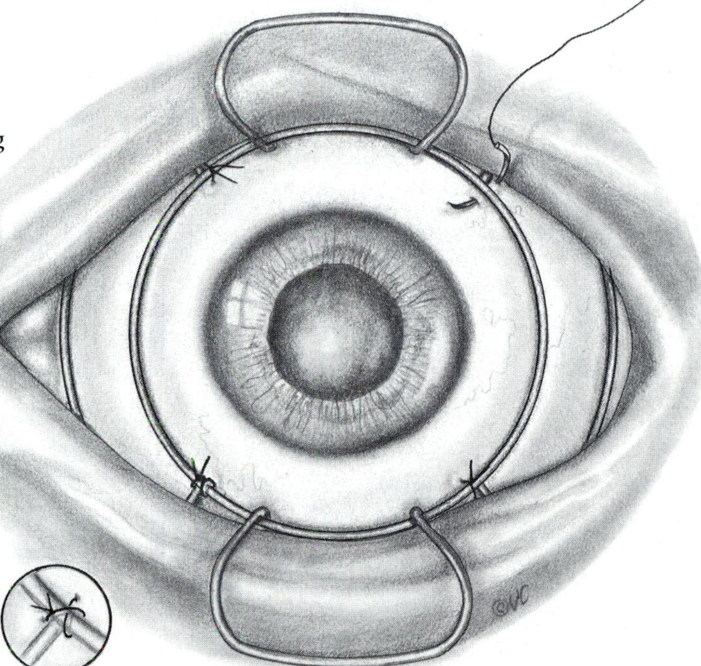

FIGURE 2-1. Suturing McNeill-Goldman ring to superficial sclera.

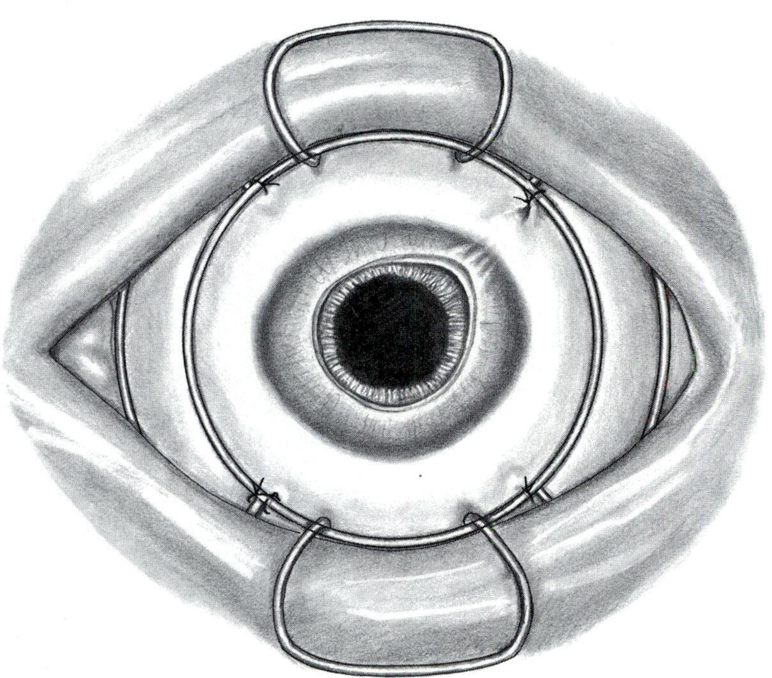

FIGURE 2-2. Corneal distortion caused by improperly sutured McNeill-Goldman ring.

Trephining the Recipient Cornea

Because an eccentric corneal graft increases the incidence of corneal graft rejection and postoperative astigmatism, we usually center the graft in the geometric center of the cornea by marking the center with a surgical marking pen (Fig. 2-3) and centering a trephine that does not have an internal obturator on this mark. A trephine that has an internal obturator can be centered on the cornea only by examination of the amount of corneal tissue surrounding the blade.

Several trephines have been developed to cut the recipient cornea. The standard trephine, to which all trephines are compared, is a tubular stainless steel blade, with or without a handle that contains an internal obturator, that is held between the thumb and index finger of the dominant hand (Fig. 2-4). We believe it is difficult to cut the cornea evenly with this type of trephine. A trephine with an internal obturator may distort the cornea if the obturator touches the apex of the cornea before the blade cuts the cornea (Fig. 2-5). This distortion frequently occurs in keratoconus and may be prevented by the use of a trephine without an internal obturator or by thermal shrinkage and flattening of the cone, which is done by light cauterization of the central cornea (Fig. 2-6).

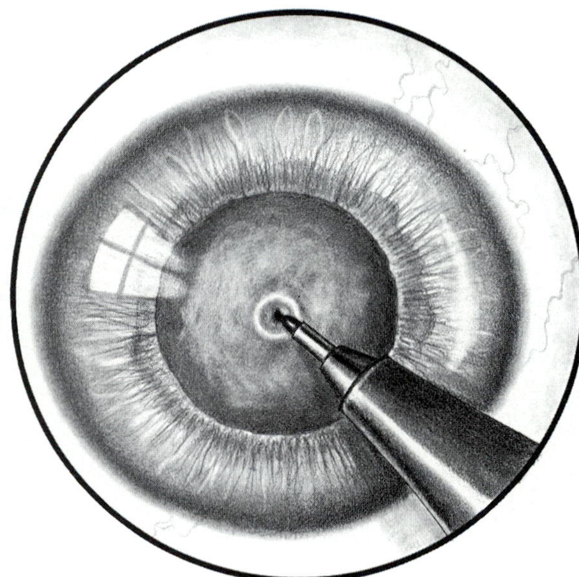

FIGURE 2-3. Marking center of cornea with marking pen.

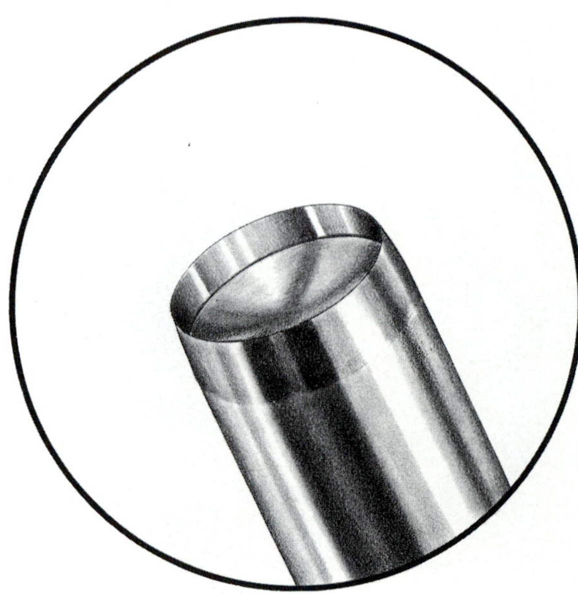

FIGURE 2-4. Standard trephine with a handle that contains an internal obturator.

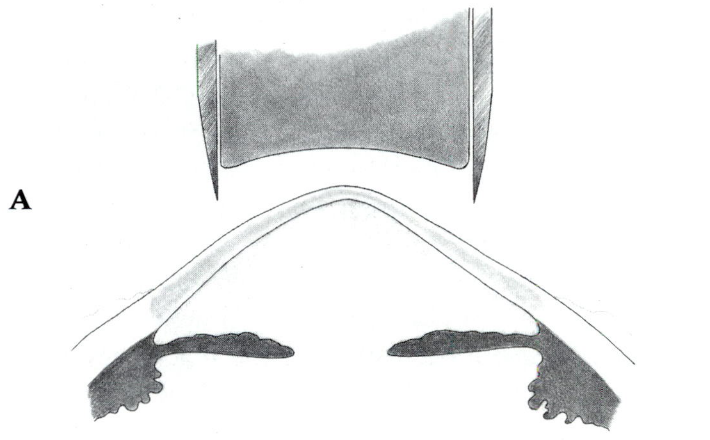

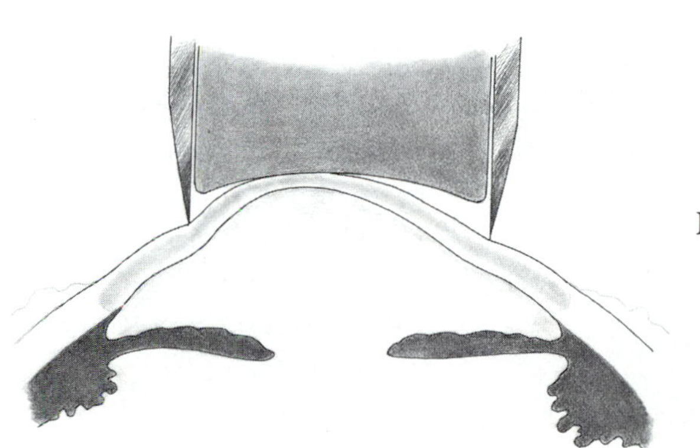

FIGURE 2-5. Corneal distortion from internal obturator.

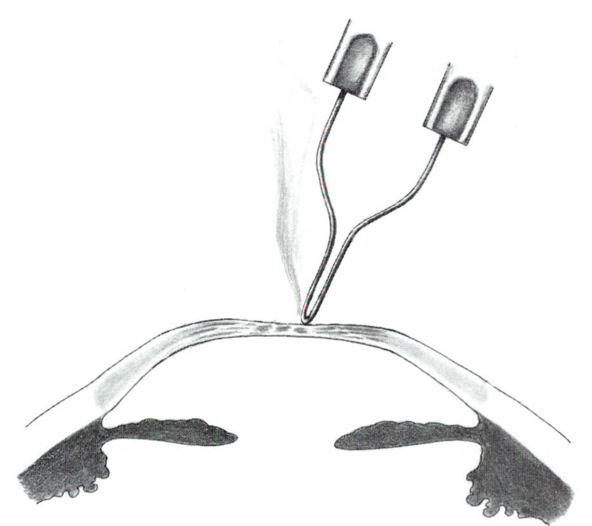

FIGURE 2-6. Shrinking cone centrally with cautery.

We prefer the Hessburg-Barron vacuum trephine to other trephines for most penetrating keratoplasties. This trephine consists of a blade assembly and a vacuum chamber connected by a silicone tube to a syringe with a spring-loaded plunger (Fig. 2-7). The vacuum chamber has an outer wall and an inner wall, between which a vacuum can be created to fixate the cornea. Inside the inner wall is a thin stainless steel blade bent in a circular fashion (Fig. 2-8). It is notched where the two ends meet. The blade is attached to a blade assembly that has a screw apparatus and can be lowered or raised by turning the plastic spokes on top of the blade assembly clockwise or counterclockwise, respectively.

Before placement of the trephine on the cornea, the edge of the blade is aligned with the inner wall of the vacuum chamber ("zeroing the blade"). The blade is then retracted (raised) so that it does not interfere with apposition of the cornea to the walls of the vacuum chamber. Although the blade may be retracted any number of turns, a total of three quarter-turns is sufficient.

After the blade has been retracted, one supports the trephine by holding the plastic platforms on top of the trephine with the thumb and index finger of the nondominant hand, looks through the center of the trephine, and aligns the crosshairs with the centration mark previously made. After the trephine is centered, the plunger of the syringe is pushed in all the way, the trephine is pressed gently and evenly on the corneal surface, and the plunger of the syringe is released abruptly. There are two ways to tell if a vacuum has been obtained and the cornea is fixated: (1) the plunger of the syringe should not extend all the way, and (2) the trephine should remain firmly on the cornea when the plastic platforms on top of the trephine are released. If a vacuum has not been obtained, the surface of the cornea is moistened with balanced salt solution and the process is repeated. Balanced salt solution should not be placed in the center of the trephine because it masks the recognition of aqueous humor should the blade perforate the cornea during trephination. It is rare for a vacuum not to be obtained if the above process is done correctly. However, pronounced irregularities of the corneal surface may prevent even apposition of the cornea to the walls of the vacuum chamber. If these irregularities are caused by edematous epithelium, the epithelium is removed or a viscoelastic substance is placed on the anterior corneal surface.

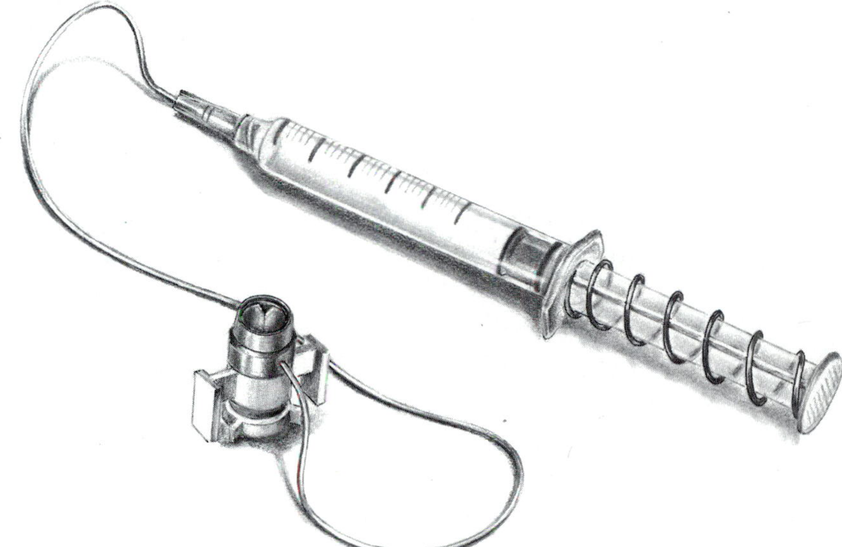

FIGURE 2-7. Hessburg-Barron vacuum trephine.

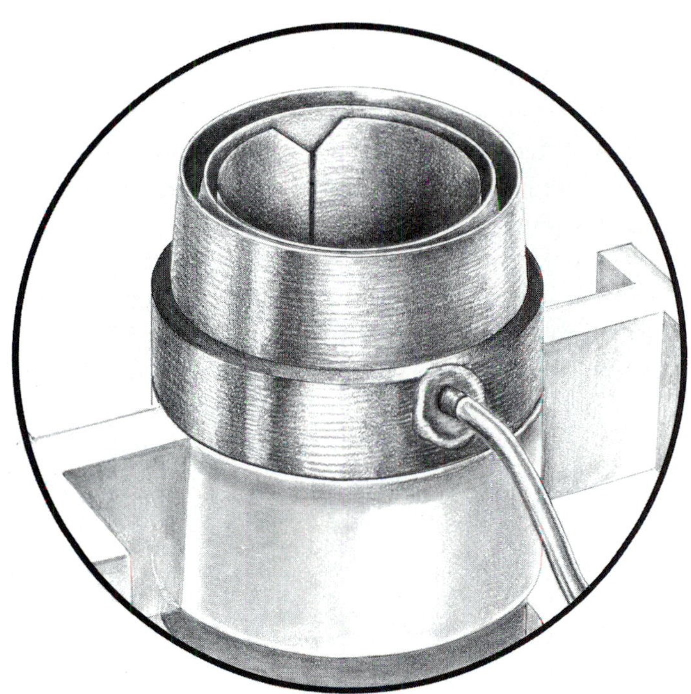

FIGURE 2-8. Vacuum chamber and blade of Hessburg-Barron vacuum trephine.

After the cornea is fixated by the vacuum, one supports the trephine by gently holding the plastic platforms on top of the trephine with the thumb and index finger of the nondominant hand without squeezing, lifting, or depressing, and lowers the blade by turning the spokes on top of the blade assembly clockwise with the index finger of the dominant hand (Fig. 2-9). One complete revolution of the blade assembly (turning the blade assembly four spokes) lowers the blade approximately 0.25 mm. Turning the blade assembly three spokes (three quarter-turns) lowers the blade to the zeroed position. Turning the spokes further results in cutting. (Actually the cornea is cut slightly as the blade is lowered to the zeroed position because of the anterior corneal curvature.) The number of spokes to turn depends on the corneal thickness and the desired depth of cut. This number is less for a thin keratoconic cornea than for a thick edematous cornea. We attempt to cut the cornea as close to Descemet's membrane as possible without perforation. However, the blade can be lowered until perforation occurs, which is recognized by the appearance of aqueous humor in the center of the trephine. Perforation with this trephine is no more risky than perforation with any other trephine. As with any trephine, once perforation occurs, one immediately removes the trephine from the eye by pressing the plunger of the syringe in all the way or cutting the silicone tube, which releases the vacuum, and lifting the trephine from the eye.

The diameter of trephine to use depends on the corneal disorder for which penetrating keratoplasty is done. We most commonly use a diameter of 7.5 mm, followed by 7.0 or 8.0 mm. A smaller diameter increases postoperative central corneal irregularities from the wound; a larger diameter increases the risk of corneal graft rejection and postoperative abnormalities of the anterior chamber angle. In an infant or child, a smaller diameter is used; in a patient with a large area of necrotic cornea, a larger diameter is used. The Hessburg-Barron vacuum trephine is currently available in diameters of 6.0 to 9.5 mm, in 0.5 mm increments. For smaller or larger diameters another type of trephine must be used.

A perforated cornea is more difficult to cut with a trephine than an intact cornea. Air or a viscoelastic substance may be placed through the perforation or through a separate limbal incision to reform the anterior chamber. Cyanoacrylate adhesive may be placed over the perforation in an attempt to seal the perforation temporarily so that trephination can be done more safely. However, this is not always possible, especially if the perforation is large. The Hessburg-Barron vacuum trephine is particularly helpful in these cases. A partial thickness cut is made; a full-thickness cut is contraindicated because of the risk of damaging the iris and lens.

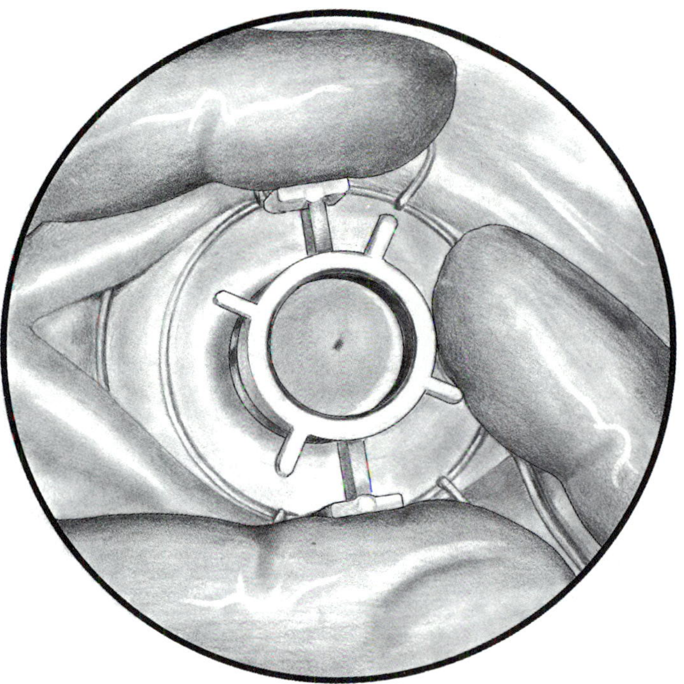

FIGURE 2-9. Lowering blade of Hessburg-Barron vacuum trephine.

Cutting the Donor Cornea

It is wise to cut the donor cornea after a partial thickness trephine cut has been made in the recipient cornea but before the anterior chamber is entered. This allows the trephine cut to be examined before the donor cornea is cut to make certain it is of appropriate diameter and the integrity of the surrounding cornea is sufficient to support sutures.

The introduction of corneal storage media, such as McCarey-Kaufman medium in 1974 and media containing chondroitin sulfate more recently, has permitted storage of the donor cornea with a rim of sclera instead of the whole eye. Although artificial anterior chambers have been designed to allow the donor cornea to be cut from the anterior surface, it is easier and less traumatic to the endothelium to cut the donor cornea from the posterior surface. Various Teflon cutting blocks have been designed with wells of various curvatures for this purpose. One removes the cornea from the storage medium by grasping the rim of surrounding sclera with a toothed forceps and placing the donor cornea, endothelial surface up, in the well of the cutting block. The donor cornea is centered in the well and is cut with a hand-held trephine (Fig. 2-10). If an internal obturator is present, it is fully retracted so that it does not touch the endothelium. The trephine is held as perpendicularly to the donor cornea as possible. Failure to hold the trephine perpendicularly may result in a beveled or oval cut. Various corneal punches have been designed to ensure that the trephine is perpendicular to the cutting block. The donor cornea is cut with a firm downward motion. Because there is resistance to cutting, the cornea is pushed into the barrel of the trephine before it is cut, which causes the donor corneal button to have a slightly larger diameter posteriorly than anteriorly. The diameter of trephine used to cut the donor cornea is usually 0.25 to 0.5 mm larger than the diameter of trephine used to cut the recipient cornea. This results in a donor corneal button that is larger than the recipient opening, which lessens the likelihood of postoperative elevation of intraocular pressure, especially in an aphakic eye. With a large recipient opening (10 mm or larger) we cut the donor cornea with a trephine 1 mm larger in diameter than the trephine used to cut the recipient cornea. In an infant, a trephine 1 mm larger in diameter than the trephine used to cut the recipient cornea is also used because of the elasticity of infant corneas, which makes wound closure more difficult.

After the donor cornea has been cut, the trephine is lifted from the cutting block. The corneal button usually remains in the well, and the peripheral cornea and scleral rim remain on the blade. If the corneal button remains in the blade, the blade is removed from the trephine handle and balanced salt solution or a viscoelastic substance is gently dripped into the center of the blade to dislodge the button. A brass cover is placed over the donor corneal button to prevent evaporation and desiccation of the tissue. It is important to ensure that the cutting block and brass cover have been cooled after autoclaving to avoid thermal damage to the tissue.

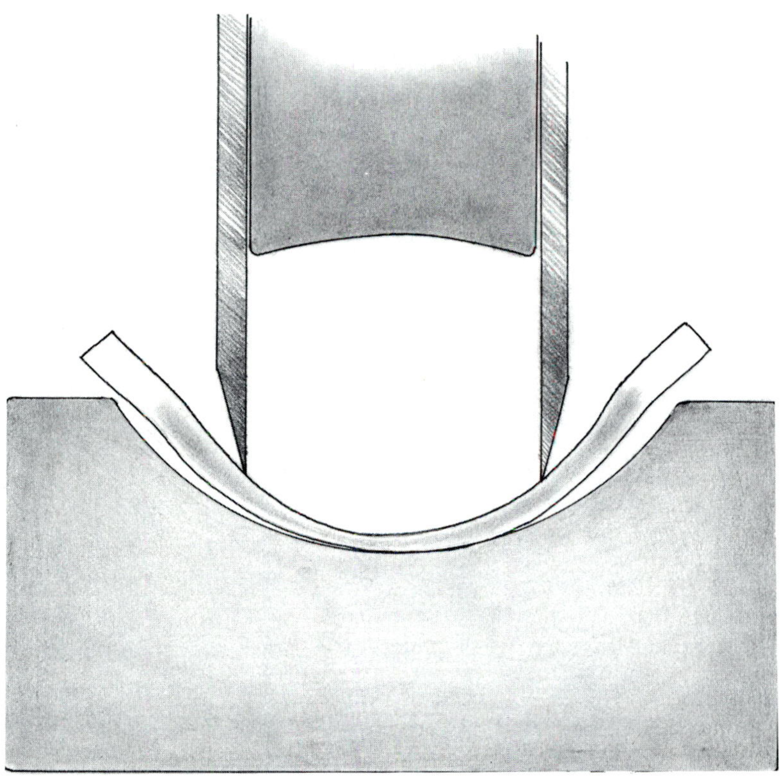

FIGURE 2-10. Cutting donor cornea.

Removing the Recipient Corneal Button

After the donor cornea has been cut, one enters the anterior chamber of the recipient eye by grasping the central lip of the trephine cut with a toothed forceps, inserting a stainless steel blade, bevel up, through the cut into the anterior chamber, and cutting upward as the blade is withdrawn (Fig. 2-11). Egress of aqueous humor must be seen to ensure that the anterior chamber has been entered. If aqueous humor is not seen, it is possible that the blade has cut down only as far as Descemet's membrane and has not entered the anterior chamber. This occurs more commonly in an edematous cornea, and it is possible to inadvertently strip Descemet's membrane from the posterior corneal stroma. Stripped Descemet's membrane is difficult to detect in a wet field; however, if the field is dried with a cellulose sponge, stripped Descemet's membrane becomes readily apparent and can be removed.

After the anterior chamber has been entered, a viscoelastic substance may be placed intracamerally to make cutting the recipient cornea with scissors easier and less traumatic, especially in a phakic eye. It is not uncommon for the lens-iris diaphragm to move anteriorly in a young phakic eye, which increases the risk of damage to the lens and iris as the recipient cornea is cut.

Removal of the recipient corneal button is completed by insertion of scissors through the perforation made by the stainless steel blade and cutting along the trephine cut (Fig. 2-12). Although some surgeons have advocated a beveled cut, with the anterior opening larger than the posterior opening (much like the opening of a jack-o-lantern), most surgeons prefer a perpendicular cut. To achieve this, the scissors must be held perpendicularly, unlike in a cataract incision, where the scissors are held at an angle. It is often easier to insert the scissors at an angle initially, with the posterior blade angled centrally, and then rotate the scissors perpendicularly. Care is taken to avoid trauma to the peripheral corneal endothelium. As the cornea is cut, the scissors are lifted anteriorly as they are closed to prevent damage to intraocular structures. If the scissors are not held perpendicularly, an uneven cut may result. Any tags of tissue should be removed with Vannas scissors to prevent irregularities of the wound. After the recipient corneal button has been removed, it is placed endothelial surface up, kept moist, and not removed from the sterile field until the donor cornea is in place. Although such cases are rare, the recipient corneal button may be used to close the eye should some disaster befall the donor corneal button.

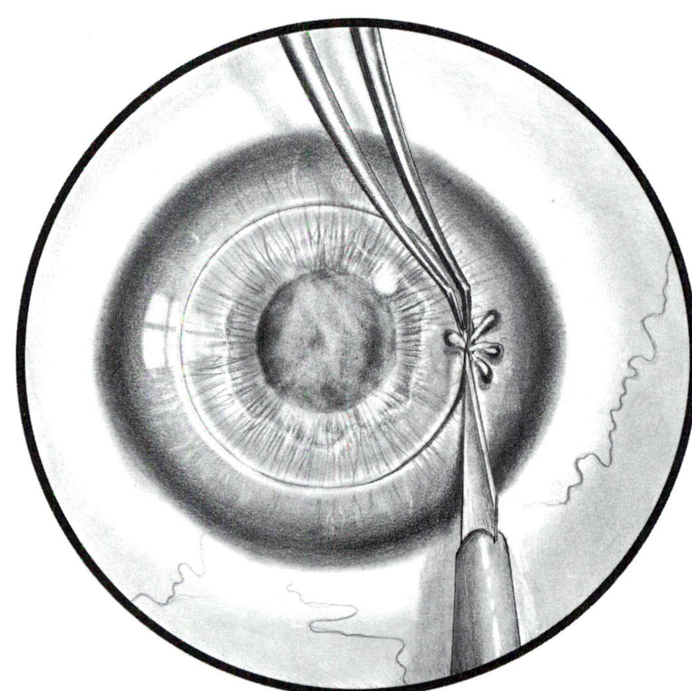

FIGURE 2-11. Entering anterior chamber with stainless steel blade.

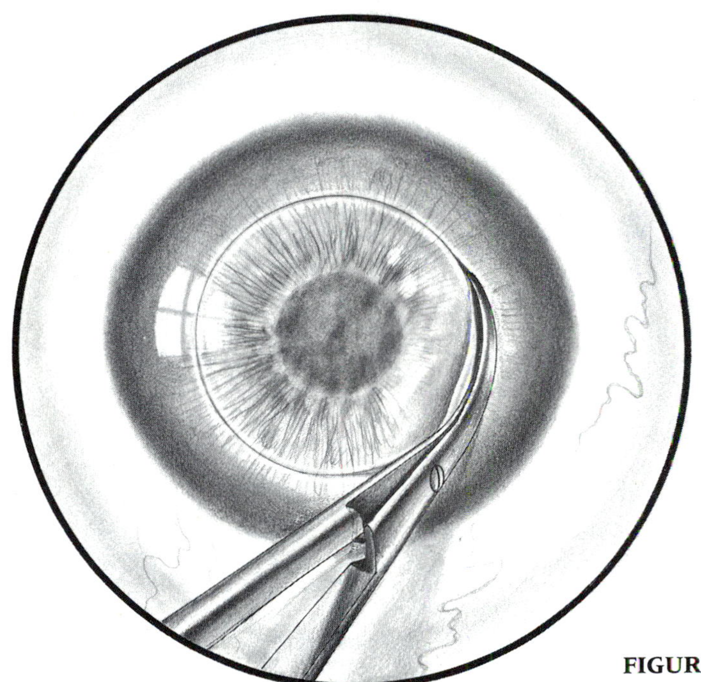

FIGURE 2-12. Cutting cornea with scissors.

A perforated cornea is more difficult to cut with scissors than an intact cornea. To enter the anterior chamber with a stainless steel blade through the trephine cut risks damaging intraocular structures. It is usually easier and safer to place the posterior blade of the corneal scissors centrally, through the perforation, and cut the cornea radially toward the trephine cut (Fig. 2-13). The cornea is then cut with scissors along the trephine cut in the usual fashion.

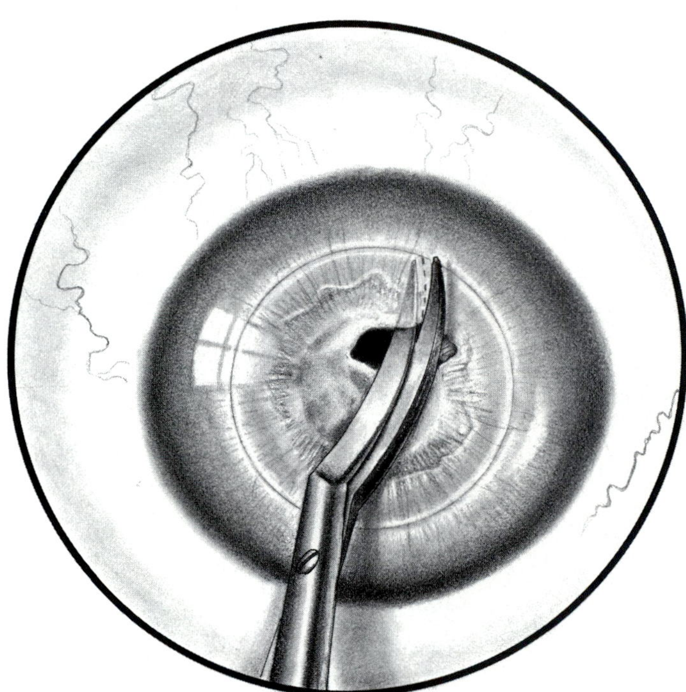

FIGURE 2-13. Cutting perforated cornea.

CONCOMITANT INTRAOCULAR PROCEDURES

Corneal disorders that necessitate penetrating keratoplasty are frequently accompanied by other anterior segment abnormalities that must be treated at the time of penetrating keratoplasty if the graft is to survive and visual rehabilitation is to be maximized. The following procedures are most often combined in this way:

Cataract extraction
Posterior chamber intraocular lens implantation
Intraocular lens removal
Vitrectomy
Iridoplasty
Anterior chamber intraocular lens implantation

Each of these are discussed here.

Cataract Extraction

In the past, there has been controversy whether to combine penetrating keratoplasty and cataract extraction in an eye with corneal disease and a cataract, or to perform the procedures separately. Separate procedures subject the patient to two operations and prolong visual rehabilitation. If the cataract is extracted before penetrating keratoplasty, an extracapsular technique usually cannot be used because of poor visibility through the diseased cornea. If the cataract is extracted after penetrating keratoplasty, the corneal graft is subjected to surgical trauma that can cause the graft to fail. With current surgical techniques, it is preferable to combine penetrating keratoplasty and cataract extraction in an eye with corneal disease and a cataract.

The cataract can be extracted through the recipient corneal opening; a separate limbal incision is not necessary. If an intracapsular cataract extraction is indicated (as for a subluxated lens), a cryoprobe tip is placed on the superior midperipheral anterior capsule after the capsule has been dried with a cellulose sponge. The lens is extracted with the cryoprobe while gentle pressure is applied at the inferior limbus with a lens loop (Fig. 2-14).

See also p. 161 for cataracts.

If an extracapsular cataract extraction is indicated, the anterior capsule may be opened in an interrupted fashion with a hypodermic needle or a stainless steel blade (Fig. 2-15). Alternatively, Vannas scissors may be used to cut the anterior capsule. In either case, the central anterior capsule is removed with forceps. The nucleus is expressed with a lens loop while gentle pressure is applied at the limbus with a muscle hook (Fig. 2-16). The lens cortex is aspirated with a manual or automated irrigation/aspiration apparatus (Fig. 2-17). The irrigation ports are directed anteriorly and posteriorly, and the aspiration port is directed horizontally. The posteriorly directed irrigation fluid helps to keep the posterior capsule away from the aspiration port. It also helps to keep the posterior capsule away from the iris and cornea so that a circumferentially closed space is not created between the peripheral posterior capsule and iris. Such a space can accumulate irrigation fluid and cause the central posterior capsule to bulge anteriorly and rupture. The posterior capsule should be gently pressed posteriorly with the irrigation/aspiration apparatus to prevent accumulation of irrigation fluid behind the iris. After the cortex has been aspirated, the posterior capsule can be polished with a wet cellulose sponge if necessary. A more detailed description of these techniques is provided in Chapter 8.

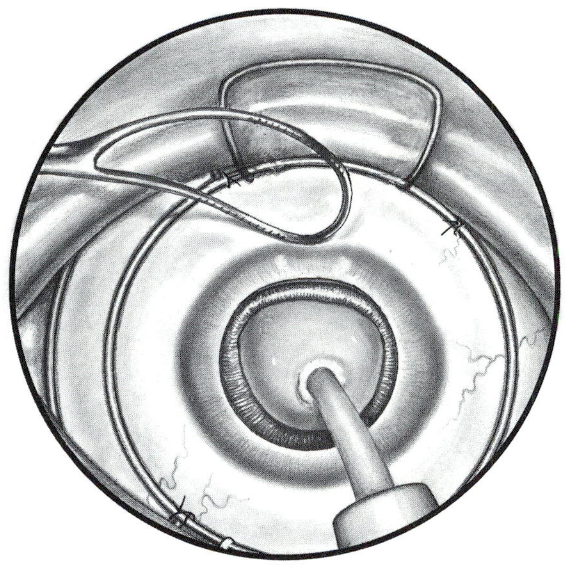

FIGURE 2-14. Extracting lens with cryoprobe.

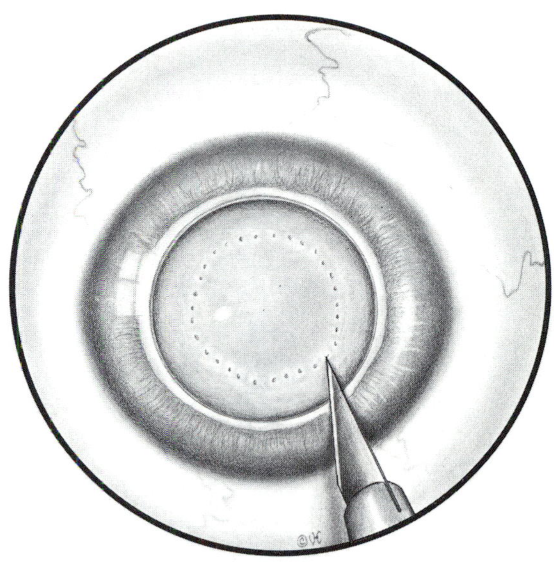

FIGURE 2-15. Anterior capsulotomy.

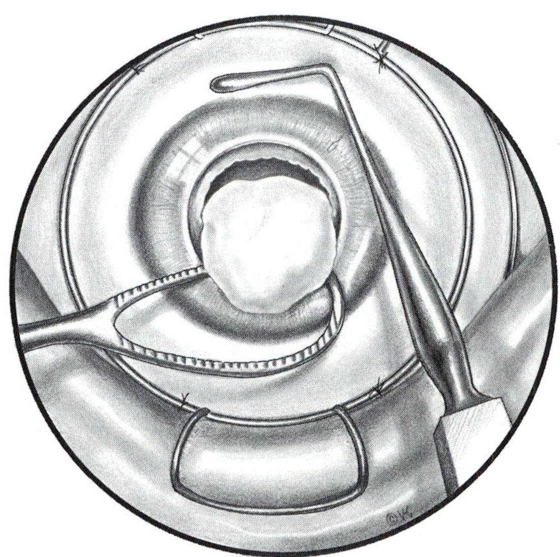

FIGURE 2-16. Delivering lens nucleus.

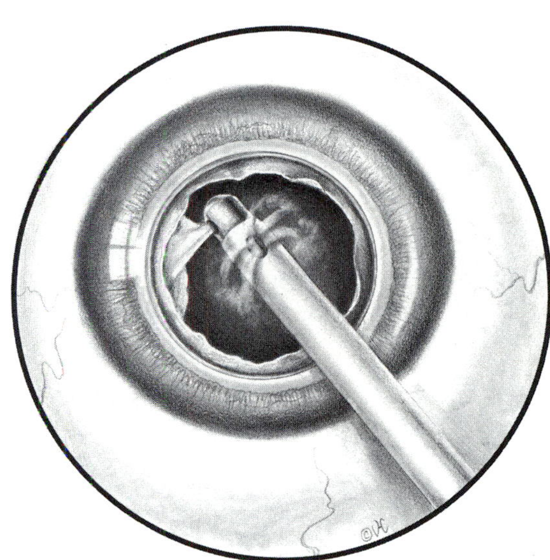

FIGURE 2-17. Aspirating cortex.

Posterior Chamber Intraocular Lens Implantation

In a patient in whom an extracapsular cataract extraction is done and an intraocular lens is indicated, a posterior chamber intraocular lens is preferred. The appropriate power of the intraocular lens is more difficult to determine for this case than for a routine cataract extraction because preoperative keratometry measurements are frequently difficult to obtain and may not correlate well with postoperative keratometry measurements. An assumed preoperative keratometry measurement, keratometry measurement of the fellow eye, or an assumed postoperative keratometry measurement based on data from previous penetrating keratoplasties have all been used in calculating the power of the intraocular lens.

It appears desirable to place a posterior chamber intraocular lens in the capsular bag if the posterior capsule and zonules are intact. A viscoelastic substance may be placed between the posterior capsule and anterior capsular flap to facilitate this placement. The optic of the intraocular lens is grasped with a smooth forceps, and the inferior haptic is placed in the capsular bag. The superior haptic is then grasped and is placed in the capsular bag (Fig. 2-18). The superior anterior capsular flap can be retracted to aid in the proper placement of the superior haptic. Repositioning of the intraocular lens can be done with a Sinskey hook if necessary. Other techniques are described in Chapter 10.

If the posterior capsule is not intact centrally but there is a peripheral rim, a posterior chamber intraocular lens can be implanted with the haptics in the iridociliary sulcus. If there is no posterior capsule, a posterior chamber intraocular lens can be sutured to the iris or sclera as shown in Fig. 22-17. This is particularly useful in a patient in whom an anterior chamber intraocular lens is contraindicated (as in a patient with glaucoma who is intolerant to contact lenses).

Contact between an intraocular lens and the cornea damages the corneal endothelium. Therefore one places a viscoelastic substance on the intraocular lens before suturing the donor corneal button (Fig. 2-19). Unlike in a routine cataract extraction, it is difficult to remove all the viscoelastic substance at the end of the procedure without damaging the donor cornea or wound; therefore some of the viscoelastic substance must usually be left in the eye. One of the complications of viscoelastic substances is elevation of intraocular pressure postoperatively; however, this elevation is usually transient and can be managed medically. Although there is controversy about the efficacy of various antihypertensive agents in the control of postoperative intraocular pressure elevation caused by viscoelastic substances, we give patients topical timolol maleate and a systemic carbonic anhydrase inhibitor at the end of the procedure if there are no contraindications. Topical pilocarpine gel and intracameral carbachol have also been reported as effective.

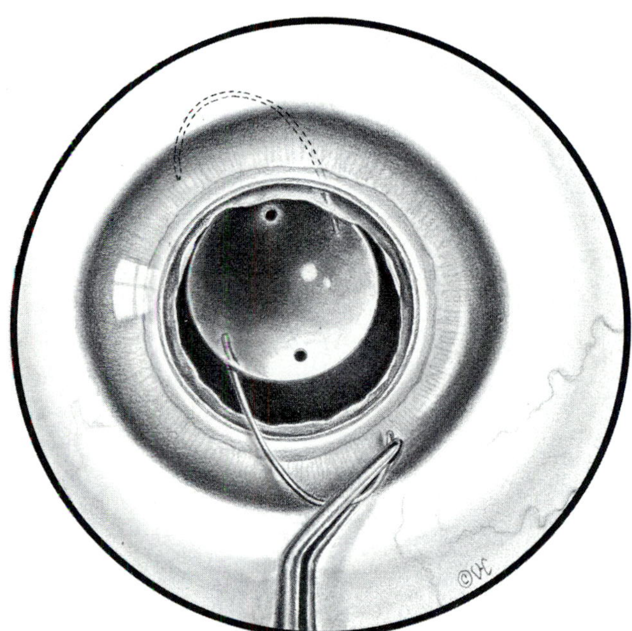

FIGURE 2-18. Implanting posterior chamber intraocular lens.

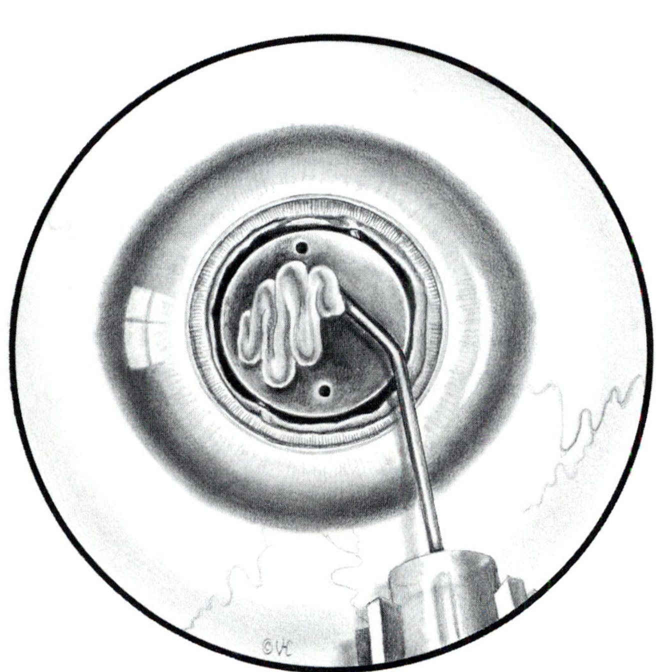

FIGURE 2-19. Placing viscoelastic substance on surface of intraocular lens.

Intraocular Lens Removal

Pseudophakic bullous keratopathy is currently the most common indication for penetrating keratoplasty in the United States. At the time of penetrating keratoplasty a decision must be made whether to remove the intraocular lens. Any lens that fits improperly or is associated with chronic inflammation, glaucoma, hyphema, or chronic cystoid macular edema should be removed. In general, we remove all iris-supported and semiflexible closed-loop anterior chamber intraocular lenses because of the high incidence of complications associated with these lenses.

The methods used to remove an intraocular lens vary with the style of the lens (see also Part Two: Cataract Surgery). A solid anterior chamber intraocular lens (such as the Choyce lens) can usually be removed through the recipient corneal opening (Fig. 2-20). Care is taken not to depress one end of the intraocular lens too much while lifting the other end. If it becomes evident that an extreme amount of force will be required to remove the intraocular lens through the corneal opening, a separate limbal incision is made through which the lens is removed. Cutting a solid anterior chamber intraocular lens in half to facilitate its removal is usually traumatic and unnecessary.

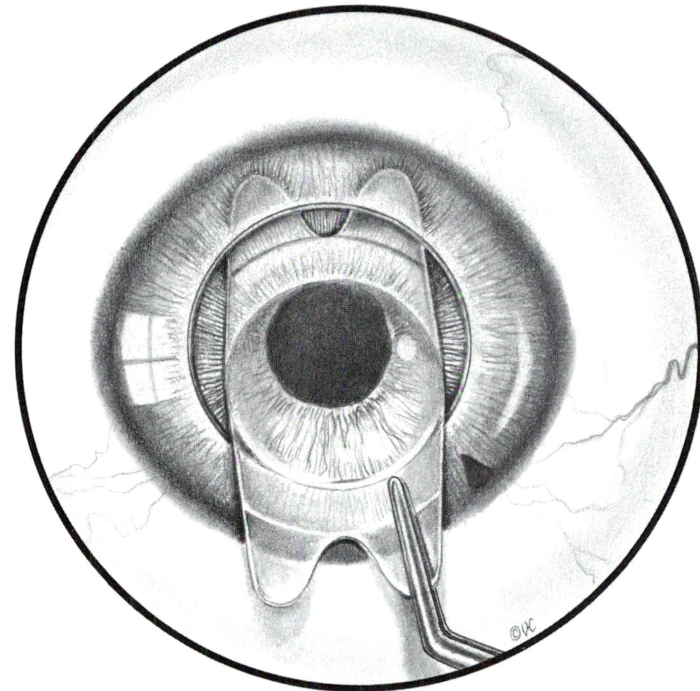

FIGURE 2-20. Removing Choyce anterior chamber intraocular lens.

A semiflexible closed-loop anterior chamber intraocular lens (such as the Leiske or Azar lens) frequently has iris synechiae around the peripheral haptics, which make removal of the lens more difficult. Simple tugging on the intraocular lens may result in tearing of synechiae, bleeding, and damage to the iris, with possible iridodialysis or cyclodialysis. One therefore removes the intraocular lens by cutting both sides of each haptic (Fig. 2-21). The optic is grasped with forceps and removed (Fig. 2-22). Each haptic is then grasped with forceps and spun through the anterior synechiae (Fig. 2-23). Removal of a Stableflex intraocular lens necessitates cutting all eight struts of the haptics, removing the optic, and spinning all four haptics through the iris synechiae (Fig. 2-24). This subject is also discussed in Chapter 10.

In a patient with pseudophakic bullous keratopathy and a posterior chamber intraocular lens, the intraocular lens is usually left in place. However, if removal is indicated (as with persistent inflammation), one removes the intraocular lens by rotating the optic in the appropriate direction with a Sinskey hook while pulling slightly anteriorly (Fig. 2-25). This usually results in prolapse of one of the haptics anterior to the cornea. The optic is then grasped with forceps, and the other haptic is spun out. If there is resistance to rotation of the intraocular lens and it is believed that the haptics are fibrosed in the capsular bag or iridociliary sulcus, the haptics are cut as far peripherally as possible (Fig. 2-26), the optic is removed, and the haptics are left in the eye. Some posterior chamber intraocular lenses have loops or notches on one haptic. Although these may have aided in implantation of the intraocular lens, they make its removal more difficult. Attempts to remove such an intraocular lens by rotation may result in trauma and bleeding if the haptic is fibrosed in the iridociliary sulcus. Therefore one should make every attempt to determine the exact style of the intraocular lens in question before attempting to remove it.

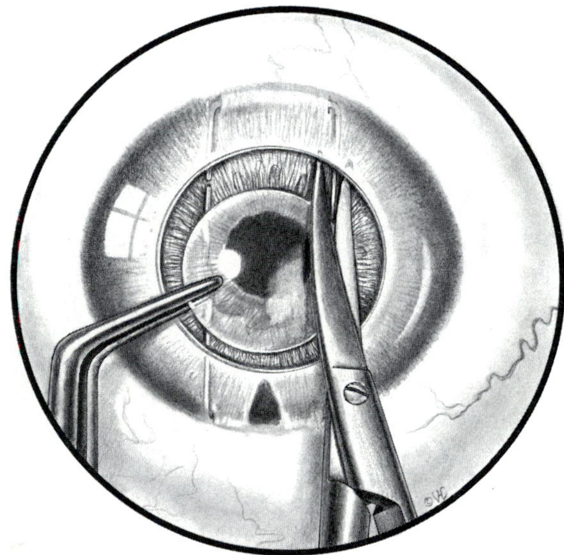

FIGURE 2-21. Cutting haptics of closed-loop anterior chamber intraocular lens.

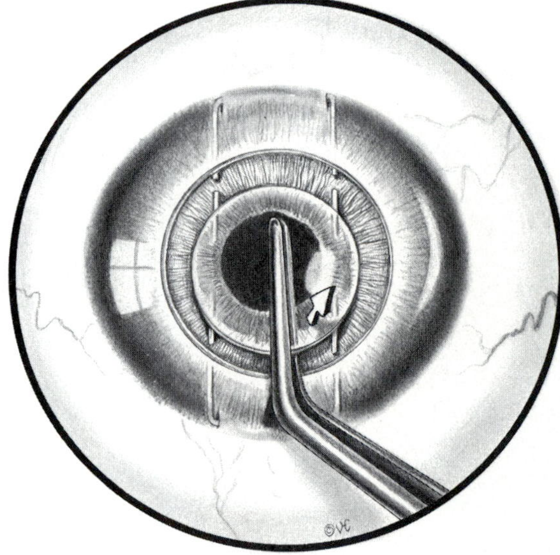

FIGURE 2-22. Removing optic of closed-loop anterior chamber intraocular lens.

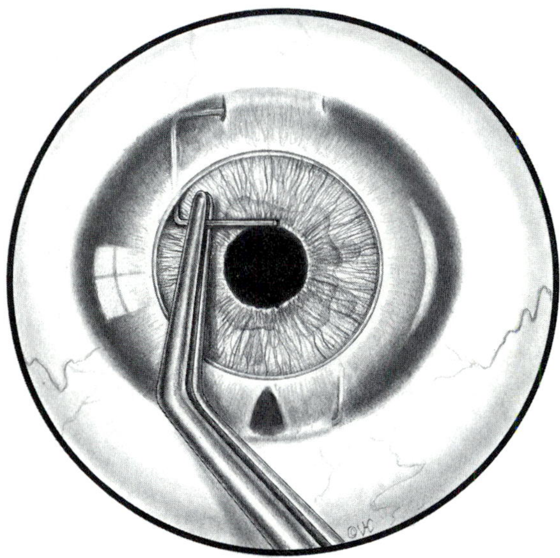

FIGURE 2-23. Rotating haptic of closed-loop anterior chamber intraocular lens through anterior synechia.

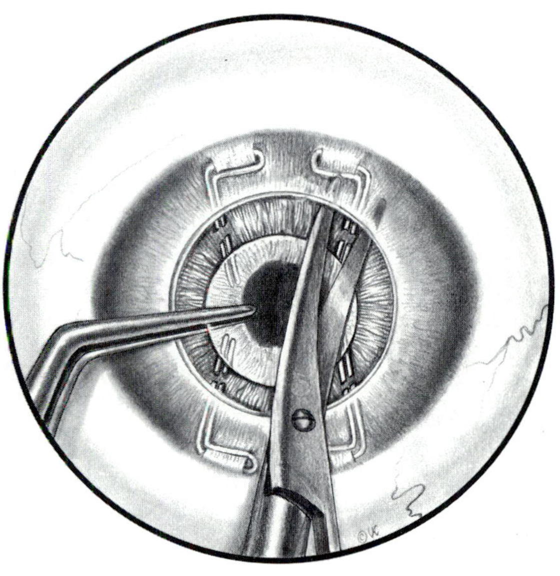

FIGURE 2-24. Cutting haptics of Stableflex anterior chamber intraocular lens.

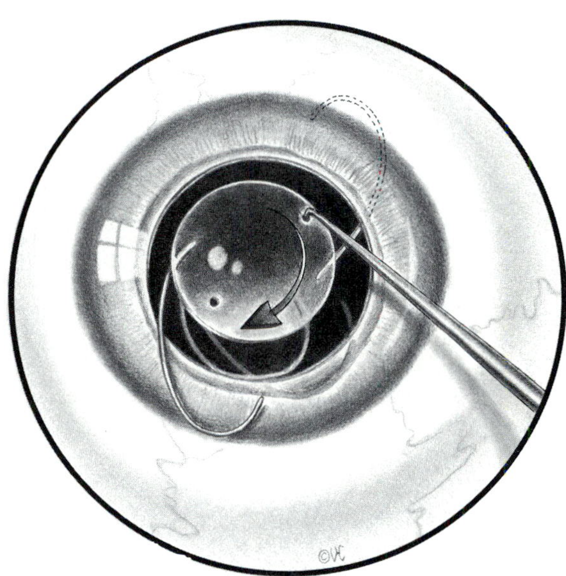

FIGURE 2-25. Rotating optic of posterior chamber intraocular lens.

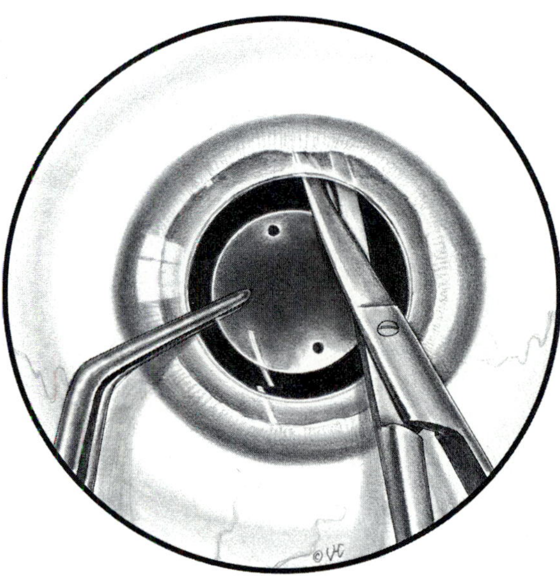

FIGURE 2-26. Cutting haptics of posterior chamber intraocular lens.

Vitrectomy

If there is vitreous in the anterior chamber, a thorough anterior vitrectomy must be done for a corneal graft to survive. Vitreous left in the anterior chamber almost certainly dooms the graft. Although aspiration of liquid vitreous with a needle or a cellulose sponge vitrectomy was acceptable in the past, a vitrectomy with an automated vitrector is preferred today (Fig. 2-27). Any of several vitrectomy instruments can be used. The most important principle is to remove all the vitreous from the anterior chamber. Because vitreous frequently prolapses anteriorly if left in the eye after surgery, the eye is filled with balanced salt solution several times to prolapse any vitreous anteriorly at the time of surgery so that it can be removed. After a thorough anterior vitrectomy, the anterior surface of the iris is checked for vitreous strands with a cellulose sponge. If any are present, they are cut with scissors. A peripheral iridectomy is made if one is not present. For further discussion of vitrectomy techniques, refer to Chapter 22.

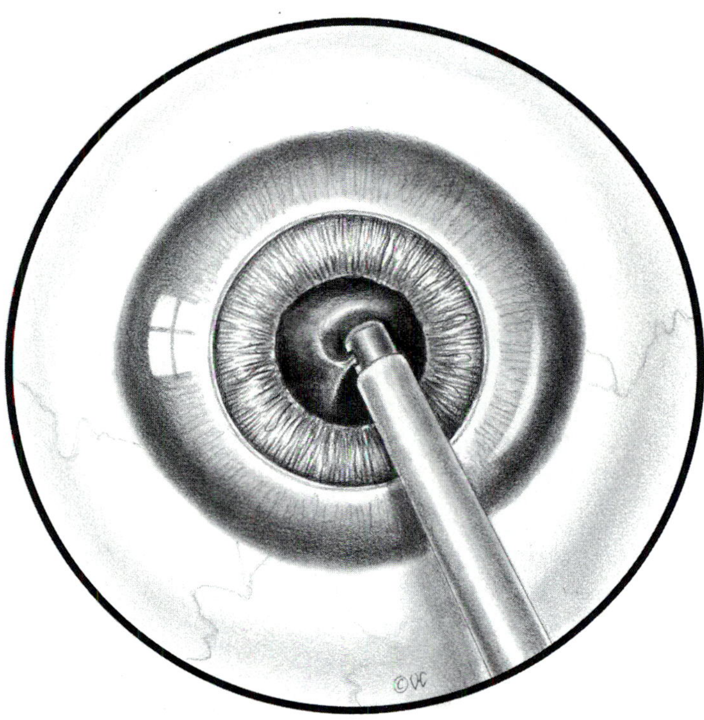

FIGURE 2-27. Anterior vitrectomy.

Iridoplasty

It is common for a floppy iris to become adherent to the peripheral cornea and penetrating keratoplasty wound, resulting in peripheral anterior synechiae, which increase the risk of glaucoma and corneal graft rejection. Such an iris is therefore repaired to restore a taut iris diaphragm that will remain posteriorly, away from the graft. If a sector iridectomy is present, it is closed with interrupted 10-0 polypropylene sutures. A smooth forceps is used to grasp the iris, and the needle is passed near the iris sphincter (Fig. 2-28). The needle should always be held with the needle holder or smooth forceps so that it will not fall into the posterior chamber. The most peripheral part of the sector is left open to function as a peripheral iridectomy (Fig. 2-29). The sutures are tied with a double-throw followed by two single-throws, and the suture ends are cut on the knot. Vannas scissors are preferred to a stainless steel blade because there is less tension on the suture as it is cut, and consequently less risk of pulling the suture through the iris. Figs. 8-15 to 8-18 and 8-20 to 8-22 also illustrate iridoplasty techniques.

If the pupil is updrawn, the inferior iris is cut (Fig. 2-30) to create a sector iridectomy (Fig. 2-31), which is then partially closed with interrupted 10-0 polypropylene sutures (Fig. 2-32).

Anterior synechiae are bluntly dissected with an iris sweep or are hydraulically dissected with a viscoelastic substance. If these maneuvers result in bleeding, it is safer to sharply dissect the anterior synechiae from the posterior surface of the cornea with scissors. If this is not possible, the edges of the iris on either side of the synechiae are cut so that the synechiae do not progress, and the edges are approximated with interrupted 10-0 polypropylene sutures, creating, in essence, several small peripheral iridectomies.

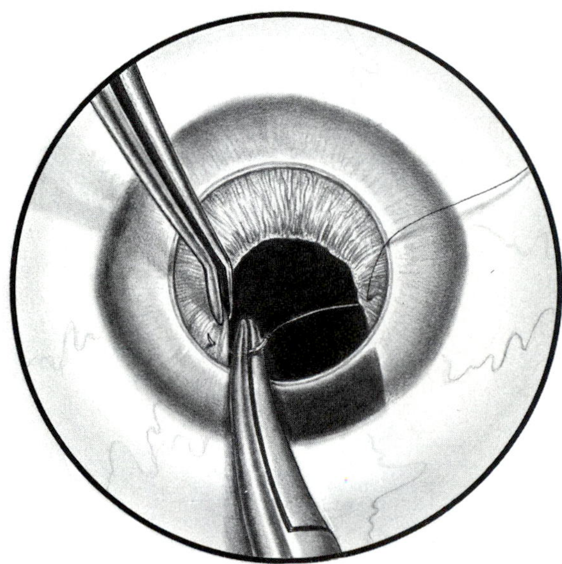

FIGURE 2-28. Closing sector iridectomy.

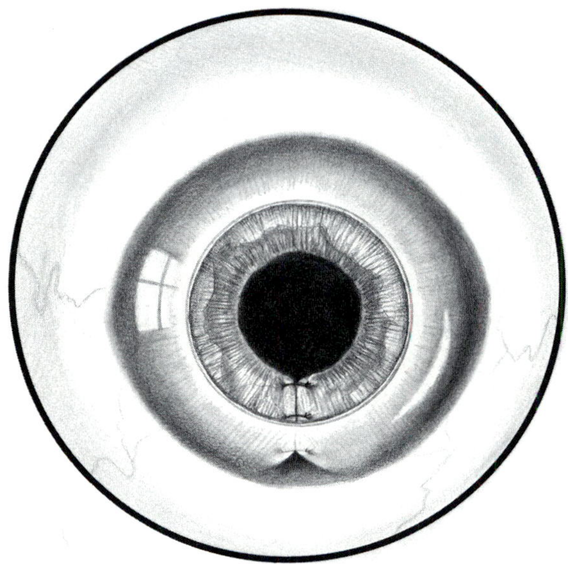

FIGURE 2-29. Partially closed sector iridectomy.

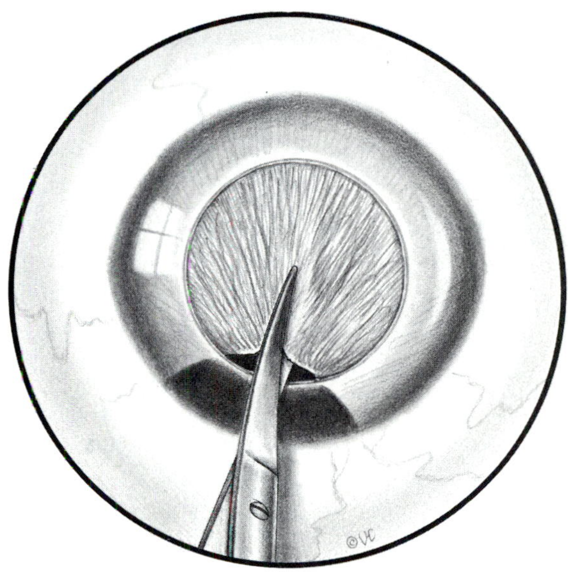

FIGURE 2-30. Cutting updrawn pupil.

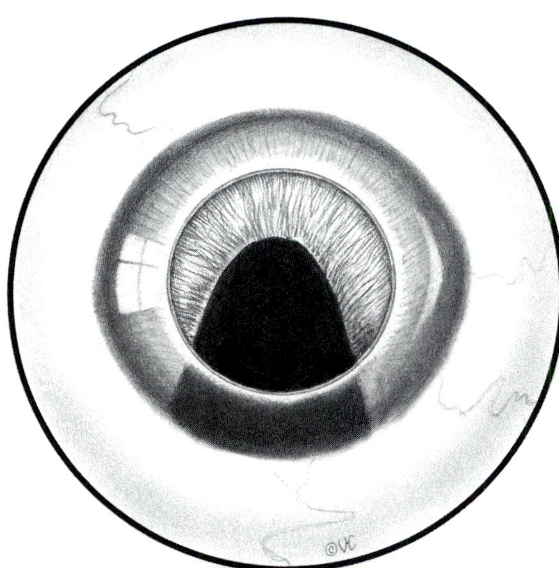

FIGURE 2-31. Sector iridotomy.

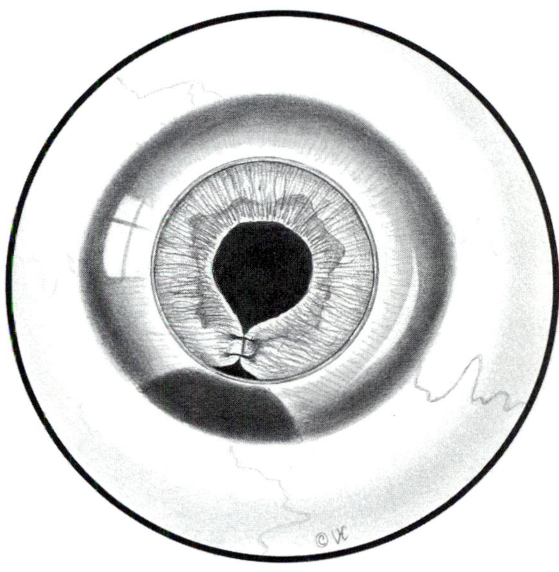

FIGURE 2-32. Partially closed sector iridotomy.

Anterior Chamber Intraocular Lens Implantation

Many aphakic patients or pseudophakic patients in whom an intraocular lens is removed are candidates for implantation of a more modern intraocular lens. Implantation of a posterior chamber lens has already been described. There appear to be many anterior chamber intraocular lenses that can be implanted safely. The most important principles in anterior chamber intraocular lens implantation are to be certain that (1) there is no vitreous in the anterior chamber, (2) there is a stable iris diaphragm on which to support the intraocular lens, and (3) the intraocular lens does not distort the iris (Fig. 2-33). As with a posterior chamber intraocular lens, one places a viscoelastic substance on the anterior chamber intraocular lens before suturing the donor cornea to prevent damage to the donor corneal endothelium. The techniques of anterior chamber intraocular lens implantation are discussed on p. 234.

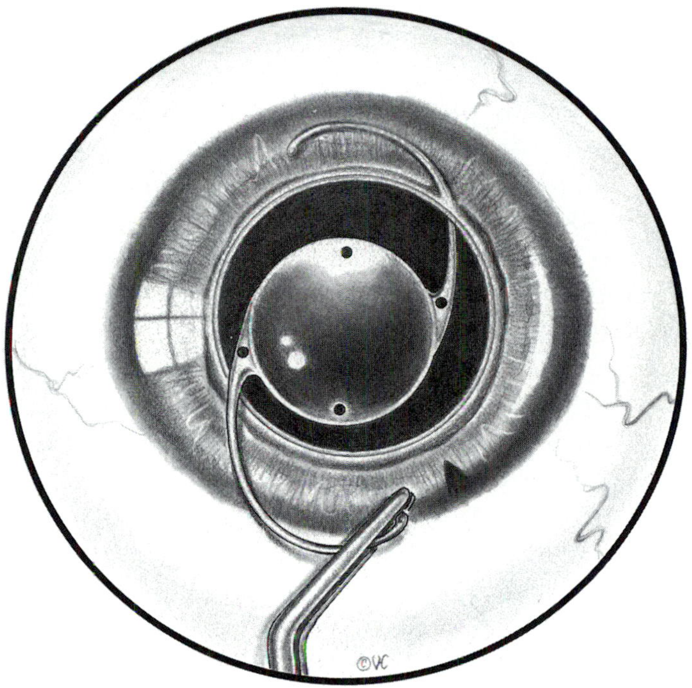

FIGURE 2-33. Implanting anterior chamber intraocular lens.

SUTURING THE DONOR CORNEA

The donor cornea should be sutured in place as quickly as possible. This is especially important in an infant or child, in whom the eye will collapse easily, even in the presence of a scleral support ring, and the lens will extrude unless the donor cornea is secured quickly.

The donor corneal button is scooped out of the well of the cutting block with a fenestrated (Paton) spatula. The fenestrations in the spatula permit drainage of the corneal storage medium so that the cornea does not slide around on a layer of fluid. The spatula is held in the surgeon's dominant hand, and the donor corneal button is brought to the inferior limbus, where it is tilted vertically so that the anterior edge can be grasped with a forceps held in the surgeon's nondominant hand (Fig. 2-34). A double-pronged (Polack) forceps provides stability of the donor cornea as the first suture is placed (Fig. 2-35). A single-pronged forceps may be used; however, the cornea may undergo torque as the first suture is placed if the needle is not placed directly beneath the forceps. If torque occurs, the assistant can stabilize the donor cornea inferiorly with another toothed forceps.

The preferred suture for penetrating keratoplasty is 10-0 nylon on a spatulated cutting needle. A stronger suture (9-0 nylon) may be used in an eye in which posterior segment manipulation is expected at the end of surgery (as in an eye with corneal disease and a retinal detachment undergoing combined penetrating keratoplasty and retinal detachment repair) or in a patient who may manipulate the eye postoperatively. The suture is placed approximately 0.75 mm from the edges of the donor and recipient corneas. If the recipient cornea is thin, a longer suture bite is taken in the recipient. The posterior layers of the two tissues are approximated by placement of the needle as close to Descemet's membrane as possible in both the donor and recipient corneas. Although full-thickness sutures have been advocated by some, they theoretically cause more endothelial trauma. Leaks around full-thickness sutures are not uncommon, and although these leaks usually seal themselves within a day or two postoperatively, there is theoretically an increased risk of postoperative hypotension or endophthalmitis.

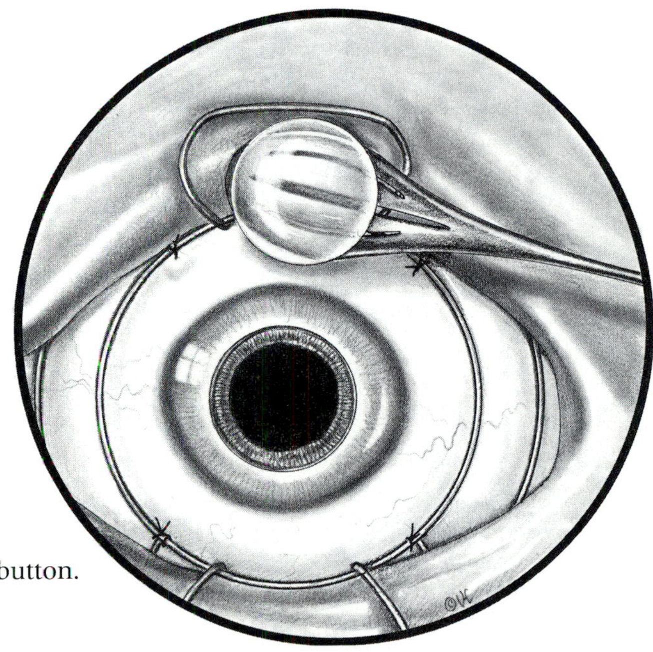

FIGURE 2-34. Transferring donor corneal button.

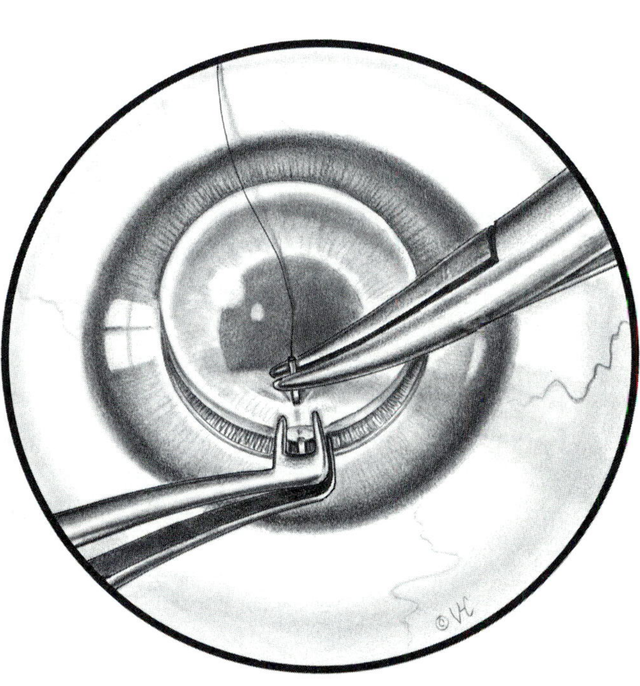

FIGURE 2-35. Placing first suture between prongs of Polack forceps.

The most important suture in penetrating keratoplasty is the second suture because it determines the distribution of the tissue. This suture should bisect the donor corneal button and recipient cornea exactly (Fig. 2-36). One best accomplishes this by first ignoring the recipient cornea and placing the suture in the donor corneal button exactly 180 degrees from the first suture and then ignoring the donor cornea and placing the suture through the recipient cornea so that it bisects the recipient cornea exactly. Before the needle is pulled through the recipient cornea, the needle is released from the needle holder and the distribution of the donor cornea is examined. The needle may need to be repositioned several times to ensure even distribution of the tissue; however, care taken at this time will prevent high postoperative astigmatism caused by uneven distribution of the tissue. Some surgeons mark the peripheral cornea with a radial keratotomy marker before the recipient corneal button is removed to aid in proper placement of sutures. After the first two sutures have been placed, the third and fourth sutures are placed 90 degrees from the first two sutures. These first four sutures are collectively called "cardinal sutures."

There are many suture patterns that may be used in penetrating keratoplasty, including interrupted, running, and a combination of interrupted and running sutures. Interrupted sutures are preferred in a cornea that is heavily vascularized because of differential healing of the wound, in an infant or child, and in a patient in whom the integrity of the wound should not depend on one suture knot (such as a patient who may manipulate the eye, a patient who may sustain trauma to the eye, an athlete, or an obese patient). The type of suture pattern does not appear to affect postoperative astigmatism if the recipient and donor corneas are cut precisely, the donor cornea is distributed evenly, and the donor and recipient corneas are approximated accurately.

With interrupted sutures, 16 sutures are usually placed; the second four sutures are placed equidistant between the first four sutures, and the last eight sutures are placed equidistant between the first eight sutures (Fig. 2-37). More sutures may be required in large grafts. The suture ends are cut on the knot, and the knot is rotated into the recipient cornea just beneath the epithelium. Rotation of the knot into the recipient cornea results in less postoperative irritation and also allows an intraoperative assessment of the stability of the knot. It is rare for a knot to unravel once it has been rotated into corneal tissue. The knot is rotated in a manner such that any suture ends point toward the corneal surface in an arrow-shaped fashion, which allows the suture to be removed more easily postoperatively.

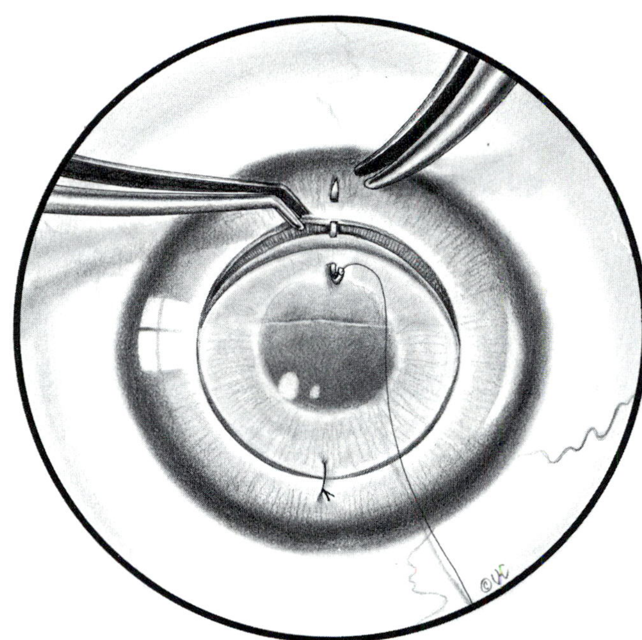

FIGURE 2-36. Placing second suture to distribute tissue evenly.

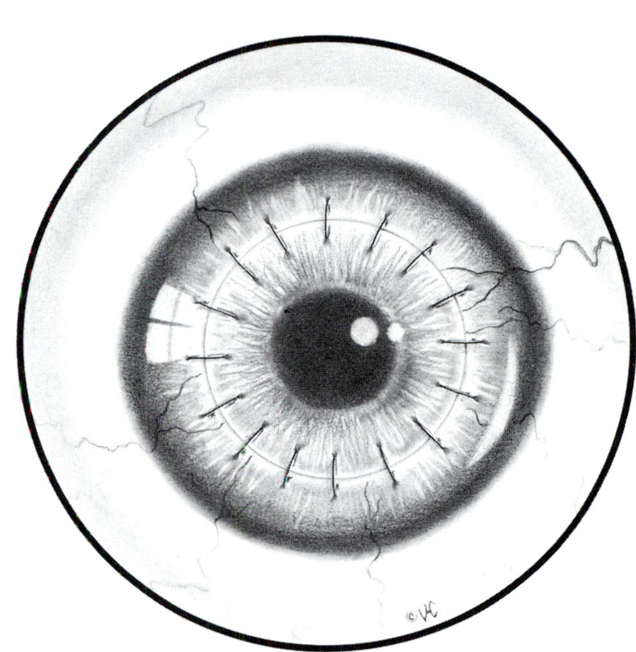

FIGURE 2-37. Interrupted sutures.

If interrupted sutures are used alone, the sutures are removed as soon as they become loose or vascularized. In an infant, the sutures may be removed as early as 1 week postoperatively. In an adult, the sutures are usually removed selectively from 6 months to 1 year postoperatively. One removes a suture by cutting it centrally with a stainless steel blade. The peripheral end is grasped with a smooth forceps, and the suture is removed through the recipient cornea with a quick motion. Removal of the suture through the graft should be avoided because it may cause elevation of the graft or dehiscence of the wound. Each suture is removed as soon as it is cut, instead of first cutting all the sutures and then removing them, so that if the wound is less stable than anticipated, there will not be a dehiscence of the entire wound.

In the running suture technique, a 10-0 nylon suture is started with the first bite through the recipient cornea only (Fig. 2-38). The suture is then run around the circumference of the wound, with three to five suture bites in each quadrant. The last suture bite goes through the donor cornea only. The suture is tightened with a smooth forceps and is tied with a triple-throw, followed by two single-throws. A triple-throw may be placed initially and the suture retightened if necessary. The suture should be taut enough to appose the wound so that it is watertight. By starting the suture in the recipient cornea and ending in the donor cornea, the knot will automatically be buried in the wound and there will be no irritating suture ends postoperatively (Fig. 2-39).

There are three disadvantages of a running suture: (1) the integrity of the suture depends on only one knot, (2) the needle may become dull if it is not properly handled, making placement of the needle difficult by the time the last quadrant of the wound is sutured, and (3) the suture may break, necessitating splicing of the suture. One splices a running suture that breaks by first placing the needle of a new suture (or the old suture if it is long enough to complete closure of the wound) through the donor and recipient corneas and pulling the suture through the tissue until the end appears (Fig. 2-40). This stabilizes the end of the suture and makes tying of the two sutures easier. After the sutures have been tied, the ends of the sutures are cut with a stainless steel blade and the knot is rotated into the corneal wound. Rotation of the knot is done at this time, instead of when the suture is tightened, to ensure that the knot is stable and is able to be rotated into the wound. One tightens a suture that has been spliced by starting from the area of the splice and tightening circumferentially away from the splice in each direction so that the knot remains buried in the wound.

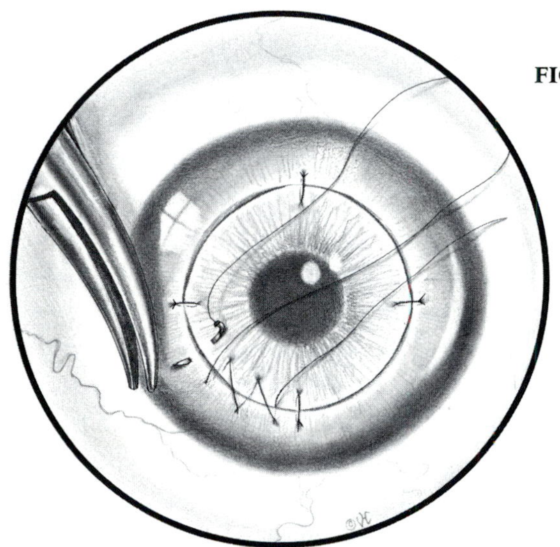

FIGURE 2-38. Running 10-0 nylon suture.

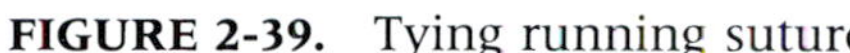

FIGURE 2-39. Tying running suture.

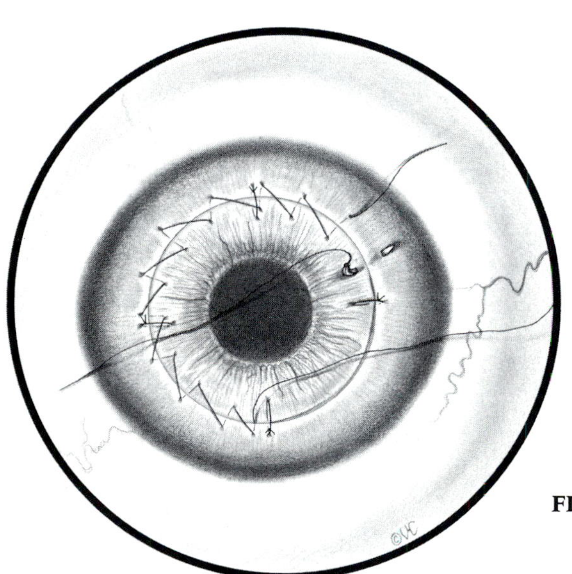

FIGURE 2-40. Splicing running suture.

In the double running suture technique, the cardinal sutures are removed after the running 10-0 nylon suture has been placed (Fig. 2-41). An 11-0 nylon suture is started in the recipient cornea midway between two 10-0 nylon suture bites and is run circumferentially around the wound (Fig. 2-42), ending with the last bite through donor cornea only. The suture is tightened just enough to remove any slack and is tied with a triple-throw followed by two single-throws (Fig. 2-43). The purpose of the 11-0 nylon suture is to provide stability of the wound after the 10-0 nylon suture has been removed; it is not intended to provide primary wound closure. An 11-0 nylon suture that is too tight can cause postoperative astigmatism.

In the double running suture technique, the 10-0 nylon suture is usually removed 3 months postoperatively. Every other suture bite is cut with a stainless steel blade (Fig. 2-44). If the blade is held parallel to the 11-0 nylon suture, the risk of accidentally cutting the 11-0 nylon suture is minimized. The pieces of 10-0 nylon suture are picked up between the cut ends and removed. The 11-0 nylon suture may be kept in place indefinitely; however, it eventually biodegrades. Sometimes during this process it can break and the ends can cause irritation and precipitate an infection or graft rejection. For this reason, some surgeons routinely remove the 11-0 nylon suture 1 year postoperatively.

Interrupted sutures may be combined with a running suture if one first places 16 interrupted 10-0 nylon sutures followed by a running 11-0 nylon suture as described above (Fig. 2-45). Some surgeons place 8 to 12 interrupted 10-0 nylon sutures followed by a running 10-0 or 11-0 nylon suture, with the intent of modifying postoperative astigmatism by selective removal of the interrupted sutures in the early postoperative period.

During suturing, the epithelium is kept moist with balanced salt solution or a viscoelastic substance. The viability of the donor corneal epithelium is especially important in a patient with dry eyes, chemical burn, pemphigoid, or Stevens-Johnson syndrome. In such a patient a bandage soft contact lens can be placed over the graft at the end of the procedure or a temporary tarsorrhaphy done to protect the epithelium in the early postoperative period.

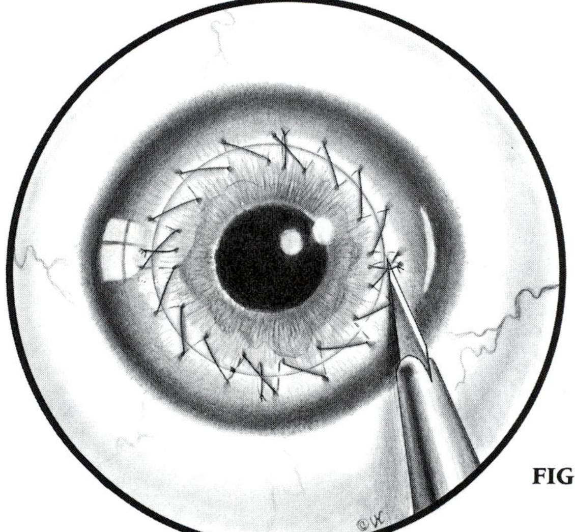

FIGURE 2-41. Removing cardinal sutures.

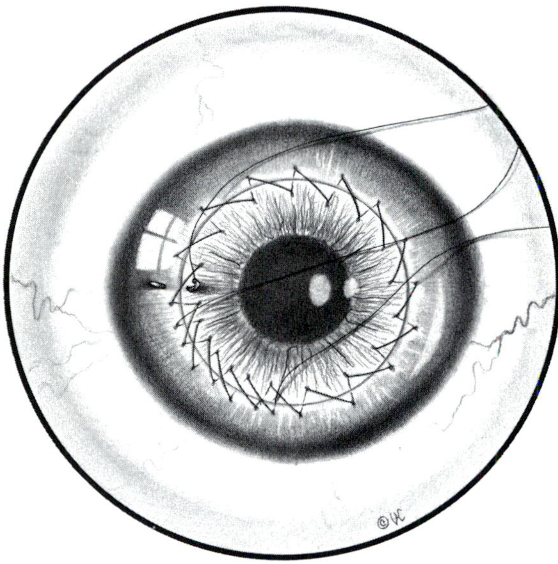

FIGURE 2-42. Running 11-0 nylon suture.

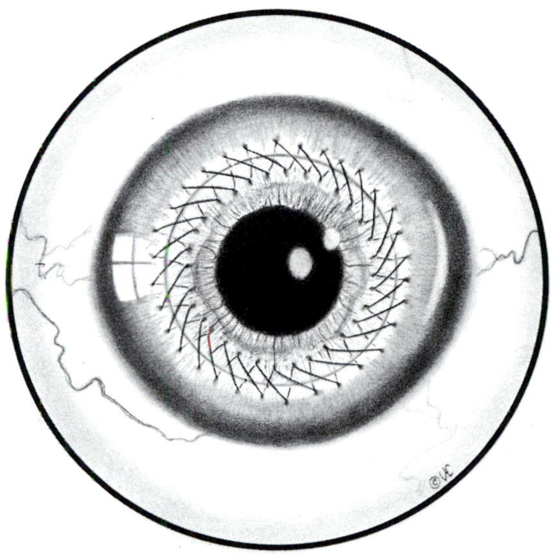

FIGURE 2-43. Double running sutures.

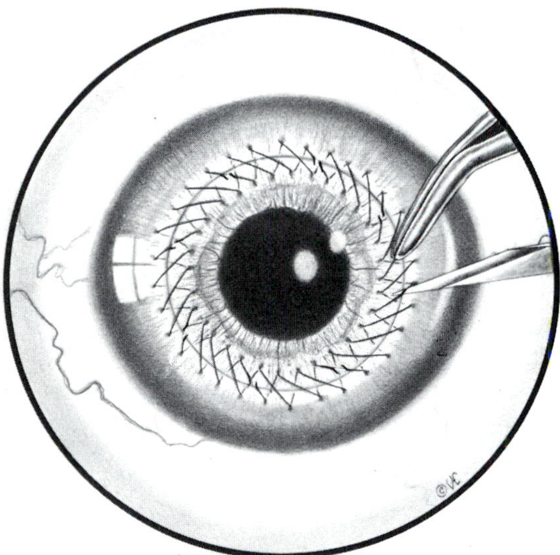

FIGURE 2-44. Removing 10-0 nylon running suture.

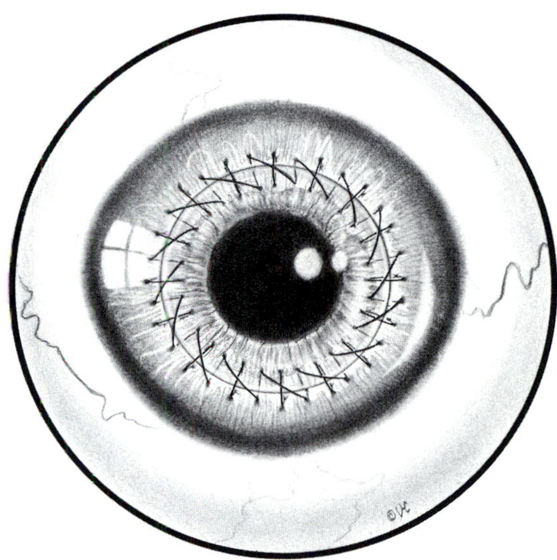

FIGURE 2-45. Interrupted and running sutures.

CHAPTER 3

Lamellar Keratoplasty

Principles of Inlay Lamellar Keratoplasty

Inlay lamellar keratoplasty is used optically to treat anterior corneal opacities or surface irregularities, and tectonically to treat corneal thinning disorders or perforations. In the late 1800s, inlay lamellar keratoplasty was more successful and consequently more commonly performed than penetrating keratoplasty for the treatment of many corneal disorders. There were several reasons for this: (1) lamellar keratoplasty is an extraocular procedure and therefore does not require closure of a perforating corneal wound, (2) survival of a lamellar graft does not depend on viable donor corneal endothelial cells, and (3) there is no risk of endothelial rejection in a lamellar graft. Inlay lamellar keratoplasty was not successful, however, for the treatment of corneal disorders with endothelial cell dysfunction, such as Fuchs' dystrophy. With the increased understanding and success of penetrating keratoplasty in the early 1900s, the number of indications for inlay lamellar keratoplasty as an optical procedure diminished. Today inlay lamellar keratoplasty is used more as a tectonic procedure than an optical procedure and for peripheral disorders more than for central disorders.

The technique of inlay lamellar keratoplasty involves removal of abnormal anterior corneal tissue by a lamellar keratectomy and replacement of that tissue with donor corneal stroma and Bowman's layer.

Optical Inlay Lamellar Keratoplasty

Preparing the recipient lamellar bed

For anterior corneal disorders that involve the visual axis, such as Reis-Bückler dystrophy, a partial-thickness trephine cut is made in the cornea that is deep enough to include all the abnormal anterior corneal tissue centrally (Fig. 3-1). A trephine with an internal obturator may be used; however, the Hessburg-Barron vacuum trephine creates a cut of more even depth. The most common diameter of trephine used is 7.5 or 8.0 mm.

A lamellar keratectomy is done when the central edge of the trephine cut is grasped with a toothed forceps and the tissue at the base of the cut is dissected with a blunt spatula or a sharp lamellar dissecting blade (Fig. 3-2). As the dissection is done, the anterior lamellae are pulled upward to help separate the tissue. The parallel arrangement of collagen fibrils aids in separation of the tissue. The dissection should be done in a dry field. As the tissue is dissected, care is taken to remain at the same depth and to avoid perforating the cornea. If perforation occurs, aqueous humor may collect between the recipient cornea and graft postoperatively. If the perforation is small, air is injected into the anterior chamber through the limbus to press the recipient cornea against the graft. If the perforation is moderate, the recipient cornea surrounding the perforation is sutured to the graft with 10-0 nylon mattress sutures. If the perforation is large, the procedure may have to be converted to penetrating keratoplasty.

The recipient bed should have an even base and steep, well-defined vertical edges (Fig. 3-3). Irregularities of the base can decrease postoperative visual acuity. Foreign material trapped in the recipient bed can also decrease postoperative visual acuity. Therefore precautions, such as removal of powder from surgical gloves and the elimination of lint-producing gauze sponges from the surgical field, are taken to minimize foreign material. The recipient bed is irrigated with filtered balanced salt solution, and the irrigant and any foreign material are aspirated with a pediatric feeding tube connected to suction.

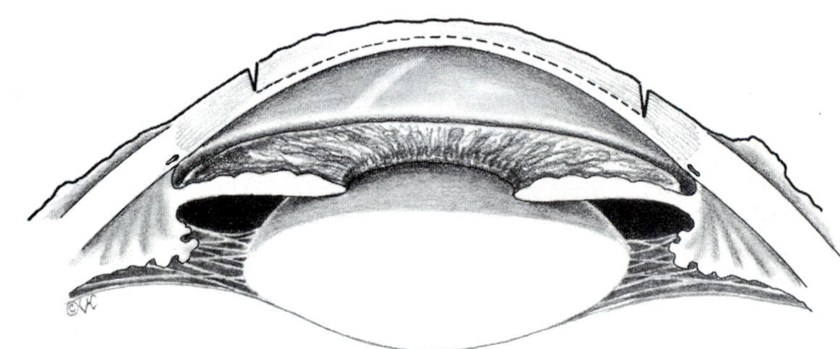

FIGURE 3-1. Partial-thickness trephine incision for lamellar keratoplasty.

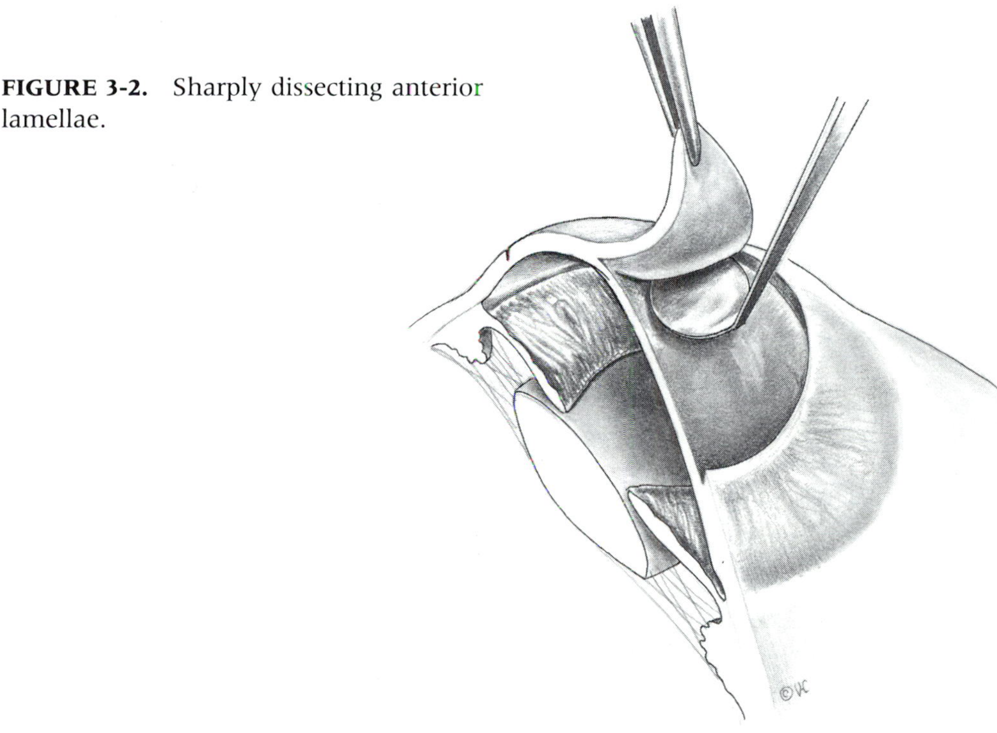

FIGURE 3-2. Sharply dissecting anterior lamellae.

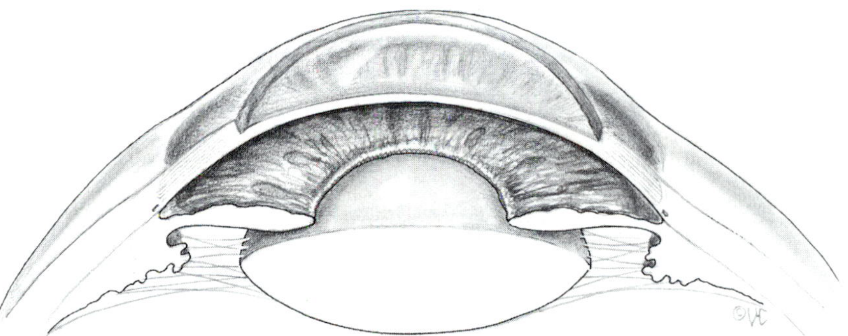

FIGURE 3-3. Recipient lamellar bed with even base and steep edges.

Preparing the donor lamellar graft

The donor lamellar graft consists of stroma, Bowman's layer, and, in some cases, epithelium. It can be obtained from a whole eye, a cornea stored in corneal preservation medium, or a cornea that has been frozen, lathed, and lyophilized.

If a whole eye is used, the eye is held with sterile gauze. A partial thickness cut is made with a trephine to the same depth as the recipient lamellar bed. A spatula or dissecting blade is inserted at the base of the cut, and the anterior and posterior corneal lamellae are separated in a manner similar to that used to prepare the recipient bed. Alternatively, a partial thickness cut can be made at the limbus with a stainless steel blade to the same depth as the recipient bed. A lamellar dissector is inserted at the base of the cut and is moved horizontally to separate the lamellae (Fig. 3-4). The lamellar graft is then cut to the appropriate diameter with a trephine (Fig. 3-5).

If a donor cornea stored in corneal preservation medium is used, the endothelium and Descemet's membrane are removed and the cornea is cut from the posterior surface with a trephine, as described in Chapter 2.

Commercially prepared donor lamellar tissue that has been frozen, lathed from the posterior surface on a cryolathe, and lyophilized is available (KeratoPatch, Allergan Medical Optics, Irvine, California). The tissue is 10 mm in diameter, is 0.3 mm thick, and has no inherent optical power. Larger diameters are available. Before use, the tissue is rehydrated in balanced salt solution with gentamicin sulfate (100 μg/ml) for 20 minutes. At the end of the rehydration period, the tissue is removed from the rehydrating solution and is placed in the Teflon well of a cutting block. A drop of the rehydrating solution is placed in the well, and the cutting block is covered with a brass cover to prevent evaporation and desiccation and contamination of the tissue with dust. The advantages of this tissue are that it is readily available, is prepared preoperatively (which decreases the length of the procedure), and has a smoother posterior surface than that of tissue that is dissected by hand.

For a recipient bed smaller than 5 mm in diameter, the donor lamellar graft should be the same diameter; for a bed 5 to 9 mm, the graft should be 0.25 to 0.5 mm larger than the bed; for a bed larger than 9 mm, the graft should be 0.50 to 1 mm larger than the bed.

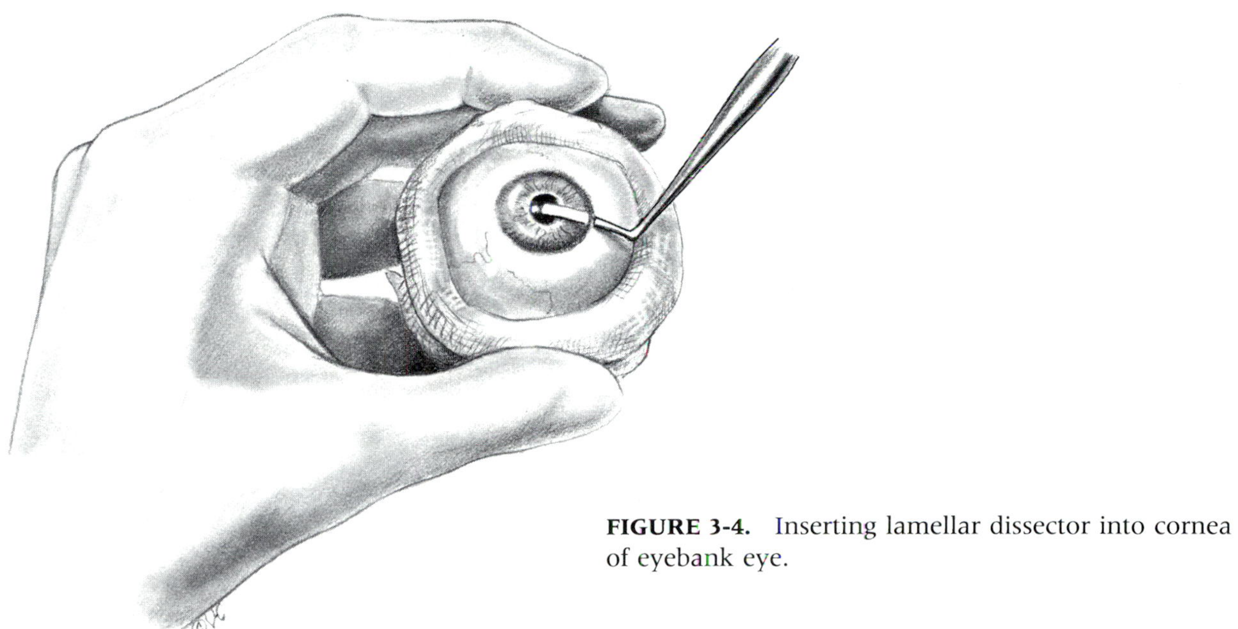

FIGURE 3-4. Inserting lamellar dissector into cornea of eyebank eye.

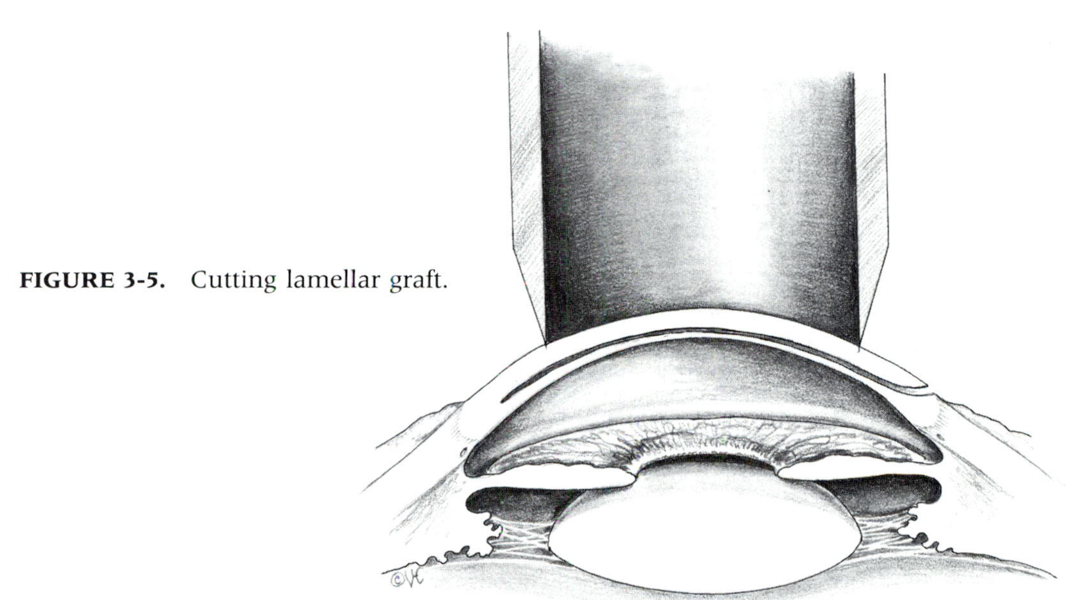

FIGURE 3-5. Cutting lamellar graft.

Suturing the donor lamellar graft

The donor lamellar graft is grasped with a double-pronged (Polack) forceps, and the surfaces are irrigated with filtered balanced salt solution; the irrigant and any debris are aspirated with a pediatric feeding tube connected to suction. The graft is placed in the recipient bed and is sutured with four interrupted 10-0 nylon sutures, as in penetrating keratoplasty. The sutures are placed 0.75 mm from the edges of the donor and recipient corneas. Twelve additional interrupted 10-0 nylon sutures or a running 10-0 nylon suture are placed (Fig. 3-6). Interrupted sutures are removed when they become loose or vascularized. Otherwise, they are removed 2 to 3 months postoperatively.

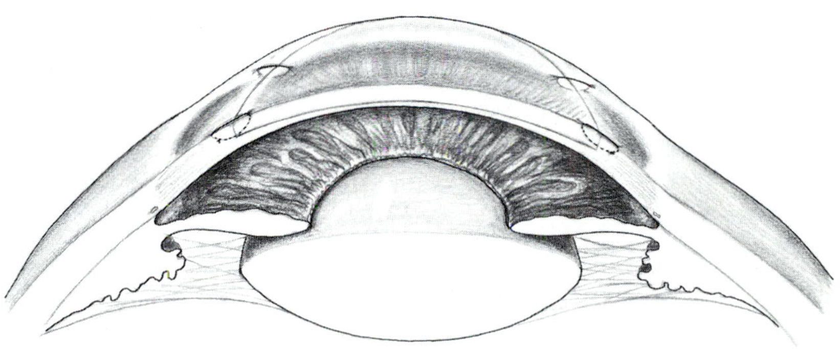

FIGURE 3-6. Inlay lamellar graft sutured in place.

Tectonic Inlay Lamellar Keratoplasty

As stated above, inlay lamellar keratoplasty is usually used today as a tectonic procedure for various corneal thinning disorders. Keratoconus used to be among these disorders; however, with the introduction of onlay lamellar keratoplasty (epikeratophakia), inlay lamellar keratoplasty has become obsolete as a treatment for keratoconus except in a patient with central anterior stromal scarring who is not a candidate for penetrating keratoplasty. Inlay lamellar keratoplasty is still a valuable procedure for peripheral corneal thinning caused by disease (such as Terrien's marginal degeneration) or surgical removal of tissue (such as excision of a pterygium) and for corneal perforations.

The treatment of a corneal perforation depends on the location and cause of the perforation. We use penetrating keratoplasty for a large central perforation involving the visual axis, cyanoacrylate adhesive for a paracentral perforation, and inlay lamellar keratoplasty for a peripheral perforation. We prefer inlay lamellar keratoplasty to cyanoacrylate for the treatment of a peripheral perforation because the results with cyanoacrylate can be unpredictable. Cyanoacrylate requires the use of a bandage contact lens, with the attendant risk of infection, and frequent office visits. Inlay lamellar keratoplasty allows the perforation to be closed definitively in a predictable manner.

At the beginning of the procedure, a tract is made into the anterior chamber at the limbus with a stainless steel blade. This tract provides a route through which the anterior chamber can be reformed with balanced salt solution, a viscoelastic substance, or air, and through which instruments can be inserted to sweep incarcerated tissue from the perforation site. Creation of the tract at the beginning of the procedure, when the anterior chamber may be partially formed, is easier than attempts to create it later, when the anterior chamber is flat. Prolapsed iris is repositioned if it appears viable. Any epithelium growing over the surface of the iris is meticulously removed to prevent intraocular implantation of epithelial cells.

The area of the perforation is outlined with a small trephine, and a partial thickness cut is made large and deep enough to include all the necrotic tissue (Fig. 3-7). An anterior keratectomy is done with a sharp lamellar dissecting blade to remove all the necrotic tissue. A donor lamellar graft ("patch graft") is sutured into the recipient bed with interrupted 10-0 nylon sutures (Fig. 3-8).

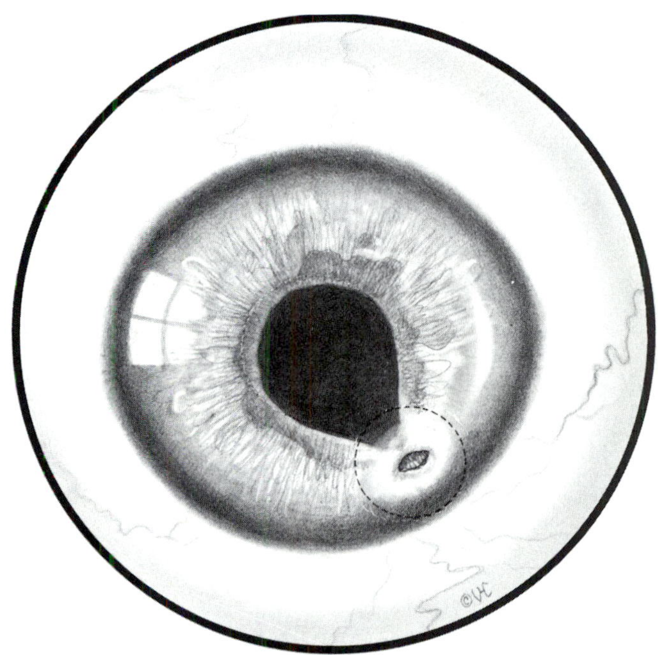

FIGURE 3-7. Corneal perforation. Area of necrotic tissue has been outlined with trephine.

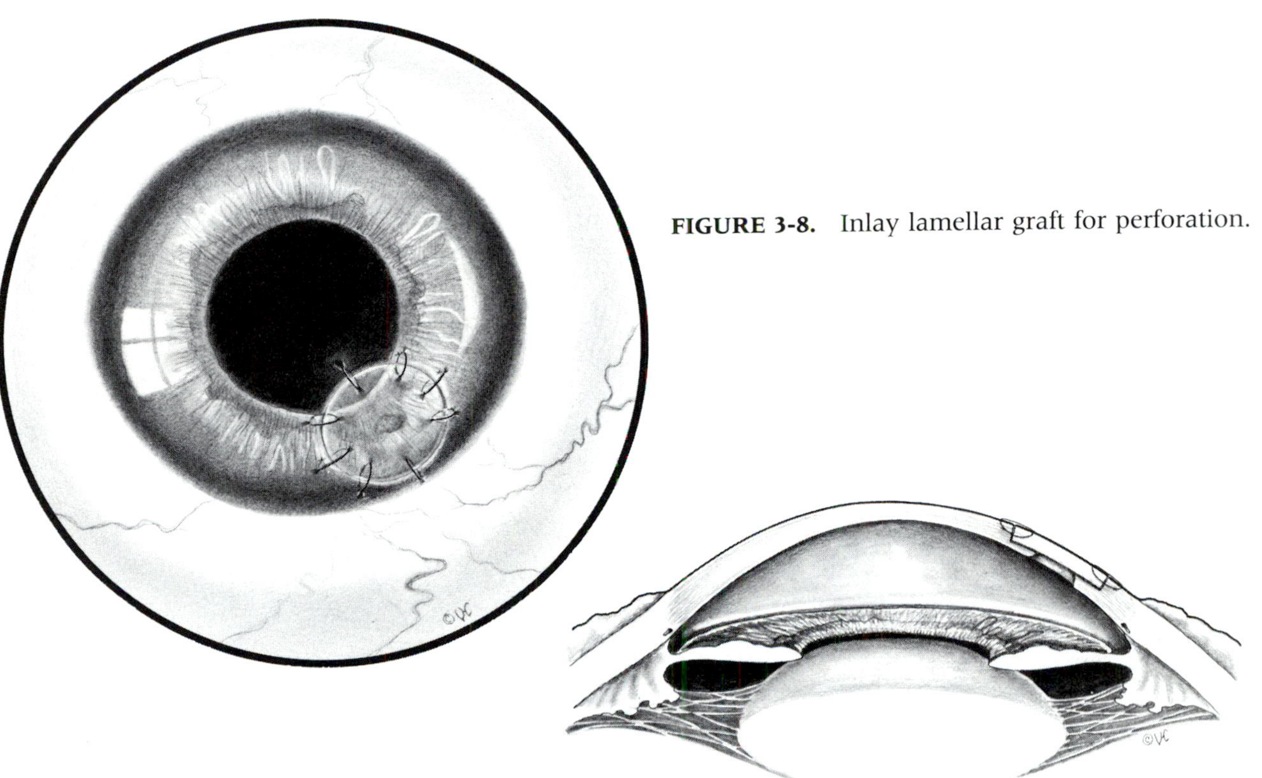

FIGURE 3-8. Inlay lamellar graft for perforation.

A perforation caused by dry eyes or exposure is likely to recur in a lamellar graft unless the underlying disorder is treated. A partial inlay conjunctival flap that covers the lamellar graft is helpful in preventing reperforation (Fig. 3-9). If a conjunctival flap is not done, the graft frequently suffers the same fate as the patient's cornea. (The techniques for conjunctival flaps are described in Chapter 4.)

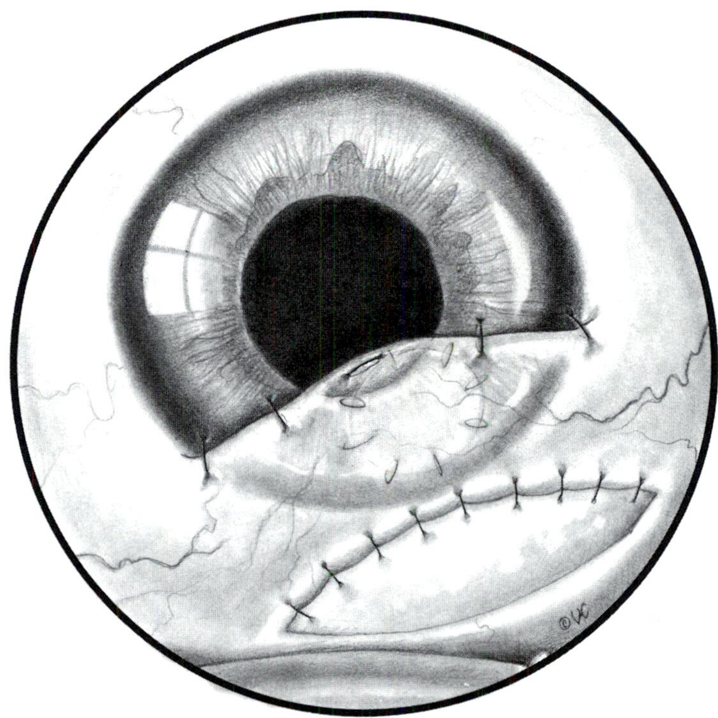

FIGURE 3-9. Partial conjunctival flap covering inlay lamellar graft.

Principles of Onlay Lamellar Keratoplasty

As stated above, inlay lamellar keratoplasty was used in the past to treat keratoconus. It requires a lamellar keratectomy of the recipient cornea, with the attendant risks of corneal perforation and an irregular lamellar bed. Onlay lamellar keratoplasty (epikeratophakia) is similar to inlay lamellar keratoplasty except that a lamellar keratectomy of the recipient cornea is not required. It can be used as a tectonic procedure for the ectatic corneal disorders of keratoconus, pellucid marginal degeneration, or keratoglobus. (The use of onlay lamellar keratoplasty strictly as a refractive procedure is described in Chapter 5.)

Onlay lamellar keratoplasty for keratoconus evolved after the introduction of epikeratophakia for aphakia. It is indicated in a patient with keratoconus who is contact lens intolerant and does not have corneal scarring within 1 mm of the visual axis. If there is central scarring, penetrating keratoplasty is indicated. The advantage of onlay lamellar keratoplasty over inlay lamellar keratoplasty for the treatment of keratoconus is that it does not require lamellar dissection of the recipient cornea; the advantages over penetrating keratoplasty are that it is an extraocular procedure and does not carry the risk of endothelial graft rejection.

The main objective of onlay lamellar keratoplasty for keratoconus is to flatten the cone (Fig. 3-10) so that the patient can resume contact lens wear. However, most patients additionally have a reduction in their myopia and may have good spectacle-corrected vision or even good uncorrected vision.

Technique of onlay lamellar keratoplasty

The techniques of onlay lamellar keratoplasty for keratoconus vary slightly from those of epikeratophakia for aphakia or myopia; the wound configuration is different and the sutures are tied tightly.

The donor lamellar graft is available from Allergan Medical Optics and consists of donor corneal stroma and Bowman's layer that has been frozen, lathed from the posterior surface on a cryolathe to a central thickness of 0.3 mm, and lyophilized. There is a 0.75 mm wing peripherally that tapers to a thickness of 0.11 mm. The diameter of the standard graft is 9.0 mm; however, larger grafts can be ordered for larger cones. There is no inherent power in the graft because the anterior and posterior surfaces are parallel centrally. The graft is rehydrated in balanced salt solution with gentamicin sulfate (100 μg/ml) for 20 minutes, after which it is removed from the rehydrating solution, placed in the Teflon well of a cutting block, and covered with a brass cover to prevent evaporation and desiccation and contamination with dust.

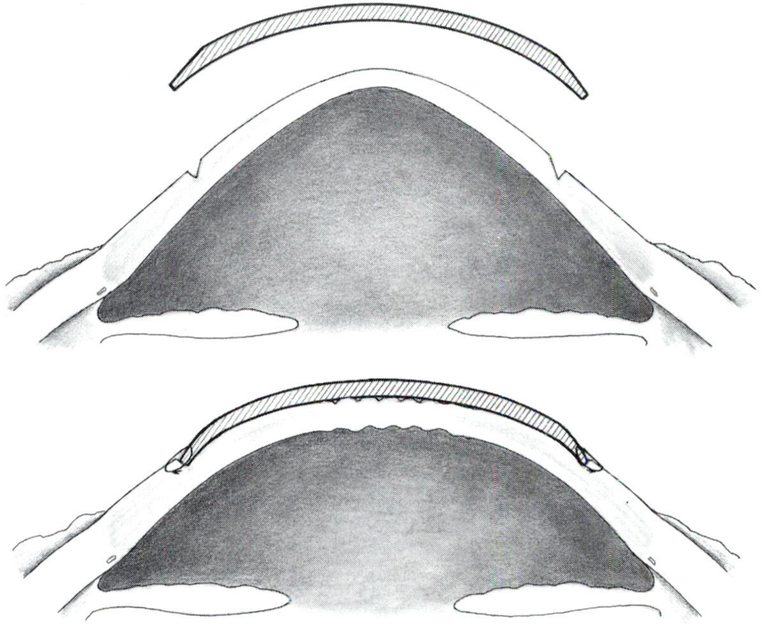

FIGURE 3-10. Onlay lamellar graft for keratoconus.

Because flattening of the cone decreases the volume of the anterior chamber and increases the intraocular pressure, the patient is usually given intravenous mannitol preoperatively. Intermittent external pressure is also applied to the eye after the anesthetic has been administered. The center of the cone is marked with a surgical marking pen to aid in centration of the trephine. A ring of epithelium is removed, as in epikeratophakia for aphakia or myopia, leaving a central island with the centration mark and a 0.5 mm rim of peripheral epithelium as a source of corneal epithelium for reepithelialization of the graft.

The Barron twin blade trephine (Fig. 3-11) is used to create two trephine cuts that delineate the area of the annular keratectomy. This trephine is similar to the Hessburg-Barron vacuum trephine (described in Chapter 2) except that it has two concentric blades. The outer blade is 8.5 mm in diameter; the inner blade is 7.5 mm in diameter and is recessed 0.3 mm from the outer blade. The trephine also has a stop that allows the blades to be lowered only a certain distance. After the outer blade has been zeroed and retracted, the trephine is centered on the centration mark to surround the cone. The entire cone must be surrounded to prevent inadvertent perforation of thin keratoconic tissue beneath the trephine. A vacuum is obtained and the blades are lowered; then the spokes on top of the blade assembly are turned until the stop is reached. The trephine is removed from the eye. The resulting concentric cuts are 0.5 mm apart (Fig. 3-12). The peripheral cut is approximately 0.25 mm in depth; the central cut is approximately 0.10 mm in depth. Currently this trephine is available in only one size for the standard 9 mm graft.

One creates an annular keratectomy by grasping the cornea between the two trephine cuts with a toothed forceps, placing the posterior blade of a Vannas scissors in the depth of the peripheral cut, angling the anterior blade of the scissors approximately 45 degrees so that it lies in the central cut, and excising a strip of cornea between the two cuts (Fig. 3-13). This results in a beveled keratectomy with a width of 0.5 mm and a depth of 0.25 mm peripherally and 0.1 mm centrally (Fig. 3-14).

The central island of epithelium is removed, and the anterior surface of the cornea and the surfaces of the graft are irrigated with filtered balanced salt solution. The irrigant and any loose epithelial cells or debris are aspirated with a pediatric feeding tube connected to suction.

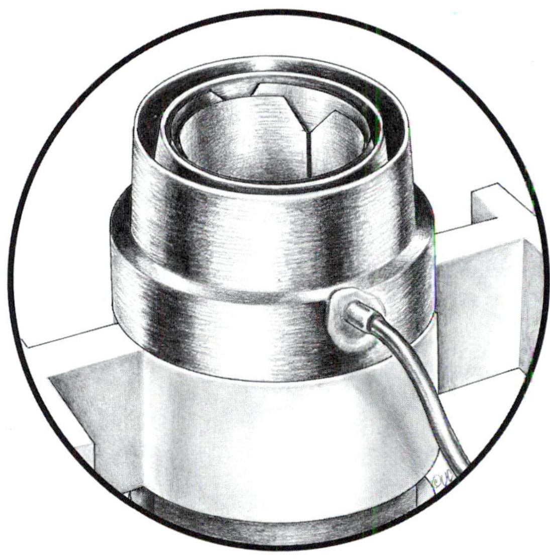

FIGURE 3-11. Barron twin blade trephine.

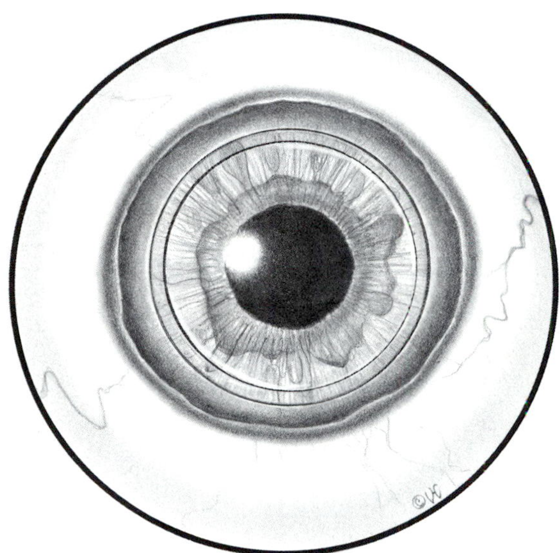

FIGURE 3-12. Concentric incisions from Barron twin blade trephine.

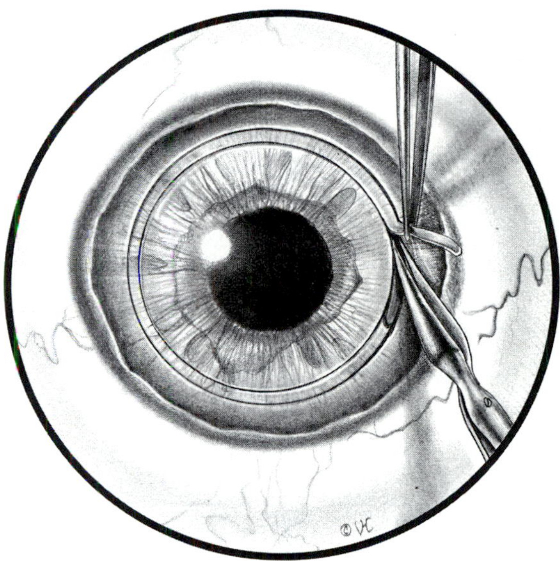

FIGURE 3-13. Removing corneal tissue between concentric incisions.

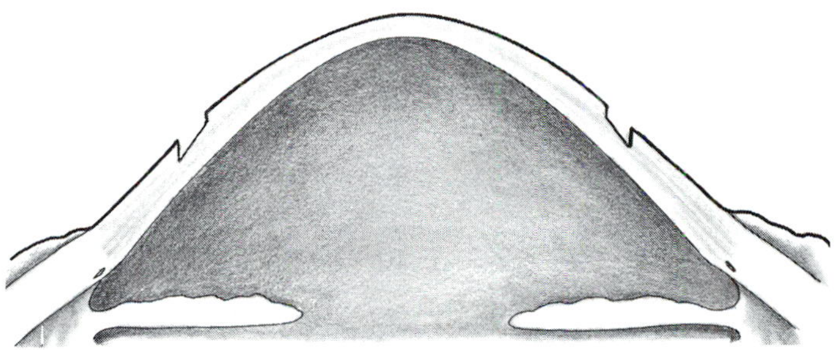

FIGURE 3-14. Peripheral annular keratectomy.

The graft is sutured with 16 interrupted 10-0 nylon sutures. The needle enters the graft 0.75 mm from the edge, passes near the posterior surface to exit through the wing, enters the recipient cornea at the peripheral edge of the keratectomy, and exits 0.75 to 1 mm peripherally. The suture is tied tightly with a triple-throw followed by two single-throws. During placement of the second suture it is not uncommon for the edge of the graft to fall short of the peripheral edge of the keratectomy because of the cone. A Paton spatula is used to push the graft and underlying cone posteriorly so that the graft can be sutured to the edge of the keratectomy (Fig. 3-15). If stress on the tissues breaks the 10-0 nylon, 9-0 nylon may be used for the first four sutures. (These sutures may either be left or replaced with 10-0 nylon sutures at the end of the procedure.) The suture ends are cut on the knots, and the knots are rotated into the recipient cornea. Any suture ends should point toward the anterior corneal surface in an arrow-shaped fashion to facilitate removal of the sutures postoperatively.

Gentamicin sulfate and methylprednisolone acetate are injected subconjunctivally, and gentamicin sulfate and cyclopentolate hydrochloride are applied topically. A bandage soft contact lens may be inserted or a temporary tarsorrhaphy done, and an eye pad and shield placed. The postoperative care is similar to that for epikeratophakia for aphakia or myopia with regard to corneal re-epithelialization (see Chapter 5). Any loose sutures or sutures that attract blood vessels are removed as soon as they are recognized; otherwise they are removed 3 months postoperatively. There are usually several striae in Descemet's membrane at the end of the procedure because of compression of the cone; however, many of these striae disappear with time.

In some patients, onlay lamellar keratoplasty is preferred to penetrating keratoplasty, but there is a scar near the visual axis that may be pushed into the visual axis when the cone is compressed. (An example is a patient with keratoconus who is uncooperative and manipulates the eye to the extent that intraocular surgery is contraindicated.) In such a case the scar can be moved peripherally with a "reefing suture," which is a mattress suture of 10-0 nylon that is placed centrally to the keratectomy adjacent to the scar, passes posteriorly to the keratectomy, and exits peripherally to the keratectomy. As the suture is tightened, it pulls the scar peripherally. The tissue lens is then sutured in place (Figs. 3-16 and 3-17).

Onlay lamellar keratoplasty can also be used to treat pellucid marginal degeneration, in which case the graft is decentered inferiorly to cover the area of thinning. A large (12 mm) onlay lamellar graft can also be used to treat keratoglobus, either as a sole procedure or to provide tissue to which a penetrating keratoplasty graft can be sutured in the future.

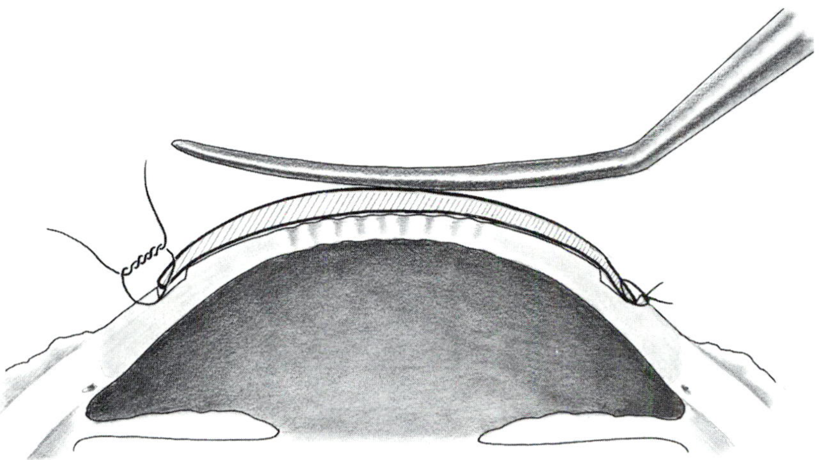

FIGURE 3-15. Flattening cone with Paton spatula.

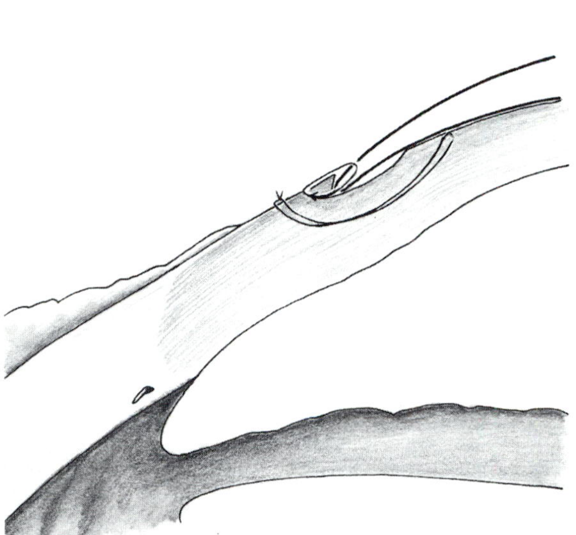

FIGURE 3-16. Reefing suture underneath onlay lamellar graft.

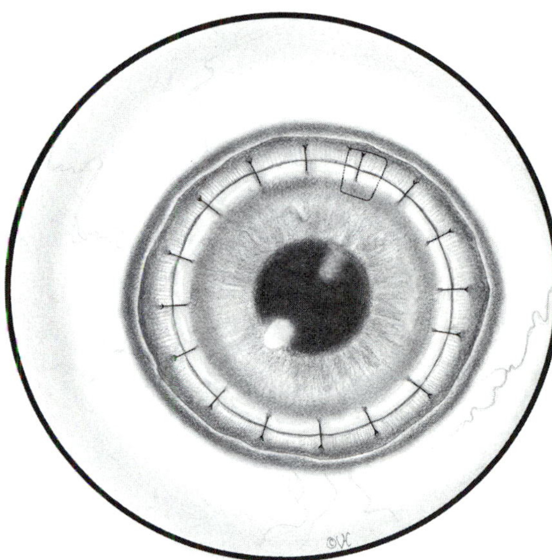

FIGURE 3-17. Onlay lamellar graft and reefing suture. The reefing suture has pulled paracentral scar out of visual axis.

CHAPTER 4

Conjunctival Flaps and Excision of Pterygium

CONJUNCTIVAL FLAPS

Conjunctival flaps are used to treat a variety of disorders of the corneal surface that are unresponsive to other modes of therapy. These disorders include chronic ulcers caused by dry eyes or exposure, certain infectious ulcers unresponsive to antimicrobial therapy, and corneal disorders in eyes with poor visual potential that would otherwise be candidates for visual rehabilitation by penetrating keratoplasty. A conjunctival flap protects the anterior corneal surface. Although it provides some integrity to the cornea, it should not be used as the sole treatment for a corneal perforation.

A conjunctival flap can be total or partial. The type of flap is determined by the extent of corneal disease. Although the techniques for total and partial conjunctival flaps vary, there are five principles common to both: (1) the entire area of diseased cornea should be covered by the flap, (2) there should be no buttonholes in the flap, (3) there should be no tension on the flap, (4) there should be no necrotic tissue beneath the flap, and (5) there should be no epithelium beneath the flap.

Total Conjunctival Flap

The technique described below for a total conjunctival flap is that of Gundersen. Because the conjunctiva is most abundant superiorly, the superior conjunctiva is preferred for a total conjunctival flap. The inferior conjunctiva and temporal conjunctiva are less abundant but can be used if necessary. The nasal conjunctiva is so sparse that it cannot be used for a total conjunctival flap.

The eye is rotated inferiorly by placement of a 6-0 silk suture at the superior limbus (Fig. 4-1), placement of 6-0 silk sutures at the nasal and temporal limbus, or placement of a 4-0 silk suture through the superior rectus muscle. If a superior rectus muscle suture is used, it is placed far enough posteriorly so that it is not in the area of conjunctiva intended for the flap.

Lidocaine hydrochloride with epinephrine is infiltrated beneath the conjunctiva to separate it from Tenon's capsule and to aid in hemostasis (Fig. 4-2). The hypodermic needle is inserted temporally or nasally, away from the area of conjunctiva intended for the flap, so that it does not create a buttonhole in the flap. The anesthetic is injected and is allowed to diffuse beneath the superior conjunctiva.

The superior extent of conjunctiva intended for the flap is determined by measurement from the limbus; it is usually 15 mm posterior to the limbus. An incision is made through the conjunctiva at this point and is extended horizontally slightly beyond the width of the cornea. Conjunctiva is dissected from Tenon's capsule from the incision toward the limbus. The flap should be as thin as possible and should not include any Tenon's capsule. The dissection is done by grasping the conjunctival edge with smooth forceps and sharply separating conjunctiva from Tenon's capsule with blunt-tipped scissors. Opened scissors are inserted beneath the conjunctiva, the conjunctiva is draped over the scissors, the scissors are visualized through the conjunctiva, and the scissors are closed (Fig. 4-3). Care is taken that conjunctiva does not fall between the blades of the scissors and is inadvertently cut. This method of dissection prevents buttonholes, which are common if the posterior surface of the conjunctiva is visualized as the scissors are closed. Blunt dissection is avoided because it may tear the conjunctiva. When the dissection reaches the limbus, a 360-degree limbal peritomy is done with sharp-tipped scissors (Fig. 4-4).

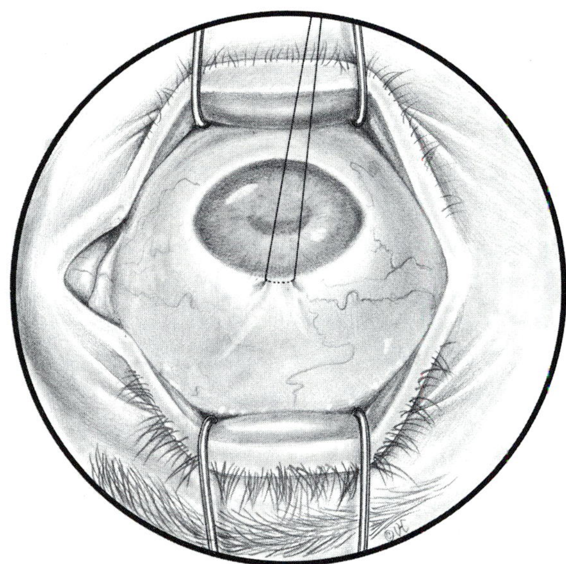

FIGURE 4-1. Traction suture at superior limbus.

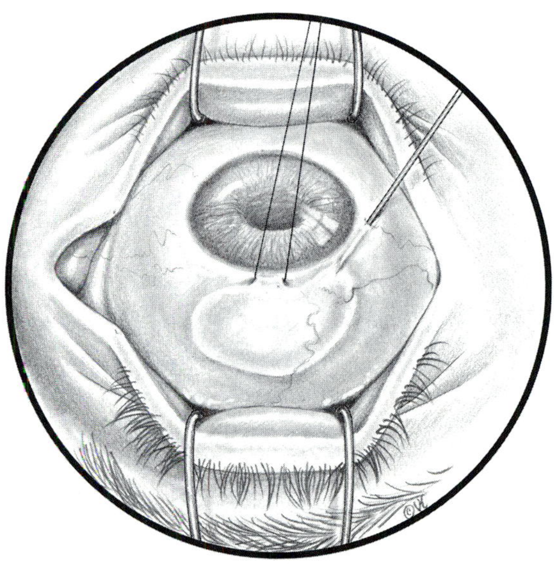

FIGURE 4-2. Infiltrating local anesthetic with epinephrine subconjunctivally.

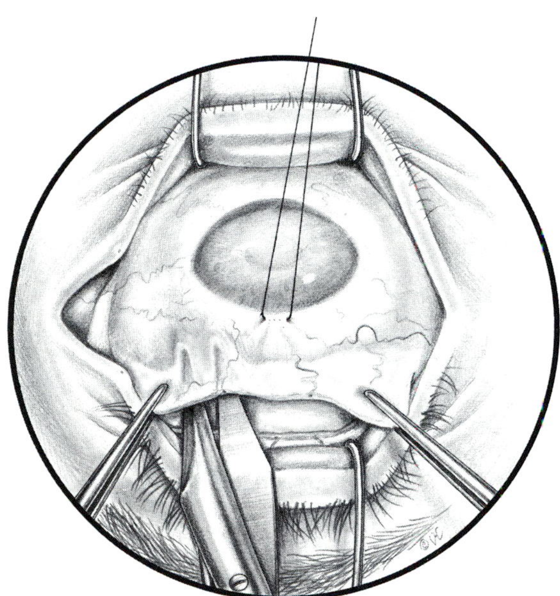

FIGURE 4-3. Dissecting conjunctiva with blunt-tipped scissors.

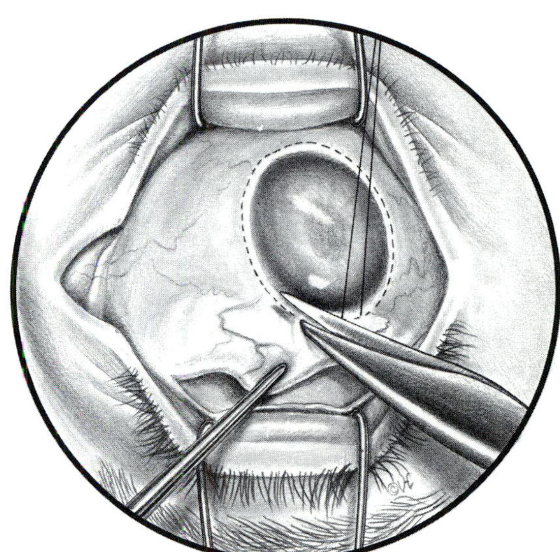

FIGURE 4-4. Creating limbal peritomy with sharp-tipped scissors.

The conjunctival dissection and limbal peritomy create a bridge flap that can be moved inferiorly to cover the cornea (Fig. 4-5). There should be no tension on the flap. Relaxing incisions are made in the conjunctiva, if necessary, to release any tension on the flap. Before placement of the flap on the cornea, all of the corneal and limbal epithelium is removed. A cellulose sponge saturated with absolute alcohol is used to scrub the anterior surface of the cornea and limbus to ensure that there are no viable epithelial cells that could become trapped beneath the flap to form epithelial inclusion cysts. The cellulose sponge is prepared by soaking it in absolute alcohol and squeezing it between the fingers to remove excess alcohol. This prevents alcohol from running over the ocular surface, which can cause irritation and destruction of the conjunctival epithelium. In addition to removal of the corneal epithelium, all necrotic corneal tissue is removed because the flap will erode if it is placed over necrotic tissue. This may necessitate a superficial lamellar keratectomy. If the underlying cornea is thin and there is no active infection, an inlay lamellar graft is placed for tectonic support.

The flap is sutured inferiorly with interrupted 8-0 or 10-0 Vicryl sutures placed through the inferior edge of the flap, the limbal episcleral tissue, and the superior edge of the inferior conjunctiva. The flap is sutured superiorly with sutures placed through the superior edge of the flap and the superior episcleral tissue. This results in coverage of the entire cornea with conjunctiva (Fig. 4-6). There is an area of Tenon's capsule superiorly that is devoid of an epithelial covering, but this area will reepithelialize postoperatively from adjacent conjunctival epithelial cells. It is important to anchor the edges of the flap to episcleral tissue so that the flap will not retract postoperatively and leave areas of bare cornea. If the inferior edge of the flap is sutured just to the superior edge of the inferior conjunctiva, the suture line can migrate superiorly to lie on the cornea (Fig. 4-7); the areas between the sutures can then enlarge and expose the cornea.

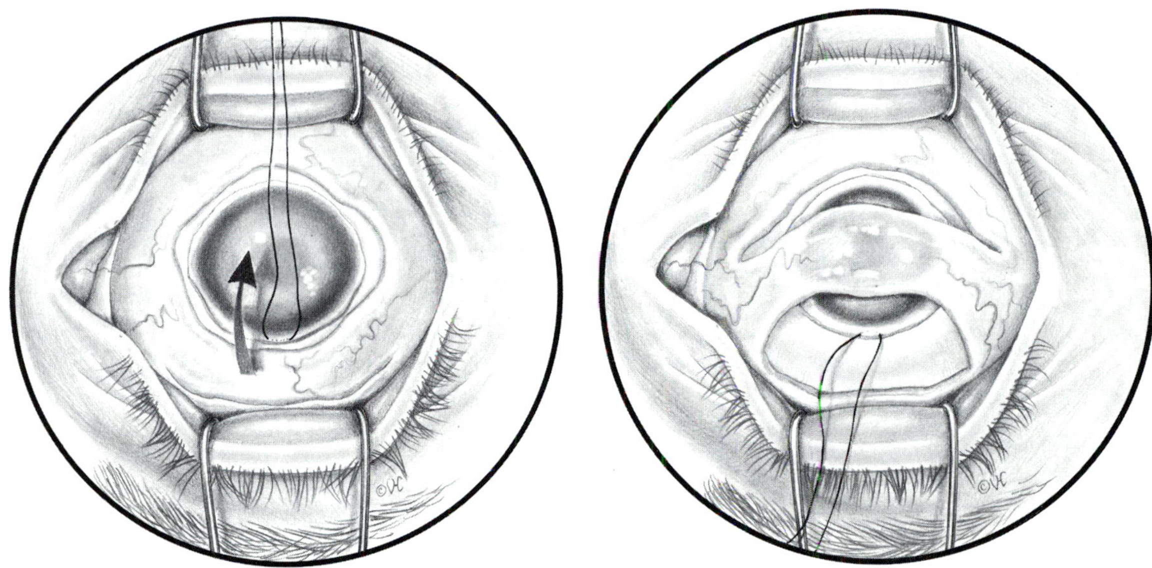

FIGURE 4-5. Moving conjunctival flap over cornea.

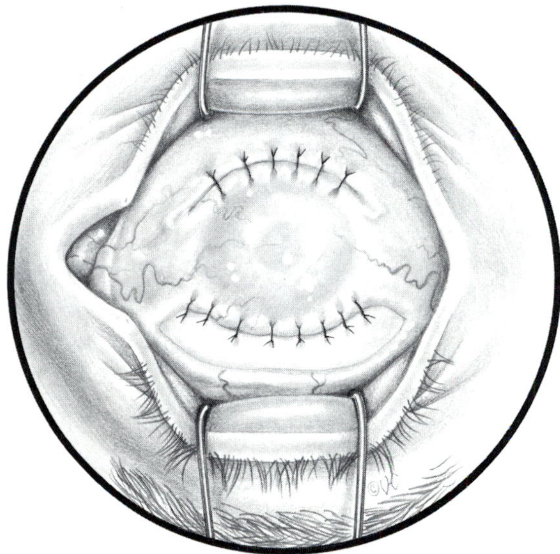

FIGURE 4-6. Total conjunctival flap sutured in place.

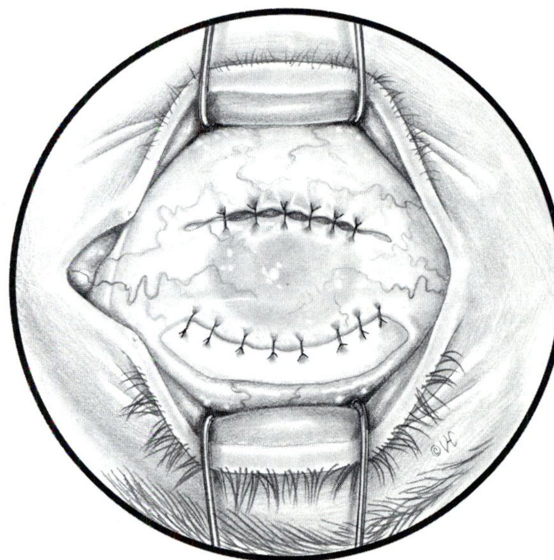

FIGURE 4-7. Migration of inferior suture line over cornea.

Buttonholes in the flap are usually the result of careless dissection. They are to be avoided because they can enlarge postoperatively and expose the cornea. Small buttonholes are moved off the cornea, if possible, or are closed with a 10-0 nylon suture placed through one edge of the buttonhole, the superficial underlying cornea, and the other edge of the buttonhole (Fig. 4-8). Large buttonholes are moved off the cornea, if possible; otherwise a new flap may have to be dissected from another area of conjunctiva.

At the end of the procedure, topical antibiotic and cycloplegic drops are instilled, and an eye pad and shield are placed. The flap is examined the first day postoperatively for buttonholes or areas of retraction, which are repaired with 10-0 nylon sutures. A topical cycloplegic agent is continued until postoperative inflammation has resolved. Vicryl sutures do not have to be removed. During the ensuing weeks the blood vessels in the flap become less congested. A thin conjunctival flap allows visualization of the iris through the flap and is cosmetically acceptable to most patients.

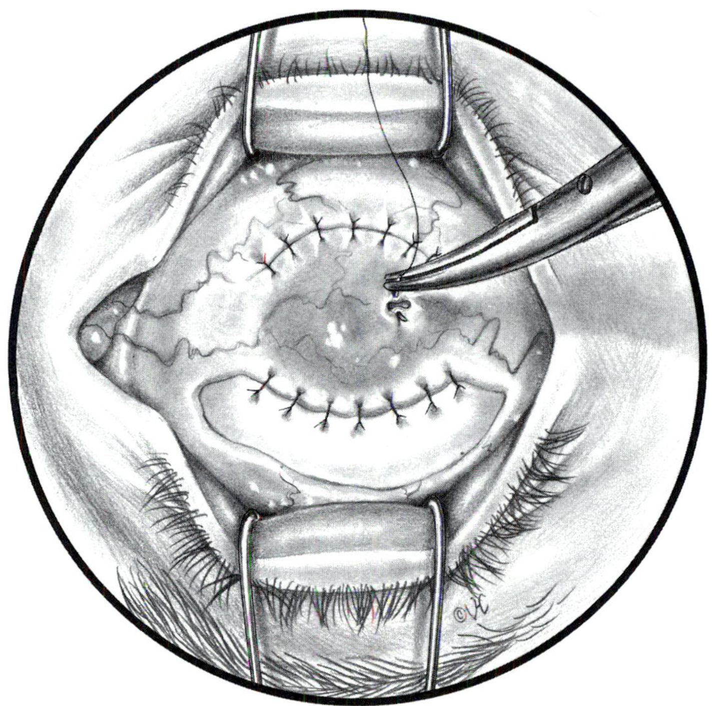

FIGURE 4-8. Closing small buttonhole in conjunctival flap.

Partial Conjunctival Flap

A partial conjunctival flap is an inlay flap and is indicated in many peripheral corneal surface disorders that are unresponsive to other modes of therapy (such as a chronic ulcer from lagophthalmos) (Fig. 4-9). In some cases, such as peripheral fungal keratitis, a partial conjunctival flap is preferred to prolonged medical therapy. The flap usually heals the diseased area, is cosmetically acceptable, and does not interfere with visual acuity.

One performs a lamellar keratectomy by outlining the area of corneal disease with a partial thickness corneal incision made with a stainless steel or gem blade, grasping the edge of the incision with a toothed forceps, and dissecting the diseased tissue with a lamellar dissecting blade (Fig. 4-10). This is done in a manner that gives well-defined vertical edges of corneal tissue to which the flap is sutured. If the underlying cornea is thin and there is no active infection, an inlay lamellar graft is placed for tectonic support.

The conjunctiva adjacent to the area of diseased cornea is used for a fornix-based flap. A limbal conjunctival peritomy is made in the area adjacent to the lamellar keratectomy, and conjunctiva is dissected from Tenon's capsule as described above (Fig. 4-11). The edge of the flap is grasped with smooth forceps and is sutured into the lamellar bed with interrupted 10-0 Vicryl sutures (Fig. 4-12). There should be no tension on the flap; if there is, a relaxing incision is made peripheral to the flap, and the peripheral edge of the flap is sutured to the superficial episclera. In some cases, a pedunculated flap may have to be fashioned to cover the affected area without tension. The postoperative care for a partial conjunctival flap is similar to that for a total conjunctival flap.

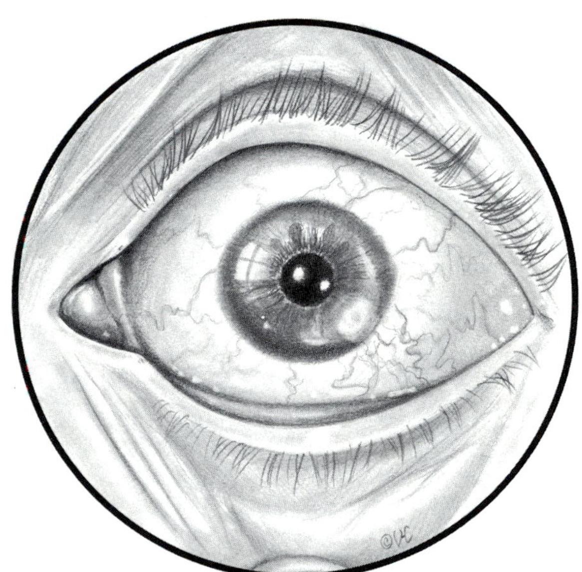

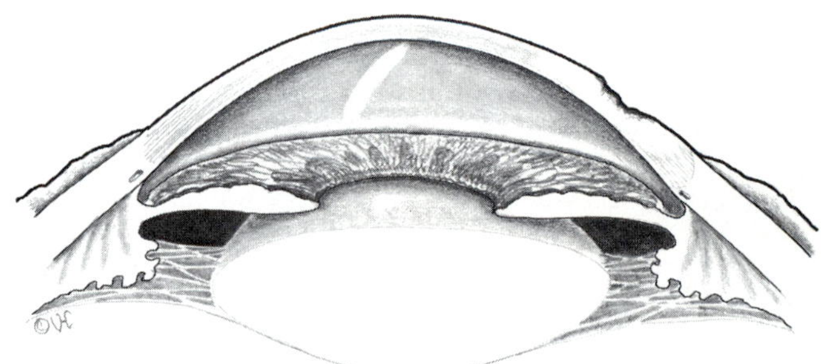

FIGURE 4-9. Abnormality of peripheral corneal surface.

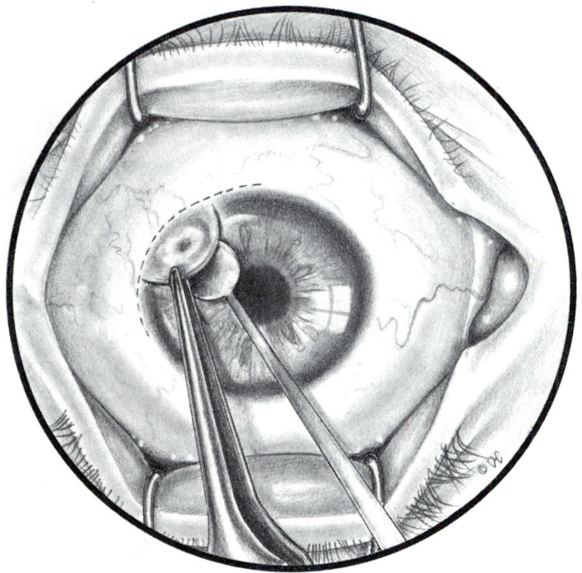

FIGURE 4-10. Sharply dissecting peripheral lamellar tissue.

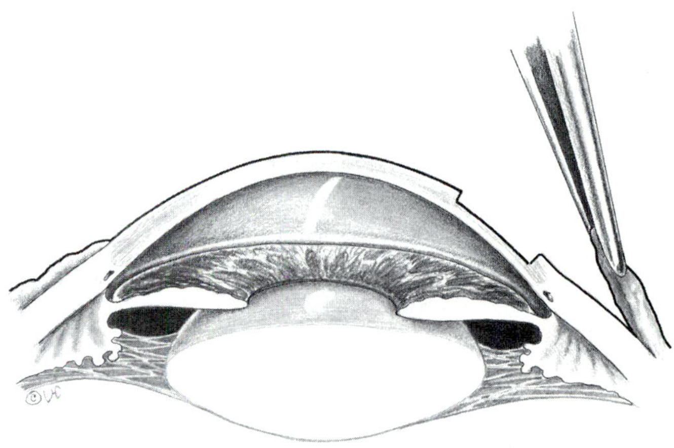

FIGURE 4-11. Conjunctiva dissected from Tenon's capsule.

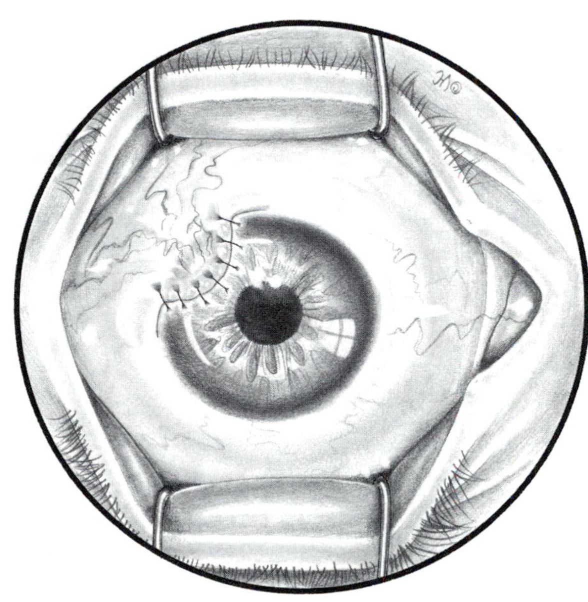

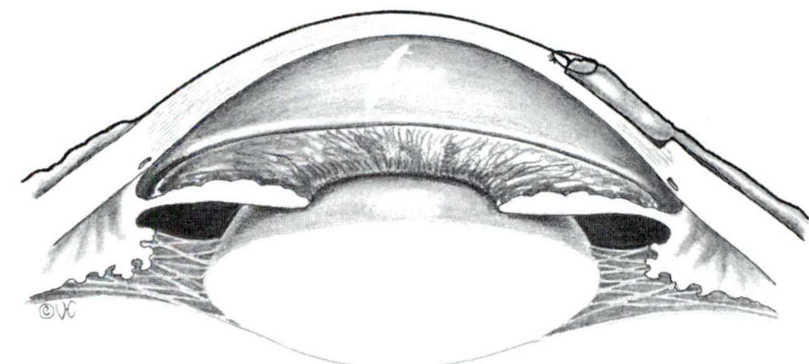

FIGURE 4-12. Partial conjunctival flap sutured in place.

Excision of a Pterygium

A primary pterygium is best left alone unless it encroaches on the visual axis, is causing increasing astigmatism, or is cosmetically unacceptable. The treatment of a primary pterygium involves removal of the abnormal tissue from the cornea and adjacent paralimbal area.

The treatment of a recurrent pterygium is more difficult because the pterygium usually extends deeper into the cornea and there is more exuberant subconjunctival fibrous tissue. There are three important objectives in the treatment of a recurrent pterygium: (1) excising the abnormal tissue in its entirety, (2) obtaining a good optical result, and (3) preventing recurrence.

One removes the head of the pterygium by outlining the edges of the pterygium with a partial-thickness corneal incision made with a stainless steel or gem blade. The shape of this incision depends on the size of the pterygium. For a small pterygium, a linear incision is made. For a large pterygium, a trapezoidal incision is made (Fig. 4-13). One performs a lamellar keratectomy by grasping the edge of the incision with a toothed forceps and dissecting the tissue with a lamellar dissecting blade (Fig. 4-14). When the dissection reaches the limbus, the head of the pterygium is excised with scissors (Fig. 4-15). This method of excision creates a steep edge at the limbus of the same depth as the rest of the lamellar bed and prevents the lamellar dissection from extending into the sclera.

One removes the body of the pterygium by incising the conjunctiva superior and inferior to the pterygium with scissors (Fig. 4-16) and dissecting and excising the subconjunctival fibrous tissue. If the subconjunctival fibrous tissue is exuberant, the horizontal rectus muscle is isolated to prevent inadvertent disinsertion of the muscle and to make identification of the plane of dissection easier. All the subconjunctival fibrous tissue must be removed to decrease the likelihood of recurrence of the pterygium. In cross section, the lamellar bed is deep, with steep distinct edges; the subconjunctival dissection is shallower (Fig. 4-17).

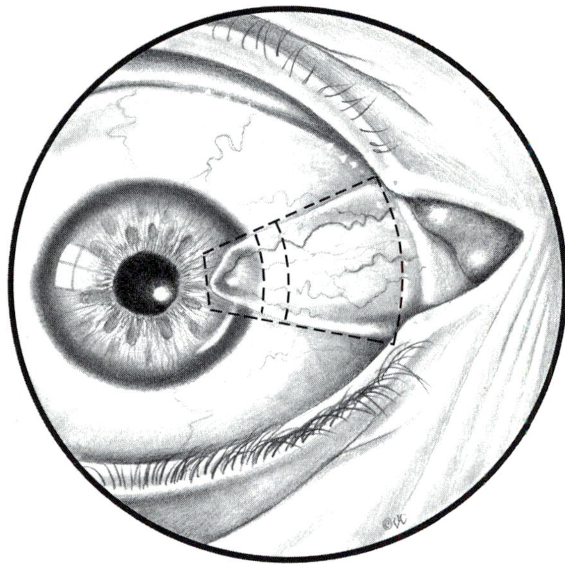

FIGURE 4-13. Area of pterygium to be excised.

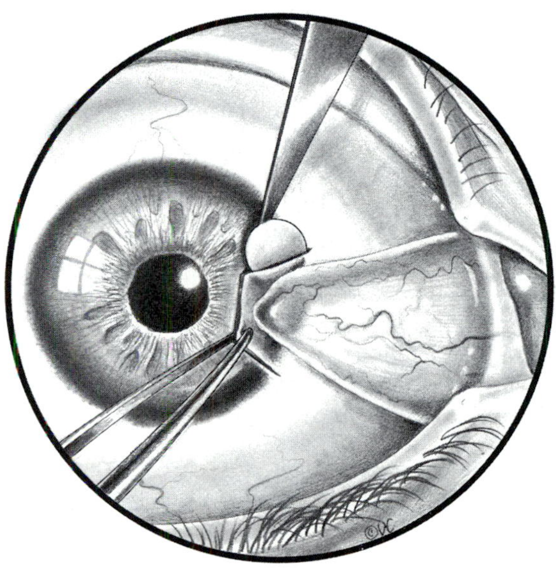

FIGURE 4-14. Sharply dissecting head of pterygium.

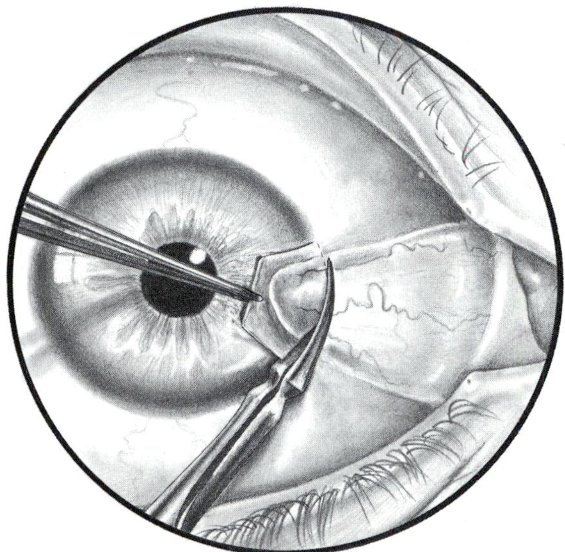

FIGURE 4-15. Excising head of pterygium at limbus with scissors.

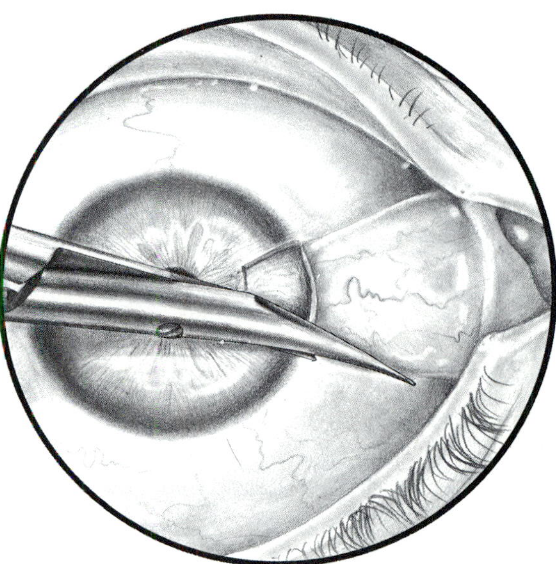

FIGURE 4-16. Excising body of pterygium.

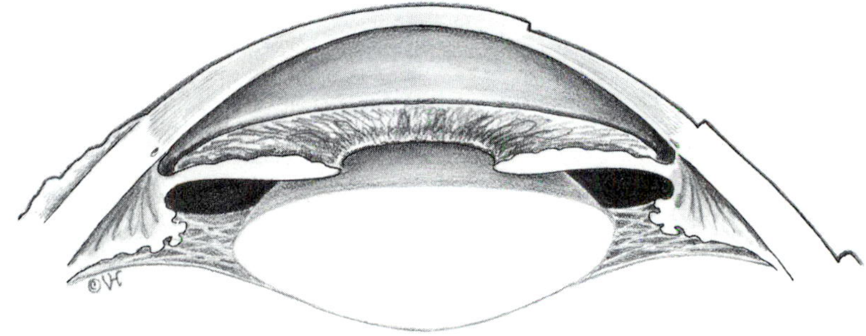

FIGURE 4-17. Cross-section of lamellar bed from pterygium removal.

If the cornea underlying the lamellar bed is thin, an inlay lamellar graft is placed. The donor lamellar graft is prepared or obtained as described in Chapter 3. It is easiest to cut the graft to fit as it is being sutured. First, the graft is sutured to the limbal edge with interrupted 10-0 nylon sutures. The curvature of a 10 mm graft usually matches that of the limbus for three or four clock hours before the differences in curvature become apparent. After the limbal sutures have been placed, the graft is cut with straight scissors to match the lamellar bed and is sutured in place. If the central edge of the graft is close to the visual axis, a horizontal suture is used in that area instead of a radial suture (Fig. 4-18).

The sclera adjacent to the limbus is meticulously cleaned and paralimbal blood vessels are cauterized. The superior conjunctiva is undermined, and a conjunctival flap is dissected, translocated, and sutured with 8-0 or 10-0 Vicryl sutures to cover the sclera (Fig. 4-19). A free conjunctival autograft from the superotemporal area can be used if necessary. There should be a 3 mm area of bare sclera adjacent to the limbus.

The postoperative care is the same as for an inlay lamellar graft, with the addition of topical corticosteroids. The limbal sutures are usually removed in 2 weeks; the remaining sutures are removed in 4 to 6 weeks.

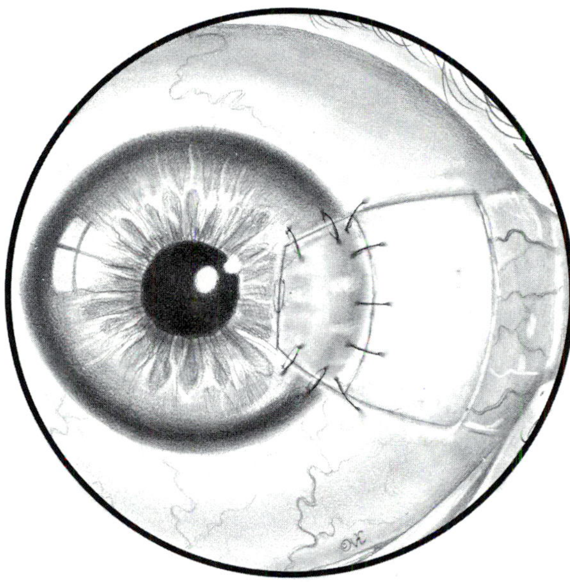

FIGURE 4-18. Inlay lamellar graft for pterygium. Central suture is out of visual axis.

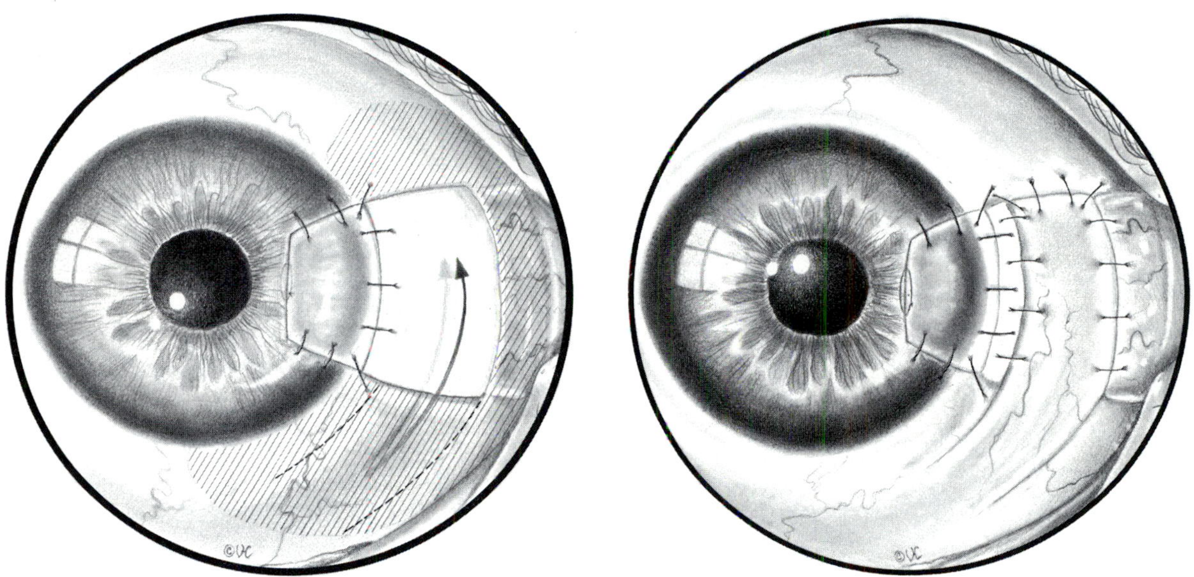

FIGURE 4-19. Moving conjunctival flap to cover area of bare sclera peripherally.

CHAPTER 5

Refractive Surgery

Refractive surgery includes a variety of corneal surgery procedures that change the refractive power of the cornea (see Table 1-1, p. 4). Some procedures whose primary goal is usually other than altering corneal power (such as restoring corneal integrity or transparency) may in certain circumstances be considered primarily refractive procedures. For example, when penetrating keratoplasty is performed in a patient with keratoconus who can no longer be successfully fitted with a contact lens, it can be thought of as a refractive procedure. Similarly, inlay lamellar keratoplasty, onlay lamellar keratoplasty, and excision of a pterygium may be primarily refractive, depending on circumstances. Such "multipurpose" procedures are described in previous chapters. In this chapter, only strictly refractive procedures, that is, procedures whose sole goal is to change the refractive power of the cornea, are described.

Refractive surgery can be classified as lamellar procedures, keratotomy procedures, and keratectomy procedures. Lamellar procedures include keratophakia, keratomileusis, epikeratophakia, and intracorneal lens implantation. Keratotomy procedures include radial keratectomy and various astigmatic keratotomy incisions. Keratectomy procedures include wedge resection and excimer laser photoablation. The placement of compression sutures is an additional refractive procedure that does not fit into this classification.

The theory on which refractive surgery is based is discussed in Chapter 1. This chapter is limited to a description of various refractive surgical techniques. Because the area of refractive surgery is rapidly evolving and changing, this chapter stresses the principles rather than the specifics of these procedures.

Epikeratophakia

Epikeratophakia for aphakia or myopia is a refractive onlay lamellar keratoplasty procedure that is designed to correct the refractive error of the eye by altering the anterior corneal curvature. It evolved from the refractive lamellar keratoplasty procedures of keratophakia and keratomileusis.

In keratophakia, an anterior lamellar section of cornea is removed, a preshaped tissue lens of donor corneal stroma is placed in the lamellar bed, and the removed section of cornea is placed on top of the tissue lens (Fig. 5-1). The tissue lens is thicker centrally than peripherally and causes steepening of the anterior corneal curvature.

There are two types of keratomileusis: autoplastic and homoplastic. In autoplastic keratomileusis, an anterior lamellar section of cornea is removed, shaped, and replaced in the lamellar bed. If more tissue is removed peripherally than centrally, the anterior corneal curvature steepens (Fig. 5-2, *A*). If more tissue is removed centrally than peripherally, the anterior corneal curvature flattens (Fig. 5-2, *B*). In homoplastic keratomileusis an anterior lamellar section of cornea is removed and a preshaped tissue lens of donor corneal stroma and Bowman's layer is placed in the lamellar bed. Homoplastic keratomileusis can correct higher amounts of ametropia than autoplastic keratomileusis. The surgical technique of homoplastic keratomileusis is simpler than that of autoplastic keratomileusis because the tissue lens is preshaped; however, donor corneal tissue is required. A modification of these procedures, called "keratomileusis in situ," is being evaluated. In this technique, an anterior lamellar section of the cornea is removed, the lamellar bed is shaped, and the removed section of cornea is replaced in the lamellar bed.

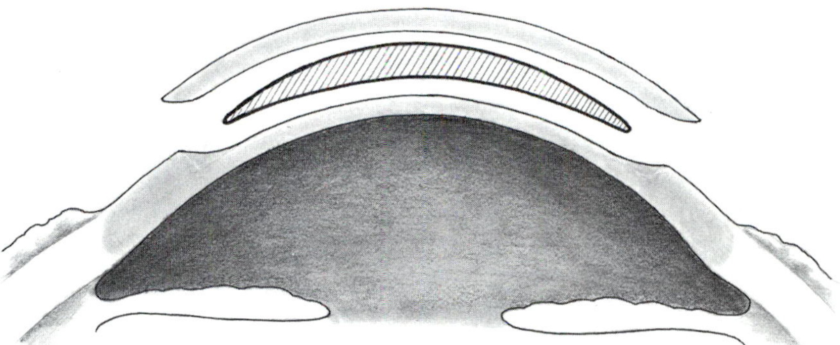

FIGURE 5-1. Keratophakia.

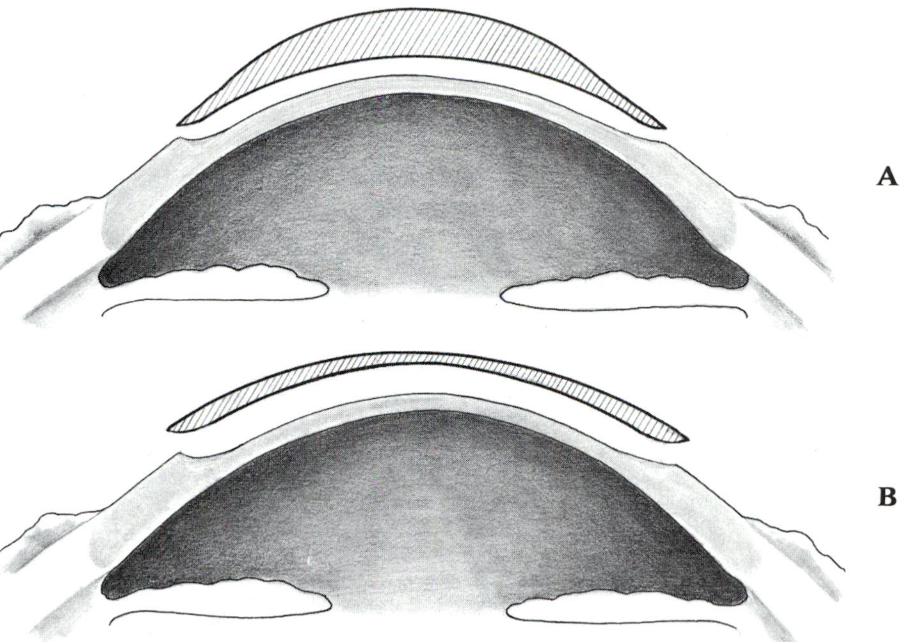

FIGURE 5-2. **A,** Keratomileusis for hypermetropia. **B,** Keratomileusis for myopia.

In epikeratophakia for aphakia or myopia, the central corneal epithelium is removed and an L-shaped peripheral keratotomy is created. A preshaped tissue lens of donor corneal stroma and Bowman's layer is placed on the anterior corneal surface. The edge of the tissue lens is tucked and sutured into the peripheral keratotomy, and an adhesion forms between the posterior surface of the tissue lens and the patient's cornea in this area. If the tissue lens is thicker centrally than peripherally, the anterior corneal curvature steepens (Fig. 5-3). If the tissue lens is thicker peripherally than centrally, the anterior corneal curvature flattens (Fig. 5-4). The advantages of epikeratophakia over keratophakia and keratomileusis are that the surgical techniques are simpler and safer, and the procedure is more reversible because Bowman's layer of the patient's cornea is not disturbed centrally.

Epikeratophakia for aphakia or myopia is considered in a patient who is spectacle and contact lens intolerant and who does not have any progressive corneal disorder. Uncontrolled blepharitis or dry eyes is a contraindication to the procedure.

Tissue lenses for epikeratophakia are available commercially (Kerato-Lens, Allergan Medical Optics, Irvine, California). One makes a tissue lens by restoring a preserved donor cornea to normal thickness in a cornea press, freezing it, and lathing it from the posterior surface on a cryolathe. For plus power, more tissue is removed peripherally than centrally; for minus power, more tissue is removed centrally than peripherally. The tissue lens has a central optical zone and a peripheral wing, much like a contact lens. After the donor cornea has been lathed, it is placed in a glass vial and lyophilized. The tissue lens contains no viable cells; it merely provides a collagen framework that alters the anterior corneal curvature. The tissue lens is repopulated with epithelial cells and keratocytes from the patient's cornea.

The tissue lens is ordered on the basis of two parameters: spherical equivalent of the refractive error at the corneal plane and average keratometry measurement. The spherical equivalent at the corneal plane is calculated from the spectacle refraction and the vertex distance of that refraction with the following formula:

$$P_c = P_s/(1 - vP_s)$$

where P_c is the power at the corneal plane in diopters, P_s is the power at the spectacle plane in diopters, and v is the vertex distance in meters. Only spherical tissue lenses are available commercially, but small amounts of astigmatism (less than 2 diopters) may be masked by these lenses. Toric tissue lenses for the correction of astigmatism are currently under investigation.

Epikeratophakia can be done under local or general anesthesia. In a cooperative patient, a centration mark is made on the cornea before anesthetic is administered. (Methods for making the centration mark are described later in the section on radial keratotomy.) This mark is used for centering the trephine and hence the tissue lens. In an uncooperative patient in whom a centration mark cannot be made, the trephine is centered on the geometric center of the pupil.

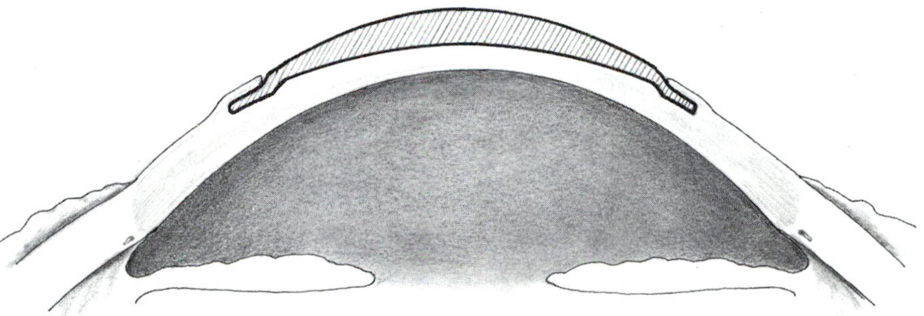

FIGURE 5-3. Epikeratophakia for hypermetropia.

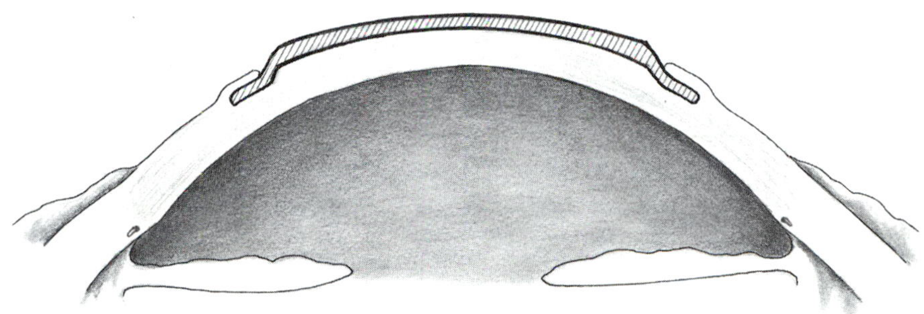

FIGURE 5-4. Epikeratophakia for myopia.

As anesthetic is administered, the tissue lens is placed in balanced salt solution with gentamicin sulfate (100 μg/ml). The tissue lens is rehydrated for 20 minutes in this solution, after which it is removed, placed in the Teflon well of a cutting block, and covered with a brass cover to prevent evaporation and desiccation and contamination with dust. The full 20-minute rehydration period is necessary before the tissue lens can be used.

After administration of anesthetic, lid specula are inserted. Sutures (4-0 silk) are placed through the superior and inferior rectus muscles for stabilization and manipulation of the eye. A ring of midperipheral epithelium is removed after an epithelial defect is created with a blunt cellulose sponge saturated with absolute alcohol or 4% cocaine solution that contains no preservatives (Fig. 5-5). One prepares the cellulose sponge by soaking it in alcohol or cocaine solution and squeezing it between the fingers to remove excess solution. Care is taken to avoid getting the alcohol or cocaine onto the peripheral cornea or conjunctiva because it will damage epithelial cells in these areas and so delay postoperative epithelialization of the tissue lens. After an epithelial defect has been created, the midperipheral corneal epithelium is removed with a blunt spatula, such as the Paton spatula (Fig. 5-6). A central island of epithelium that contains the centration mark and a 0.5 mm rim of peripheral epithelium are left. The central epithelium with the centration mark is used to center the trephine; the peripheral epithelium provides a source of corneal epithelial cells to cover the tissue lens postoperatively. If the peripheral epithelium is removed, conjunctival epithelium must migrate and transdifferentiate to cover the tissue lens. A sharp instrument is not used to remove the epithelium because it may damage Bowman's layer and cause scarring between the central cornea and tissue lens, which can impair postoperative visual acuity and decrease the reversibility of the procedure. Loose epithelial cells are removed from the field so that they will not become trapped between the cornea and the tissue lens and form inclusion cysts.

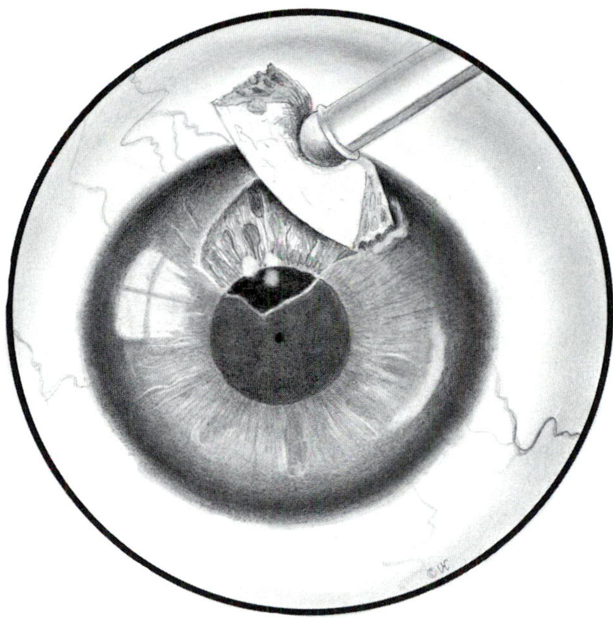

FIGURE 5-5. Creating epithelial defect with blunt cellulose sponge saturated with cocaine solution.

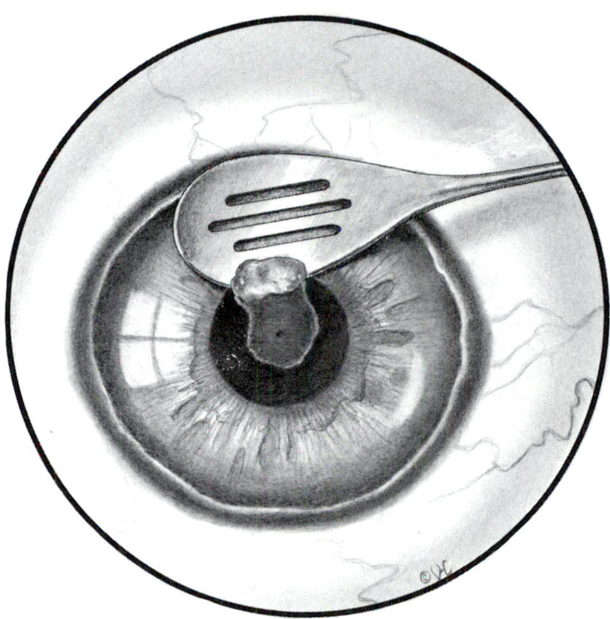

FIGURE 5-6. Removing midperipheral epithelium with Paton spatula.

A Hessburg-Barron vacuum trephine (described previously in Chapter 2) is used to create a partial-thickness corneal incision. This trephine is preferred because it creates an incision of uniform depth. The diameter of the trephine is 1.5 mm smaller than the diameter of the tissue lens. The blade of the trephine is zeroed in and is retracted three quarter-turns (Fig. 5-7). The anterior corneal surface is moistened with balanced salt solution, and the crosshairs of the trephine are centered on the centration mark or pupil as one looks through the center of the trephine. The plunger of the syringe is pushed in all the way, the trephine is pressed gently on the corneal surface, and the plunger of the syringe is released abruptly. After a vacuum has been obtained and the cornea is fixated, one lowers the blade by turning the spokes on top of the blade assembly five quarter-turns (1¼ full turns) (Fig. 5-8). Quarter-turns must be differentiated from full turns to prevent inadvertent perforation of the cornea. Care is taken not to lift, depress, or tilt the trephine as the spokes are turned. After the incision is made, the plunger of the syringe is pushed in all the way, and the trephine is removed from the eye. A modification of this trephine that contains a stop that limits the distance the blade can be lowered is available. The trephine cut is examined with a cellulose sponge for depth and uniformity. The depth of the cut should be just posterior to Bowman's layer, or approximately 0.10 to 0.15 mm. A stainless steel blade may be used to deepen the cut, if necessary.

After the trephine cut has been made, the central island of epithelium is removed and the anterior surface of the cornea is irrigated with filtered balanced salt solution (Fig. 5-9). A pediatric feeding tube connected to suction is used to remove the irrigation fluid and any loose epithelial cells or debris from the anterior surface of the cornea. Clarity of the interface between the cornea and tissue lens is dependent on the absence of epithelial cells and debris in the interface. Powder from surgical gloves and lint from gauze sponges are major sources of foreign material. Therefore all members of the surgical team should rinse their gloves before beginning the procedure, and gauze sponges should not be used.

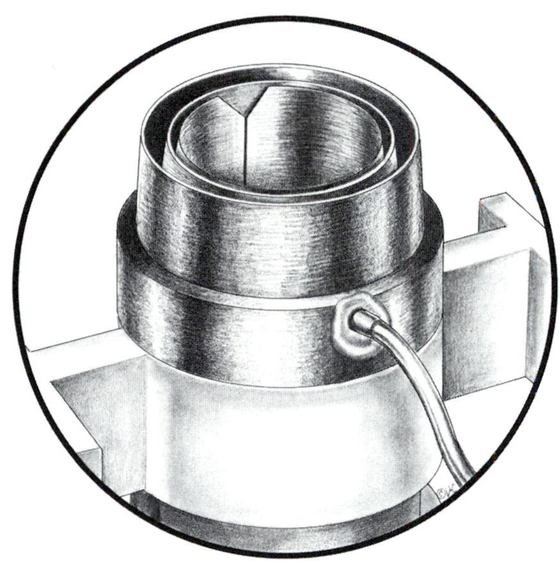

FIGURE 5-7. Blade of Hessburg-Barron vacuum trephine retracted from inner wall of vacuum chamber.

FIGURE 5-8. Lowering blade of Hessburg-Barron vacuum trephine.

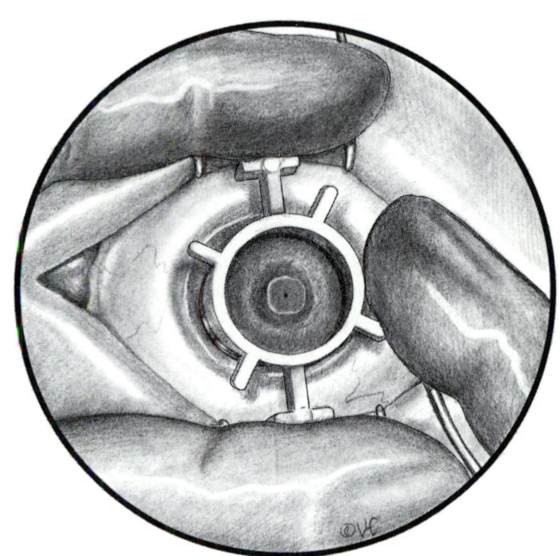

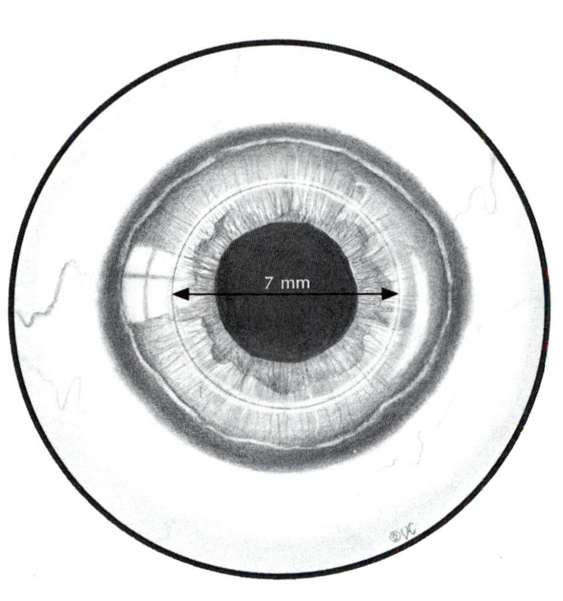

FIGURE 5-9. Partial-thickness trephine cut.

One makes a peripheral 1 mm lamellar dissection with a lamellar dissecting blade by grasping the peripheral edge of the trephine cut with a toothed forceps, inserting the blade into the depth of the cut, and dissecting the peripheral lamellae parallel to the anterior corneal surface (Fig. 5-10). The trephine cut and lamellar dissection create an L-shaped pocket into which the wing of the tissue lens is inserted (Fig. 5-11). This pocket should be continuous and even around the entire circumference of the cornea.

The rehydrated tissue lens is grasped with a double-pronged (Polack) forceps for stabilization, and both surfaces of the tissue lens and the anterior surface of the patient's cornea are irrigated with filtered balanced salt solution. The irrigation fluid is aspirated with a pediatric feeding tube connected to suction. The rehydrated tissue lens assumes a shape much like a contact lens, with a convex anterior surface and a concave posterior surface. The surfaces can also be differentiated by their appearances; the anterior surface is shinier than the posterior surface.

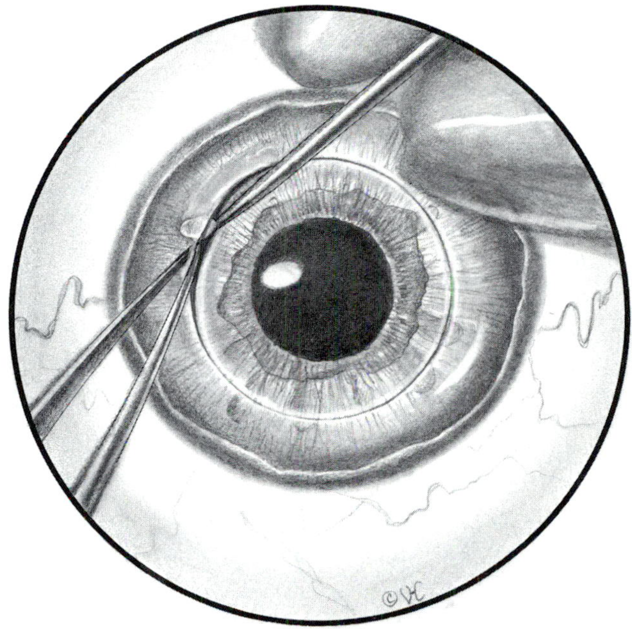

FIGURE 5-10. Dissecting peripheral lamellae.

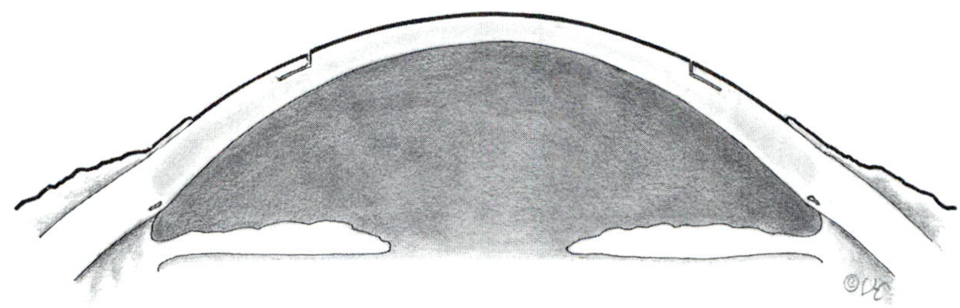

FIGURE 5-11. L-shaped pocket created by trephine cut and peripheral lamellar dissection.

The tissue lens is sutured with 16 interrupted 10-0 nylon sutures. For the first suture, the tissue lens is placed on the cornea and the needle is placed between the two prongs of the forceps, approximately 0.75 mm from the edge of the tissue lens (Fig. 5-12). The needle splits the wing of the tissue lens; it does not pass through the full thickness. The peripheral edge of the trephine cut is grasped with a single-pronged toothed forceps, and the needle is passed into the pocket created by the lamellar dissection to exit 1 mm peripheral to the trephine cut. This method of suturing permits the wing of the tissue lens to be tucked into and fixated in the pocket created by the lamellar dissection (Fig. 5-13). The suture is tied with a triple-throw followed by two single-throws that are just tight enough to secure the tissue lens to the cornea. There is an urge to tie sutures too tightly in epikeratophakia because of the custom of using sutures to close wounds. A conscious effort must be made to avoid this. Tight sutures cause compression and distortion and can lead to postoperative astigmatism and undercorrection in both aphakia and myopia.

As in penetrating keratoplasty, the second suture is the most important suture in epikeratophakia because it determines the distribution of the tissue lens. For the second suture, the tissue lens is grasped with a toothed forceps, and the needle is placed exactly 180 degrees from the first suture. The peripheral edge of the trephine cut is then grasped, and the needle is passed into the pocket created by the lamellar dissection to exit 1 mm peripheral to the cut. Before the needle is pulled through the cornea, one evaluates the distribution of the tissue lens by examining the trephine cut through the tissue lens. The tissue lens is usually translucent enough so that the cut can be seen through it (Fig. 5-14). If the distribution is uneven, the needle is removed from the cornea and replaced. The distribution is reevaluated, and the needle is replaced again, if necessary. When the distribution is even, the needle is pulled through the cornea and the suture is tied.

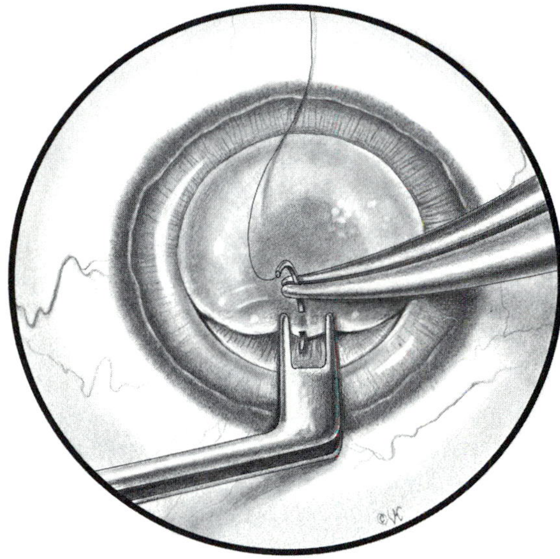

FIGURE 5-12. Placing first suture between prongs of Polack forceps, with needle splitting wing of tissue lens.

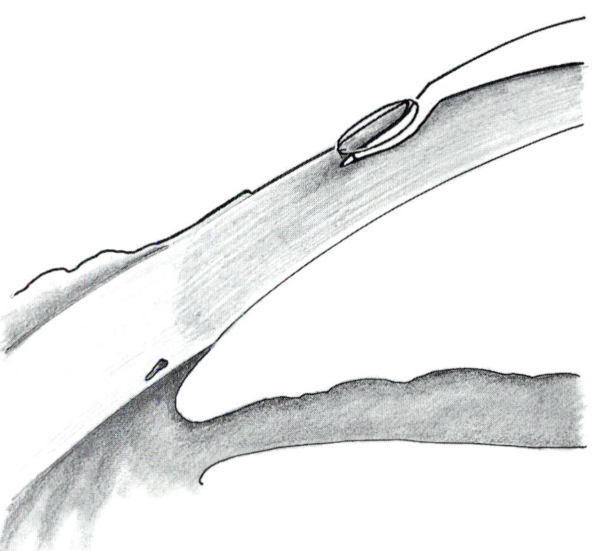

FIGURE 5-13. Wing of tissue lens sutured into lamellar pocket.

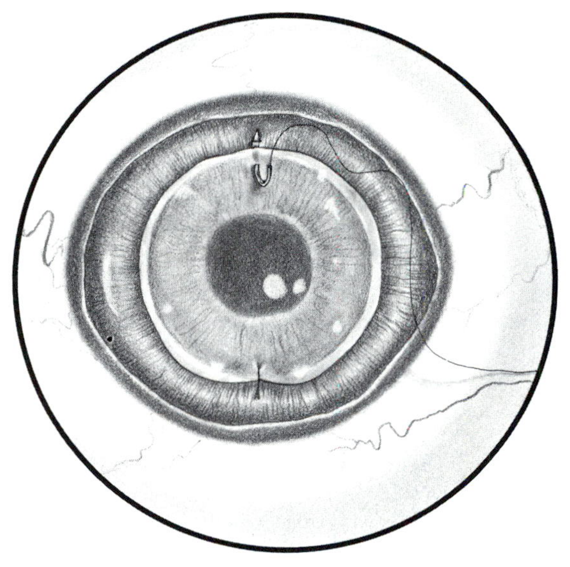

FIGURE 5-14. Placing second suture to distribute tissue lens evenly.

The third and fourth sutures are placed 90 degrees from the first two sutures, and the next four sutures are placed equidistant between the first four sutures. The last eight sutures are placed equidistant between the first eight sutures. These sutures may be placed either by direct visualization, with the needle splitting the wing of the tissue lens, or the tissue lens can be tucked into the pocket created by the lamellar dissection (Fig. 5-15) and the sutures placed through the entire thickness of the tissue lens, entering at the edge of the trephine cut and exiting 1 mm peripheral to the cut.

After placement of all sixteen sutures, the wing of the tissue lens is tucked into the pocket created by the lamellar dissection. It is important that the entire wing is tucked beneath the corneal surface to prevent postoperative astigmatism. The suture ends are cut on the knots, and the knots are rotated into the peripheral cornea. Any suture ends should point toward the corneal surface in an arrow-shaped fashion, which makes postoperative removal of the sutures easier.

At the end of the procedure a qualitative surgical keratoscope is used to evaluate sphericity of the anterior corneal surface. Although the end of a safety pin or a circular opening in a piece of plastic or metal can be used, we prefer a qualitative surgical keratoscope, such as the Troutman keratoscope. Care is taken to ensure that the patient's eye is parallel to the keratoscope and that the lid specula are not pressing on the eye. The shape of the reflection of lights from the anterior corneal surface indicates whether the surface is spherical. A circular reflection indicates little or no astigmatism (Fig. 5-16). An oval reflection indicates astigmatism, with the steep axis in the area where the oval is narrowest, and the flat axis in the area where the oval is widest. Astigmatism can be caused by a tight suture in the steep axis (Fig. 5-17), or a loose suture or dehiscence of the wing of the tissue lens in the flat axis. Intraoperative evaluation for astigmatism allows these flaws to be corrected at the time of surgery.

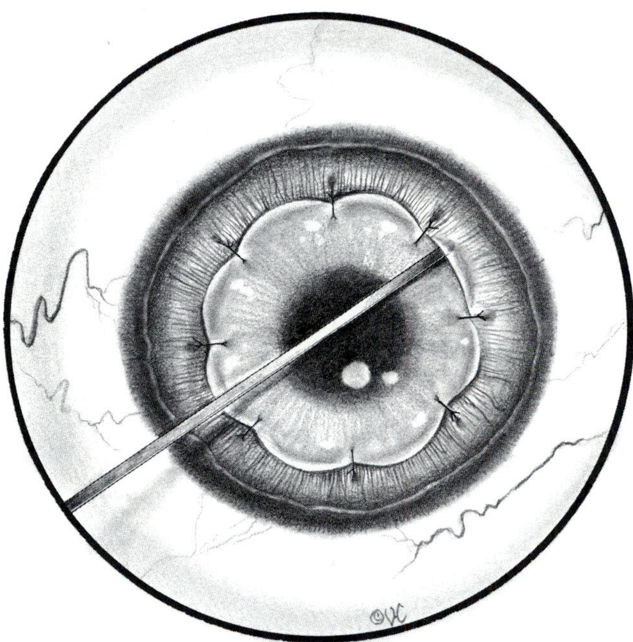

FIGURE 5-15. Tucking wing of tissue lens into lamellar pocket.

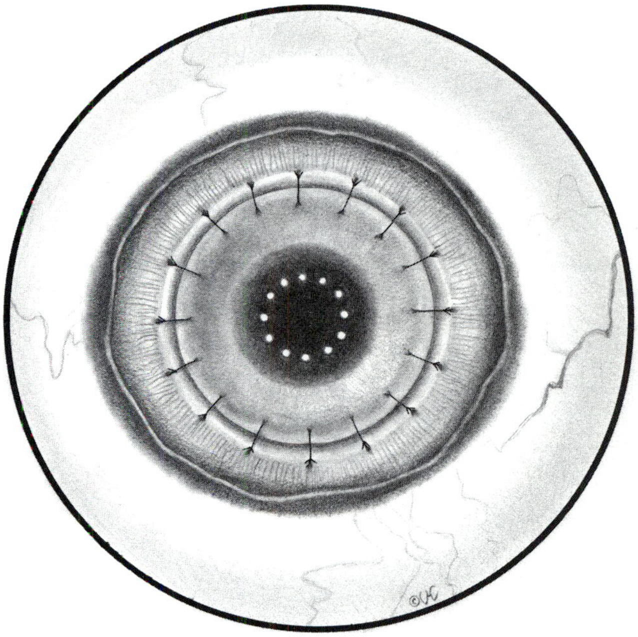

FIGURE 5-16. Properly sutured tissue lens. Circular reflection from surgical keratoscope indicates little or no astigmatism.

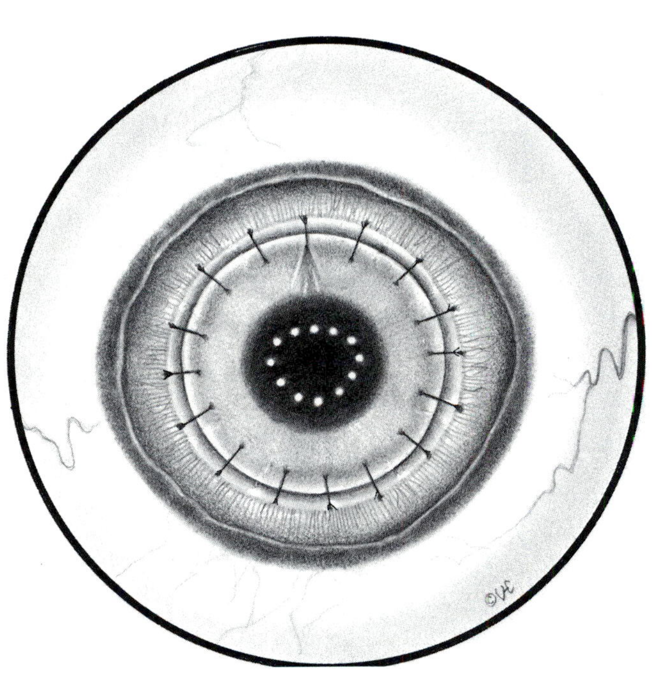

FIGURE 5-17. Improperly sutured tissue lens. Oval reflection from surgical keratoscope is caused by a tight suture.

Gentamicin sulfate and methylprednisolone acetate are injected subconjunctivally, and gentamicin sulfate and homatropine sulfate drops are applied topically. No corticosteroids are injected in children.

In an adult, there are three methods for promoting postoperative epithelialization of the tissue lens: (1) semipressure patch, (2) bandage soft contact lens, or (3) temporary tarsorrhaphy. The method depends on the patient's and surgeon's preferences. We have used all three methods but have found that a temporary tarsorrhaphy promotes epithelialization rapidly, is well tolerated by most patients, and requires less frequent office visits than the other methods (see p. 1018 and also Part Seven: Ophthalmic Plastic Surgery). One performs a temporary tarsorrhaphy by closing the lids with two or three 5-0 nylon mattress sutures. The needles enter the skin of the lower lid 5 mm below the lid margin, exit the lower lid margin posterior to the meibomian gland orifices, enter the upper lid margin posterior to the meibomian gland orifices, and exit the skin of the upper lid 5 mm above the lid margin. Pieces of a sterile rubber band can be used as bolsters. The sutures are tied with a double-throw, followed by a bowknot. The suture ends are taped to the patient's forehead. This method allows the sutures to be untied, the lids opened, the eye examined, the lids closed, and the sutures retied.

On the first postoperative day the surface of the tissue lens is examined for epithelialization. This examination is enhanced by the application of topical fluorescein. If a bandage lens is used, topical proparacaine hydrochloride is instilled and the lens is moved to the side with a sterile cotton applicator. This allows the fluorescein to flow under the bandage lens and over the tissue lens to stain areas devoid of epithelium. This technique is less traumatic than removal and reinsertion of the bandage lens. Although the bandage lens is stained with fluorescein, this does not interfere with the function of the lens.

If a semipressure patch is used, topical homatropine hydrobromide drops and gentamicin sulfate ointment are applied, a new patch is placed, and the eye is examined every 24 to 48 hours until epithelialization is complete. If a bandage lens is used and it fits well and is tolerated by the patient, topical homatropine and gentamicin drops are applied twice a day and the eye is examined every 24 to 48 hours until epithelialization is complete. If a temporary tarsorrhaphy is used, the lid sutures are retied. Homatropine and gentamicin drops are placed over the medial canthus and allowed to trickle onto the eye twice a day. The tarsorrhaphy is opened and the eye examined at weekly intervals until epithelialization is complete.

The tissue lens is usually covered with epithelium during the first postoperative week. After the tissue lens has epithelialized, an ointment that contains no preservatives is used 4 times a day and tapered over the next month. Delayed epithelialization must be treated aggressively; otherwise the tissue lens will melt. As stated above, in our experience a temporary tarsorrhaphy is the best method for promoting epithelialization. Therefore, if the tissue lens does not epithelialize progressively with a semipressure patch or bandage lens, a tarsorrhaphy is done. If there is no progression of epithelialization with a tarsorrhaphy, the tissue lens is removed.

Early refraction is important for detection of large amounts of astigmatism or undercorrection. Astigmatism caused by tight sutures is treated by removal of those sutures, even if this is done the first day postoperatively. One treats astigmatism caused by dehiscence of the wing of the tissue lens by tucking the wing back into the pocket created by the lamellar dissection. This can be done at the slitlamp under topical anesthesia. One treats a recurrent dehiscence by resuturing the wing in that area. Excessive undercorrection is usually indicative of tight sutures and is treated by the immediate removal of at least half if not all the sutures. As with penetrating keratoplasty, loose sutures or sutures that attract blood vessels are removed as soon as they are recognized. Otherwise the sutures are removed at 3 weeks. Sutures are removed through the peripheral cornea to avoid passing the knot through the tissue lens and risking dehiscence of the wing of the tissue lens.

Astigmatism or undercorrection caused by tight sutures may be irreversible if it is not recognized early and the tight sutures are removed. Persistent astigmatism can be treated by surgical dehiscence of the wing of the tissue lens for 45 degrees on either side of the steep axis. The wing is reinserted into the lamellar pocket but is not sutured. Persistent undercorrection can be treated with a 360-degree relaxing incision of the wound.

In children, a bandage lens is inserted at the end of the procedure, and a plastic eye shield with holes is placed. Oral amoxicillin is given for 2 to 3 weeks. Gentamicin sulfate and atropine sulfate ointments are squirted through the holes of the eye shield onto the lids twice a day and are allowed to melt and run onto the eye. This is less traumatic than attempting to instill medications directly onto the eye. The bandage lens is left in place for 2 to 3 weeks postoperatively, at which time an examination under anesthesia is done and the bandage lens and all the sutures are removed.

If medical or optical complications necessitate removal of the tissue lens, the trephine cut is reopened in one area with a stainless steel blade (Fig. 5-18), and the pocket created by the lamellar dissection is entered by separation of the anterior surface of the tissue lens from the overlying cornea with an iris sweep (Fig. 5-19). This is easily done because there is no scarring between Bowman's layer of the tissue lens and the stroma of the cornea overlying it. When the edge of the wing is reached, the sweep is directed posteriorly, and the posterior surface of the tissue lens is separated from the underlying cornea (Fig. 5-20). This is the only area where the tissue lens is adherent to the cornea because there are two stromal surfaces apposed to one another. The sweep is then passed across Bowman's layer of the patient's cornea to the other side of the wound, where it is popped out of the wound (Fig. 5-21) and swept along the entire circumference of the wound. Care is taken during this maneuver not to dissect corneal lamellae. Another tissue lens may be placed; if not, the patient is treated as for a large corneal abrasion.

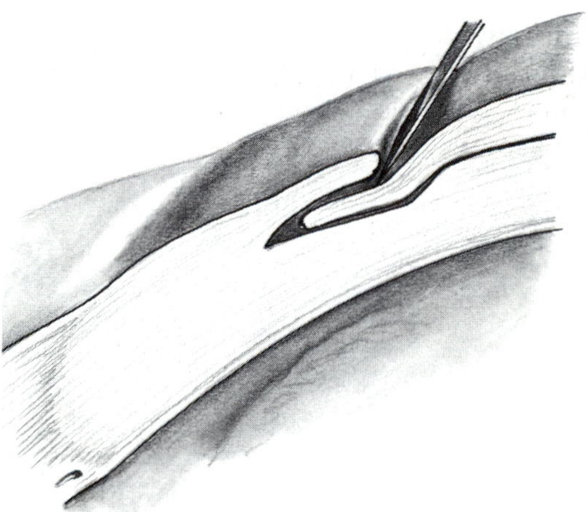

FIGURE 5-18. Reopening trephine cut.

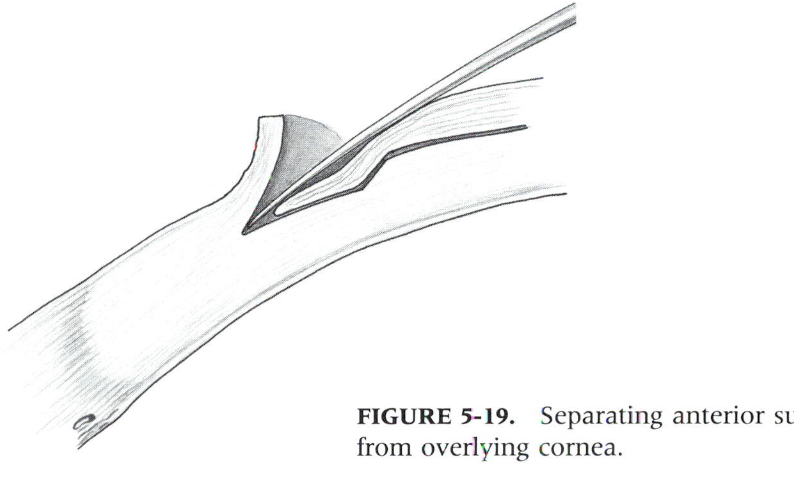

FIGURE 5-19. Separating anterior surface of tissue lens from overlying cornea.

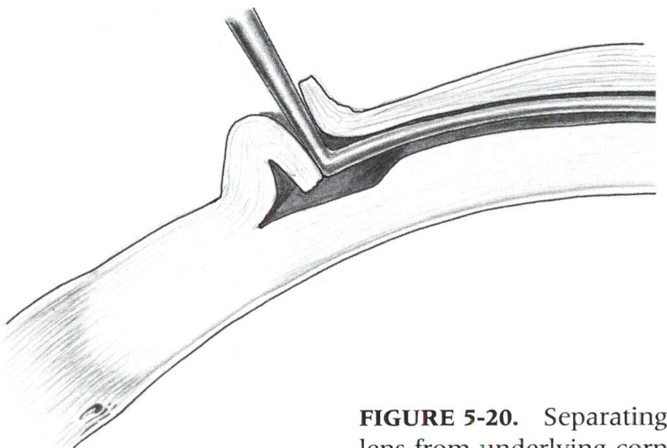

FIGURE 5-20. Separating posterior surface of tissue lens from underlying cornea.

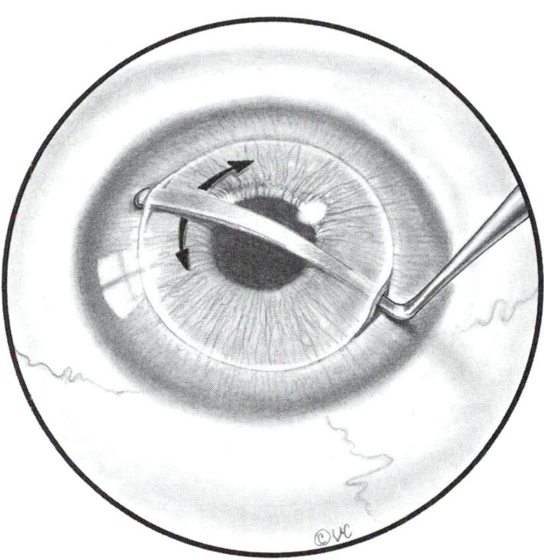

FIGURE 5-21. Separating tissue lens from cornea with iris sweep.

Radial Keratotomy

In radial keratotomy, radial incisions are made in the cornea to flatten the cornea and correct myopia. In the 1950s, anterior and posterior incisions were made; however, endothelial damage from the posterior incisions caused late bullous keratopathy. Radial keratotomy was essentially abandoned after the development of contact lenses. It was revived in the late 1970s in the Soviet Union and was introduced into the United States in the early 1980s.

Radial keratotomy can correct mild to moderate degrees of myopia. It may be considered in a spectacle and contact lens intolerant adult with 2 to 5 diopters of myopia. The myopia should be stable, and there should be no underlying corneal disorder. Major drawbacks to radial keratotomy are unpredictability and instability. A patient considering radial keratotomy should be informed that, although surgical parameters are selected to achieve emmetropia, undercorrection, overcorrection, or a fluctuating refraction is possible postoperatively. A patient with presbyopia should realize that near vision will be exchanged for distance vision and that reading glasses will be required if radial keratotomy is done bilaterally.

The techniques for radial keratotomy vary. However there are two principles common to all the techniques: the amount of myopic correction depends on (1) the diameter of the optical clear zone and (2) the depth of the incisions. The smaller the diameter of the optical clear zone and the deeper the incisions, the greater is the correction. The technique recommended here is a modification of that of the Prospective Evaluation of Radial Keratotomy (PERK) study.

The center of the optical clear zone may be the geometric center of the cornea, the center of the entrance pupil (the virtual image of the pupil formed by light from the real pupil refracted by the cornea), or the point where the visual axis (the line from the fovea to the point of fixation) intersects the cornea. It appears that the center of the entrance pupil, or more appropriately, the point where the line of sight (the line from the center of the entrance pupil to the point of fixation) intersects the cornea, is preferred for centering corneal refractive procedures. Accurate marking of the center of the optical clear zone is important because a misplaced mark may result in postoperative glare from misplaced incisions. The patient must have a natural pupil for optimal centering; therefore miotics or mydriatics are not given for the procedure. Topical proparacaine hydrochloride is applied, the patient fixates on a fixation light on the microscope that is coaxial with the surgeon's sighting eye, and a mark is made on the epithelium with a 25-gauge hypodermic needle at the center of the patient's entrance pupil (Fig. 5-22). The corneal light reflex is not used because of error arising from the angle lambda (the angle formed at the center of the entrance pupil by the pupillary axis and the line of sight). The fixation light varies with the type of microscope, and the method for its use should be obtained from the manufacturer of the microscope. One should take care not to damage Bowman's layer by applying too much pressure with the needle. One checks the placement of the mark by having the patient look away and refixate. Another mark is made in the center and is checked to make sure it is coincident with the first mark.

Topical proparacaine is applied again to the eye, and cellulose sponges soaked in proparacaine are held at the limbus to obtain good anesthesia because this is the area that is used for stabilizing the eye as the incisions are made.

An optical zone marker of appropriate diameter is chosen. This marker consists of a dull circular metal ring, a centering device (either crosshairs or a point), and a handle. A diameter of 3.0 mm, 3.5 mm, or 4.0 mm is most commonly used. There are various nomograms that specify the diameter of the optical zone marker, but, in general, the smaller the diameter, the greater is the correction. A diameter of less than 3 mm is not recommended because of the increased risk of postoperative glare from incisions that are too close to the line of sight. The optical zone marker is centered on the mark previously made in the epithelium, pressed gently on the corneal epithelium, and rotated 90 degrees (Fig. 5-23). One should take care not to damage Bowman's layer by applying too much pressure.

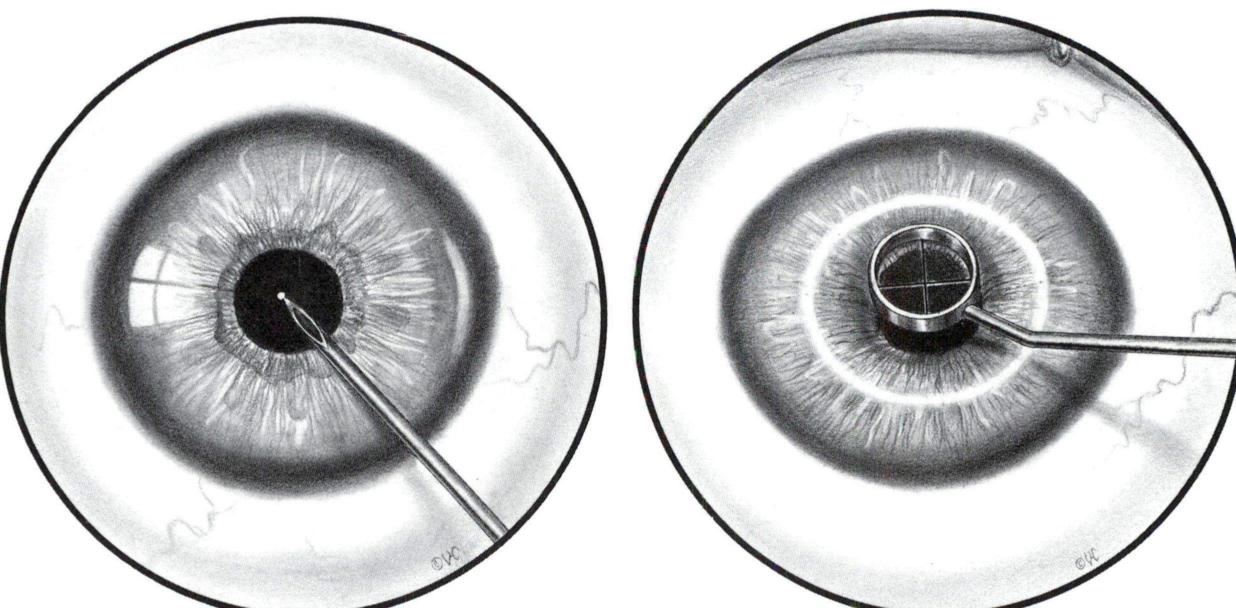

FIGURE 5-22. Marking epithelium at center of entrance pupil with hypodermic needle.

FIGURE 5-23. Marking optical zone.

The corneal thickness is measured paracentrally at the 3, 6, 9, and 12 o'clock meridians at the peripheral edge of the optical zone mark (Fig. 5-24). A variety of ultrasonic pachymeters are available with fluid-filled, jelly-filled, or solid tips. The tip of the pachymeter is held perpendicularly to the corneal surface, and measurements are taken at each location until two identical measurements are obtained at each location. Thereafter, care is taken to keep the anterior corneal surface moist, but not flooded, with balanced salt solution. If the cornea is allowed to dry, it may thin, increasing the risk of corneal perforation as the incisions are made; if the cornea is kept too moist, it may swell, resulting in shallow incisions and undercorrection. After pachymetry is completed, the incisions are made expediently to minimize any fluctuations in corneal hydration.

Although stainless steel razor blade fragments were used in the past, the current knife of choice for radial keratotomy is a diamond blade knife. This knife consists of a handle with a micrometer, a footplate, and a diamond blade with a dull vertical edge and an angled cutting edge. There are several nomograms for selecting the length of the blade. The PERK study uses a diamond blade set at 100% of the thinnest paracentral measurement. The length of the knife is set initially with the micrometer on the handle; however, the length should be double-checked with a gauge (Fig. 5-25). There are many types of gauges; however, the risk of damaging the blade is lessened if the gauge has a holder for the handle of the knife. The handle of the knife is placed in the holder, and the edge of the gauge is abutted against the footplate of the knife. The gauge is aligned with the tip of the blade, and the blade is adjusted under high magnification of the microscope to the appropriate length, with care being taken to avoid parallax.

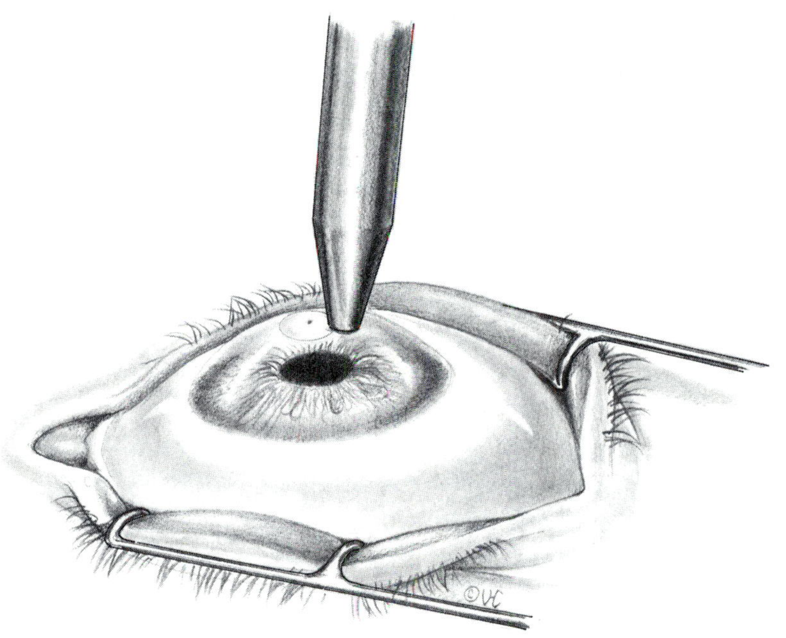

FIGURE 5-24. Measuring corneal thickness with ultrasonic pachymeter.

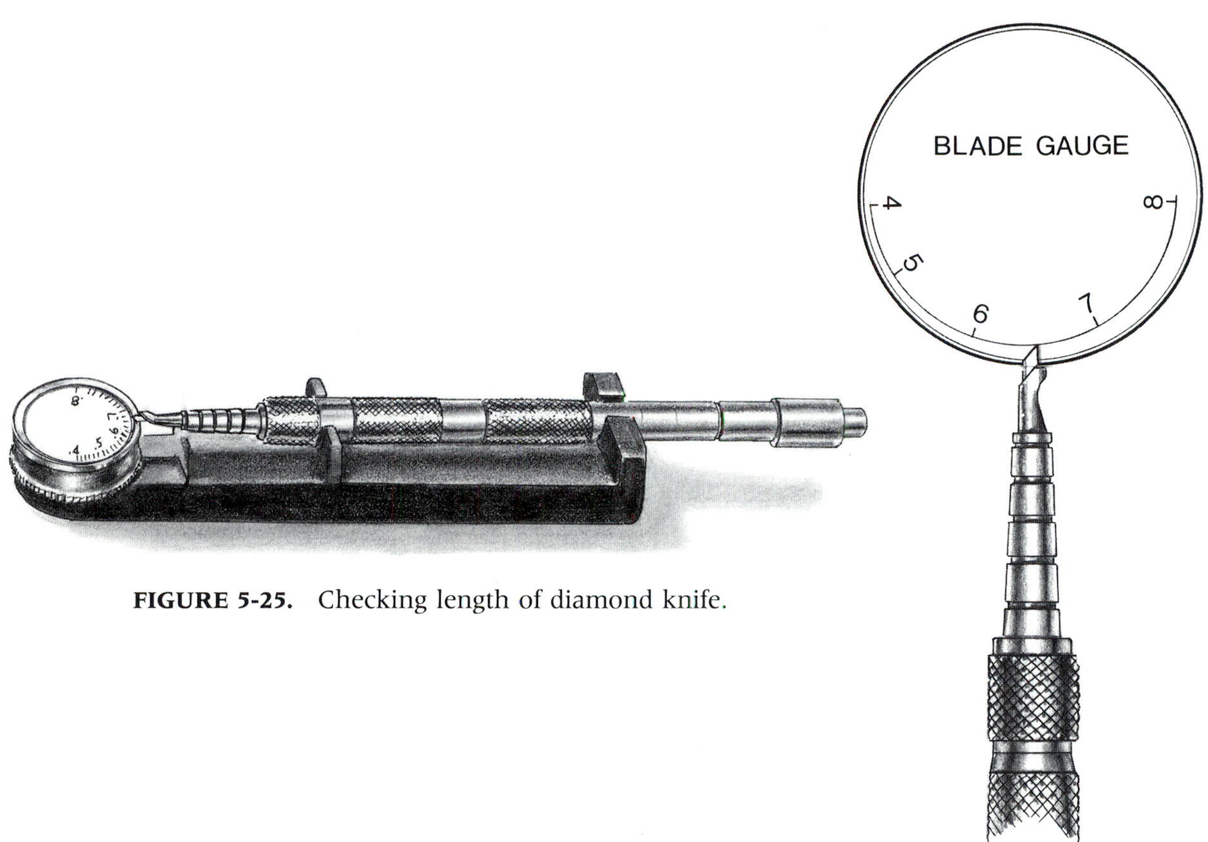

FIGURE 5-25. Checking length of diamond knife.

There are various nomograms for the number of incisions that should be made to achieve various amounts of myopic correction. In general, the greater the number of incisions, the greater the correction; however, most of the correction is obtained with the initial incisions. There has been a tendency therefore to decrease the number of incisions from 16 to 8, or even 4. This decreases the risk of overcorrection and allows the surgeon to perform a staged procedure, adding more incisions later if there is undercorrection.

Although the incisions can be made from the limbus to the optical zone mark, this method risks accidental crossing of the mark and cutting into the optical clear zone. It is safer to make the incisions from the optical zone mark to the limbus. The eye is stabilized with double-pronged forceps, and the knife is inserted perpendicularly to the cornea at the optical zone mark. Firm pressure is applied, and the knife is slowly drawn toward the limbus, stopping just short of the limbal blood vessels (Fig. 5-26). Since most of the correction of radial keratotomy results from incisions placed close to the optical zone mark, it is important that the incision at the optical zone mark be of adequate depth. One best accomplishes this by waiting one or two seconds after the knife has been inserted before drawing it toward the limbus. It is also important that the knife be held perpendicularly to the corneal surface as the incision is made; otherwise the incision will be too shallow (Fig. 5-27).

The pattern of incisions should be such that if the procedure has to be aborted (as with macroperforation) there will be minimal astigmatism. For eight incisions, the incisions are placed as indicated in Fig. 5-28.

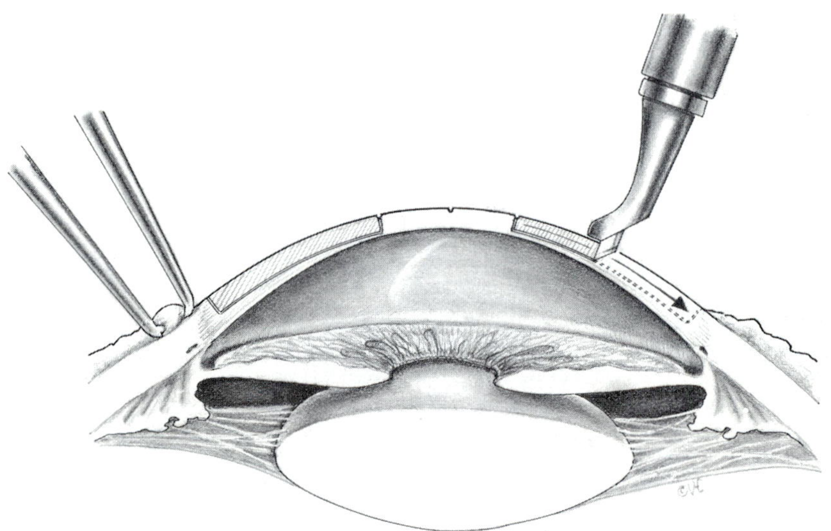

FIGURE 5-26. Correctly incising cornea with diamond knife.

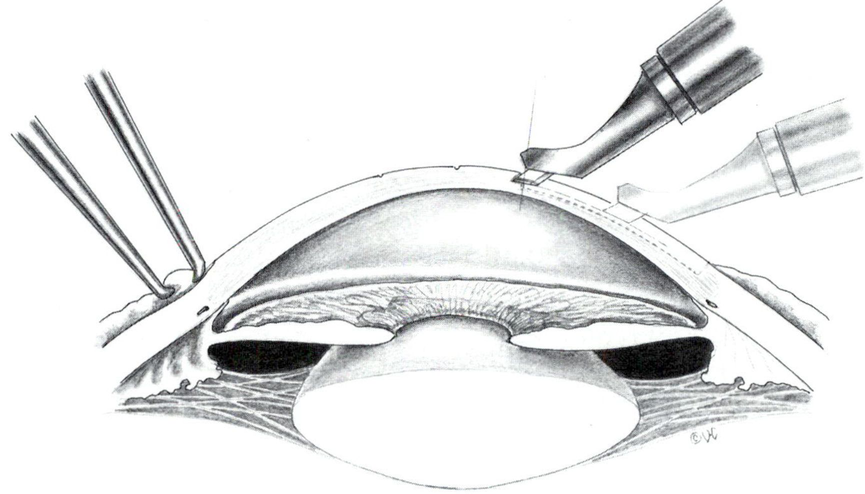

FIGURE 5-27. Incorrectly incising cornea with diamond knife. The knife is not perpendicular to the corneal surface.

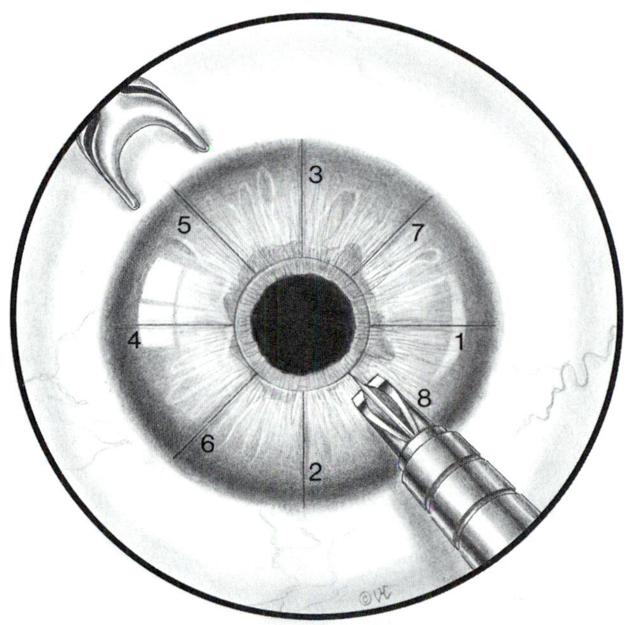

FIGURE 5-28. Order of incisions for radial keratotomy.

The depth of the incisions are less than the length of the blade because tissue is displaced by the knife. Although an attempt can be made to check the depth of the incisions with a depth gauge, it is not very accurate because the depth gauge can push the posterior layers of the cornea posteriorly, creating the impression that the incisions are deeper than they actually are (Fig. 5-29). A more practical method is to examine the incisions along their entire length with an instrument that spreads open the incisions (Fig. 5-30). If incision is shallow or irregular, the blade can be inserted into the incision, with care being taken to hold the blade perpendicularly, and the tissue is recut. Freehand dissection of the tissue down to Descemet's membrane is not recommended because of the high risk of perforation. Although some surgeons advocate routinely deepening the incisions in the corneal periphery, the effect of this on the correction appears to be minimal.

There is usually a mild amount of bleeding from limbal blood vessels even though an attempt has been made to avoid these vessels with the knife. The blood and any epithelial cells or debris are irrigated with balanced salt solution on a cannula held parallel to the incision so that Descemet's membrane is not detached by the stream of irrigating solution (Fig. 5-31). If there is a moderate amount of bleeding from the limbal blood vessels, one can stop it by holding a cellulose sponge at the limbus. The sponge may be saturated with epinephrine solution to provide better hemostasis.

Microperforations that occur during the procedure usually seal themselves without the need for sutures. If there is a macroperforation, the procedure must be aborted and the incision closed with interrupted 10-0 nylon sutures (Fig. 5-32).

Although the postoperative care varies, a topical antibiotic solution should be applied at the end of the procedure. A cycloplegic agent may be used to decrease inflammation. An eye pad and shield may be placed; however some surgeons prefer to leave the lids open. The patient is seen the first day postoperatively, at which time the visual acuity is measured, the integrity of the epithelium assessed, and the incisions inspected. We prescribe a topical antibiotic and cycloplegic agent four times a day for the first week after surgery.

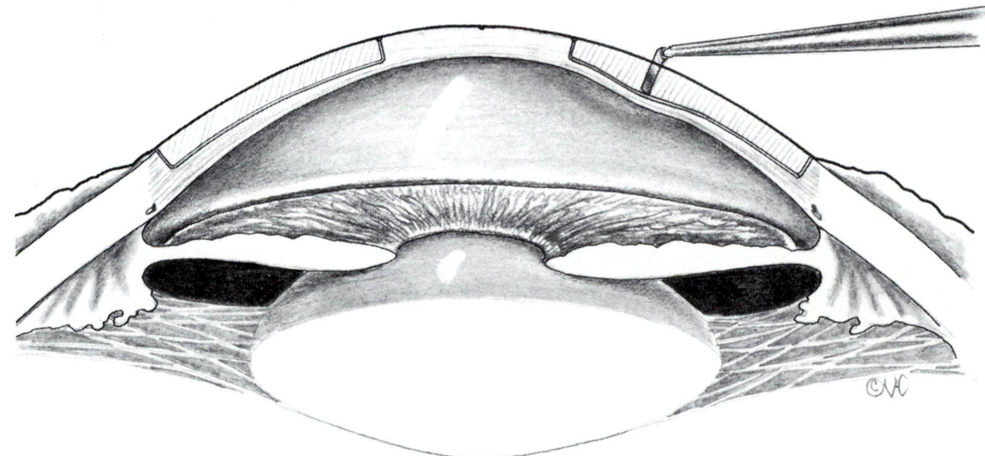

FIGURE 5-29. Checking depth of wound with depth gauge.

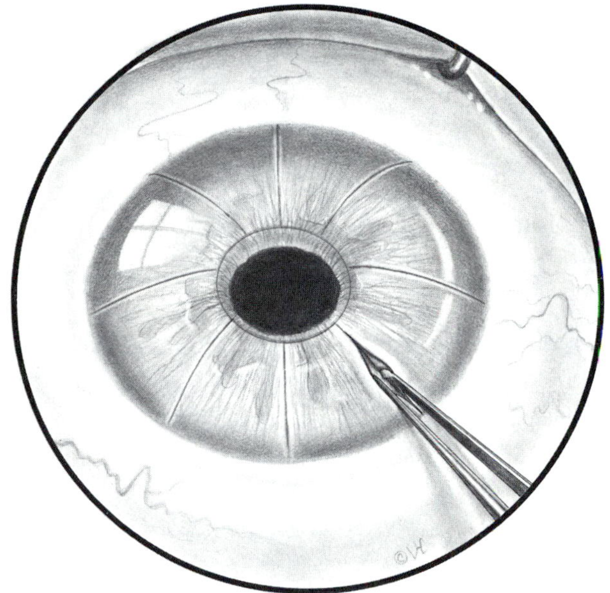

FIGURE 5-30. Inspecting incisions with wound spreader.

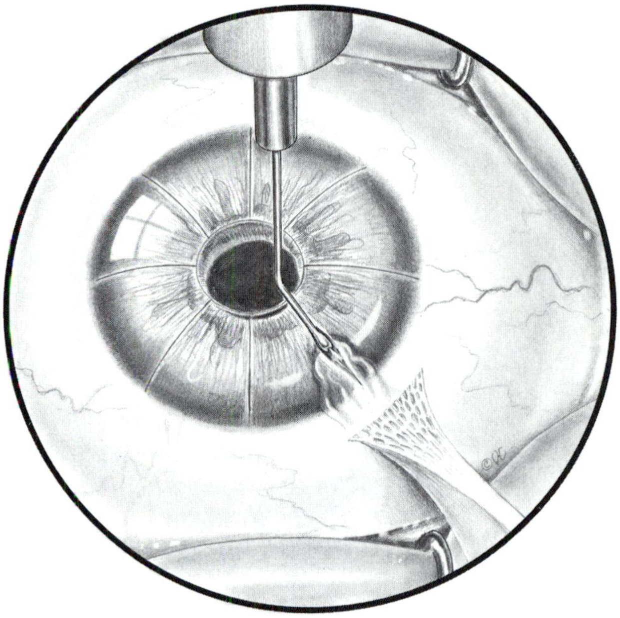

FIGURE 5-31. Irrigating incisions with blunt-tipped cannula held parallel to incisions.

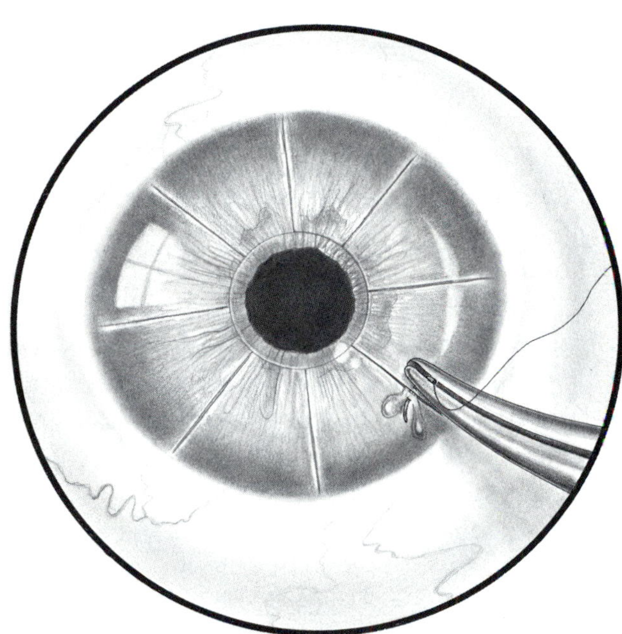

FIGURE 5-32. Suturing perforation.

PRINCIPLES IN TREATING ASTIGMATISM

Astigmatism is, perhaps, the most difficult corneal disorder to correct surgically. The surgical procedures for astigmatism are not difficult to perform, but the results can be unpredictable. Reasons for this unpredictability include the underlying corneal disorder causing the astigmatism and variable wound healing from patient to patient. A procedure that works for one patient may not work for another patient. Nevertheless, there are patients who are visually incapacitated by astigmatism in whom a surgical procedure for astigmatism may be indicated.

Preoperative evaluation includes qualitative and quantitative assessment of the astigmatism with refraction, keratometry, and keratoscopy. Refraction reveals the magnitude and axis of central astigmatism at the spectacle plane, the patient's best corrected visual acuity with spectacles, and the tolerance of the patient to spectacles; however it does not reveal peripheral astigmatism or astigmatism at the corneal plane. Keratometry quantitates the central astigmatism at the corneal plane and allows a qualitative assessment of central corneal irregularity; however it does not provide an assessment of the cornea peripheral to the central 3 mm. Keratoscopy evolved from the Placido disc and involves the reflection of rings of light from the anterior corneal surface. Photographic documentation of the reflection and, more recently, computer analysis of these photographs have greatly aided in the evaluation of astigmatism. These more recent methods allow quantitation of astigmatism along several meridians from the center to the periphery of the cornea. Because central astigmatism can be the result of several vectors in the peripheral cornea, it is necessary to examine the entire cornea when one is evaluating astigmatism.

Astigmatism may be regular or irregular, symmetric or asymmetric. Fig. 5-33 illustrates regular symmetric astigmatism, as demonstrated by a qualitative surgical keratoscope, such as the Troutman keratoscope. In the figure, the reflection of lights from the anterior corneal surface is a symmetric oval. The short diameter of the oval is vertical and indicates the steep meridian; the long diameter of the oval is horizontal and indicates the flat meridian. For consistency, the surgical procedures for astigmatism described in this chapter are for the correction of such astigmatism (that is, steep vertical axis and flat horizontal axis), unless otherwise indicated.

Before any surgical procedure for astigmatism is considered, the cause of the astigmatism should be determined. These causes include surgery (such as cataract extraction or penetrating keratoplasty), ectatic corneal disorders (such as keratoconus, pellucid marginal degeneration, or keratoglobus), corneal degenerations (such as pterygium or Terrien's marginal degeneration), and trauma. Astigmatism occurring after cataract extraction can be caused by tight sutures (steep vertical meridian) or a wound dehiscence (flat vertical meridian). It is important to recognize such causes because the astigmatism may be corrected by removal of the tight sutures in the first case or by repair of the wound in the second case.

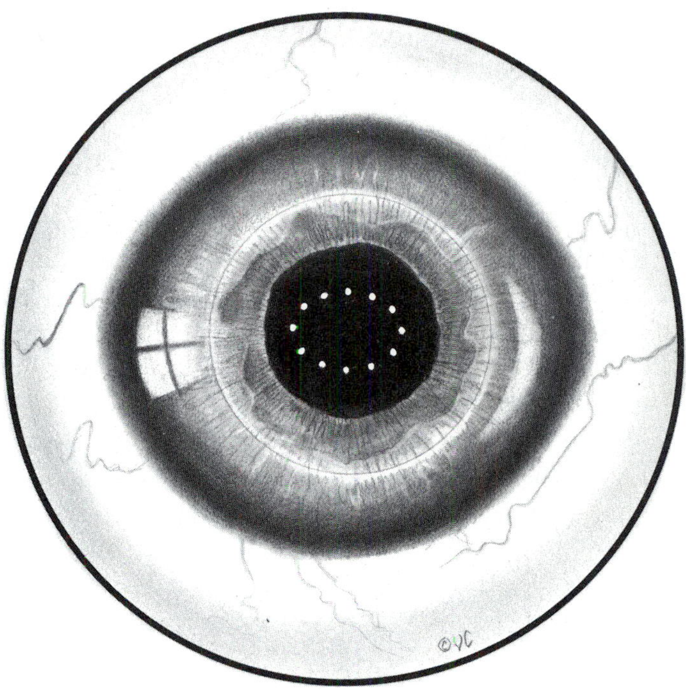

FIGURE 5-33. Regular symmetric astigmatism.

Astigmatism occurring after penetrating keratoplasty can be caused by several factors, including the underlying corneal disorder, faulty cutting of the recipient or donor cornea, and poor apposition of the tissue. Astigmatism caused by wound dehiscence can be recognized by elevation of the edge of the graft (Fig. 5-34); the cornea is steep in the area immediately adjacent to the dehiscence but is flat centrally. Wound dehiscence is repaired by placement of 10-0 nylon sutures across the wound at either end of the dehiscence. These sutures limit progression of the dehiscence as the wound is surgically opened. A stainless steel blade is inserted, bevel up, through the wound into the anterior chamber, and the wound is opened in the abnormal area (Fig. 5-35). The wound is then closed properly with interrupted 10-0 nylon sutures, as in penetrating keratoplasty.

If astigmatism is not caused by abnormal sutures or an abnormal wound, one of the surgical procedures described below may be considered. Before considering any surgical procedure for astigmatism, however, one should determine that the astigmatism cannot be corrected satisfactorily with spectacles or contact lenses. As stated above, refraction should always be done. In some patients (such as those with high hypermetropia), the amount of cylinder at the spectacle plane is less than the amount of cylinder at the corneal plane, and spectacles may be tolerated. Trial frames are invaluable when one is assessing tolerance to cylinder correction in spectacles. If spectacles are not tolerated, a trial of contact lenses should be initiated.

The surgical procedures for astigmatism can be divided into those that steepen the flat meridian and those that flatten the steep meridian. Most of the procedures affect both meridians ("coupling effect"); however, they will be grouped in this chapter as if they affected only one meridian. Procedures that steepen the flat meridian include compression sutures and wedge resection; procedures that flatten the steep meridian include relaxing incisions of various shapes and sizes.

Except for wedge resection, the procedures described below can usually be done with topical anesthesia. One can mark the area of the steep meridian preoperatively by instilling topical anesthetic, having the patient look through a phoropter, and marking the limbus at the steep or flat meridian with a marking pen. An anatomic landmark on the keratoscope photograph can be useful in orientation. The area of the steep or flat meridian should always be checked intraoperatively with a surgical keratoscope. Care is taken that the eye is parallel to the surgical keratoscope and that the lid specula are not pressing on the eye.

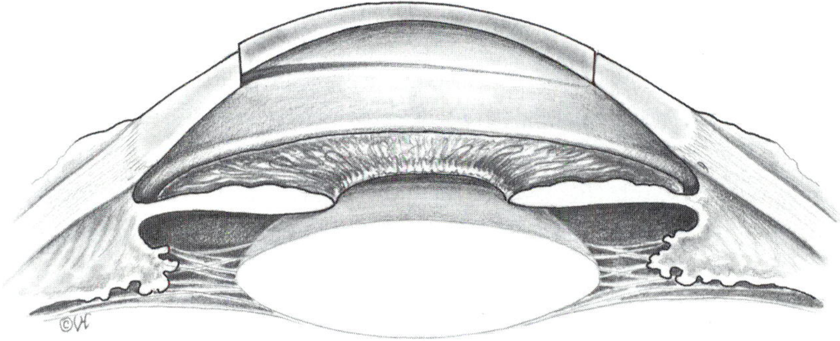

FIGURE 5-34. Graft override causing flattening of central cornea in that meridian.

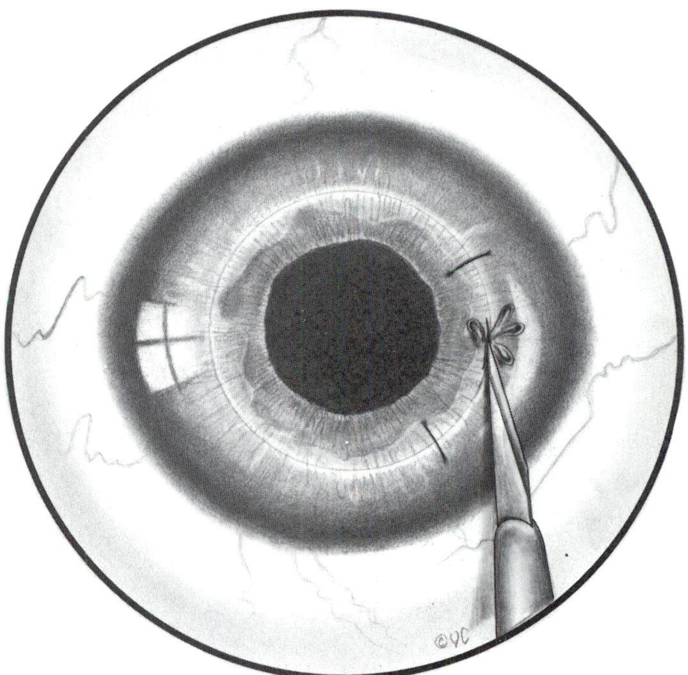

FIGURE 5-35. Opening keratoplasty wound. Sutures prevent dehiscence of entire wound.

Procedures that Steepen the Flat Meridian

Compression sutures

One or two compression sutures can be placed across a penetrating keratoplasty wound in the flat meridian to steepen that meridian. The preferred suture for this is 9-0 nylon; 10-0 nylon does not have enough tensile strength, polypropylene is too elastic, and mersilene tends to cheesewire through the tissue. The sutures are placed 1 mm from the wound margin, at a depth of approximately three fourths of the corneal thickness (Fig. 5-36). They are tightened under keratoscopic control until a slight overcorrection is achieved. The sutures are left in place indefinitely unless they loosen or attract blood vessels.

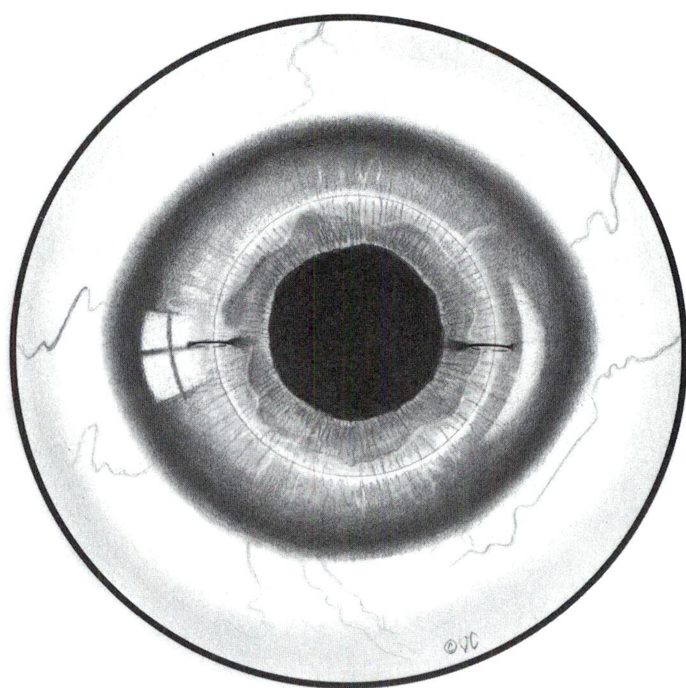

FIGURE 5-36. Compression sutures.

Wedge resection

A corneal wedge resection may be considered in a patient who has a large amount of astigmatism after penetrating keratoplasty. The procedure requires local anesthesia (that is, retrobulbar or peribulbar). A triangular wedge of corneal tissue is removed in the flat meridian, and the edges of the keratectomy are sutured with interrupted sutures. This results in steepening of that meridian. One incision is made in the keratoplasty wound for 3 clock hours straddling the flat meridian (Fig. 5-37); the other incision is made either central or peripheral to the keratoplasty wound, depending on the size of the graft. In a large graft the second incision is made central to the wound; in a small graft the second incision is made peripheral to the wound (Fig. 5-38). The distance between the two incisions, and hence the amount of tissue to be resected, is determined by the amount of astigmatism. In general, for the first 5 diopters, 0.1 mm of tissue is resected for each diopter; for each subsequent 2 diopters, 0.1 mm of tissue is resected. No more than 1.5 mm of tissue should be resected, and tissue should be resected from only one side of the graft. The incisions are made down to Descemet's membrane with a stainless steel blade or a Gem blade. The first incision is made perpendicularly to the anterior corneal surface. The second incision is angled to connect with the ends and base of the first incision. Vannas scissors are used if necessary to complete the incisions and to remove corneal tissue between the incisions (Fig. 5-39). The edges of the keratectomy are closed with several tightly tied interrupted 10-0 nylon sutures (Fig. 5-40). If intraoperative keratoscopy shows an undercorrection, the sutures are replaced with ones tied more tightly. If there is an overcorrection, two compression sutures are placed across the keratoplasty wound 90 degrees from the wedge resection. If there is a persistent overcorrection postoperatively, the sutures used to close the keratectomy are selectively removed beginning 6 weeks after surgery. Otherwise the sutures are left in place indefinitely. A wedge resection is a more involved surgical procedure and requires a longer visual rehabilitation period than some of the other surgical procedures for astigmatism; we therefore reserve the procedure for patients with large amounts of astigmatism unresponsive to other surgical procedures.

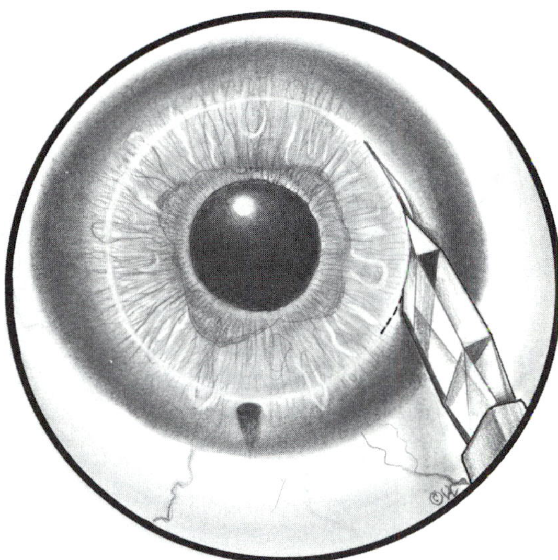

FIGURE 5-37. Incising keratoplasty wound for wedge resection.

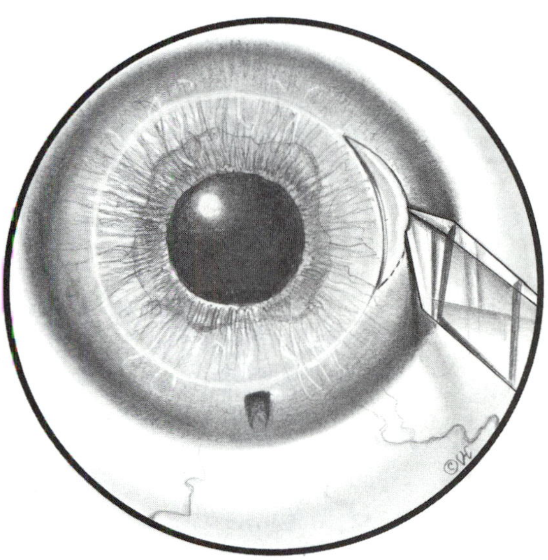

FIGURE 5-38. Incising cornea peripheral to keratoplasty wound.

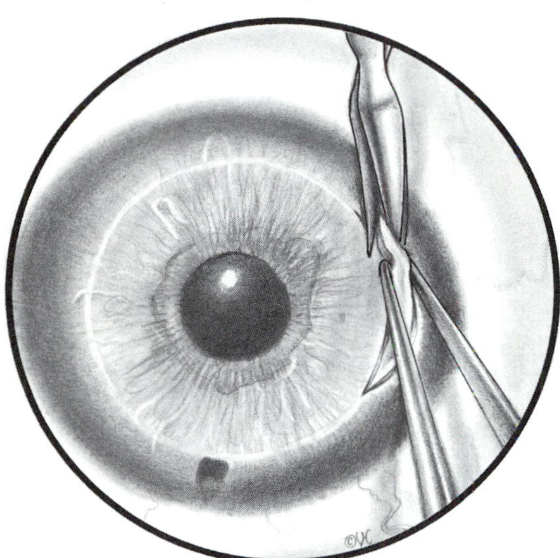

FIGURE 5-39. Excising corneal tissue with Vannas scissors.

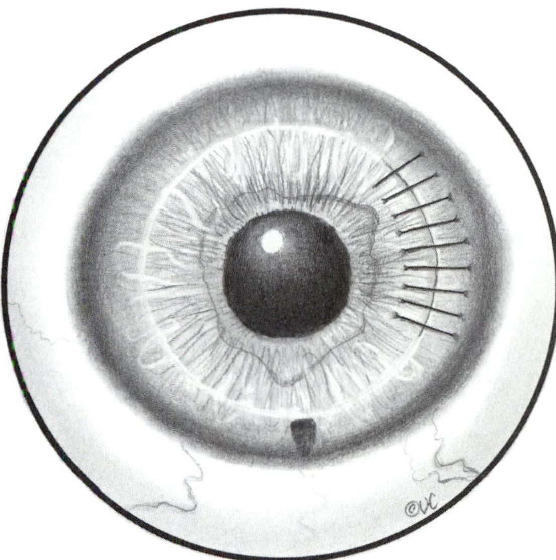

FIGURE 5-40. Closing edges of keratectomy.

Procedures that Flatten the Steep Meridian

Arcuate relaxing incisions

Arcuate relaxing incisions are placed in the steep meridian to flatten that meridian. The incisions may be placed in the keratoplasty wound; because of irregularities of the wound, however, the risk of perforation is lessened if the incisions are placed central to the wound. Incisions placed peripheral to the wound have less effect than incisions placed central to the wound. If the astigmatism is symmetric, a relaxing incision is placed at each end of the steep meridian. The incisions are made 1 mm central to the wound for 3 clock hours straddling the steep meridian (Fig. 5-41). The incisions may be made with a stainless steel blade or a Gem blade set to a predetermined length after the corneal thickness is measured intraoperatively with an ultrasonic pachymeter. We prefer to dissect the corneal tissue with a stainless steel blade under direct visualization and intraoperative keratoscopic control until a reversal of the astigmatism is achieved. If the corneal tissue is dissected down to Descemet's membrane and the astigmatism has not reversed, two compression sutures are placed across the keratoplasty wound 90 degrees from the relaxing incisions to achieve more effect (Fig. 5-42). These sutures may be removed postoperatively if there is excessive overcorrection. Otherwise they are left in place indefinitely. If the astigmatism is asymmetric, as shown in Fig. 5-43, only one relaxing incision is made at the steepest end of the steep meridian (Fig. 5-44).

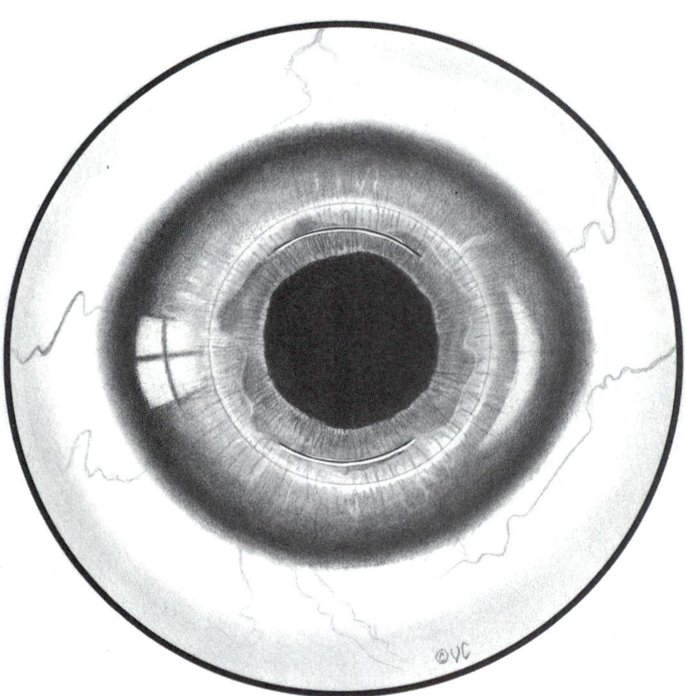

FIGURE 5-41. Arcuate relaxing incisions for symmetric astigmatism.

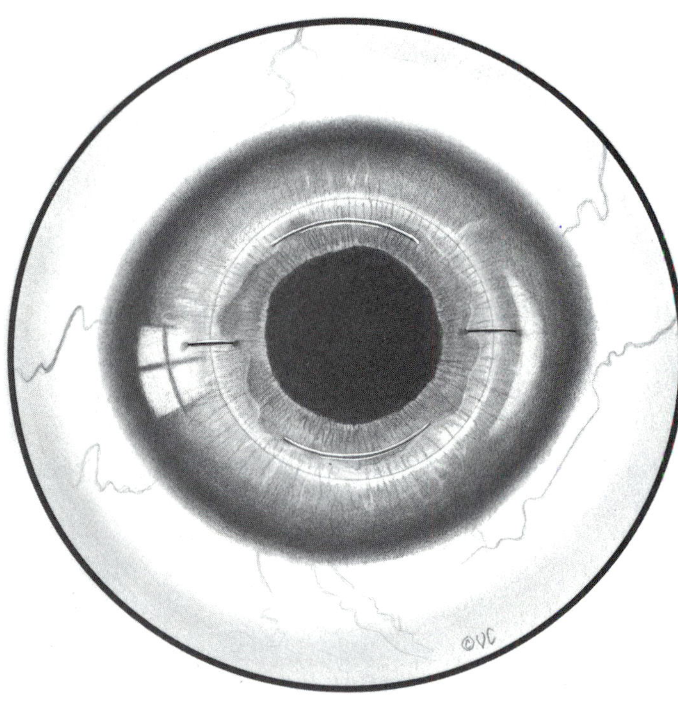

FIGURE 5-42. Arcuate relaxing incisions and compression sutures.

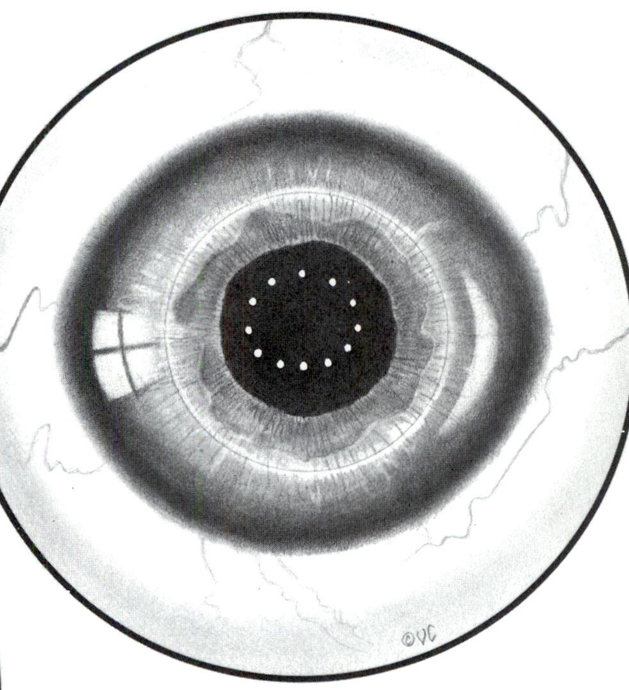

FIGURE 5-43. Moderately asymmetric astigmatism.

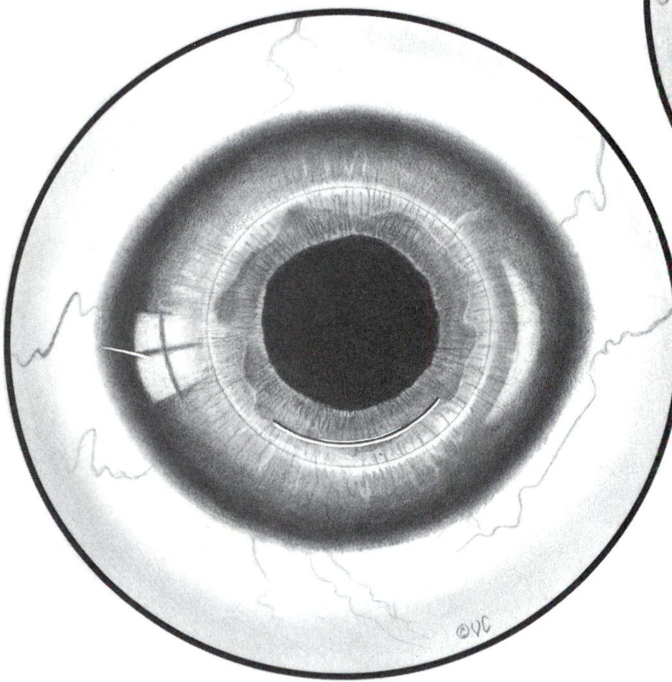

FIGURE 5-44. Arcuate relaxing incision for asymmetric astigmatism.

Trapezoidal keratotomy

Trapezoidal keratotomy (Ruiz procedure) combines transverse and semiradial incisions at each end of the steep meridian to flatten that meridian (Fig. 5-45). As in radial keratotomy, the amount of correction depends on the diameter of the optical clear zone. The techniques for trapezoidal keratotomy are similar to those described previously in the section on radial keratotomy. The center of the entrance pupil is marked on the corneal epithelium. An optical zone marker with a diameter of 3 to 6 mm is centered on this mark and is pressed gently and rotated 90 degrees. The corneal thickness at the peripheral edge of the optical zone mark is measured, and a diamond blade is set to 80% to 100% of this thickness. Two sets of four transverse incisions 2 to 3 mm in length are made at each end of the steep meridian. The first incision of each set is made tangential to the optical zone mark. The remaining three incisions of each set are spaced equally between the first incision and the limbus. The semiradial incisions are made from the optical zone mark just to but not crossing the limbus. One should take care to avoid intersecting the transverse incisions to avoid healing problems (chronic epithelial defect or stromal melt or both). Nomograms are available for determining the diameter of the optical clear zone and the length of the transverse incisions. Trapezoidal keratotomy tends to be more unpredictable than the other surgical procedures, especially for postkeratoplasty astigmatism.

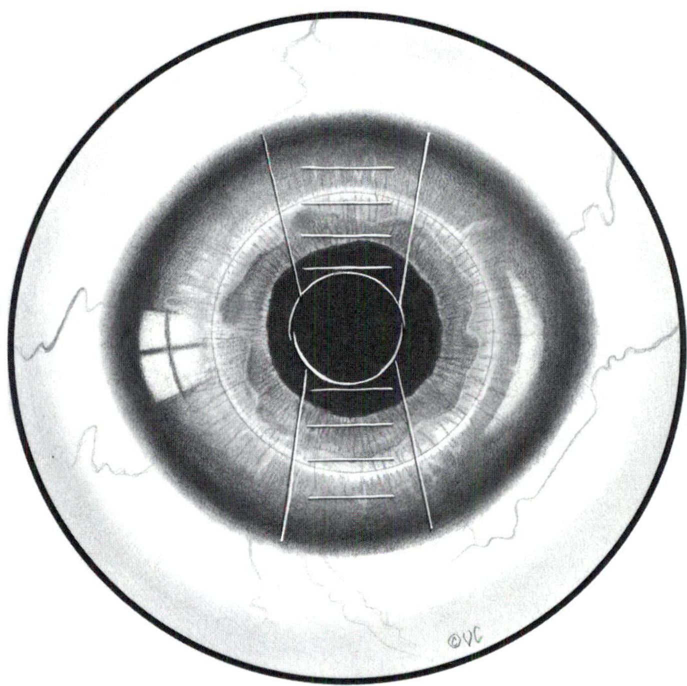

FIGURE 5-45. Trapezoidal keratotomy.

Transverse incisions

One or two sets of transverse incisions can be made in the midperipheral cornea at each end of the steep meridian to flatten that meridian (Fig. 5-46). The incisions are usually made at optical zone diameters of 5 to 8 mm and are 1 to 3 mm in length.

Transverse incisions combined with radial keratotomy

In patients who have astigmatism and myopia, one can combine astigmatic keratotomy with radial keratotomy by making transverse incisions in addition to the radial incisions. The radial incisions are placed such that transverse incisions can be made in the steep meridian without intersecting the radial incisions (Fig. 5-47). Nomograms are available for the placement and length of transverse incisions. The transverse incisions should not intersect the radial incisions because of poor wound healing where two incisions intersect (Fig. 5-48).

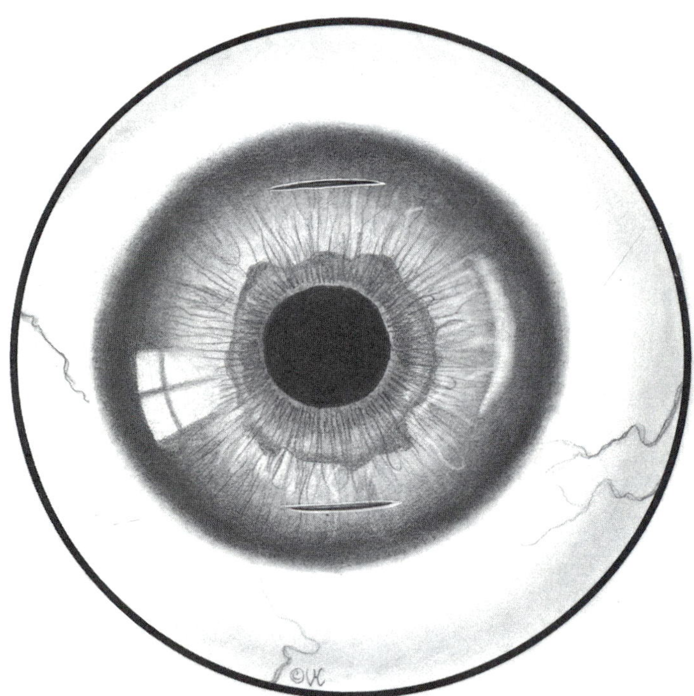

FIGURE 5-46. Transverse relaxing incisions.

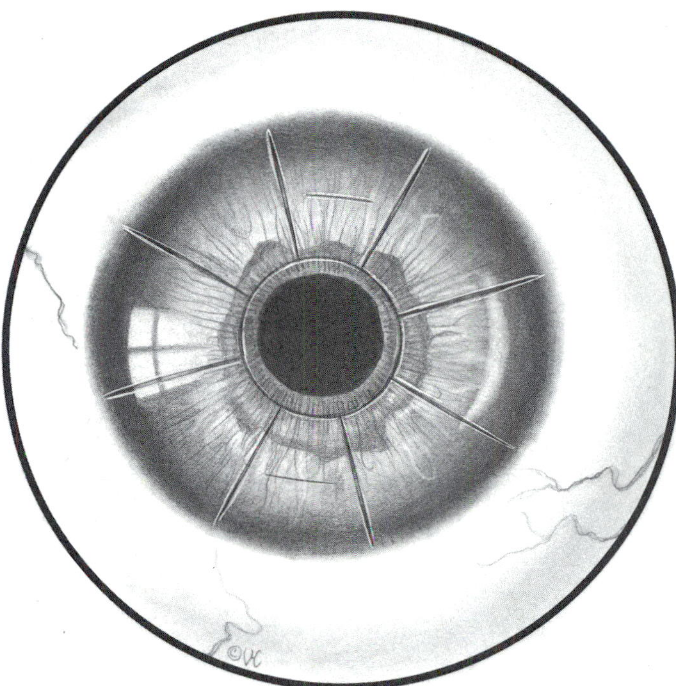

FIGURE 5-47. Transverse relaxing incisions combined with radial keratotomy.

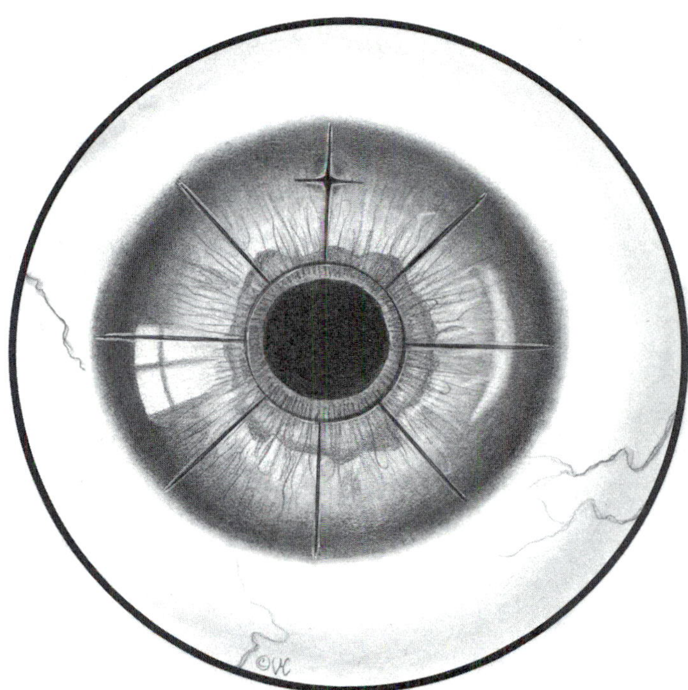

FIGURE 5-48. Corneal irregularity from poor wound healing where transverse incision crosses radial incision.

CHAPTER 6

Anterior Segment Reconstruction with Keratoprosthesis

The idea of replacing the cornea with alloplastic material was first conceived by Pellier de Quengsy, who suggested replacing scarred corneas with glass. In 1853 Nussbaum reported implantation of glass into rabbit corneas. Subsequent investigators unsuccessfully implanted quartz, celluloid, and glass in human corneas. After World War II it was observed that the human cornea tolerated imbedded Plexiglas, that is, polymethylmethacrylate (PMMA), well. This observation stimulated ocular alloplastic research into the use of PMMA for prosthetic corneal replacement and for use in intraocular lens implantation.

The terms "keratoprosthesis" and "prosthokeratoplasty" are often used interchangeably to describe alloplastic reconstruction of the anterior segment. However, "keratoprosthesis" refers to the device and "prosthokeratoplasty" refers to the surgical procedure of keratoprosthesis insertion.

Current keratoprosthesis designs have features common to the prototype developed by Stone in 1965. Stone's original device, illustrated in Fig. 6-1, had an optical cylinder and a supporting plate, both of PMMA. The supporting plate had fenestrations to allow attachment to the host cornea and to permit adequate nutrition of the anterior cornea. Current designs may be regarded as having evolved from this original design. Stone's design allowed for a two-stage operation, which is still advocated by some. The two stages are (1) implantation of the supporting plate in a lamellar pocket in the cornea and allowing it to heal and (2) trephination through the posterior cornea and insertion of the optical cylinder through the entire cornea (Fig. 6-2).

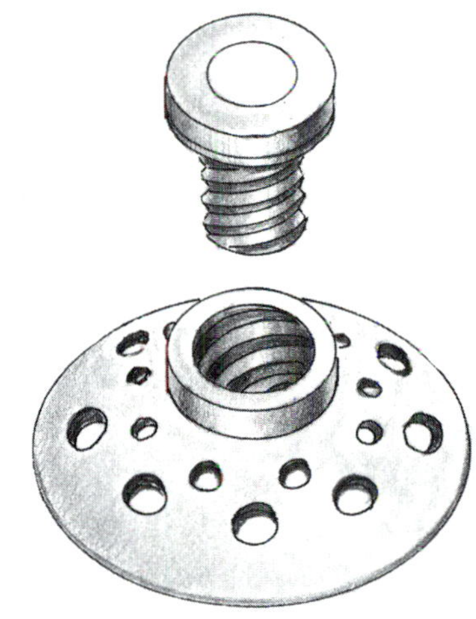

FIGURE 6-1. Stone keratoprosthesis.

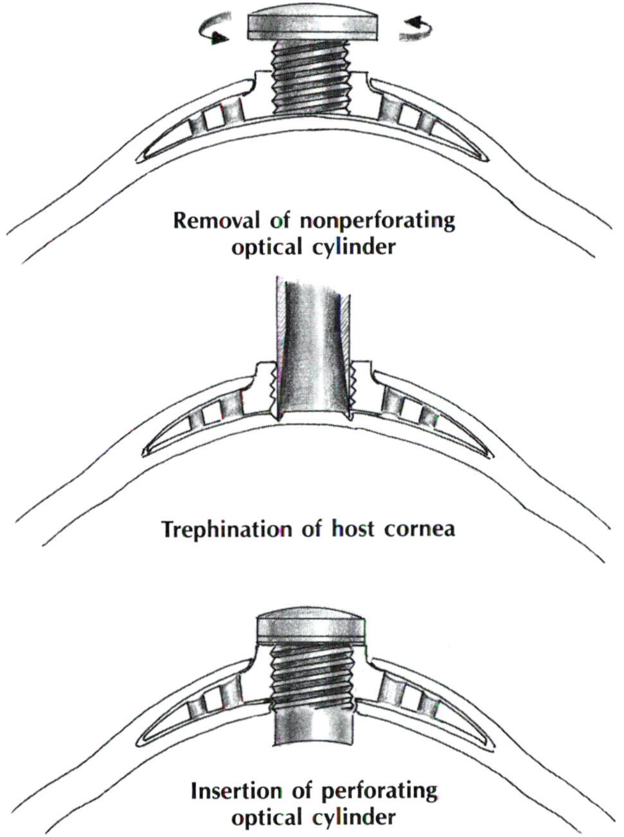

FIGURE 6-2. Second stage of Stone keratoprosthesis procedure.

CARDONA KERATOPROSTHESIS

The Cardona keratoprosthesis, referred to as the through-and-through keratoprosthesis (model TT), is the most widely used keratoprosthesis in the United States today, and the procedures described in this chapter relate specifically to it. As a result of the work of Cardona and his associates, including years of laboratory, animal, and human studies related to materials, design, and surgical technique, this keratoprosthesis is successful in many eyes otherwise considered hopeless.

The keratoprosthesis (Fig. 6-3) consists of an optical cylinder of PMMA and a supporting Teflon plate. The optical cylinder has a diameter of 3.5 mm and a length of either 6.5 or 9.5 mm. The 6.5 mm device is used if the eyelids are to remain open, whereas the 9.5 mm device is used when prosthokeratoplasty is combined with a total tarsorrhaphy and the optical cylinder projects through the eyelid. Both sizes of optical cylinders have an internal pigmented ring to reduce unwanted reflections and glare.

The Teflon skirt is 8.5 mm in diameter. It has eight fenestrations 1.8 mm in diameter and 16 fenestrations 0.4 mm in diameter. The large fenestrations are used for suturing the skirt to the cornea. Additional sutures can be placed through the small outer row of fenestrations.

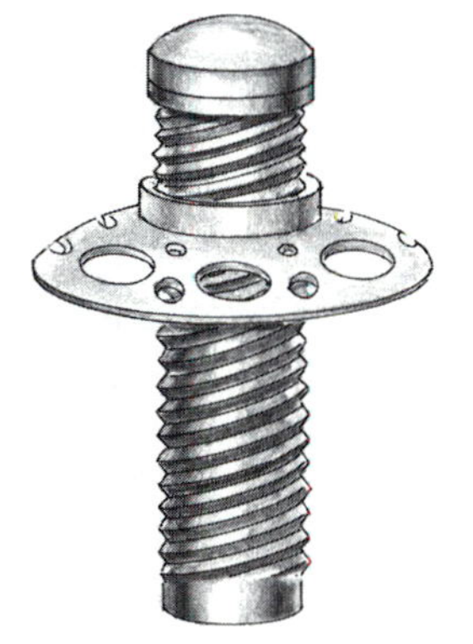

Fully assembled keratoprothesis

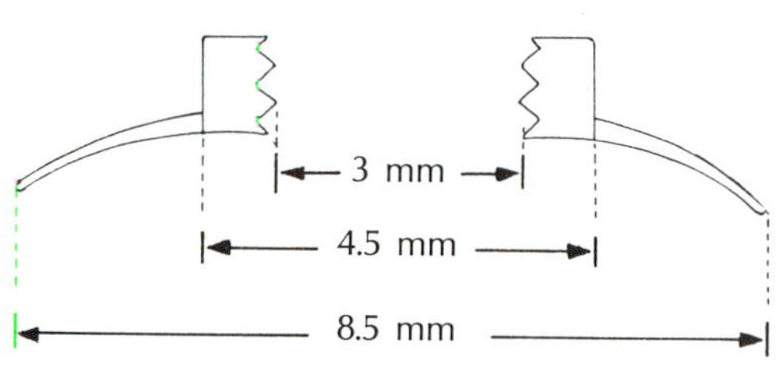

Cross section of supporting plate

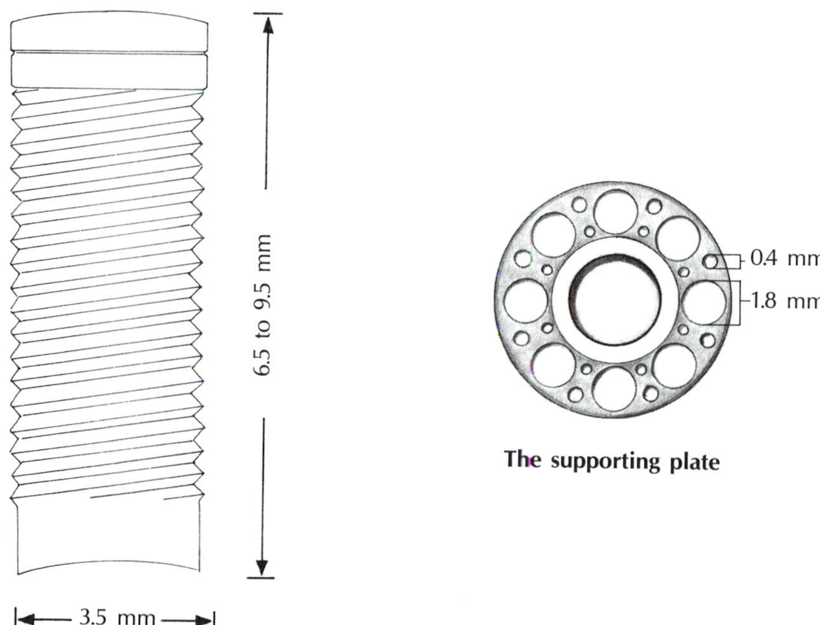

The optical cylinder

The supporting plate

FIGURE 6-3. Cardona through-and-through (TT) keratoprosthesis.

POLACK KERATOPROSTHESIS

The Polack keratoprosthesis (Fig. 6-4) is made of aluminum oxide (Al_2O_3) ceramic. The supporting plate is an opaque 8.5 mm ring fabricated of Al_2O_3 with a rough surface. This special feature enhances the bioadhesive properties of aluminum oxide, an improvement over PMMA devices. The optical cylinder is fabricated from a single Al_2O_3 crystal (refractive index 1.767) and is 3.5 mm in diameter and 10 mm in length. The cylinder is threaded and its power is 60 diopters. Waring has indicated that the Polack keratoprosthesis has a relatively low success rate when compared to the Cardona keratoprosthesis.

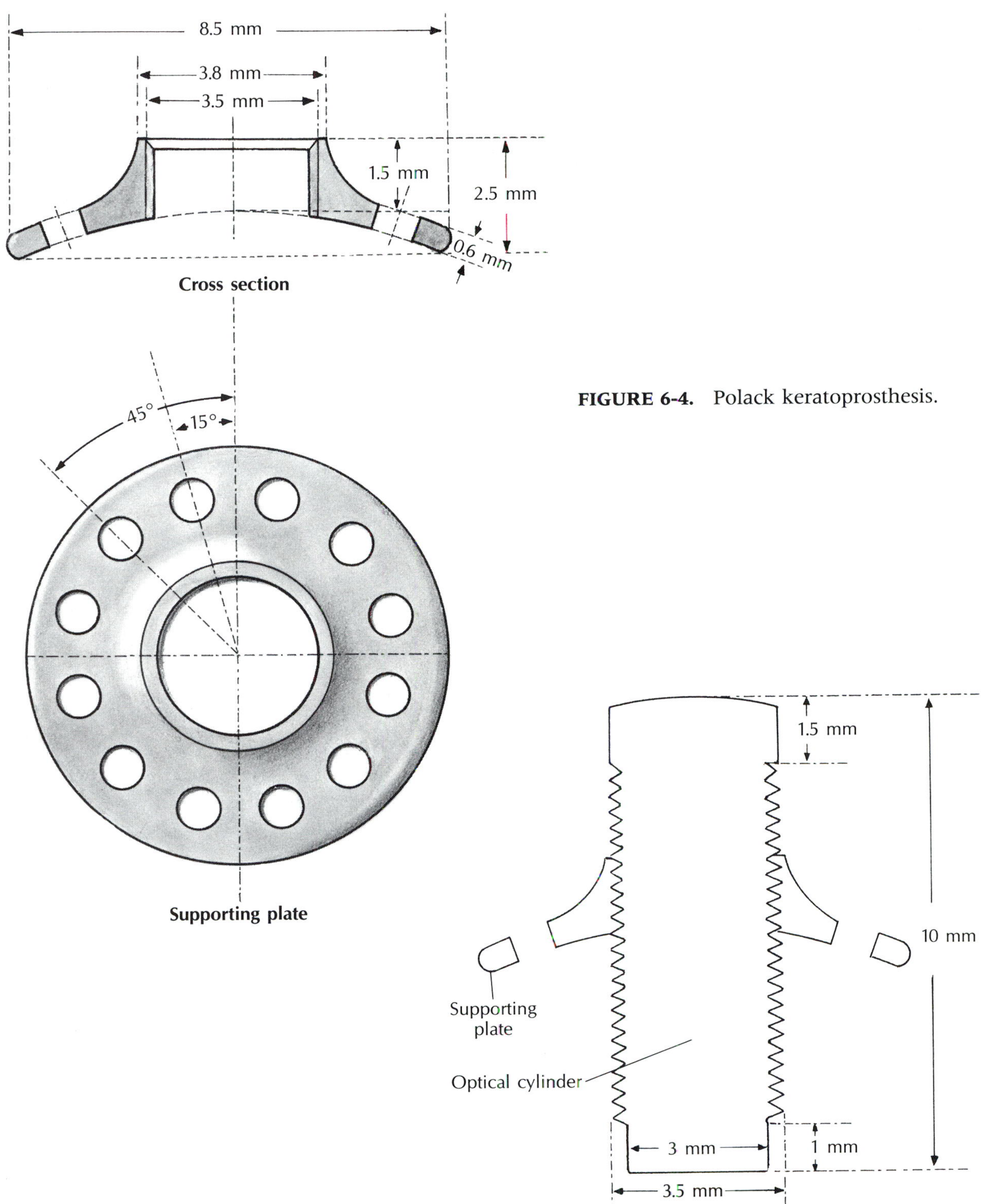

FIGURE 6-4. Polack keratoprosthesis.

GIRARD KERATOPROSTHESIS

The Girard keratoprosthesis is a three-piece keratoprosthesis (Fig. 6-5) consisting of an optical cylinder (PMMA Perspex C.Q.), supporting plate (Proplast), and a retaining nut (PMMA Perspex C.Q.). The retaining nut holds the cornea between it and the supporting plate, thus improving retention and fixation of the keratoprosthesis. The optical cylinder is 4.19 mm in diameter and 4 mm long. This wider optical cylinder increases the visual field. The success rate of the Girard keratoprosthesis is comparable to that of the Cardona keratoprosthesis.

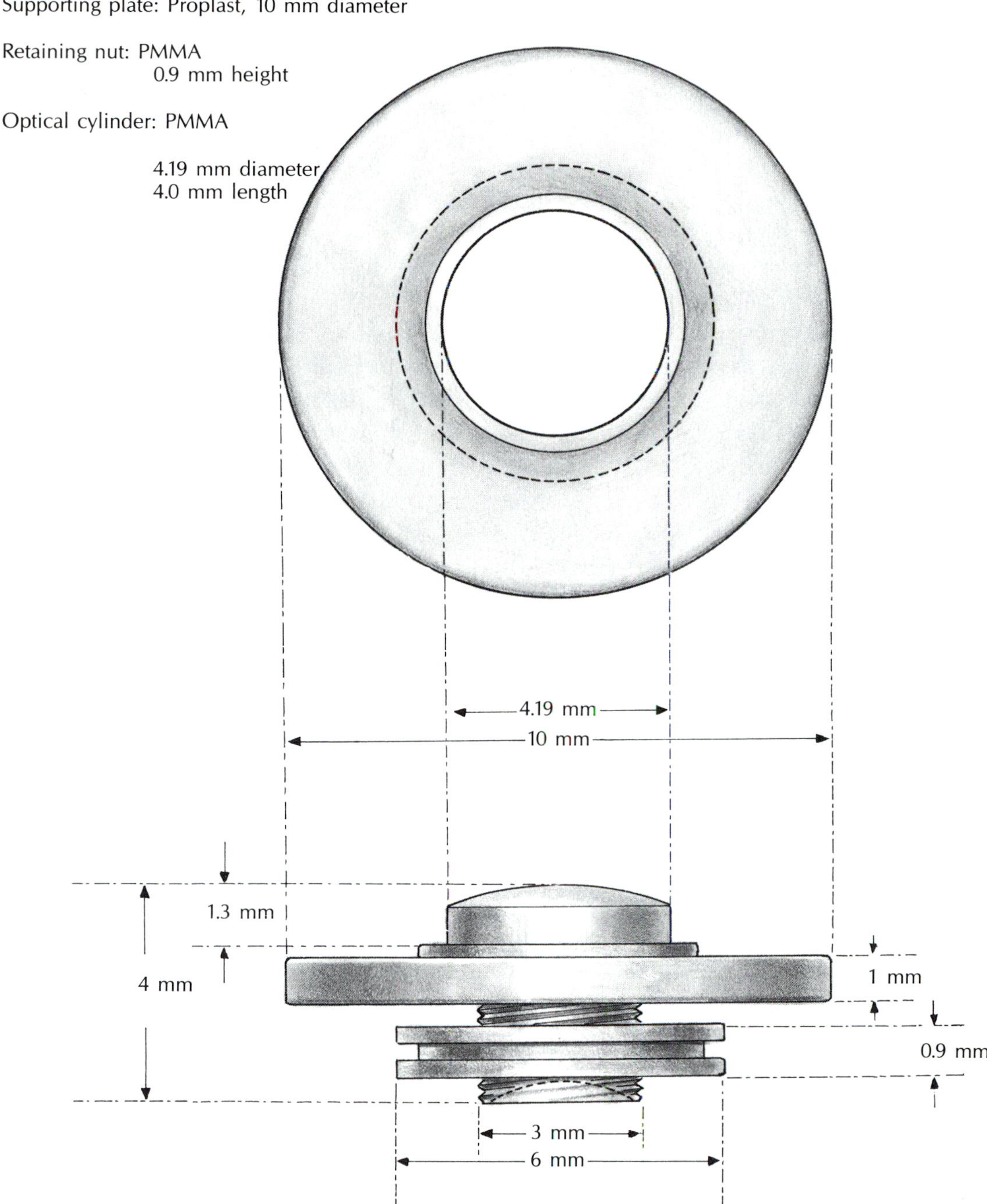

FIGURE 6-5. Girard keratoprosthesis.

PATIENT EVALUATION AND PREPARATION

Indications and contraindications

Keratoprosthesis is reserved for patients in whom penetrating keratoplasty is generally unsuccessful. These include patients with the following conditions:

1. Severe dry eyes
2. Cicatricial conjunctivitis (such as trachoma, Stevens-Johnson syndrome, or pemphigoid)
3. Severe chemical burn
4. Severe destructive corneoscleral disease with loss of anterior segment integrity (such as a blast injury)

If any of these conditions exists and the patient has a visual acuity of 20/200 or worse in the better eye and evidence of macular function, prosthokeratoplasty may be considered. Prosthokeratoplasty is contraindicated if functional vision is present in one eye, if a keratoprosthesis is successful in one eye, or if there are any posterior segment abnormalities that limit visual rehabilitation. In addition, the procedure is not recommended in children because there are no favorable long-term safety and efficacy data for any current model extending 10 to 20 years. A national multicenter prospective study is currently in progress to collect data on the comparative safety and efficacy of various models.

Preoperative care

In addition to the routine tests performed on any patient about to undergo ophthalmic surgery, the following procedures have particular importance in patients undergoing prosthokeratoplasty:

1. Assessment of macular function. It is advisable that some evidence of macular function be demonstrated.

1.1 Gross perception to color light (red, blue, green).

1.2 Two-point light discrimination (note distance).

1.3 Entoptic response.

2. Assessment of visual field. Goldmann or automated perimetry should be attempted; however, if the patient is unable to perform this, light projection may be used. Prosthokeratoplasty is not recommended if severe visual field constriction or only a small temporal field exists.

3. Assessment of retinal status.

3.1 B scan. Since it is impossible to visualize the retina in keratoprosthesis candidates, B-scan ultrasonography is mandatory. These results will determine the presence or absence of a lens, intravitreal opacification, retinal detachment, and other abnormalities of the posterior segment.

3.2 A scan. A-scan ultrasonography is essential to determine and compare the axial lengths of the two eyes. Phthisis bulbi, atrophia bulbi, or prephthisical changes are poor prognostic factors in a prospective candidate for prosthokeratoplasties. Although reduced axial length is not a contraindication for prosthokeratoplasty, it is an important prognosticator both preoperatively and postoperatively. It is important to note that at least one eye that carried a diagnosis of phthisis bulbi underwent prosthokeratoplasty with successful visual rehabilitation. The eye in question had an axial length of 17 mm in comparison with the fellow normal light-perception eye of 22 mm. Reduced axial length is a common finding preoperatively because of the extensive anterior segment damage in these eyes. Flattening of the corneal curvature and anterior segment collapse coexist and result in the typical "pancake" deformity of the anterior segment. In addition, significant increase in the thickness of the retrochoroidal layer as determined by A scan is an important parameter in the prediction of the success of prosthokeratoplasty.

4. Ophthalmic photography. The extent of ocular surface disease must be thoroughly documented to justify the medicolegal indication for prosthokeratoplasty. Conjunctival scarring in the fornices should be demonstrated by photos in various fields of gaze.

5. Assessment of ocular surface status.

5.1 Schirmer tests.

5.2 Tear-film break-up time test.

6. Assessment of corneal thickness.

6.1 Retroillumination and use of slitlamp (biomicroscopy).

6.2 Pachymetry. In totally opaque corneas preoperative pachymetry is essential for determination of corneal thickness. A thinned cornea will not support a keratoprosthesis. Evidence of a thinned or staphylomatous cornea necessitates a tectonic graft before or at the time of prosthokeratoplasty.

Reconstructive Procedures

Currently there are two choices for keratoprosthesis surgery depending on the projection of the optical cylinder through the eyelid (blepharokeratoplasty) or between the eyelids (prosthokeratoplasty). The choice is based on whether the ocular surface will support a keratoprosthesis. In general, if the ocular surface is moist (wet eye), the eyelids are left open. If the ocular surface is dry (dry eye), the eyelids are closed and the optical cylinder projects through the eyelid. If the eyelids are left open, the 6.5 mm optical cylinder is used; if the eyelids are closed, the 9.5 mm optical cylinder is required.

Fig. 6-6 illustrates the major steps of prosthokeratoplasty. Prosthokeratoplasty is a lengthy procedure and is best performed by a team of surgeons. While the cosurgeons harvest the periosteum, the primary surgeon assembles the keratoprosthesis and begins the ocular component of the procedure.

The first step is to harvest periosteum. The pretibial area is preferred because the absence of muscle in this area makes the dissection easy. The anterior tibial crest is palpated, and 1% lidocaine with epinephrine is infiltrated in a 4 cm area to provide hydrodissection and hemostasis. A no. 15 blade is used to incise the skin for 4 cm along the anterior tibial crest. The ends of this incision are extended 2 cm medially.

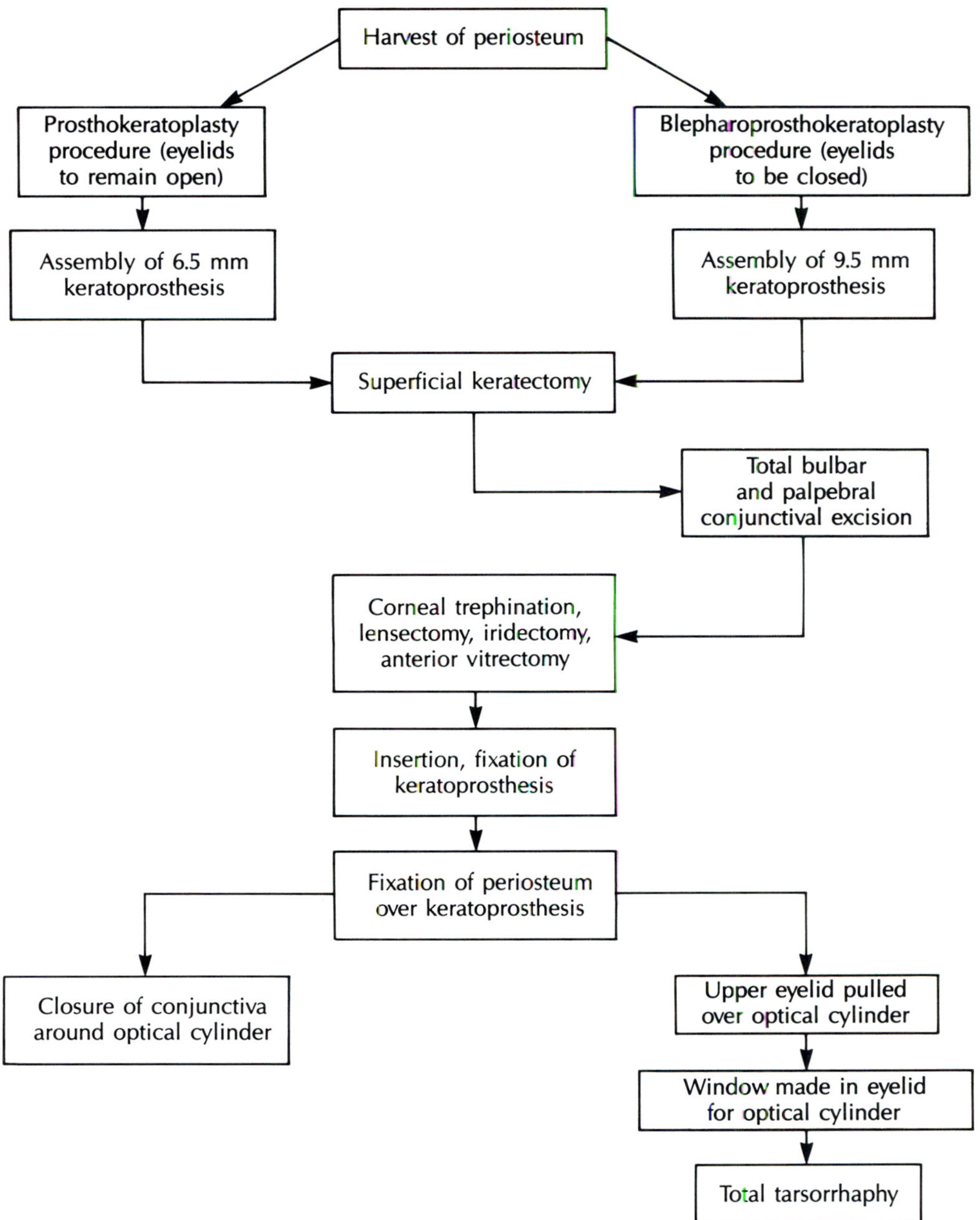

FIGURE 6-6. Flow chart for prosthokeratoplasty.

Any subcutaneous fat is excised and the periosteum is identified. An incision is made along the anterior tibial crest through the periosteum. The surgeon strips the periosteum from the tibia with a periosteal elevator. A rectangular strip of periosteum (approximately 3 by 2 cm; Fig. 6-7) is excised and placed in a sterile petri dish filled with balanced salt solution.

Before performing the superficial keratectomy, the surgeon assembles the keratoprosthesis by threading the optical cylinder into the Teflon skirt. This assembly must be done before intraocular surgery to avoid assembly problems intraoperatively when the procedure cannot be aborted. The keratoprosthesis is then placed in a sterile petri dish filled with balanced salt solution.

The ocular component of prosthokeratoplasty begins with the determination of the visual axis. Proper alignment of the optical cylinder, with the visual axis, should be attempted because there is a potential for 20/20 vision in some keratoprosthesis patients whose ocular disease is restricted to the anterior segment. The determination of the visual axis is usually a gross approximation because of the extensive corneal scarring present in most keratoprosthesis patients. In general, it is not possible to identify the pupil or iris details because of the extensive anterior segment disease present. Transillumination may be helpful in identifying the pupil through an opaque cornea. To avoid visual axis misalignment, it is recommended that the insertions of the four rectus muscles be identified. The limbus is then located based on the insertion distances of the muscles from the limbus (Fig. 6-8). Calipers are used to identify a point 6 mm from the medial limbus and 5.5 mm from the inferior limbus. These numbers are based on a corneal horizontal diameter of 12 mm and a vertical diameter of 11 mm. A 3.5 mm trephine is centered over a point slightly inferior and nasal to the middle of the cornea. The trephine is rotated so that the location for the optical cylinder can be marked.

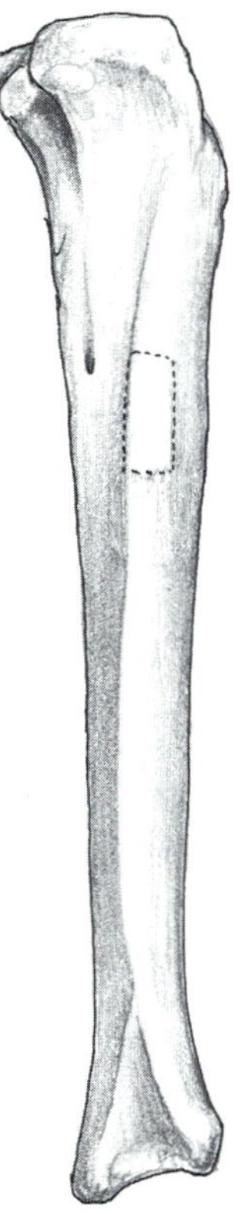

FIGURE 6-7. Harvest of periosteum from tibia.

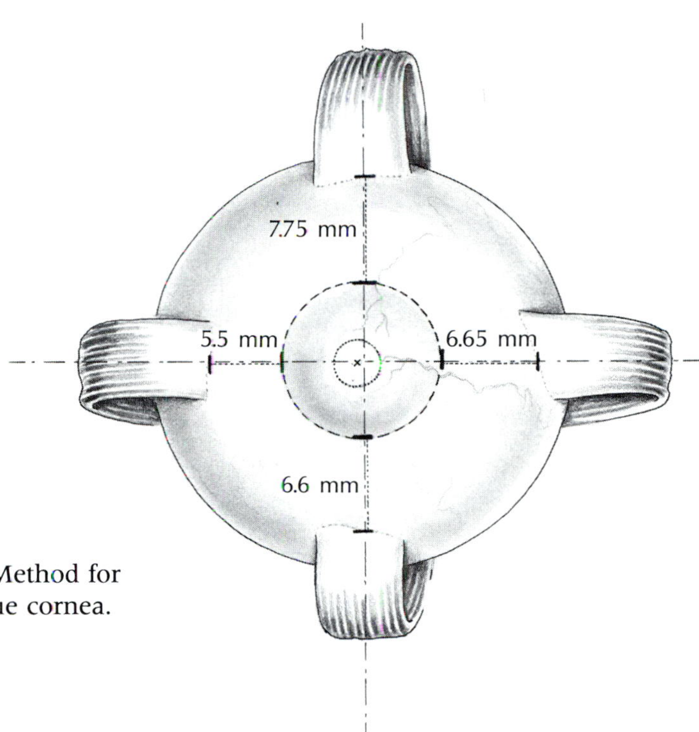

FIGURE 6-8. Estimation of visual axis. Method for determining visual axis in a totally opaque cornea.

A total superficial keratectomy is performed to remove corneal epithelium and Bowman's layer (Fig. 6-9). If the eyelids are to remain open, care is taken to preserve the bulbar conjunctiva adjacent to the limbus. If the eyelids are to be closed, the surgeon excises all the bulbar conjunctiva. The dissection of bulbar conjunctiva is continued beyond the superior and inferior fornices onto the tarsal plates. It is critical to excise all conjunctiva at the lateral canthus and medial canthus, including the plica semilunaris, to prevent postoperative formation of epithelial inclusion cysts. Stevens scissors are used to dissect and excise the palpebral conjunctiva, tarsal plate, and orbicularis muscle (Fig. 6-10). The levator is purposefully disinserted and allowed to retract. Similarly the inferior palpebral conjunctiva, tarsal plate, and orbicularis muscle are excised. The excision of the tarsal plates allows more pliable tissue to surround the optical cylinder, and the excision of the orbicularis muscle and disinsertion of the levator decrease movement of the eyelid against the optical cylinder. Next, the eyelid margins are clamped with a curved hemostat and excised with straight scissors or a stainless steel blade (Fig. 6-11). Application of the hemostat limits any hemorrhage that may result from the excision. The excision of the upper and lower eyelid margins results in the removal of meibomian gland tissue that could contribute to a chalazion, a lid abscess, or annoying debris on the optical cylinder. The excisions described above create bare surfaces between the eye and eyelids that scar together postoperatively (Fig. 6-12).

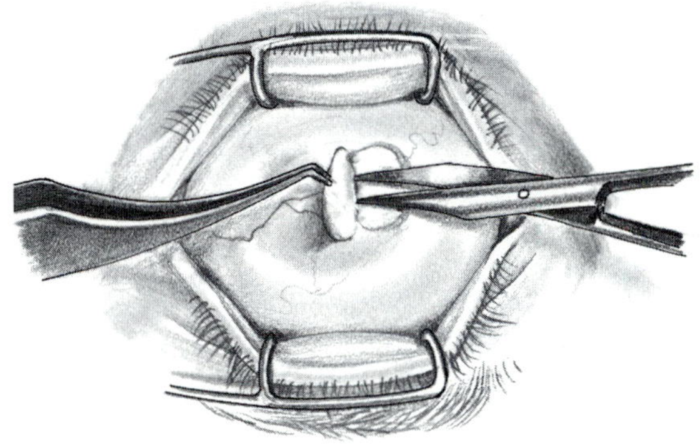

FIGURE 6-9. Superficial keratectomy.

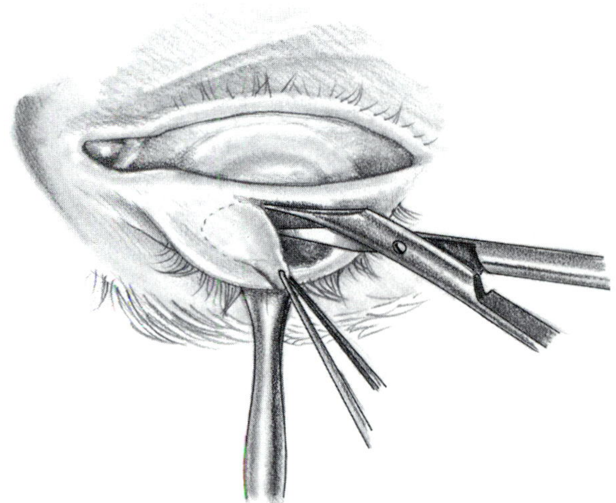

FIGURE 6-10. Excision of palpebral conjunctiva and tarsal plates.

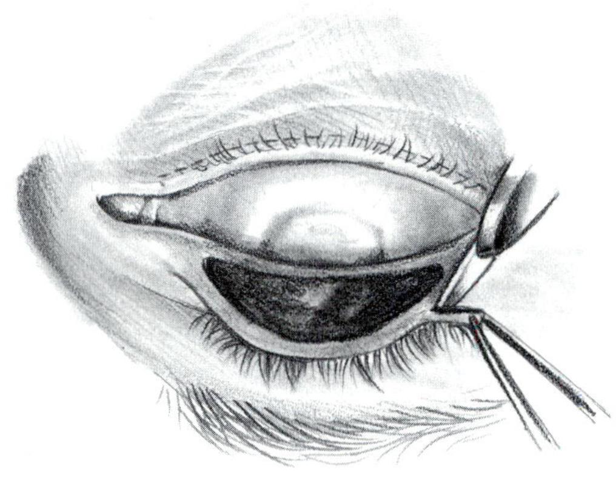

FIGURE 6-11. Excision of eyelid margin with a stainless steel blade.

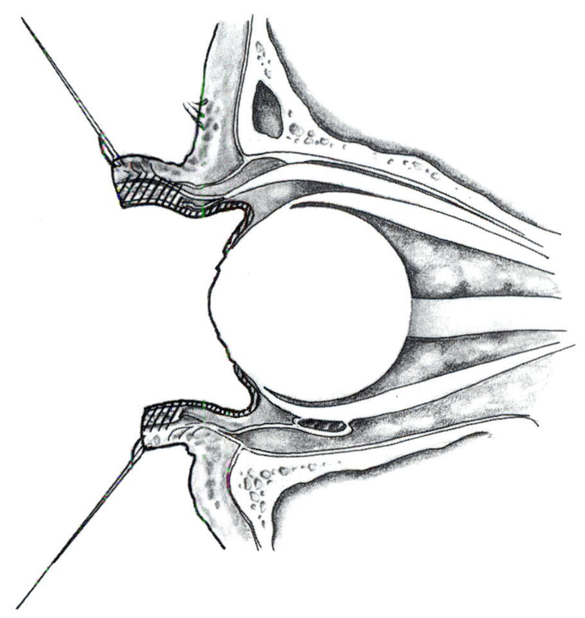

FIGURE 6-12. Resection of bulbar and palpebral conjunctiva, tarsal plate, eyelid margins, and orbicularis muscle.

A 3.5 mm corneal trephine is placed at the site previously marked and is rotated three fourths through the corneal thickness (Fig. 6-13). Since a lensectomy incision must be made, it is not advisable to complete the corneal trephination at this stage because it would be difficult to make and suture the limbal incision with a full-thickness corneal trephine incision present.

A standard 11 to 13 mm limbal cataract incision is made, and the lens is extracted whether cataractous or not because the optical cylinder of the keratoprosthesis will project beyond the lens plane. If there has been no previous lens surgery, an intracapsular cryoextraction is performed (Fig. 6-14). If lens or capsular remnants remain from previous lens surgery, they are removed as completely as possible with a vitrector. To minimize the postoperative complication of retroprosthetic membrane formation, all lens and capsular remnants must be completely excised.

A copious amount of a viscoelastic substance is placed over the vitreous face to act as a barrier to the dispersion of blood before the iridectomy is done. A peripheral iridotomy is done and converted to a keyhole iridotomy with DeWecker scissors. Endocautery is applied to any bleeding iris vessels. The iris is sharply dissected from the iris root circumferentially for 360 degrees with Vannas scissors. It is important to maintain hemostasis during this procedure because hemorrhage into the vitreous not only may retard visual rehabilitation but also may set the stage for retroprosthetic membrane formation, intravitreal fibrosis, and tractional retinal detachment. A vitrector is then inserted, and a total anterior vitrectomy is done.

The cataract incision is closed with interrupted 10-0 nylon sutures (Fig. 6-15). Balanced salt solution is instilled via an irrigation cannula through the limbal incision to restore the intraocular pressure.

The trephine incision is completed by inserting a 15-degree blade into the incision and entering the anterior chamber. The corneal button is excised with corneal scissors or the 15-degree blade. Since these corneas are heavily vascularized, it is important to anticipate hemorrhage during this stage of the procedure and maintain hemostasis with cauterization.

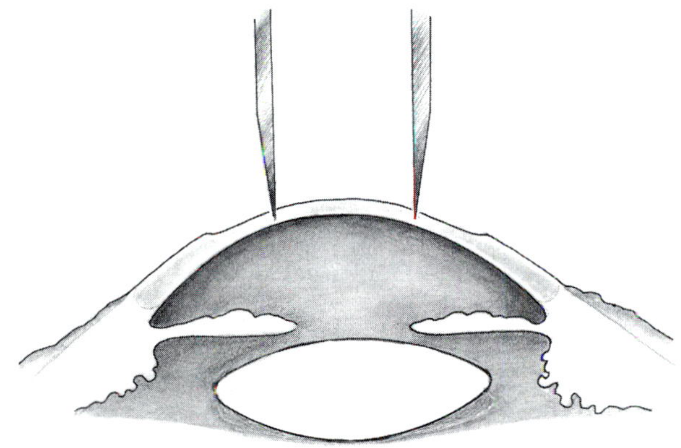

FIGURE 6-13. Centering of 3.5 mm trephine over visual axis of cornea.

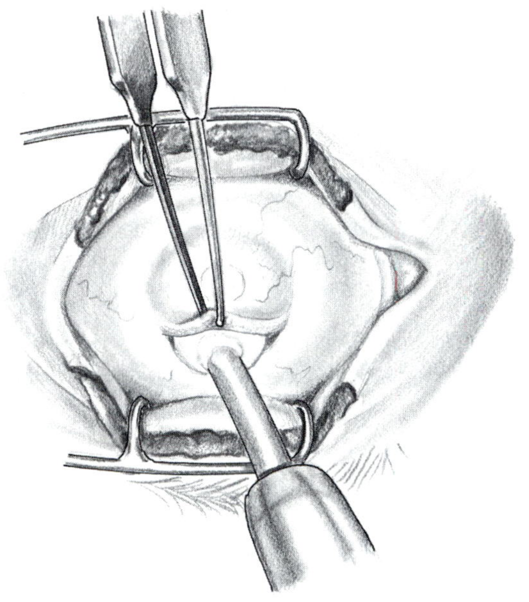

FIGURE 6-14. Intracapsular lens extraction.

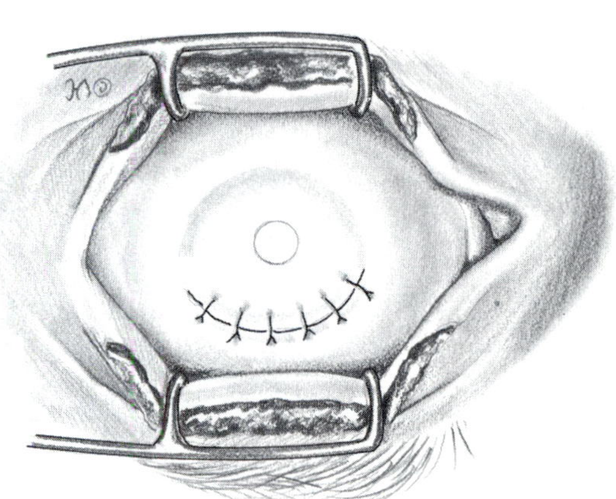

FIGURE 6-15. Closure of limbal incision.

The previously assembled keratoprosthesis is retrieved from the petri dish and placed into the sterile field. The neck of the Teflon skirt is grasped with Aquavella forceps, and the optical cylinder is placed through the corneal opening. The surgeon should use a clockwise twisting motion to help ease the optical cylinder threads into the opening. The optical cylinder is inserted posteriorly until the neck of the Teflon skirt is flush against the cornea.

The Teflon skirt is sutured to the cornea through each of the eight large fenestrations with 8-0 nylon sutures. Cardinal sutures at 12, 6, 3, and 9 o'clock are placed initially as with a standard corneal graft. Each of the eight smaller peripheral fenestrations are similarly sutured with 8-0 nylon sutures. At this point the keratoprosthesis is securely fixed to the cornea (Fig. 6-16).

The next steps involve covering the Teflon skirt with a protective layer of periosteum and conjunctiva or periosteum and eyelid tissue. In anticipation of these steps the height of the optical cylinder is adjusted (that is, unthreaded, counterclockwise motion) using a microrasp so that it projects a few millimeters above the Teflon skirt.

The periosteum is retrieved and situated over the globe. It should cover the insertions of the rectus muscles. The point of projection of the optical cylinder of the keratoprosthesis is noted and marked with a methylene blue pen. Then the periosteum is placed in a dry petri dish and a linear slit incision approximately 4 mm in length is made through the periosteum with a no. 11 Bard-Parker blade. The periosteum (shiny side up) is then fitted over the optical cylinder and aligned over the four rectus muscles.

Multiple interrupted 5-0 chromic sutures are used to fix the periosteum to episclera (Fig. 6-17). Secure fixation adjacent to the rectus muscles promotes good blood supply, which is important to the viability of the periosteal graft.

If the eyelids are to be closed, the upper eyelid is pulled over the keratoprosthesis and the point of projection of the optical cylinder is noted (Fig. 6-18). A chalazion clamp is placed on the eyelid centered over this point, and a no. 11 blade is used to make a horizontal linear incision approximately 4 mm in this area (Fig. 6-19).

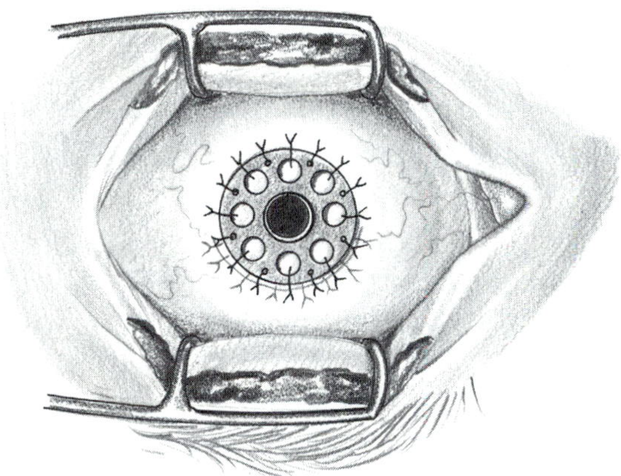

FIGURE 6-16. Fixation of supporting plate to cornea.

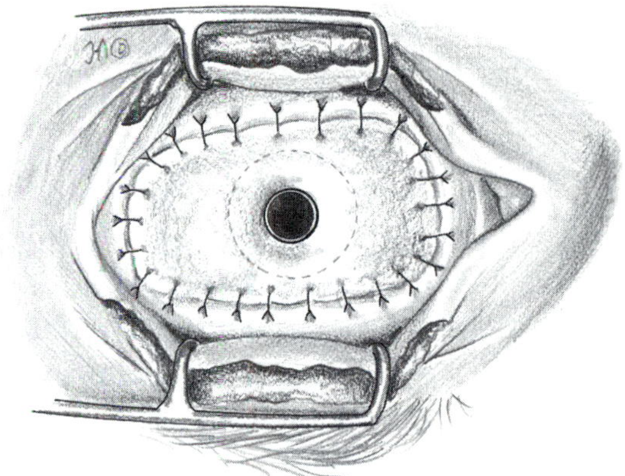

FIGURE 6-17. Fixation of periosteum over supporting plate.

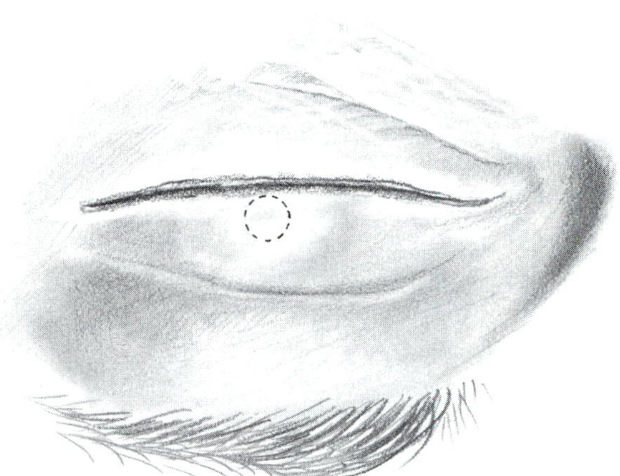

FIGURE 6-18. Localization of projection site of optical cylinder through upper eyelid.

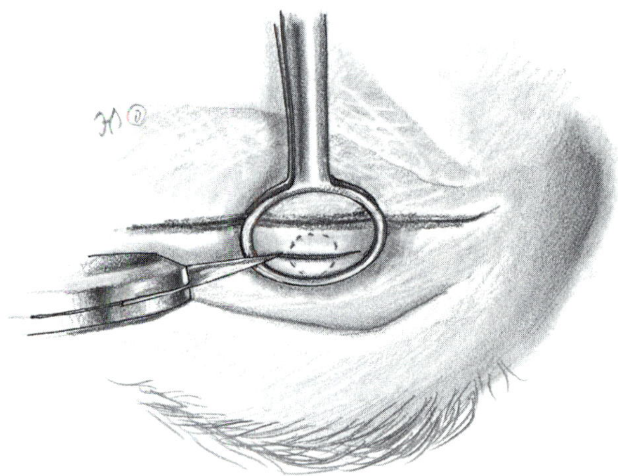

FIGURE 6-19. Creation of upper eyelid "window" for optical cylinder.

The optical cylinder is fitted through this incision, and 6-0 silk is used to close the incision around the cylinder. Finally the upper and lower eyelid margins are sutured with 6-0 silk to create a total permanent tarsorrhaphy (Figs. 6-20 and 6-21).

If the eyelids are to remain open, the conjunctiva is sutured over the periosteum and snuggly coapted around the optical cylinder using 6-0 plain suture (Figs. 6-22 and 6-23). It is important that the conjunctiva not be under tension because this can lead to postoperative erosion of the conjunctiva and dehiscence of the keratoprosthesis. It may be necessary to place a relaxing incision in the superior and inferior fornices in order to adequately drape the conjunctiva around the optical cylinder.

Antibiotic ointment is applied, and a patch and shield are placed. The leg wound is dressed with Telfa and an elastoplast compressive dressing. The use of postoperative prophylactic systemic antibiotics is optional.

POSTOPERATIVE CARE

Keratoprosthesis patients are generally admitted after the procedure and are hospitalized for 2 or 3 days postoperatively. Topical antibiotics are given postoperatively. The use of corticosteroids is contraindicated in keratoprosthesis patients given the permanent vulnerability of their eyes to infection and the risk of extrusion. In general, mild analgesics are sufficient to control postoperative pain in these patients. Eyelid and leg sutures are generally removed at the end of 2 weeks.

Visual acuity of 20/20 has been recorded as early as 3 to 7 days postoperatively in some keratoprosthesis patients. However, in general, optimal visual rehabilitation may not occur for 1 to 3 months.

The surface of the optical cylinder commonly is covered with mucus, or eyelid secretion. This material may reduce visual acuity from 20/20 to 20/200. Since debris may accumulate daily, patients are instructed in the technique of cleaning the surface of the optical cylinder with sterile saline solution and a cotton applicator. It is important that clockwise wiping motions be utilized to avoid unthreading of the optical cylinder. Periodically adherent deposits may accumulate on the optical cylinder surface. These may be removed with a cotton applicator soaked in a standard contact lens cleaning solution. Care is taken to avoid contact with the conjunctiva.

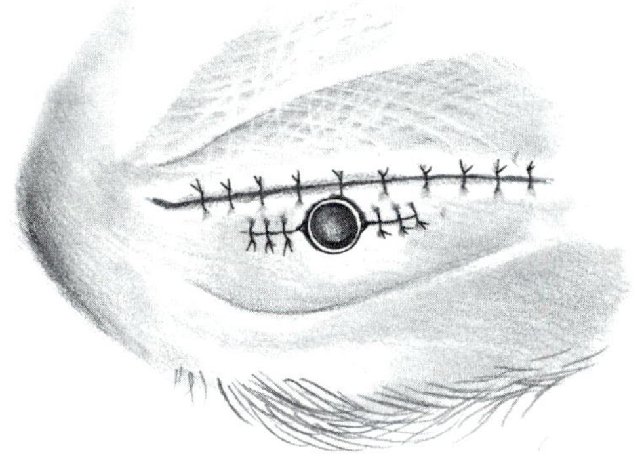

FIGURE 6-20. Closure of skin around optical cylinder and total tarsorrhaphy.

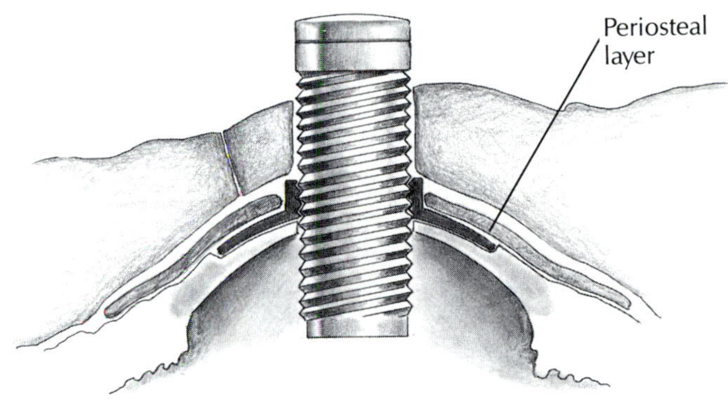

FIGURE 6-21. Sagittal section illustrating keratoprosthesis in situ through the eyelid.

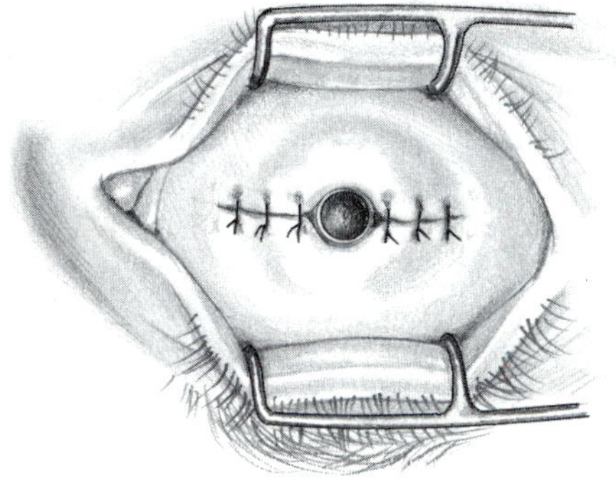

FIGURE 6-22. Closure of conjunctiva over periosteum.

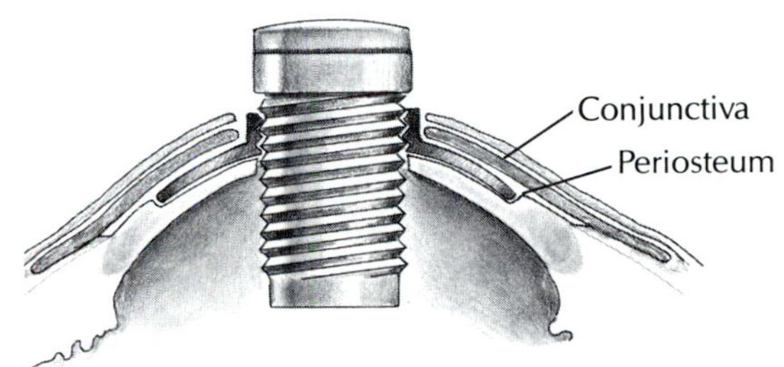

FIGURE 6-23. Sagittal section illustrating keratoprosthesis in situ with the eyelids left open.

INTRAOPERATIVE COMPLICATIONS

1. Visual axis misalignment
2. Scratched optical cylinder
3. Intraoperative hemorrhage

Visual axis misalignment

As stated previously, there is a potential for 20/20 vision in some keratoprosthesis patients. Careful intraoperative determination of the visual axis will maximize this potential. If the steps described in the previous section are followed, the keratoprosthesis should be properly centered. If, however, it becomes evident later in the procedure that the partial-thickness trephine incision has been incorrectly placed, it can be closed with 10-0 nylon sutures and another incision made in the correct location.

Scratched optical cylinder

The keratoprosthesis is affixed to the globe with the optical cylinder in situ. During the suturing of the supporting plate care must be taken to avoid inadvertent scratching of the optical cylinder with forceps or suture needles. Scratching of the cylinder can lead to visual aberrations such as distortion and glare and thus is to be avoided.

Intraoperative hemorrhage

Hemorrhage is, perhaps, the most frequent operative complication of prosthokeratoplasty because of the severe vascularization of the ocular surface in these eyes. Hemostasis of bleeding conjunctival and eyelid vessels must be achieved before the eye is opened. Cauterization of corneal and iris vessels that bleed is required during the surgical procedure. It is important to prevent anterior segment bleeding into the vitreous, which can preclude early visual rehabilitation and set the stage for intravitreal fibrosis, retroprosthetic membrane formation, vitritis, and tractional retinal detachment. Blood in the anterior vitreous can easily be removed during the vitrectomy; blood more posteriorly is more difficult if not impossible to remove in this setting and is best avoided.

POSTOPERATIVE COMPLICATIONS

Glaucoma

Glaucoma is a frequent complication in patients with a keratoprosthesis both before and after surgery. Since these patients have extensive anterior segment disease, they frequently have glaucoma preoperatively. It is important to attempt glaucoma assessment and control before surgery because with the keratoprosthesis in place, either through the eyelid or between the eyelids, there is no accurate method of measuring intraocular pressure. The intraocular pressure must be assessed by periodic visual fields and observation of the optic nerve head. Fig. 6-24 illustrates a typical visual field obtained in a keratoprosthesis patient. The visual field is constricted to 20 to 30 degrees because of the optical cylinder design. Consequently, early field loss may be impossible to detect, a situation emphasizing the importance for thorough glaucoma assessment and control before surgery. When the keratoprosthesis is through the eyelid, topical medications cannot be administered. Therefore glaucoma must be controlled before surgery.

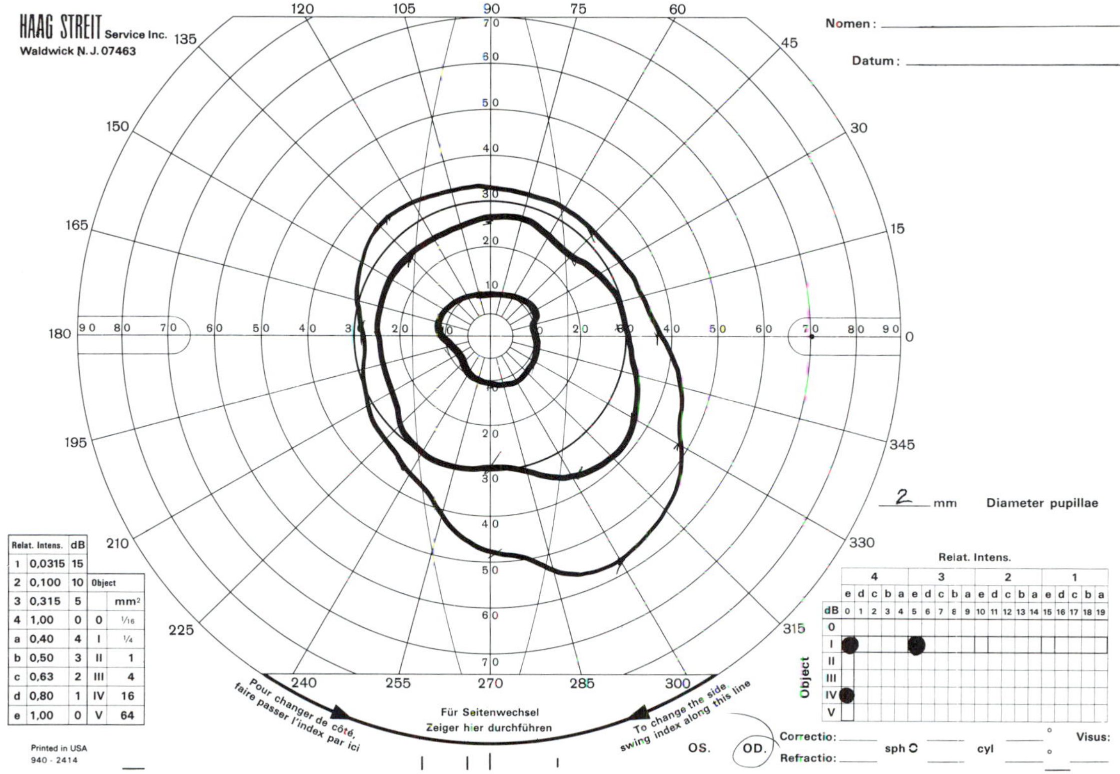

FIGURE 6-24. Goldman visual field of a through-the-lid keratoprosthesis subject who had 20/15 visual acuity. Notice the visual field constriction resulting from the keratoprosthesis. (Traces: *outer* at IV; *middle* at I4e; *inner* at I3e.)

Intraocular infection

The evaluation of the interior of the eye after prosthokeratoplasty is complex because of the common communication of the anterior chamber, posterior chamber, and vitreous cavity. The procedure creates a unicameral eye; thus any cells or flare visualized may represent predominantly anterior segment inflammation, posterior segment inflammation, or a combination of the two. In general, the use of topical or periocular corticosteroids is not recommended because of the possibility of inhibiting wound healing leading to extrusion. The presence of intraocular inflammation requires careful assessment and follow-up observation. At the time of initial presentation, culture and sensitivity is recommended because endophthalmitis may result from such innocuous conditions as conjunctivitis or chalazion. The presence of tenderness or ocular discharge in association with intraocular inflammation represents endophthalmitis and should be treated as such until proved otherwise.

Dehiscence

The earliest stage of dehiscence is thinning of the skin-periosteal or conjunctival-periosteal layer over the supporting plate. If the keratoprosthesis projects through the upper eyelid, thinning or retraction of the skin may be noted. When dehiscence is established, the neck of the supporting plate is visible.

There are two basic approaches to the management of dehiscence depending on whether the eyelids have been left open or are closed.

Prosthokeratoplasty eyes

When dehiscence occurs in a prosthokeratoplasty eye, it is important to assess the fixation status of the keratoprosthesis. Dehiscence may be graded in terms of the number of clock hours of exposure of the supporting plate or neck. In early dehiscence there is 1 clock hour of exposure (Fig. 6-25). In late dehiscence there are 3 clock hours of exposure (Fig. 6-26). When exposure of the supporting plate or neck is present, tectonic graft materials are necessary. Either periosteum, fascia lata, or temporalis fascia is sutured over the area of dehiscence with 6-0 chromic sutures. Conjunctiva is then used to cover the tectonic graph. The conjunctiva must not be under tension. Buccal mucous membrane may be used as an alternative to conjunctiva in order to avoid tension on the conjunctiva.

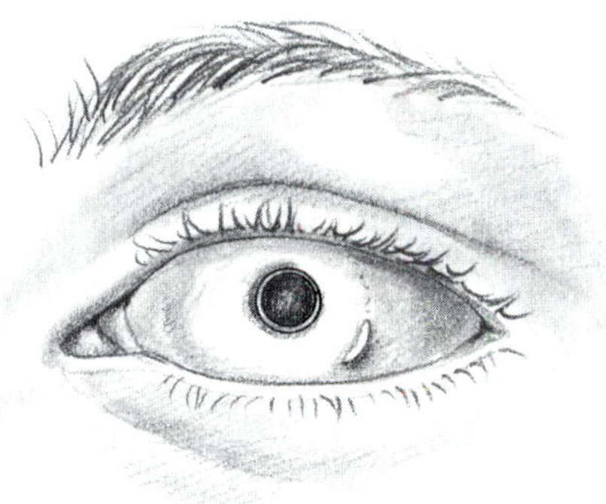

FIGURE 6-25. Early dehiscence.

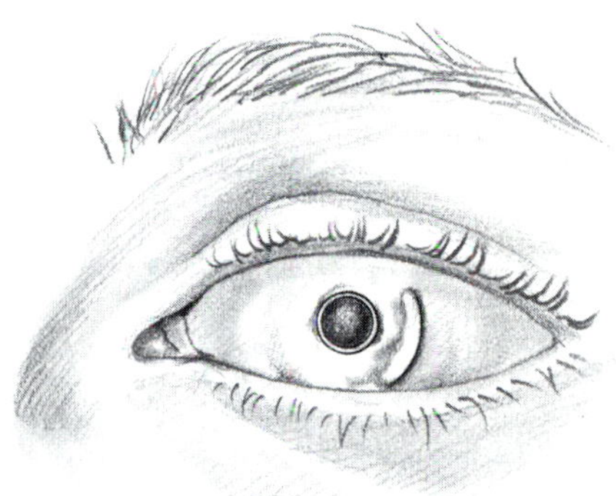

FIGURE 6-26. Late dehiscence.

Blepharoprosthokeratoplasty eyes

When dehiscence occurs in a blepharoprosthokeratoplasty eye, it is important not to underestimate the degree of dehiscence particularly because most of the supporting plate is not visible (Fig. 6-27, *A* and *B*). It is important at the time of surgical repair to explore the dehiscence to determine the stability of the supporting plate. If most of the supporting plate is well fixated and no tilt of the optical cylinder is observed, tectonic overlay grafting is recommended. Tilt of the optical cylinder is an ominous sign and indicates extensive loss of fixation of the supporting plate (Fig. 6-27, *C*). The first layer should be periosteum (or fascia lata or temporalis fascia), which is sutured with 6-0 chromic to the episclera. It is important that the skin not be under tension. A free skin graft from the opposite eyelid or the preauricular area may be obtained. Since vascularization of the tectonic material is essential to success, a bucket-handle skin graft from the brow area may be advisable. These procedures are summarized in Figs. 6-28 to 6-32.

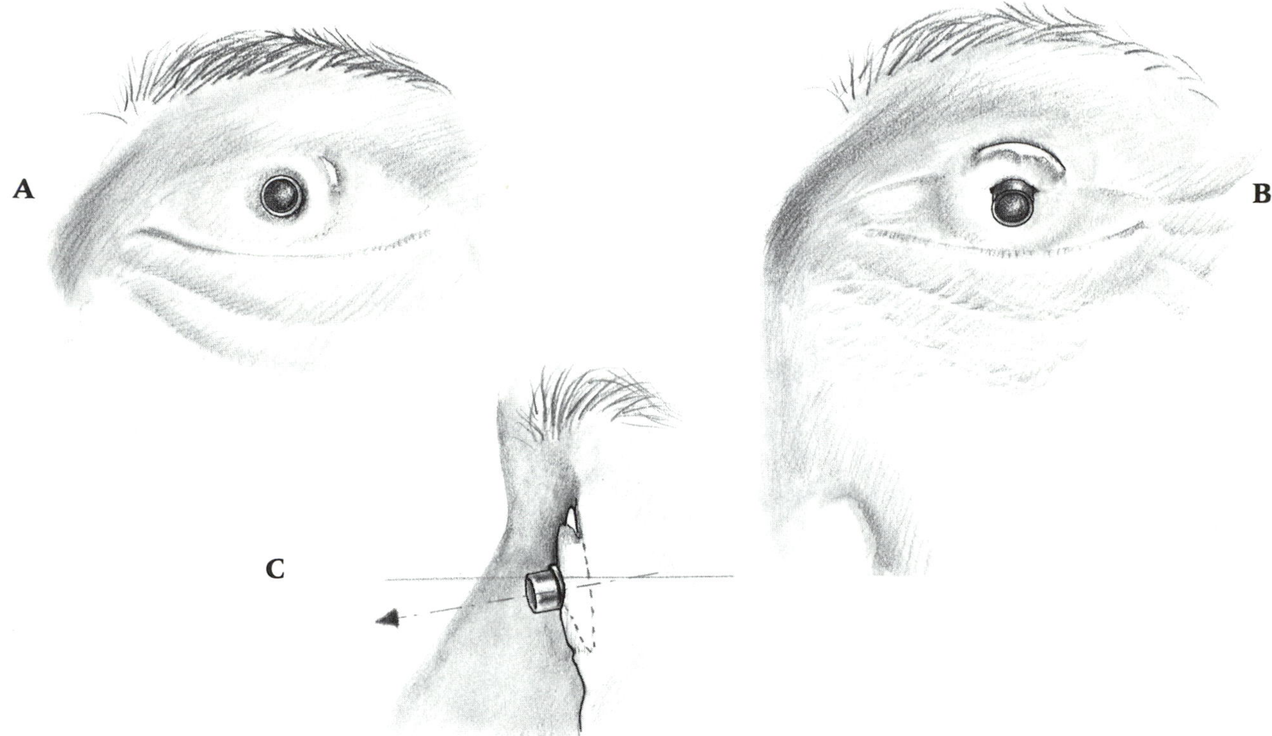

FIGURE 6-27. Progression of dehiscence in a through-the-lid keratoprosthesis. **A,** Early dehiscence. **B,** Late dehiscence. **C,** Late dehiscence with tilt of optical cylinder.

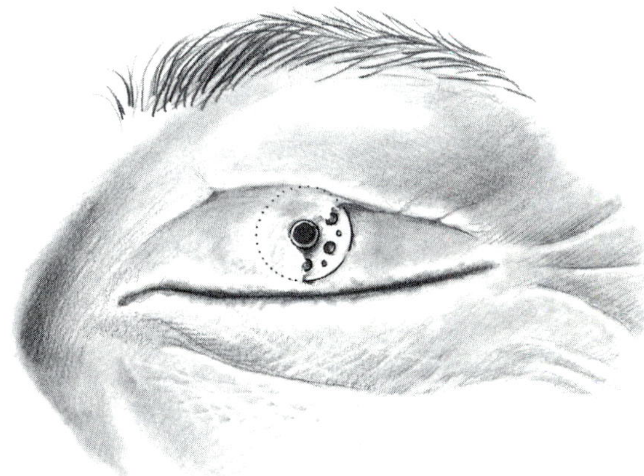

FIGURE 6-28. Late dehiscence.

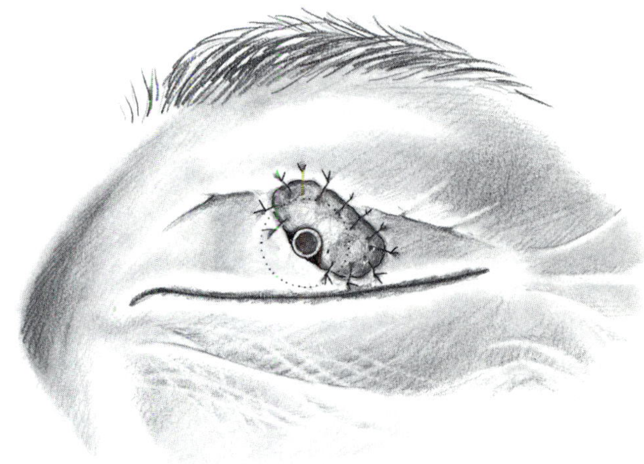

FIGURE 6-29. Management of dehiscence. Periosteal graft over area of dehiscence.

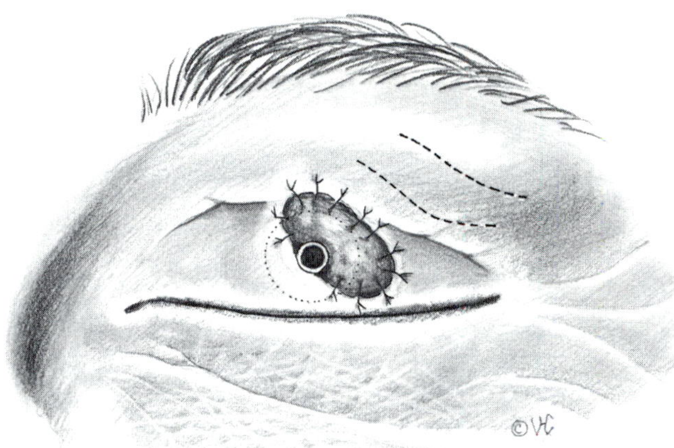

FIGURE 6-30. Marking of incision of bucket-handle graft.

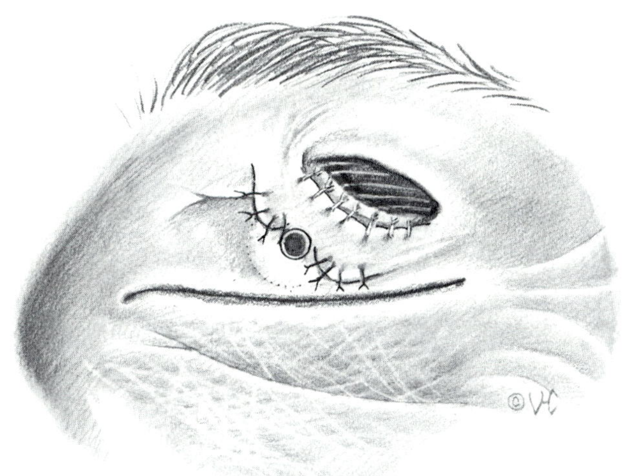

FIGURE 6-31. Mobilization of bucket-handle graft.

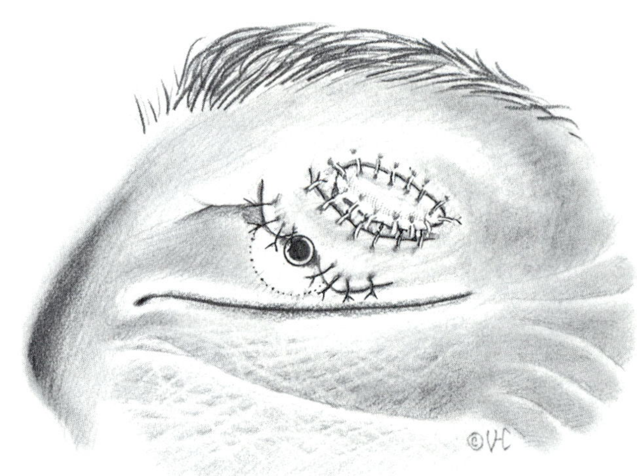

FIGURE 6-32. Final position of bucket-handle graft and free skin graft.

Giant papillary conjunctivitis

Giant papillary conjunctivitis (GPC) is a complication of contact lenses, ocular prostheses, and keratoprostheses. A case of GPC in which the tarsal plates contained amyloid was recently observed by me. Unusual instances of giant papillary nodules involving the bulbar conjunctiva adjacent to the optical cylinder have been observed. These giant papillary masses may reduce visual acuity. These nodules of the bulbar conjunctiva and papillae of the palpebral conjunctiva are regarded as variants of the allergic response of the conjunctiva to constant mechanical alloplastic irritation. Unless these giant papillae obstruct the optical cylinder no treatment is recommended. When treatment is required, surgical excision rather than topical corticosteroids is recommended. In general, topical corticosteroids are contraindicated in the presence of a keratoprosthesis because their use may lead to tissue melting, poor wound healing, and ultimate complications such as extrusion or dehiscence.

Retroprosthetic membrane

The growth of tissue behind the posterior surface of the optical cylinder of the keratoprosthesis is known as "retroprosthetic membrane formation." Before routine anterior vitrectomies were done, the incidence of retroprosthetic membrane formation was as high as 50%. The range of this complication is now between 10% and 15%. The formation of a retroprosthetic membrane is correlated with decreasing visual acuity and observation of an opaque membrane on the posterior surface of the optical cylinder. Removal of the membrane is a formidable operative procedure because it requires unthreading of the optical cylinder followed by membranectomy-vitrectomy under conditions of suboptimal visualization. The potential for hemorrhage or damage to the retina with these procedures is ever present. Recently, Nd:YAG (neodymium–yttrium-aluminum-garnet) laser photodiscission has been a suggested method for removal of a retroprosthetic membrane; however, damage to the posterior surface of the optical cylinder can occur.

Extrusion

The most dreaded complication of prosthokeratoplasty is extrusion. Before development of current techniques and models of keratoprostheses, extrusion rates of 20% to 50% were common. However, with the current Cardona TT model the rate of extrusion has been reduced. Extrusion is a complication of current alloplastic corneal devices because of the lack of bioadhesion. Design features such as fenestrations have been added to allow tissue ingrowth and metabolic exchange. The use of periosteum, fascia lata, or temporalis fascia has been effective in promoting fixation of the alloplastic device to the cornea. Supporting plates of aluminum oxide and Proplast have been designed to promote bioadhesion and reduce extrusion. Despite these technologic advances, extrusion remains ubiquitous, and a patient with a successful keratoprosthesis must be followed indefinitely at intervals of 3 to 6 months. Extrusion may be associated with tissue necrosis and melting, which typically has a precipitous presentation.

Extrusion is managed by removal of the keratoprosthesis, tectonic penetrating keratoplasty, and insertion of a new keratoprosthesis through the graft. A two-stage operation with either the Choyce or the Girard keratoprosthesis may be advisable if substantial necrosis, melting, or loss of tissue integrity is present. The two-stage approach is also preferable if any possibility of intraocular infection exists. A buccal mucous membrane graft is an important adjunct to the successful management of extrusion in some cases because it hastens the establishment of a good blood supply to the tectonic graft in addition to acting as a tectonic graft itself.

Vitreous hemorrhage

Vitreous hemorrhage is an uncommon postoperative complication of prosthokeratoplasty. When it occurs, trauma should be suspected. Because the optical cylinder must project 1 to 2 mm above the conjunctiva or skin, the opportunity for inadvertent trauma to the keratoprosthesis exists during routine cleansing of the optical cylinder or during sleep. It is therefore recommended that a patient place a protective metal shield over the eye before going to sleep. When a vitreous hemorrhage is suspected clinically, it should be confirmed with ultrasonography. A vitreous hemorrhage may be associated with a retinal tear or may be the first step in the development of a tractional retinal detachment. A vitreous hemorrhage in a patient with a keratoprosthesis is best managed by observation, including sequential ultrasonography, because the risks of surgical removal of the blood in this situation are great.

Conjunctival overgrowth

The growth of conjunctiva over the optical cylinder can result in decreased visual acuity. Conjunctival overgrowth can typically be managed by surgical excision of the abnormal tissue. However, recurrence is likely unless a conjunctivoplasty is performed at the time of the excision. Care must be taken to avoid trauma to the surrounding tissue and to remove the least amount of tissue necessary lest the complication of overgrowth be replaced by the complication of atrophy and dehiscence. Occasionally advancement of the height of the optical cylinder is required to get the anterior surface of the optical cylinder above the surrounding tissue. Conjunctival filtration blebs and cysts that communicate with the anterior chamber may masquerade as conjunctival overgrowth. Thus any excision must be approached with caution.

Retinal detachment

The occurrence of a retinal detachment in the presence of a keratoprosthesis forebodes a grave prognosis. Visualization of the posterior pole through the optical cylinder is difficult, and visualization of the equator or ora is virtually impossible. Thus identification of the tear or other topographic features of the retinal detachment are unsuccessful. A 360-degree high buckle can be placed as a blind procedure because of the inability to identify precise aspects of the tear. It is important that ultrasonography be performed to identify vitreous traction, and, if present, it is recommended that the keratoprosthesis surgeon assist the retinal surgeon with the vitrectomy and retinal detachment surgery. Despite heroic attempts, the occurrence of a retinal detachment is frequently the coup de grace for an eye with a keratoprosthesis.

Eyelid infections

Eyelid infections and inflammations in the presence of a keratoprosthesis are an ominous and potentially sight-threatening complication because they can progress to endophthalmitis. This is a particular risk when the keratoprosthesis projects through the eyelid. An eyelid abscess may exist alone or in association with lid inflammations such as a chalazion or external hordeolum, and any induration of the eyelid should be considered an abscess until proved otherwise. An eyelid infection represents a therapeutic emergency in a keratoprosthesis patient. Prompt surgical incision and drainage is recommended as well as systemic antibiotics, topical antibiotics, and close observation. These patients need to be observed closely for signs of endophthalmitis because of the communication of the intraocular contents with the optical cylinder. Any decrease in vision associated with globe tenderness represents endophthalmitis until proved otherwise.

VARIANTS ON PROCEDURE

Tectonic grafting

Occasionally a tectonic lamellar keratoplasty must be performed before prosthokeratoplasty or as a component of the procedure if the preoperative workup indicates a thinned or staphylomatous cornea. It is generally preferable to perform the tectonic graft before prosthokeratoplasty in order to assure that the cornea will support the keratoprosthesis. If the tectonic graft is performed as a component of prosthokeratoplasty, it should follow the superficial keratectomy or conjunctival excision.

Adjustment of optical cylinder height

The height of the optical cylinder above the neck of the supporting plate may require adjustment postoperatively when eyelid edema or conjunctival chemosis resolves. Additionally, routine surface cleansing of the optical cylinder may result in gradual unthreading of the optical cylinder, and this excessive projection of the optical cylinder requires immediate attention. The technique of height adjustment using microrasps is illustrated in Fig. 6-33.

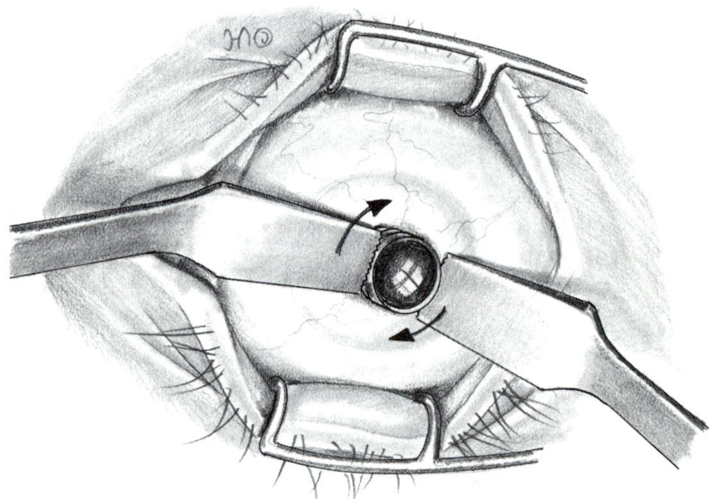

FIGURE 6-33. Adjustment of level of projection of the optical cylinder. The cylinder is rotated clockwise to lower its level and counterclockwise to raise its level.

PART TWO

CATARACT SURGERY

Henry M. Clayman

CHAPTER 7

Essentials of Cataract Surgery

Cataract surgery is an ancient operation that has evolved from couching to extracapsular surgery, thence to intracapsular surgery and back to extracapsular surgery in contemporary usage. Phacoemulsification, of course, is a variant of extracapsular surgery. Future horizons appear to be endocapsular surgery, whereby the capsule is punctured and the cataractous contents are evacuated and replaced with a synthetic substance acting in place of the crystalline lens, perhaps with some retention of accommodation. Presumably, this surgery will either be carried out from a 1 mm limbal or pars plana incision with minimal postoperative astigmatism. This technique is not currently feasible in human subjects.

The decision to operate on a cataract is made on the basis of an eye examination; Fig. 7-1 is an attempt to describe the preoperative evaluation and the steps to surgery. It is becoming apparent that visual acuity as measured by the Snellen test is only one of the criteria to be evaluated before cataract surgery. This test addresses itself to the quantity of vision in the dim light of the surgeon's examining room where black letters are viewed against a bright white background. It does not define the quality of vision, a concept that is still in its infancy. Glare testing is a welcome evolutionary step toward vision quality testing.

INTRACAPSULAR VERSUS EXTRACAPSULAR CATARACT SURGERY

If one arbitrarily dates the evolution of contemporary cataract surgery from Daviel (1696-1762), the ensuing years have seen the popularity of both extracapsular and intracapsular cataract surgery wax and wane. In the past 15 years, ophthalmic surgeons in the United States have again favored extracapsular techniques, a phenomenon greatly influenced by the advent of posterior chamber intraocular lenses (IOLs).

The advantage of an intracapsular extraction is that it is easier inasmuch as one maneuver is required to extract the cataract. In contrast, extracapsular surgery requires several steps to achieve the same end, that is, anterior capsulectomy, extraction of the nucleus, and evacuation of the residual cortex. Moreover, intracapsular surgery is cheaper because the only instrument of sophisticated technology that is required is the cryosurgical probe. Extracapsular surgery is generally performed with an automated irrigation/aspiration device, or sometimes with ultrasound, which is a significant capital expense. Furthermore, an apparatus-specific, nonreusable pack containing irrigation and aspiration tubing with irrigation fluid adds further expense.

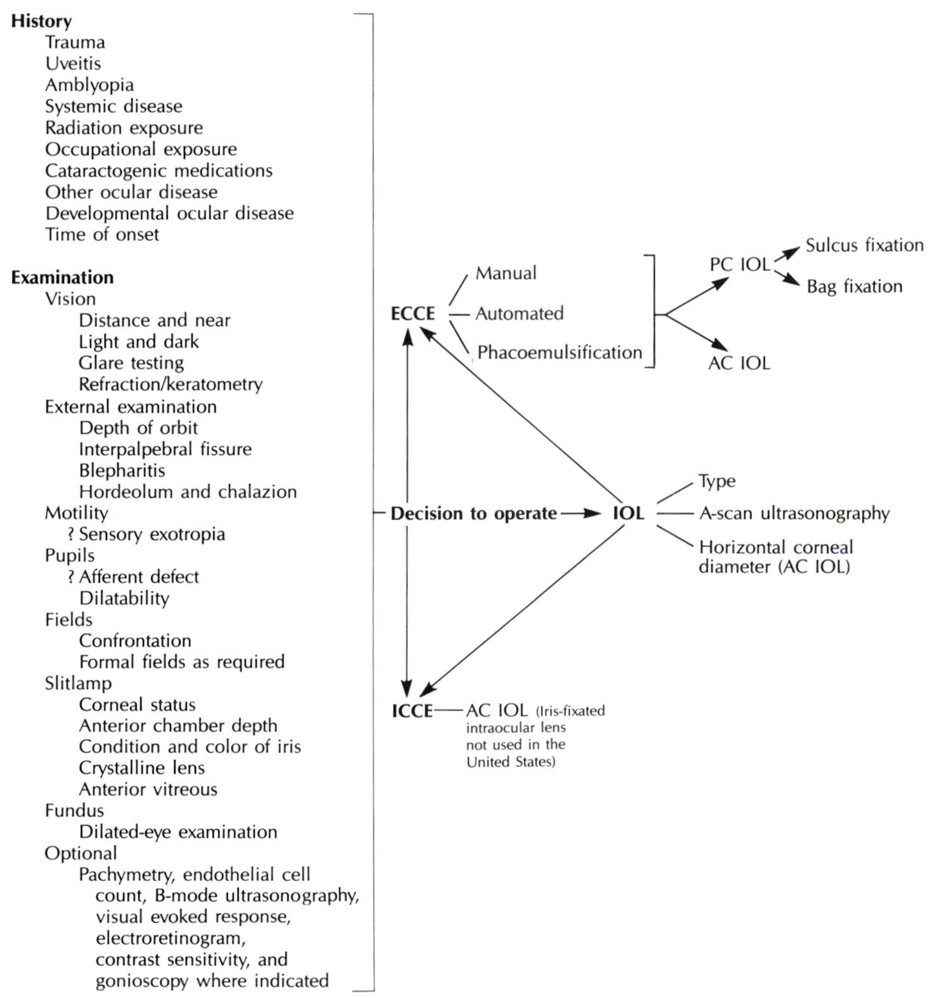

FIGURE 7-1. Factors involved in a decision to operate and surgical choices. *AC,* Anterior chamber; *ECCE,* extracapsular cataract extraction; *ICCE,* intracapsular cataract extraction; *IOL,* intraocular lens; *PC,* posterior chamber.

After reading the above comments, one may well ask, Why bother with extracapsular surgery? The answer is that there are substantial long-term patient benefits. The incidence of cystoid macular edema (CME) and retinal detachment (RD) is significantly less than with the intracapsular technique, and this is also probably true for postoperative keratopathy. Additionally, a posterior chamber IOL, whether sulcus or capsular bag fixated, requires an extracapsular technique. Posterior chamber IOLs have shown their superiority over iris and anterior chamber IOLs, and this has accelerated the evolution to extracapsular techniques.

PATIENT EVALUATION AND PREPARATION

Intraocular pressure

I do not routinely use preoperative medication to reduce intraocular pressure though many surgeons do. The exception is patients with glaucoma who are

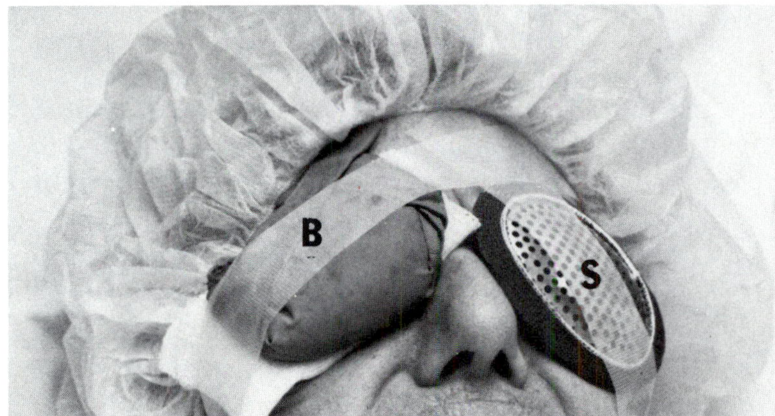

FIGURE 7-2. Mercury bag, *B*, is used to induce ocular hypotension in the operative eye. A protective shield, *S*, covers the nonoperative eye for identification and intraoperative protection.

already taking ocular hypotensive medications. In these cases, carbonic anhydrase inhibitors and topical beta adrenergic receptor blockers are continued at their normal dose to the point of surgery. Miotics and epinephrine derivatives are discontinued, the former because of miosis and the latter because of rebound hyperemia, which causes bleeding from the conjunctival flap and sometimes the incision. I use neither balloons nor "superpinkie" devices to induce ocular hypotension. I rely on a mercury bag applied in the holding area (Fig. 7-2).

Preoperative sedation

There is wide variation in surgeon and anesthesiologist preference for postoperative sedation. Personally, I prefer midazolam hydrochloride (Versed), 1 mg, intramuscularly, 90 minutes preoperatively. Less would be given in debilitated patients and more, under an anesthesiologist's supervision, for excessively anxious or hyperactive patients. My patients have no nourishment (NPO) after midnight before surgery. Exceptions are made, as required, in diabetic patients on whom I prefer to operate early in the schedule. For a long schedule, where a given patient may be operated on at noon or later, I permit an early clear liquid breakfast.

Mydriasis

Over the years, I have used various combinations of mydriatics. Currently, I favor cyclopentolate 1% and phenylephrine 10%, one drop of each 5 minutes apart, for three doses. I have recently added topical flurbiprofen (Ocufen) to this regimen, giving one drop simultaneously with the mydriatics. Topical flurbiprofen is not a mydriatic but rather maintains intraoperative mydriasis by inhibiting miosis-producing prostaglandin secretion, which is incited by intracameral manipulations. Flurbiprofen is highly efficacious, especially in light irides, and is a useful adjunct to cataract surgery, as are the other topical prostaglandin inhibitors that have recently been introduced.

Facial scrub

There is not a specific scrub for the face and operative field that has the approbation of all surgeons. Some surgeons advocate a facial scrub with hexachlorophene (pHisoHex) the night before surgery; others do not. In the operating room a povidone-iodine (Betadine) detergent scrub is often used, being applied to the adnexa and adjacent facial area. Whatever type of scrub is favored, it is desirable to leave the solution on the skin for about a minute to enhance bacteriostasis.

Positioning and draping

The patient should obviously be comfortable on the operating table. Elderly patients may have accompanying musculoskeletal disease, and every effort should be made to avoid discomfort from hard surfaces, restraining straps, and monitoring devices. From the surgeon's point of view, the patient's head should be as close to the end of the table as possible to avoid the surgeon having to reach too far forward, a position that compromises fine hand movements. Where a hand rest is used, the patient's head should abut the inner aspect of this device. The face should be looking straight up without the chin excessively elevated. A head turned to the left or the right causes fluid pooling at the canthi and also compromises the orange reflex. It can also cause misplacement of the limbal incision (see p. 176). I place an eye shield over the nonoperative eye, first, for identification and, second, to protect this eye from hand pressure during surgery on the fellow eye (Fig. 7-2). To provide adequate aeration under the drapes and mitigate any claustrophobia, I routinely use a nasal oxygen cannula at a flow rate of 4 liters per minute. Many draping routines are available. My preference is a split sheet, which drapes the body as the apex of the split is pulled up above the nose. Part of the split covers the nonoperative eye while the other portion is placed just lateral to the lateral canthus of the operative eye (Fig. 7-3). I do not drape over the Mayo stand. An adhesive head drape is applied to the forehead to demarcate the sterile field, and a plastic adhesive eye drape is then positioned so that the globe is visible.

Perioperative antibiotics

The usage of prophylactic antibiotics and preoperative cultures is controversial and has medicolegal ramifications. I personally give a drop of neomycin-polymyxin solution each time the preoperative mydriatics are instilled and dress the eye with a similar ointment at the conclusion of the operation. Intraoperatively, at the last step, I inject cephalosporin and gentamicin subconjunctivally at the inferior cul-de-sac.

Anesthesia

In the United States, most anterior segment intraocular procedures on adult patients are performed under local anesthesia, customarily with an anesthesiologist monitoring the patient and providing intravenous medication as re-

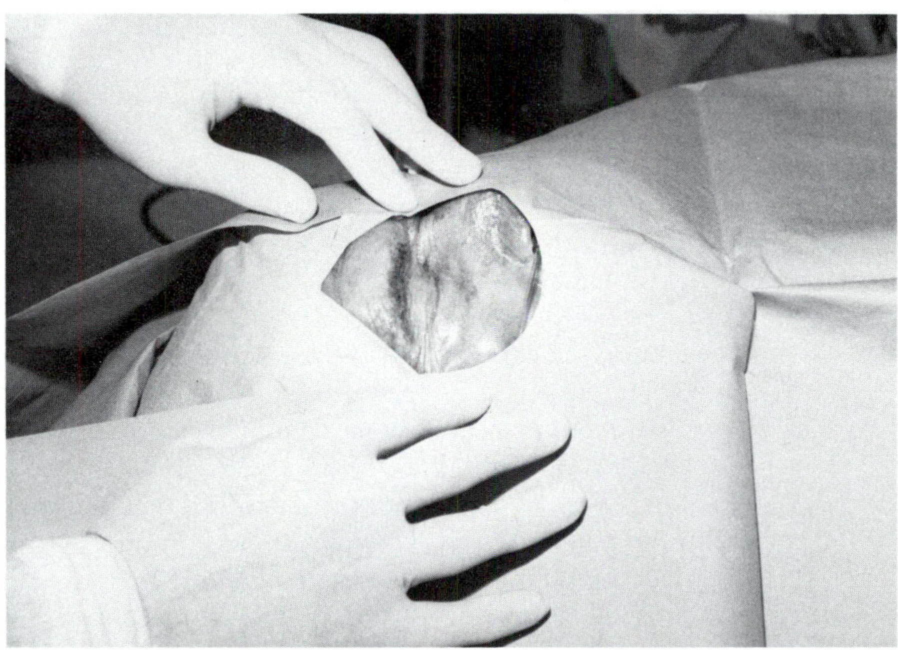

FIGURE 7-3. The eye and adnexa isolated within the operative fields by drapes.

quired. Usually, the ophthalmologist administers the local anesthetic injection, but in some facilities this is also performed by the anesthesiologist. This mode of anesthesia avoids the systemic effects of general agents and is especially efficacious in the elderly and those patients with systemic disease. Traditionally, the globe and adnexa are anesthetized, but variants to this have emerged in contemporary ophthalmology, such as periocular block and eschewing lid and facial blocks. Even though local anesthesia is used, appropriate medical clearances should be obtained where applicable.

Retrobulbar injection

Various anesthetic agents and additives have been proposed for retrobulbar injection, and currently a mixture of 2% Xylocaine (lidocaine hydrochloride) and 0.5% Marcaine (bupivacaine hydrochloride) are widely used. Sometimes epinephrine is added on the premise that it will help hemostasis and prolong the duration of the anesthesia by vasoconstriction with concomitant decreased diffusion of the anesthetic mixture, albeit with the risk of arrhythmias. Hyaluronidase (Wydase) has also been added to the injection in the expectation that it will increase diffusion of the anesthetic and therefore enhance the onset of action. To some extent, epinephrine and hyaluronidase have contradictory purposes, and their necessity could be questioned. With the use of a long-acting anesthetic, such as bupivacaine hydrochloride, the speculative anesthesia prolongation effect of epinephrine may not be necessary, and, though time-hallowed, it is doubtful that hyaluronidase has any merit.

The injection may be administered with a variety of needles, and a dull-tipped 23-gauge is popular. This should be 1¼ to 1½ inches in length. The patient is asked to look up and slightly nasally as a preliminary step for the injection, and this position is with the presupposition that preoperative and intraoperative sedation have not tranquilized the patient at the expense of cooperation (Fig. 7-4). The needle is introduced at the junction of the medial and lateral thirds of the inferior orbital rim and angled posteriorly, superiorly, and slightly medially to the orbital apex. The experienced physician will feel a "give" as the muscle cone is entered. Sometimes aspiration is applied to the syringe at this point to avoid intravascular injection of the anesthetic. The anesthetic mixture is injected slowly but purposefully, with usually 3 ml being sufficient. There is no objection to small aliquots of anesthesia being injected as the needle is directed to the orbital apex. However, if too much anesthesia is injected prematurely (especially anterior to the orbital septum), considerable infiltration and swelling of the palpebral conjunctiva will occur.

There are variations to the retrobulbar method, described above, often called the "up-and-in" technique, referring to the position of the eye as the retrobulbar injection is being administered. For example I prefer the patient to look up but not "in." A recent editorial and publication in a major ophthalmic journal deprecates the "up-and-in" technique as predisposing the globe, orbital vessels, and optic nerve to injury. It is suggested that a "straight ahead" or "down-and-out" position of the globe may be safer. The problem with this strategy is incomplete anesthesia in the upper portion of the globe where the superior rectus suture is placed (see p. 171) and the cataract section is customarily made.

Peribulbar anesthesia

As an alternative to retrobulbar anesthesia, peribulbar (or periocular) anesthesia has found favor in the past few years. Its advocates claim there is less risk of ocular damage, and an anesthesiologist can easily master the technique. Moreover, vision does not "gray out." Disadvantages are incomplete anesthesia, sub-

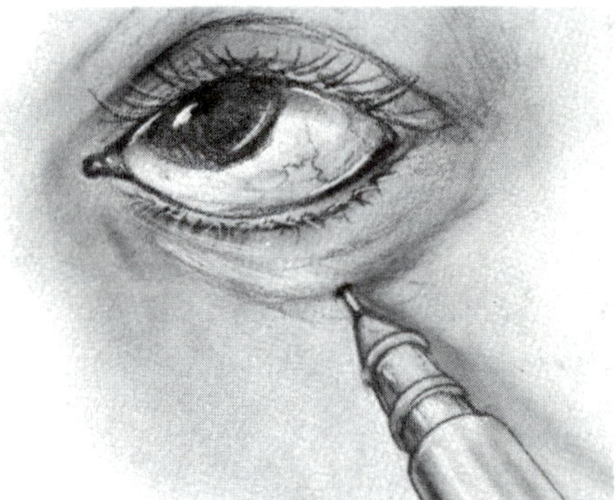

FIGURE 7-4. With the patient looking "up and in," the retrobulbar injection is administered with the needle directed to the apex of the orbit.

conjunctival anesthetic infiltration, and sensitivity to the light of the operating microscope.

Various methods have been proposed, and one of these is described here. An injection to anesthetize the skin is made subcutaneously just medial to the lateral canthus at the inferior orbital rim, with use of approximately 0.5 ml of lidocaine without epinephrine. An additional 1 ml is injected into the orbicularis oculi muscle in the same area. The upper lid is similarly infiltrated immediately inferior to the supraorbital notch. Digital pressure is applied with a sterile gauze to decrease the risk of lid ecchymosis.

The next step is the peribulbar injection, and for this a semiblunt 23-gauge, 1¼-inch retrobulbar needle is used on a 10 ml syringe with an anesthetic mixture of bupivacaine hydrochloride and hyaluronidase. The inferior lid is entered at the site of the initial subcutaneous injection, and 1 ml is injected immediately posterior to the orbicularis oculi muscle. The needle is then insinuated along the inferior orbit, and another 1 ml bolus is injected at the equator of the globe, after one first aspirates to avoid an intravascular injection. The needle is then advanced to its full extent in a slightly superior-medial direction, and a further 2 ml is injected, again with aspiration before injection.

The superior injection is similar. The lid is entered in the area of the subcutaneous anesthetic injection, and 1 ml of anesthetic solution is injected posterior to the orbicularis oculi, whereupon the needle is inserted farther posteriorly, and 1 ml of anesthetic solution is injected over the superior nasal equator of the globe, before one advances the needle to the area of the superior orbital fissure, where a further 1 ml is injected (Fig. 7-5). The needle is withdrawn. It will be

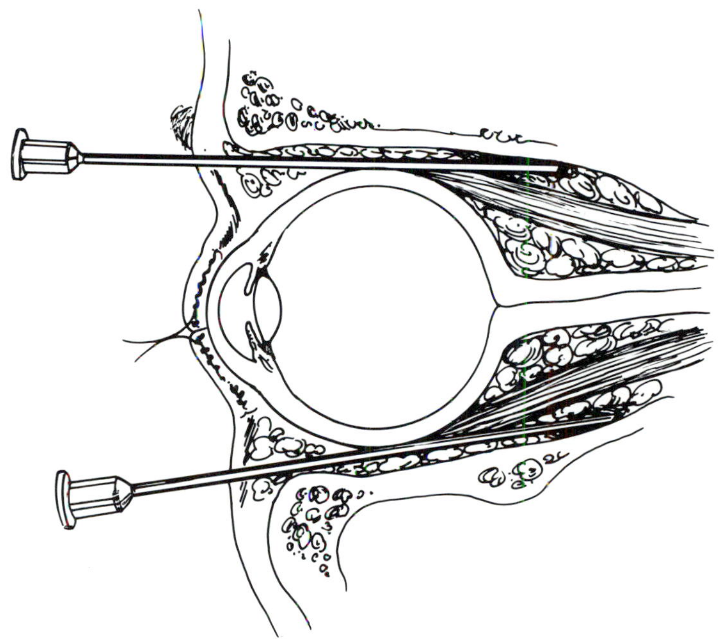

FIGURE 7-5. The position of the peribulbar needles in relation to the globe. Notice that the needles are inserted sequentially, not simultaneously as shown.

observed that the lids are tense. Digital pressure is applied to the globe through closed eyelids with a sterile gauze, and then a balloon or "superpinkie" device is applied. This presupposes that this block is applied in the holding area and not after the sterile preparation and drape.

Local anesthesia of adnexa

Van Lint block (lid block). The Van Lint block technique is to achieve anesthesia and akinesia of the eyelids. The inferior injection of approximately 2 ml of anesthetic solution is accomplished subcutaneously along the inferior orbital rim, passing the needle from a lateral entrance site in a nasal direction. The superior orbital rim is similarly injected, and a small bolus is injected just distally to the lateral canthus by angulation of the needle posteriorly.

O'Brien block. The O'Brien block anesthetizes the facial nerve at its egress from the stylomastoid foramen. This point may be palpated as a depression below the zygoma, more apparent when the patient's mouth is closed. It is more specifically identified anterior to the ear at a point 2 cm anterior and 1 cm below the external auditory meatus. Other seventh nerve blocks include the Nadbath and Atkinson techniques.

I do not use any lid block for routine cataract surgery and rely solely on the retrobulbar block. The patients experience less pain from injection and have less ecchymosis and possibly less postoperative ptosis. The block is also given sterilely, that is, on the operating table after the patient has been draped. I prefer this to blocking the patient in the holding area because in the operating room vital functions are being constantly monitored and the anesthesiologist is physically present in contradistinction to being available.

SURGICAL ANATOMY

Limbus

Except for the infrequent case of a clear corneal cataract section and pars plana lensectomy (p. 420), all cataract surgery is performed in the limbus. This is a transitional area between cornea and sclera delineated anteriorly by the vertical line joining the termination points of Bowman's and Descemet's membranes, which in turn corresponds to the most anterior extent that a limbus-based conjunctival flap can be reflected. Posteriorly the limbus extends to the insertion of Tenon's capsule, variably about 1 mm posterior to the conjunctival insertion. The limbus varies in width, being wider superiorly, less wide inferiorly, and narrowest temporally and nasally (Fig. 7-6). The anterior limbus has a bluish hue that changes to slate gray and then to white as one moves posteriorly. The limbus overlies the angle structures, and the middle blue zone, where the blue-gray transcends to white, corresponds to Schwalbe's line, though there may be variations according to the ocular axial length. The relatively avascular nature

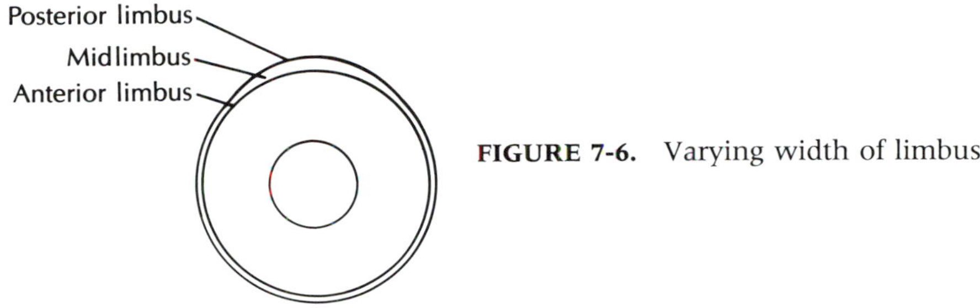

FIGURE 7-6. Varying width of limbus.

of the superior limbus is an obvious advantage to the cataract surgeon who should be mindful that eccentric sections where the limbus is narrow, such as temporally, can result in excessive bleeding if they are done too posteriorly.

Lens and zonules

The lens consists of a capsule, a cortex, and a nucleus. The ratio of the softer cortex to the harder nucleus varies widely between patients. Generally the nucleus becomes harder and better defined as the patient becomes older. The anterior capsule is not of uniform thickness, being thicker at the midperiphery of the anterior capsule, which is the reason that this location is suggested for the application of the cryoprobe (see Fig. 8-3, p. 179).

The zonules, sometimes called the "suspensory ligament," support the lens and are the mediators of ciliary muscle action (Fig. 7-7). They originate from the ciliary body (and occasionally the pars plana) inserting into the lens capsule. The location of insertion is variable with attachments to the anterior capsule, lens equator, and posterior capsule. In intracapsular surgery, placement of the cryoprobe too peripherally can result in freezing of anteriorly inserted zonules, which will compromise cataract extraction and cause undesirable traction on the ciliary body. This is a second reason for placing the cryoprobe as shown in Fig. 8-3. The zonules weaken with age and so make intracapsular cataract extraction generally feasible after 40 years of age though with the aid of alpha chymotrypsin. Before that age, extracapsular surgery or one of its variants is indicated.

Another reason for selecting extracapsular surgery in younger patients is the lenticular-vitreous attachment. This is a circular attachment of the vitreous to the posterior surface of the lens capsule, variously known as Weigert's ligament, or the ligamentum hyaloideocapsularium (Fig. 7-8). This attachment weakens with age, about 40 years, permitting intracapsular cataract extraction, though cases of persistent attachments are sometimes encountered. Before 40 years of age, attempts at intracapsular extraction of nonsubluxated cataracts result in a substantial risk of vitreous loss.

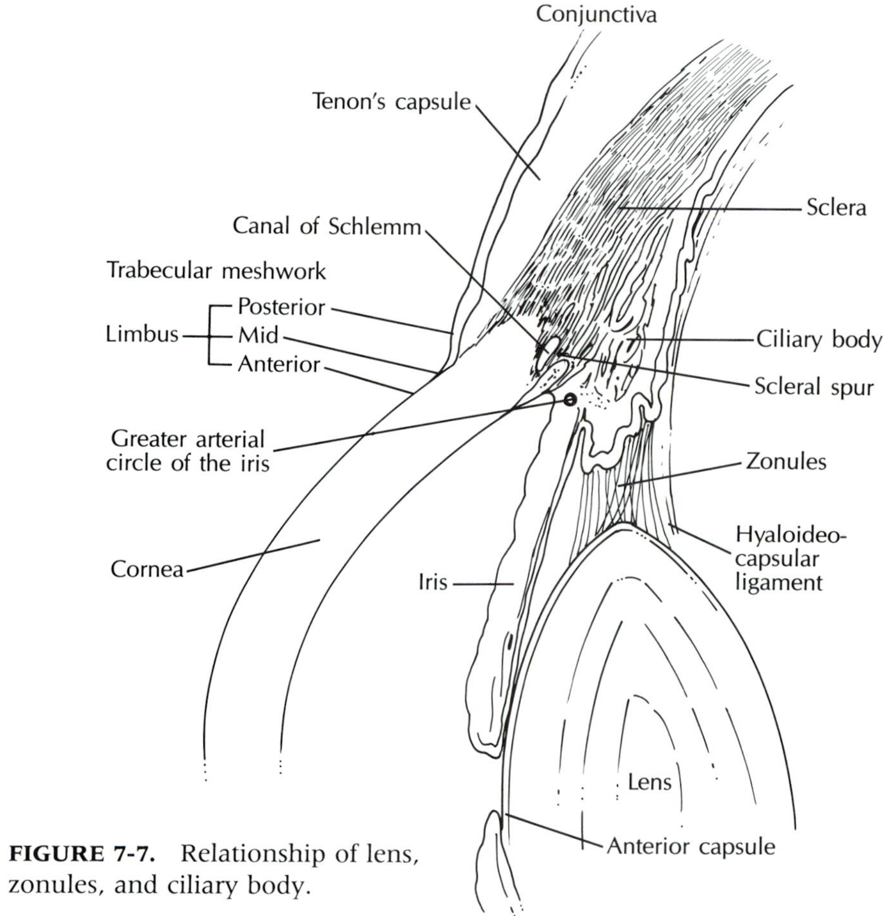

FIGURE 7-7. Relationship of lens, zonules, and ciliary body.

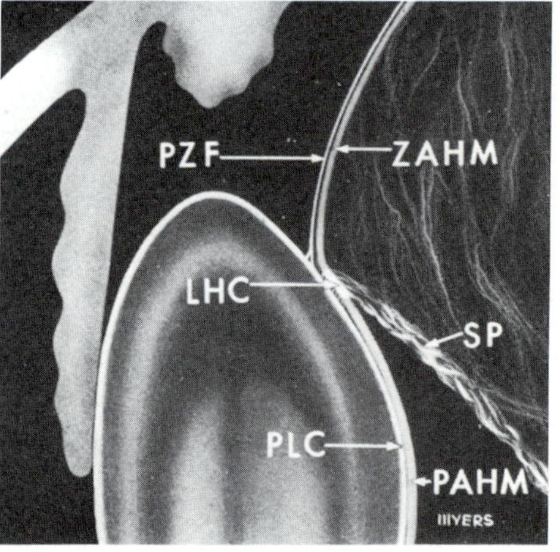

FIGURE 7-8. Relationship of ligamentum hyaloideocapsularium to crystalline lens. *LHC,* Ligamentum hyaloideocapsularium; *PAHM,* patellar portion of anterior hyaloid membrane; *PLC,* posterior lens capsule; *PZF,* posterior zonular fibers; *SP,* superior plica; *ZAHM,* zonular portion of anterior hyaloid membrane. (From Jaffe NS: The vitreous in clinical ophthalmology, St Louis, 1969, The CV Mosby Co.)

SUPERIOR RECTUS SUTURE PLACEMENT

The purpose of the superior rectus suture is twofold. First, it partially immobilizes the globe in cases of incomplete akinesia. Second, it rotates the globe inferiorly exposing the superior limbus, which is the customary site for the cataract surgical incision.

To place the superior rectus muscle suture, a muscle hook held in the right hand is placed at the inferior conjunctival cul-de-sac and the globe is rotated downwards. Tooth forceps held in the left hand grasp the muscle whereupon a 4-0 block silk suture is placed under the muscle (Fig. 7-9). This is a seemingly innocuous manuever. However, reports of perforated globes caused by the passage of this suture appear in the literature, and caution should be exercised. Placement of the suture is enhanced, and the risk of scleral penetration is minimized if the grasped muscle is slightly elevated with the left hand as the right hand passes the traction suture. After the needle has been passed under the muscle, the two ends may be slipped under the lid retractor or clamped to the drape, at the surgeon's discretion. If the suture is clamped to the drape, excessive traction, which might cause elevated intraocular pressure, should be avoided. The superior rectus suture can be placed either transconjunctivally or directly into the muscle after the conjunctival flap has been dissected.

An inferior rectus muscle suture may be helpful when the globe is enophthalmic or an incision at an atypical limbal incision is contemplated.

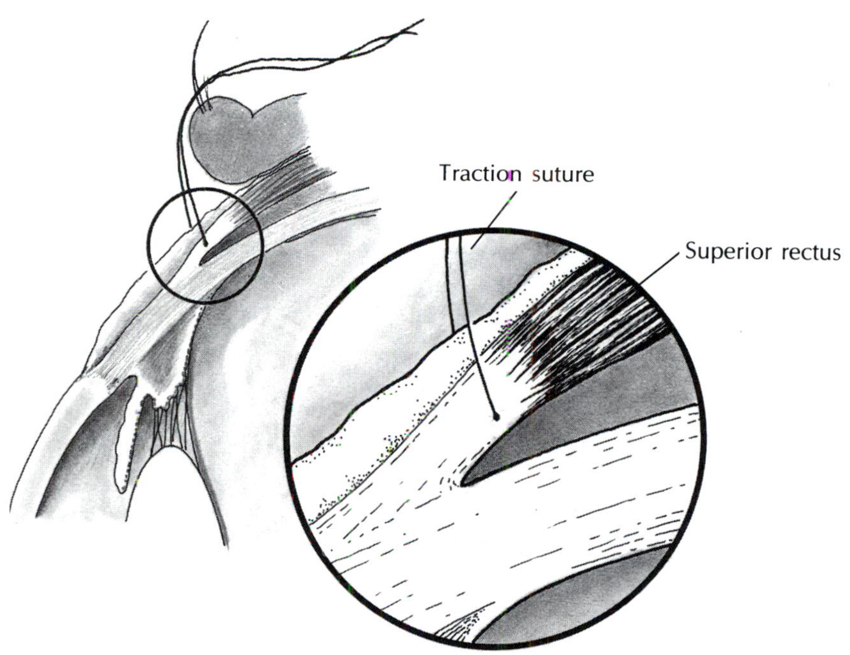

FIGURE 7-9. Superior rectus suture.

CONJUNCTIVAL FLAP

There is no consensus on whether a fornix-based flap is better than a limbal-based flap, though I prefer the former for cataract surgery. I prepare a fornix-based flap by grasping both conjunctiva and Tenon's capsule with fine forceps held in the left hand at the 12 o'clock position close to the surgical limbus. The tissues are excised to bare sclera, and the closed scissors are passed laterally through the aperture created and permitted to expand to lyse adhesions. Then the scissors are removed, and one blade is placed back through the aperture, resting against bare sclera, while the other blade hugs the conjunctival insertion and a lateral incision is performed. This maneuver is repeated in the opposite direction to fashion a conjunctival flap of the desired size (Fig. 7-10). The flap created may be excised at its lateral extremities to increase exposure.

To create a limbus-based flap, the conjunctiva and Tenon's capsule are similarly grasped with fine forceps held in the left hand. However, the incision down to bare sclera is performed from 2 to 7 mm posterior to the limbus, according to the surgeon's preference. As with a fornix-based flap, closed scissors are introduced through the aperture created in both directions laterally and permitted to open to lyse the adhesions. Then the scissors are removed and reinserted with one blade hugging the sclera and the other external to fashion the flap (Fig. 7-11). A limbus-based flap requires dissection to the surgical limbus to lyse the proximal adhesions (Fig. 7-11, *inset*), and various instruments have been proposed for this. I use a no. 64 Beaver blade aided by a cotton-tipped applicator held in the left hand.

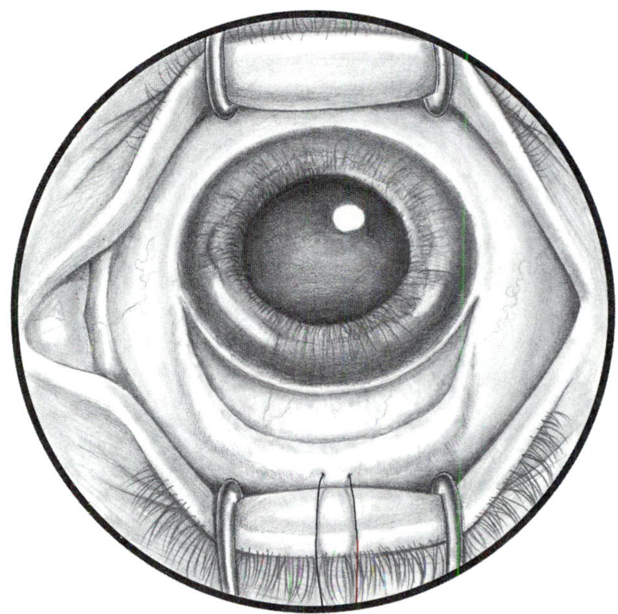

FIGURE 7-10. Fornix-based conjunctival flap.

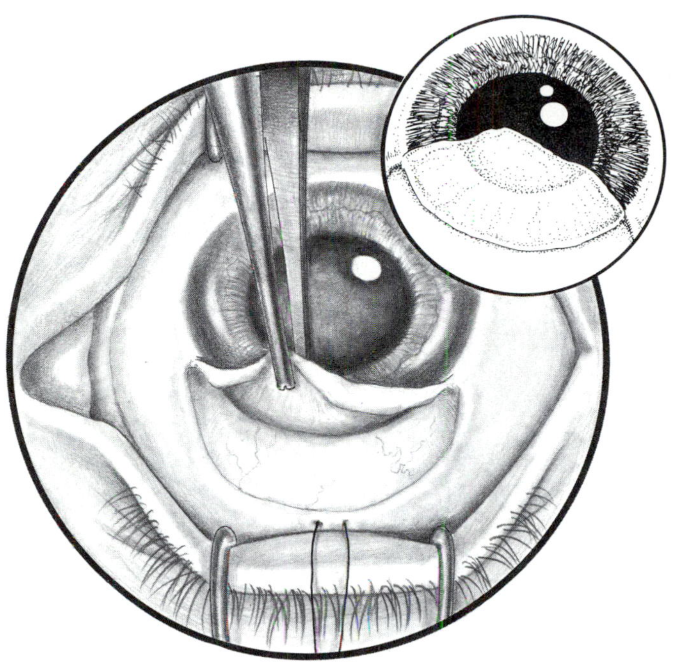

FIGURE 7-11. Limbus-based conjunctival flap. *Inset,* Limbus-based conjunctival flap after dissection.

CHAPTER 8

Cataract Extraction

A cataract is an opacity of the crystalline lens, and cataract surgery involves the removal of all or part of the lens. Although this is obvious to contemporary medicine, the function and anatomic location of the crystalline lens are of relatively recent knowledge, and the concept of *removing* the cataractous lens from the eye dates from Daviel (1696-1762), as noted in Chapter 7. Before Daviel's description of cataract extraction in 1753, the preferred management of cataract was couching, wherein the cataractous crystalline lens was displaced out of the visual axis but *remained* within the eye. Daviel's technique was extracapsular, and more or less contemporaneously Sharp described the intracapsular method. Both techniques are described in this chapter, but the methodology would seem incredible to the pioneering eighteenth century ophthalmic surgeons.

Intracapsular Cataract Extraction

Initial incision

The sclera should be grasped with tooth forceps close to the site of the contemplated incision, which is then performed with either a razor knife or a diamond knife. This initial incision should be large enough to permit the introduction of corneoscleral scissors. Moreover, there is disagreement as to whether the incision should be multiplanar or uniplanar. Among the numerous considerations are apposition of the incision, style of suturing, and axis and magnitude of postoperative astigmatism. Succinctly, it may be stated that the more corneal the incision, the more there is astigmatism, and the more scleral, the greater is the possibility of hyphema. The initial incision is in the surgical limbus in the posterior aspect of the gray-blue portion, as illustrated (Fig. 8-1). A uniplanar incision simplifies this maneuver.

Corneoscleral incision

The corneoscleral scissors are introduced intitially to the left, so that one blade is within the anterior chamber and the other blade is external to it. The incision is made to the left in the surgical limbus and is run slightly corneal at the lateral extremities. This is to avoid hemorrhage from the long choroidal artery or its tributaries. At this point, I place a safety suture of 8-0 Vicryl or Dexon through the section at the 12 o'clock position in case the eye has to be closed precipitously or for later use as a traction suture. This suture is looped out the field. The incision is then enlarged similarly to the right (Fig. 8-2).

Peripheral iridectomy

The technique of peripheral iridectomy is described on p. 188. If it is the surgeon's intention to subsequently place an anterior chamber intraocular lens (IOL), the position of the iridectomy should be such that there is no risk of the proximal feet of the IOL subluxating through the iridectomy. Some have advocated that the peripheral iridectomy should be midstromal when an anterior chamber IOL is to be placed; this concept has merit.

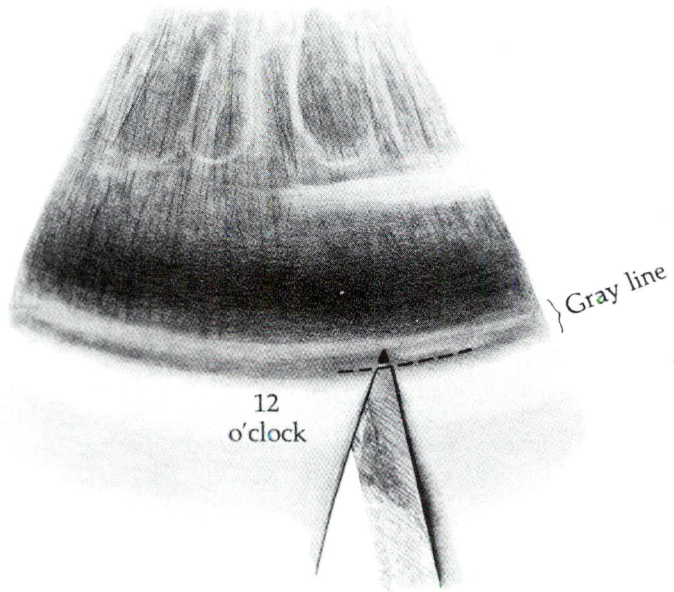

FIGURE 8-1. Initial incision in surgical limbus.

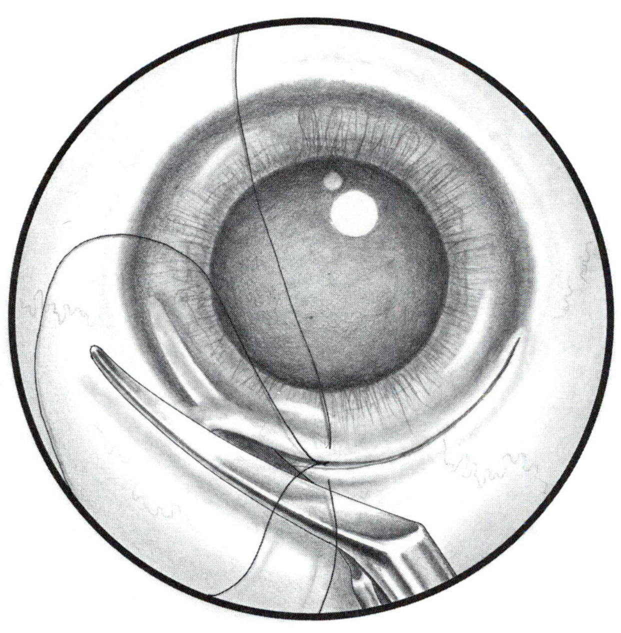

FIGURE 8-2. Incision for cataract extraction enlarged to left and right.

Extraction of the cataract

Capsule forceps are rarely used nowadays in the United States, and the cryotechnique of intracapsular extraction is described here.

The extraction of the cataract may be assisted by enzymatic zonulolysis with intracameral alpha chymotrypsin, though this is not absolutely necessary in older patients. The enzyme is injected with a fine cannula into the anterior chamber and allowed to remain for at least 60 seconds. The cornea is elevated with the preplaced 12 o'clock suture, and the anterior chamber is dried with a cellulose sponge placed against the anterior lens capsule. With an assistant retracting the cornea, the surgeon grasps the iris with forceps held in the left hand while the cryoprobe held in the right hand is placed on the anterior capsule; then the freezing mechanism is activated. The probe should be placed at the junction of the superior one third and lower two thirds of the crystalline lens, as shown in Fig. 8-3. A gentle lateral rocking motion is used to break zonular attachments, and the cataract is gently withdrawn from the eye (Fig. 8-4). An excessively large ice ball should be avoided because this can adhere to the adjacent iris. Some surgeons use an iris retractor or a cellulose sponge in the left hand for exposure before placement of the cryoprobe. I believe that a pair of forceps is preferable because these could be used to strip zonules, clear a suture from the field, or lift a dropped cornea.

After extraction of the cataract, any prolapsed iris is swept back into the anterior chamber and the 12 o'clock suture is tied and trimmed. The anterior chamber is re-formed with air or balanced saline solution and the section is closed. Of course, if it is the surgeon's intention to place an anterior chamber lens, the suturing technique is modified and the anterior chamber is re-formed with a viscoelastic substance (see p. 234).

Closure of incision

No agreement exists on the suturing after cataract extraction or whether preplaced sutures are desirable. Furthermore, it would be tedious to debate the pros and cons of the various techniques. When interrupted sutures are used at the conclusion of the suturing, the knots may be buried in the needle track by sliding the sutures appropriately. It is generally easier to bury a knot by sliding it through the corneal aspect of the wound rather than through the scleral portion.

In considering postoperative astigmatism that may result from various suture techniques, one needs an accurate knowledge of the patient's preoperative keratometry. Under the assumption that a given patient has no astigmatism by keratometry preoperatively, it can be reliably stated that absorbable sutures will produce against-the-rule astigmatism. Nonabsorbable sutures, such a 10-0 nylon, will produce with-the-rule astigmatism, which tends to diminish in time. It is also clear that the more anterior the incision and the suture placement, in the case of nonabsorbable sutures, the greater is the with-the-rule astigmatism; this astigmatism decreases as the incision is placed more posteriorly. I have been unimpressed with attempts to place sutures at various depths in the incision or various styles of suturing as a means to reduce astigmatism in the long run.

The conjunctiva may be closed with interrupted absorbable sutures, such as 8-0 Vicryl or Dexon. My personal preference is to use the wet-field cautery and coaptation forceps. The adjacent margins of incised conjunctiva are grasped and the cautery is activated; this produces a sealing effect.

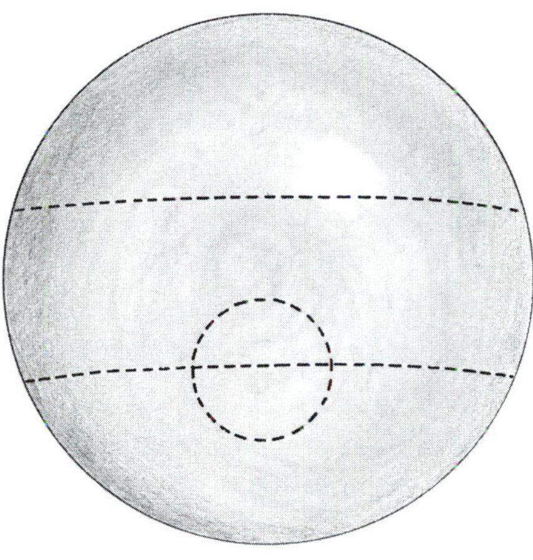

FIGURE 8-3. Position of placement of cryoprobe on cataract.

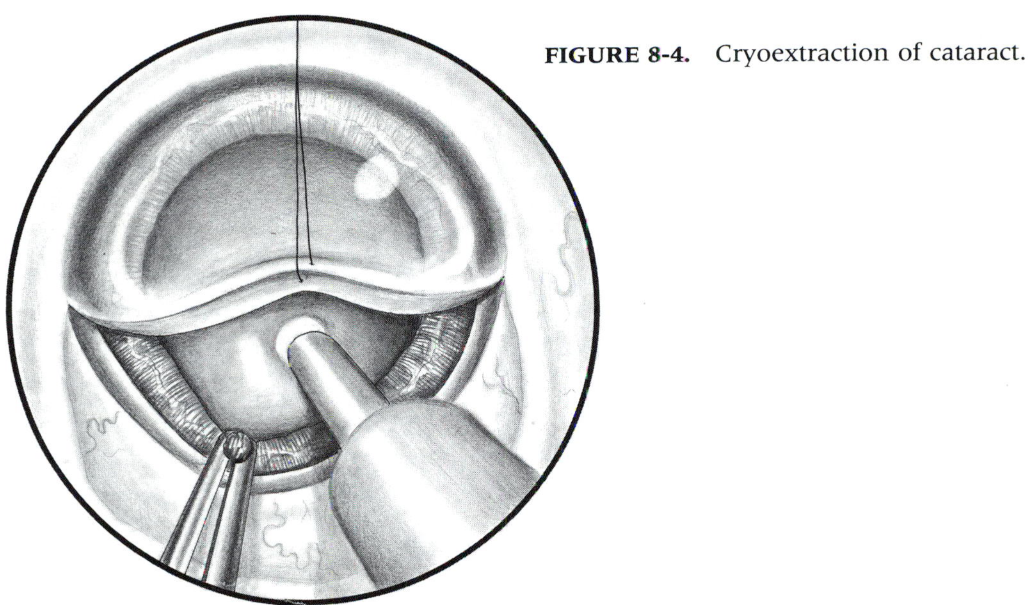

FIGURE 8-4. Cryoextraction of cataract.

Extracapsular Cataract Extraction

Initial incision

The initial incision should not be bigger than 2 mm lest the contents of the anterior chamber escape during the subsequent anterior capsulectomy. The surgeon should also be mindful to make the internal dimensions of this initial incision the same size as the external dimensions to avoid a wedge-shaped initial incision. This could cause the point of the cystotome to snag on the inner aspects of the incision, risking a detachment of Descemet's membrane.

Anterior capsulectomy

Various instruments are advocated for an anterior capsulectomy, and I use a disposable 22-gauge needle on which is fashioned a hook. The anterior capsulectomy may be performed either under air, with continuous irrigation, or with a viscoelastic substance (VES) in the anterior chamber. Air somewhat obscures the visualization but is cheap and readily available. Continuous irrigation has its merits, in that visibility is excellent and, as the anterior capsule is cut, the resultant flap can be seen to curl up and show that the incision is complete. A VES coats the cornea and the cystotome, affording additional protection, and usually does not leak out the incision. Its viscous bulk can prevent the anterior capsule from scrolling and inhibit the ready identification of potential capsular tags. Again, there is no agreement on the merits of one technique versus another, but since the advent of the viscoelastic materials, there is a movement away from using air for this maneuver.

When phacoemulsification was first advocated a "Xmas tree" anterior capsulotomy was performed. This was named for the shape of the resultant anterior capsulotomy, which ideally resembled the triangular outline of the foliage of a well-formed Christmas tree. In this technique the anterior capsule was engaged at the 6 o'clock position with a cystotome (Fig. 8-5) that was gently withdrawn superiorly ripping the anterior capsule and forming a triangular opening (Fig. 8-6). The proximal flap of the anterior capsule thus formed was usually externalized and excised. The problem with the "Xmas tree" anterior capsulectomy was its capriciousness, sometimes extending beyond the lens equator and compromising the posterior capsule. The "can-opener" method, described on p. 182, has largely superseded the former technique for this reason, but variants of the "Xmas tree" concept are currently being resurrected as *capsulorrhexis*. Capsulorrhexis involves the surgeon ripping the anterior capsule in a few deft rotatory maneuvers that leave a circular anterior capsular opening. There is a knack to capsulorrhexis, and at this time no standardized technique that is within the capabilities of most surgeons can be advocated.

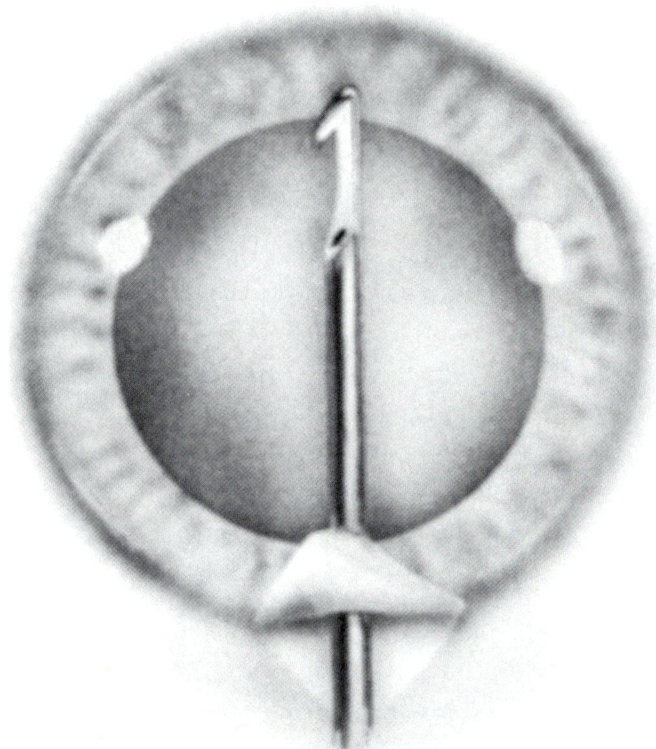

FIGURE 8-5. The anterior capsule is engaged with a cystotome at the 6 o'clock position. (From Jaffe NS: Cataract surgery and its complications, ed 3, St. Louis, 1981, The CV Mosby Co.)

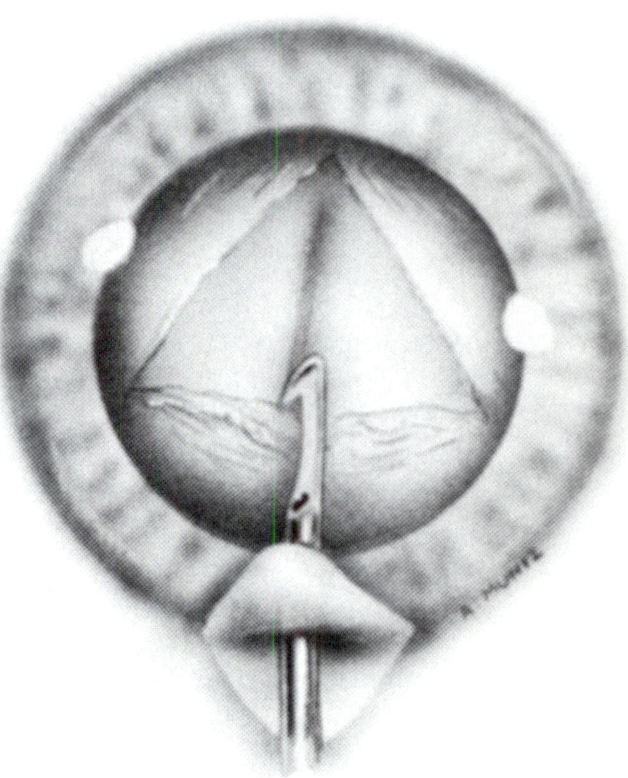

FIGURE 8-6. A triangular anterior capsulotomy is obtained when one tears the anterior capsule with the cystotome as it is being withdrawn. (From Jaffe NS: Cataract surgery and its complications, ed 3, St. Louis, 1981, The CV Mosby Co.)

In the "can-opener" technique the cystotome is placed into the anterior chamber and the anterior capsule is engaged according to the surgeon's preference. I begin the anterior capsulectomy inferiorly and perform a can-opener capsulectomy in a D configuration. The needle traverses first from 6 o'clock to 12 o'clock in a clockwise direction and then the capsulectomy is completed from 6 o'clock to 12 o'clock in a counterclockwise direction. At the conclusion of this, the capsular flap is maneuvered free with a cystotome, and the cystotome is then removed from the eye (Fig. 8-7). It is wise to place the capsular cuts quite close together to avoid flaps, and a helpful concept is to have the anterior capsulectomy almost a mirror of the corona ciliaris in the closeness of the incisions and resultant grooves in the underlying nucleus. A more efficient cut is performed when the cystotome instrument is moved from the center peripherally. The tendency is to perform smaller diameter anterior capsulectomies to clearly define the anterior capsular margin for subsequent "in-the-bag" IOL placement. (See also Fig. 14-9, *A*.)

Corneoscleral incision

The incision is then enlarged in a similar fashion to an intracapsular cataract extraction though the incision may be somewhat smaller, approximately 150 degrees. A 12 o'clock safety suture is also advisable with an extracapsular technique, using either 8-0 Vicryl or Dexon.

Expression of nucleus

Several techniques are available to express the nucleus, including the Daviel spoon, the Pearce-Knolle loop, and the Sheets loop (vectis).

When the Daviel spoon is used, it is placed at the posterior scleral lip of the incision, and gentle pressure is exerted, which causes the superior pole of the nucleus to prolapse (Fig. 8-8, *A*). The spoon is slid just under the prolapsed superior pole of the nucleus, and counterpressure is applied on the limbus at the 6 o'clock position (Fig. 8-8, *B*), which will cause the nucleus to deliver itself, with its egress out of the posterior chamber and out of the eye being guided by the spoon, which is customarily held in the right hand (Fig. 8-8, *C*). If the surgeon has an assistant available, that assistant not only retracts the cornea but also can help the delivery of the nucleus by spearing it with a fine needle to facilitate its removal from the eye. When there is a relative miosis of the pupil, the superior pole of the nucleus may be covered by a sheet of anterior capsule, which will impede its delivery. The left-hand instrument is a pair of forceps, and these may be used to retract the capsule so that the superior pole will present. The surgeon is reminded that the capsule has a shiny appearance and the nucleus has a semimatte consistency, which can help in differentiation.

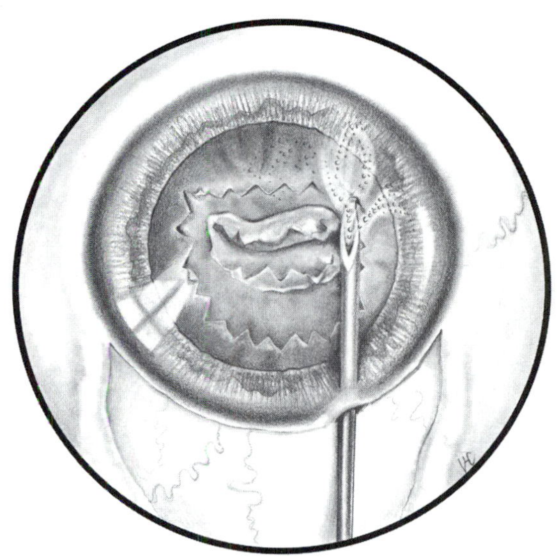

FIGURE 8-7. Anterior capsulectomy performed under irrigation.

A

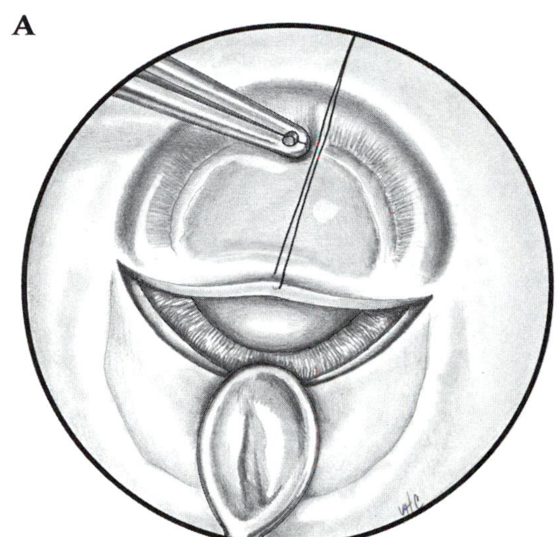

B

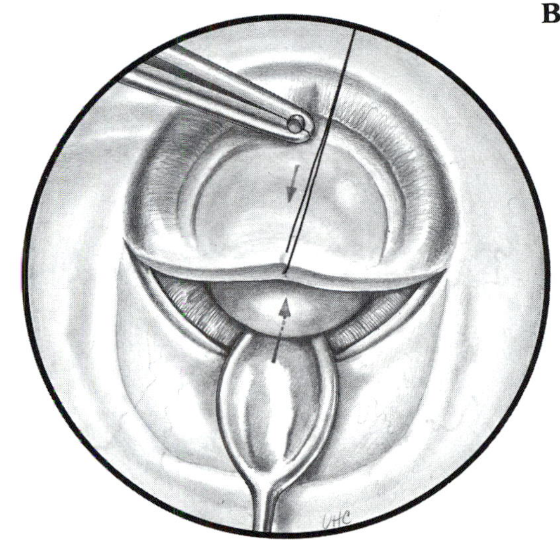

C

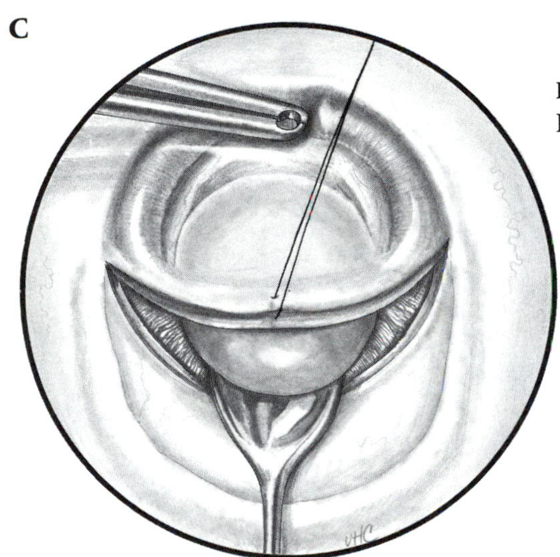

FIGURE 8-8. **A,** Initial position of Daviel spoon. **B,** Counterpressure inferiorly. **C,** Nucleus delivers.

The Sheets irrigating vectis is a sturdy irrigating loop that is positioned at the scleral portion of the incision, and pressure is applied. The irrigation through the vectis insinuates itself around and behind the nucleus, breaking the cortical adhesions, and the pressure on the posterior scleral lip will cause the nucleus to deliver itself (Fig. 8-9). Any reluctance on the nucleus's part can be countered by pressure with an instrument on the inferior limbus at 6 o'clock, as described for the Daviel spoon technique.

When the Pearce irrigating vectis is used, it is slid under the nucleus, and the irrigation acts in the same manner as that with the Sheets vectis. Moreover, it provides a cushion of fluid with which the vectis delivers the nucleus from the eye in a manner similar to the usage of a shovel (Fig. 8-10).

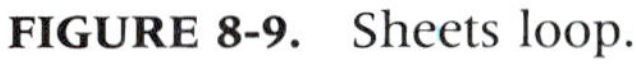

FIGURE 8-9. Sheets loop.

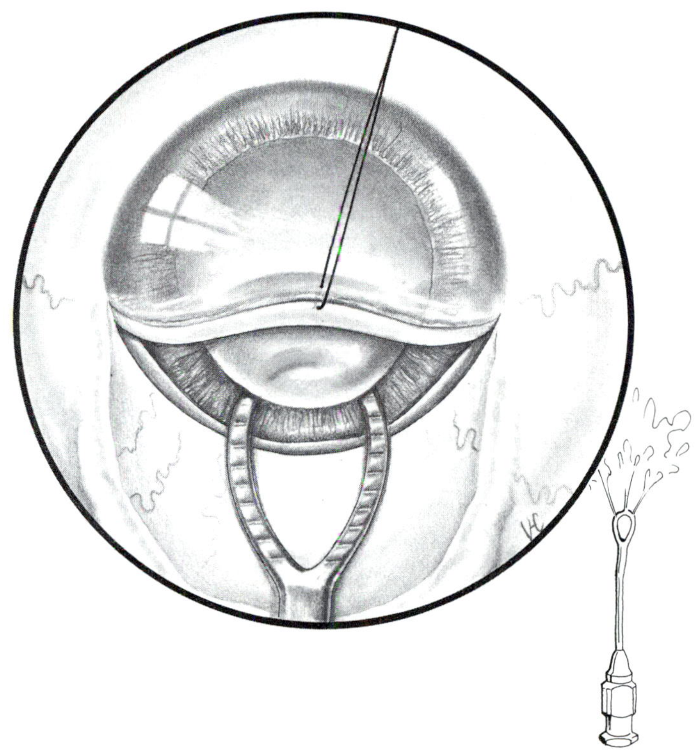

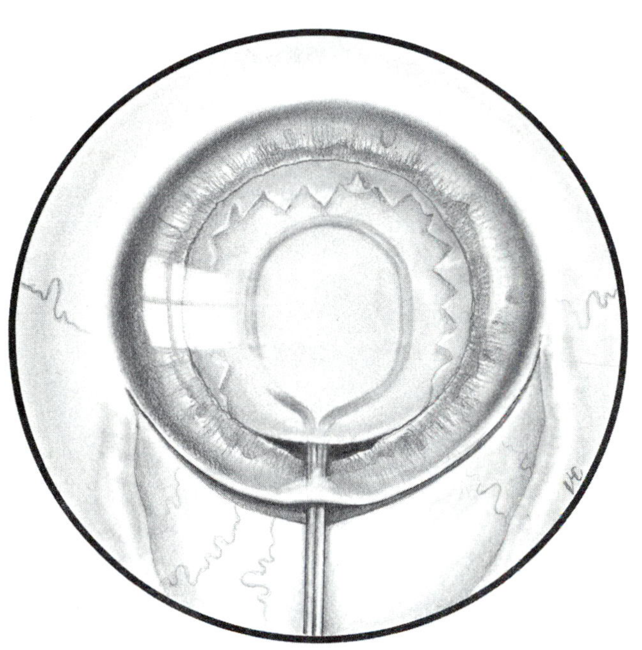

FIGURE 8-10. Pearce loop.

Aspiration of cortex

To perform the irrigation/aspiration (I/A) phase of an extracapsular cataract extraction, using an automated technique, one must suture the incision to form a closed chamber. Generally speaking, a 12 o'clock suture and two sutures, one 3.0 mm to the right and the other 3.0 mm to the left of the cardinal 12 o'clock suture, will suffice. Sometimes, to avoid continuous iris prolapse during I/A, additional sutures are placed. With a phacoemulsification technique, no sutures are obviously required because the I/A handpiece is inserted through the 3 mm incision, which was used to introduce the phacoemulsification handpiece.

The residual cortex, after the nucleus has been removed, can be conceptualized as the flesh of a peach after the pit has been disposed of. The analogy is that the skin of the peach is the capsule, and the flesh is the cortex. Considering this example, the cortex is three-dimensional and somewhat U-shaped. A more efficient I/A can be obtained if the leading edge of the cortex (peach flesh) were secured with the I/A handpiece. This would provide aspiration at a level superior to the posterior capsule for safety's sake and moreover would be more efficient because portions of cortex may be mechanically stripped out of the capsular cul-de-sac and aspirated by gentle withdrawal of the probe toward the center of the pupil.

The I/A handpiece is introduced into the eye. Most surgeons favor the tip with a 0.3 mm aspiration orifice. This handpiece is inserted in the irrigation mode, and then when the superior leaf of cortex is off, aspiration is activated, and the vacuum is built up, the cortex is gently stripped out of the capsular cul-de-sac and aspirated (Fig. 8-11). This procedure is repeated 360 degrees until the eye is devoid of cortex (Fig. 8-12). The 12 o'clock position may be difficult to aspirate because of exposure, and if this occurs, a microhook can be inserted between adjacent sutures to retract both iris and capsule. If the surgeon inadvertently aspirates the posterior capsule, striae will be seen radiating from the aspiration orifice (Fig. 8-13), and the vacuum should be released. Generally, this will not rupture the posterior capsule if the vacuum is low and the handpiece is not abruptly removed. If a residual fragment of nucleus is drawn to the aspiration orifice but is too hard to be aspirated, it may be held at the orifice with suction (Fig. 8-14) and manually crushed with a spatula or nucleus rotator introduced into the anterior chamber with the left hand. This is in fact manual emulsification. When the aspiration phase is concluded, the handpiece is withdrawn from the eye.

FIGURE 8-11. Superior edge of cortex engaged with aspiration handpiece.

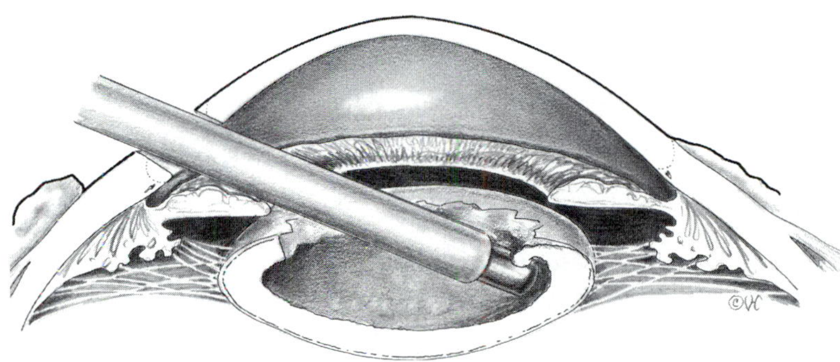

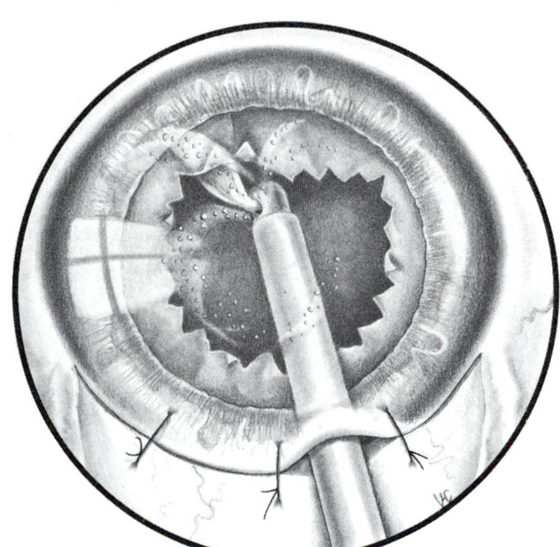

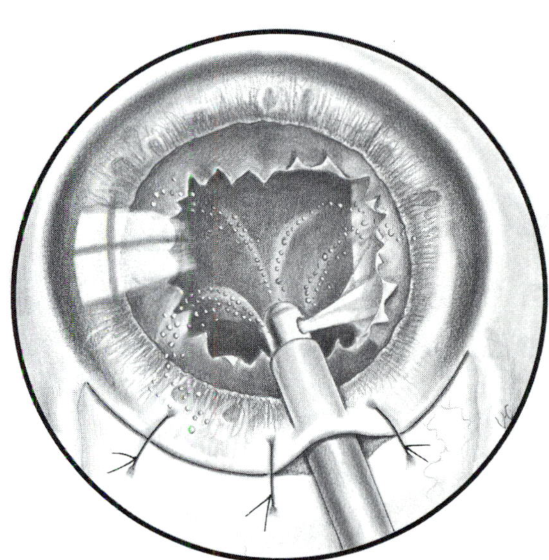

FIGURE 8-12. Cortical remnants aspirated from capsular cul-de-sac.

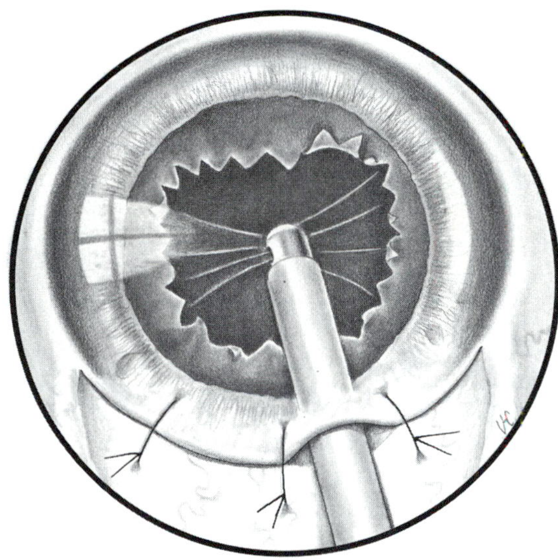

FIGURE 8-13. Inadvertent aspiration of posterior capsule with production of striae.

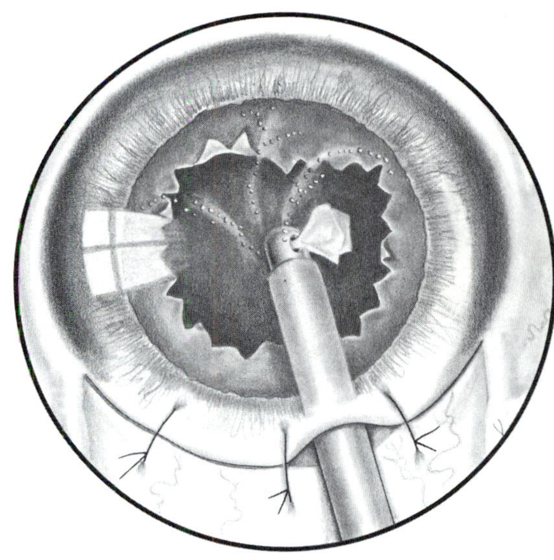

FIGURE 8-14. Residual fragment of nucleus entrapped at aspiration orifice.

Extracapsular cataract extraction and the miotic pupil

When intracapsular surgery was dominant, the surgeon could manipulate and stretch the iris sufficiently to allow placement of the cryoprobe, even in pupils as small as 4 mm in diameter. Extracapsular surgery, of course, requires several steps for cataract extraction, and an adequate pupillary diameter is mandatory. The principal technique of extracapsular cataract extraction (ECCE) is modified when persistent miosis is present, the principal modification being the creation of an iris coloboma. My preference is a superior peripheral iridectomy, subsequently connected to the pupil by a radial iridotomy. Intraoperatively a radial iridotomy preserves iris tissue if the surgeon wishes to suture the iris. If the iris is not sutured, the postoperative appearance is cosmetically more pleasing than the iris defect secondary to a sector iridectomy.

A 3 mm superior incision is made, and a knuckle of iris is grasped with fine forceps held in the left hand. Westcott scissors, in the right hand, excise the grasped iris to form the peripheral iridectomy (Fig. 8-15). When the scissors are held horizontally as in the diagram, a broader based iridectomy is obtained than when the scissors are introduced vertically *(inset)*. After this maneuver the iris is reposited as required. (See also pp. 280 and 316.)

A viscoelastic substance (VES) is now introduced into the anterior chamber, re-forming it. The VES is injected through a 27-gauge cannula, which can also be used to simultaneously lyse posterior synechiae and verify the patency of the iridectomy (Fig. 8-16).

Fine scissors, such as Vannas or micro-Westcott scissors, are inserted into the anterior chamber. Initially the scissors are inserted closed and horizontal. They are then turned slightly obliquely and opened. One blade is passed through the aperture of the iridectomy and under the iris while the other blade is passed over. When the scissors are closed, the radial iridotomy is now complete, and the scissors are withdrawn from the eye (Fig. 8-17).

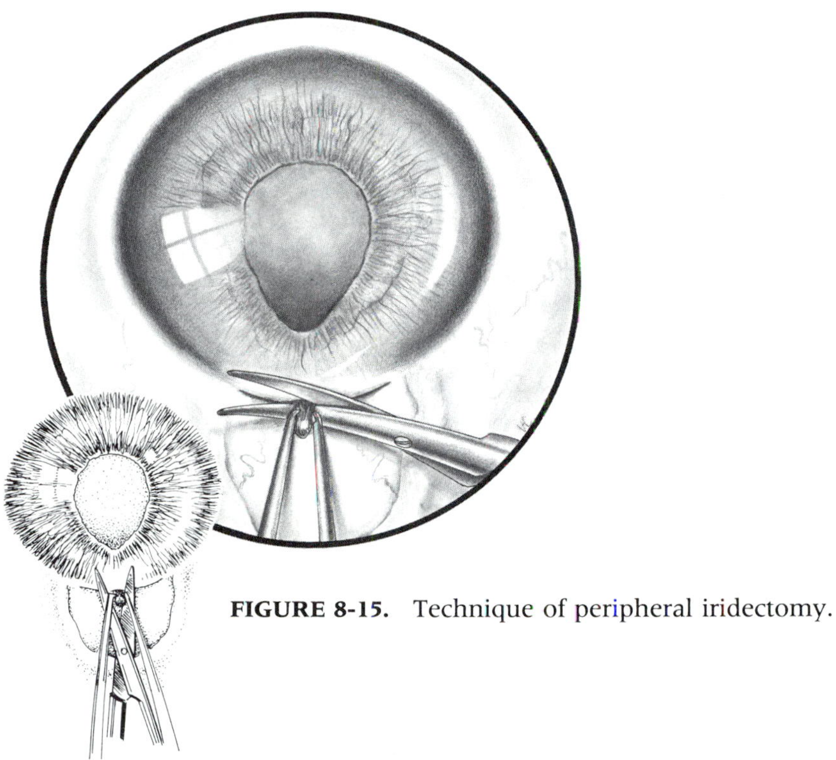

FIGURE 8-15. Technique of peripheral iridectomy.

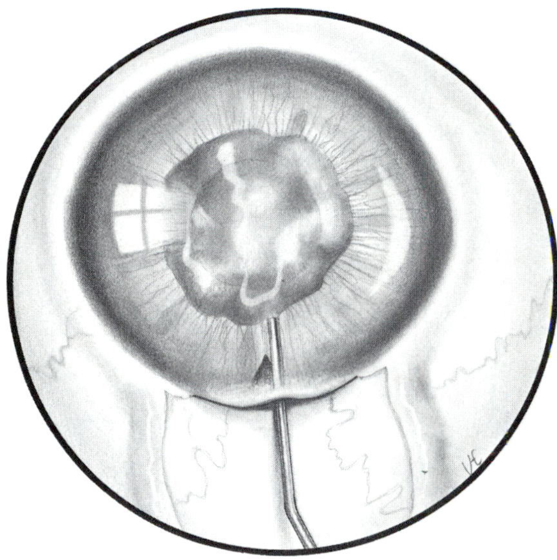

FIGURE 8-16. Reforming anterior chamber with a viscoelastic substance (VES).

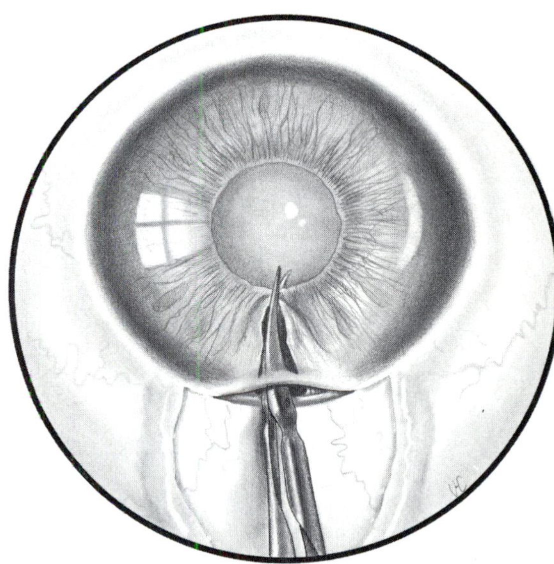

FIGURE 8-17. Technique of radial iridotomy.

It is advantageous to engage the iris at the apex of the peripheral iridectomy. This position avoids an iris tag, which can impede the irrigation/aspiration phase of the operation. In this manner the resultant iris coloboma has neat edges as illustrated (Fig. 8-18).

The next step is the anterior capsulectomy, and before insertion of the cystotome another bolus of VES may be required on the premise that some leaked out during the radial iridotomy. The cystotome needle is now inserted, and beginning inferiorly, an anterior capsulectomy is performed. The inferior flap may be made slightly centrally (1) because it defines the capsular flap for subsequent IOL insertion and (2) because an inferior flap is not an impediment to subsequent nuclear expression. Laterally the surgeon may reach under the iris with the cystotome while performing the capsular cuts (Fig. 8-19). This enhances the diameter of the anterior capsulectomy and is aided by the injection of a small bolus of VES under the iris. Superiorly the capsulectomy can be more peripheral because the iris coloboma provides exposure and the expression of the nucleus is aided. The resultant anterior capsulectomy has a conical form. The operation then proceeds as previously described for an extracapsular extraction.

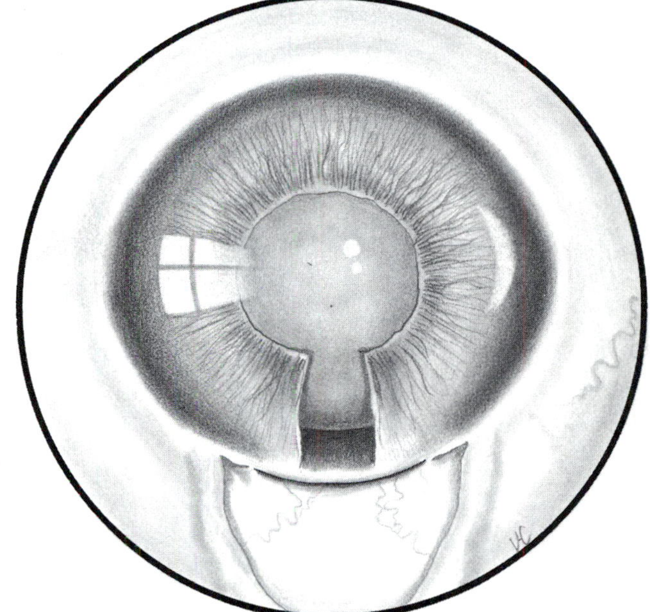

FIGURE 8-18. Surgical coloboma.

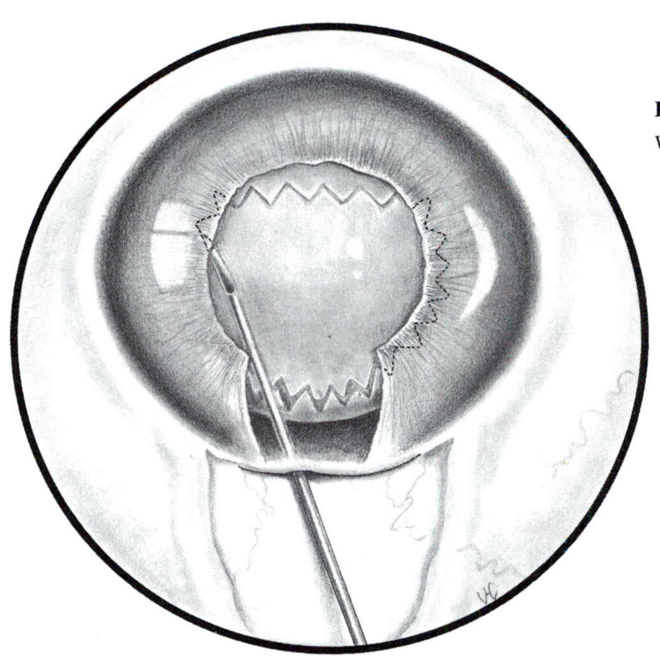

FIGURE 8-19. Technique of anterior capsulectomy with surgical coloboma.

Repair of iris coloboma

If it is the surgeon's intent to repair the surgical coloboma, this should be performed *after* the posterior chamber IOL or *before* an anterior chamber IOL is inserted. When a 10-0 polypropylene suture is placed through the margins of the iris coloboma just distal to the iris sphincter (Fig. 8-20), one should use a VES (see also p. 320). The loops of a posterior chamber lens should be rotated away from the coloboma (Fig. 8-21) to prevent a loop from prolapsing into the anterior chamber postoperatively. Similarly an anterior chamber lens should be rotated such that the footplates are remote from the coloboma to prevent postoperative subluxation. The suture is tied and trimmed (Fig. 8-22).

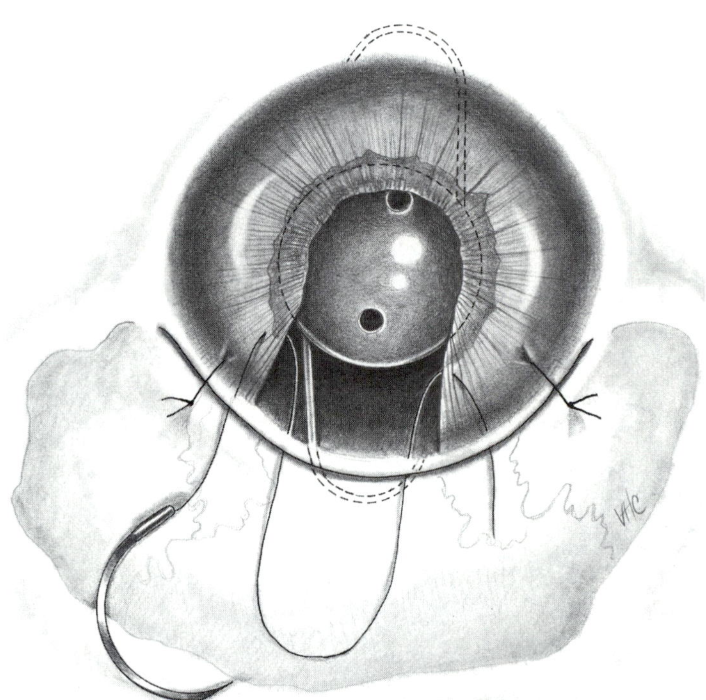

FIGURE 8-20. A suture is placed in the margins of the iris coloboma just distal to the iris sphincter.

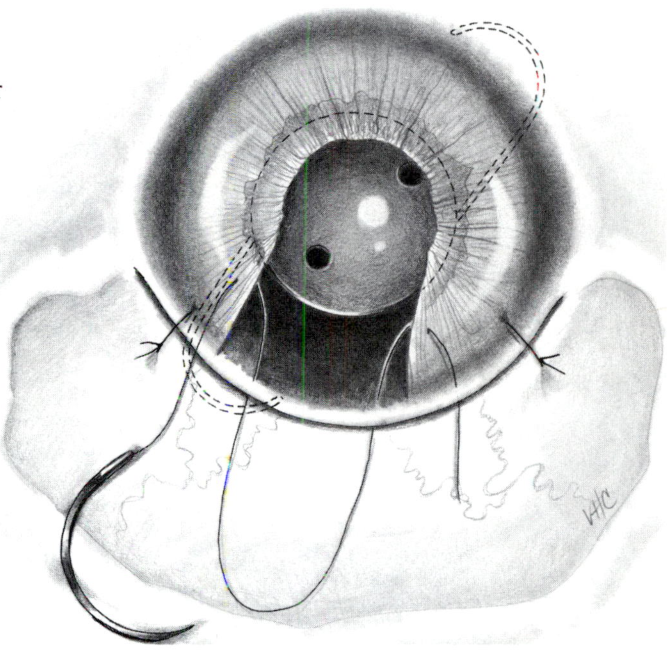

FIGURE 8-21. The posterior chamber intraocular lens (IOL) is rotated so that the superior loop does not coincide with the coloboma.

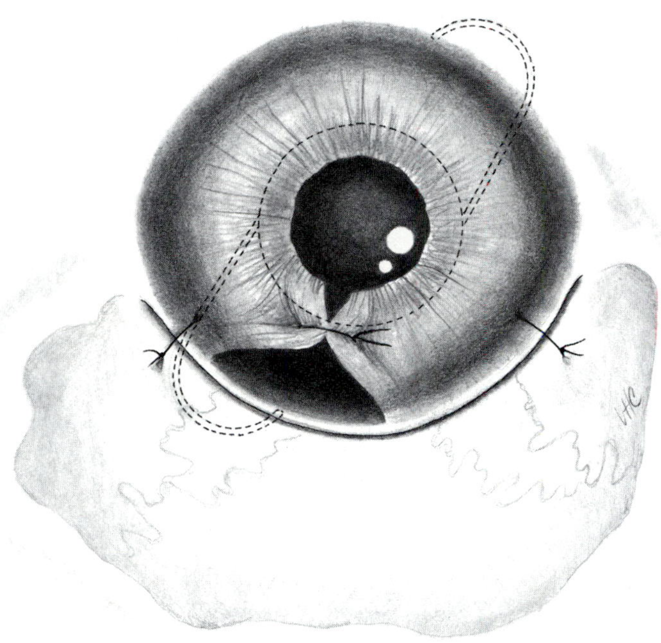

FIGURE 8-22. The suture is tied and trimmed. The unsutured distal portion of the coloboma functions as a peripheral iridectomy.

Manual techniques

The principal difference between a manual technique and an automated technique of extracapsular cataract extraction lies in the management of the cortical aspiration. In an automated technique, it is done with a formed anterior chamber with an instrument that provides simultaneous irrigation and aspiration at various vacuums. The manual technique utilizes a syringe. Illustrated is one method where cortex is aspirated with a cannula on a small syringe filled with a small aliquot of balanced saline solution (Fig. 8-23). The technique of McIntyre is a hybrid between the automated technique and the manual technique. He has an ingenious stopcock device that provides continuous infusion from an irrigation bottle while cortex is manually aspirated by a syringe attached to this stopcock valve.

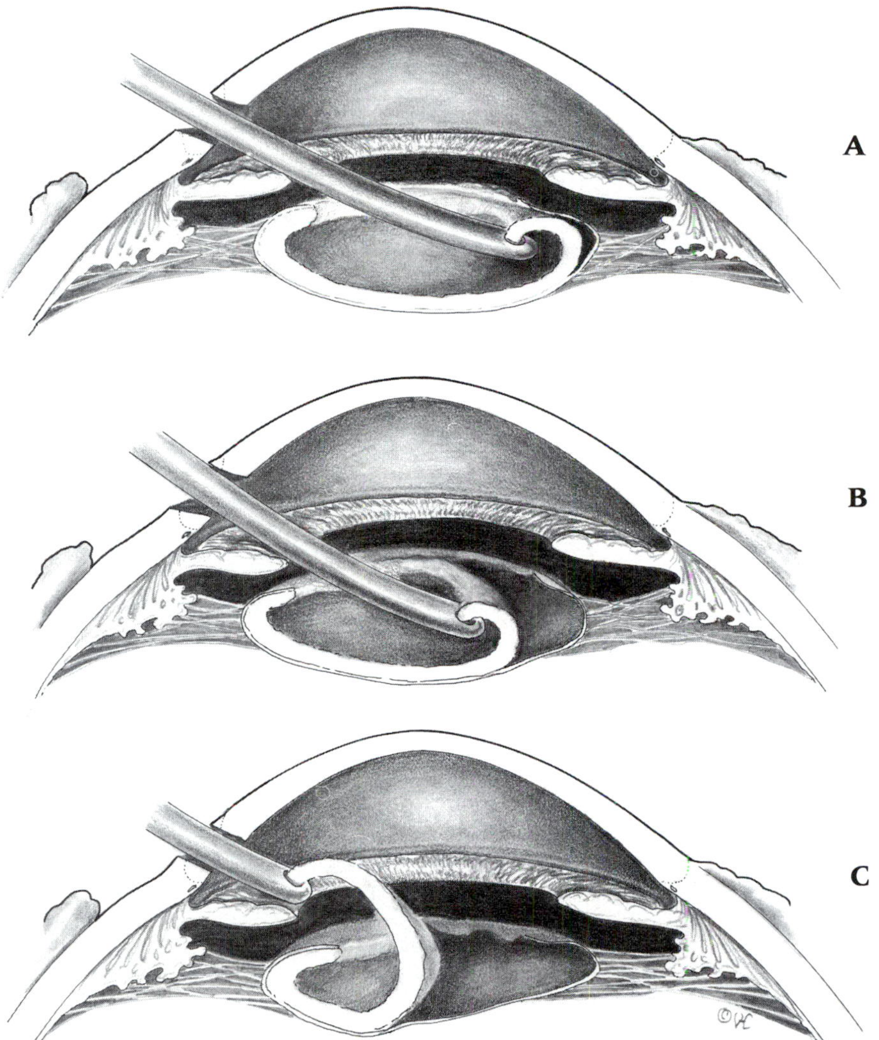

FIGURE 8-23. **A,** Superior aspect of cortex engaged with aspiration syringe. **B,** Cortex aspirated and stripped out of cul-de-sac. **C,** Aspiration and manual removal of cortex from eye.

CHAPTER 9

Phacoemulsification

Phacoemulsification (KPE) is a variant of extracapsular cataract extraction and was introduced by Kelman in 1967. It is estimated that 20% to 30% of cataract extractions in the United States are currently performed with KPE, a technique by which a cataract may be extracted through a 3 mm incision. Kelman's innovation was greeted with considerable opposition from certain segments of the profession, and it is to the inventor's credit and perseverance that KPE has become an invaluable part of the ophthalmic surgeon's armamentarium and enjoys ever-increasing usage. Since Kelman's initial description of the technique, the equipment has improved dramatically with more ultrasonic power and vacuum being available. The delivery of the ultrasonic power has been enhanced by piezoelectric crystal handpieces, and linear controls have been developed whereby graduated amounts of ultrasonic power and vacuum are delivered to the eye by increments of pressure on the foot pedal, much like an automobile accelerator. These advancements have made KPE safer and faster. As a form of extracapsular cataract extraction, KPE shares the initial incision and anterior capsulectomy described in the previous chapter, and I am beginning with the management of the nucleus, which is the principal distinguishing feature of KPE.

Nucleus Procedures

After the anterior capsulectomy has been completed, the initial incision is enlarged to 3.0 mm to accommodate the ultrasonic handpiece. It is important that the internal dimensions of the enlarged incision be the same as the external dimensions to avoid a funnel-shaped incision, which could compress the irrigation sleeve (see p. 180).

Before phacoemulsification, the surgeon selects a suitable ultrasonic tip, the choice ranging from a 15 degree to a 65 degree bevel. Different tip configurations, such as round, oval, and elongated, can also be obtained. After the selection has been made, a viscoelastic substance (VES) is used as required, the ultrasonic handpiece is introduced into the anterior chamber, and irrigation is begun followed by irrigation/aspiration (I/A), which usually removes from the eye the portion of anterior capsule excised in the anterior capsulectomy. Ultrasound (U/S) is activated, and the nucleus is saucerized with a step at the inferior third being left (Fig. 9-1). This saucerization may be performed down to the level of the posterior Y suture, which is usually visible if any degree of nuclear sclerosis is present. The ultrasound is used much like a wood plane, with the ultrasonic power activated with forward motion, removing fragments of the nucleus. As the ultrasonic handpiece is withdrawn to make the next stroke of saucerization, no ultrasonic power is required, just as a wood plane does not cut when pulled backwards.

To digress for a moment, let us consider the hardness of the nucleus, which is customarily evaluated on the degree and color of the nuclear sclerosis, such as 1+, 2+, 3+, 4+, and amount of brunescence. This is a guide, in my view, but not a "go, no-go" criterion. A much better indication is the ease with which the ultrasonic tip saucerizes the nucleus and also the birefringence of the grooves created in the nucleus with this maneuver. If the nucleus proves to be excessively hard, the surgeon may convert to a planned extracapsular cataract extraction (ECCE). Therefore I usually set up for a phacoemulsification in most cases, unless the preoperative examination presents an obvious contraindication, such as cataracta nigra or subluxation of the crystalline lens.

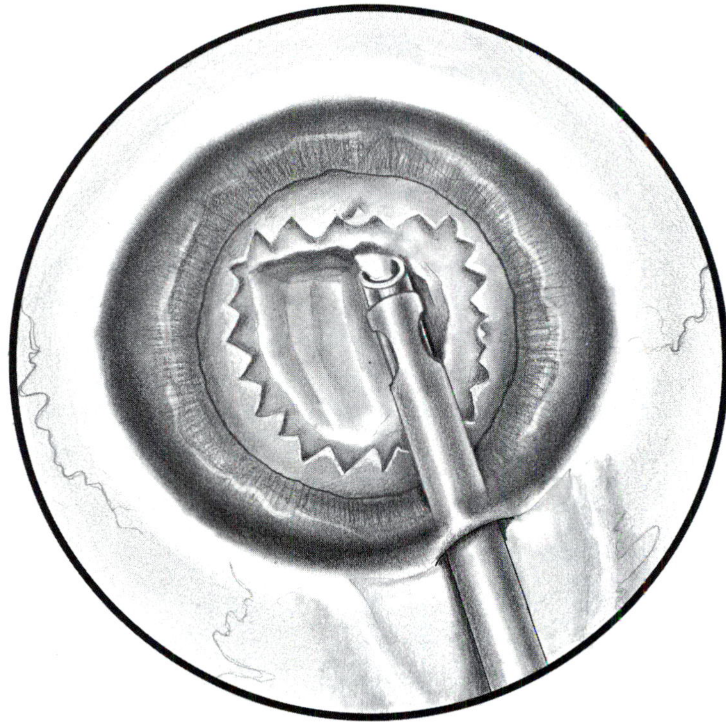

FIGURE 9-1. Sculpting of nucleus leaving step at inferior third.

With saucerization of the nucleus complete, the surgeon must now bring the superior pole of the nucleus to the iris plane where it can be emulsified. To effect this, a nucleus rotator, held in the left hand, is introduced through the second incision and placed against the inferior ledge of nucleus, fashioned as noted above, while continuous irrigation maintains a formed anterior chamber, (Fig. 9-2). The ultrasonic handpiece is withdrawn to the superior pupillary margin. The surgeon terminates the irrigation mode whereupon the anterior chamber *slowly* shallows because the incision is partially tamponed by the silicone sleeve of the ultrasonic handpiece. As the anterior chamber collapses, the contents of the posterior chamber move anteriorly, but not uniformly because the nucleus rotator presses gently inferior and slightly posterior, providing an impediment. This results in the anterior movement of the posterior chamber's contents, primarily superiorly, and it is this action that pushes the superior pole of the nucleus anteriorly. As this occurs, it is trapped by the ultrasonic handpiece, and irrigation is immediately activated, which reforms the anterior chamber and lyses many of the nuclear and cortical adhesions. The result is that the nucleus is "stranded" at the iris plane, much like a boat on the beach as the tide recedes. The nucleus rotator is reposited at the left margin of the nucleus, and emulsification is begun (Fig. 9-3).

The rotator, as its name implies, rotates successive portions of the nucleus to the ultrasonic handpiece; it then emulsifies these in short bursts (Fig. 9-4). The rotation of the nucleus is easier in the irrigation mode because the anterior chamber is more vacuous; hence, during the rotation emulsification of the nucleus, the surgeon is alternating between irrigation and ultrasound. As successive portions of the nuclear periphery are emulsified, the nuclear diameter will be reduced, and the nuclear remnants will spontaneously prolapse into the anterior chamber where the emulsification is completed. Small fragments of nucleus have a tendency to ricochet around the anterior chamber during the final phases of emulsification. This phenomenon can be minimized by reduction of the ultrasonic power and use of the nucleus rotator to guide nuclear fragments to the ultrasonic tip and steady them there. At the conclusion of emulsification, the ultrasonic handpiece is withdrawn from the eye.

Access to the superior pole of the nucleus can be obstructed in several contingencies. The most preventable is when there is an excessively wide border of residual anterior capsule superiorly; that is, the superior border of the anterior capsulectomy is too centrad. This places a leaf of anterior capsule between the superior nucleus and the ultrasonic handpiece, making trapping of the superior nuclear pole difficult and possibly risky, inasmuch as a superior zonular dialysis can result. The best treatment is prevention by the execution of an adequate anterior capsulectomy (see p. 180). Admittedly, when pupillary dilatation is marginal, an anterior capsulectomy of adequate dimensions may be impossible, and the surgeon may reconsider his strategy and perform a sector iridectomy as a prelude to the anterior capsulectomy (see p. 188) or convert to a planned ECCE (see p. 180), or do both. An excessively soft eye is another impediment to the surgeon's access of the superior nuclear pole, and this is discussed on p. 202.

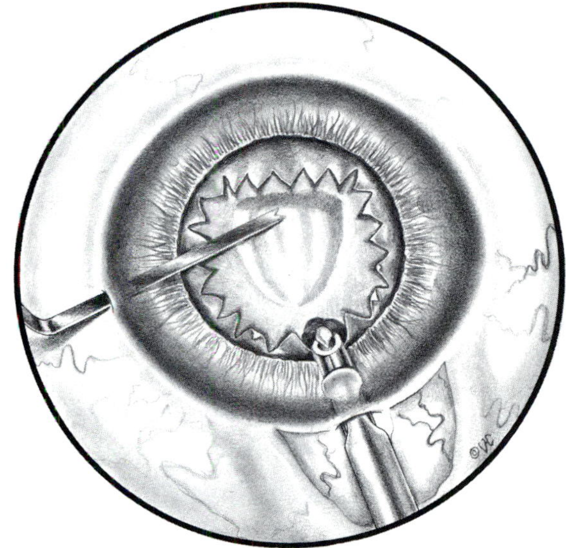

FIGURE 9-2. Placement of nucleus rotator against sculpted nucleus.

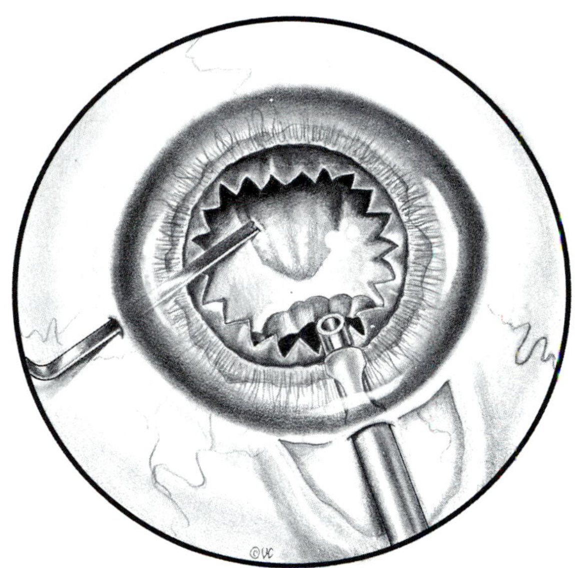

FIGURE 9-3. Superior pole of nucleus is prolapsed.

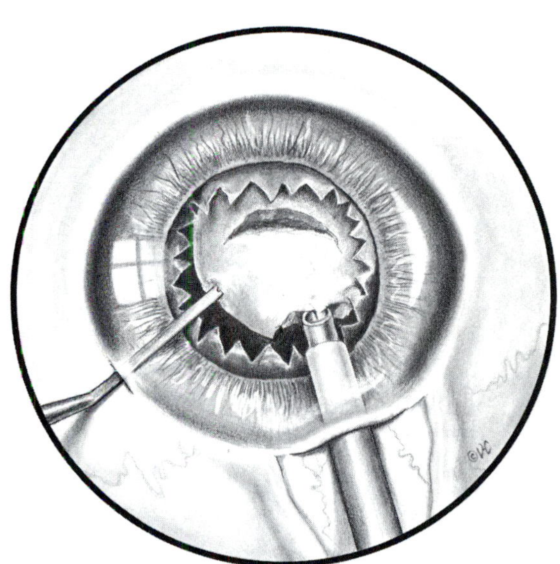

FIGURE 9-4. Periphery of nucleus is emulsified as second instrument provides support.

When performing a bimanual Kelman phacoemulsification (KPE), one should take care to avoid overworking the instrument held in the left hand. This usually involves pushing the nucleus into the right inferior quadrant of the capsular bag. The tension or vibration of a jagged piece of nucleus can produce a capsular rupture in this quadrant.

Avoid letting the nucleus tip into an anteroposterior position. This can occur as the nucleus, partially emulsified and reduced in size, becomes more mobile. Characteristically the margins of the nucleus are roughened by emulsification, and vibration of the superior pole of the nucleus by the ultrasonic tip causes a countervibration of the inferior pole against the posterior capsule, with rise of capsular rupture (Fig. 9-5).

The adage that "soft" cataracts are easier to emulsify than "hard" cataracts is true once the surgeon has isolated the nucleus in a position suitable for emulsification. However, to reach this stage can be quite difficult because the softness advantageous to emulsification is a disadvantage to intracameral manipulation. In a two-handed technique, the second instrument will slice through the nucleus in the same way as the cystotome if an anterior chamber prolapse is attempted. Moreover, "soft" cataracts often have ill-defined nuclei with tenacious attachments to the cortex, which, in turn, is adherent to the capsular bag, compounding the difficulties of nucleus exposure.

A variety of methods can be used when this problem arises. In the first, the aspiration is used in the ultrasound mode. This gives low vacuum but an aspiration orifice of approximately 0.9 mm with a 15-degree bevel. With aspiration activated, the surgeon insinuates the ultrasonic handpiece tip into the inferior capsular bag, under the iris, and engages the cataract, which is allowed to occlude the tip for maximum aspiration. Then it is gently pulled out of the capsular cul-de-sac (Fig. 9-6). This maneuver is repeated until a substantial portion of the cataract is in the anterior chamber, whereupon it is emulsified, usually at a low ultrasonic power setting.

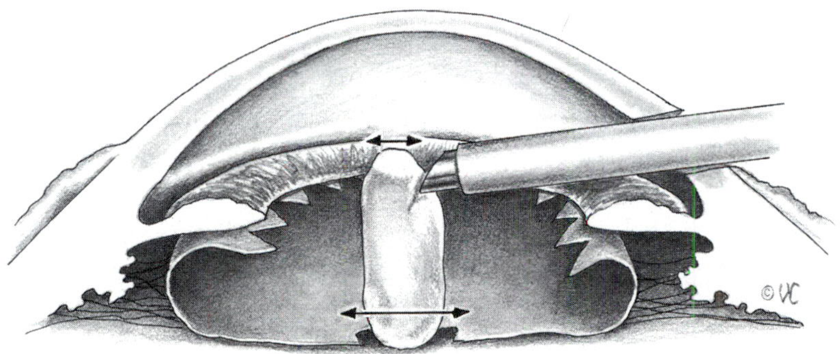

FIGURE 9-5. Nucleus in anteroposterior plane.

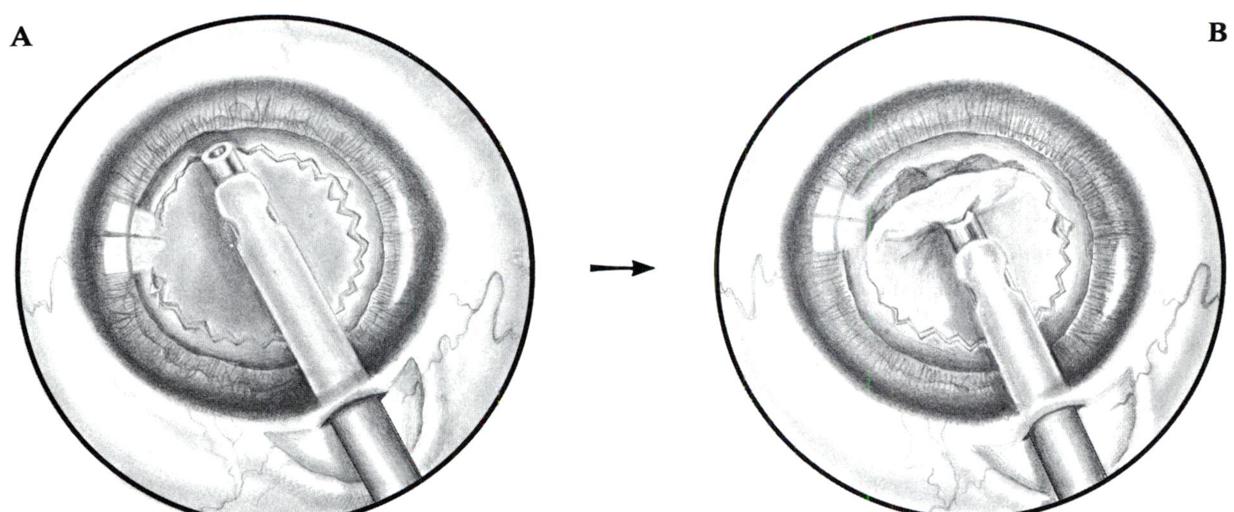

FIGURE 9-6. **A,** Phaco tip is embedded into inferior nucleus while in irrigation/aspiration. **B,** Soft nucleus is aspirated out of capsular cul-de-sac.

This maneuver does not always succeed, and a second method utilizes a VES to isolate the nucleus. A small bolus of VES is injected into the anterior chamber through a 25-gauge cannula, and then the iris and anterior capsule are retracted with a microhook inserted through the second incision. The cannula is then insinuated around the nucleus, and the VES is injected under it in small aliquots, tipping the nucleus anteriorly (Fig. 9-7). As much of the nucleus as possible is prolapsed in this manner and then emulsified.

External pressure may also be used to prolapse the soft cataract. All instruments are withdrawn from the eye, and the surgeon gently presses on the limbus in a convenient location (Fig. 9-8). This pressure will, one would hope, cause the nucleus to come forward. If the ultrasonic handpiece is now inserted in irrigation mode, the fluid flow will push the nucleus back in the capsular cul-de-sac, and so it is important to secure the prolapsed nucleus before reinsertion of the ultrasonic handpiece. One may accomplish this with VES under the nucleus or "tire-levering" the nucleus into the anterior chamber. All the above techniques are under the presupposition that the surgeon has not damaged the zonules or broken the posterior capsule during repeated attempts to prolapse the nucleus before realizing it was too soft to handle in a conventional manner.

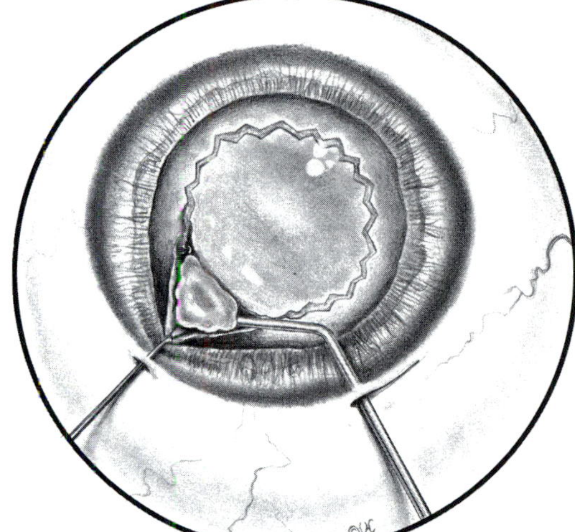

FIGURE 9-7. Soft nucleus is prolapsed anteriorly by a bolus of viscoelastic substance (VES).

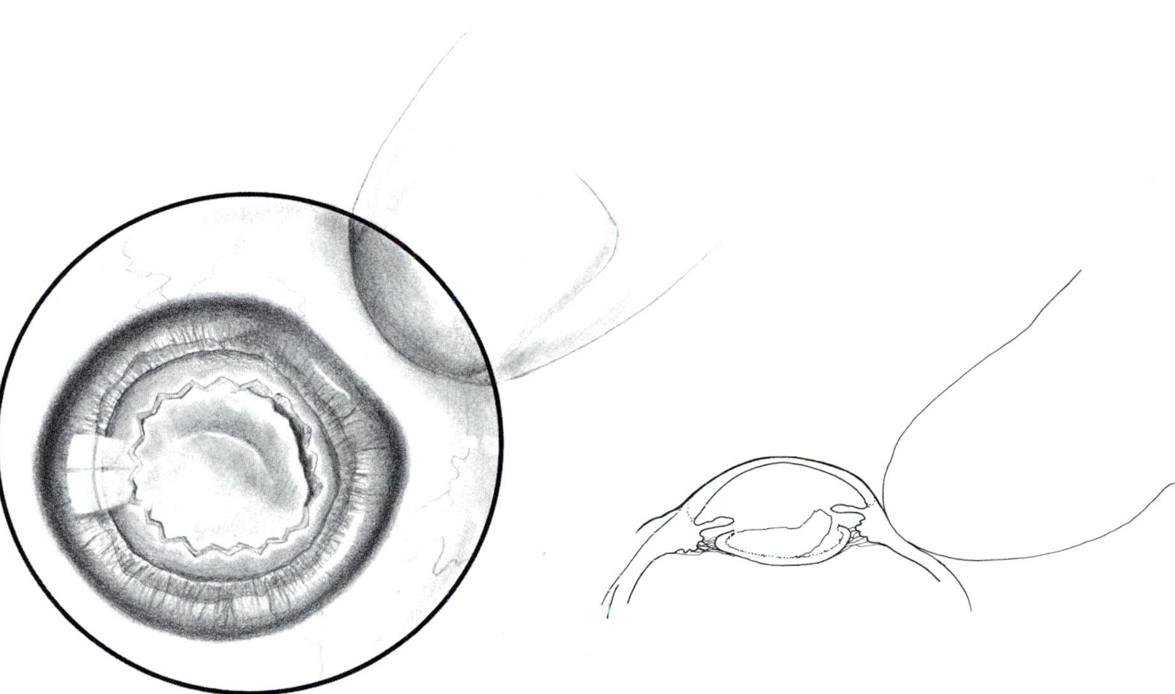

FIGURE 9-8. External pressure is used to prolapse nucleus.

Posterior Capsule Procedures

Numerous salutary effects have been attributed to the intact posterior capsule. However, a few cases will have fibrosis and opacification of the posterior capsule that will not be aspiratable at surgery. If visually significant, the patient will not see well and a neodymium-YAG posterior capsulectomy will be required in the immediate postoperative period.

The surgeon should be circumspect in deciding to use discission on these plaques intraoperatively. If the capsule is engaged as shown in Fig. 9-9, the posterior capsulectomy will often tear around the fibrotic margins, leaving a dense capsular defect from whose margin a pendular flap of the original opacification may remain. On the other hand, piercing the area of opacification with an instrument can be difficult.

In my opinion, the last word has not been written on the merits of an intact posterior capsule versus a surgical or laser capsulectomy, and techniques or philosophy will likely change.

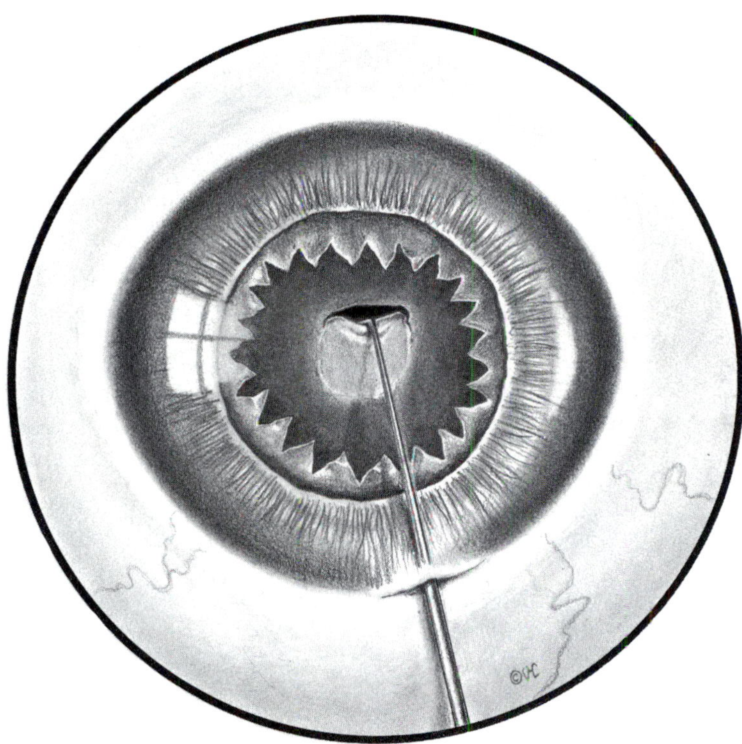

FIGURE 9-9. Discission of adherent plaque.

Intraoperative Complications—Rupture of Posterior Capsule

Rupture of the posterior capsule can occur at various times during an extracapsular cataract extraction or Kelman phacoemulsification. When it occurs before aspiration of residual cortex, a decision must be made on whether to proceed with irrigation/aspiration. A small amount of cortex may be left; however, a substantial amount should be aspirated (Fig. 9-10).

Aspiration should be in a direction that will not put stress on the capsular tear and hence will not cause it to enlarge. Generally the aspiration should therefore be centrad (in the direction from the periphery to the center) (Fig. 9-11). For automated techniques, it is advisable to lower the irrigation bottle and use a lower vacuum level.

Areas of residual cortex too precarious to aspirate may be stripped from the posterior capsule by injection of a bolus of VES between the cortex and the capsule (Fig. 9-12). This strips the cortex, which is now amenable to aspiration. On the other hand, it may be maneuvered into the capsular cul-de-sac where, one would hope, it will be sequestered and out of the visual axis.

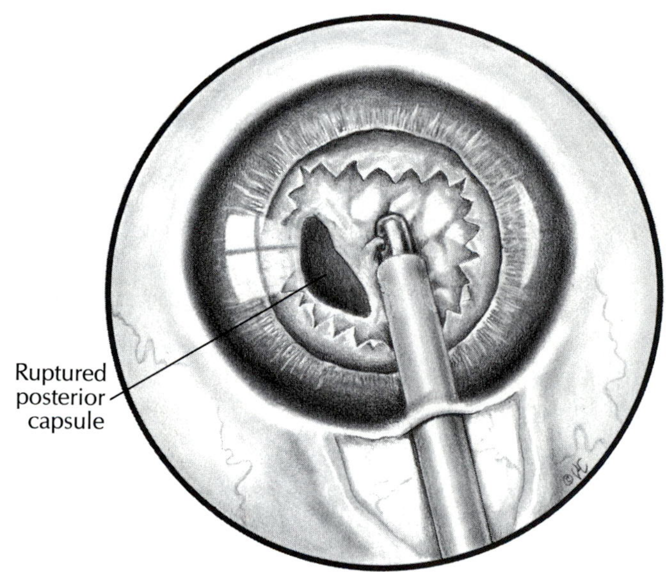

FIGURE 9-10. Intraoperative rupture of posterior capsule.

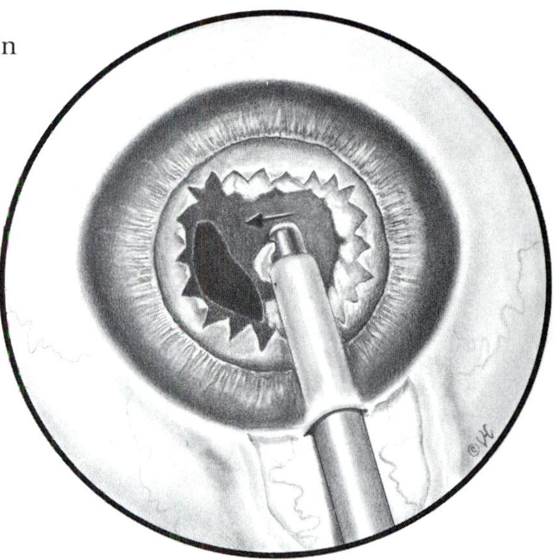

FIGURE 9-11. Technique of aspiration in presence of posterior capsular defect.

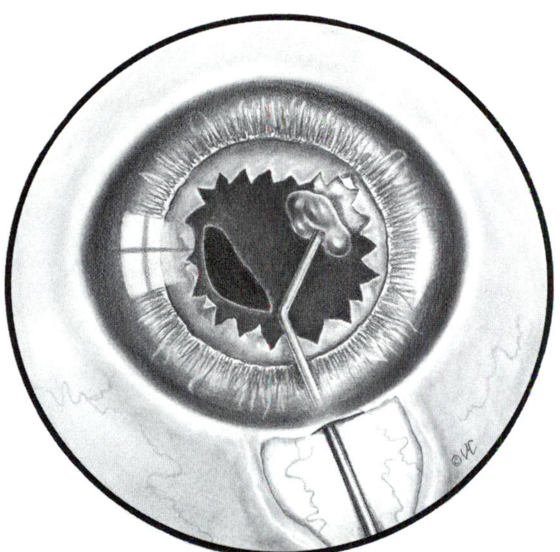

FIGURE 9-12. Bolus of VES used to maneuver residual cortex.

The surgeon may be undecided if the posterior capsule is intact, and the "halo sign" is useful in this contingency. A smooth, bright metallic instrument is gently pressed against the posterior capsule, producing a shallow depression. The incident light from the operating microscope is reflected from the metallic instrument to the rim of the depression (Fig. 9-13). The *intact* posterior capsule reflects when it is stretched, and the surgeon will see a halo of light surrounding the metallic instrument, reflected from the capsule (Fig. 9-14).

A posterior vitreous detachment may mimic a floating cortical remnant, and small pieces of cortex may be washed into the vitreous cavity during the procedure. A surgeon, unsure of the position of the posterior capsule, may try to aspirate these, inevitably rupturing the posterior capsule and disrupting the vitreous. The halo sign is useful in delineation of the position of the posterior capsule *before* any questionable maneuver.

With a small capsular defect, conventional intraocular lens (IOL) insertion may be performed. It is advisable to cover the area of the defect with a bolus of VES and then fill the capsular bag and the anterior chamber before IOL insertion (Fig. 9-15).

When there is a significant defect in the posterior capsule, the axis of IOL insertion should be changed to avoid any IOL manipulation over the defect. Furthermore, the IOL should be positioned such that it is supported by intact capsule (Fig. 9-16). In an extracapsular cataract extraction, pertinent sutures are removed to facilitate insertion (Fig. 9-17), whereas after a Kelman phacoemulsification the incision is enlarged *(inset)* in the appropriate direction.

With a large capsular defect, ciliary sulcus placement is preferable to capsular fixation to avoid further enlargement of the defect by tension on the capsular bag.

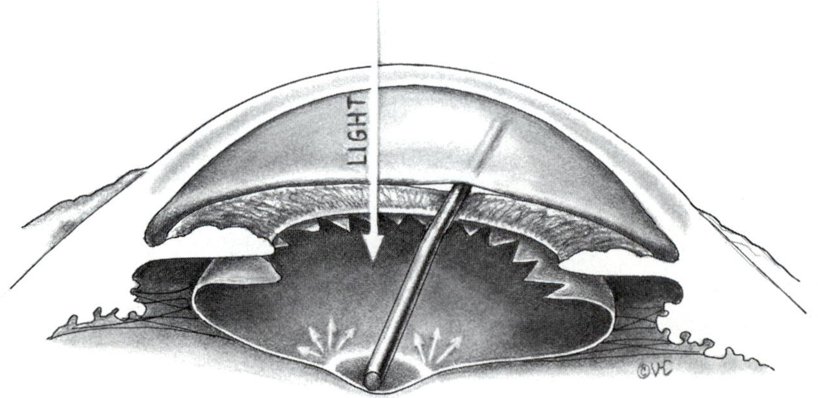

FIGURE 9-13. Mechanism of "halo sign."

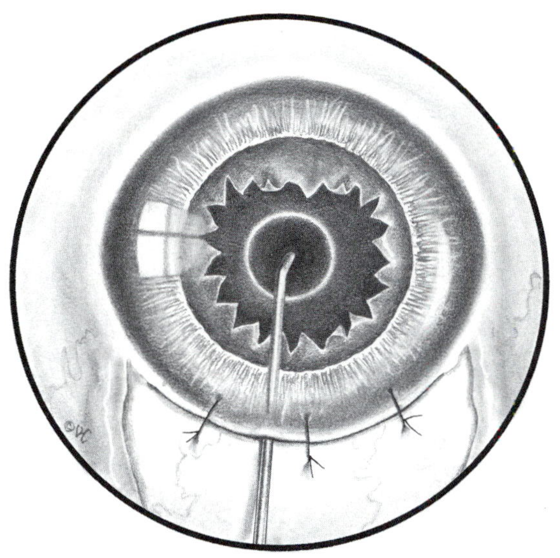

FIGURE 9-14. Appearance of "halo sign."

FIGURE 9-15. Insertion of posterior chamber intraocular lens over posterior capsular defect cushioned by VES.

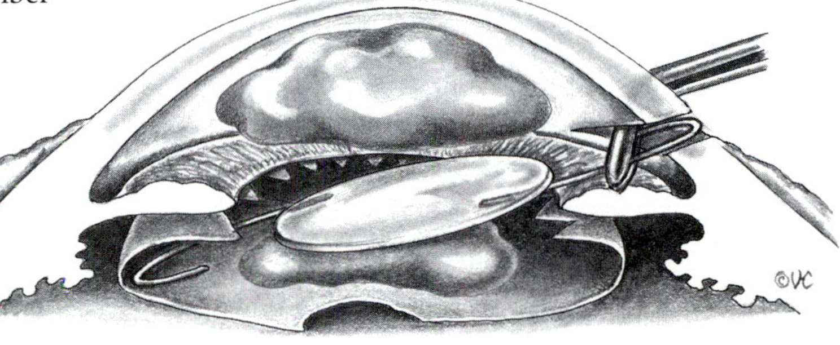

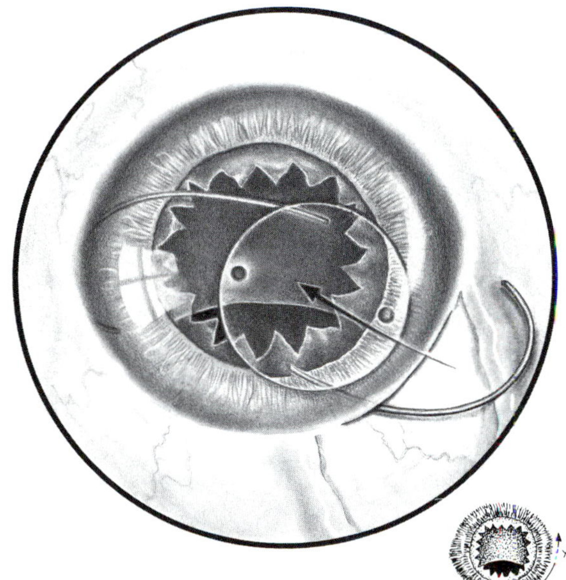

FIGURE 9-16. Change in axis of posterior chamber intraocular lens insertion to avoid posterior capsular defect.

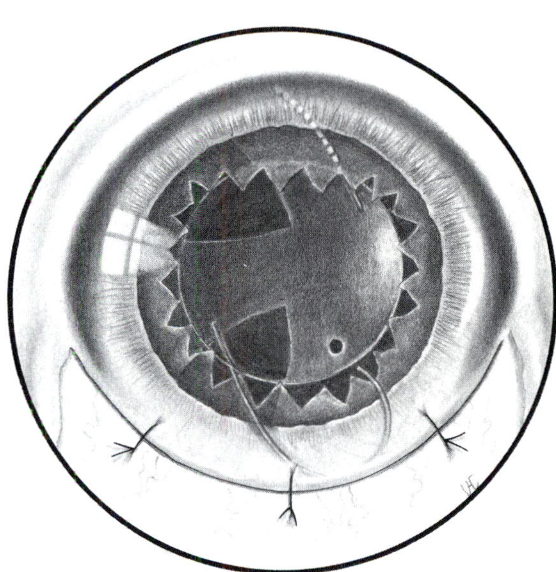

FIGURE 9-17. Posterior chamber intraocular lens in situ in presence of capsular defects.

Intraoperative Complication—Residual Capsular Flap

When there is a residual capsular flap (Fig. 9-18) that could impinge on the visual axis, it should be managed, if technically feasible.

A superior flap may be grasped with suitable forceps and excised (Fig. 9-19). Avoid excessive traction on the flap, lest a tear result and expand around the equator into the posterior capsule.

A sessile flap, nonamenable to externalization, can be excised as shown (Fig. 9-20). The anterior chamber is re-formed with VES, with care being taken to unfold the flap, and scissors are then introduced. The flap is excised and removed with forceps.

A pedunculated flap in a suitable position may be removed with a maneuver some have called the "toilet-tissue" technique. The flap is grasped with forceps, and with an abrupt snapping motion is broken free from its pedunculated base and removed from the eye (Fig. 9-21).

A residual flap inaccessible to either of these techniques can be folded out of the visual axis. With VES in the anterior chamber, the cannula used for injection can also be used to fold the flap upon itself and into the capsular cul-de-sac (Fig. 9-22).

Recalcitrant cases of residual flaps that are visually significant are treatable with the neodymium-YAG laser postoperatively. Some flaps need no treatment.

Other flaps, though not impairing vision, can distort the pupil. A portion of the pupil will often appear horizontal, corresponding to the width of the offending flap.

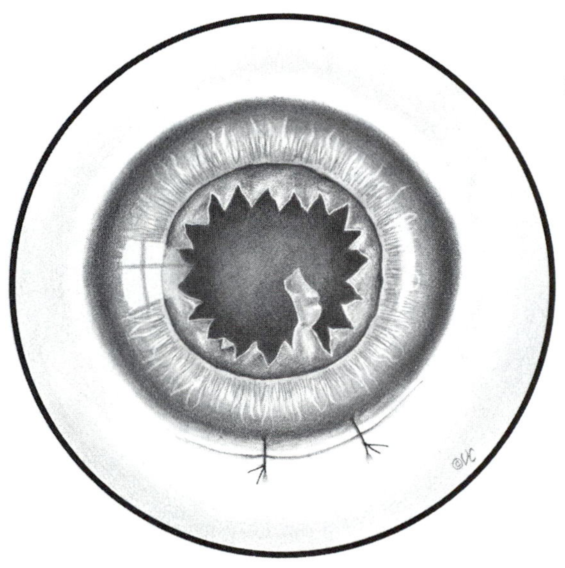

FIGURE 9-18. Residual superior tag.

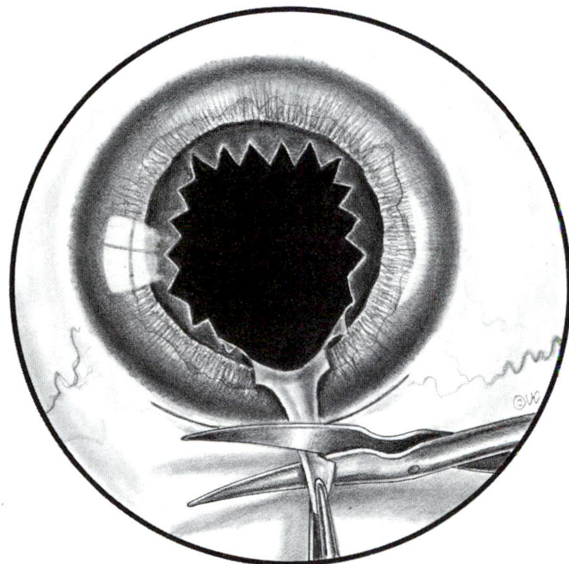

FIGURE 9-19. Excision of superior tag.

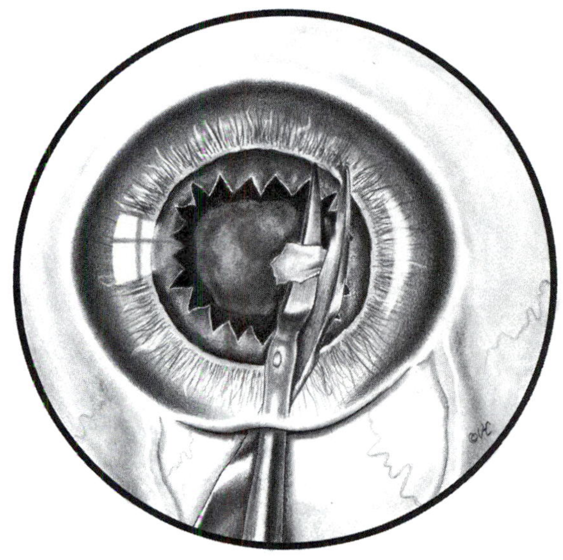

FIGURE 9-20. Management of lateral sessile tag.

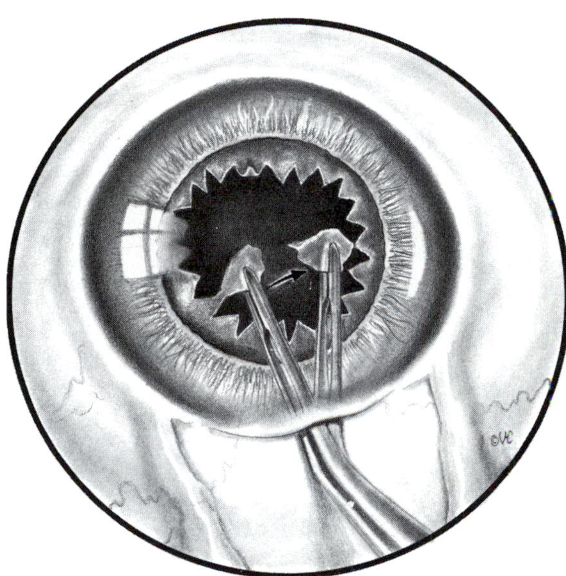

FIGURE 9-21. "Toilet paper" maneuver to remove pedunculated tag.

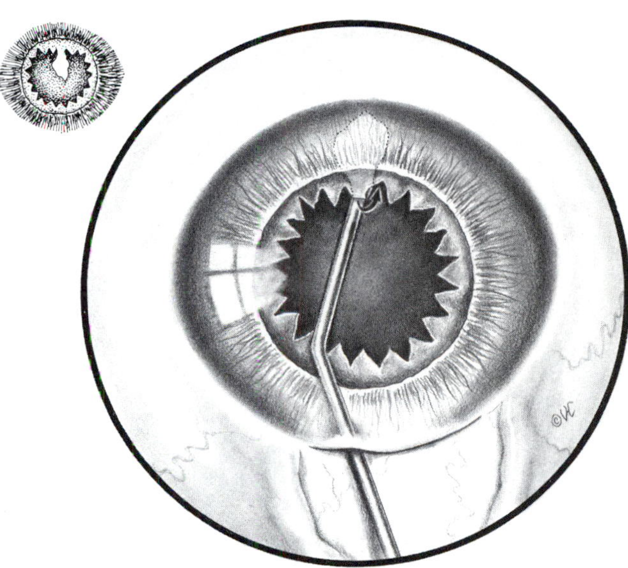

FIGURE 9-22. Folding flap out of visual axis with VES.

Intraoperative Complication—Decentered Posterior Capsulotomy

There is no surgical treatment for decentered posterior capsulectomy if a primary discission is the surgeon's intention (Fig. 9-23). Prevention by meticulous technique is the sure cure but a postoperative laser capsulectomy may also be considered.

A

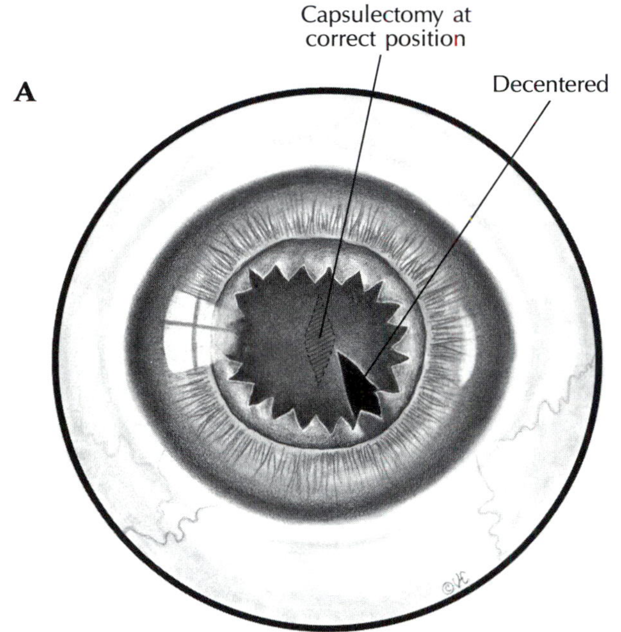

B

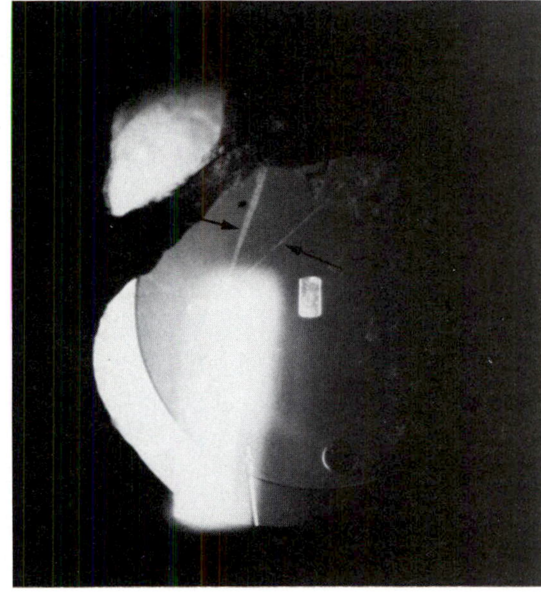

FIGURE 9-23. A, Decentered posterior capsulectomy. **B,** Decentered posterior capsulotomy behind posterior chamber intraocular lens.

Intraoperative Complication—Iridodialysis

An intraoperative iridodialysis can be caused by any intracameral instrumentation and usually occurs in the proximity of the incision. A small iridodialysis is of no consequence and functions as a peripheral iridectomy. However, a large iridodialysis can be cosmetically distasteful and cause an aberrant position of the pupil. Iridodialysis repair can be performed with a McCannel suture (see p. 244) where the needle engages the midportion of the dialysed iris (Fig. 9-24), which is sutured to the adjacent scleral margin (Fig. 9-25), by use of a 10-0 polypropylene suture.

An alternative method may be employed when a larger corneal incision is contemplated as in intracapsular or extracapsular cataract extraction. A traction suture is placed in the corneal side of the incision at the 12 o'clock position, and two interrupted 10-0 polypropylene sutures are placed in the dialysed iris (Fig. 9-26), which is then sutured to the scleral incision (Fig. 9-27). Fig. 9-28 shows the postoperative appearance.

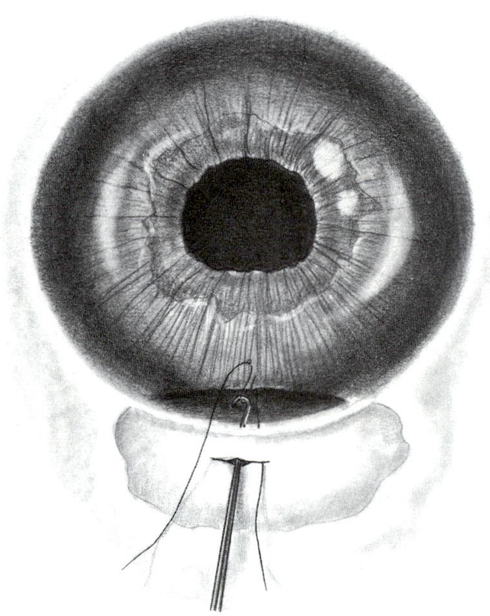

FIGURE 9-24. After McCannel suture has been passed through the margin of dialysed iris and cornea, it is drawn back through the incision with a microhook.

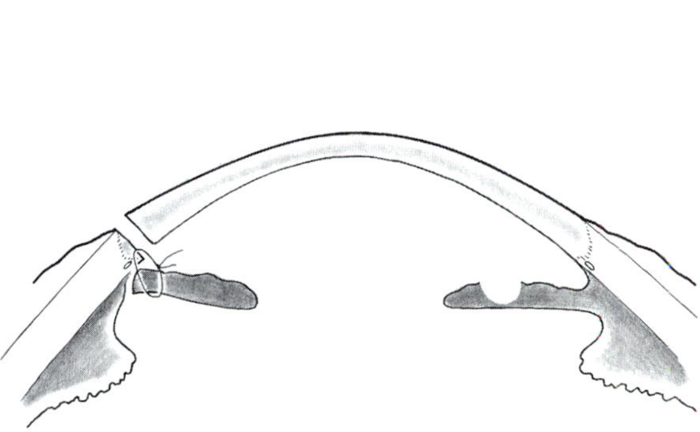

FIGURE 9-25. The dialysed iris is sutured to the scleral margin of the incision.

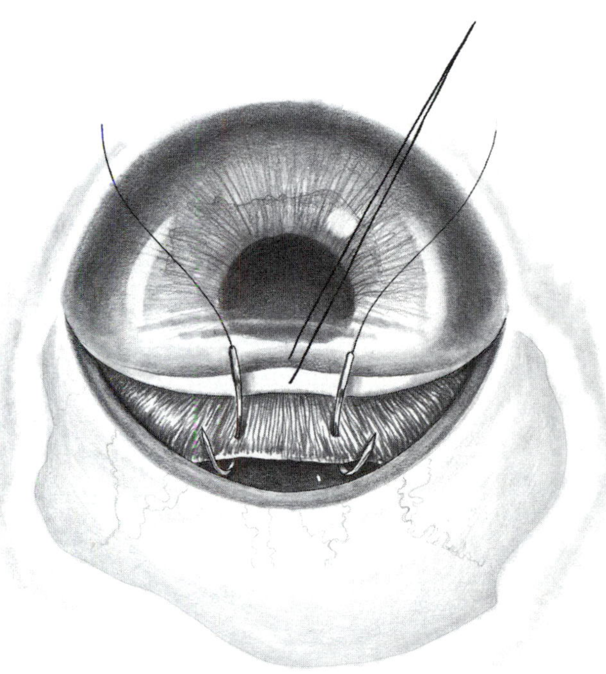

FIGURE 9-26. With an assistant retracting the cornea, sutures are placed in the dialysed iris.

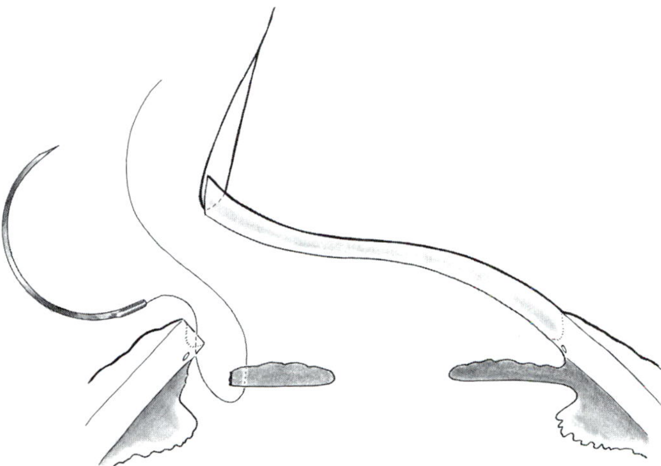

FIGURE 9-27. Iris is sutured to sclera.

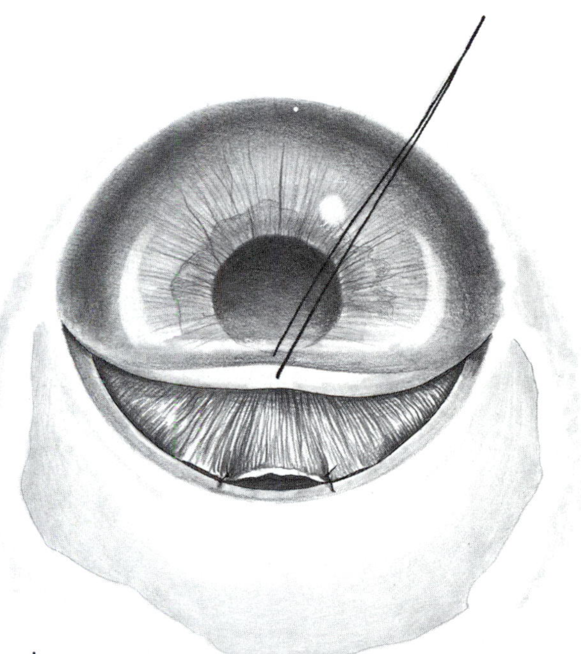

FIGURE 9-28. Appearance of iridodialysis after repair.

Intraoperative Complication—Vitreous Loss

Intracapsular surgery

When intracapsular surgery was the preferred technique of cataract extraction, vitreous loss was usually seen immediately after the cryoextraction and was heralded by instant reformation of the anterior chamber and presentation of vitreous at the wound. Formally, an anterior vitrectomy was performed with a cellulose sponge and scissors (Fig. 9-29), until this technique was largely superseded by a mechanized vitrectomy technique.

In either technique, the purpose of vitrectomy is to remove vitreous from the wound and to relieve iris distortion caused by vitreous strands, that is, an anterior vitrectomy, which entails removal of all vitreous anterior to the iris (see Fig. 9-30). Specifically, when the diagnosis of vitreous loss is made, the surgeon should ascertain whether any external pressure, such as lid retractors or a superior rectus suture, is aggravating the situation. After this, the vitreophage is inserted, and the cutting mechanism is activated concomitant with gentle aspiration (Fig. 9-30). Copious irrigation is undesirable because it can displace vitreous from the posterior chamber into the anterior chamber.

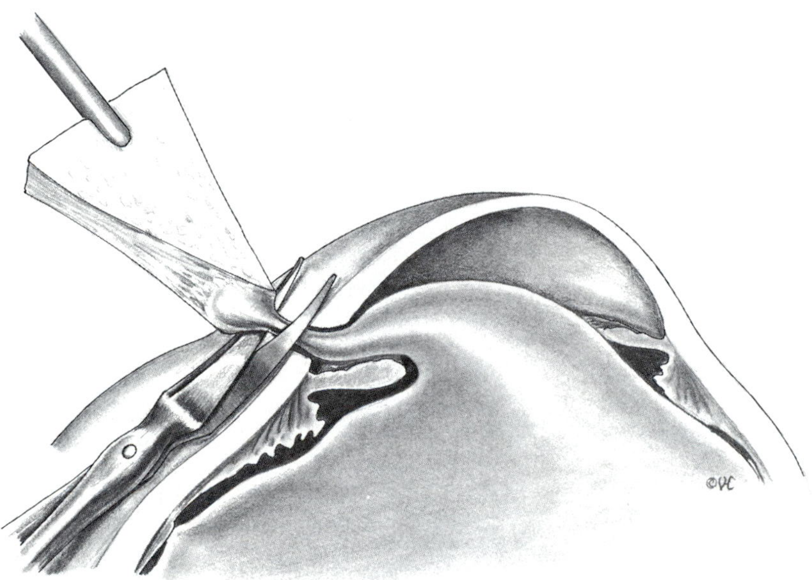

FIGURE 9-29. Cellulose sponge technique of anterior vitrectomy.

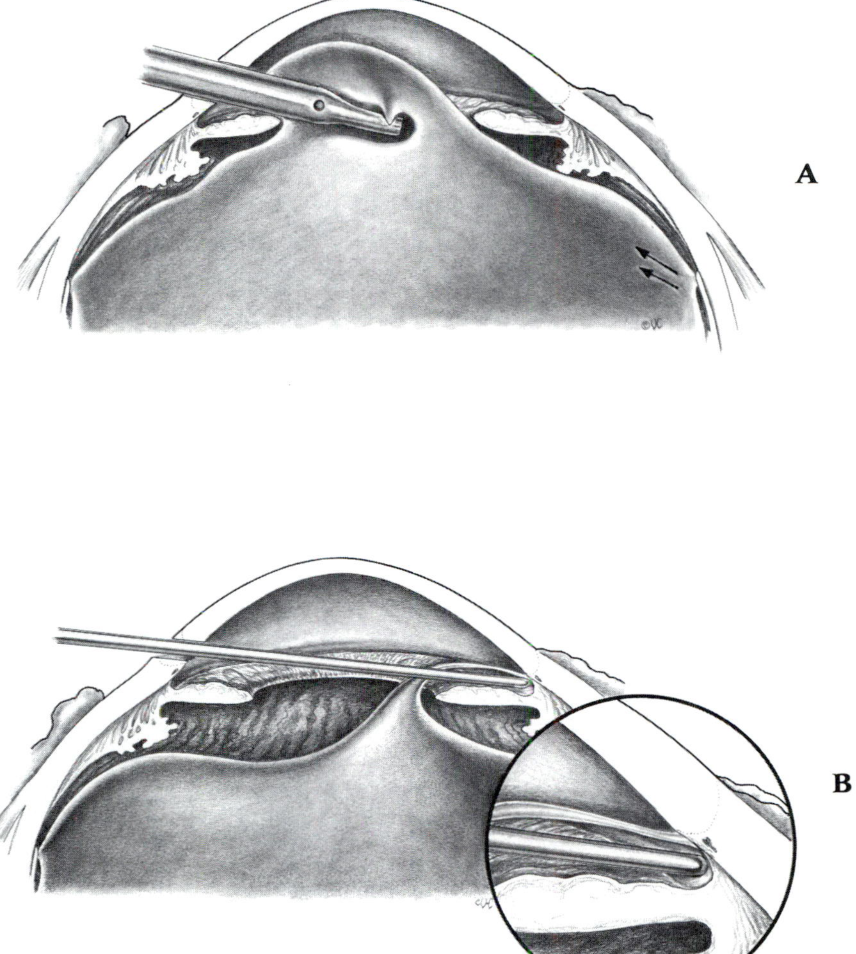

FIGURE 9-30. **A,** Mechanized anterior vitrectomy. **B,** Removal of residual vitreous strand to avoid pupillary distortion.

As the anterior vitrectomy proceeds, scleral collapse is often seen, and the iris plane falls posteriorly (Fig. 9-31). An air bubble is sucked into the anterior chamber. These are useful signs that the anterior chamber is now devoid of vitreous; therefore the anterior vitrectomy is terminated, and the instrument is withdrawn from the eye. The incision is inspected, and the margins are swept with the cellulose sponge (Fig. 9-32) to allow detection of any residual vitreous strands, which are excised with scissors. It is useful to temporarily tie the safety suture and instill an air bubble into the anterior chamber. A septate air bubble is suggestive of residual vitreous within the anterior chamber, which may be swept with a spatula or be mechanically removed (Fig. 9-33). Another useful maneuver is to instill an intracameral miotic into the anterior chamber and observe for distortion of the pupil, which indicates a residual vitreous strand, which may be manipulated with the spatula (Fig. 9-34).

In the case of an intracapsular cataract extraction, a peripheral iridectomy is performed, and the incision is closed. If an anterior chamber lens is to be inserted, the technique is not unique and is as described on p. 234. The surgeon should be careful that the iris plane is not concave before anterior chamber IOL insertion because such a concavity could cause a reverse "iris tuck" where the iris is invaginated posteriorly against the ciliary body (see p. 236).

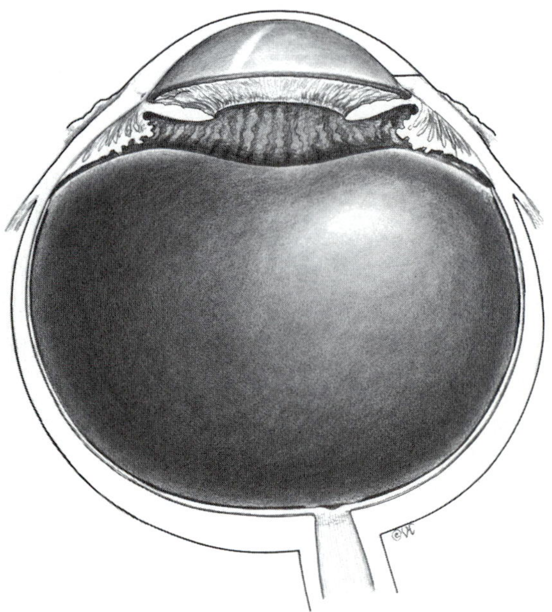

FIGURE 9-31. Position of vitreous and iris after adequate anterior vitrectomy.

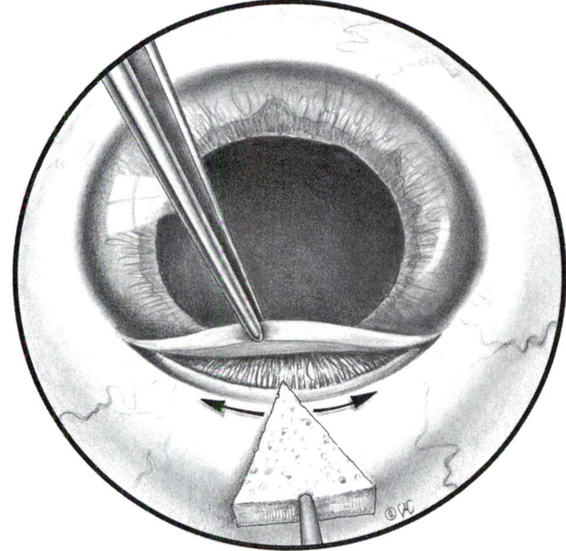

FIGURE 9-32. Wound is swept with cellulose sponge to detect any residual vitreous.

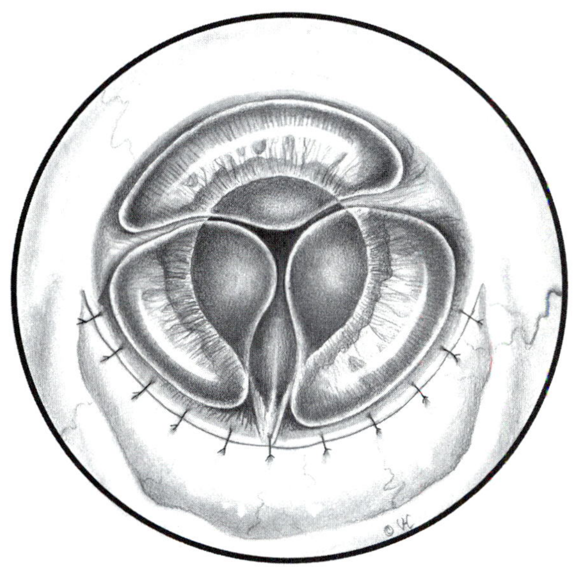

FIGURE 9-33. Septate appearance of air bubble in presence of residual vitreous strand.

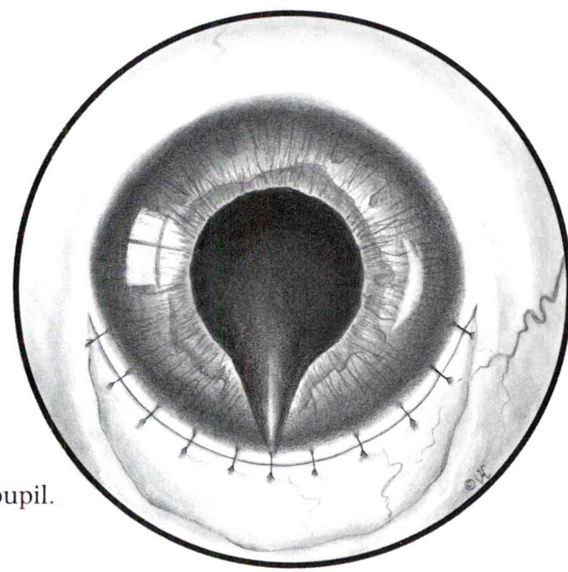

FIGURE 9-34. Residual vitreous strand distorting pupil.

Extracapsular surgery

Vitreous loss in extracapsular surgery presents a special opportunity and special problems (Fig. 9-35). The opportunity is preservation of sufficient posterior capsule and intact zonules to make posterior chamber IOL insertion feasible (see p. 226). Part of this is fortuitous and depends on how the capsule ruptures and when vitreous is lost. However, the other part is in the hands of the surgeon who, by a fastidious anterior vitrectomy, will avoid further damage to the residual posterior capsule and zonules, hopefully making subsequent posterior chamber IOL insertion possible.

The special problems are twofold and involve, first, the possible loss of the nucleus into the posterior chamber. The surgical management of this loss is discussed on p. 426. Not every surgeon is capable of performing a bimanual pars plana vitrectomy at the time of occurrence, and in my experience, not every nucleus needs to be removed. I do not believe that the surgeon will err if the patient is observed, in this contingency, for subsequent ocular reaction. Of course, if the nucleus can be entrapped and removed from the eye before posterior chamber prolapse, in the event of posterior capsule rupture, then the necessity for a pars plana procedure is obviated.

The second problem is management of the cortex. Most of the mechanized vitreophages will remove cortex well, and the trick is to accomplish this with preservation of posterior capsule as noted above, if possible. Generally, cortex in the posterior segment will reabsorb without surgical intervention, though with some inflammatory response.

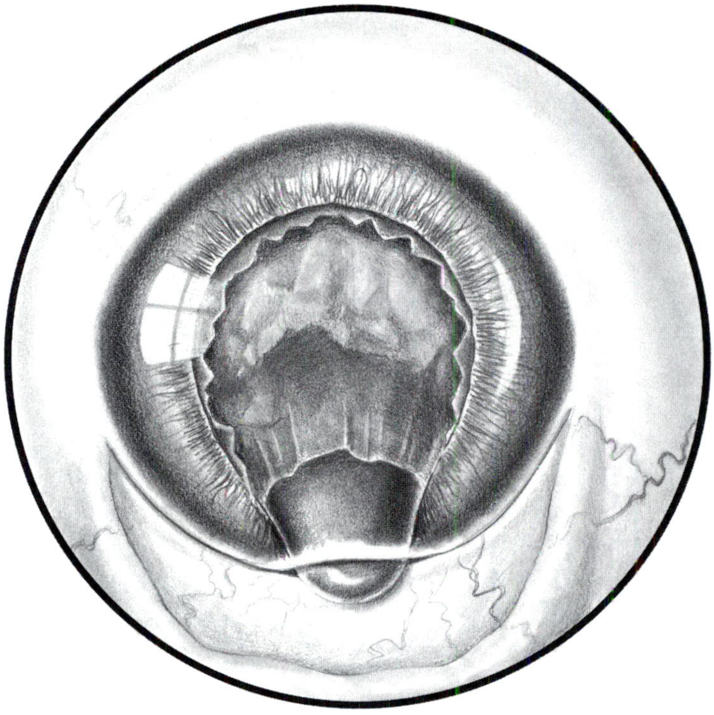

FIGURE 9-35. Loss of vitreous during extracapsular surgery.

CHAPTER 10

Intraocular Lens Implantation

It has been stated that aphakia was the primary complication of cataract surgery. Aphakic spectacles magnified the image, produced a ring scotoma, and required frequent adjustment. Contact lenses were often not tolerated by the elderly aphake, were sometimes lost, and produced their own set of complications. To extract the crystalline lens and not provide a tolerated optical correction would be analogous to amputating a limb without contemplating a subsequent prosthesis. Intraocular lenses (IOLs) are the optimum prosthesis for cataract surgery, providing the patient with a quantity and quality of vision so superior to other optical modalities that they defy rational debate. Posterior-chamber IOLs are inserted in over 90% of cataract patients in the United States, and anterior-chamber IOLs are estimated at 8% of the IOL market. I discuss first posterior-chamber IOLs, for which there are numerous variants to the basic insertion techniques.

Posterior Chamber Intraocular Lenses

Viscoelastic substance (VES) should be used strategically to expand desired tissue planes (Fig. 10-1). For example, when "in-the-bag" insertion is desired, the capsular cul-de-sac should be expanded with VES to create a space to facilitate insertion (Figs. 10-2 and 10-3). Merely filling the anterior chamber could collapse the anterior capsular flap against the posterior capsular flap, thus impeding insertion.

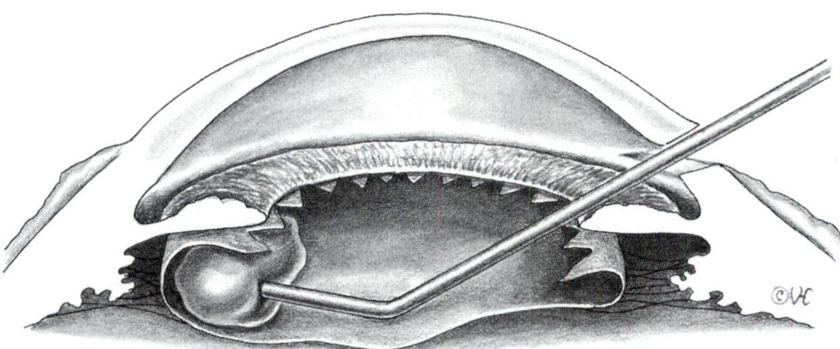

FIGURE 10-1. Filling inferior cul-de-sac with viscoelastic substance (VES).

FIGURE 10-2. Strategic filling of posterior chamber with VES as prelude for posterior chamber intraocular lens insertion.

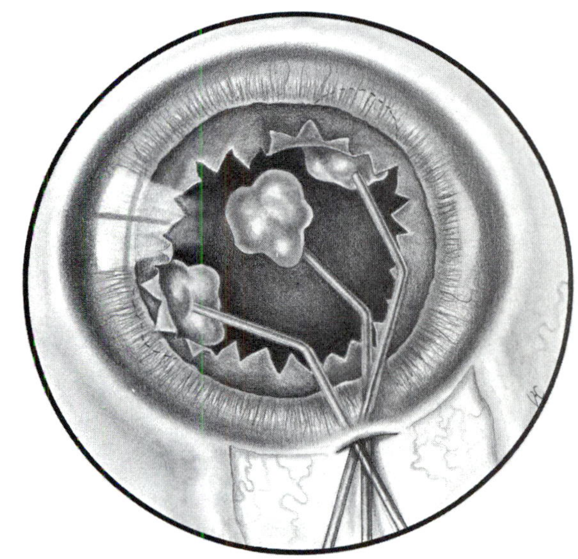

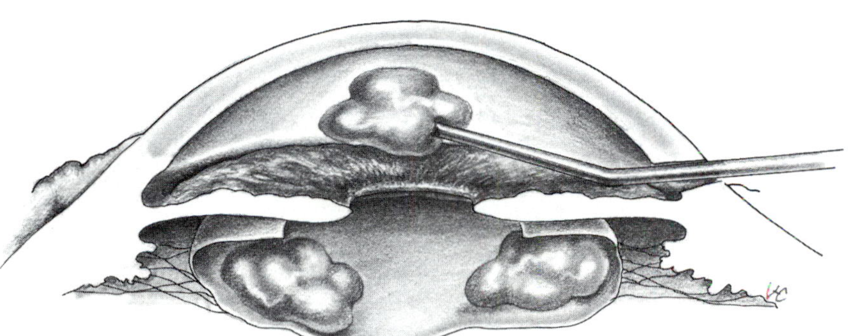

FIGURE 10-3. A bolus of VES anterior to iris to reform anterior chamber and protect endothelium.

The incision of the J-looped posterior chamber lens falls into two generic categories: dialing and nondialing techniques. The placement of the inferior loop is the same in both techniques. Under air or a VES, the intraocular lens (IOL) (optic and inferior loop) is inserted into the anterior chamber, and the inferior loop is placed under the iris or under the iris and inferior anterior capsular flap, depending on whether sulcus or "in-the-bag" fixation is desired (Fig. 10-4).

In the dialing technique, the superior loop is now placed within the eye *anterior* to the iris (Fig. 10-5).

Under the assumption that the surgeon's intention to place the IOL "in the bag," a microhook is inserted with the left hand, either through the second portal with Kelman phacoemulsification or through the left lateral aspect of the incision in an extracapsular cataract extraction (ECCE) (Fig. 10-6).

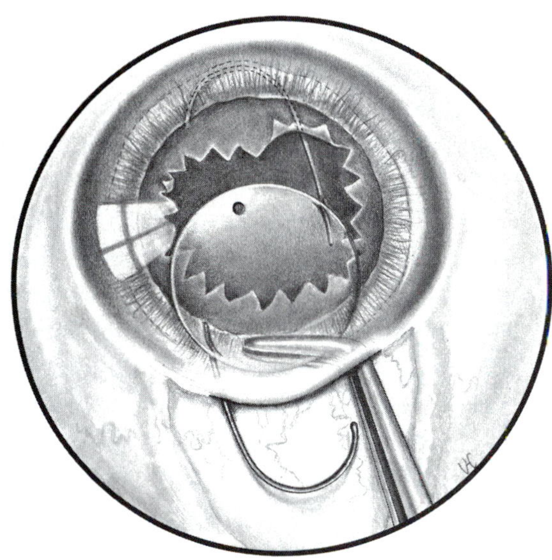

FIGURE 10-4. Initial maneuver for posterior chamber intraocular lens insertion. Inferior haptic inserted in capsular bag.

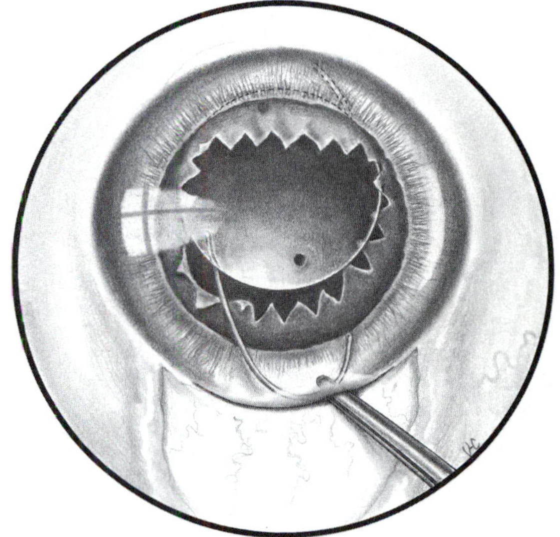

FIGURE 10-5. Superior haptic placed under the shelf of incision anterior to iris.

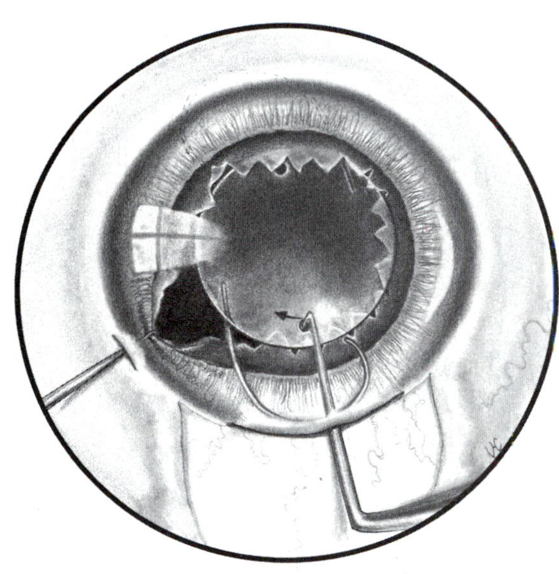

FIGURE 10-6. Microhook in left hand retracts both iris and anterior capsule.

This hook retracts both iris and anterior capsule (Fig. 10-7) as the IOL is dialed into the capsular bag with a lens guide (Fig. 10-8). There is a tendency to use intraocular lenses without positioning holes, in which case the lens guide or other suitable instrument is placed at the junction of the superior haptic and the optic for the dialing maneuver.

When the nondialing technique of posterior chamber IOL insertion is used, the insertion of the inferior loop is as noted in Fig. 10-4. After the inferior loop is positioned, the superior loop is left external to the eye (Fig. 10-9). It is then grasped with a suitable forceps, such as the Kelman-McPherson, and with a microhook in the left hand optionally retracting both iris and capsule, the superior loop is bent and placed directly within the capsular bag (Fig. 10-10). If it is the surgeon's intent to place it in the sulcus, the microhook grasps only iris for this maneuver. After the superior loop is positioned, both instruments are withdrawn, and the implant may be rotated to a horizontal position if this is the surgeon's desire (Fig. 10-11).

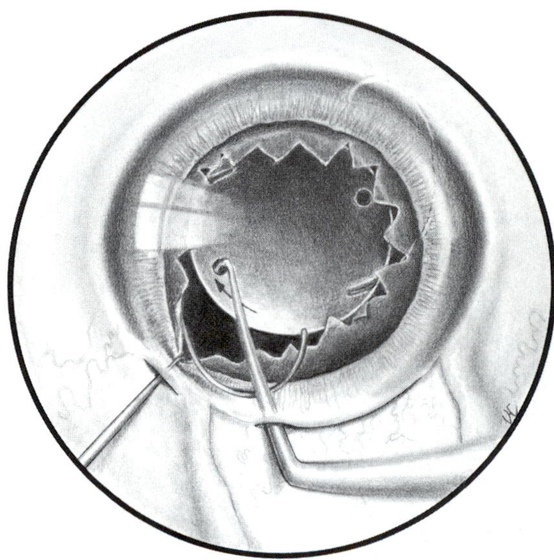

FIGURE 10-7. Superior haptic of posterior chamber intraocular lens is dialed into capsular bag.

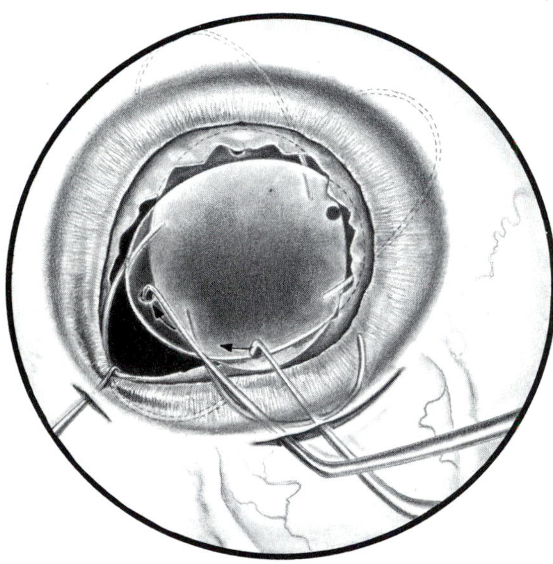

FIGURE 10-8. Rotatory motion used in dialing technique.

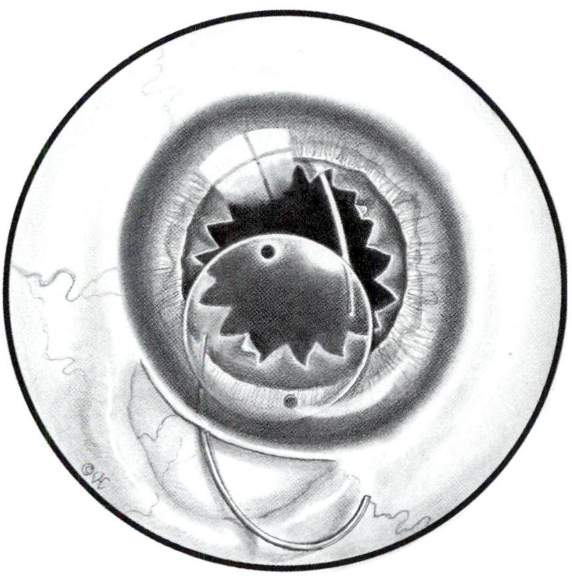

FIGURE 10-9. Superior haptic is left external as a prelude to nondialing technique.

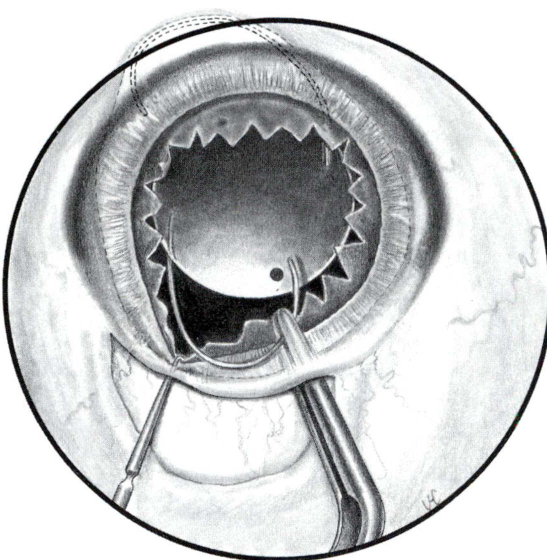

FIGURE 10-10. Superior haptic grasped with forceps and placed directly in capsular bag as iris and anterior capsule are retracted.

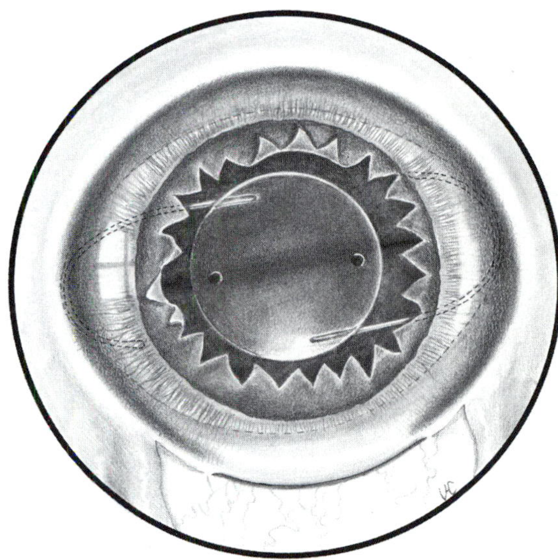

FIGURE 10-11. Posterior chamber intraoculaı lens is rotated to horizontal position as required.

When the pupil is widely dilated and the surgeon has correctly placed the implant in the capsular bag, the optic may seem to locate itself slightly nasal (Fig. 10-12). The reason is that the capsular bag is located such that the optical center of the crystalline lens will correspond with the physiologic pupil, which is frequently somewhat nasal; hence the correctly placed optic appears nasal. The surgeon will often see stress lines in the posterior capsule after correct in-the-bag placement of a posterior chamber J-looped lens. These are striae induced at the apex of each J loop and are indicative of correct positioning.

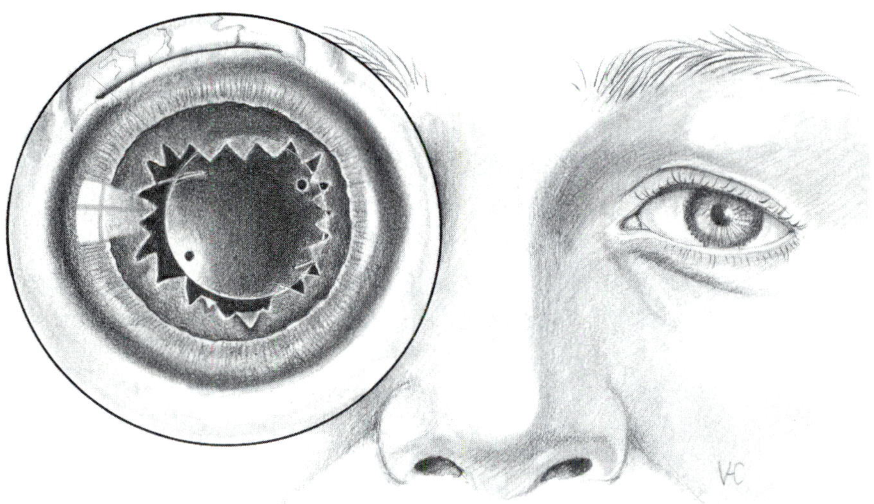

FIGURE 10-12. J-looped posterior chamber intraocular lens correctly in capsular bag appears slightly nasal when pupil is dilated.

Anterior Chamber Intraocular Lenses

The rigid type of Choyce anterior chamber intraocular lenses (AC IOLs) are rarely used nowadays in the United States, and the semiflexible closed-loop IOLs have had unacceptable complications and seem consigned to oblivion. The Kelman type of flexible AC IOLs dominate the IOL market of the United States, and it is this type of IOL that is illustrated here, though the design varies somewhat between manufacturers.

The technique for insertion of an anterior chamber intraocular lens is the same for an extracapsular or intracapsular cataract extraction. In a Kelman phacoemulsification, of course, the incision has to be enlarged to about 6 mm. The pupil should be constricted with an intracameral miotic and the anterior chamber filled with a VES. Overfilling should be avoided because this will make the iris diaphragm concave, predisposing to iris tuck, which is described on p. 236. The first maneuver (1) is the insertion of the inferior loop. The "toe" *(A)* of the foot is obliquely inserted through the incision until the "heel" *(B)* clears the right margin of the incision, at which point the IOL is straightened to the vertical position (2). It is then slid across the anterior chamber, avoiding entrapment by the pupil, until the inferior haptic is in the angle. The IOL is released from the insertion forceps, and the "superior loop" *(C)* is placed in the superior angle (Fig. 10-13). A peripheral iridectomy is desirable and should be placed remote from the superior haptic to minimize the risk of prolapse through the aperture of the iridectomy. Some surgeons advocate a midstromal iridotomy when an AC IOL is used.

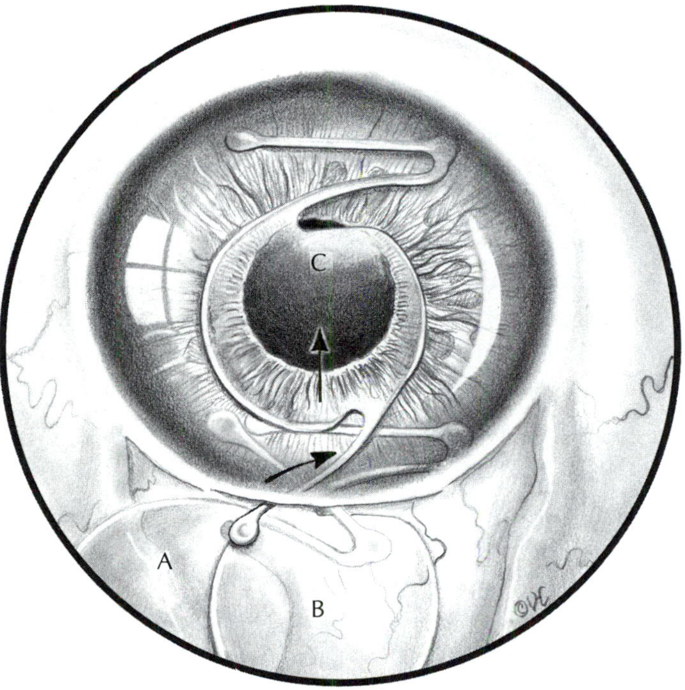

FIGURE 10-13. Technique of insertion of anterior chamber intraocular lens.

Secondary Intraocular Lens Implantation

A secondary IOL refers to insertion remote from the original cataract extraction. The usual contingency is a patient who had a previous unilateral intracapsular cataract extraction and is now contact lens intolerant. Assuming the anterior chamber is devoid of vitreous, a secondary insertion is the same as a primary insertion, though the surgeon may select a temporal incision to avoid the conjunctival fibrosis from the previous surgery. This strategy can also minimize the risk of vitreous loss through previously placed peripheral iridectomies, which are customarily superiorly located.

When the anterior hyaloid face is intact but prolapsing into the anterior chamber, it can usually be pushed posteriorly by a bolus of viscoelastic substance, whereupon the secondary insertion proceeds after pupillary constriction by instillation of an intracameral miotic. The problem occurs when there is a substantial amount of free vitreous in the anterior chamber. Under these circumstances, an anterior vitrectomy is inevitable and is usually innocuous, though the increased risk of retinal detachment cannot be denied.

Iris tuck, alluded to previously, occurs when the inferior haptic of an anterior chamber IOL is slid across the anterior chamber trapping the inferior iris between it and the adjacent angle, resulting in an oval pupil (Fig. 10-14). I call this "anterior" iris tuck in contradistinction to "posterior" iris tuck, which occurs when the superior haptic is positioned and pushed posteriorly too forcefully. The result is invagination of the iris between the superior haptic and ciliary body (Fig. 10-15). This "posterior" iris tuck is more ominous than the anterior variety. Iris tuck is iatrogenic and should be avoided or corrected at the time of surgery.

Secondary insertion into posterior chamber

When a posterior chamber IOL is inserted secondarily, it infers that the posterior capsule is intact or almost intact. The lens cannot be inserted into the capsular bag because the anterior leaflet of anterior capsule has become fibrosed to the posterior capsule; hence sulcus fixation is the only means available to the surgeon. The surgeon should ascertain that there is access to the sulcus in the desired axis of insertion. Sometimes fibrosis between the posterior iris stroma and posterior capsule can impair this access, and the potential space for insertion should be tested with a spatula. Assuming that it is feasible, the technique is the same as for the nondialing primary insertion technique. I say nondialing because any rotary motion inserting the upper loop of the lens may encounter iris capsular adhesions, as noted previously.

I have the clinical impression that there is less capsular fixation of a posterior chamber IOL after a secondary insertion than with a primary insertion.

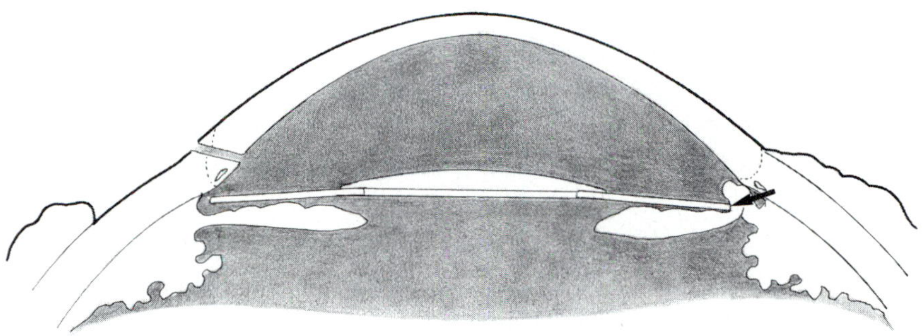

FIGURE 10-14. Anterior iris tuck, *arrow*.

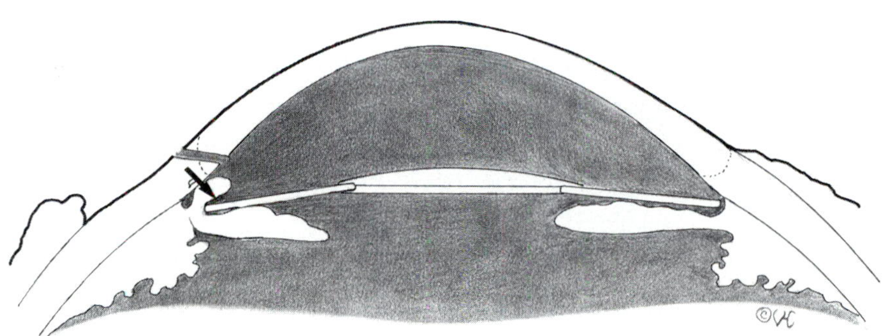

FIGURE 10-15. Posterior iris tuck, *arrow*.

Soft Intraocular Lenses

In an attempt to insert an IOL through a 3 mm phacoemulsification incision, the profession has seen the introduction of IOLs fabricated from soft plastic materials, which may be folded. Current materials include silicones, polymethylmethacrylate (PMMA), hydrogels, and xerogels, the last hydrating within the eye.

Foldable IOL designs in clinical use at this time are posterior chamber IOLs of either the conventional J-loop design (see Fig. 10-19, *A*) or a one-piece design reminiscent of earlier anterior chamber IOLs. Neither design is capable of insertion through a 3 mm incision; at least 4 mm is required, and more in higher dioptric powers. Insertion requires mandatory use of a VES and a lens-folding instrument. The lens is folded (Fig. 10-16), the instrument is then turned horizontally and inserted through the incision (Fig. 10-17), and in this position the inferior haptic is placed in the posterior chamber. The instrument is now rotated to a vertical position and disengaged from the IOL, which unfolds (Fig. 10-18), whereupon the lens holder is withdrawn from the eye. The superior haptic is maneuvered into position by iris retraction and manipulation of the IOL (see p. 228).

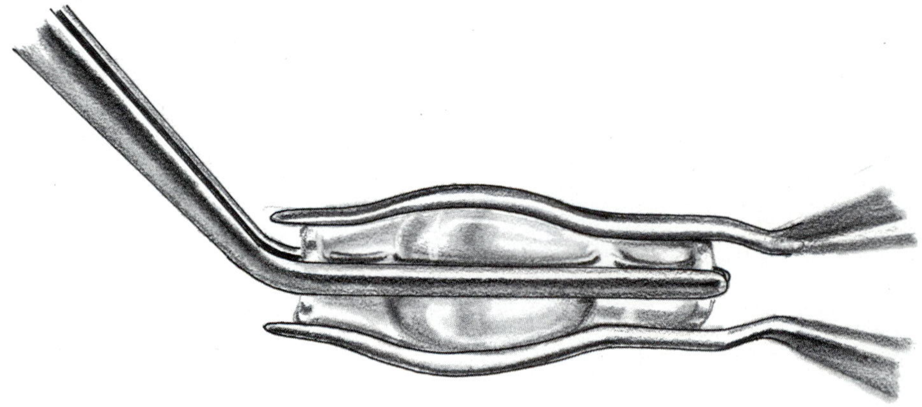

FIGURE 10-16. Implant being folded.

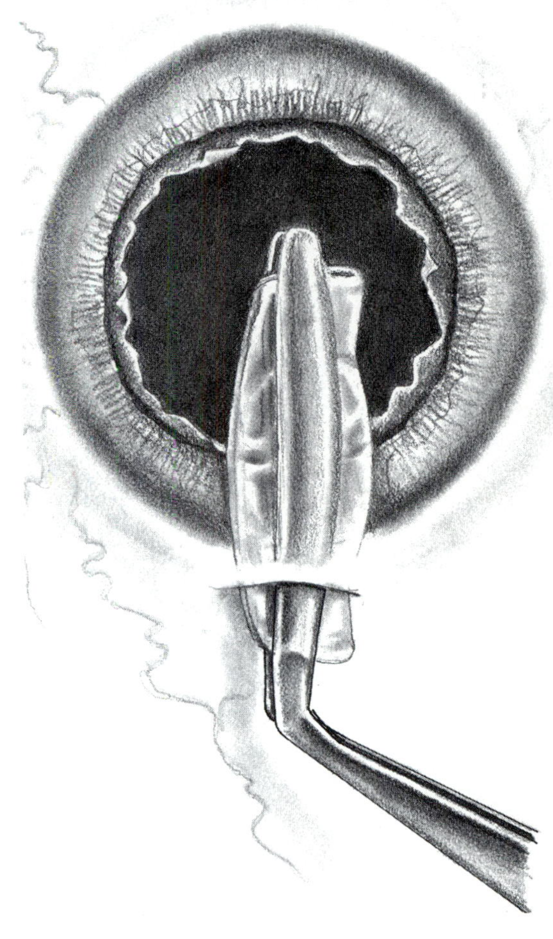

FIGURE 10-17. Implant being inserted through small insertion.

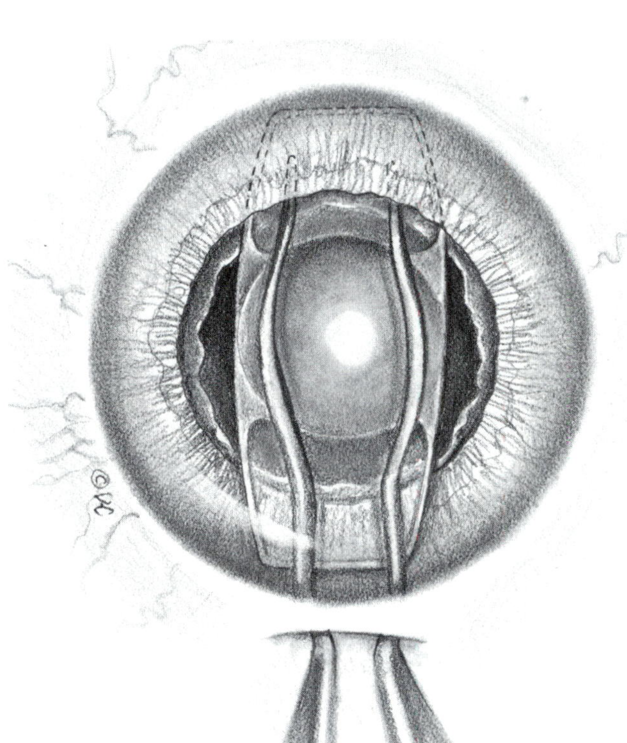

FIGURE 10-18. Implant inserted.

An alternative folder is shown in Fig. 10-19.

There is some debate as to whether foldable posterior chamber IOLs should be placed "in the bag" or in the ciliary sulcus. There are cases where capsular fibrosis has caused soft IOLs to tilt within the eye and spontaneously extrude into the anterior chamber. This is more common with one-piece designs, since the "J loops" generally absorb the compressive forces of the capsule. As yet, there is no consensus.

Whether soft intraocular lenses, *in their present status,* offer any significant advantage over conventional posterior chamber IOLs is debatable, especially given the excellent results achieved with the latter. The inability of foldable IOLs to pass through a 3 mm phacoemulsification incision and the maneuvers involved in the intracameral unfolding and positioning are, in my view, an impediment to their general use. The profession also needs to be reassured, by long-term results, that such IOLs are a real patient benefit. On the other hand, if by selection of thinner materials (that is, of higher refractive index) and reduction of the horizontal IOL diameter this lens could be inserted through a phacoemulsification incision, such lenses would be a great advantage. Additionally, if the lens were to be provided prefolded in an inserter, this would significantly assist the surgeon. This presumes that the lens is nondeformable and will return to its intended shape, even with maximum shelf life.

Soft IOLs and associated surgical techniques will need to evolve in the same way that conventional IOLs have done before the best design and technique become apparent.

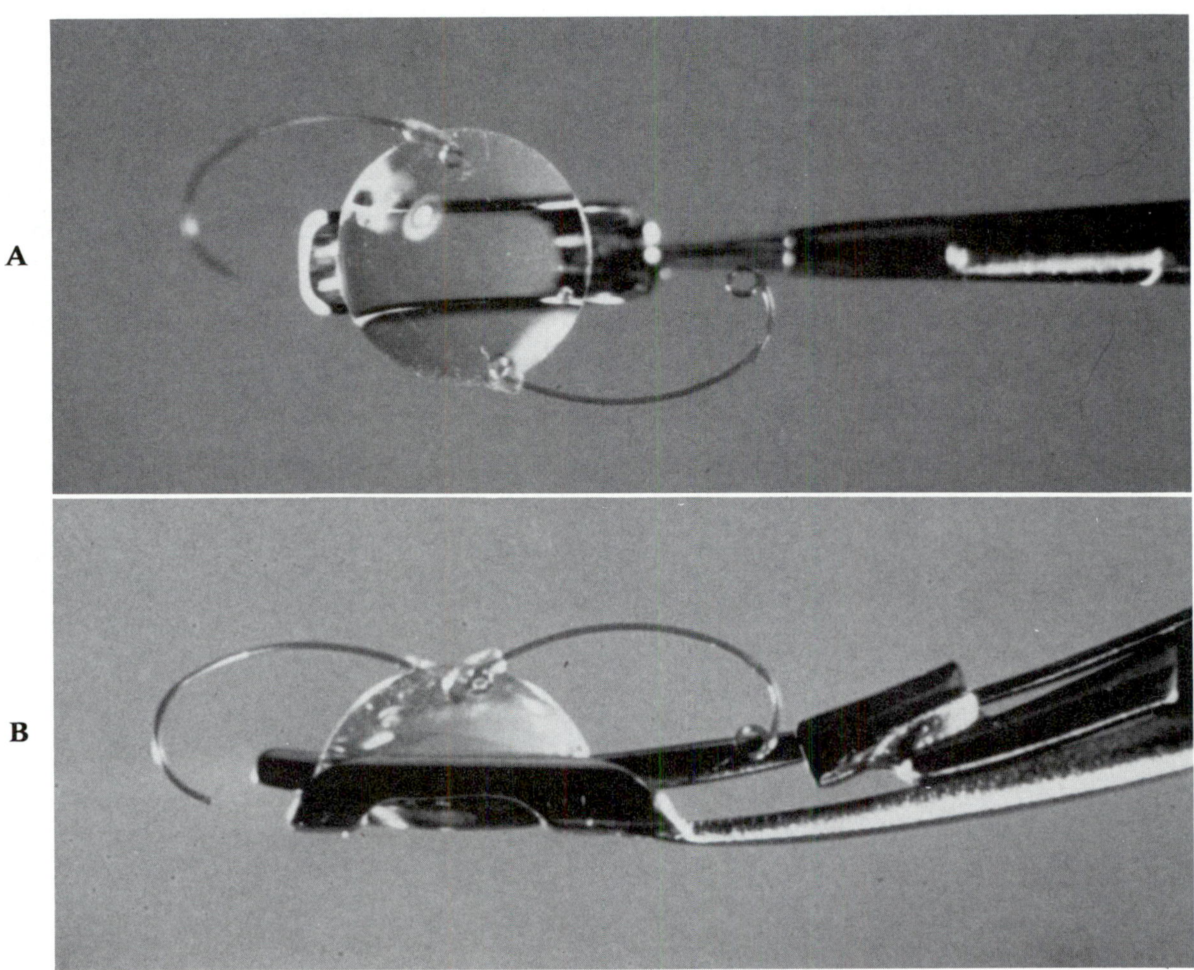

FIGURE 10-19. Alternative type of folder. (Courtesy Allergan Medical Optics, Irvine, Calif.)

Intraocular Lens Complications

The most common reason for removal of a posterior chamber lens is incorrect power. If the lens was fixed within the capsular bag, it is imprudent to remove the lens in toto in one maneuver because this may deliver the capsular bag as well. Since it is usually the power of the lens that is the cause for removal, my preferred technique is to amputate the optic from the loops and remove it from the eye. Sometimes the loops will slide out of a fibrous tunnel in the bag, and sometimes they will not. If the case is the latter, the replacement intraocular lens is placed in the ciliary sulcus, a position avoiding the axis of the original haptic loops, which are left within the eye.

Intraoperative Complication—Sunset Syndrome

The sunset syndrome generally occurs in the immediate postoperative period after posterior chamber lens insertion. The lens, initially correctly centered, on subsequent visits appears lower and lower in the pupillary aperture, like the sun sinking below the horizon, hence the "setting-sun syndrome" (Fig. 10-20). The reason is a capsular or zonular defect occurring at surgery either undiagnosed or concealed from the surgeon's view. The posterior chamber IOL slowly sinks through this defect into the vitreous cavity.

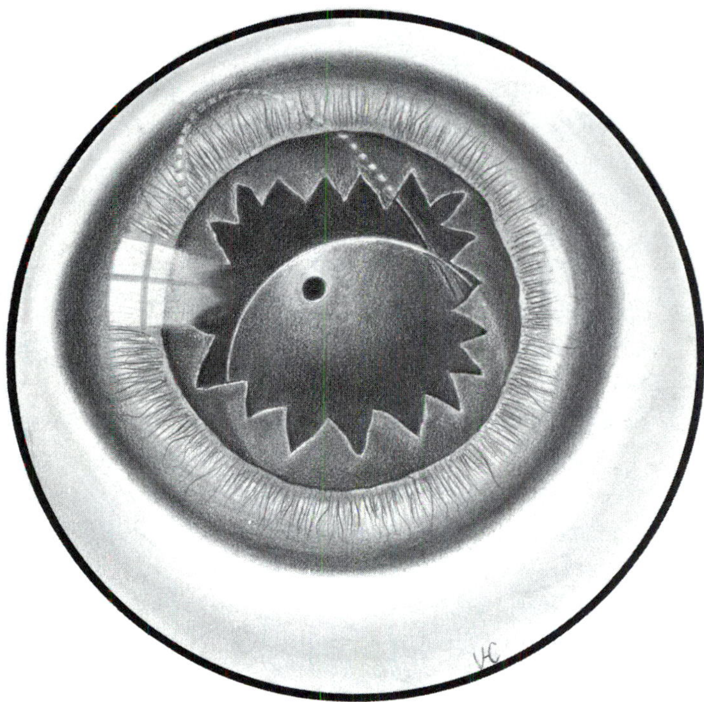

FIGURE 10-20. Sunset syndrome.

When the diagnosis is made, intervention should be prompt. The easiest corrective maneuver, if the lens can be grasped, is to induce an iatrogenic pupillary capture. The lens is brought up into the pupillary aperture and positioned so that the optic is anterior to the iris but the haptic loops remain posterior (Fig. 10-21, *A*). The iris fixates the lens in position (Fig. 10-21, *B*). As the lens is brought into the pupillary aperture, it may be rotated with a dialing hook if required to achieve this capture. A second possibility is to remove the lens entirely and replace it with an anterior chamber lens, there already being presumptive evidence of inadequate capsular fixation. A third possibility is the use of the McCannel suture. With a McCannel suture, bring the implant to the pupillary aperture to secure the suture there. A stab wound is made in the limbus just peripherally to clear the cornea in a position closest to the superior loop, which in the case of a posterior chamber lens is behind the iris. A 9-0 or 10-0 polypropylene suture on a half-curve cutting needle is passed through this incision, avoiding penetration of the lips of the incision. The needle is then passed through the iris, around the loop, and out through the anterior surface of the iris. The lens may have to be steadied with an instrument in the left hand as this is done. The needle is then regrasped and passed through clear cornea (Fig. 10-22). The needle is excised from the suture, a hook is inserted through the incision, and the portion of suture that has penetrated the cornea is pulled back through the original incision (Fig. 10-23). The suture then is tied and trimmed, with the net effect being that the superior loop of the lens is sutured to the iris. This whole procedure is facilitated by the use of a VES. The McCannel suture technique can be used for any mobile intraocular lens using the appropriate haptic loop. See p. 432 for posterior segment techniques.

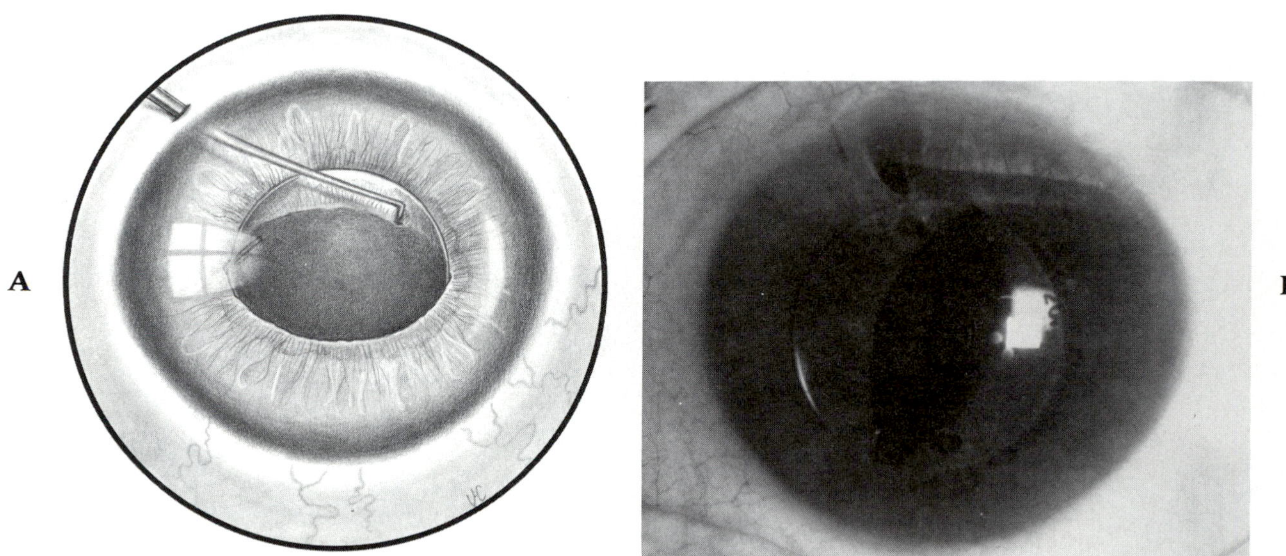

FIGURE 10-21. **A,** Induction of iatrogenic pupillary capture. **B,** Pupillary capture of posterior chamber intraocular lens.

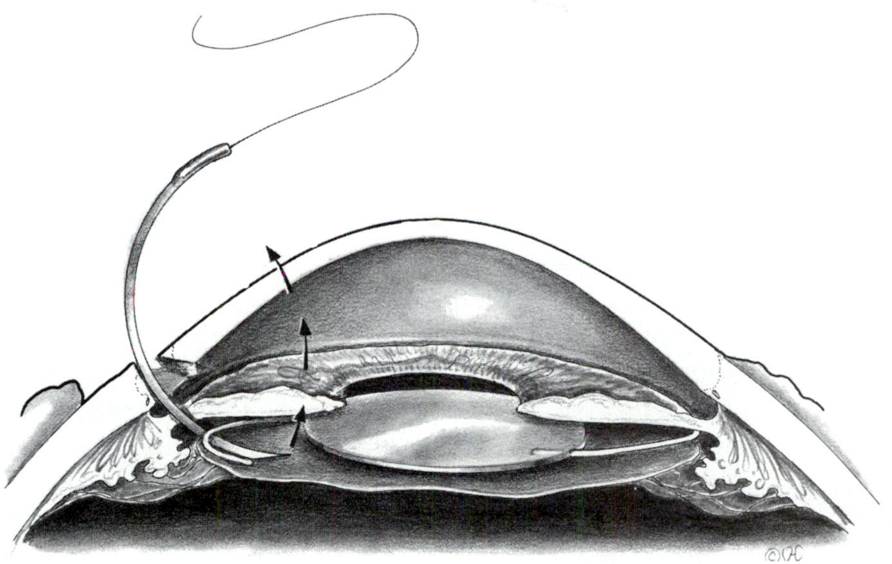

FIGURE 10-22. McCannel suture technique—initial passage of needle.

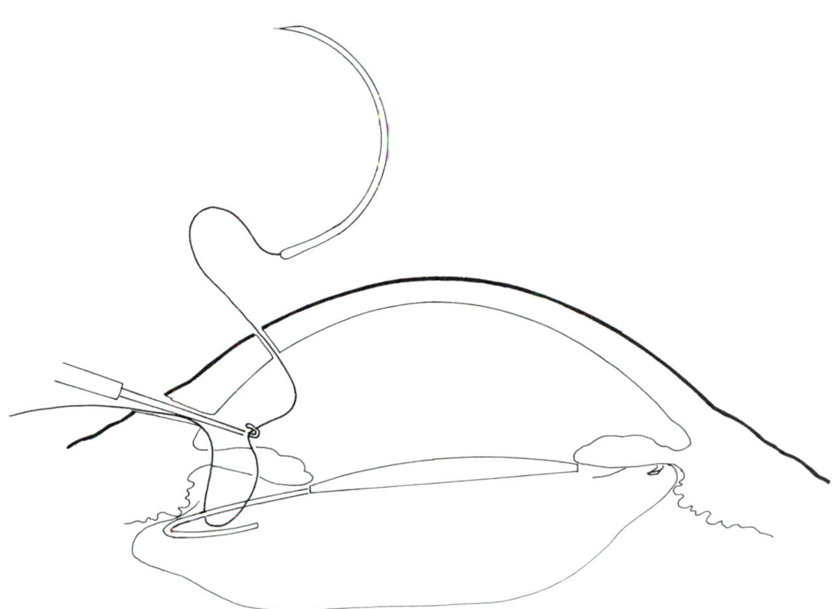

FIGURE 10-23. Retrieval of McCannel suture before tying.

Intraoperative Complication—Windshield-Wiper Syndrome

In the windshield-wiper syndrome a posterior chamber intraocular lens oscillates with the patient's head movements (Fig. 10-24). The cause is inadequate IOL fixation possibly compounded by an IOL that is too short. The treatment is IOL fixation with a McCannel suture as noted on p. 244. The superior loop of the implant is pulled into the peripheral iridectomy (Fig. 10-25), where it is secured by the McCannel suture. In cases where there is no peripheral iridectomy, one can be made adjacent to the stab incision for the McCannel suture. Alternatively, a viscoelastic substance can be injected into the anterior chamber, anterior to the iris overlying the superior haptic loop. This has the effect of depressing the iris against the loop, thus defining its outline through the iris. A McCannel suture is now placed, fixating the haptic loop to the iris.

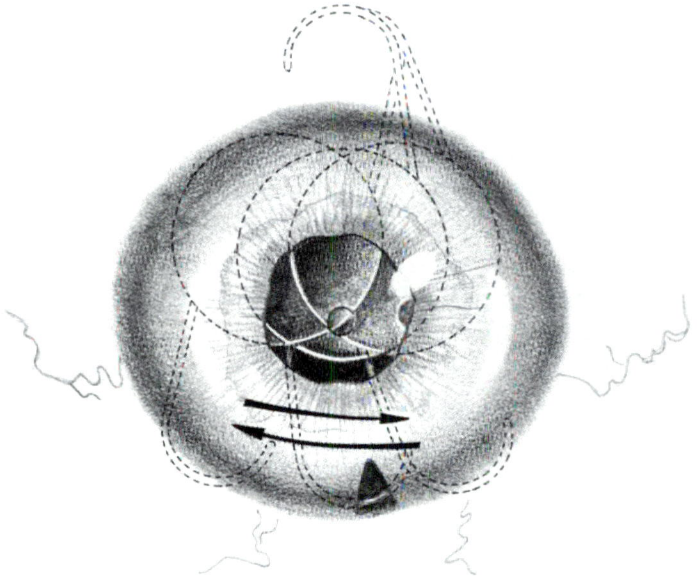

FIGURE 10-24. Posterior chamber intraocular lens exhibiting "windshield wiper" movement.

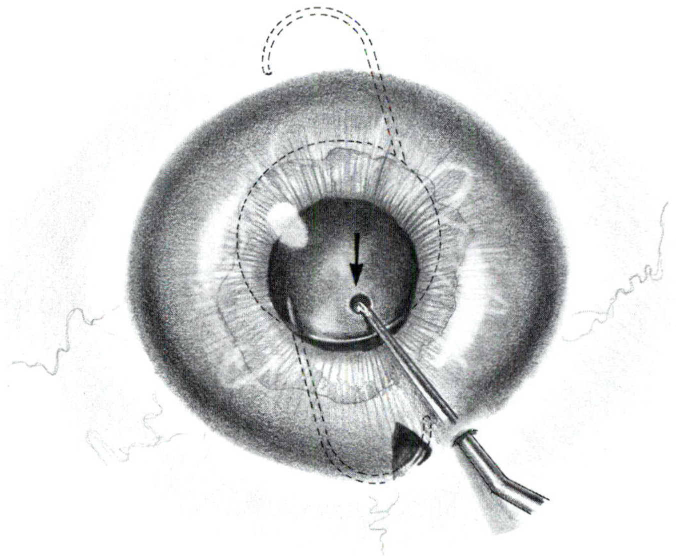

FIGURE 10-25. Intraocular lens is positioned so that the superior haptic is adjacent to the peripheral iridectomy as a preliminary step to the passage of a McCannel suture.

Intraoperative Complication—Descemet's Detachment

Frequently a small detachment of Descemet's membrane may be seen in the area of the limbal corneal cataract incision, and this is of no concern. A sizable detachment of Descemet's membrane is clinically significant and will result in persistent corneal edema in the area over the detachment if left untreated. Trauma to Descemet's membrane can be caused by any intracameral instrumentation; however its incidence has been lessened by the availability of viscoelastic substances. When this complication does occur, prompt recognition is desirable so that it may be rectified while the patient is still in the operating room. Late recognition necessitates a second operation.

Repair of a Descemet's detachment may be accomplished by an intracameral injection of air or a VES at a site remote from the detachment (Fig. 10-26). The purpose is to unfurl the detachment, and with a VES the viscosity of the injected bolus is sufficient. The use of air often requires the globe to be rotated superiorly to prevent air from getting between the detachment and the residual cornea. As the air bubble comes into contact with the Descemet's flap, the globe is rotated inferiorly so that the air bubble is caused to rise, floating the detachment back into its correct position. Through-and-through 10-0 nylon or polypropylene sutures may be required to fix a large Descemet's detachment (Fig. 10-27).

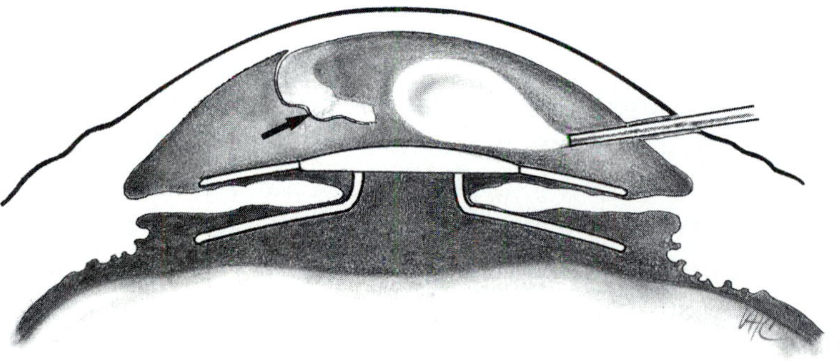

FIGURE 10-26. Injection of air or a viscoelastic substance (VES) to unfurl and reposition a detached Descemet's membrane.

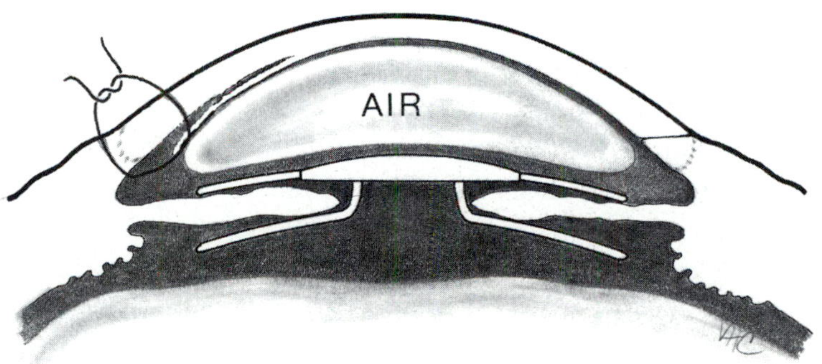

FIGURE 10-27. Full-thickness corneal suturing to reattach a large detachment of Descemet's membrane. The air or VES is left in situ and so requires monitoring of the intraocular pressure.

Intraoperative Complication—Removal of Intraocular Lenses

The most common reason nowadays for the removal of an intraocular lens is the low-grade uveitis with macular edema and sometimes corneal edema seen with closed-loop semiflexible anterior chamber intraocular lenses. These lenses have now had additional core restrictions placed on them by the Food and Drug Administration and have fallen into disuse within the profession. When a closed-loop lens has to be removed, one makes a superior incision that corresponds generally to the location of the superior loop. It is advisable first to make a small stab incision, drain a small quantity of aqueous, and then insert a bolus of VES. It is also helpful to inject a small quantity of intracameral acetylcholine for miosis. The superior incision is then enlarged, and an attempt is made to deliver the superior loop. Sometimes iris must be dissected free from this loop, but generally it can be lifted out of the angle and delivered to the incision. The problem is with the delivery of the inferior loop, which is often fibrosed to the inferior angle (Fig. 10-28). If the lens will not deliver with gentle traction, one or both inferior loops must be amputated. In this maneuver, with the chamber formed with a VES, Wescott scissors are introduced, and each individual loop is excised as required. The intraocular lens is then removed from the eye (Fig. 10-29). The residual portion of the inferior loop frequently can be grasped with forceps and then slid out of the angle, where it is encased in a fibrous tunnel of tissue (Fig. 10-29). It is also removed from the eye. When manipulation of the inferior loop is hazardous and if a hyphema occurs, it is prudent to leave the loop in situ. The surgeon is cautioned that the original amputation should be such that residual tips of the loop do not excoriate the cornea. If it is the surgeon's intention to insert another model anterior chamber lens, reference should be made to the secondary technique, which is described on p. 236. Special problems occur with semiflexible closed-loop anterior chamber lenses where there are four individual closed loops. The superior loops can usually be freed from the angle, but the inferior loops are invariably fibrosed. The technique is as described previously. However, the surgeon has to do it twice, once for each individual inferior loop. Semiflexible, anterior chamber intraocular lenses are also discussed on pp. 34 and 434.

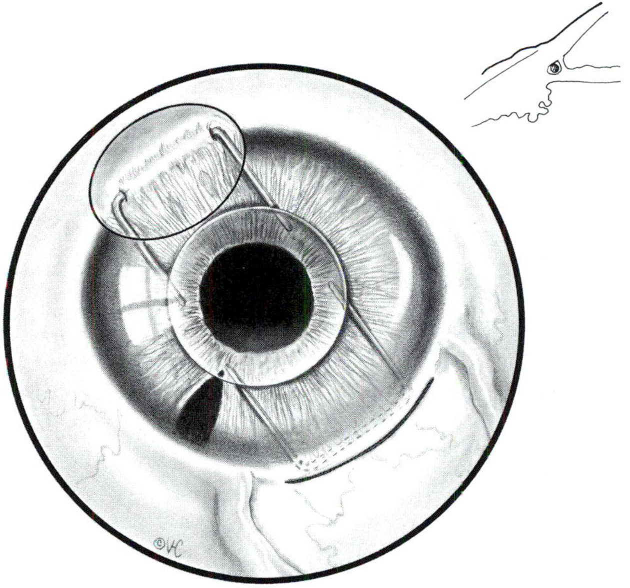

FIGURE 10-28. Semiflexible anterior chamber intraocular lens in situ with fibrosis of inferior loop in angle.

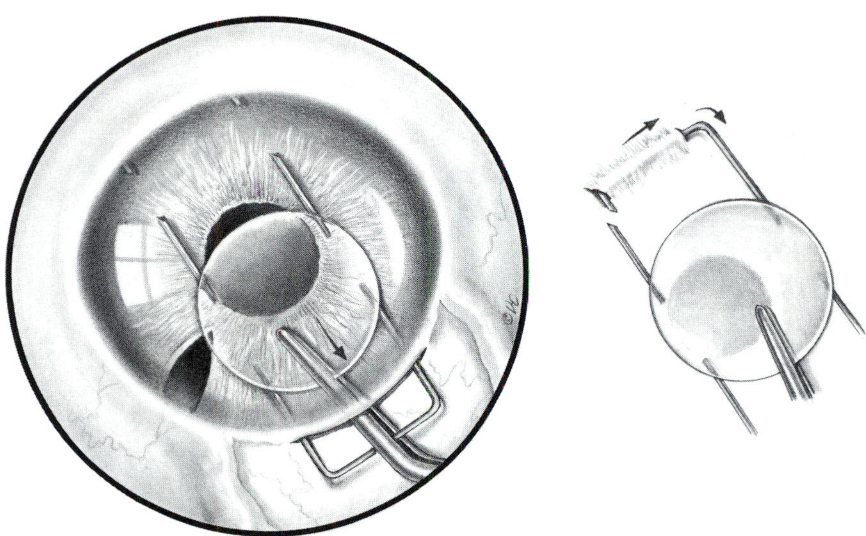

FIGURE 10-29. Amputation of inferior loop.

PART THREE

GLAUCOMA SURGERY

Raymond Harrison
Maurice H. Luntz

CHAPTER 11

Essentials of Glaucoma Surgery

DEFINITION

The term "glaucoma" denotes a variety of pathologic conditions in which the optic nerve is eventually damaged and loss of visual field ensues because of intolerance of intraocular pressure. A vulnerable optic nerve head can suffer glaucomatous damage despite intraocular pressures within the usual accepted normal range. However, intraocular pressures above that range may never damage an optic nerve. In general, the aim of treatment of glaucoma is to lower the intraocular pressure enough to arrest the progress of the disease. Surgical intervention is indicated when tolerated medical treatment is ineffective or when the mechanism of the increased intraocular pressure is attributable to closure of the angle.

PATIENT EVALUATION AND PREPARATION

In glaucoma surgery, the patient's general medical condition is of great significance. A thorough preoperative medical history and physical examination are essential. Tests should include complete blood count, blood chemistry profile, urinalysis, electrocardiogram, and chest x-ray examination. Control of diabetes and hypertension and correction of hypokalemia in patients taking carbonic anhydrase inhibitors or diuretics are commonly needed. Long-term use of cholinesterase inhibitors should alert the anesthesiologist to danger of succinylcholine-induced apnea. Preoperative hyperosmotic therapy may be contraindicated if the patient has cardiac disease. These are but a few examples of the importance of medical evaluation.

Local or general anesthesia may be chosen, depending on the patient's medical status and temperament, as well as the surgeon's preference. With local anesthesia, a Van Lint block is sufficient for lid akinesia. A retrobulbar or peribulbar block with lidocaine (Xylocaine) 2.0% and bupivacaine (Marcaine) 0.5%, mixed in equal parts, is usually effective. Lidocaine 1.0% alone is adequate for short procedures. Subconjunctival injection of local anesthetic is not necessary, though it may aid in dissection of a conjunctival flap to display unscarred conjunctiva if there has been previous surgery. General anesthesia is preferred for combined cataract surgery and glaucoma filtration, as well as for aphakic eyes undergoing filtering surgery. A more detailed description of local anesthesia is given in Chapter 7.

Preparation of the operative field is begun by free irrigation of both eyes and cleansing of the skin with saline. A soap solution is then applied to the skin. After removal of the soap, Betadine (povidone-iodine complex) is applied. Finally, the skin is wiped with alcohol. If local anesthesia is used, tetracaine is instilled in both eyes before the preparation. A Barraquer wire speculum or adjustable Pierse speculum is applied. A plastic drape (Steridrape) is applied to cover the eyelids, skin, and eyelashes, exposing only the conjunctiva. Antibiotic ophthalmic solution (such as gentamicin) is instilled before the surgery is started.

Fig. 11-1 shows the limbal area with a half-thickness scleral flap reflected. The surgical landmarks are transparent cornea, a bluish gray band of trabecular meshwork, and a white opaque sclera. The junction of trabecular meshwork and sclera is the external indication of the deeper lying scleral spur. Schlemm's canal is in proximity to the scleral spur. The canal may be just anterior to the scleral spur or just posterior or at the scleral spur. This point is usually 2 to 2.5 mm behind the surgical limbus.

Fig. 11-2 outlines the chamber angle anatomy. The trabecular meshwork is not morphologically uniform. The uveal meshwork originates within connective tissue of the iris root. Radially oriented strands encompass large polygonal holes. The corneoscleral meshwork forms the bulk of the trabecular meshwork. Equatorially oriented plates form a lattice of rhombic spaces. Each plate is covered with endothelial cells and has a core of collagenous and elastic fibers under tension. The cribriform portion is the outermost trabecular meshwork and supports the inner wall of Schlemm's canal with a loosely arranged fiber system.

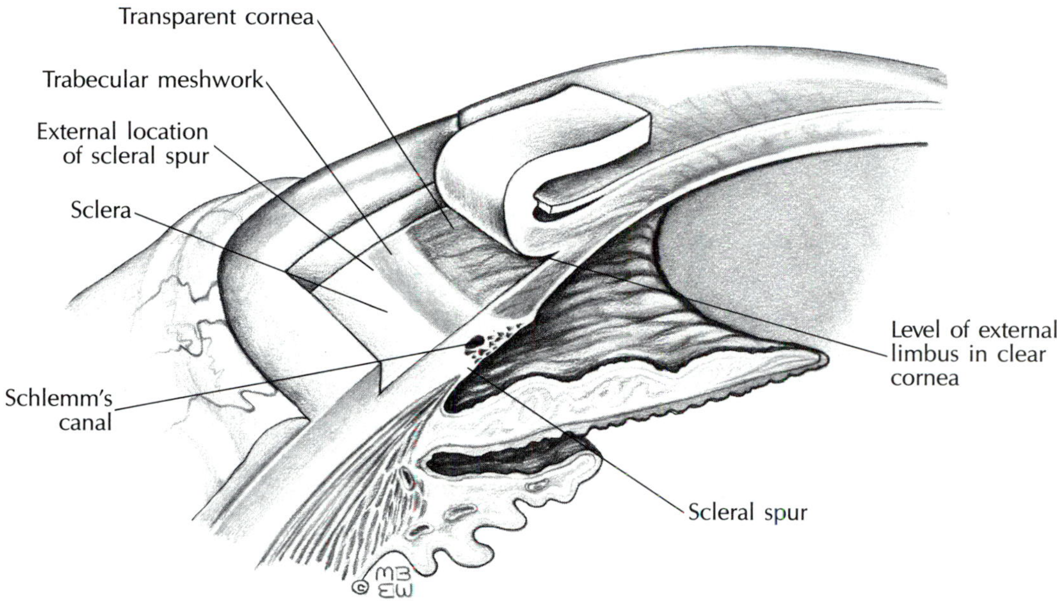

FIGURE 11-1. Limbal area and scleral flap.

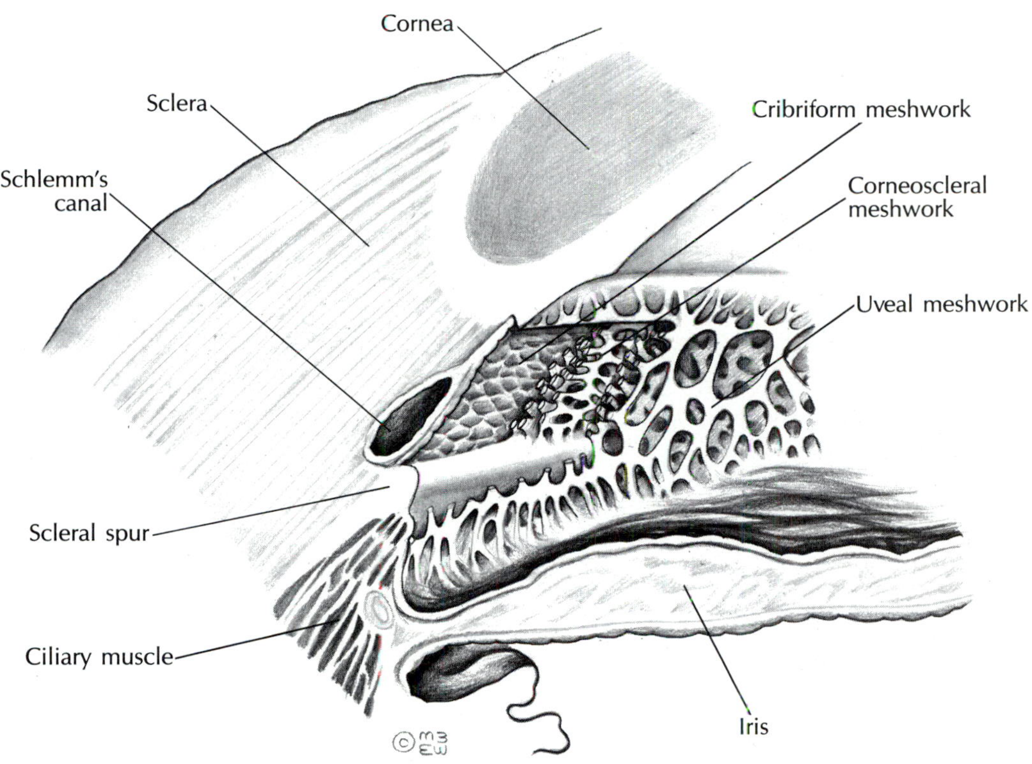

FIGURE 11-2. Chamber angle anatomy.

CHAPTER 12

Congenital Infantile and Juvenile Glaucoma

The following procedures will be considered in this chapter: (a) goniotomy, (b) trabeculotomy, and (c) combined trabeculotomy and trabeculectomy. Other filtering procedures are described in Chapter 13, cyclocryotherapy in Chapter 14, and seton implantation in Chapter 14.

CHOICE OF SURGERY AND PROGNOSIS

The earlier in life developmental glaucoma presents, the worse is the prognosis. On the other hand, surgery is generally more successful when performed as early as possible.

The corneal diameter is of no prognostic significance, but the appearance of the anterior chamber angle can be related to success of surgery.

Angle anomalies are divided into three groups:

Group 1. Presumed mesodermal anomaly (Luntz) or trabecular dysgenesis (Hoskin). The trabecular meshwork alone is involved. The cornea and iris are normal. The angle anomaly may be the result of a deposit of mesodermal tissue. These eyes have the best prognosis for surgery, either goniotomy or trabeculotomy, with intraocular pressure control of 90%.

Group 2. Cicatricial angle (Luntz) or iridotrabecular dysgenesis (Hoskins). The anomaly involves trabecular meshwork and peripheral iris, possibly the result of a cicatrizing process in the periphery of the anterior chamber angle. These eyes have a far poorer prognosis with surgery, particularly goniotomy or trabeculotomy, which have a success rate of approximately 30%, compared with those in group 1. Trabeculectomy or combined trabeculotomy-trabeculectomy has a success rate of approximately 50%. In those that fail with filtration surgery, a seton, such as a Molteno plastic implant, is indicated.

Group 3. Iridotrabecular-corneal dysgenesis (Luntz, Hoskins) in which the anomaly involves cornea, trabecular meshwork, and iris. Examples of this group are Rieger's phenomenon and Peter's anomaly. These eyes have a poor prognosis with trabeculotomy or goniotomy. They do better with trabeculectomy. Many, however, eventually require a seton.

Even with implantation of a seton, the prognosis in groups 2 and 3 probably does not exceed a 60% success rate.

Trabeculotomy is preferred to goniotomy for the following reasons:

1. Trabeculotomy has a higher success rate than goniotomy, controlling intraocular pressure in over 90% of eyes with congenital glaucoma of all degrees of severity.
2. Trabeculotomy does not require the introduction of sharp instruments across the anterior chamber, with attendant risk of damage to other ocular tissues. It can be performed with undiminished accuracy in advanced cases where the cornea is edematous or scarred, with poor visibility in the anterior chamber.
3. A trabeculotomy is anatomically more precise in creating an opening between the anterior chamber and Schlemm's canal. The radius of the arc swept by the goniotomy knife is twice that of the chamber angle.
4. The surgeon does not have to adapt to the visual distortion produced by the operating gonioprism.

Anesthesia

The patient is usually a child, and general anesthesia is preferred. Ketamine should be avoided, because it may increase intraocular pressure.

Before surgery is begun, a careful measurement of the intraocular pressure and corneal diameter, evaluation of the clinical state of the cornea and of the appearance of the iris and lens, and gonioscopy must be done. The optic disc is examined, if not already described. The axial length of the eye is measured by A-scan ultrasonography. The electrophysiologic activity of the retina and optic nerve is determined by photopic and scotopic electroretinogram and visual-evoked potential, if available.

Surgical Technique for Goniotomy

Goniotomy lenses

The most frequently used goniotomy lenses are the Worst, Barkan, and Swan-Jacob lenses (Fig. 12-1, *A*).

Technique

The goniotomy lens is placed on the cornea and, in the case of the Worst lens, secured with 7-0 silk sutures to the perilimbal episcleral tissue. (A Barkan lens is not sutured.) A suitable goniotomy knife, usually the Barraquer or Worst goniotomy knife, is selected, and the cannula is connected to a polyvinyl chloride (PVC) tube to a 5 ml syringe or an intravenous infusion bottle containing balanced salt solution. All air bubbles are removed from the system. The bottle is hung approximately 100 to 150 cm above the eye, and the knife is checked for a suitable rate of infusion, adjusted by the height of the bottle or the force with which the syringe plunger is depressed. Using a surgical microscope at a magnification of 10, one inserts the knife into the anterior chamber through the cornea immediately anterior to the limbus. Under direct visualization, the surgeon ensures a deep anterior chamber and advances the knife across the anterior chamber parallel to the plane of the iris but clear of the iris and lens surface until reaching the trabecular meshwork in the angle area opposite to the point of insertion (Fig. 12-1, *B*). The knife is farther advanced until its point enters the trabecular meshwork, and it is then rotated to the left and to the right, incising an area of approximately one third the circumference of the angle. The incision should be into the trabecular meshwork just anterior to the insertion of the iris (Fig. 12-1, *C*). As the knife incises the trabecular meshwork, the iris falls backwards, and the angle deepens. Great care should be taken to avoid incarcerating the iris in the knife edge or damaging the lens. If iris is incarcerated, the knife should be withdrawn and then replaced. When bleeding occurs, the rate of fluid infusion into the chamber should be increased to clear the bleeding from the area of surgery and to tampon the bleeding vessel. If the saline infusion leaks too rapidly from the anterior chamber and fails to tampon the bleeder, a large air bubble is introduced into the anterior chamber to stop the bleeding. Once the incision is completed and the chamber is deepened, the knife is carefully withdrawn from the eye, with care being taken to avoid injury to the iris or lens. At the end of the procedure, the anterior chamber is filled with balanced salt solution or air to maintain a deep chamber. The goniotomy lens is removed from the eye. A viscoelastic substance may be used in this procedure.

A drop of an antibiotic-corticosteroid preparation is instilled into the conjunctival sac, and a patch and shield are applied to the eye.

The eye is dressed the day after surgery, when the anterior chamber should be deep and the pupil active. Topical antibiotic-corticosteroid drops are continued until the anterior chamber reaction resolves.

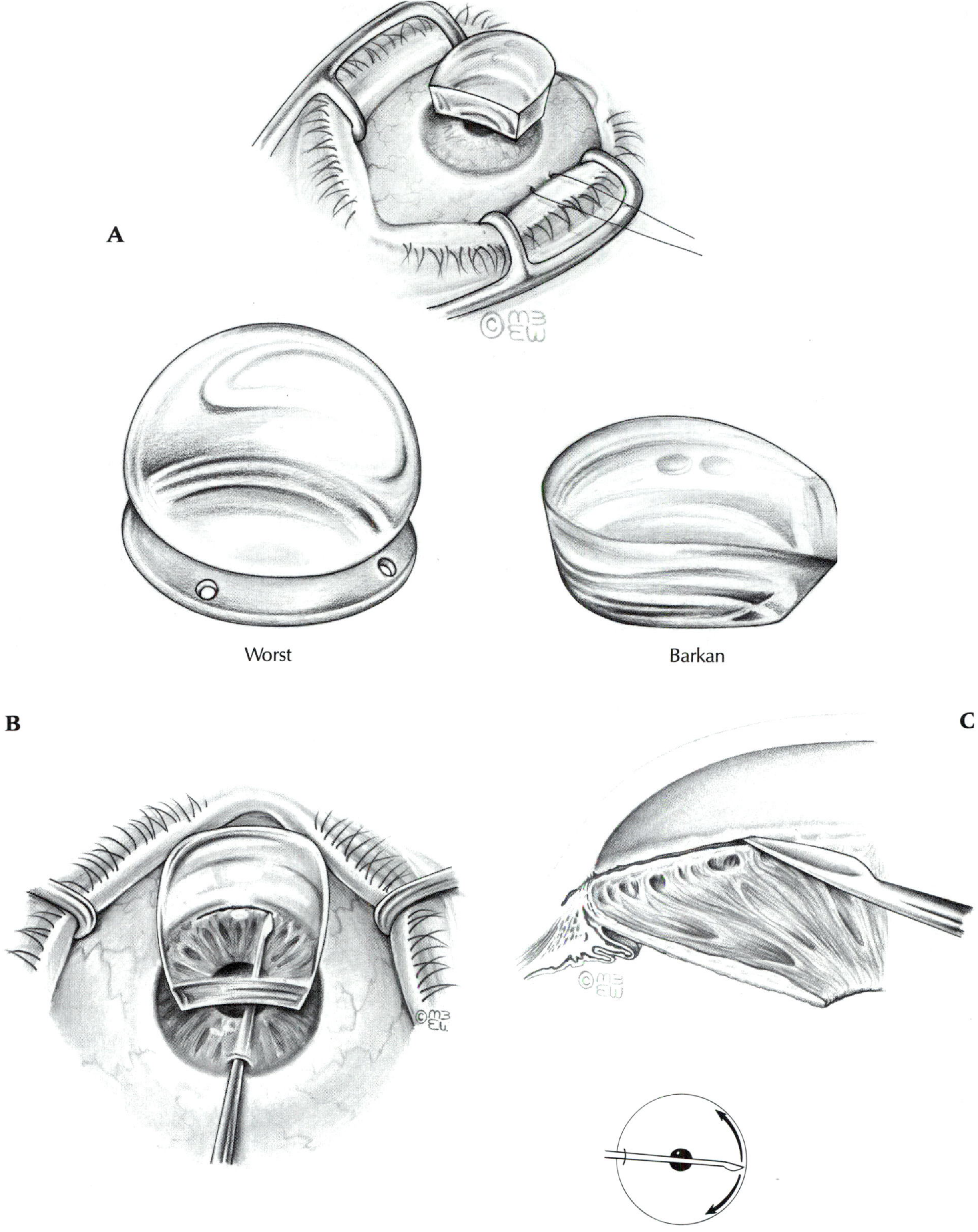

FIGURE 12-1. **A,** Goniotomy lenses. **B,** Incision into trabecular meshwork. **C,** Incision into anterior meshwork. (From Ritch R, Shields MB, Krupin T: The glaucomas, St Louis, 1989, The CV Mosby Co.)

Surgical Technique for Trabeculotomy

Conjunctival flap (magnification of 5)

The fornix-based 7 mm length conjunctival flap is raised at the limbus (see also p. 172). The dissection is continued to the sclera, raising the conjunctiva, Tenon's fascia, and episclera. In this manner, a triangular portion of sclera is exposed, at a measure of at least 3 mm from its base at the surgical limbus to its apex (Fig. 12-2). The surface of the sclera is cleaned.

Rotation of the globe may be facilitated when 4-0 Mersilene sutures are passed through the lamellar thickness of sclera at each edge of the conjunctival flap at the surgical limbus.

Scleral dissection (magnification of 10)

Using a microblade or a diamond knife, one makes an incision through half the scleral depth, extending from the surgical limbus at the midpoint of the exposed sclera posteriorly for 3 mm (Fig. 12-3, *A*). Holding one edge of this incision with forceps and rotating it outward to allow greater visibility, one deepens the scleral incision until deep corneal lamellae become visible in the depths of the anterior half of the incision (Fig. 12-3, *B*). At this point, the incision is undermined on each side to increase the surgical exposure (Fig. 12-3, *C*). Once the undermining has been completed, the surgeon has a view of the external surgical landmarks and can proceed to the next step, which is the dissection of the external wall of the canal of Schlemm. These surgical landmarks are illustrated in Fig. 11-1.

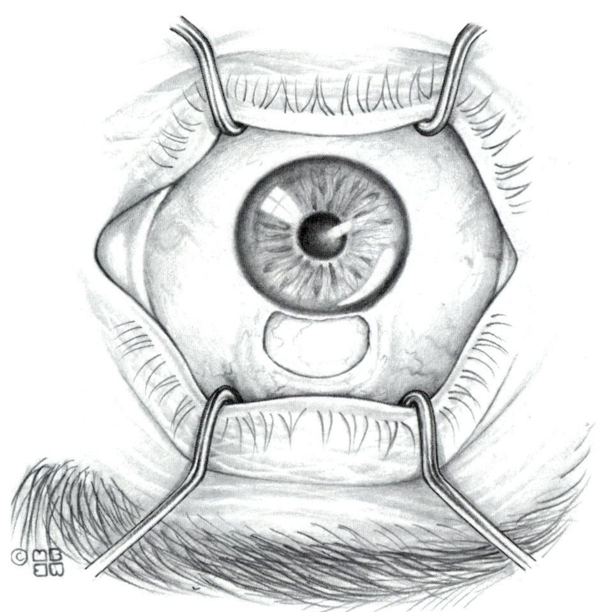

FIGURE 12-2. Fornix-based conjunctival flap.

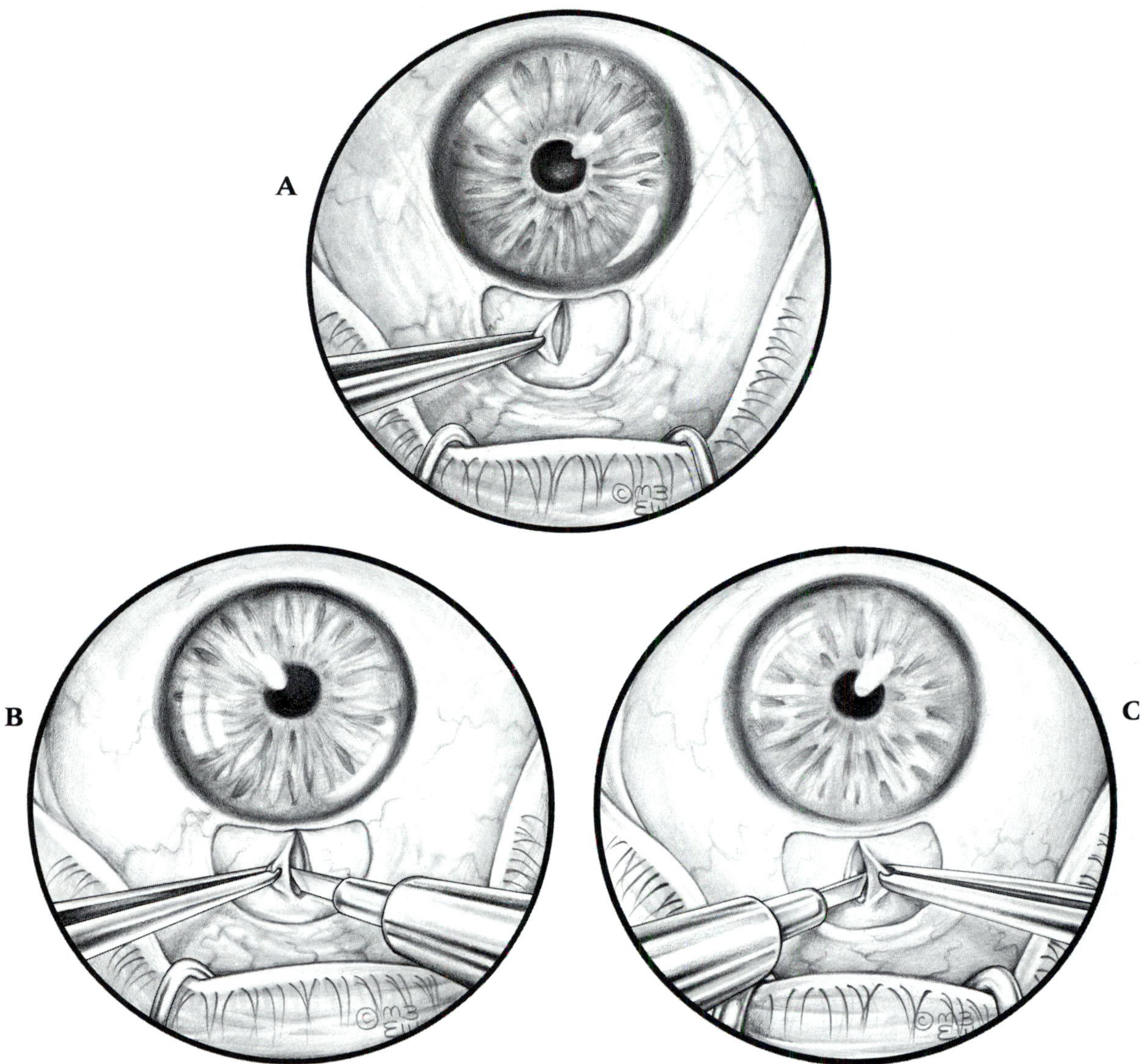

FIGURE 12-3. **A,** Scleral incision. **B,** Deepening scleral incision. **C,** Undermining sclerotomy incision. (From Ritch R, Shields MB, Krupin T: The glaucomas, St Louis, 1989, The CV Mosby Co.)

Dissection into canal (magnification of 15)

Having recognized these landmarks, the next step is to make a vertical incision using a diamond knife or a microblade (such as a no. 75 Beaver blade) across the scleral spur at the junction of the lower margin of the trabecular band and the scleral tissue (Fig. 12-4, *A*). This incision is carefully deepened until it is carried through the external wall of Schlemm's canal, at which point there is a flow of aqueous humor and occasionally aqueous mixed with blood. The dissection is carefully continued through the external wall until the inner wall of the canal becomes visible. The inner wall is characteristically slightly pigmented. Once this point is reached, one blade of a Vannas scissors is passed along the canal, with the other blade lying superficial to the external wall. When the blade of the Vannas scissors is introduced, it should enter with ease and slide along the canal. Otherwise, further dissection through the entered wall is required to avoid production of a false passage. Two parallel cuts are made, and a strip of the external wall of the canal is excised. The canal is opened for 1 to 1.5 mm circumferentially (Fig. 12-4, *B* and *C*). The inner wall of the canal is characteristically pigmented.

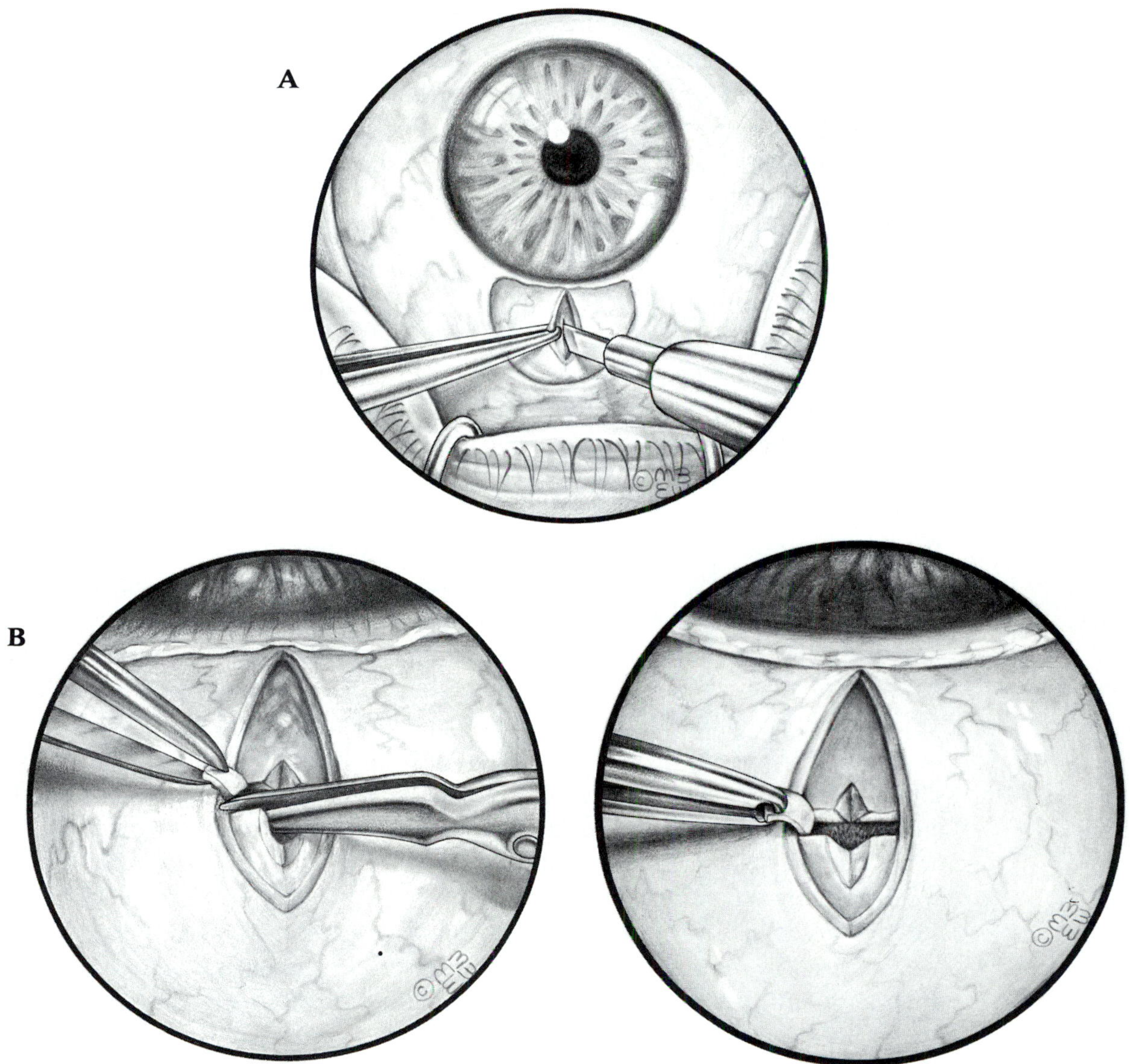

FIGURE 12-4. **A,** Vertical incision across scleral spur. **B,** Vannas scissors blade passed along canal. **C,** Schlemm's canal unroofed. (From Ritch R, Shields MB, Krupin T: The glaucomas, St Louis, 1989, The CV Mosby Co.)

Introduction of trabeculotomy probe (magnification of 5)

A trabeculotomy probe we prefer is shown in Fig. 12-5, *A*. The lower blade has a diameter of 0.20 mm and fits into the canal; the upper blade runs over the limbus and is separated by 1 mm from the lower blade. The upper blade is kept resting on the cornea, thereby ensuring that the lower blade does not press downward through the inner wall of the canal or ride upward, creating a false passage. The shaft of the probe is divided into three segments, so that the central third can be stabilized with the left hand while the right hand rotates the upper and lower thirds around the central third, rotating the probe into the anterior chamber (Fig. 12-5, *B*). This method will avoid anterior or posterior movement of the probe tip and so avoid iris trauma or disruption of corneal lamellae.

The probe is passed along the canal to the nasal side and rotated into the anterior chamber, thus opening this portion of the inner wall of the canal (Fig. 12-5, *C*). The same process is repeated on the other side, again with the probe rotated into the anterior chamber (Fig. 12-5, *D*). The probe is withdrawn, and, if the procedure has been adequately performed, a bridge of the inner wall of the canal of Schlemm remains intact across the area of canal that was unroofed. This bridge prevents the iris from prolapsing into the surgical incision, and so a peripheral iridectomy is not necessary (Fig. 12-5, *E*). If the iris does prolapse into the incision, a peripheral iridectomy should be performed.

During the procedure, the anterior chamber should be present at all times. As the probe passes into the anterior chamber, disrupting the inner wall of the canal, there may be a little intracameral bleeding from the inner wall.

As the probe is swung from the canal into the anterior chamber, the surgeon should carefully watch the iris for movement. Movement of the iris implies that the probe is catching onto the iris surface and may induce an iridodialysis. The probe should be immediately withdrawn without continuing its entry into the anterior chamber and replaced, with the tip of the probe being kept slightly anterior so that it does not prematurely rupture the inner wall. The cornea should also be carefully monitored to ensure that the probe is not intrascleral and ripping through sclera, cornea, and Descemet's membrane. This movement is easy to detect because small air bubbles appear in the cornea as the probe ruptures through corneal lamellae. In that case, the probe needs to be repositioned, pushing the tip a little posteriorly.

Most important, the probe should pass with ease along the canal and from the canal into the anterior chamber without force being used.

Trabeculotomy may be performed under a one-third to one-half thickness lamellar scleral flap. This technique is described on p. 272 under "Combined Trabeculotomy and Trabeculectomy." The advantage of the radial incision without a scleral flap is that if the anterior chamber has been accidentally entered another radial incision can be made in an adjacent area of sclera without the conjunctival flap having to be enlarged.

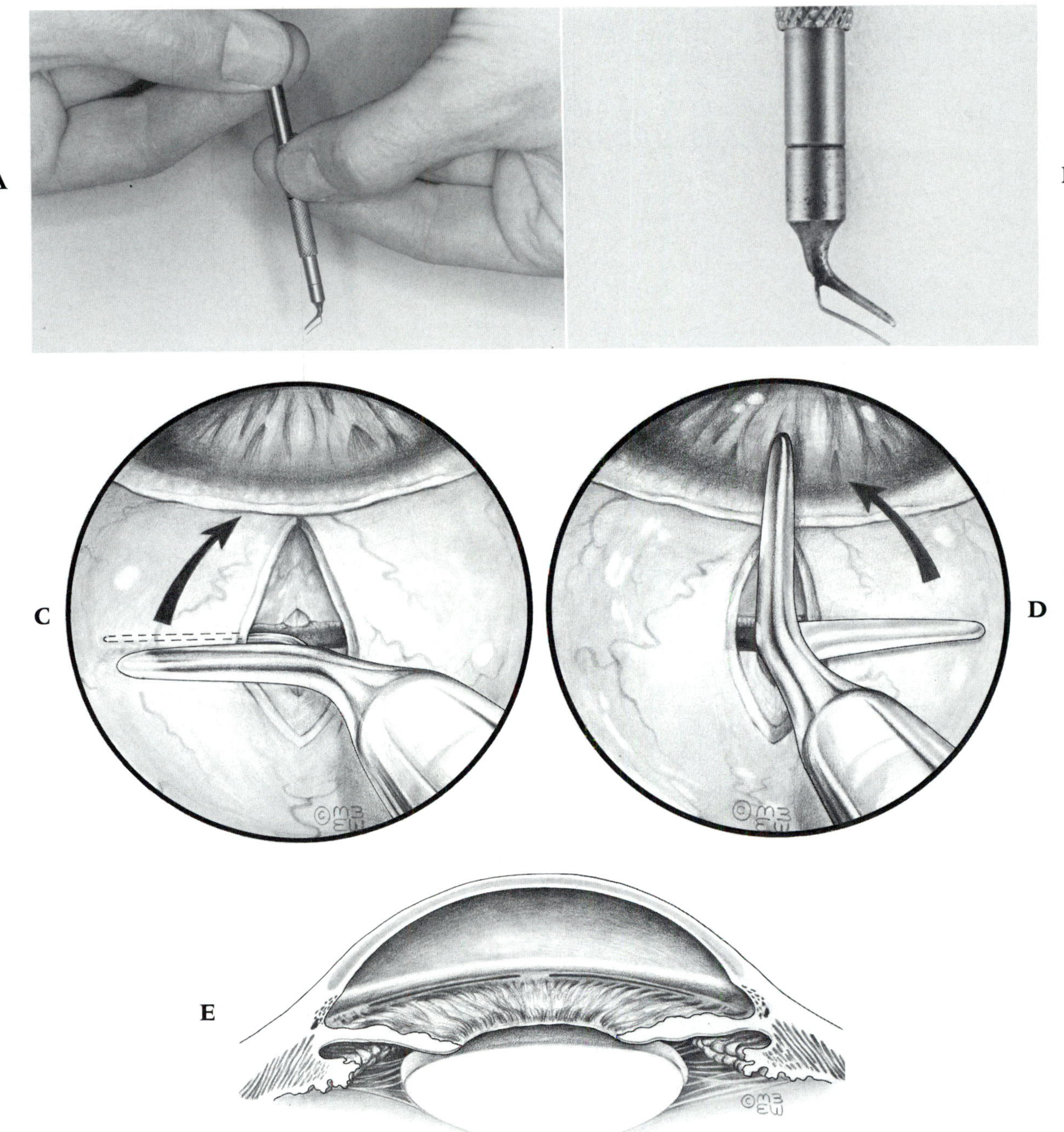

FIGURE 12-5. **A,** Trabeculotome (Luntz). **B,** Segments of shaft of trabeculotome. **C,** Blade enters Schlemm's canal. **D,** Same process repeated on temporal side. **E,** Intact inner bridge. (From Ritch R, Shields MB, Krupin T: The glaucomas, St Louis, 1989, The CV Mosby Co.)

Closure of the incision

Closure of the procedure is achieved with three virgin silk sutures in the scleral incision (Fig. 12-6, *A*). The conjunctival flap is rotated forward to the limbus and secured with a 10-0 nylon suture at each edge of the flap (Fig. 12-6, *B*).

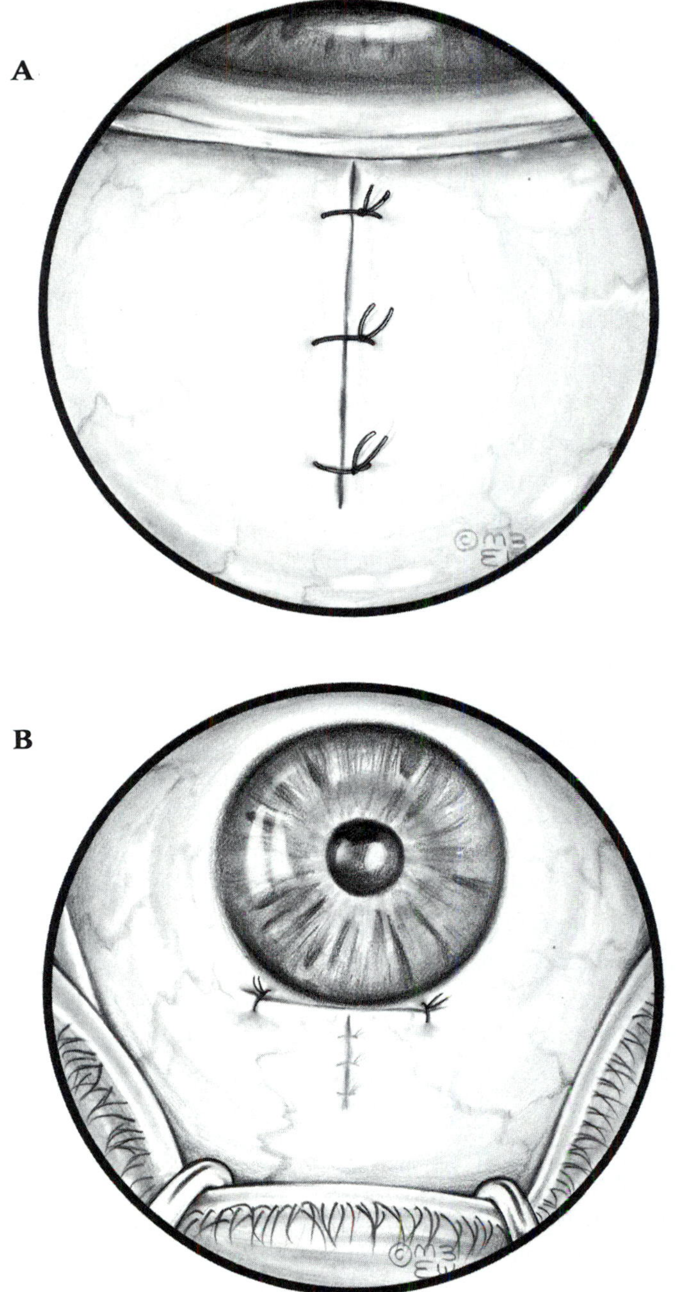

FIGURE 12-6. A, Closure. **B,** Securing conjunctival flap. (From Ritch R, Shields MB, Krupin T: The glaucomas, St Louis, 1989, The CV Mosby Co.)

Combined Trabeculotomy and Trabeculectomy

In eyes with cicatrized angles or frank iridocorneal dysgenesis, trabeculotomy gives poor results. The results are somewhat better with trabeculectomy (see Chapter 13) or combined trabeculotomy and trabeculectomy. The combined operation is performed with a 7 mm fornix-based conjunctival flap at the superior limbus. A 3 mm square scleral flap of half thickness is hinged at the limbus and rotated anteriorly to expose the surgical landmarks, that is, deep corneal tissue anteriorly and then trabecular band and sclera seriatim. The technique for trabeculectomy is initially followed as described later. A 2 mm square block is outlined in the deep corneal and trabecular tissue at the base of the scleral flap extending posteriorly to the scleral spur. This block is incised to the deep layers without the posterior chamber being entered. A radial incision is made across the scleral spur and trabecular band and dissected down until Schlemm's canal is identified (Fig. 12-7, *A*). The canal is 2 mm behind the surgical limbus and at the external landmark of the scleral spur. The outer wall of the canal is dissected into its lumen, and a small sinusotomy is made on each side with Vannas scissors. A trabeculotomy is performed on each side, as described earlier. The anterior chamber should still be intact.

The 2 mm square block of cornea and trabecular tissue is now excised to complete the trabeculectomy (Fig. 12-7, *B*). The conjunctival flap is secured later as shown in Fig. 12-6. If trabeculectomy alone is chosen, the operation as described is followed.

Filtration surgery in a severely buphthalmic eye has a poor prognosis for success, and there is a significant risk of vitreous loss because of zonular degeneration. Vitreous adherence to the incision, contraction of the vitreous, retinal detachment, and phthisis may ensue. Ciliodestructive procedures are probably less traumatic in these eyes but should be applied with caution, and parents should be warned of the high risk of phthisis bulbi.

Plastic drainage devices (seton)

Implantation of a seton is reserved for those eyes in which the previously described operations have failed to control intraocular pressure. We favor the Molteno drainage device. The surgical technique is described in Chapter 14.

Cyclocryotherapy

When all other surgical procedures have failed, resort is made to the ciliodestructive procedure called "cyclocryotherapy." The surgical method is described in Chapter 14.

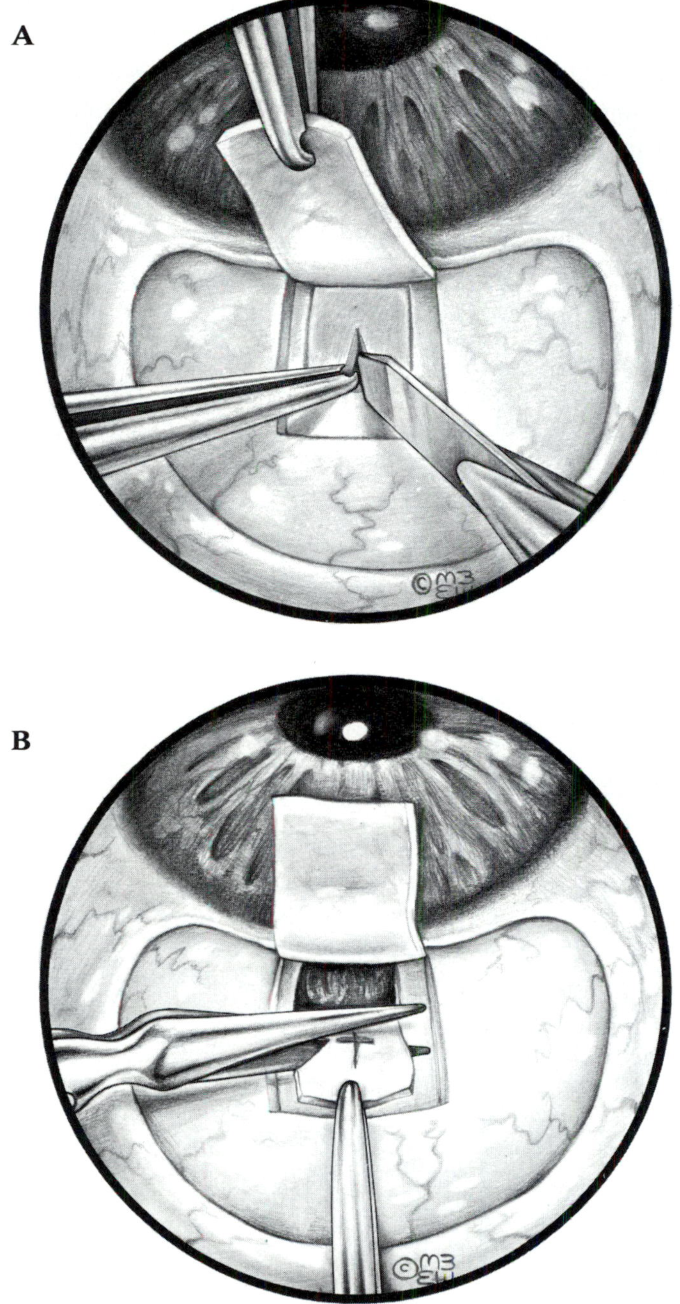

FIGURE 12-7. Combined trabeculotomy and trabeculectomy. **A,** Radial incision across scleral spur and trabecular band. **B,** Two-millimeter square deep block of cornea and trabecular tissue excised. (From Ritch R, Shields MB, and Krupin T: The glaucomas, St Louis, 1989, The CV Mosby Co.)

Visual rehabilitation

Visual rehabilitation is just as important in the management of the disease as surgical control of the intraocular pressure. Strabismus, anisometropia, and amblyopia are common. Removal of media opacities (such as corneal transplant for corneal scarring and cataract extraction) is necessary for visual rehabilitation, which also includes refractive correction and orthoptic training. Often, successful surgical lowering of intraocular pressure is marred by dense amblyopia. These measures should be undertaken at as early an age as possible.

CHAPTER 13

Angle-Closure, Primary and Secondary Open-Angle, and Chronic Closed-Angle Glaucoma Procedures

The first operation of choice in angle-closure glaucoma is laser peripheral iridotomy. The need for surgical peripheral iridectomy arises infrequently. Laser iridotomy has the great advantage of not requiring an incision into the globe in an operating room setting.

Argon Laser Iridotomy

Anesthesia is obtained with proparacaine (0.5%) drops. Pilocarpine (2%) is instilled 1 hour before the operation if the pupil is more than 2 mm, to place the iris on stretch. The Abraham lens (Fig. 13-1, *A*) is applied to the cornea after the cup is filled with gonioscopic solution free of air bubbles. The lens is a modified Goldmann fundus lens with a +66D button and has an antireflective coating. The button reduces the power density of the laser beam as it passes through the cornea by one-fourth and increases it at the point of photocoagulation on the iris by four times. The minimal diameter of the beam at the cornea is twice that with the Goldmann lens without the button and one half that seen at the iris outside the button. An economy of time and energy is obtained, thereby reducing corneal burns and anterior chamber reaction. Precision of placement of the laser energy and recognition of the end point, that is, a clear opening through the iris, are aided by the magnification. The lens also stabilizes the eye and acts as a lid speculum. The surgeon should have comfortable elbow supports.

Extreme peripheral sites should be avoided to prevent endothelial burns. Arcus senilis should also be avoided. Ideally one should use a location one half to one third of the distance from the periphery to the pupil in the superior half of the iris, avoiding the 12 o'clock area where gas bubbles collect (Fig. 13-1, *B*). Blue-green light is selected. Penetration is facilitated at an iris crypt or where the stroma is thinnest. In a blue iris, a good site is an iris freckle.

Preliminary stretch burns may be created at a 200 μm spot size with 0.5-watt power for 0.2 second. Three or four such spots at the edge of crypt contract the iris and stretch the crypt. In our experience, stretch burns are not generally necessary when the Abraham lens is used. An initial burn of 500 μm at 0.5 W for 0.2 second is used (the "hinge"). The spot size is then reduced to 200 μm and then 100 μm, and energy levels are increased to 0.75 W from 0.1 or 0.2 second. A rapid succession of burns is made at the center of the initial burn or crypt, with the lowest energy levels being used at which progression is evident. When penetration of iris stroma and the pigment epithelium is reached, dense bursts of pigment ("smoke signals") appear in the anterior chamber. A mushroom cloud of aqueous and pigment slowly balloons through the iridotomy site when the pigment epithelium is penetrated. The anterior chamber deepens. At this stage, one should enlarge the pinpoint iridotomy by "chipping away" at the margin, using settings of 50 μm at 0.75 to 1.0 W for 0.1 second. The iridotomy is usually enlarged by elimination of loose pigment clumps and strands of iris stroma. The laser beam is directed well away from the macula once penetration is seen as a black pinpoint hole. Adequate patency is ascertained by observation of the lens capsule and a red reflex on retroillumination on direct slitlamp examination.

The procedure should be stopped at any stage if (1) no visible response occurs, (2) corneal epithelial burns appear as milky spots, (3) endothelial burns are seen as opalescent areas, (4) pigment dispersion renders the anterior chamber turbid, and (5) 100 to 150 burns have been applied in one session.

The patient should remain 2 to 3 hours for postoperative checks of intraocular pressure. The anterior chamber depth is compared with the preoperative assessment and the fellow eye, if untreated. Gonioscopy will confirm that the angle has opened. Elevated intraocular pressure is treated with appropriate medical therapy, including carbonic anhydrase inhibitors and oral hyperosmotic agents if necessary. The intraocular pressure is checked the following morning.

Postoperative care with topical steroid drops (prednisolone 1%) every 2 hours on the same day usually suffices. A mild iritis rarely persists beyond the day of laser surgery. Cycloplegics are unnecessary. Complications are rare. Localized lens opacification at the site of iridotomy does not spread. Corneal epithelial burns resolve in a few days. Pupil distortion is insignificant. The chief problem is transient rise of intraocular pressure within hours after completion of the iridotomy. Pressure levels may reach 40 to 50 mm Hg. Miotics are continued for at least 3 weeks until permanent patency of the iridotomy is established. Pigment hyperplasia may block an iridotomy after 2 to 3 weeks. Retreatment is usually brief and very successful. In uninflamed eyes, a satisfactory iridotomy can be attained in almost all cases. Laser iridotomy is much less likely to be achieved in an acute phase of angle-closure glaucoma because of corneal edema and unclear anterior chamber. A surgical peripheral iridectomy may be required in acute congestive angle closure.

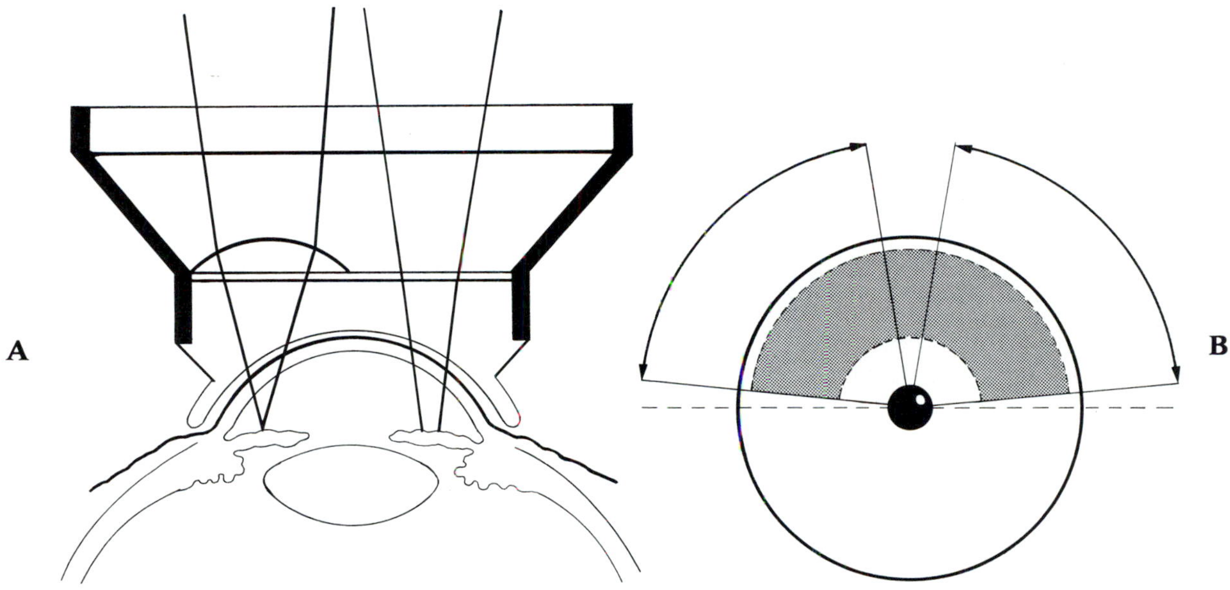

FIGURE 13-1. **A,** Abraham lens. **B,** Optimal locations for argon laser iridotomy.

Neodymium-YAG Laser Iridotomy

The neodymium–yttrium-aluminum-garnet laser (Nd:YAG) creates an iridotomy by the photodisruptive effect of extremely high energy delivered in a very short time to the selected site. The microexplosion produces a patent iridotomy independent of iris color. This is a great advantage in the light blue iris, where argon laser is often inefficacious. The very thick brown iris is also more readily penetrated by the neodymium-YAG laser. The exceedingly short time for delivery of the laser energy is also an advantage with patients who are unable to maintain a still position at the slitlamp as required with the argon laser. In general, neodymium-YAG iridotomies do not close, unless there is uveitis or neovascularization. Hyphema can complicate the procedure but is rarely more than trivial. Pretreatment with argon laser at the chosen site will prevent bleeding.

Technique

The Abraham lens is used with gonioscopic fluid free of air bubbles. Anesthesia is topical. A crypt or thin area of peripheral iris is selected. Basal iris is preferred in order to avoid injury to the lens capsule, if possible. Four to 8 mJ with three or four pulses per burst is usually adequate. On penetration, a stream of aqueous-containing pigmented particles enters the anterior chamber. The lens capsule is not seen at the end point, and transillumination is also not always observed through the characteristically small iridotomy. Gonioscopy will confirm that the angle has opened. Postoperative care is similar to that of argon laser iridotomy.

Surgical Peripheral Iridectomy

A corneal incision or a limbal incision under a conjunctival flap may be utilized. The corneal incision has the advantage of leaving the conjunctiva in its pristine state. A scarred conjunctiva adherent to sclera is a complicating factor if a filtering operation becomes necessary in the future. Local anesthesia is used.

Technique with corneal incision

The operating microscope is used at a magnification of 10. A 3 mm length incision is made with a diamond knife or microblade (Beaver no. 75) into the cornea just anterior to the limbus and at the anterior edge of limbal corneal vessels. The superonasal quadrant is preferred. Corneal stroma is dissected down to Descemet's membrane. The corneal side of the incision is grasped with a Hoskin no. 28 forceps (Keeler). With the cornea pulled slightly upwards and away from the iris, the anterior chamber is entered with the knife for the full 3 mm (Fig. 13-2, *A*).

Iris prolapse is facilitated by pressure on the scleral side of the incision with a flat iris spatula (Fig. 13-2, *B*). Care must be exercised if the iris is grasped through the incision with the Hoskin forceps. While the peripheral iris is being held with the forceps, a second similar pair of forceps is applied beneath the first to obtain a grasp nearest to the pupil before iris is pulled out of the incision. Failure to carry out this "double grasping" maneuver may result in tearing the iris base, iridodialysis, and intraocular bleeding. It is important to ensure that both stromal and pigment layers are held. DeWecker scissors are used to cut iris parallel to the limbus in one snip. The portion of iris held in the forceps is removed (Fig. 13-2, *C*). The iridectomy is at the junction of the peripheral and middle thirds of the iris, thus avoiding major iris vessels. (See also p. 188.)

Pressure on the scleral side of the incision allows the iris to slip back into the anterior chamber if it has not already done so. A jet of balanced saline solution directed into the incision aids in dislodging incarcerated iris. Full-thickness patency should be ascertained by retroillumination. Two 10-0 nylon sutures at full corneal depth are placed across the center of the incision and tied with firm apposition without being too tight. The knot is buried on the corneal side (Fig. 13-2, *D*). The suture can be retained indefinitely. Postoperatively, antibiotic-corticosteroid drops are used for about 5 days. A short-acting mydriatic is given once daily for a few days. No patch is required the day after surgery. Results are very satisfactory.

Technique with limbal incision and conjunctival flap

A conjunctival flap including Tenon's fascia is made 5 mm in length and 4 mm from the cornea. Incision through the limbus into the anterior chamber is done with a diamond knife or microblade for 3 mm. The knuckle of iris that protrudes is grasped with Hoskin forceps and excised with DeWecker scissors, using the technique of actual iridectomy similar to that described with a corneal incision. The incision is repaired with a single 10-0 nylon suture, and one should test it for watertight closure by pressing with the tip of a fine forceps. The anterior chamber is not usually lost. It must be seen to be formed before the patient is allowed to leave the operating room. The conjunctival flap may be left unsutured or closed with a short continuous 6-0 plain catgut suture. The postoperative management is similar to that with the corneal incision. If the limbal incision is made too posterior, injury to ciliary body may result and cause bleeding. If the incision is made too anterior, iris prolapse may be difficult, especially if the pupil is miotic. A postoperative flat chamber requires immediate surgical repair of a leaking incision.

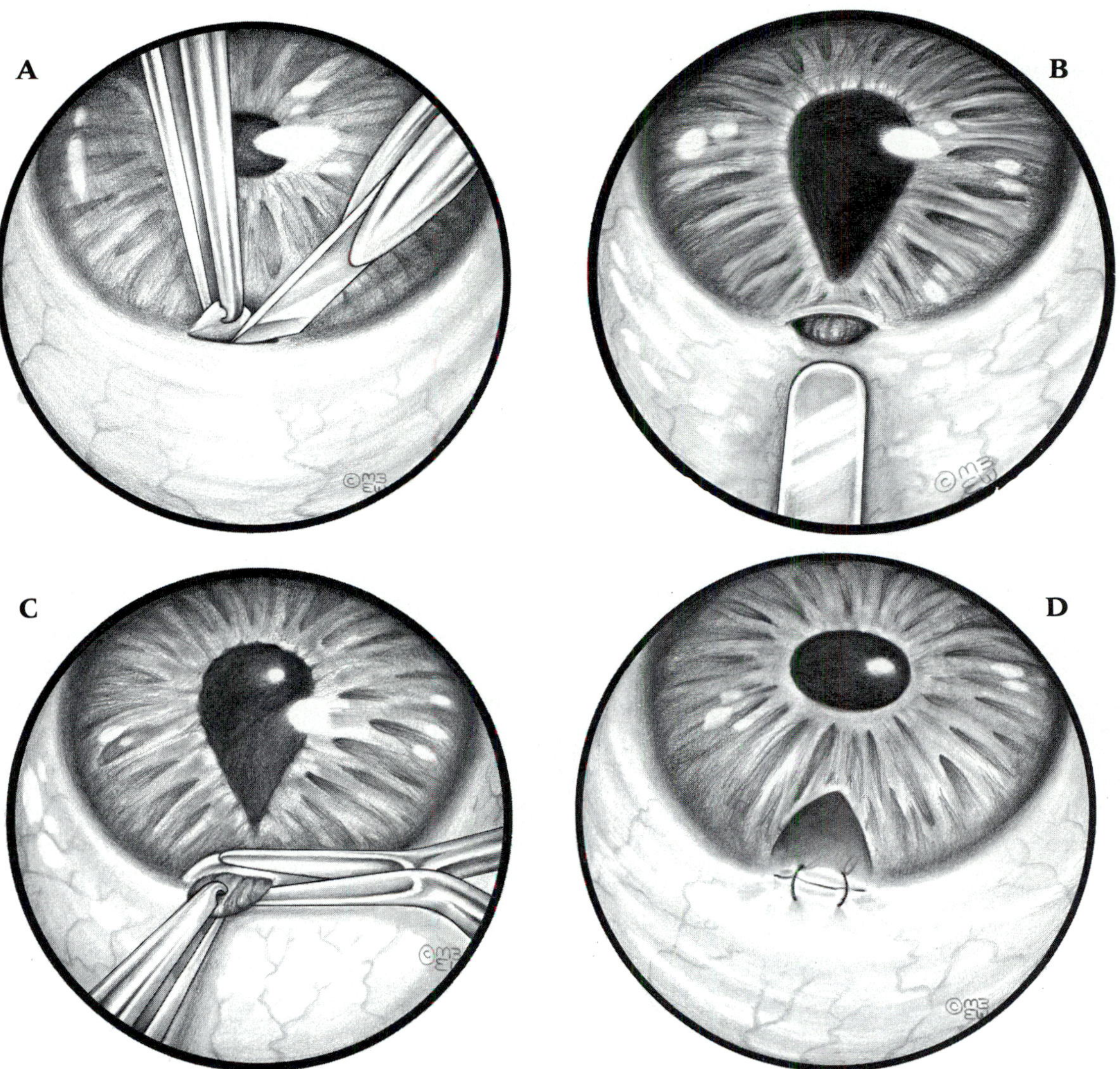

FIGURE 13-2. **A,** Corneal incision. **B,** Applying pressure to facilitate iris prolapse. **C,** Removal of portion of iris. **D,** Suture placement.

Argon Laser Trabeculoplasty

Indications

Indications for argon laser trabeculoplasty (ALT) are as follows:

1. Primary open-angle glaucoma when full, appropriate medical treatment fails to control the intraocular pressure adequately, or side effects of medications are not tolerated.
2. Mixed glaucoma (combined mechanism) if peripheral iridotomy fails to permit medical control, despite opening of the angles.
3. Poor compliance with medical therapy.
4. Borderline or questionable control on medical therapy before cataract surgery.
5. Secondary open-angle glaucoma, including pseudoexfoliation and pigmentary dispersion, as in (1).

Contraindications

1. Active iritis.
2. Lack of clarity of cornea or of anterior chamber, or of both.
3. Angle closure by peripheral anterior synechiae for more than 75% circumference.
4. Inability of the patient to cooperate at the slitlamp.
5. Congenital, infantile, and juvenile glaucoma (the contraindication is not absolute in the juvenile subgroup).

Technique

Topical anesthesia with proparacaine suffices. The Goldmann three-mirror or Ritch goniolens is used (Fig. 13-3, *A* and *B*). With the latter lens, there are two pairs of basic mirrors, one inclined at 59 degrees (round top) to afford a face-on view of the inferior angle, and the other at 64 degrees (flat top) to allow a similar view of the superior angle. The superior angle is often narrower than the inferior angle and can be better visualized with the round-top mirror. One mirror in each pair has a 17-diopter planoconvex button lens aligned and bonded over it. The button lenses provide magnification of 1.4, reducing the spot size to 35 μm and increasing the laser power density.

The gonioscopy fluid (hydroxypropyl methylcellulose 2.5%) must be free of air bubbles when applied to the goniolens. Standard settings are 50 μm for 0.1 second and initial power at 0.75 W. Increased power may be needed to obtain a visible response of blanching without or with a small gas bubble. Large gas bubbles indicate excessive photocoagulation, and one should avoid them by reducing power accordingly. One places the spots on the anterior trabecular meshwork overlapping on the pigment band, using 25 spots per quadrant evenly spaced. Only two quadrants are treated at an initial session. The remaining 180 degree area is treated at an undetermined future time if deemed necessary (Fig. 13-3, *C*). It is convenient to start temporally and work around counterclockwise.

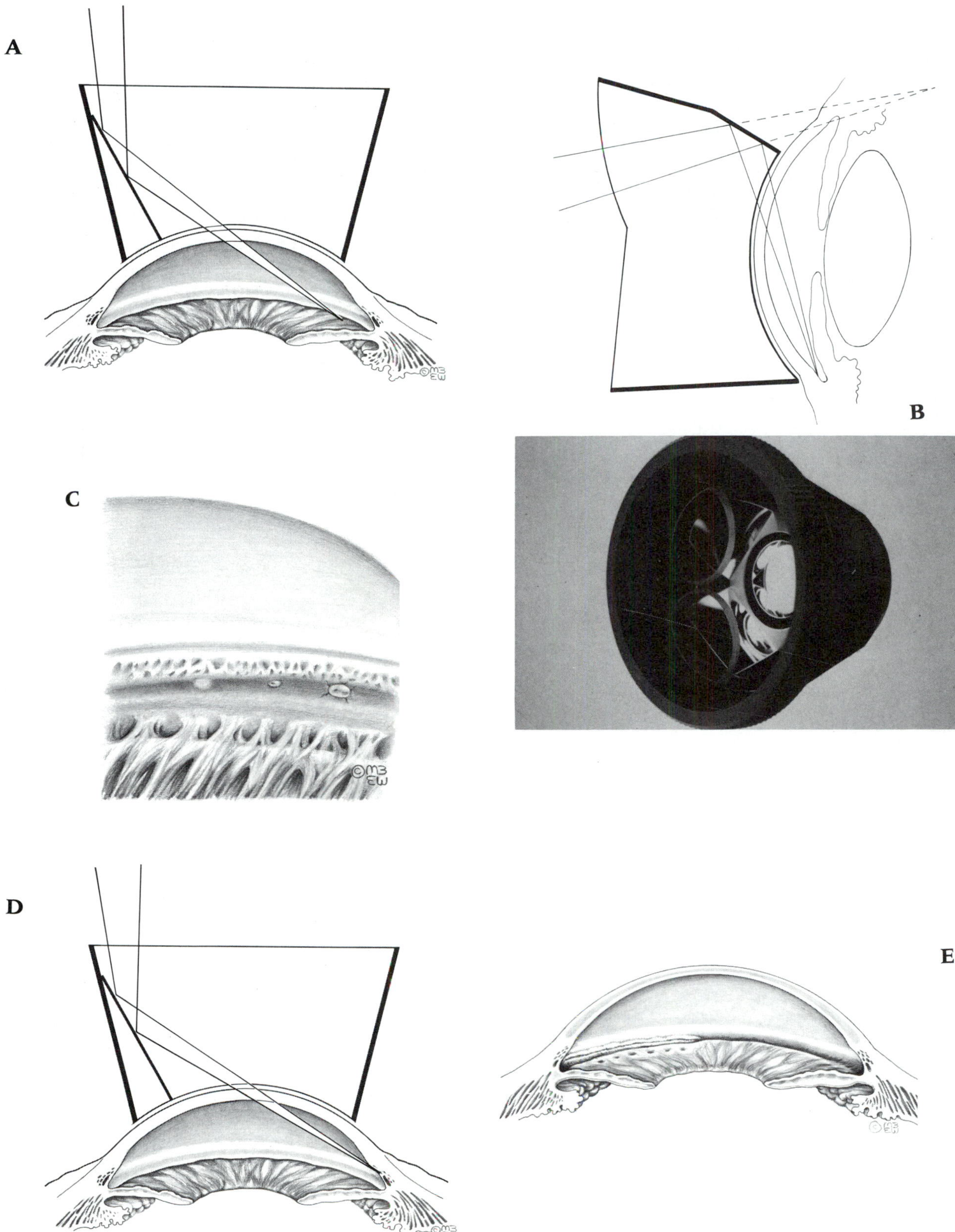

FIGURE 13-3. **A,** Goldmann three-mirror antireflection-coated goniolens. Notice that the 59-degree mirror (round-top) is used to visualize trabecular meshwork. **B,** Ritch trabeculoplasty lens. **C,** Laser spots on anterior meshwork and trabecular pigment band. **D** and **E,** Peripheral iris retraction (iridoplasty).

One can facilitate visualization of the angle by having the patient look in the direction opposite to that of the angle being treated.

The angle may be too narrow to permit adequate visualization of the entire trabecular meshwork, especially in the superior quadrants. It is expedient then to utilize the technique of peripheral iris retraction or tangential photocoagulation. This can be helpful in opening a narrow angle if no peripheral anterior synechiae have formed. (This technique can be of value in treating plateau iris angle closure.) Four to six burns are placed per quadrant. Settings are 100 to 200 μm at 0.5 W for 0.2 second. The iris shrinks away from the cornea to display angle architecture. Settings are adjusted according to response (Fig. 13-3, *D* and *E*).

Postoperative care

A postoperative rise of intraocular pressure is very common. Pressures are checked at 1 and 2 hours postoperatively and the following morning. Appropriate medical treatment is given to abort a rise. This is of great importance if advanced loss of visual field is present. In these circumstances, oral acetazolamide or oral 50% glycerol, or both, may be used immediately before argon laser trabeculoplasty (ALT) is carried out and repeated 6 hours afterwards.

A mild postoperative inflammatory reaction is usually very transient. We routinely give topical prednisolone 1.0% qid for 5 days. Peripheral anterior synechiae and iritis are usually avoided when one does not place the spots on the posterior trabecular meshwork. Corneal epithelial burns form a ring in the central cornea but are transient and require no treatment. Preoperative medical treatment is maintained.

Filtering Surgery

Filtering surgery is indicated when full medical treatment and ALT, when feasible, have failed to control the intraocular pressure. One must evaluate each patient on an individual basis, bearing in mind general health and status of the fellow eye. The following general guidelines are used:

1. Progressive loss of visual field, despite good compliance and tolerance of medications.
2. Intraocular pressure over 35 or 40 mm Hg without progression of field defect.
3. Intraocular pressure over 40 mm Hg with no definite visual field defect.
4. Advanced visual field loss and intraocular pressure over 15 mm Hg.
   a. Central "tubular" field.
   b. Field loss to within 10 degrees of fixation.
   c. Extension of field defect into fixation of the fellow eye at similar pressure levels.
5. Progressive enlargement of the cup, especially vertically, to a cup-disc ratio of 0.7 or more.

Trabeculectomy

Trabeculectomy is the most commonly performed filtering operation and is the procedure of choice in primary and secondary open-angle glaucoma. It has the merit of a lamellar scleral flap that covers the fistulized area, reducing free egress of aqueous from the anterior chamber into the subconjunctival space. There is less likelihood of bleb rupture, flat anterior chamber, hypotony, and early cataract formation than in full-thickness fistulizing operations. General anesthesia is our choice, but local anesthesia may be suitable. There is no single trabeculectomy but various modifications of the original technique (Cairns).

A fornix-based or limbus-based conjunctival flap may be used. The advantages of a fornix-based flap are (1) better exposure of the operative field, facilitating dissection of the scleral flap into the cornea; (2) elimination of "buttonhole" damage to the conjunctiva; (3) easier dissection if conjunctiva has been scarred by previous surgery; and (4) adherence of the conjunctival flap at the limbus, resulting in a posteriorly situated, diffuse, thicker-walled bleb that does not overlie the limbus.

A limbus-based conjunctival flap allows the replaced scleral flap to be more loosely sutured, thus permitting freer drainage. In practice, the overall results are similar whichever type of conjunctival flap is used. The fornix-based flap is obligatory when extracapsular cataract extraction with posterior chamber intraocular lens implantation is combined with trabeculectomy.

Technique

Fornix-based conjunctival Tenon's flap (magnification of 5 to 7)

A fornix-based conjunctival Tenon's flap 7 mm long is raised at the limbus (Fig. 13-4). The conjunctiva and Tenon's fascia are dissected back in a natural surgical plane between themselves and the sclera. There is less dissection of Tenon's fascia compared to a limbus-based flap. Any bleeding points on the flap or episclera are dealt with at this stage. (See also p. 172.)

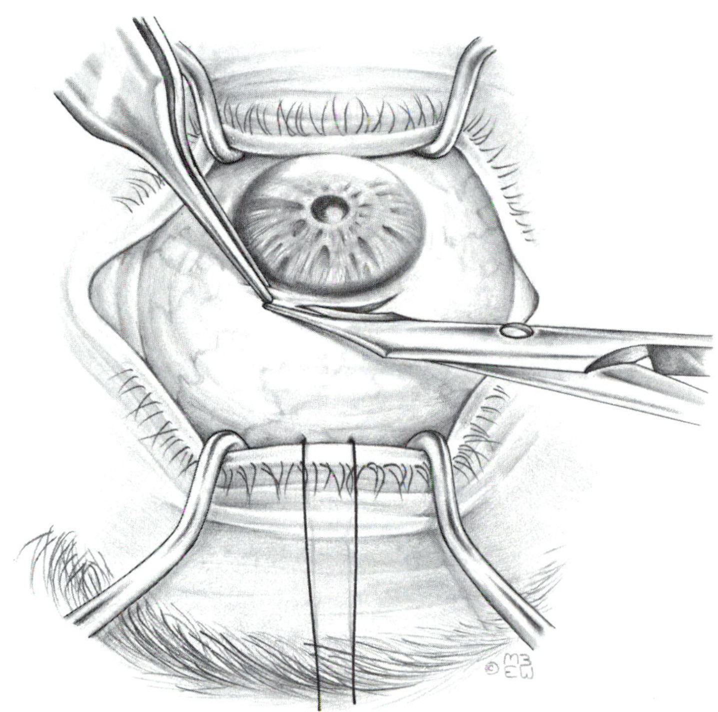

FIGURE 13-4. Fornix-based conjunctival flap.

Scleral flap (magnification of 5 to 7, no. 75 Beaver blade with 15-degree angle or diamond knife)

The scleral surface is cleaned, and a flap 3 mm long and extending 2.5 mm posteriorly from the limbus is outlined with one or two cautery marks in the exposed sclera. This flap is hinged at the limbus to ensure that the conjunctival and scleral suture lines are separated.

The scleral flap is incised initially along the posterior incision, which is 2.5 mm posterior to the limbus, and this incision is dissected down to the surface of the pars plana (Fig. 13-5, *A*). Next, two half-thickness radial scleral incisions are made 3 mm apart from the limbus to join each end of the prepared posterior incision (Fig. 13-5, *B*). The thickness of the sclera can be estimated from the full-thickness posterior incision, allowing accurate dissection of a one-third-thickness lamellar scleral flap. Staying in the same surgical plane, one carries the flap forward to the cornea to just within the surgical limbus (Fig. 13-5, *C*) using a hockey stick–shaped disposable Grieshaber blade no. 68-101 (Beaver blade equivalent no. 66) or a diamond knife (Fig. 13-5, *D*).

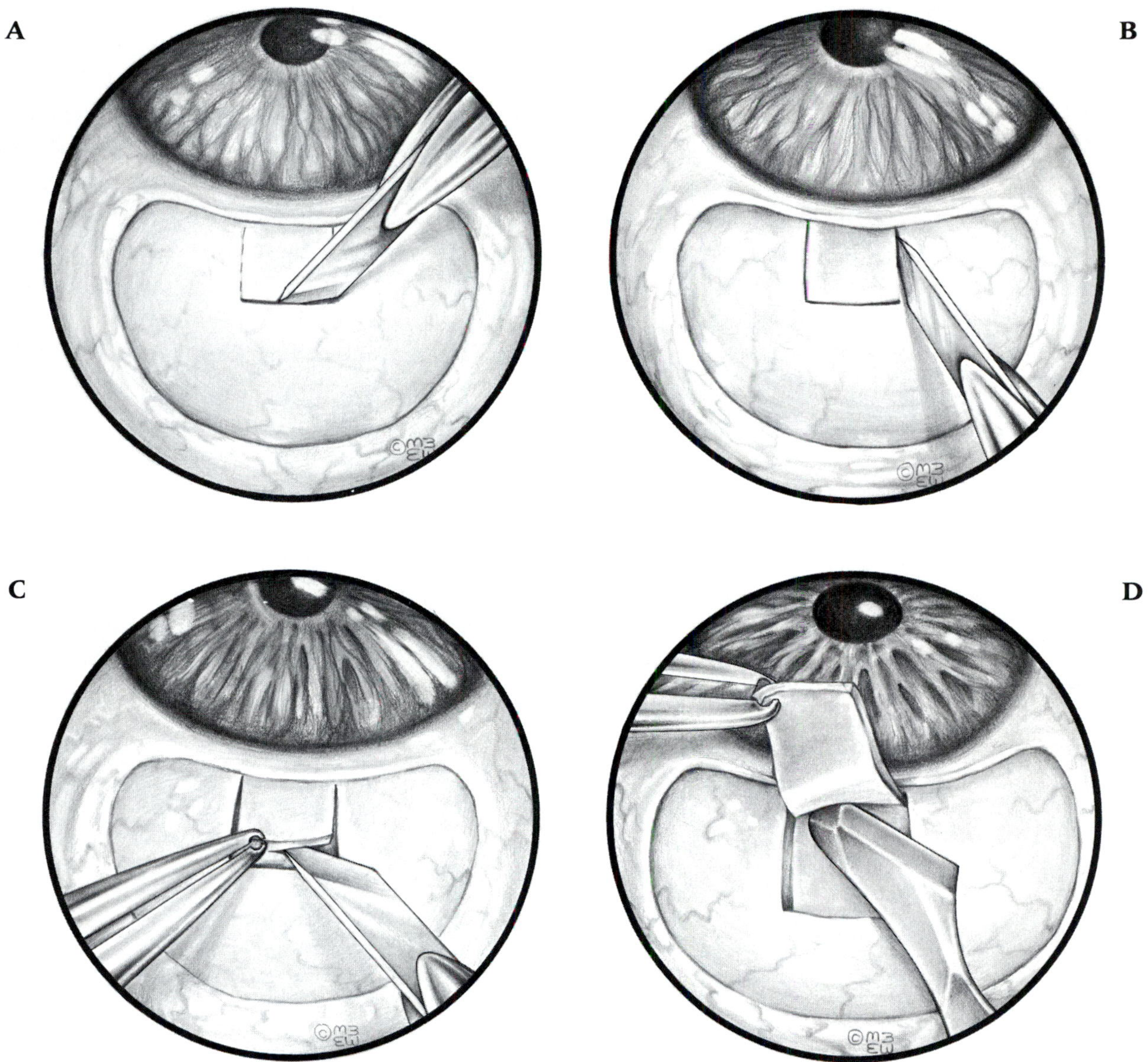

FIGURE 13-5. **A,** Scleral flap dissection. **B,** Radial incisions in sclera. **C,** Exposure of full thickness of sclera. **D,** Dissection of lamellar scleral flap. (From Ritch R, Shields MB, Krupin T: The glaucomas, St Louis, 1989, The CV Mosby Co.)

Anatomic landmarks

With the lamellar scleral flap retracted, the salient external landmarks are easily recognized in the deeper undissected tissues (Fig. 11-1). Anteriorly, there is transparent deep corneal tissue; behind, there is a gray band of parallel-fibered trabecular tissue that merges posteriorly into white, opaque sclera with crisscrossing fibers. At the junction of the gray trabecular band and the sclera is the scleral spur and Schlemm's canal. This external landmark for the scleral spur and of Schlemm's canal is by far the most important surgical landmark. It indicates the posterior limit of the dissection of corneotrabecular tissue, which is removed in a Cairns' type of trabeculectomy. Two 10-0 nylon sutures are placed from the posterior corners of the scleral flap to the posterior corners of the flap bed and pulled out of the way.

Fig. 13-6 shows that with a limbus-based conjunctival flap (see also p. 172) one can bring the operation to this stage of exposure of the landmarks in the scleral trapdoor bed according to the following successive steps:

1. Securing hemostasis on sclera with a wet-field "eraser" cautery.
2. Cleaning limbal episcleral fascia with a Tooke blade.
3. Outlining scleral flap as for technique with fornix-based conjunctival flap.
4. Fashioning lamellar scleral flap at one-third thickness, using diamond knife or pointed 15-degree microblade.
5. Carrying out dissection of lamellar scleral flap forward to deep cornea, exposing surgical landmarks in trapdoor bed, as in Fig. 13-5, *D*.

Then the trabeculectomy is performed in the same fashion as follows.

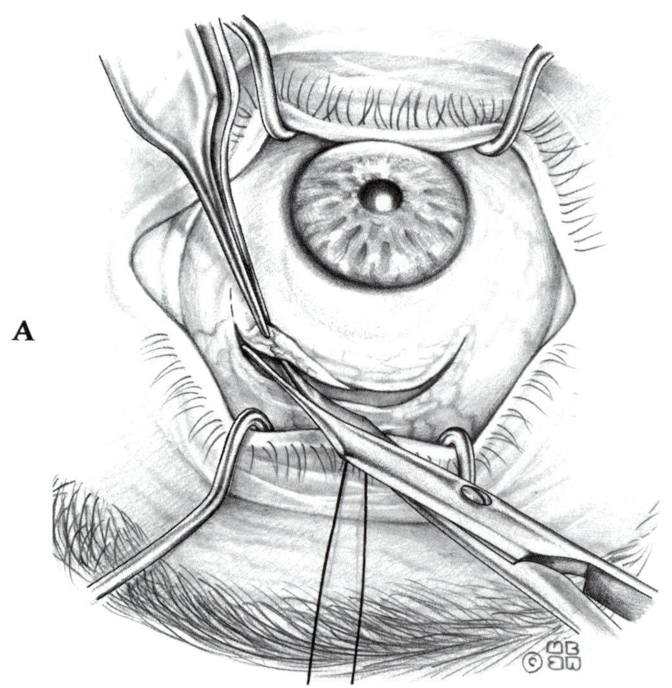

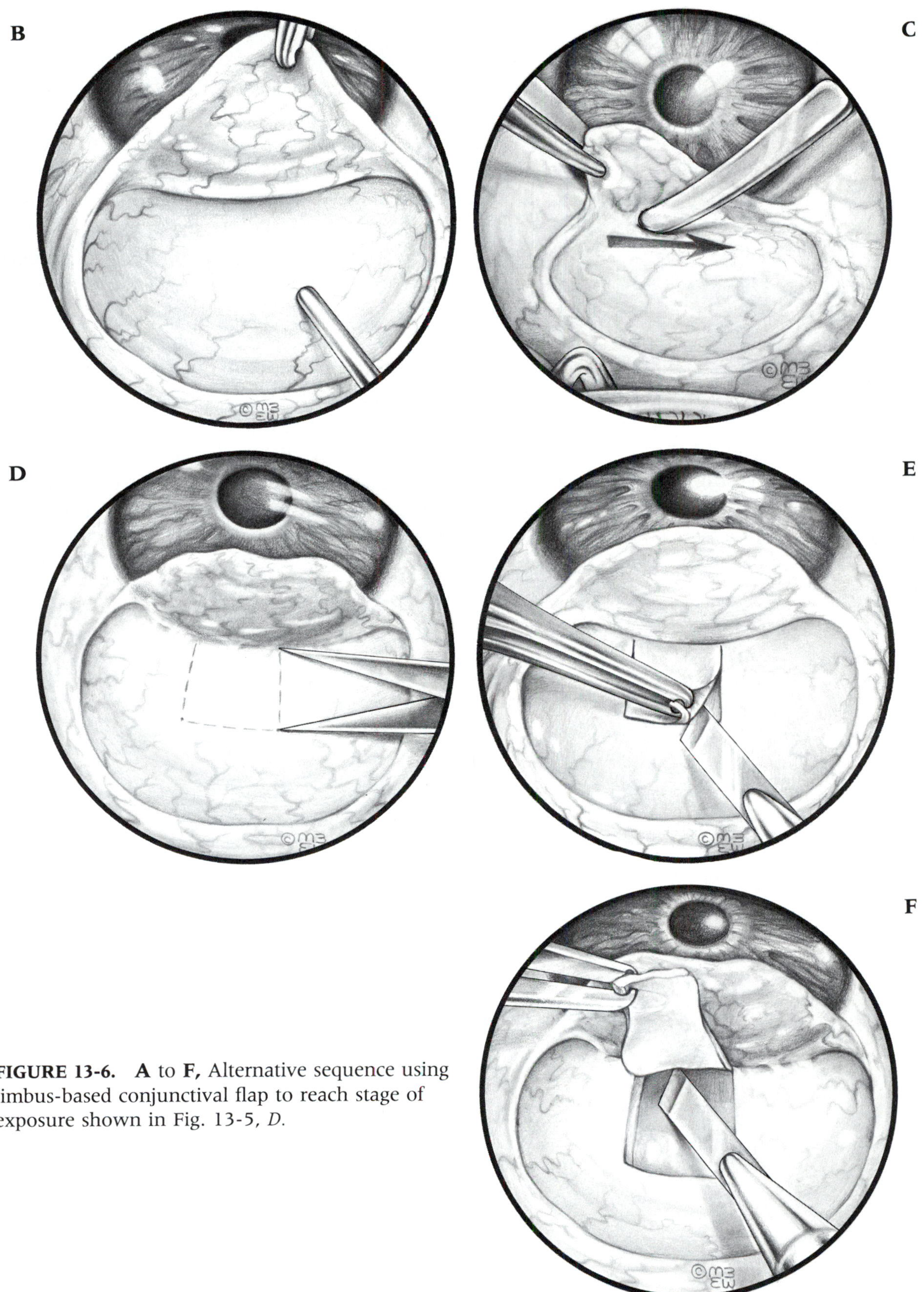

FIGURE 13-6. **A** to **F,** Alternative sequence using limbus-based conjunctival flap to reach stage of exposure shown in Fig. 13-5, *D.*

Trabeculectomy (magnification of 10)

Using a no. 75 Beaver blade with a 15-degree angle or a diamond knife, the next step is to outline a square flap of approximately 2 mm in the scleral bed (Fig. 13-7, *A*).

With the internal flap outlined, the anterior incision is dissected through Descemet's membrane into the anterior chamber. It should be noted that the chamber is not lost at this stage because iris will plug the incision.

The dissection into the anterior chamber is made slowly, using a sharp, pointed microblade with a 15-degree angle (such as a no. 75 Beaver blade) or a diamond knife, allowing aqueous humor to seep slowly out until the eye becomes soft but without loss of the anterior chamber. Once the eye has softened, air is injected into the anterior chamber to maintain a moderate depth. The incision into the anterior chamber is enlarged by careful dissection with a microblade until the opening is large enough to introduce a blade of a straight Vannas scissors with which the anterior incision is completed, still without loss of the anterior chamber (Fig. 13-7, *B*). One similarly completes the radial incisions on each side by incising posteriorly until the previously described landmark for the scleral spur is reached. The block so formed is removed by a posterior incision at the scleral spur, which runs parallel to the limbus (Fig. 13-7, *C*).

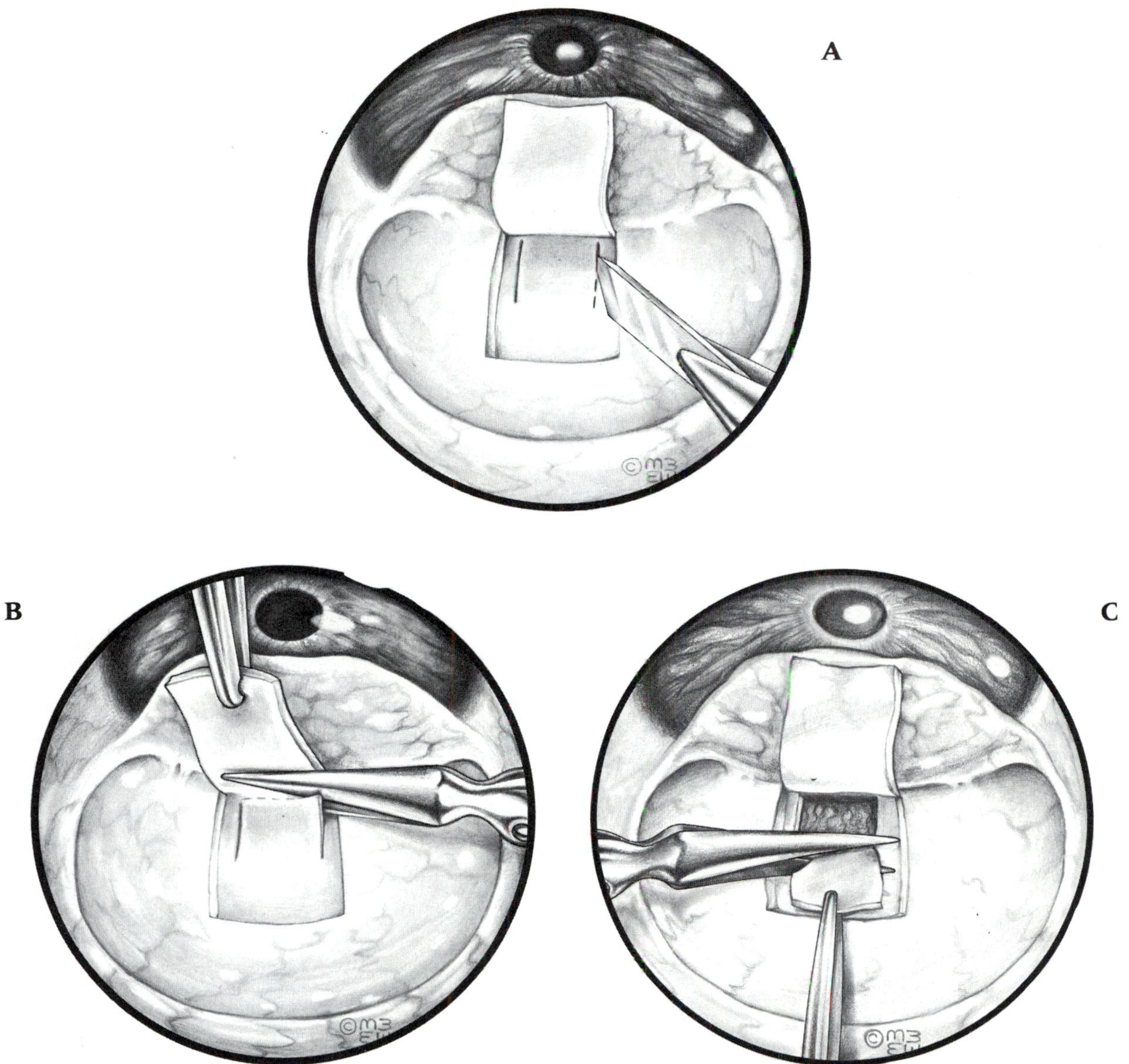

FIGURE 13-7. A, Square flap outlined in trapdoor bed. **B** and **C,** Completing anterior incision.

Iridectomy (magnification of 10)

An iridectomy is now made. It is imperative that the iridectomy is wider than the trabeculectomy opening to prevent the iris pillars from being pushed into this opening postoperatively. One achieves this by grasping the iris with Hoskin forceps, moving it to the surgeon's left side and beginning an iridectomy incision with DeWecker scissors from the right side (Fig. 13-8, *A*). As this incision approaches the midway point of the iridectomy, the iris is moved across to the right side and put on stretch and the iridectomy completed (Fig. 13-8, *B*).

The iridectomy is carefully made because vitreous may prolapse through a stretched and ruptured zonule and erupt through the iridectomy. If this occurs, a limited vitrectomy must be done, with removal of all vitreous from the iridectomy and anterior chamber anterior to the iridectomy.

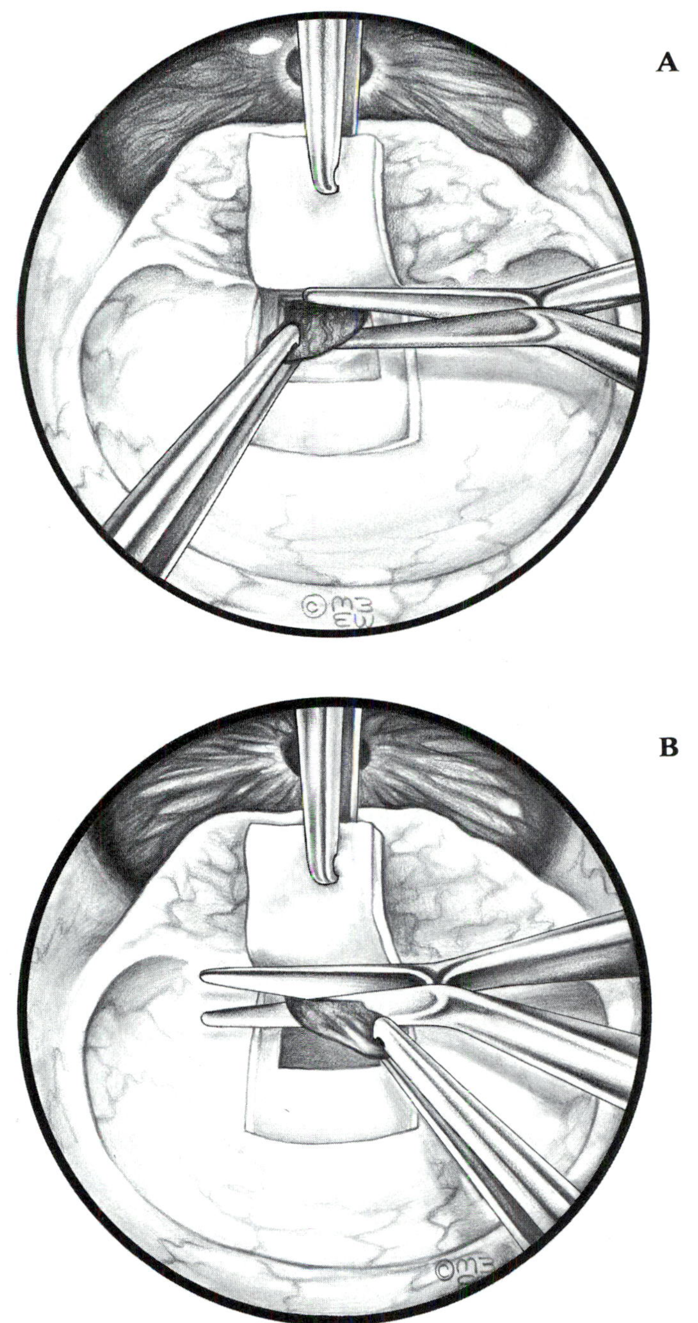

FIGURE 13-8. **A,** Peripheral iridectomy. **B,** Completing peripheral iridectomy.

Closure (magnification of 5)

As the iridectomy is completed, one repositions the lamellar scleral flap by tying the preplaced 10-0 nylon sutures at the posterior edges of the scleral flap (Fig. 13-9, *A*). Balanced salt solution is injected into the anterior chamber to replace the air bubble. The partial-thickness scleral flap is sutured by use of two additional interrupted 10-0 nylon sutures if a limbus-based conjunctival flap has been used (Fig. 13-9, *B*). The pair of sutures is placed at each side of the flap near the limbus. If a fornix-based conjunctival flap has been used, a second pair of sutures is placed midway along the flap on each side (Fig. 13-9, *C*). A limbus-based conjunctival flap is repaired with a continuous 6-0 plain catgut suture (Fig. 13-9, *D*). A fornix-based flap is rotated anteriorly to the limbus and sutured to the episclera and sclera with two 10-0 nylon sutures, one at each end of the conjunctival flap, and the conjunctival edge is pulled taut (but not tight) across the limbus (Fig. 13-9, *E*). The anterior chamber remains formed.

Balanced salt solution or air is injected under the conjunctival flap to lift it from the sclera. Methylprednisolone sodium succinate (Solu-Medrol) 0.5 ml and gentamicin sulfate (Garamycin) 0.5 ml are injected subconjunctivally into the inferior fornix.

The "Watson" modification of trabeculectomy uses a 4 mm square scleral flap under which a block of deep sclera is dissected to the pars plana, with placement of the posterior incision 3 mm behind the limbus. Two radial incisions 2 mm apart are cut toward the limbus with Vannas scissors until the ciliary body attachment to the scleral spur is reached. A cyclodialysis spatula is inserted to detach ciliary body by blunt dissection. The deep scleral flap is then excised, with a corneoscleral opening that extends back to 1 mm behind the scleral spur being left. An iridectomy is then performed.

Another modification (Harrison) of standard trabeculectomy is to apply the wet-field cautery to the margins of the window produced by removal of the block of trabecular meshwork and also to the distal margin of the lamellar scleral flap to cause a gape. Cauterization enlarges the fistula and facilitates subscleral filtration.

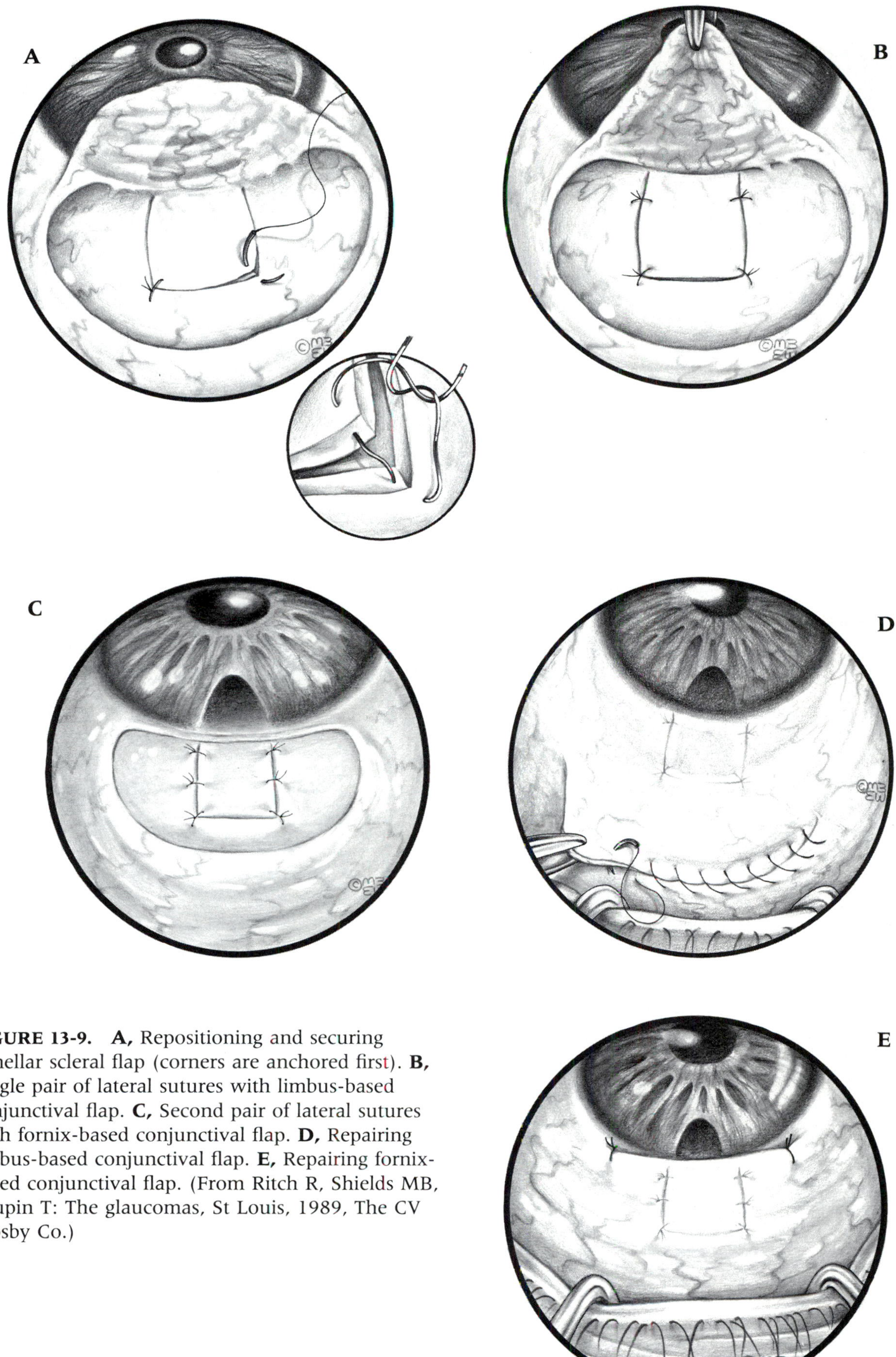

FIGURE 13-9. A, Repositioning and securing lamellar scleral flap (corners are anchored first). **B,** Single pair of lateral sutures with limbus-based conjunctival flap. **C,** Second pair of lateral sutures with fornix-based conjunctival flap. **D,** Repairing limbus-based conjunctival flap. **E,** Repairing fornix-based conjunctival flap. (From Ritch R, Shields MB, Krupin T: The glaucomas, St Louis, 1989, The CV Mosby Co.)

Intrascleral Thermosclerostomy ("Subscleral Scheie")

Intrascleral thermosclerostomy is a more radical drainage procedure than trabeculectomy but with advantages over a full-thickness fistulizing operation. A narrow scleral flap guards the fistulous area, strengthens the limbal conjunctiva at the base of the bleb, and deflects aqueous flow posteriorly.

The principal indications for this procedure are as follows:

1. Previous failed trabeculectomy.
2. Intraocular pressure over 45 mm Hg on full medication.
3. Advanced visual field loss with intraocular pressure over 35 mm Hg.
4. Secondary glaucoma from uveitis.
5. Angle closed by peripheral anterior synechiae in over 75% of the circumference.
6. Glaucoma in aphakic eyes.
7. Young black adults with visual field loss.

Technique

Unscarred conjunctiva is selected, preferably in the upper nasal quadrant. A 9 mm conjunctival incision is made in the fornix parallel to the limbus and carried through to bare sclera (Fig. 13-10, *A*). The dissection is continued forward to the limbus, which is cleaned with a Tooke blade. Hemostasis is obtained. A scleral flap is marked with a cautery 1 mm from the limbus and 5 mm in length (Fig. 13-10, *B*). The lamellar flap is cut with a diamond knife at half thickness and hinged anteriorly (Fig. 13-10, *C*). An incision is made with the diamond knife into deep sclera under the base of the anteriorly rotated flap (Fig. 13-10, *D*). A row of cautery burns is applied to the posterior wall of the incision with a bipolar cautery (Fig. 13-10, *E*). The incision is then deepened to Descemet's membrane, and another row of cautery burns is applied. The anterior lip of the deep incision is lifted with Pierse no. 28 forceps and the anterior chamber entered at one end with the diamond knife (Fig. 13-10, *F*). The opening is enlarged the full length of the deep incision (5 mm) by straight Vannas scissors (Fig. 13-10, *G*). A wide-based peripheral iridectomy is then performed, as described for trabeculectomy (Fig. 13-10, *H*). The iridectomy should extend the length of the entry into the anterior chamber.

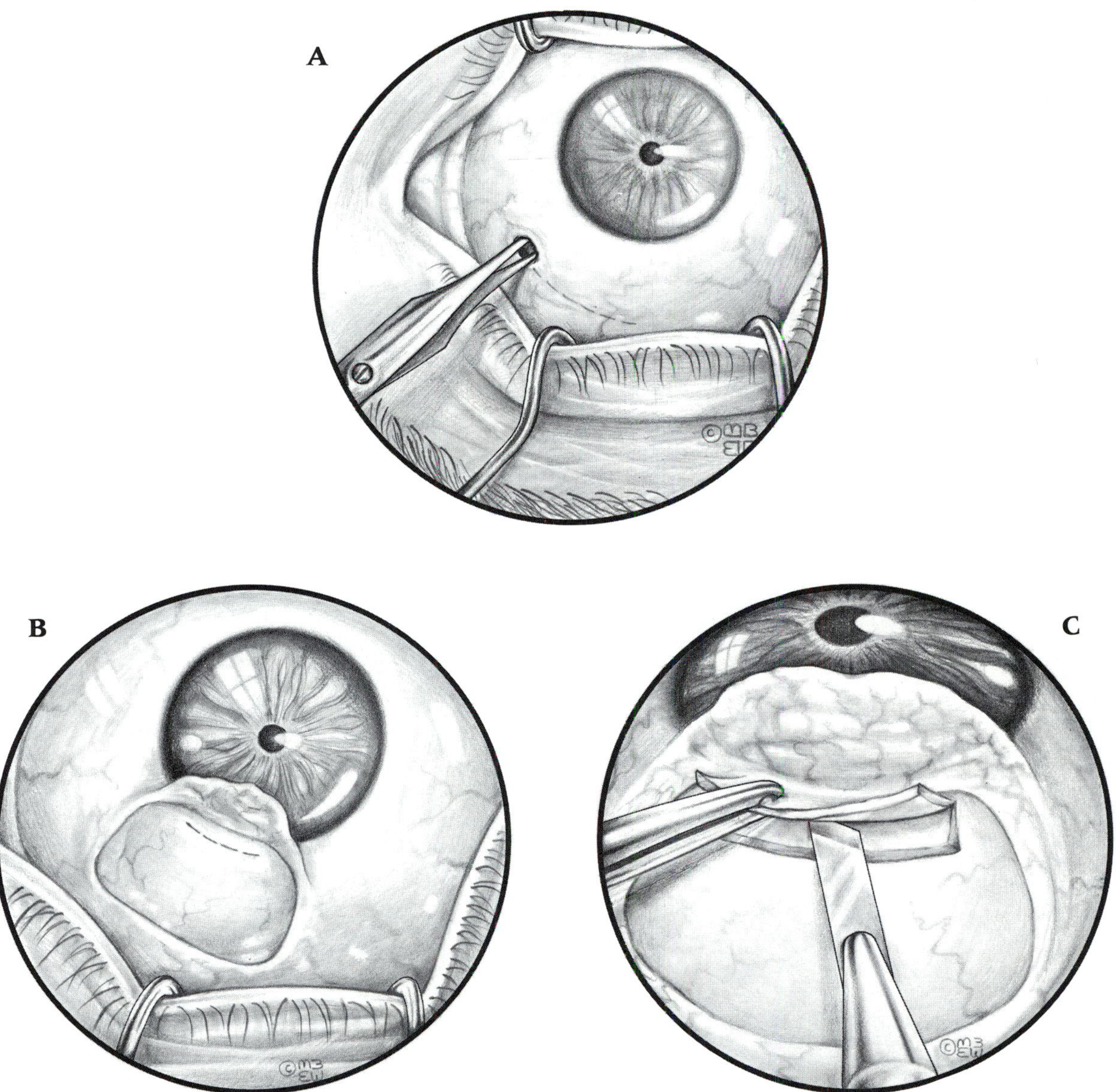

FIGURE 13-10. **A,** Conjunctival incision. **B,** Marking scleral flap. **C,** Cutting lamellar scleral flap.

Continued.

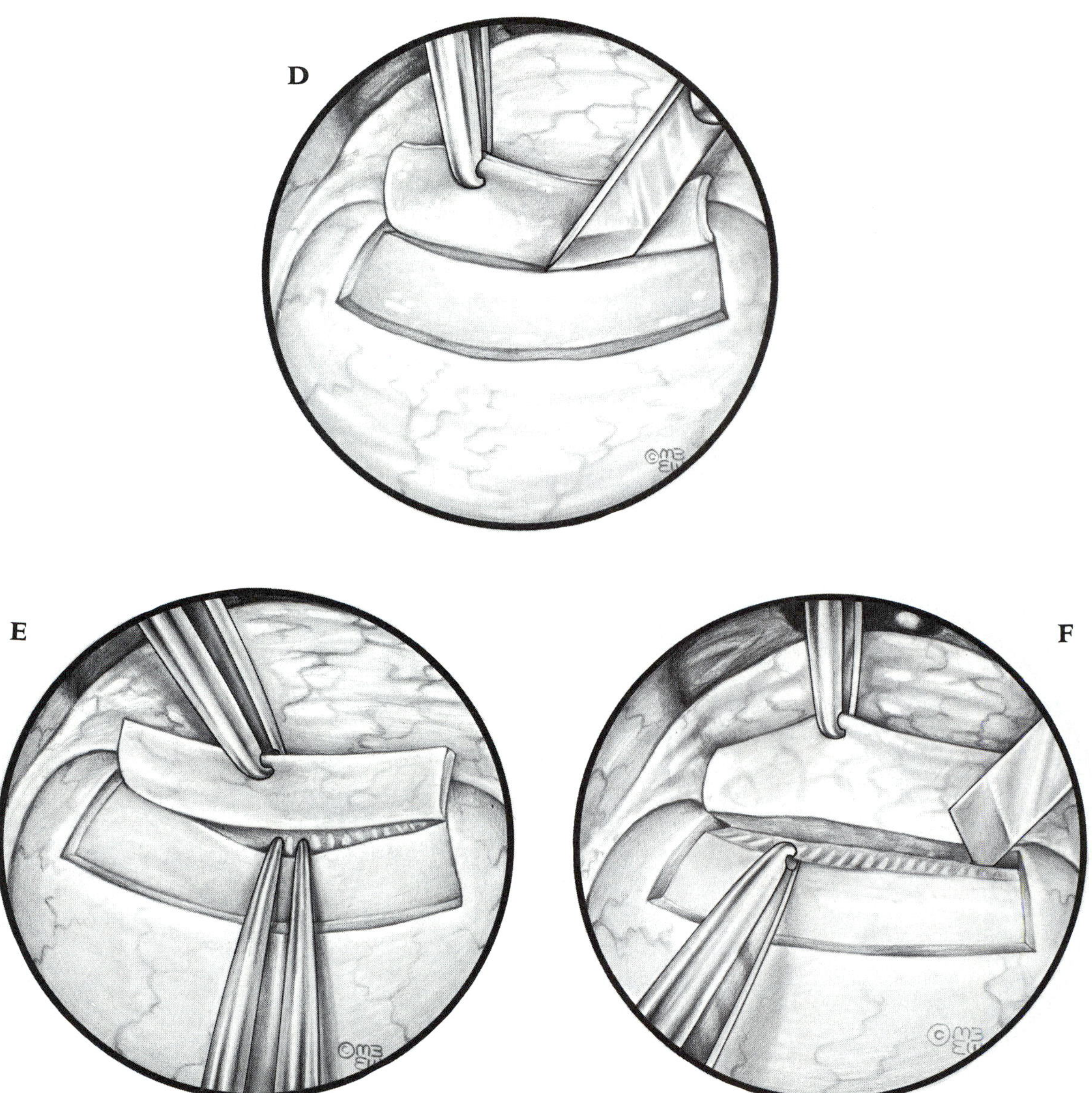

FIGURE 13-10, cont'd. D, Incision into deep sclera. **E,** Applying cautery burns. **F,** Deepening incision and applying another row of cautery burns.

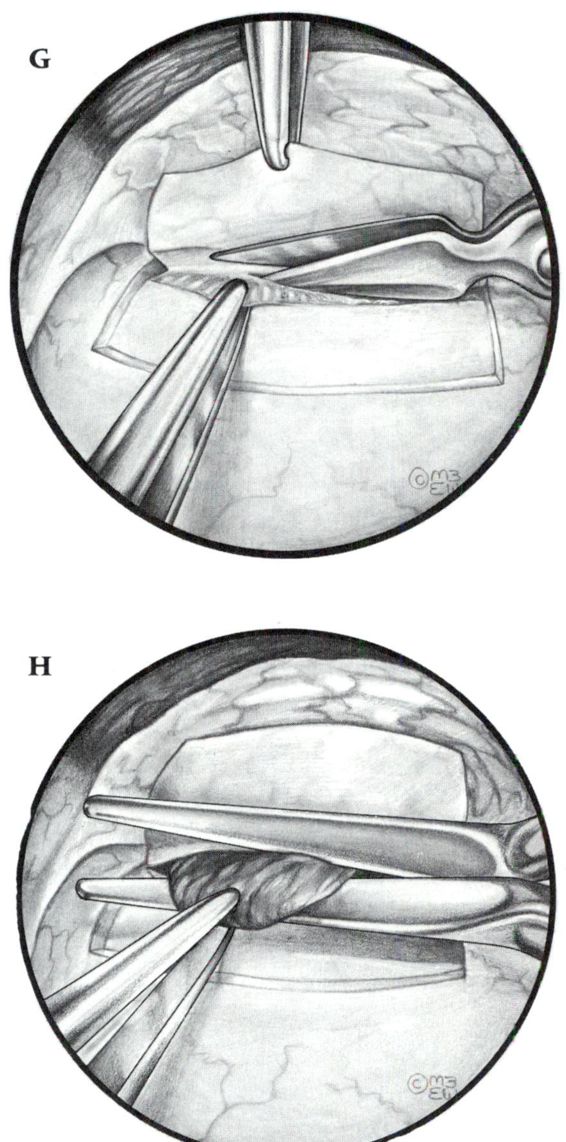

FIGURE 13-10, cont'd. **G,** Enlarging opening. **H,** Wide-based peripheral iridectomy.

Continued.

A modification of technique is to apply cautery to the scleral base before incising deeper (Fig. 13-10, *I*). The deep incision is then made in a cauterized bed (Fig. 13-10, *J*). Subsequent cautery is applied to the deep posterior lip (Fig. 13-10, *K*). After first repairing Tenon's fascia with a continuous 10-0 suture (Fig. 13-10, *L*), one repairs the edges of the conjunctival flap with a continuous 6-0 plain catgut suture (Fig. 13-10, *M*). The operation is terminated by subconjunctival injections of methylprednisolone sodium succinate (Solu-Medrol) 0.5 ml and gentamicin sulfate (Garamycin) 0.5 ml in the inferior fornix. The postoperative management is similar to that of trabeculectomy.

Unguarded full-thickness fistulizing procedures are rarely necessary but may prove effective when intrascleral thermosclerostomy has failed. A posterior lip-punch sclerectomy is chosen in these circumstances. Alternatively, a cilio-ablative procedure or seton is considered.

Subconjunctival injections of the antimetabolite 5-fluorouracil reduce postoperative scarring and may be valuable after reoperation. Persistent corneal epithelial defects may ensue, and close monitoring is necessary. Postoperative digital massage is carried out if the intraocular pressure rises to the high teens after 1 or 2 weeks. Pressure is applied to the globe through the lower lid for 10 seconds, released momentarily and repeated from 1 to 4 minutes four times a day. It may be necessary to continue massage for several months.

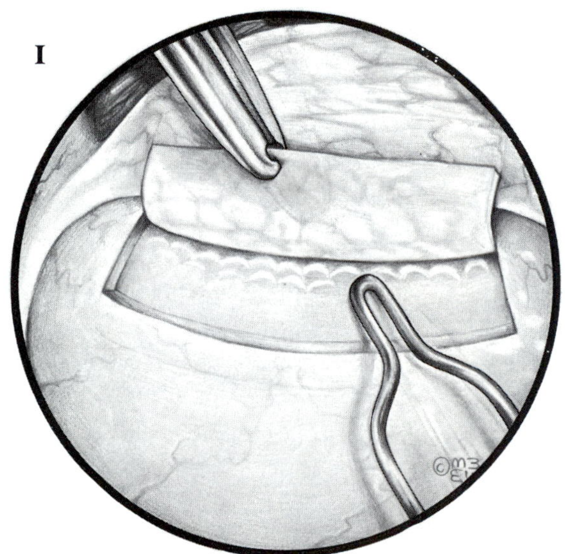

FIGURE 13-10, cont'd. **I,** Modification of technique.

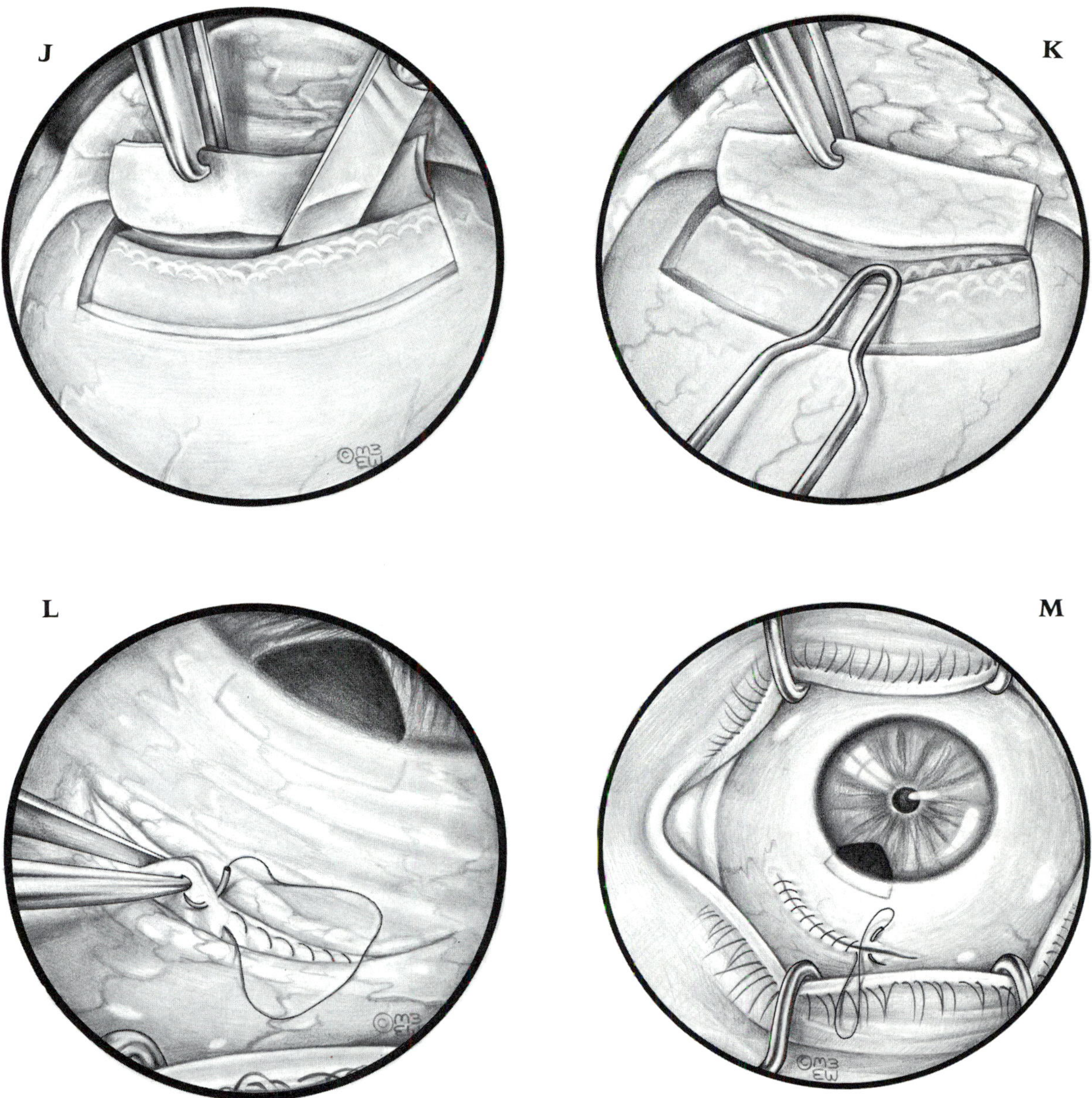

FIGURE 13-10, cont'd. **J,** Deep incision in cauterized bed. **K,** Further cautery to deep posterior lip. Procedure shown in **F** through **H** completes peripheral iridectomy. **L,** Repairing Tenon's fascia. **M,** Repairing conjunctival incision.

Therapeutic ultrasound

Focussed high-intensity ultrasound is effective in producing selective destruction of sclera over the pars plana and contiguous focal damage to ciliary epithelium. The intraocular pressure is reduced without an invasive surgical procedure being required (Coleman et al.). Therapeutic ultrasound is also a modality for restoration of failed trabeculectomies (Yablonski et al.).

Excimer laser

Excimer laser is currently under investigation for use in performing trabeculostomies. This is not a completely nonsurgical procedure, since a conjunctival flap must be made before the application of laser energy.

CHAPTER 14

Aphakic Eyes, Combined Procedures, Setons, and Other Procedures

In this chapter, combined cataract extraction and trabeculectomy, Molteno implant, cilioablative surgery, cyclodialysis, and other procedures are discussed.

Glaucoma Surgery in Aphakic Eyes

Filtering surgery

In aphakic eyes with uncontrolled glaucoma, filtering is performed when argon laser trabeculoplasty has failed or is not feasible because of extensive peripheral anterior synechiae. The filtering operation of choice is intrascleral thermosclerostomy ("subscleral Scheie"). This procedure is described in Chapter 13. The presence of vitreous in the anterior chamber reduces the chance of successful filtration. Anterior vitrectomy may be necessary to prevent vitreous blocking the fistulized area. Trabeculectomy (see Chapter 13) is less efficacious than the thermosclerostomy but lends itself to combined anterior vitrectomy if necessary. Adequate vitrectomy is carried out through the trabeculectomy window by use of a vitreophage/suction/irrigating system. Pars plana vitrectomy may be carried out followed by the guarded thermosclerostomy. Massive choroidal hemorrhage is a major feared complication in filtering surgery on aphakic eyes.

Cyclodialysis

Some surgeons still perform cyclodialysis, though the overall success rate (25% to 40%) is poorer than with filtering operations. The main virtue of cyclodialysis is the lower incidence of complications, especially vitreous loss. The intraocular pressure–lowering effect is unpredictable. Local anesthesia is sufficient. Increased uveoscleral flow or reduced aqueous formation (or both) may explain the mechanism of action of cyclodialysis.

Technique

A superior quadrant is preferred. Under a conjunctival flap made 5 mm back from the limbus, a scleral incision is made 3 mm in length, 3.5 mm behind and parallel to the limbus. The incision is deepened to the ciliary body. This level is seen to be reached when a shiny black surface appears. A 7-0 Mersilene suture is placed at half-scleral thickness across the middle of the sclerotomy and looped aside. The anterior loop is used to elevate the scleral lip to facilitate entry of a narrow cyclodialysis spatula. The latter is entered radially, passing between ciliary body and scleral spur until the tip is seen in the anterior chamber. It is most important to keep the heel of the spatula against the globe and not to damage the ciliary body with the tip, which should hug the inner sclera and glide over the scleral spur (Fig. 14-1, *A*). The blade should be depressed slightly on entering the anterior chamber to avoid stripping Descemet's membrane. It is then withdrawn and slid parallel to the limbus before being rotated into the anterior chamber (Fig. 14-1, *B*). This procedure is then repeated in the contiguous portion of ciliary body. An alternative technique employs a round-bodied spatula, which is passed into the anterior chamber with multiple thrusts (Fig. 14-1, *C*). Blood in the anterior chamber is flushed out with saline through the cyclodialysis cleft. An air injection may be made into the anterior chamber to block further entry of blood. The sclerotomy suture is tied, and the conjunctival incision repaired with 6-0 plain catgut. A miotic is instilled.

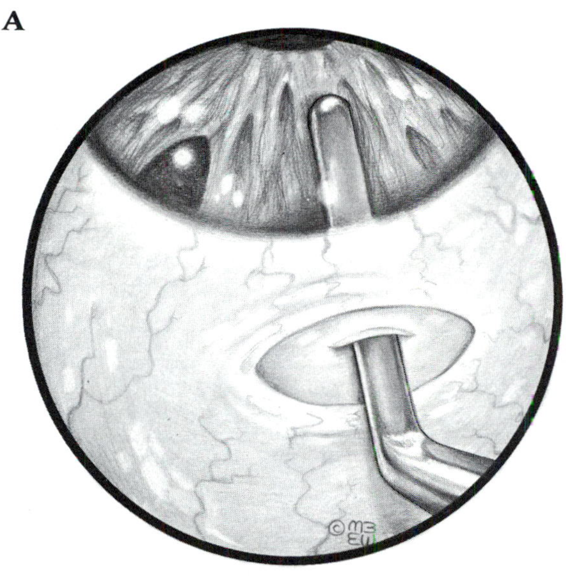

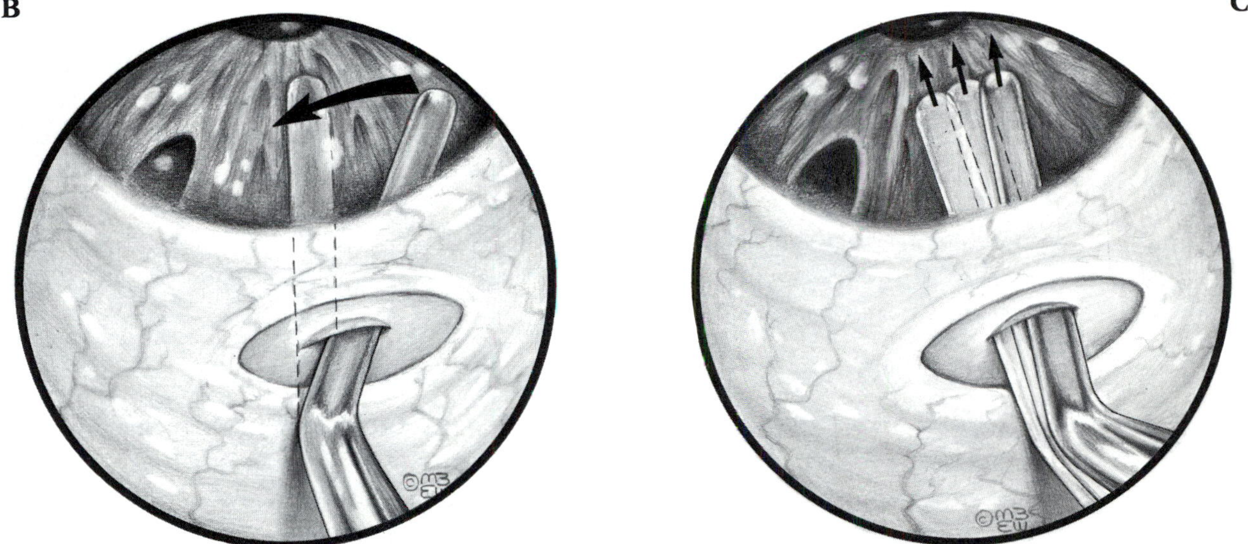

FIGURE 14-1. **A,** With scleral incision, light resistance is felt as tip of spatula separates scleral spur before entering anterior chamber. **B,** Classic Heine method. **C,** Modified procedure to separate ciliary body. There is less tendency for significant bleeding with this method.

Ciliodestructive procedures

Destruction of ciliary body tissue by diathermy, freezing, or Nd:YAG laser energy is not restricted to aphakic eyes but is reserved for severe glaucomatous eyes in which multiple surgical procedures have failed.

Diathermy applied to the pars plicata of the ciliary body under a thick scleral flap about 90 to 120 degrees can be effective (Naumann). Diathermy through full-thickness sclera can cause necrosis and staphyloma. Severe uveitis is prone to follow cyclodiathermy.

Cyclocryotherapy is commonly utilized. The procedure is most likely to be successful if the following conditions are met:

1. Probe tip 2.5 mm.
2. Probe temperature $-80°$ to $-90°$ C.
3. Each application for 60 seconds.
4. Three applications per quadrant.
5. Single freeze (not freeze-thaw-freeze) cycles.
6. The anterior edge of the probe tip should be placed 3 mm back from the anterior border of the limbus.
7. The ice ball should not freeze the cornea (Fig. 14-2).
8. Repeat cyclocryotherapy should not be undertaken sooner than 1 month, since the intraocular pressure–lowering effect is delayed.

Local anesthesia is usual. It is prudent to undertreat at the first session and repeat cyclocryotherapy in single quadrants rather than risk excessive ciliodestruction. Not more than two quadrants are treated initially. Extra caution must be exercised in neovascular glaucoma because massive hyphema can result. Hypotony and phthisis are well-recognized complications. Post-operative treatment with topical steroids is given until the reactive uveitis subsides. This is usually 1 to 2 weeks. Choroidal effusion usually resolves spontaneously. The results are often not long lasting. Cyclocryotherapy is useful as an adjunct procedure if the intraocular pressure has been greatly but inadequately reduced by an invasive procedure.

Nd:YAG cilioablation (thermal photocoagulation)

Transscleral application of the Nd:YAG laser to the ciliary body in the thermal mode has proved effective. Retrobulbar anesthesia is necessary. When the Lasag Microruptor is used, 40 applications are made for 360 degrees, with each point being 3 mm from the limbus. The energy is 3.5 to 5 joules. Exposure time is 20 msec. Instrumentation and techniques are currently in evolution. A Nd:YAG laser solid sapphire-tip fiberoptic delivery system is now the preferred method of ciliodestruction. Forty to 75 applications are made over 360 degrees, with each point of direct contact being 2 mm from the limbus. The power setting is 5 watts. Exposure time is 0.7 second. The number of applications depends on the preoperative intraocular pressure.

Argon laser photocoagulation

Argon laser photocoagulation of ciliary processes usually has limited effect. It may be carried out if at least 25% of the circumference is visualized through a sector iridectomy or a maximally dilated pupil. It can be of value as an adjunct procedure. The Goldmann three-mirror lens with antireflective coating is used. Power is 500 to 800 mW, depending on response; size is 200 μm, and the time is 0.2 second. The ciliary processes shrivel and turn white. No postoperative treatment is necessary.

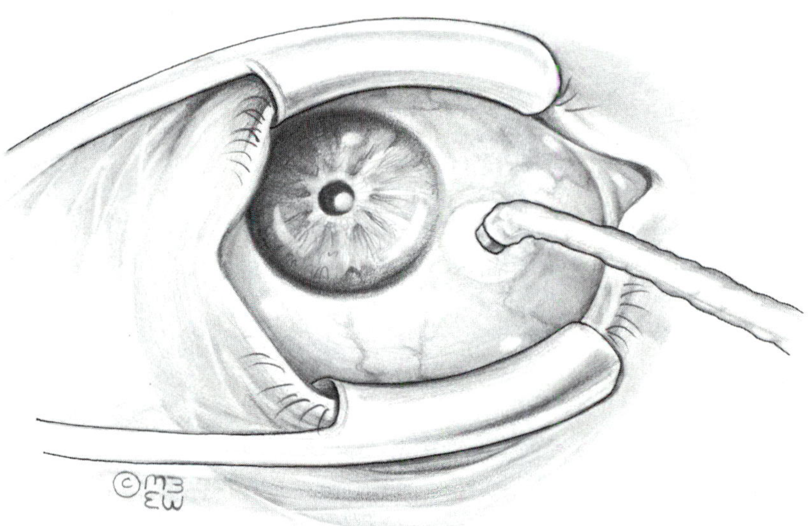

FIGURE 14-2. Ciliodestructive procedure performed with a 2.5 mm cryoprobe. The anterior edge of the probe tip is placed 3 mm behind the anterior border of the limbus. The temperature setting is between −80° and −90° C. Single-freeze applications for 60 seconds each are given at three sites per quadrant.

Combined Cataract Extraction and Trabeculectomy

In circumstances where both glaucoma drainage surgery and cataract extraction are indicated, a combined operation is usually satisfactory. The alternative option is to perform glaucoma surgery first and delay cataract surgery. This course has the disadvantage of requiring two separate intraocular procedures, each with attendant risks. It is preferable to take the latter course if the intraocular pressure is over 40 mm Hg. Glaucoma filtering surgery should be avoided on aphakic and pseudophakic eyes generally. The combined procedure is technically more complex than cataract extraction alone.

We favor extracapsular cataract extraction with posterior chamber implant combined with trabeculectomy.

Preoperative preparation

Miotic therapy should be withdrawn 24 hours before surgery to allow for maximal dilatation of the pupil. Miotics given for a long period usually prevent adequate pupil dilatation. Carbonic anhydrase inhibitors should be stopped because aqueous formation must not be reduced. Topical steroids (prednisolone 1% qid) are introduced 1 day before surgery. General anesthesia is preferred.

Technique

A superior rectus bridle suture is optional. A fornix-based conjunctival-Tenon's flap is created for 135 degrees at the superior limbus (14 mm). The flap is dissected posteriorly to expose sclera (Fig. 14-3).

Scleral flap and groove for cataract incision (magnification of 7 to 10)

In the center of the exposed sclera, a scleral flap extending 2.5 mm posteriorly from the limbus and 3 mm wide is outlined, and the posterior incision is made with a diamond knife, dissecting this through the sclera until the surface of the pars plana is just visible. The next step is to create a half-thickness scleral groove for the cataract incision, beginning 4 mm from the edge of the posterior scleral incision and cutting the groove toward the center of the exposed area and along the surgical limbus until a position at the limbus corresponding to the ipsilateral edge of the posterior incision in the sclera is reached. At this point, the scleral groove is turned at right angles and the cut continued as a radial incision extending from the limbus to the edge of the cut scleral incision. A similar limbal-radial incision is fashioned on the other side of the posterior trabeculectomy incision. The result is a 3 mm wide scleral trabeculectomy flap outlined by a cut groove with two radial incisions extending to the limbus and flaring out along the posterior limbus, thus creating a cataract incision. The total width of the cataract incision will be 9 mm (Fig. 14-4).

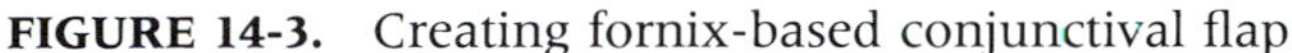

FIGURE 14-3. Creating fornix-based conjunctival flap.

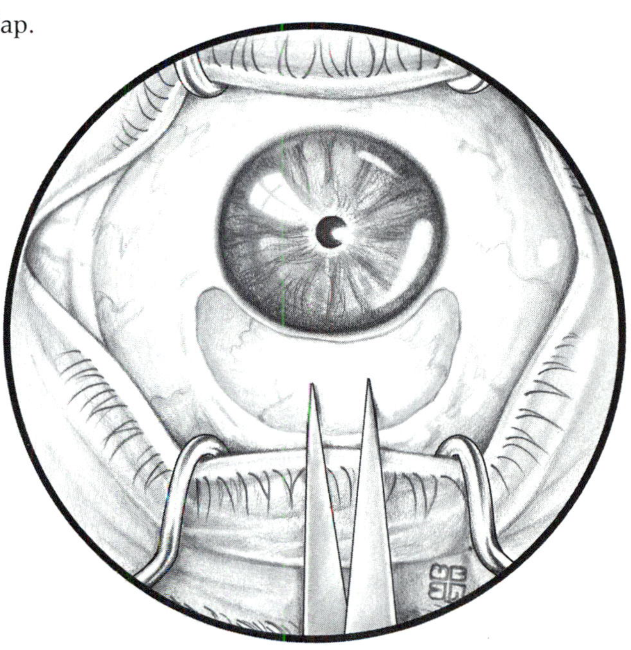

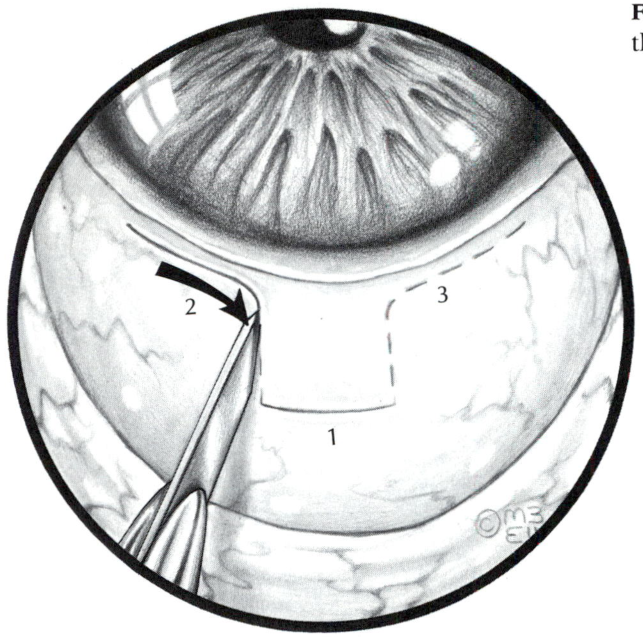

FIGURE 14-4. Scleral flap incorporated in half-thickness scleral groove.

Trabeculectomy (magnification of 10)

Returning to the posterior incision of the trabeculectomy flap, the surgeon inspects the flap and notes the thickness of the sclera from the surface of the sclera to the surface of the pars plana (Fig. 14-5, *A*). At one-third thickness, a surgical plane is formed at this level with a diamond knife. A scleral flap is dissected from the posterior incision forward to just within the surgical limbus (Fig. 14-5, *B*).

Under this lamellar scleral flap, the salient external landmarks are easily visible in the undissected scleral bed, as previously described for the trabeculectomy procedure. A 2 by 2 mm square of corneal-trabecular zone is outlined in the scleral bed hinged at the scleral spur. The anterior border of this flap is situated at the base of the lamellar scleral flap, and it is incised to half the depth of the cornea, followed by similar radial incisions to the sclera (Fig. 14-5, *C*). With this internal flap outlined, the anterior chamber is entered through the anterior incision through a small opening, and the anterior chamber is slowly decompressed. With the eye suitably softened, air is injected into the anterior chamber, and the anterior incision is completed when the two radial incisions are joined by a diamond knife (Fig. 14-5, *D*). While this is done, iris will be pushed into the incision to plug it. Using a Vannas scissors, one completes the trabeculectomy by incising the two radial incisions and rotating the flap formed in this way forward hinged at the scleral spur (Fig. 14-5, *E*). It is excised just anterior to the scleral spur (Fig. 14-5, *F*). During this entire dissection the anterior chamber remains formed because iris will follow the scissors to block the opening, and the preplaced air remains in the chamber. Preplaced 10-0 nylon anchoring sutures are placed at each corner of the lamellar scleral flap and at the posterior corners of the scleral dissection. These are moved out of the way (Fig. 14-5, *F inset*). For simplicity, the sutures will not be shown in the subsequent illustrations.

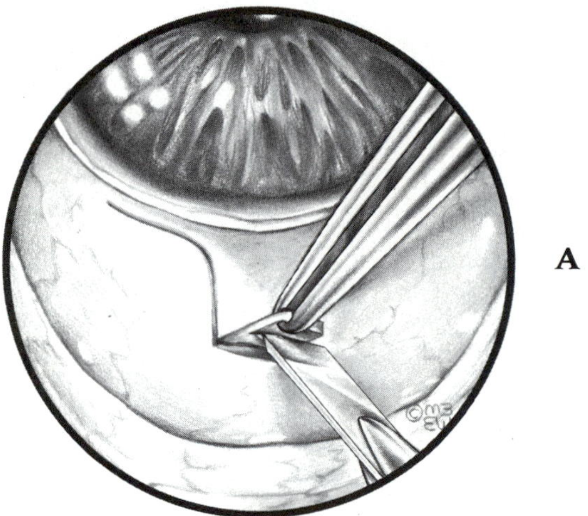

A

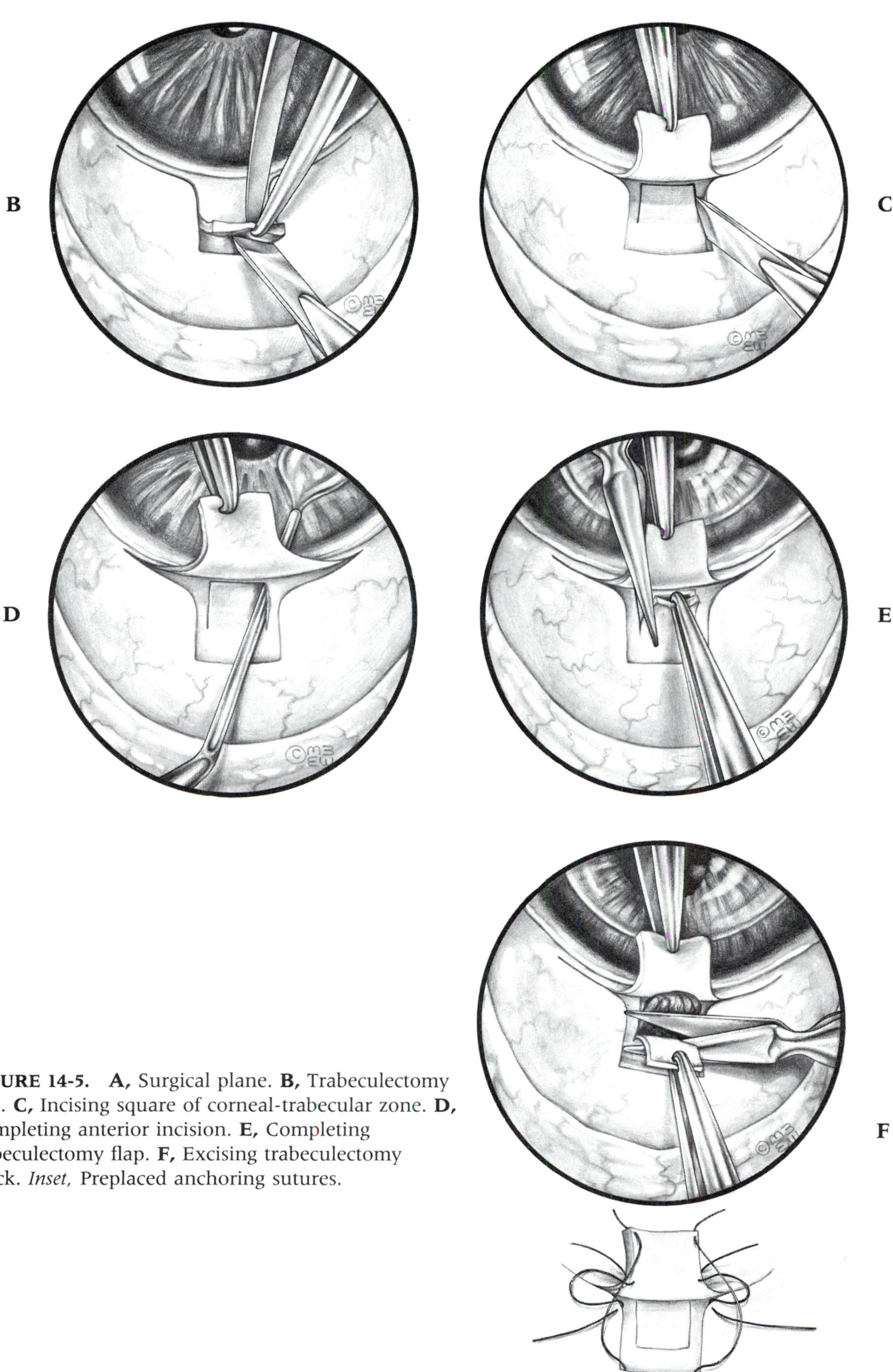

FIGURE 14-5. **A,** Surgical plane. **B,** Trabeculectomy flap. **C,** Incising square of corneal-trabecular zone. **D,** Completing anterior incision. **E,** Completing trabeculectomy flap. **F,** Excising trabeculectomy block. *Inset,* Preplaced anchoring sutures.

Iridectomy (magnification of 10)

Peripheral iridectomy wider than the trabeculectomy opening is now made so that the marginal iris pillars will not protrude through the trabeculectomy opening postoperatively. Iris is grasped with forceps from the center of the trabeculectomy opening, stretched to the left side, and cut midway from the right and then completed by stretching the iris to the right side and completing the cut (Fig. 14-6).

Cataract incision (magnification of 10)

Corneal cataract scissors are now introduced to the trabeculectomy opening. With the deep blade of the scissors in the anterior chamber and avoidance of the iris, the outer blade follows the previously dissected limbal groove, completing the cataract incision on each side of the trabeculectomy opening. A smooth vertical cut is obtained with a bevel on the cornea facing the corneal side of the incision (Fig. 14-7).

Preplaced sutures (magnification of 10)

Two additional 10-0 nylon sutures are placed across the cataract incision precisely at the junction of the limbal side of the trabeculectomy flap and the cataract incision. These sutures run obliquely at 45 degrees to the radial incisions of the scleral flap, placed just anterior to Descemet's membrane on the corneal side in full scleral thickness. They then show correct apposition of the cataract-trabeculectomy incision after their removal. The sutures are looped away from the incision.

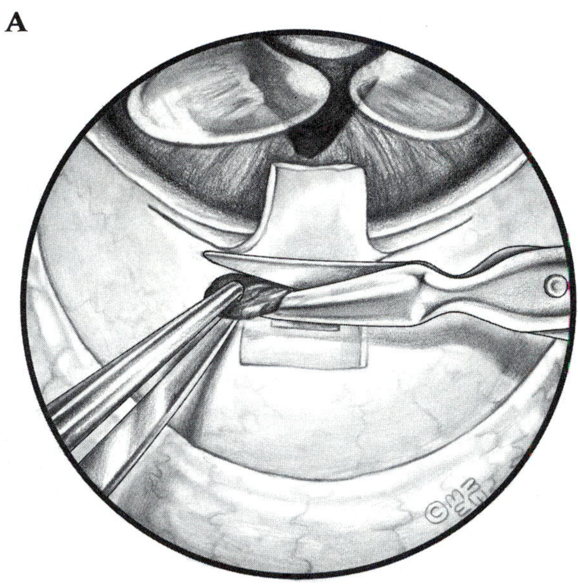

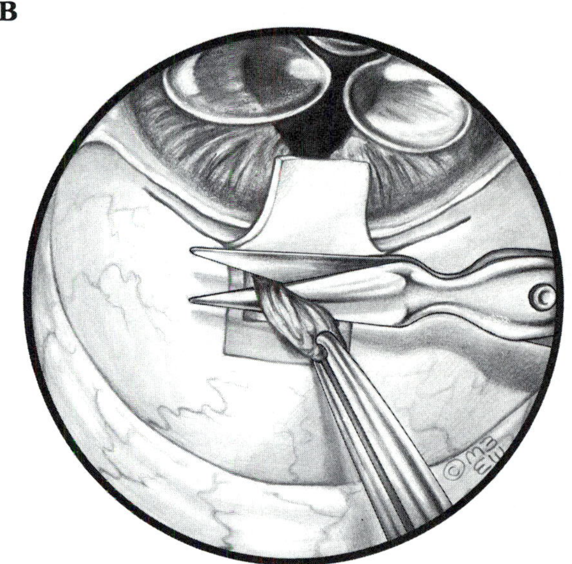

FIGURE 14-6. **A,** Beginning peripheral iridectomy. **B,** Completing peripheral iridectomy.

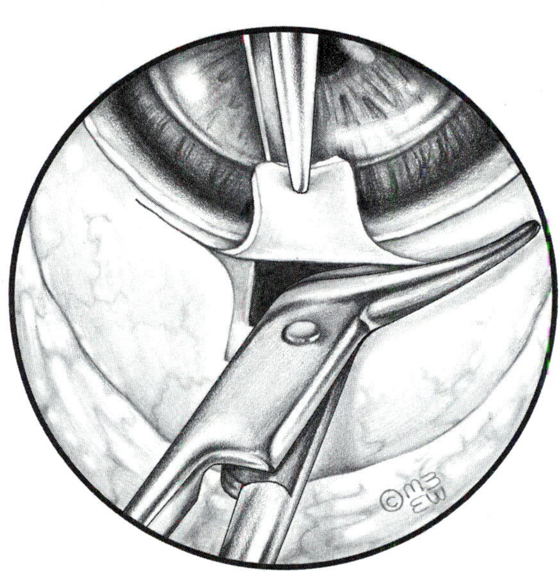

FIGURE 14-7. Cataract incision.

Evaluation of the pupil and iris adhesions (magnification of 7 to 10)

The iris and pupil are inspected for posterior synechiae. If iris adhesions are present to the anterior lens capsule, mechanical separation using an iris spatula is necessary. One should perform separation through the pupil, sweeping the spatula from the pupil under the iris. It should not be performed through the iridectomy, and it should not be performed by sweeping from the iris into the pupil. In this way, synechiae are broken, and pigment loosened by the spatula is swept under the iris and not into the pupil; thus a clear pupil is maintained.

The pupil should now be evaluated. If the pupil is adequately dilated to perform the surgery comfortably, no further pupil surgery is required. However, if the pupil is not adequately dilated, a regular iridectomy should be made from the peripheral iridectomy through to the center. The anterior chamber is filled with a viscoelastic substance such as Healon (Fig. 14-8, *A*). Straight Vannas scissors are introduced, with the inferior blade deep to the iris at the inferior edge of the iridectomy. With the scissors, a regular incision in the iris is then made through to the sphincter so that an increased area of the anterior lens capsule becomes visible. We prefer this technique to using multiple sphincterotomies (Fig. 14-8, *B*). (See also p. 188.)

Anterior capsulotomy (magnification of 10)

The anterior chamber is once again filled with a viscoelastic substance. A 25-gauge needle is suitably bent and a capsulotomy performed using the can-opener technique. The capsulotomy is completed, with the superior portion of the capsule between 10 and 2 o'clock being left intact. With a fine forceps, the capsule is then grasped and rotated superiorly, hinged at the 10 to 12 o'clock position. Using Vannas scissors, the capsulotomy is completed between 10 to 12 o'clock, and the anterior capsule so separated is removed (Fig. 14-9). (See also p. 180.)

A

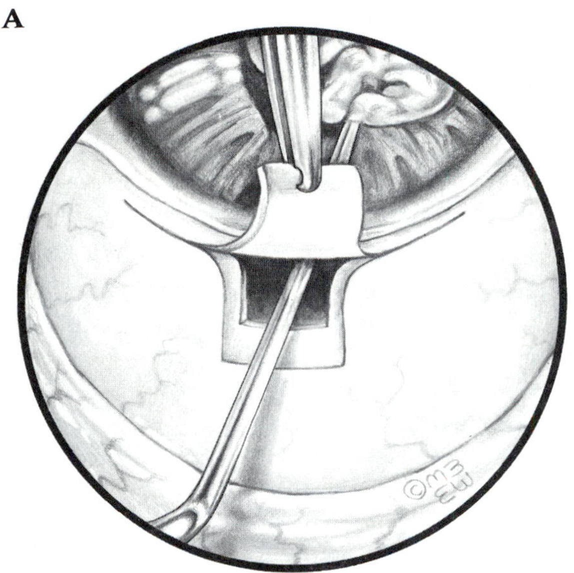

B

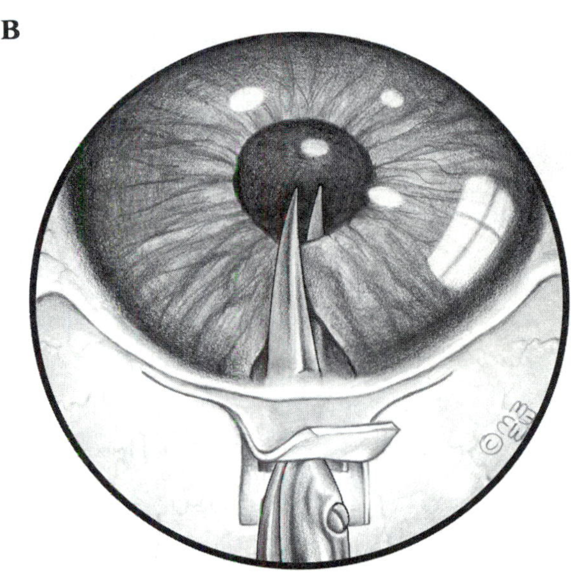

FIGURE 14-8. **A,** Filling anterior chamber with Healon. **B,** Iris is cut to the pupil with straight Vannas scissors if dilatation is inadequate.

A

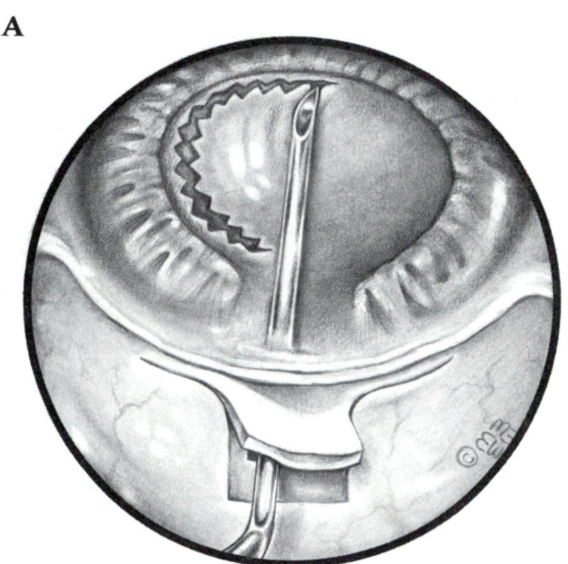

B

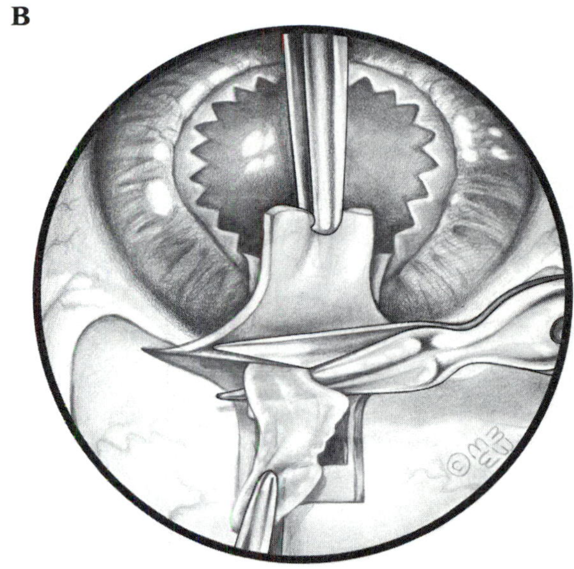

FIGURE 14-9. **A,** Capsulotomy with 25-gauge needle suitably bent, leaving superior capsule intact. **B,** Grasping capsule inferiorly with long Kelman-McPherson forceps and rotating it exteriorly.

Nuclear expression and cortical removal (magnification of 10)

The nucleus is expressed through the capsule with pressure at the 6 o'clock position on the cornea using a muscle hook, and pressure at the 12 o'clock position behind the posterior lip of a limbal incision with the lens loop (irrigating vectis) (Fig. 14-10, *A*). (See also p. 182.) The preplaced 10-0 nylon sutures at the juncture of the regular trabeculectomy and cataract incisions are then tied on each side. Further interrupted 10-0 nylon sutures are placed across the wound and tied to create a formed anterior chamber, and the cortical remnants are aspirated from the posterior chamber using mechanical irrigation/aspiration (Fig. 14-10, *B*). (See also p. 186.)

Insertion of intraocular lens (magnification of 7)

Sufficient interrupted 10-0 nylon sutures are removed to produce a 7 mm wound opening. An air bubble is introduced into the anterior chamber, and a posterior chamber lens is introduced through the 7 mm incision in the standard fashion and fixed in the ciliary sulcus. The inferior loop is inserted under the inferior rim of the pupil and under the inferior iris. Further downward movement of the implant will push the optic under the inferior iris down, and approximately half of the optic is inserted under the iris. The superior haptic is held with a Kelman-McPherson forceps and rotated over the optic, and the implant is then dialed so that the superior loop can be released under the superior iris. The implant is then further dialed into a horizontal position using a Sinsky hook. Acetylcholine chloride (Miochol) is injected into the anterior chamber to constrict the pupil (Fig. 14-11). (See also p. 228.)

A

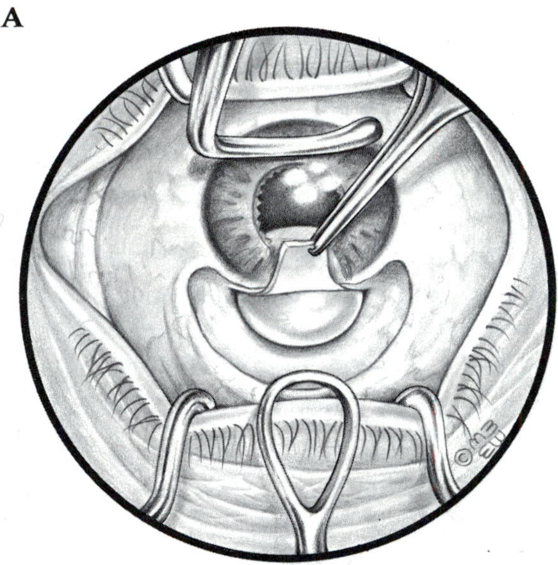

B

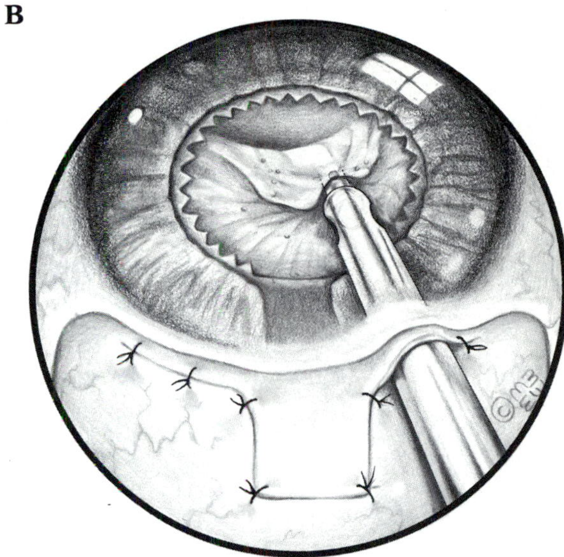

FIGURE 14-10. **A,** Expressing nucleus. **B,** Cortical removal.

A

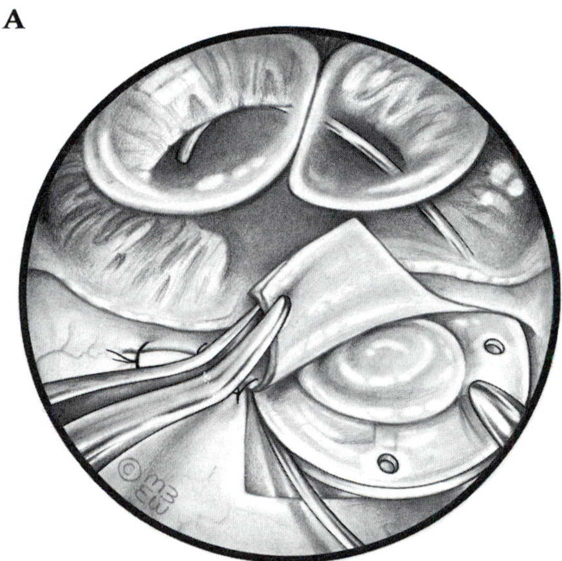

B

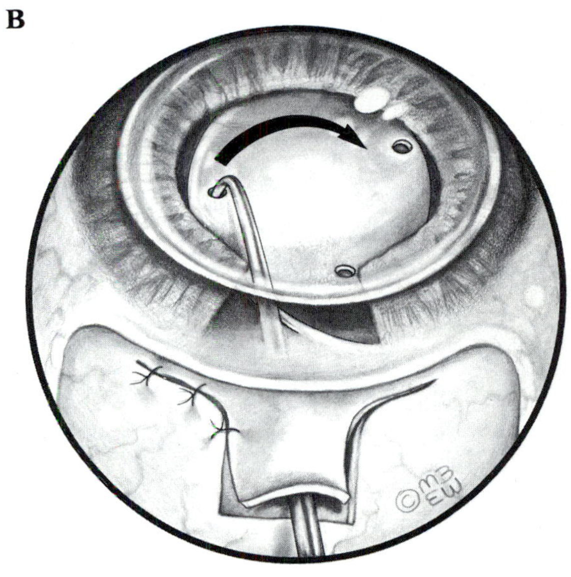

FIGURE 14-11. **A,** Introducing posterior chamber intraocular lens implant with Healon on its anterior surface. **B,** Dialing implant into horizontal position using Sinsky hook.

Repair of radial iridotomy (magnification of 10)

Using a 10-0 probing suture with a "ski," one repairs the radial iridotomy with one interrupted suture at the sphincter and one at the tip of the iridectomy (Fig. 14-12, *A*). Before the iris is repaired, the air in the anterior chamber is replaced by a viscoelastic substance, such as Healon. (See also p. 192.) The trabeculectomy-cataract incision is resutured with 10-0 interrupted sutures, with use of a total of four 10-0 nylon sutures on each side of the incision, that is, one suture at the posterior lip of the trabeculectomy lamellar scleral flap, one suture at the junction of the radial trabeculectomy-cataract incision, and two additional sutures along the cataract incision. An irrigation/aspiration is now entered into the chamber to remove the remaining viscoelastic substance (Fig. 14-12, *B*).

Conjunctival repair (magnification of 5)

The conjunctival-Tenon's flap is now rotated anteriorly until it lies snugly across the limbus. It is secured at the limbus with one 10-0 nylon suture at each edge of the incision and one 10-0 nylon suture immediately adjacent to each radial incision of the trabeculectomy flap (Fig. 14-13).

Balanced saline solution is injected under the conjunctival flap to form a bleb. Solu-Medrol and gentamicin are injected subconjunctivally into the inferior fornix. Tropicamide (Mydriacyl) drops are instilled before a patch and shield is applied.

A

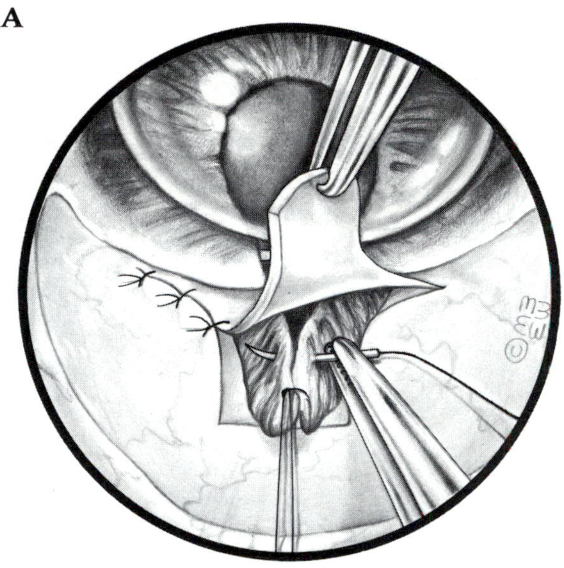

B

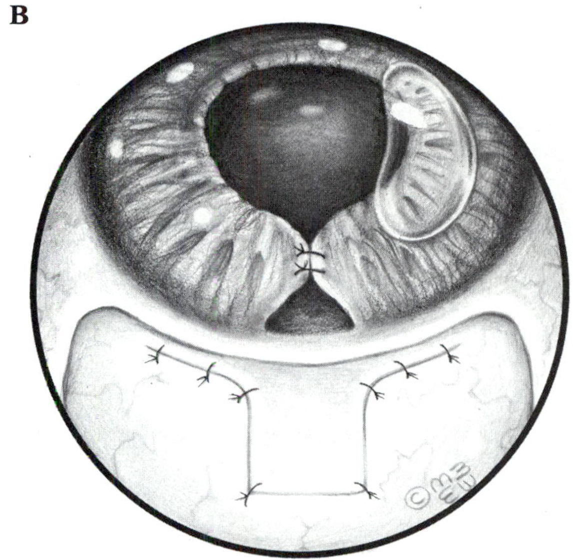

FIGURE 14-12. **A,** Repairing radial iridotomy. **B,** Repairing trabeculectomy–cataract incision.

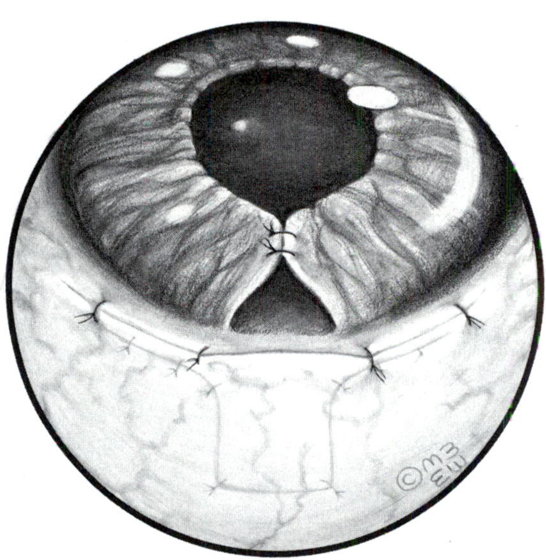

FIGURE 14-13. Securing conjunctival–Tenon's flap edge at limbus.

Setons

Setons should be considered in those eyes where filtering surgery has failed to control high intraocular pressure. The seton that we prefer is the Molteno implant, which consists of a biconcave silicone base plate of 13 mm in diameter and a long silicone tube that enters the anterior chamber (Fig. 14-14).

Technique

General anesthesia is preferred. The inferotemporal area is most suitable for implanting the seton, but any quadrant can be used.

Conjunctival flap (magnification of 5 to 7)

A fornix-based conjunctival flap is created from 6 o'clock with use of a no. 75 Beaver blade (Fig. 14-15). Scar tissue is excised, the conjunctiva undermined, and the inferior rectus muscle isolated with a muscle hook. A 4-0 silk suture is passed backward under the muscle hook and used to control the position of the globe.

Insertion of the prosthesis plate (magnification of 5)

The conjunctiva is undermined posteriorly toward the equator, extending as far back into the fornix as possible. The plate is placed on the sclera under the conjunctiva and pushed toward the fornix until the anterior border lies at least 6 mm behind the limbus. The positions of the anterior holes are marked with cautery on the sclera. Hemostasis of the entire area is obtained with wet-field electrocautery.

A 9-0 nylon suture is placed through each anterior hole in the plate, and an episcleral bite is then taken where each cautery mark was made on the sclera. The sutures are tied, thus securing the plate to the sclera (Fig. 14-16).

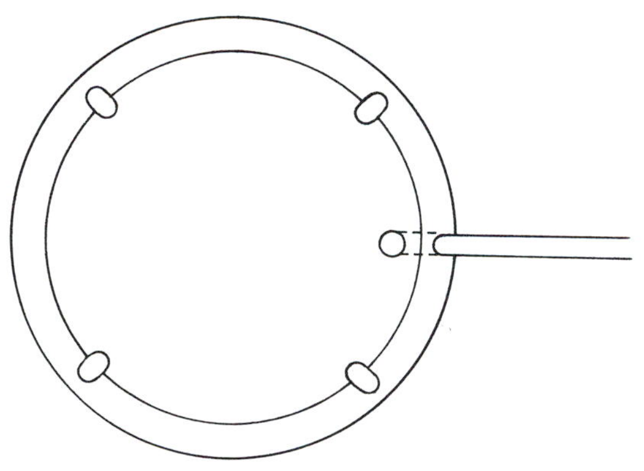

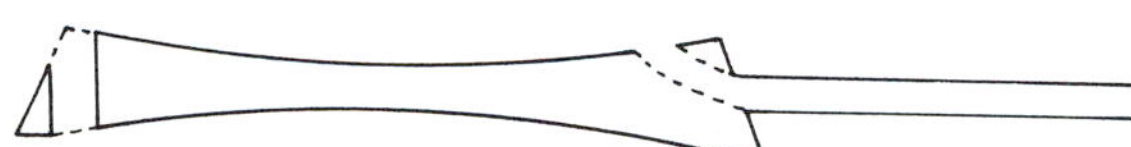

FIGURE 14-14. The Molteno implant consists of a biconcave silicone base plate 13 mm in diameter and a long silicone tube. The external diameter of the tube is 0.63 mm. The internal diameter is 0.20 mm. The uncut length is 16 mm. Aqueous humor drains subconjunctivally over the base plate, which separates conjunctiva from sclera.

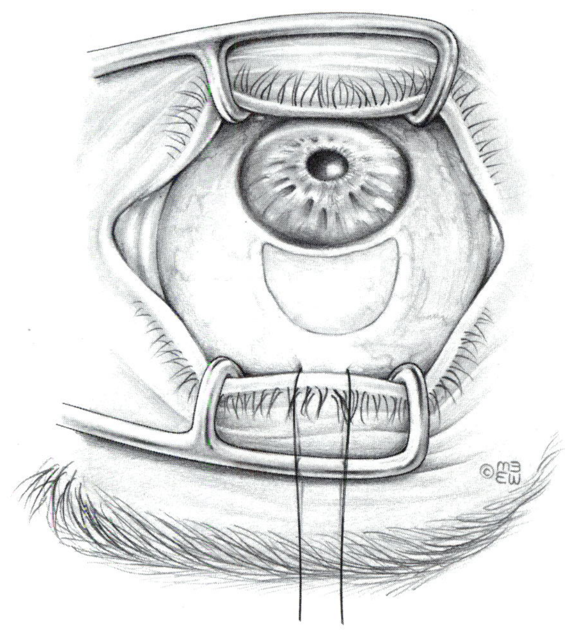

FIGURE 14-15. Fornix-based conjunctival flap.

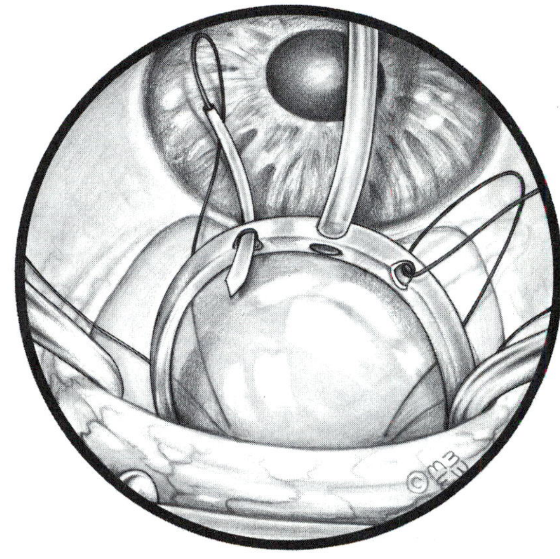

FIGURE 14-16. Positioning the Molteno implant.

Scleral flap (magnification of 5 to 7)

A 4 mm square of sclera is outlined with a wet-field electrocautery in front of the plate and extending from the limbus posteriorly in the inferotemporal quadrant. A one-half-thickness scleral lamellar flap hinged on the cornea is dissected as for a trabeculectomy (Fig. 14-17, *A*). The dissection of the flap is carried to just inside the limbus (Fig. 14-17, *B*). 10-0 nylon sutures are preplaced (Fig. 14-17, *C*).

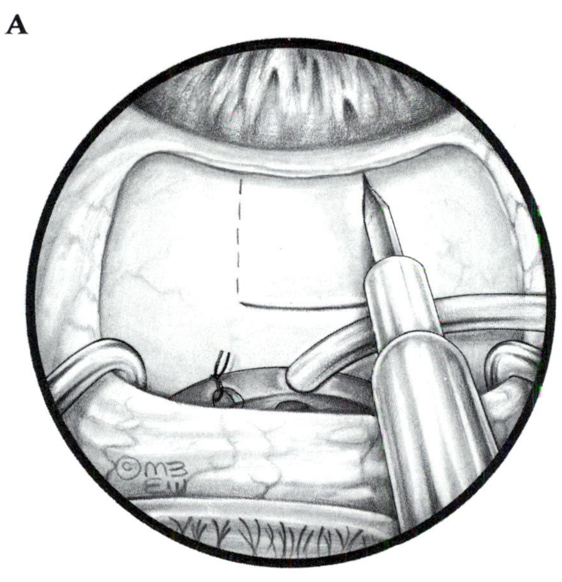

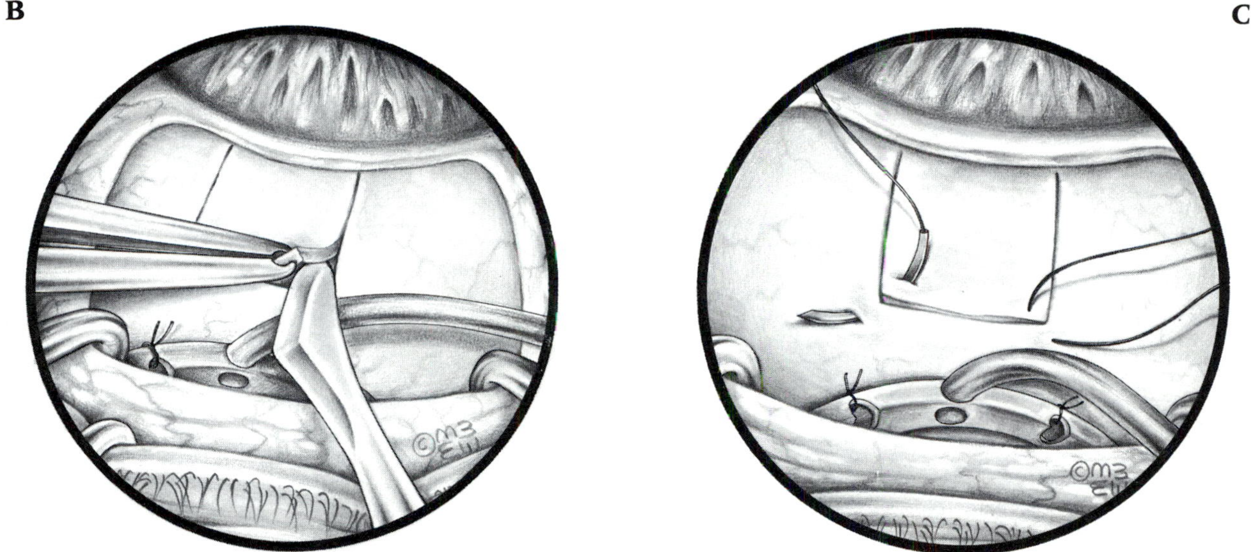

FIGURE 14-17. A, Scleral flap. **B,** Hinging scleral flap. **C,** Preplaced anchoring sutures.

Insertion of the prosthesis tube (magnification of 5 to 7)

The anterior chamber is entered at the anterior border of the scleral flap through an entry incision made with a 19- or 20-gauge needle (Fig. 14-18, *A*). The incision runs parallel to the plane of the iris. The tube is extended onto the cornea, measured, and then cut obliquely 3.5 mm from the surgical limbus (Fig. 14-18, *B*). The tube is pushed into the anterior chamber through the limbal incision (Fig. 14-18, *C*) and protrudes for about 3.5 mm into the anterior chamber. It is fixed by a 9-0 nylon mattress suture through the underlying sclera (Fig. 14-18, *D*). The anterior chamber depth is maintained with air injection. The lamellar scleral flap is closed at the sides with four interrupted 9-0 nylon sutures. The tube is then fixed to the sclera behind the scleral flap with one mattress 9-0 nylon interrupted suture, taking a bite of sclera on each side of the tubing (Fig. 14-18, *E*). The tube should lie freely in the anterior chamber in front of the iris without touching the corneal endothelium.

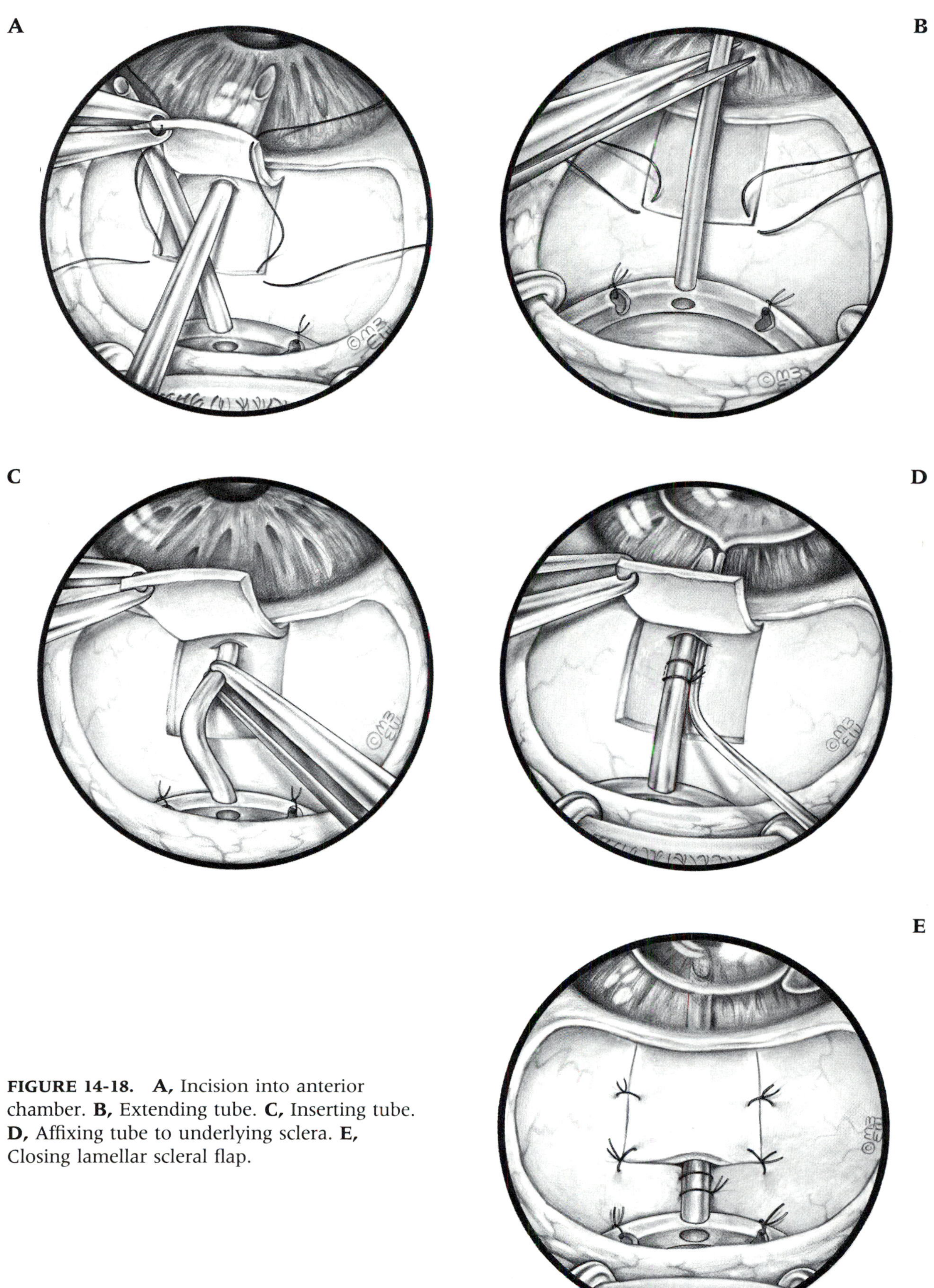

FIGURE 14-18. A, Incision into anterior chamber. **B,** Extending tube. **C,** Inserting tube. **D,** Affixing tube to underlying sclera. **E,** Closing lamellar scleral flap.

Closure (magnification of 5)

The conjunctiva is closed with interrupted 6-0 plain sutures, one at 9 o'clock and one at 4 o'clock (Fig. 14-19). Neo-Decadron (neomycin with dexamethasone) drops are instilled. A pad and shield are taped over the eye.

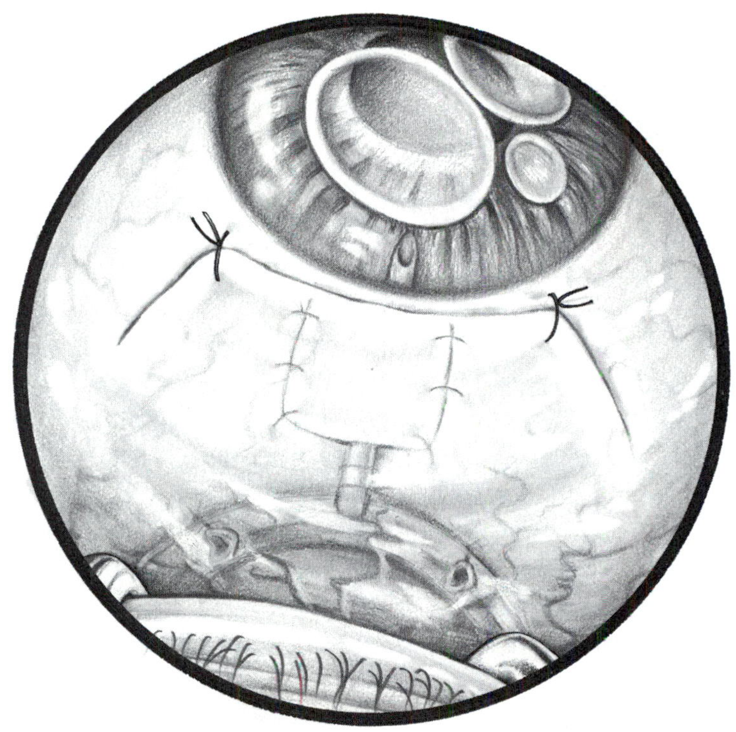

FIGURE 14-19. Closing conjunctival flap.

Surgery for Flat Anterior Chamber After Filtering Surgery

A single mechanism or multiple factors may contribute to cause a flat anterior chamber after filtering surgery. With low intraocular pressure (below 10 mm Hg), a conjunctival leak if present can usually be identified and repaired. Excessive filtration is very uncommon after trabeculectomy but is encountered not infrequently after intrascleral thermosclerostomy. It was more prevalent after unguarded full-thickness fistulizing surgery. Choroidal detachment attributable to accumulation of suprachoroidal fluid may require drainage and reformation of the anterior chamber. Lens-corneal contact mandates surgical intervention within 24 hours to prevent cataract.

With high-normal intraocular pressure (or above 21 mm Hg), pupil block can usually be differentiated from malignant glaucoma (ciliolenticular block or ciliovitreous block) by absence of a patent iridectomy in the former. A laser iridotomy is done if the anterior chamber is very shallow but not dead flat peripherally. A successful iridotomy is immediately appreciated when the intraocular pressure falls and the anterior chamber deepens. Major surgical intervention is otherwise necessary. Pupil block, ciliary block, and suprachoroidal fluid accumulation can all coexist.

The surgical procedure is by posterior sclerotomies, peripheral iridectomy, and removal of fluid from the suprachoroidal space or vitreous, or both.

Technique

A preliminary 3 mm incision is made in the cornea just within the limbus at 6 o'clock with a no. 75 Beaver microblade. The dissection is carried to Descemet's membrane, but the anterior chamber is not entered at this point. A peripheral iridectomy will be done here later.

A 3 mm conjunctival incision is made 3.5 mm behind and parallel to the surgical limbus in the lower nasal quadrant and a similar incision is made in the lower temporal quadrant (Fig. 14-20, *A*). A 2 mm incision is made down to the surface of the pars plana in each of the two quadrants (Fig. 14-20, *B*). Alternatively, two 3 mm sclerotomies may be made radially, centered 3.5 mm from the surgical limbus.

Immediate escape of suprachoroidal fluid may occur. One explores the suprachoroidal space by introducing a flat spatula in each sclerotomy and pushing under the sclera for about 0.5 mm to search for localized fluid (Fig. 14-20, *C*). Localized pressure at points around the sclerotomy often allows fluid to drain.

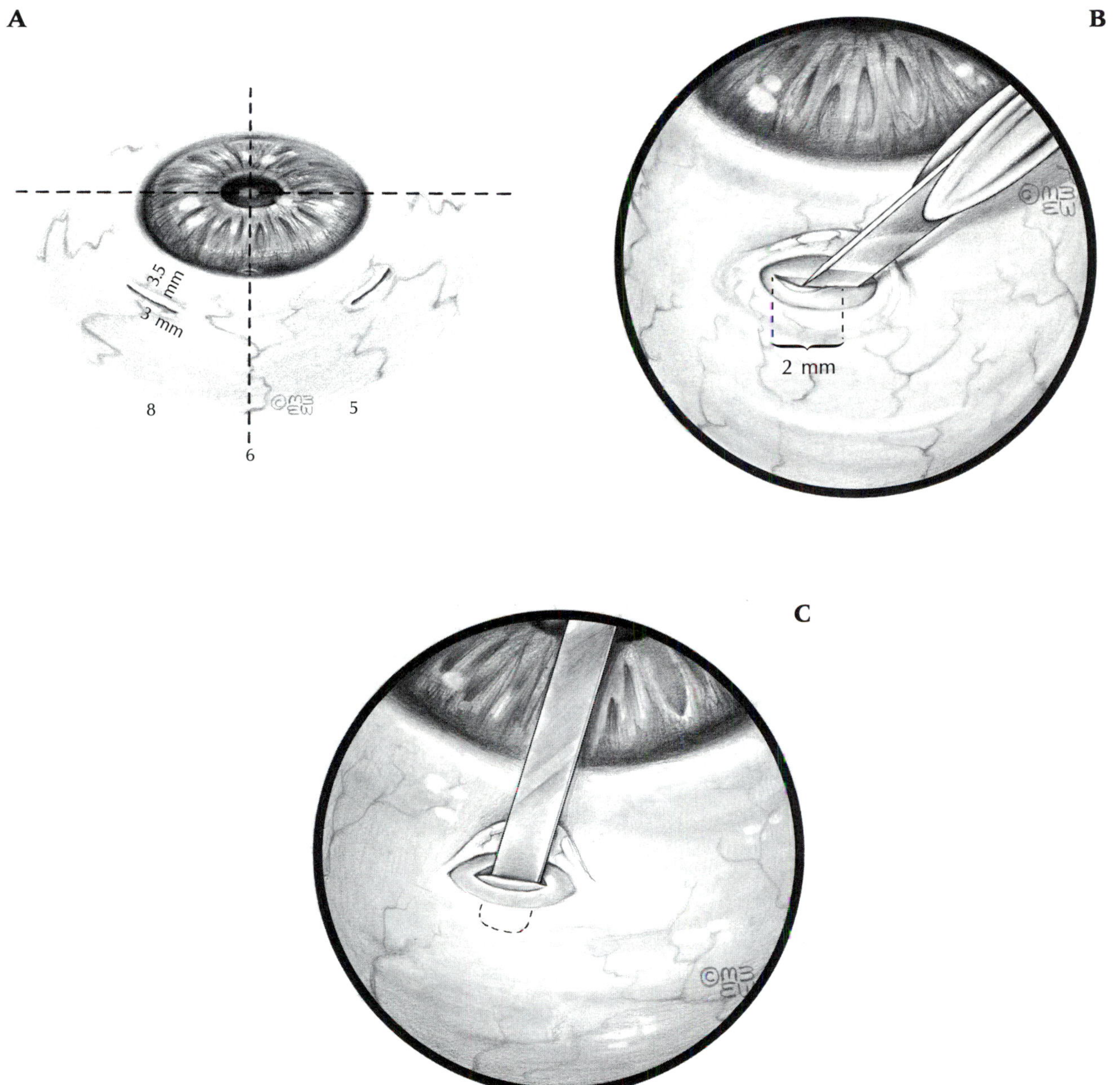

FIGURE 14-20. A, Making conjunctival incision (5× to 7×). **B,** Making scleral incision. **C,** Exploring suprachoroidal space.

Continued.

Multiple spear-shaped sponges are used to absorb the fluid (Fig. 14-20, *D*). If no fluid is found, the lower nasal sclerotomy is closed with a single 7-0 Mersilene suture. One should loosely tie a mattress suture in the lower temporal sclerotomy incision, throwing only one knot. The suture in the incision is withdrawn and placed aside.

A paracentesis is made in the cornea superiorly to allow admission of an air cannula (Fig. 14-20, *E*). The peripheral iridectomy is now completed (see Chapter 13). Failure of iris to prolapse is suggestive of posterior chamber obliteration by iris-lens or iris-vitreous adhesion. This is confirmed when one finds no aqueous drainage after completing the iridectomy. Removal of fluid from the vitreous then becomes mandatory. The corneal incision is closed with one or two 10-0 nylon sutures.

Aspiration of fluid from the vitreous is done through a 25-gauge straight cannula attached to a 2 ml syringe. The cannula is marked off at 12 mm from the tip by a piece of Steridrape. The cannula is pointed toward the center of the globe and not advanced beyond 10 or 12 mm. An air cannula is attached to another 2 ml syringe filled with air and introduced into the anterior chamber through the previous paracentesis incision. Air is injected into the anterior chamber as fluid is withdrawn from the vitreous cavity (Fig. 14-20, *F*). After 1.5 to 2 ml of fluid are withdrawn, the cannula is removed, and the sclerotomy is tightly closed (Fig. 14-20, *F inset*). The conjunctival incisions are closed with continuous 6-0 plain catgut sutures.

The air filling the anterior chamber is now replaced with balanced saline solution. The paracentesis does not require a suture. Subconjunctival injections of steroid and gentamicin may be given. Postoperative steroid-antibiotic drops and a short-acting mydriatic are used.

A more radical approach for intractable malignant glaucoma is a pars plana complete vitrectomy. When a cataract is present, it may be extracted immediately upon completion of the vitrectomy (see p. 430).

D

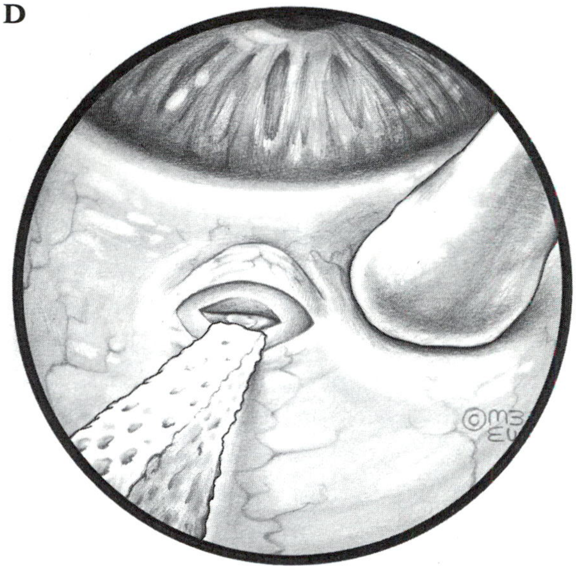

E

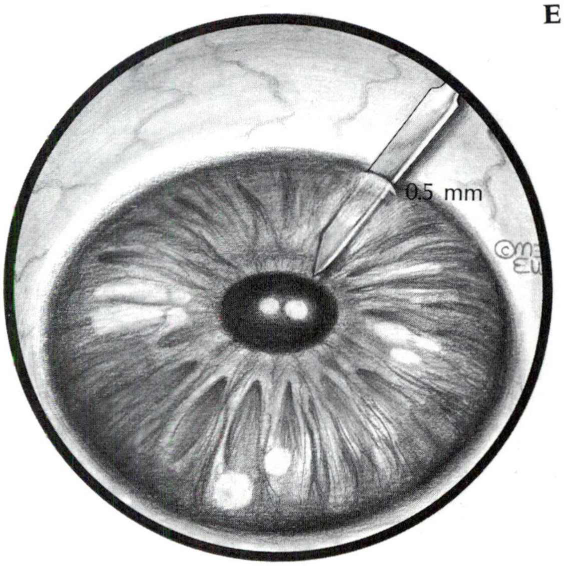

0.5 mm

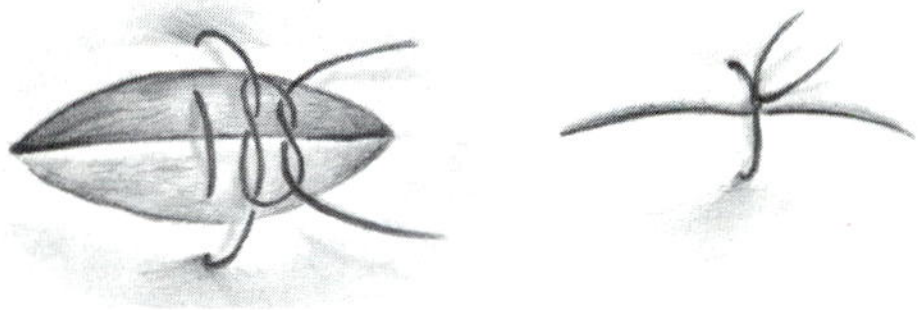

F

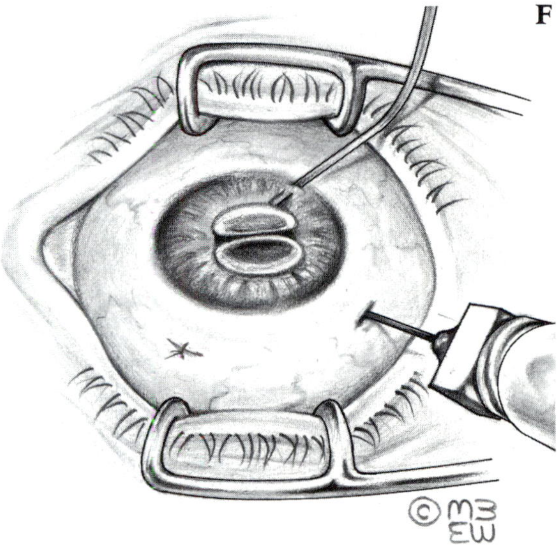

FIGURE 14-20, cont'd. D, Applying pressure locally to facilitate fluid egress. **E,** Paracentesis (7× to 10×). **F,** Withdrawing fluid. *Inset,* Cannula is removed, and the mattress suture is tied securely.

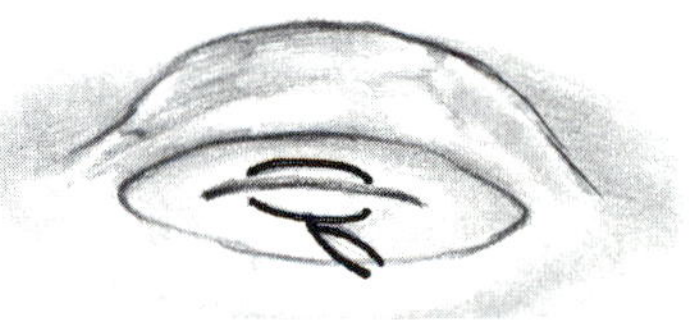

Repair of Ischemic Bleb with Late Leakage

Surgical repair becomes mandatory if a conjunctival fistula fails to close spontaneously after a few days of patching and expectant treatment, including antibiotic drops.

Technique

The conjunctiva is incised at the edge of the ischemic area, and the fistula is included. The incision is carried to the limbus and extended 3 or 4 mm on either side, so that a fornix-based hood of conjunctiva is raised. A corneal incision at half-thickness is made just anterior to the limbus corresponding to the length of the conjunctival flap. Cautery is lightly applied to the base of the corneal incision. The conjunctival flap is attached with interrupted 10-0 nylon sutures to the corneal groove, as shown in Fig. 14-21, *A*. The sutures pass through conjunctiva, scleral side of the corneal incision, conjunctiva again, and cornea again, seriatim. The sutures are tied over the conjunctiva (Fig. 14-21, *B*).

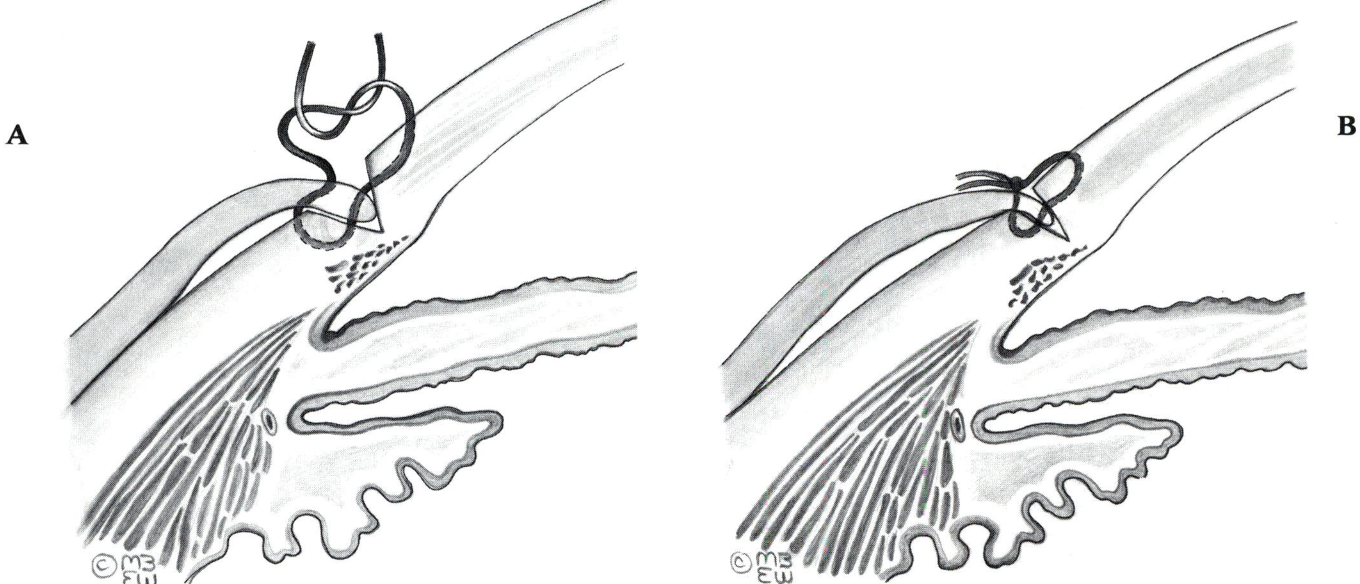

FIGURE 14-21. A, Technique of repairing ischemic bleb with late leakage. **B,** Sutures tightened and tied.

PART FOUR

STRABISMUS SURGERY

Eugene M. Helveston

CHAPTER 15

Essentials of Strabismus Surgery

PATIENT EVALUATION AND PREPARATION

Diagnosis

The proper diagnosis is an essential beginning to effective strabismus treatment. As with any area of medicine, the adage is valid: "You don't find what you don't look for—you don't diagnose what you don't know." The ophthalmologist undertaking the treatment of strabismus should be aware of the diagnostic possibilities and therapeutic alternatives from abducens palsy to Z-tenotomy. This is done initially by careful study producing an awareness of the types of strabismus that can be found. Then the ophthalmologist should develop a thorough mechanism for extracting meaningful data through a systematic approach to the work-up of a patient. This work-up begins with the history.

History

Why is the patient coming for examination? Questions to ask include the following:

1. When did the problem first occur?
2. Is diplopia noted?
3. Is the strabismus constant or changing?
4. Is the problem getting better or worse?
5. Has there been any prior treatment?
6. Have glasses been worn?
7. Has surgery been done?
8. Have other family members been affected in a similar manner?
9. What is the status of the patient's general health?
10. In children, what was the birthweight and have milestones been normal?

Depending on the specific case, many other questions can be asked about things such as preference for fixation, presence or absence of nystagmus, head nodding, ptosis, closing one eye in bright sunlight, asthenopia, and so on. Each ophthalmologist will develop his own set of exploratory questions that he finds useful in beginning and directing the examination.

Sensory status

Visual acuity should be measured for distance and near with and without correction. Special consideration should be given to binocular testing in cases of latent nystagmus. When amblyopia is present or suspected, visual acuity should be tested with single optotypes or with a neutral-density filter. Patients with amblyopia have improved visual acuity when single optotypes are used. Visual acuity also decreases less in the amblyopic eye compared to the normal eye when a neutral-density filter is placed over an amblyopic eye.

One may test stereoacuity with local or global stereopsis tests using the Titmus or various types of random-dot patterns. The Worth four-light test may be used to allow assessment of binocular awareness at the patient's angle. When tested at different distances, the Worth four-light test can give some information on the size of a central scotoma in a strabismic patient. The Bagolini glasses can determine retinal correspondence in casual seeing. The four-diopter base-out prism test will allow detection of a scotoma in an amblyopic eye with microtropia when no shift is present on the cover test.

Fusional amplitudes may be tested with the amblyoscope. Testing of the objective and subjective angle done initially on the amblyoscope can give information regarding retinal correspondence. After that, evaluation is made of the fusional divergence and fusional convergence amplitudes.

Motility examination begins with the assessment of ductions, versions, and screen comitance testing in the diagnostic positions to compare the yoke activity of the muscles. This allows overaction and underaction responses of the obliques to be noted as well as overaction and underaction responses of the rectus muscles.

In special instances, passive duction testing may be carried out with a variety of techniques. This test is important in determining whether a limited duction is based on mechanical or possibly neurogenic factors. Generated muscle force testing further differentiates mechanical from neurogenic limitations. The pneumotonograph, which may determine differential intraocular pressure, is another technique used to differentiate neurogenic from mechanical limitations of movements. One can observe saccadic velocity by comparing the speed of saccadic movements between the two eyes. The slower the saccadic movement, the more is it likely that a neurogenic deficit is present.

Prism and cover testing is carried out at distance and at near point with and without glasses. The prism and cover test may also be carried out at a fixed distance in the diagnostic positions with either eye fixing. Special attention is paid to the deviation of the straight up and straight down gaze while accommodation is controlled. This is preferably done at distance to determine the presence or absence of an A or V pattern.

The double Maddox rod test is used to measure cyclodeviations. The Bielschowsky head-tilt test with cover, used while the patient is sitting, can point to the presence of a superior oblique palsy.

A refraction is done after cycloplegia. The media are also evaluated, and the fundus is studied.

Treatment recommendations

A careful analysis of the data obtained from the evaluation will usually allow the examiner to arrive at a diagnosis. After that, a treatment program is outlined. The first aim of treatment is to provide the patient with eyes that are straight in the primary position and free of diplopia. Second, the examiner will do whatever is possible to give the patient comfortable vision with functionally fusing vision in all fields of gaze, or at least eyes that appear straight and produce a satisfactory appearance. Before undertaking surgical treatment, one should take care of non-surgical considerations. This includes treatment of refractive errors, especially hyperopia, which may lead to refractive or refractive-accommodative esotropia. Other treatment modalities include the use of both horizontal and vertical prisms, orthoptic exercises for near point of convergence improvement, and fusional vergence enhancement, in some cases through diplopia awareness followed by the stimulus to fusion. Patching for amblyopia should be carried out in young patients, and surgery is visually deferred until alternation is achieved or the maximum benefit from occlusion therapy has been obtained.

The surgical plan should answer the following questions:

1. When is the best time for surgery?
2. Which eye or eyes should be operated on?
3. Which muscle or muscles should be treated surgically?
4. Which operative approach is most suitable?
5. Should an adjustable suture be used?
6. Is botulinum toxin A therapy suitable?
7. What is the best type of anesthesia?

Depending on the individual circumstances, other possibilities may also need to be considered.

Most extraocular muscle surgery is done on an outpatient basis. Rarely is inpatient surgery done. I have treated patients surgically who required dantrolene (Dantrium) preparation because of a history of malignant hyperthermia. This requires hospitalization. Either pediatric or adult patients who have other systemic problems that make hospitalization necessary are scheduled for inpatient strabismus surgery procedures. Of course, any patient scheduled as an outpatient can be admitted if postanesthetic or surgical complications occur.

After surgery is completed, decisions are made about the time and technique that will be used for the adjustment of adjustable sutures. The use of a patch and antibiotics or steroids, or both, is also discussed.

SURGICAL ANATOMY

The eyes are framed by the *palpebral opening* (Fig. 15-1). The purposes of eye muscle surgery are to straighten the eye or eyes in the primary position, produce single binocular vision when attainable, and maintain free movement of the eyes in the physiologic range. This is done while one is maintaining normal lid contours, unscarred conjunctiva, and appropriate anatomic placement of the plica semilunaris and caruncle.

The *globe* is cushioned in orbital fat along its posterior and inferior aspects. The rectus muscles and inferior oblique project anteriorly beneath anterior Tenon's capsule in the plane of posterior Tenon's capsule to insert on the globe. Surgery on the anterior approximately one third of the rectus muscles and on the distal portion of the inferior oblique muscle can be carried out without disturbance to the fat. Likewise, the superior oblique tendon can be treated surgically without fat being encountered up to the cuff of tissue distal to the trochlea. Extraocular muscle surgery should be carried out without disturbance of this fat compartment (Fig. 15-2).

The *superior, lateral,* and *medial rectus muscles* (Fig. 15-3) are approximately 10 mm wide at their insertion. The medial rectus inserts about 5 mm from the limbus. The range is from 3 to 6 mm in patients with essential esotropia. The superior rectus inserts 7.7 mm from the limbus and the lateral rectus 6.9 mm from the limbus. The anterior corner of the superior oblique tendon is inserted about 10 mm posterior to the temporal corner of the superior rectus insertion. This insertion site is the most variable of the extraocular muscles. The tendon inserts in a curvilinear manner going posteriorly and medially for 10 to 14 mm.

The *inferior rectus muscle* (Fig. 15-4) inserts 6.5 mm from the limbus. The inferior oblique, encased in Lockwood's ligament, passes beneath the inferior rectus on a temporalward and posterior course. The superior oblique tendon passes from its insertion under the superior rectus muscle and courses superiorly and medially toward the trochlea.

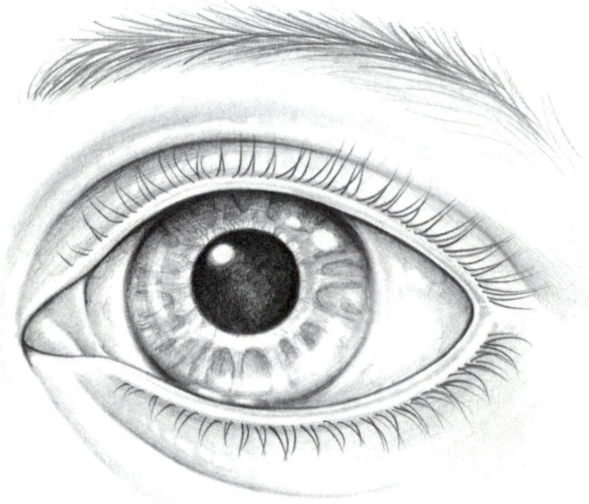

FIGURE 15-1. The palpebral opening.

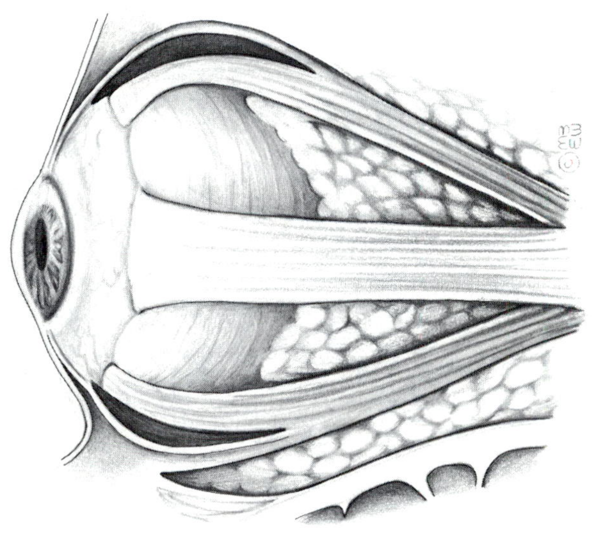

FIGURE 15-2. The globe.

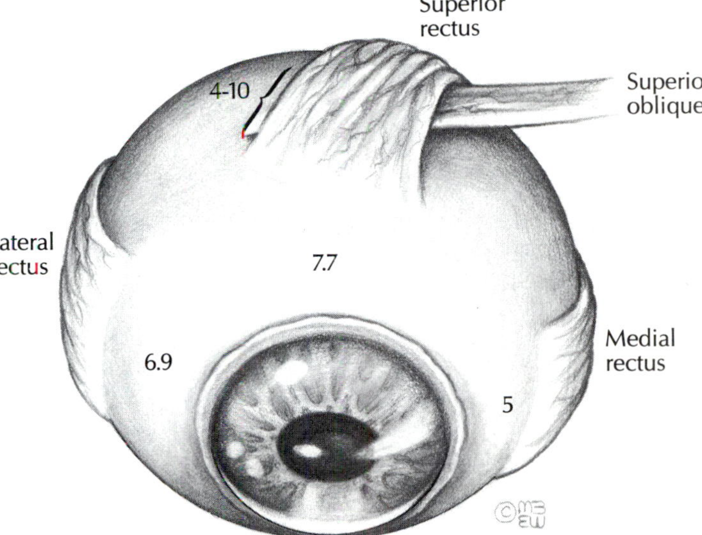

FIGURE 15-3. The rectus muscles.

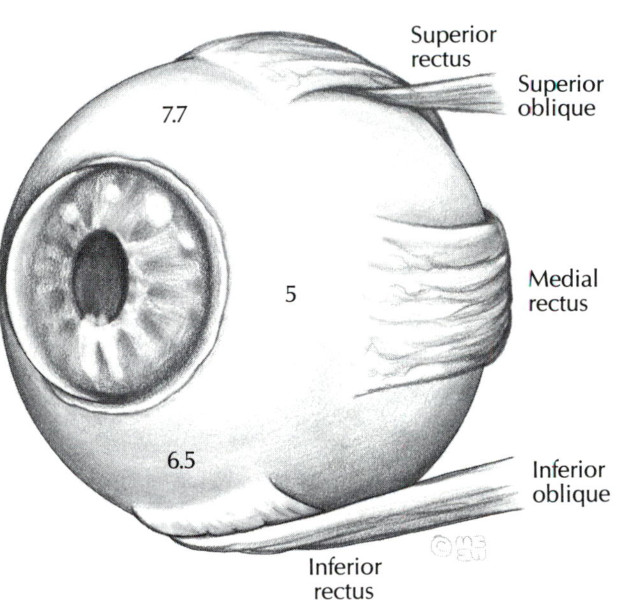

FIGURE 15-4. Inferior rectus muscle.

The *inferior oblique muscle* (Fig. 15-5) inserts into sclera just under the inferior edge of the lateral rectus muscle. The anterior corner of the inferior oblique insertion is approximately 10 mm posterior to the inferior insertion of the lateral rectus muscle. The innervation to the inferior oblique enters the muscle from the posterior direction, just after the inferior oblique muscle passes the lateral border of the inferior rectus. All other rectus muscles receive their innervation from the undersurface at a point coinciding with the junction of the middle and posterior third.

The *scleral thickness* (Fig. 15-6) varies according to location. The thinnest sclera is found just posterior to the insertion of the rectus muscles. It is 0.3 mm at this point. At the insertion, scleral thickness increases to 0.6 mm and to 0.8 mm at the limbus. At the equator the sclera is 0.5 mm thick, and in the posterior pole it is 1 mm thick or greater.

The insertion of the *superior rectus muscles* is shown in Fig. 15-7 with a limbal incision. This is the most difficult of the rectus muscles to engage on a muscle hook. The proximity of the superior oblique tendon causes it to be included when the superior rectus muscle is hooked. Care must be taken to rehook the superior rectus muscle excluding the superior oblique tendon.

Fig. 15-8 shows the inferior rectus muscle as seen from below with a limbal incision. The outer surface of the inferior rectus muscle blends into a dense condensation of fibrous tissue, Lockwood's ligament.

With the eye elevated in adduction using a forceps at the limbus, the inferior fat pads can be seen projecting forward from the cul-de-sac (Fig. 15-9). This fat pad should be avoided when one is making transconjunctival incisions to expose the inferior oblique or when doing a cul-de-sac incision to expose the lateral rectus.

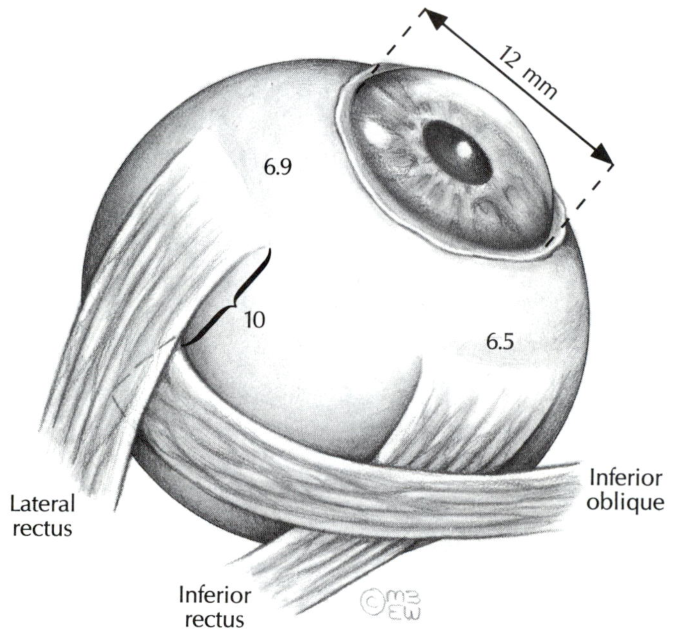

FIGURE 15-5. Inferior oblique muscle.

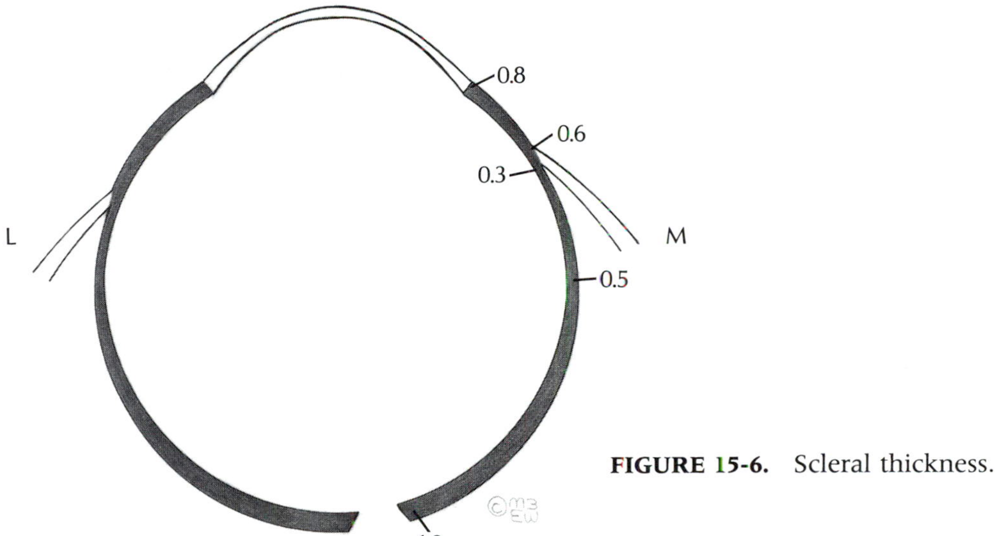

FIGURE 15-6. Scleral thickness.

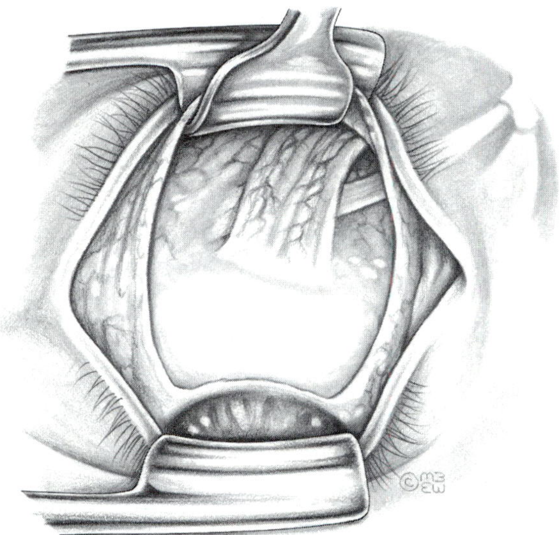

FIGURE 15-7. Superior rectus muscle.

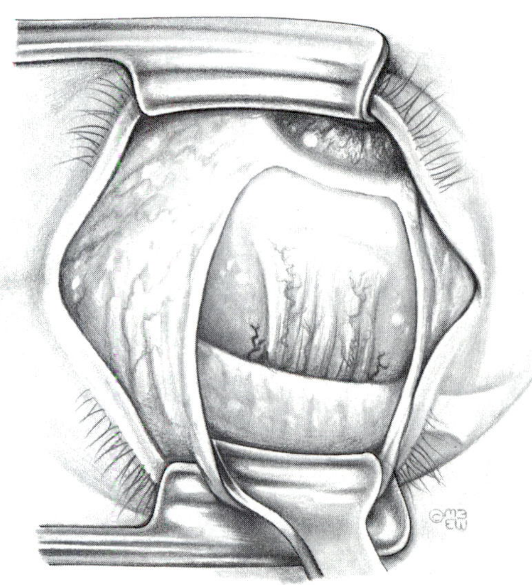

FIGURE 15-8. Inferior rectus muscle.

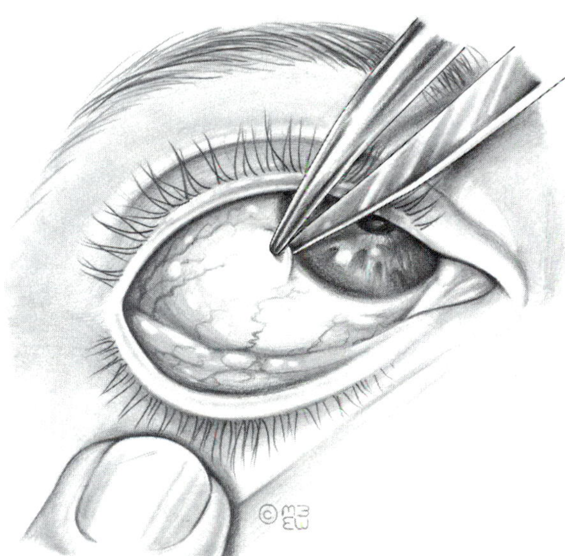

FIGURE 15-9. Inferior fat pads.

A limbal incision exposes the medial rectus muscle in Fig. 15-10. A Desmarres or similar flat-bladed retractor is useful for exposing the rectus muscles. The limbal incision also exposes the lateral rectus muscle (Fig. 15-11).

The area of surgical activity on the inferior oblique muscle is in the inferior temporal quadrant (Fig. 15-12). The innervation from the inferior branch of the oculomotor nerve enters the undersurface of the inferior oblique muscle as it passes the lateral border of the inferior rectus muscle. The inferior oblique muscle can be seen encased superficially in posterior Tenon's capsule during surgical dissection. It can be removed from posterior Tenon's capsule with careful dissection without exposure of fat. The inferior oblique muscle normally inserts approximately 10 mm posterior to the inferior corner of the lateral rectus insertion. The inferior oblique and lateral rectus may be connected by a common muscle sheath near the insertion of the inferior oblique.

Fig. 15-13 shows that the superior oblique muscle is approximately 30 mm long and the tendon is about equal length. The superior oblique tendon passes through the trochlea, which is located at the junction of the medial and upper orbital rim. The trochlea provides for a sliding mechanism of the superior oblique tendon while redirecting the pull of the superior oblique tendon. During contraction of the superior oblique muscle, the tendon is shortened and the eye is pulled downward, intorted, and abducted. With relaxation of the superior oblique muscle, the superior oblique tendon passes backward through the trochlea in a telescoping fashion. Under the influence of the inferior oblique, the eye is elevated, abducted, and extorted. Anatomic studies indicate that the superior oblique tendon can move approximately 8 mm in either direction around the primary position.

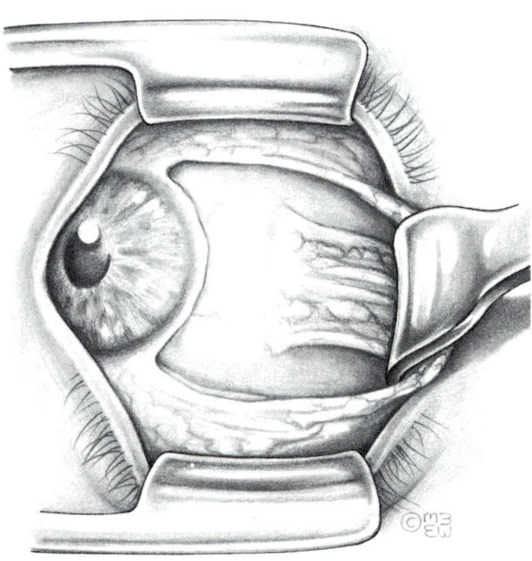

FIGURE 15-10. Medial rectus exposure.

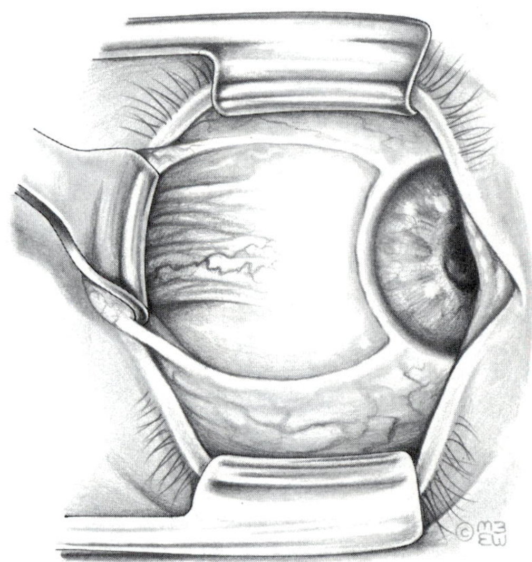

FIGURE 15-11. Lateral rectus exposure.

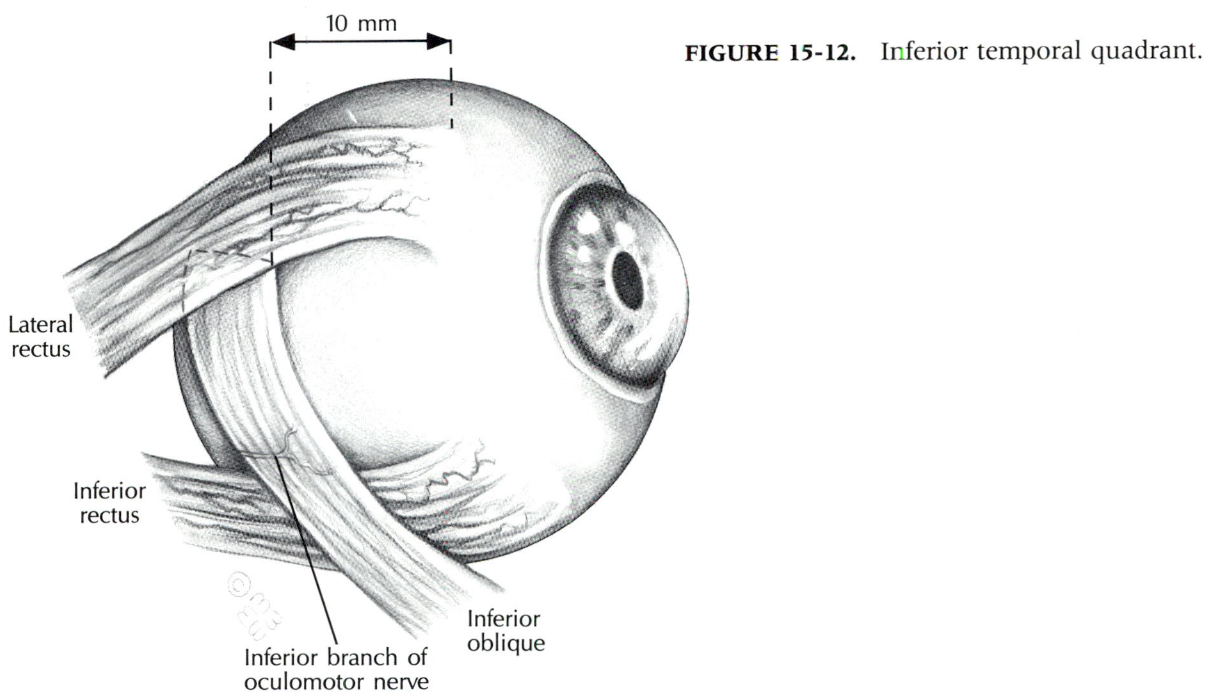

FIGURE 15-12. Inferior temporal quadrant.

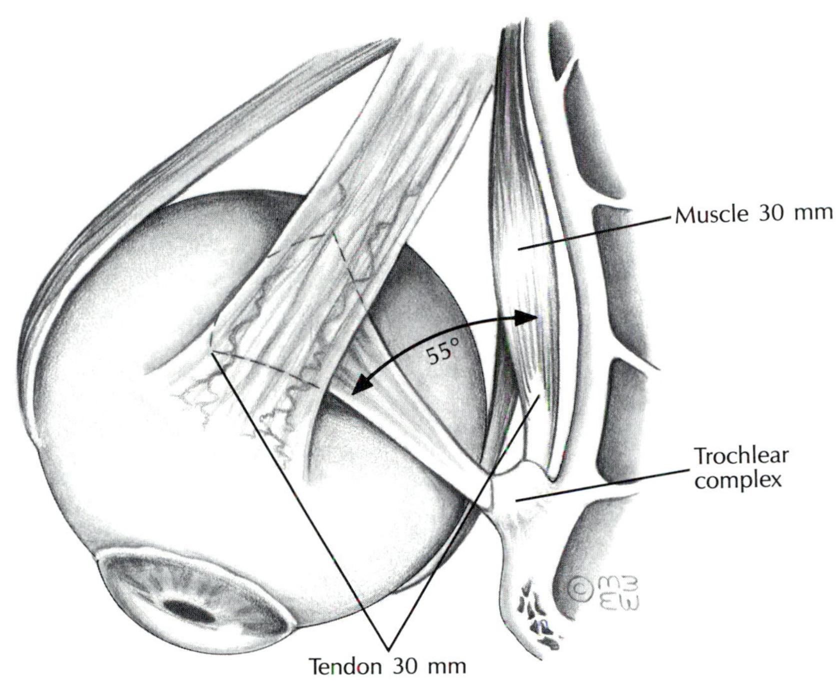

FIGURE 15-13. Superior oblique muscle and tendon.

The superior oblique tendon is made up of approximately 270 discrete fibers (Fig. 15-14). Because of scant lateral connections, a Z-lengthening tonotomy of this tendon invariably results in complete separation of the tendinous fibers. How far these tendinous fibers separate is related to the amount of dissection carried out around the tendon.

Fig. 15-15 shows that the trochlea, which serves as the turning point for the sliding superior oblique tendon action, *A*, is made up of five parts, *B*:

1. Cartilage saddle
2. Bursa-like space between the saddle and the superior oblique tendon
3. Fibrovascular structure surrounding the tendon
4. Tendon itself
5. Fibrous strap that connects the trochlear structure to the orbital rim

The superior oblique tendon passes beneath the superior rectus muscle (Fig. 15-16). In most instances this tendon has a connection to the superior rectus muscle capsule (Fig. 15-17). For the superior rectus muscle and the superior oblique tendon to be treated separately, this union must be surgically freed.

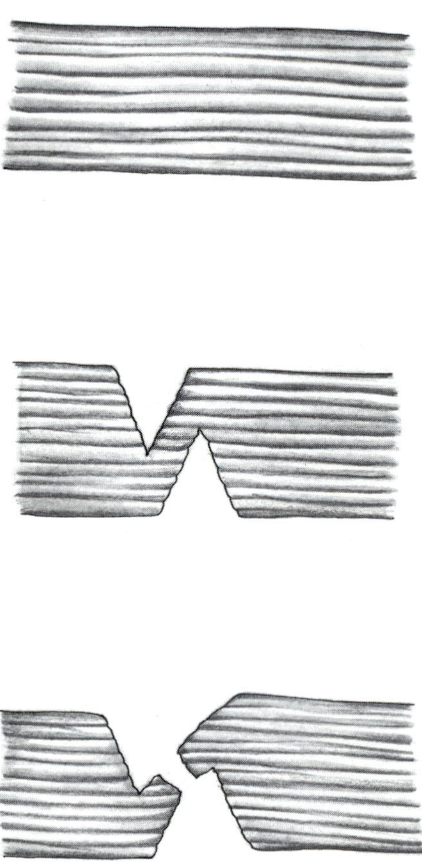

FIGURE 15-14. Z tenotomy for superior oblique tendon.

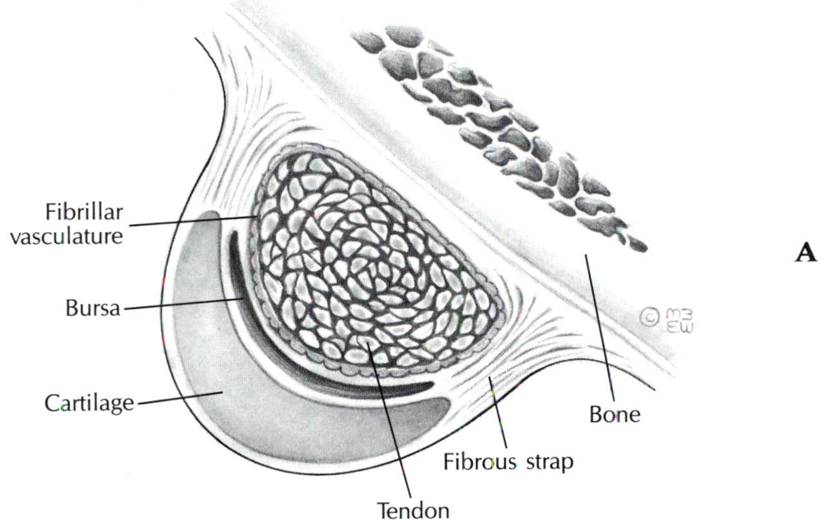

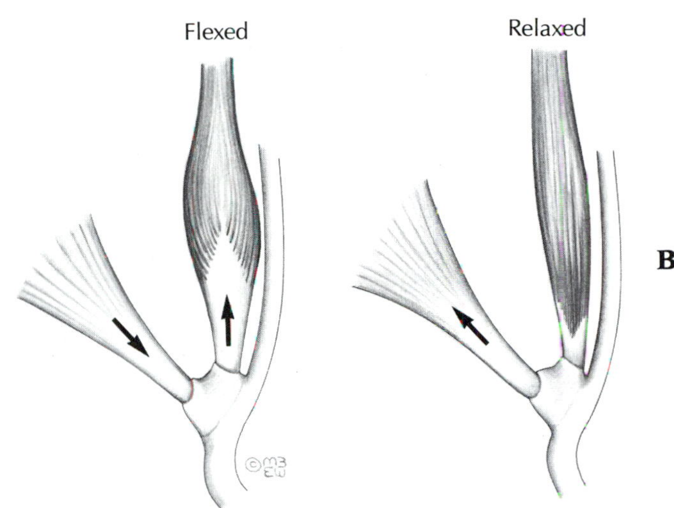

FIGURE 15-15. Trochlea.

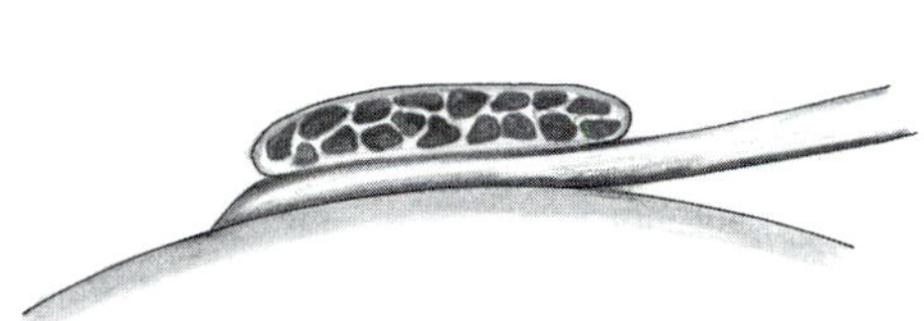

FIGURE 15-16. The superior oblique tendon beneath the superior rectus muscle.

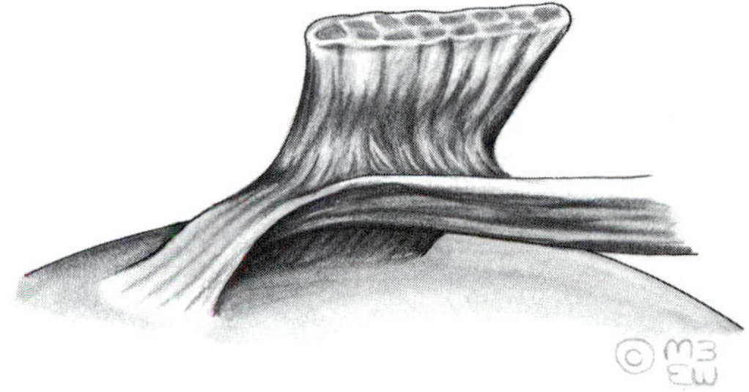

FIGURE 15-17. Connected superior oblique tendon and superior rectus muscle capsule.

CHAPTER 16

Duction Tests and Surgical Exposure

Proper design of strabismus surgery begins with an assessment of the static ocular alignment in the primary position and in the diagnostic positions of gaze. Equally as important is the question, How do the eyes get to any given position? Proper evaluation of active and passive forces are essential. Knowledge of both passive and active ocular movements is essential *every* time strabismus surgery is done.

Exposure to the extraocular muscles is obtained by incising conjunctiva and Tenon's capsule. The three commonly employed techniques are limbal, cul-de-sac or fornix, and Tron's conjunctival approach behind the lids. This last technique simply employs an incision through conjunctiva and Tenon's capsule down to bare sclera carried out away from the limbus. Exposure of the superior oblique at the insertion and of the inferior oblique in the inferior temporal quadrant can be carried out with this incision. Each technique has its place in the surgeon's armamentarium, and many surgeons use all three in appropriate situations. The ideal conjunctival incision should be like a good referee. In each case, things go better when after the fact you were not aware of their presence.

Duction Tests

Mechanical restrictions to ocular movement are measured by use of the passive duction test. For example, in Fig. 16-1, *A,* the patient has a right esotropia. In Fig. 16-1, *B,* notice that the right eye does not abduct fully. Is the restriction in abduction of the right eye attributable to mechanical restrictions, paresis of the right lateral rectus muscle, or both?

To obtain the answer to this question, the surgeon performs the passive duction test. After obtaining adequate topical anesthesia with anesthetic drops or with 4% cocaine on a cotton swab placed over the medial aspect of the eye, the surgeon grasps the medial limbal area with forceps and then, while the patient attempts to look in right gaze, the examiner attempts to complete this gaze by rotating the eyeball with the forceps (Fig. 16-1, *C*). If the examiner can freely and passively abduct the right eye, no apparent mechanical restriction exists and one may infer that there is a paresis of the right lateral rectus muscle.

If, as shown in Fig. 16-1, *D,* the attempt to abduct the right eye is met with resistance, a mechanical restriction to abduction exists.

Paresis of a given extraocular muscle may exist with or without mechanical restriction. This is evaluated by two techniques, observation or recording of saccadic velocity and estimation of muscle pull against a stabilized globe, the muscle-force generation test (Fig. 16-2).

For example, if a patient with limited abduction of the right eye as shown (Fig. 16-2, *A*) has a slow, "floating" saccade in the direction of restricted movement when movement is compared with the normal eye, paresis of the agonist muscle can be inferred. However, if the limited motion is accomplished with a brisk though limited saccade, normal or nearly normal agonist muscle innervation can be inferred. This can be confirmed by the muscle-force generation test (Fig. 16-2, *B*). In this test, the conjunctiva is anesthetized with topical anesthesia as is done with passive duction testing. The conjunctiva and Tenon's capsule are grasped while the patient is looking away from the field of action of the muscle to be tested. The patient is then asked to look slowly in the direction of the muscle to be tested. The amount of muscle-force generation can be estimated by the amount of pull on the forceps used to stabilize the globe (Fig. 16-2, *C*). This force may be in the neighborhood of 90 to 110 grams. The difference between a normal and a paralyzed muscle is very easy to determine. Various degrees of paresis require more practice on the part of the examiner and can be measured more accurately by the use of quantitative devices.

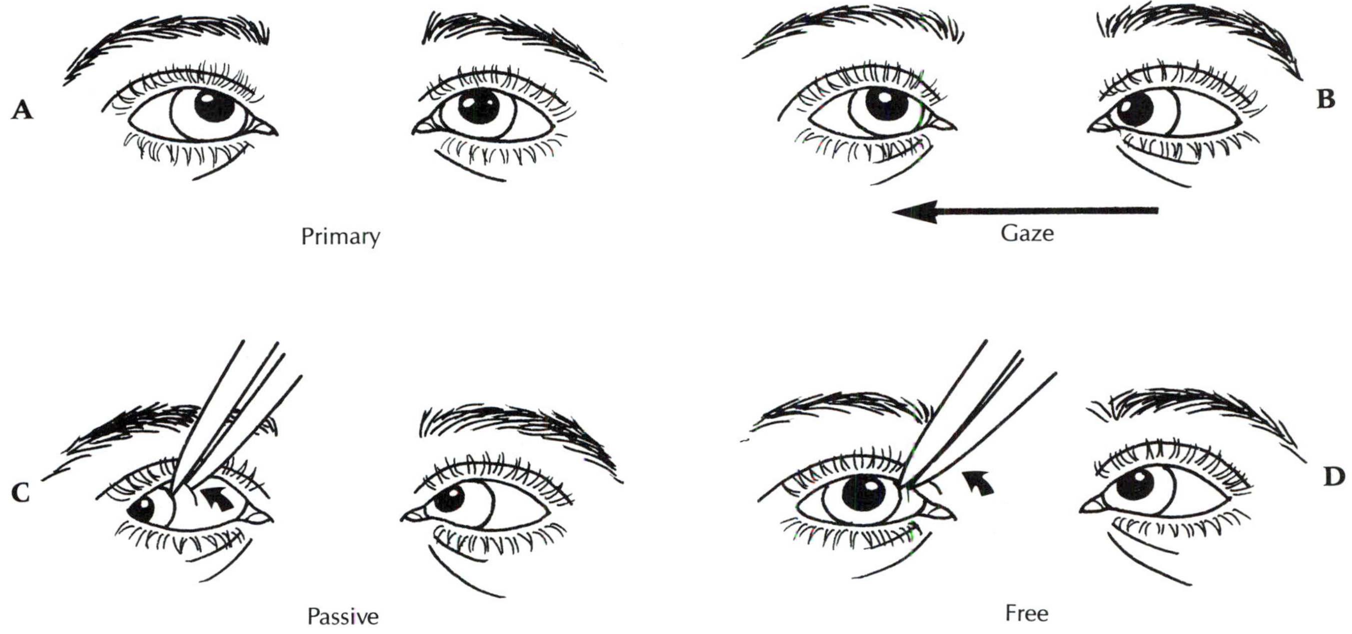

FIGURE 16-1

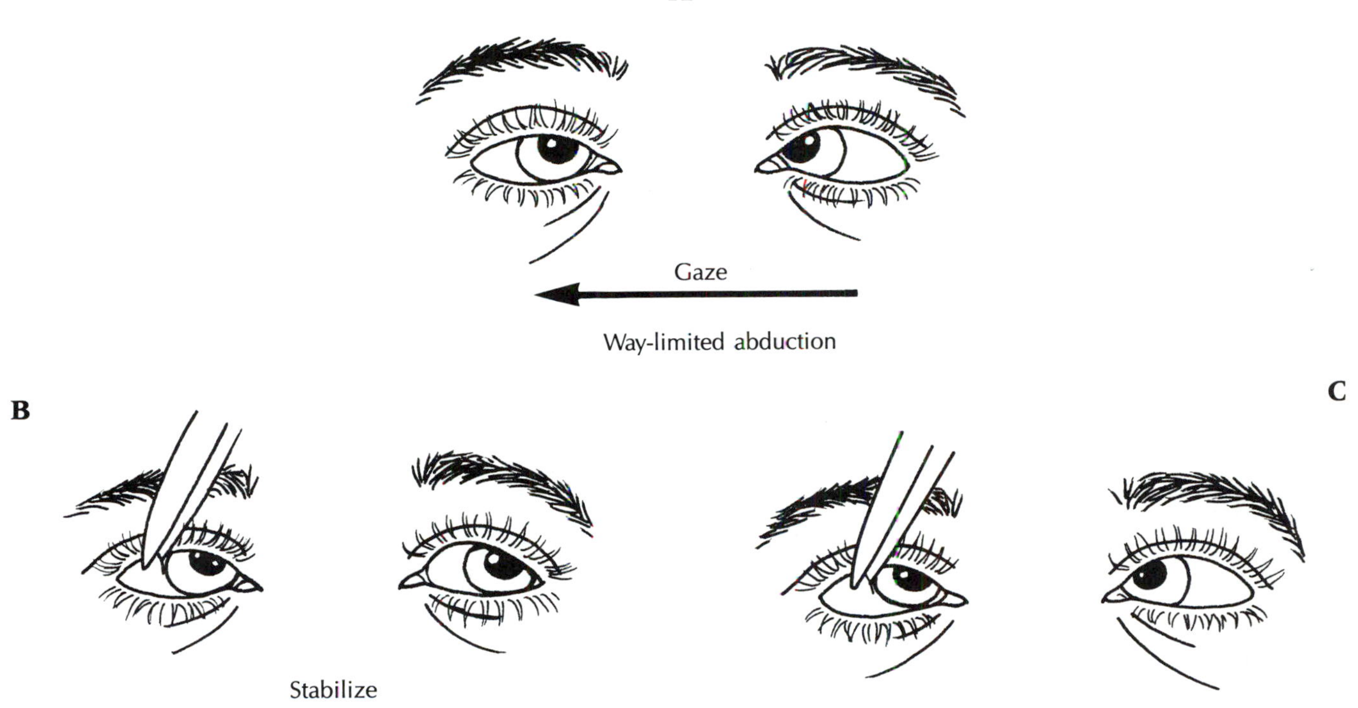

FIGURE 16-2

Surgical Exposure

Exposure to any of the four rectus muscles can be obtained by use of the limbal incision (Fig. 16-3). This incision is made at the limbus for approximately 2 to 3 clock hours centered over the rectus muscle insertion. A radial relaxing incision may be made on one or both sides of the muscle. It extends posteriorly several millimeters behind the insertion of the rectus muscle. The flap of tissue raised includes conjunctiva and anterior Tenon's capsule.

If surgery is carried out on adjacent rectus muscles or on the lateral rectus muscle and inferior oblique, an enlarged limbal incision can be made (Fig. 16-4).

After completion of the limbal incision to expose the insertion of the rectus muscles, these muscles are observed embedded in their sheath, which is a continuation of posterior Tenon's capsule. Before engaging the rectus muscle, one enters the posterior Tenon's capsule adjacent to the muscle border and slightly behind its point of insertion with a buttonhole incision and bare sclera is observed (Fig. 16-5). This is stark white in appearance compared to the pinkish appearance of the episcleral covering of sclera anterior to the muscle's insertion.

The tip of the muscle hook is placed into the buttonhole very slightly indenting sclera, and the muscle hook is passed behind the insertion of the rectus muscle (Fig. 16-6).

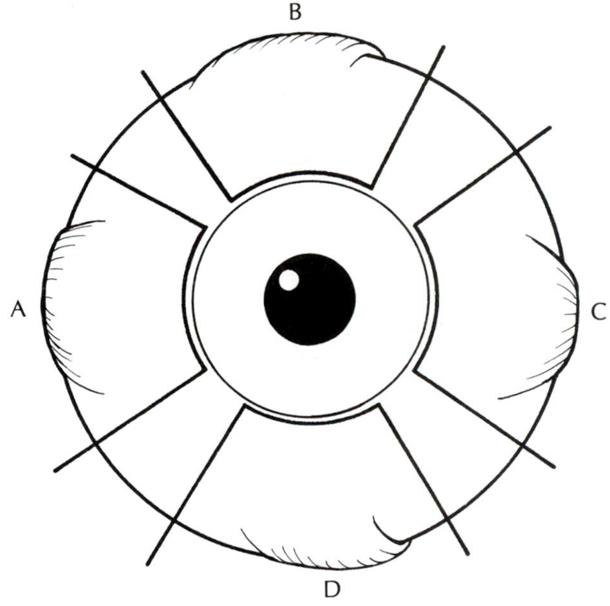

FIGURE 16-3

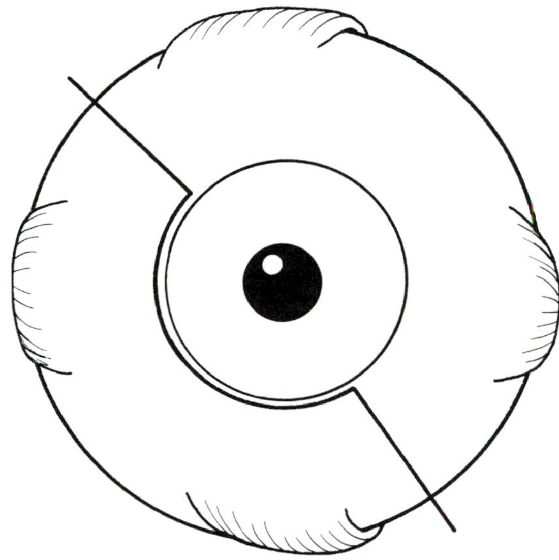

FIGURE 16-4

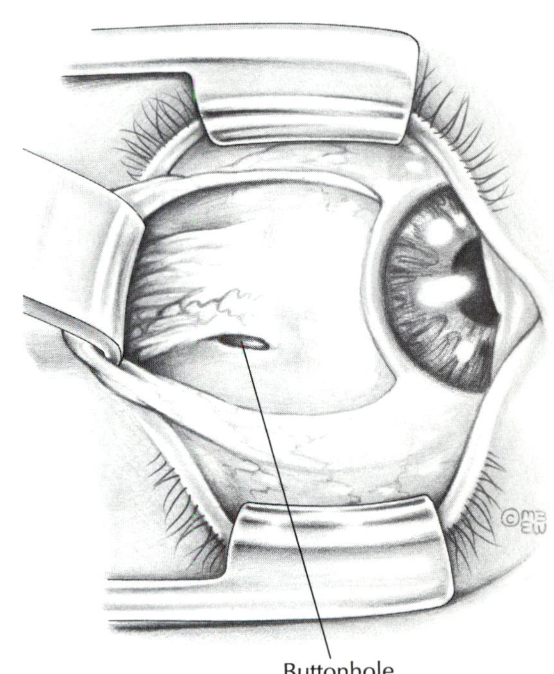

FIGURE 16-5

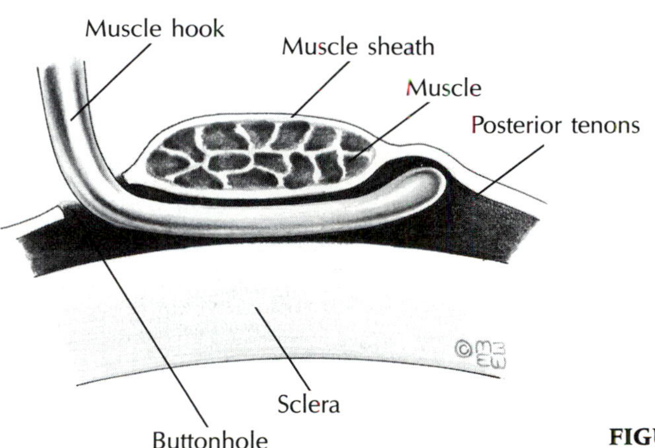

FIGURE 16-6

As the muscle hook passes completely behind the rectus muscle, its tip is located indenting the intramuscular membrane (Fig. 16-7).

The tip of the muscle hook is freed with careful dissection, and the intermuscular membrane on either border of the rectus muscle may be dissected (Fig. 16-8). For the lateral rectus, the insertion of the inferior oblique will be seen on the inferior border. For the superior rectus, the superior oblique tendon is often included in the initial engagement of the rectus muscle on the muscle hook. Careful repassing of the hook should be carried out to free the superior oblique tendon from the superior rectus. Dissection along the lateral borders of the superior rectus should be carried out with care so that the superior oblique tendon is avoided. For the inferior rectus, dissection should be carried out to free the muscle from the Lockwood's ligament. The inferior rectus passes through a tunnel of fascia as it crosses the inferior oblique. Care should be taken to avoid the vortex veins, which are usually found at one or both borders of the inferior rectus 10 to 12 mm posterior to the insertion.

The inferior oblique muscle is approached in the inferior temporal quadrant through an incision that parallels the limbus and is approximately 8 mm from the limbus (Fig. 16-9). The incision is carried through conjunctiva and anterior and posterior Tenon's capsule and exposes the sclera.

The superior oblique tendon is approached at its insertion by transconjunctival incision paralleling the superior rectus muscle and approximately 1 to 2 mm lateral to it (Fig. 16-10). The superior oblique tendon may be approached medial to the superior rectus muscle by an incision parallel to the limbus beginning just nasal to the superior rectus muscle. A limbal incision exposing the superior rectus muscle first and then the superior oblique tendon may also be used.

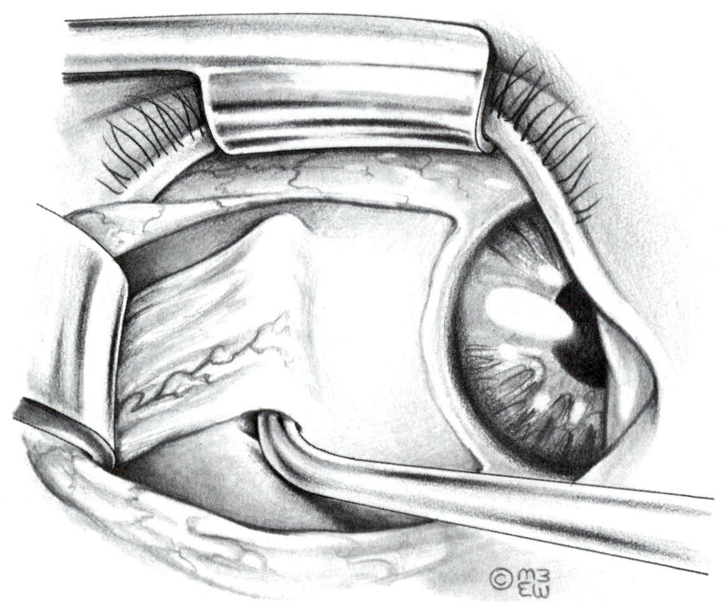

FIGURE 16-7

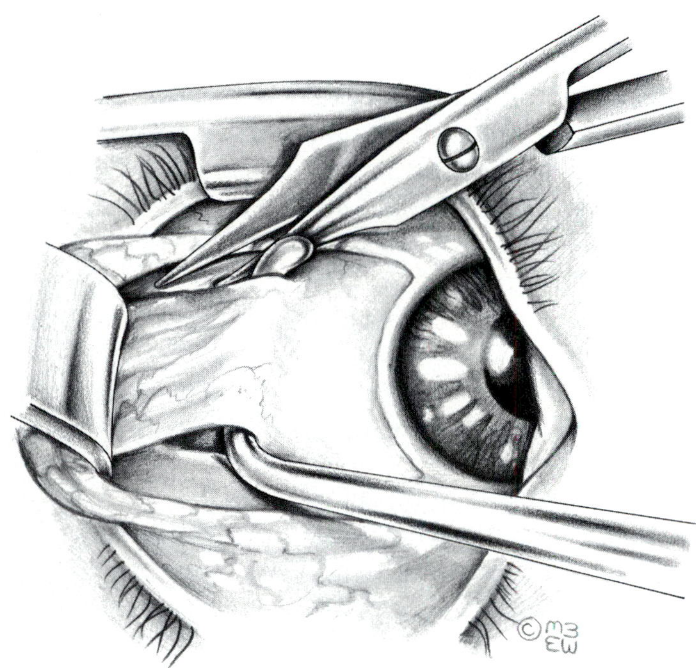

FIGURE 16-8

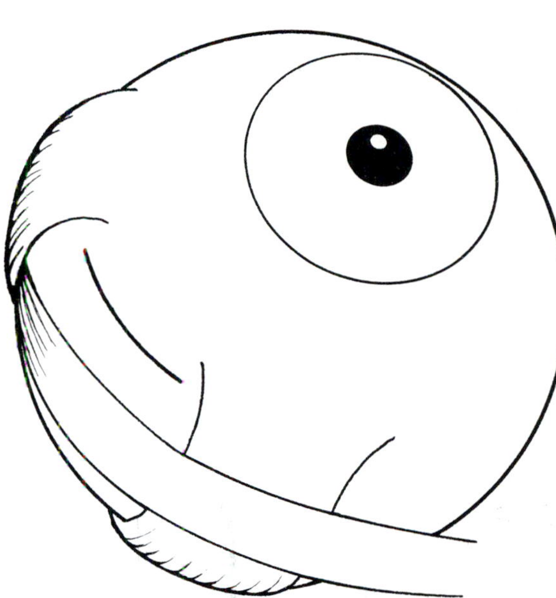

FIGURE 16-9

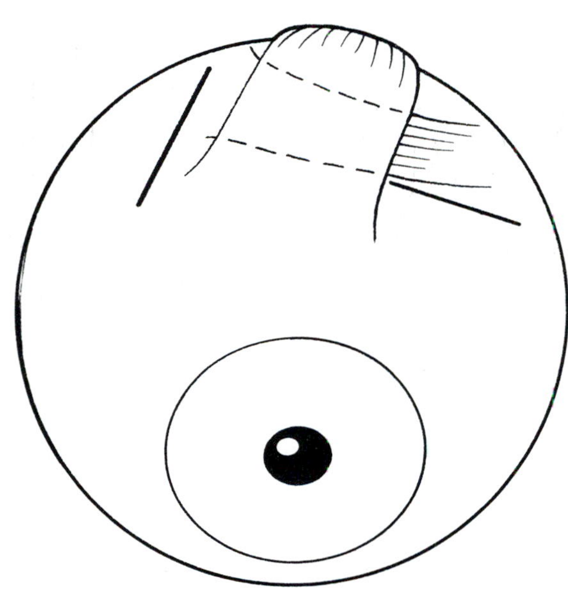

FIGURE 16-10

The cul-de-sac incision described by Parks may be used to expose any of the rectus muscles (Fig. 16-11). The incision is carried out transconjunctivally behind the upper or lower lid. It is carried out to parallel the roof or floor of the orbit and begins at the junction of the middle and either lateral or medial third of the cornea. Incision is carried through conjunctiva and anterior and posterior Tenon's capsule down to bare sclera. Especially with the inferior cul-de-sac incision, care should be taken to avoid the inferior fat pad.

The inferior cul-de-sac incision for exposure of the right medial rectus is shown in Fig. 16-12. The technique for the lateral rectus is similar. Bare sclera is exposed after dissection with blunt-tipped spring-action scissors.

A large muscle hook preferably with a knobbed or hooked end is placed with the tip on bare sclera, and the hook is guided upward just behind the insertion of the medial rectus muscle (Fig. 16-13).

With the large muscle hook remaining behind the insertion of the medial rectus muscle, a smaller muscle hook is placed just beneath anterior Tenon's capsule and is swept toward the limbus and then backward toward the muscle's origin over the larger muscle hook (Fig. 16-14). The medial rectus muscle and its sheath are between the two muscle hooks.

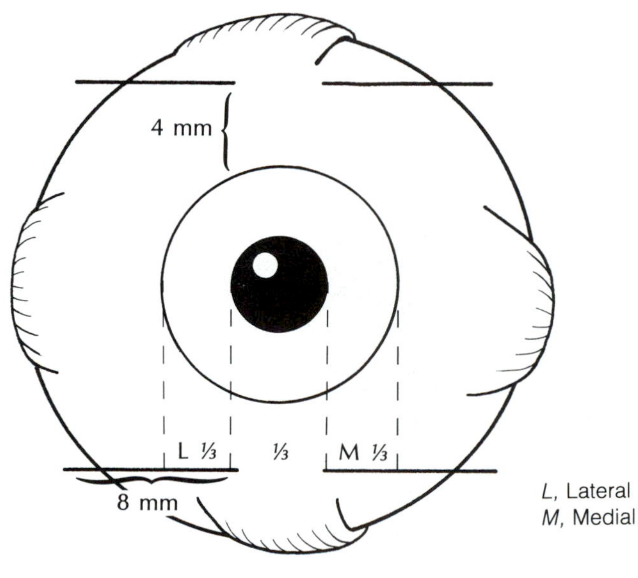

FIGURE 16-11

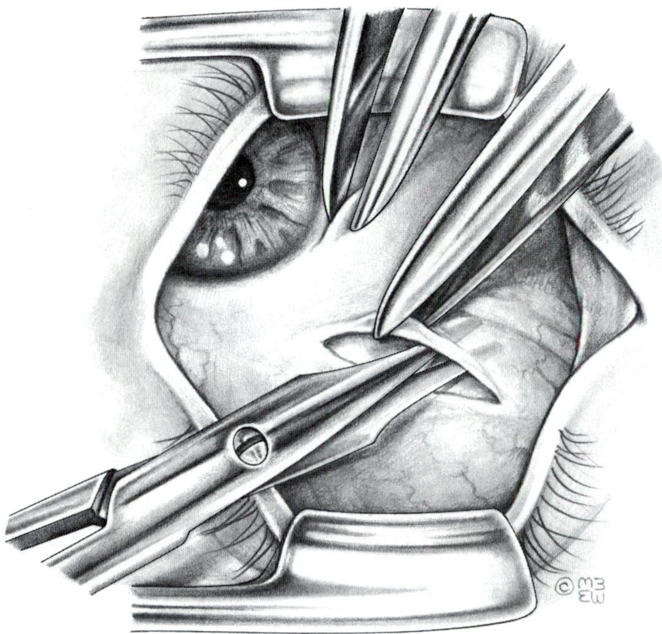

FIGURE 16-12

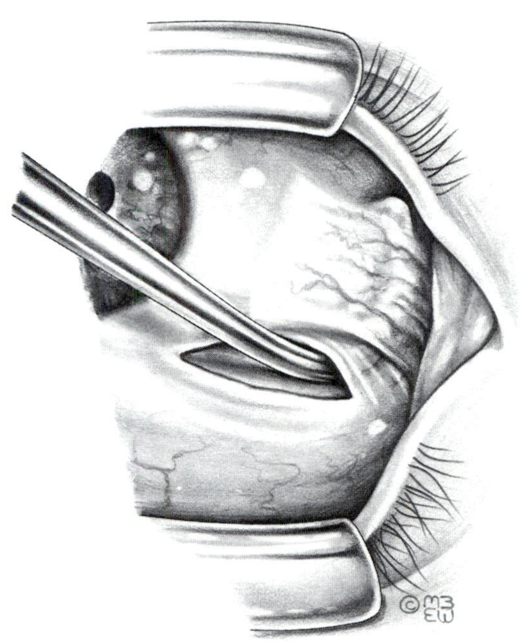

FIGURE 16-13

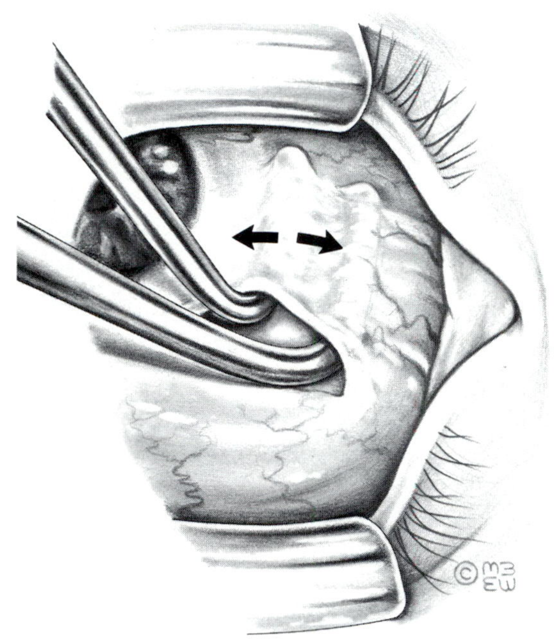

FIGURE 16-14

The small muscle hook then retracts the conjunctiva and anterior Tenon's capsule to expose the tip of the large muscle hook (Fig. 16-15). This hook is usually covered with intramuscular membrane. Dissection is carried out to free the tip. At this point the intramuscular membrane and overlying anterior Tenon's capsule may be dissected according to the plan of the surgeon. Some surgeons prefer very little intramuscular membrane dissection, and some prefer more.

Sutures are then placed just posterior to the muscle's insertion (Fig. 16-16). Either a single double-arm suture or two single-arm sutures may be used. In the case of a resection, a Desmarres retractor may be placed in the incision, and the sutures may be placed farther from the insertion in order to carry out the resection.

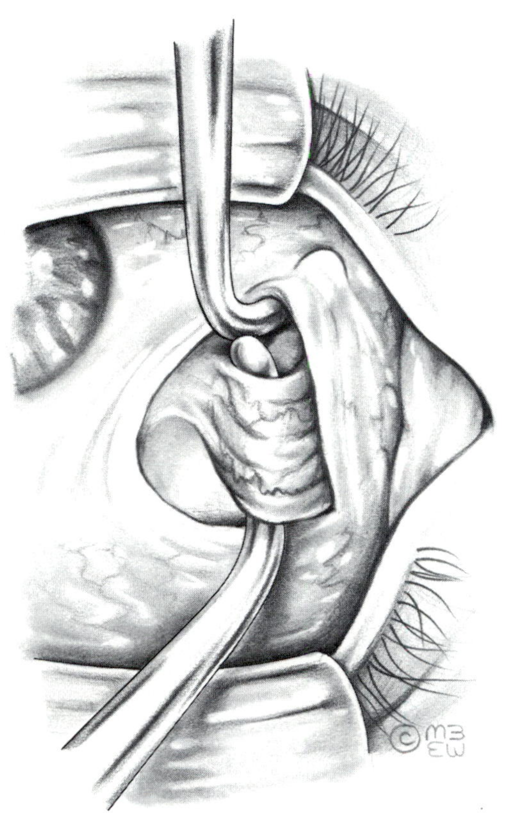

FIGURE 16-15

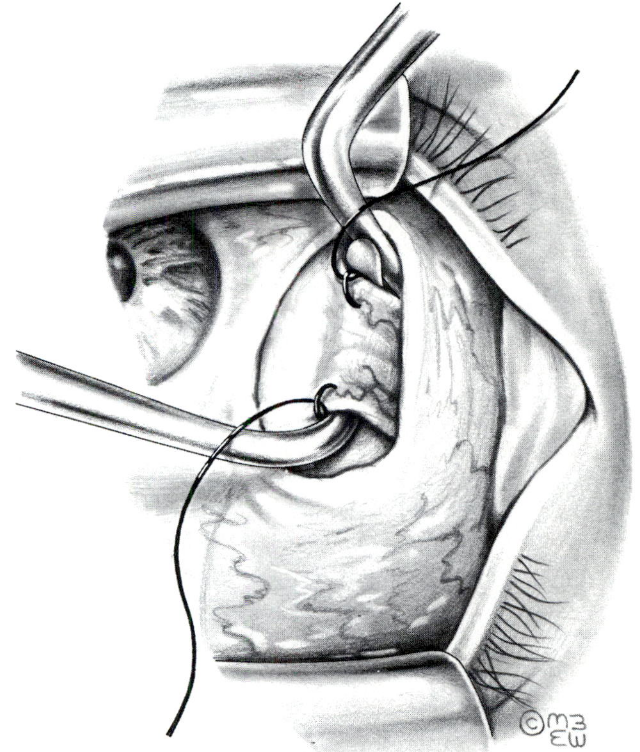

FIGURE 16-16

CHAPTER 17

Muscle Recession and Weakening Procedures

Retroplacement of an extraocular muscle alters its arc on contact and at least temporarily creates redundancy in the muscle-tendon architecture. Both of these factors reduce the effect of muscle contraction on the globe position so that the visual axis is shifted *opposite* the direction of the muscle insertion shift. Recession of a medial rectus produces a relative exo shift of the visual axis. Excessive recession of the medial rectus produces reduced adduction with an accompanying relative exo shift. As a rule, weakening procedures of the extraocular muscles are more effective millimeter for millimeter in both the short and the long term. An additional positive factor is that with weakening procedures there is tissue sparing, which in turn means that an "unoperation" can be carried out readily. Recession procedures are the most physiologic of all strabismus surgical procedures.

Muscle Recession

The essence of a recession is simply detaching and reattaching the muscle to a new point on the sclera (Fig. 17-1, *A*). The muscle must be secured with a suture (Fig. 17-1, *B*) and then securely attached to the sclera (Fig. 17-1, *C*).

Rectus muscle recession may be carried out using the limbus as a reliable landmark (Fig. 17-2). Between 1 and 2 years of age, the corneal diameter is consistent at about 11.5 to 12 mm. The anterior posterior diameter is also consistent at 21 to 22 mm. This means that the functional equator will also be a stable landmark. Medially the functional equator or the most posterior point of rectus muscle tangency is slightly anterior to the anatomic equator; for the lateral rectus the functional equator is slightly posterior to the anatomic equator. Since the rectus muscle insertion, especially the medial rectus, is variable and not related to the angle of strabismus, the limbus is a more reliable landmark than the original insertion. Therefore, especially for medial rectus recession, the limbus is an ideal reference.

The special anatomy adjacent (Fig. 17-3) to the vertical recti must be considered during recession. The superior rectus is related to the levator palpebrae and superior oblique tendon. Excessive recession of the superior rectus or the inferior rectus muscles can cause retraction of the adjacent tissues and widening of the palpebral fissure. Likewise, resection of either vertical rectus muscle can cause advancement of the adjacent lid and narrowing of the palpebral fissure. Palpebral fissure width alteration can be avoided if one limits the amount of vertical rectus recession and by thorough dissection of the intermuscular membrane around the muscles.

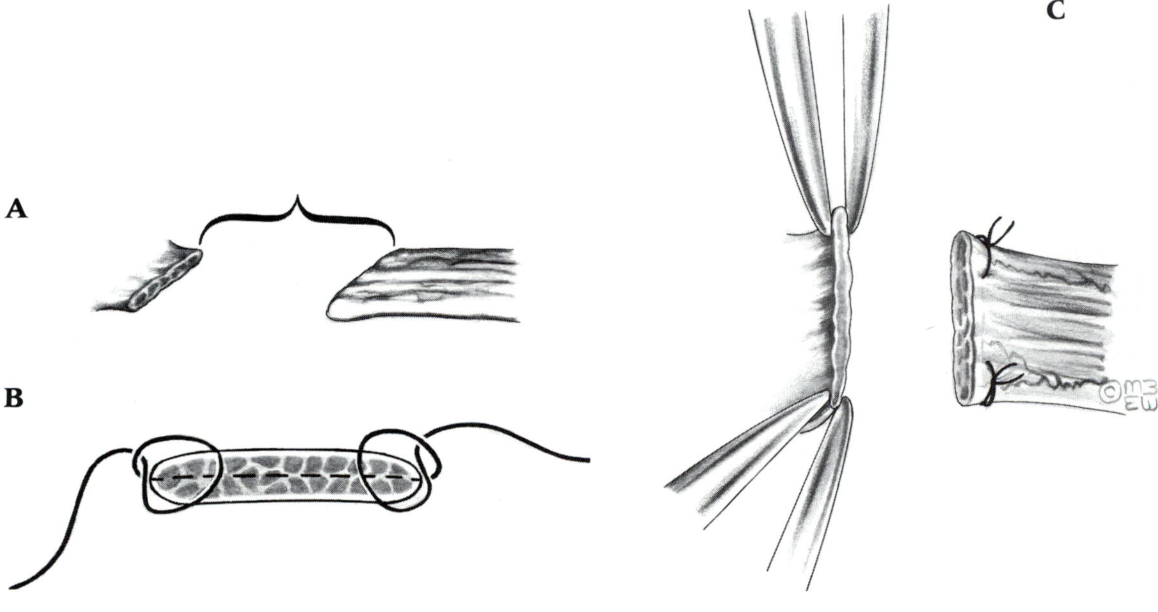

FIGURE 17-1

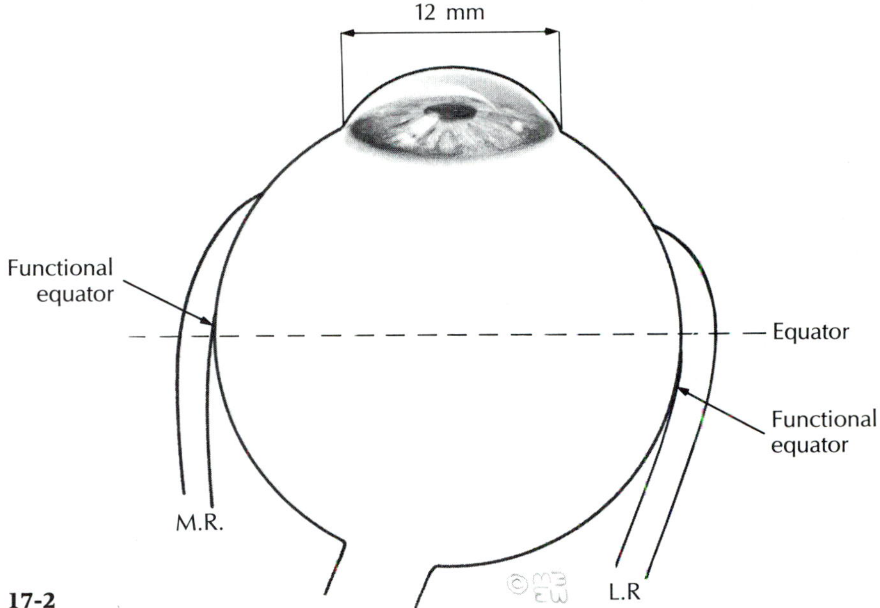

FIGURE 17-2

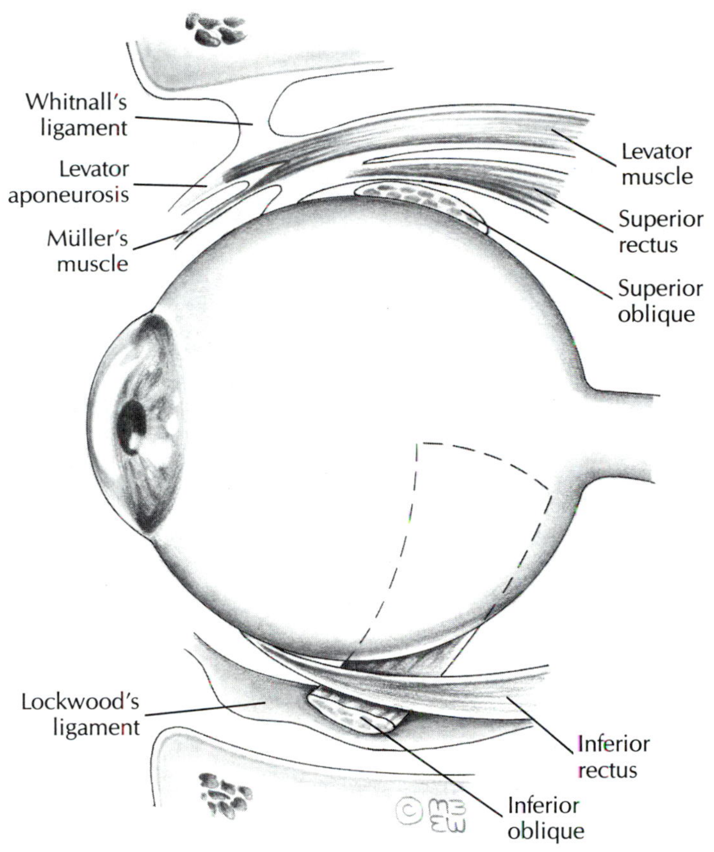

FIGURE 17-3

Before either recession or resection of a rectus muscle, the muscle may be secured with a single double-arm suture (Fig. 17-4). This suture is threaded through the thickness of the muscle, and then at each border a second loop is taken and locked. When possible, the anterior ciliary vessels should be included in the second loop and ligated.

Two single-arm sutures may be passed in two loops through the borders of the rectus muscles and then either locked or secured with a square knot (Fig. 17-5).

When the inferior oblique muscle is recessed, it is placed adjacent to the lateral border of the inferior rectus muscle (Fig. 17-6). Precise placement of this recessed inferior oblique is said to provide a graded weakening effect. If the inferior oblique is reattached anteriorly, the inferior oblique is said to become a depressor.

Sutures for recession are placed just posterior to the rectus muscle's insertion (Fig. 17-7). This placement may be done anterior to the stabilizing muscle hook or just posterior to the muscle hook. The suture should include the anterior ciliary vessels so that they may be ligated to control bleeding.

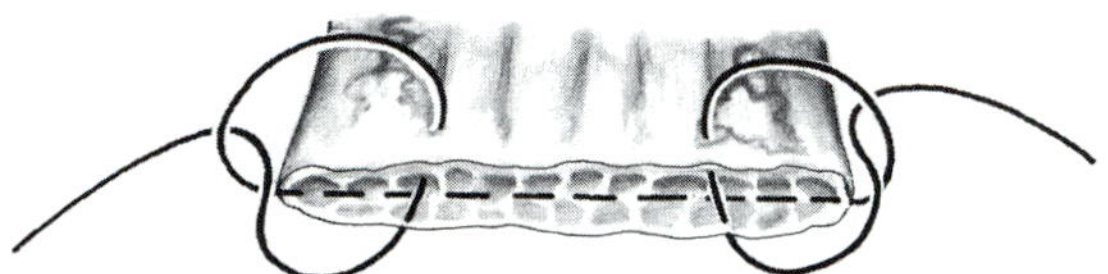

Double arm suture

FIGURE 17-4

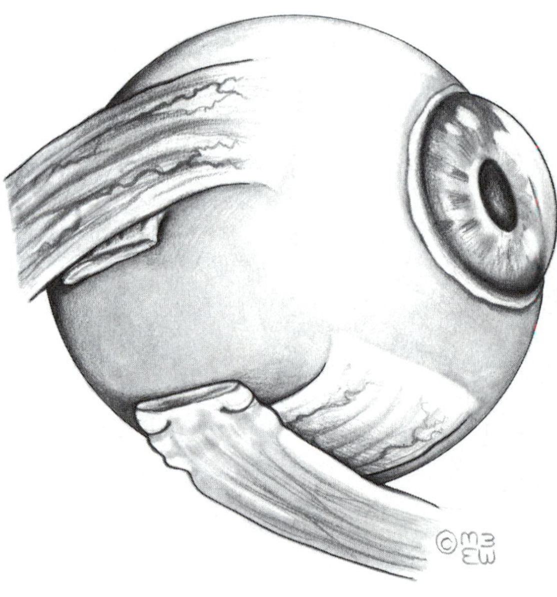

FIGURE 17-6

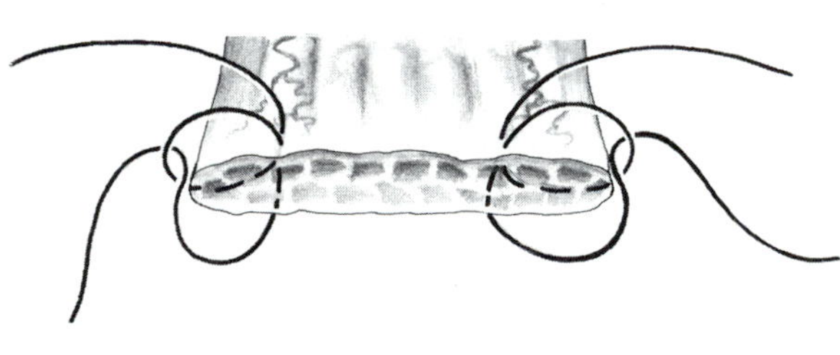

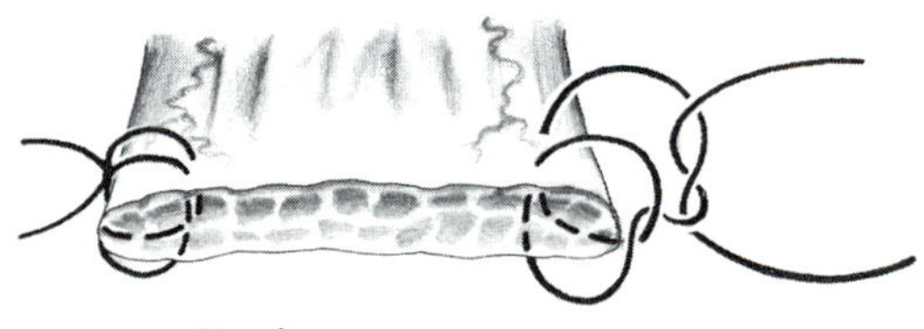

Single arm suture

FIGURE 17-5

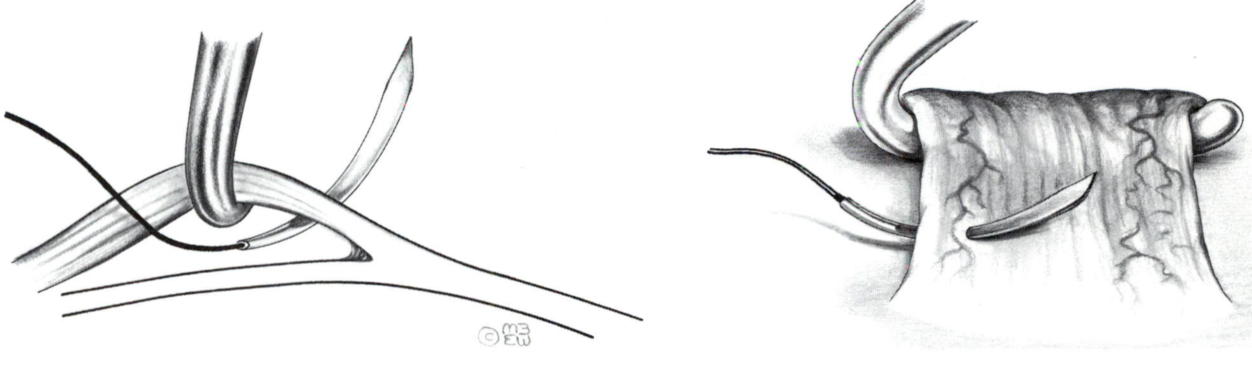

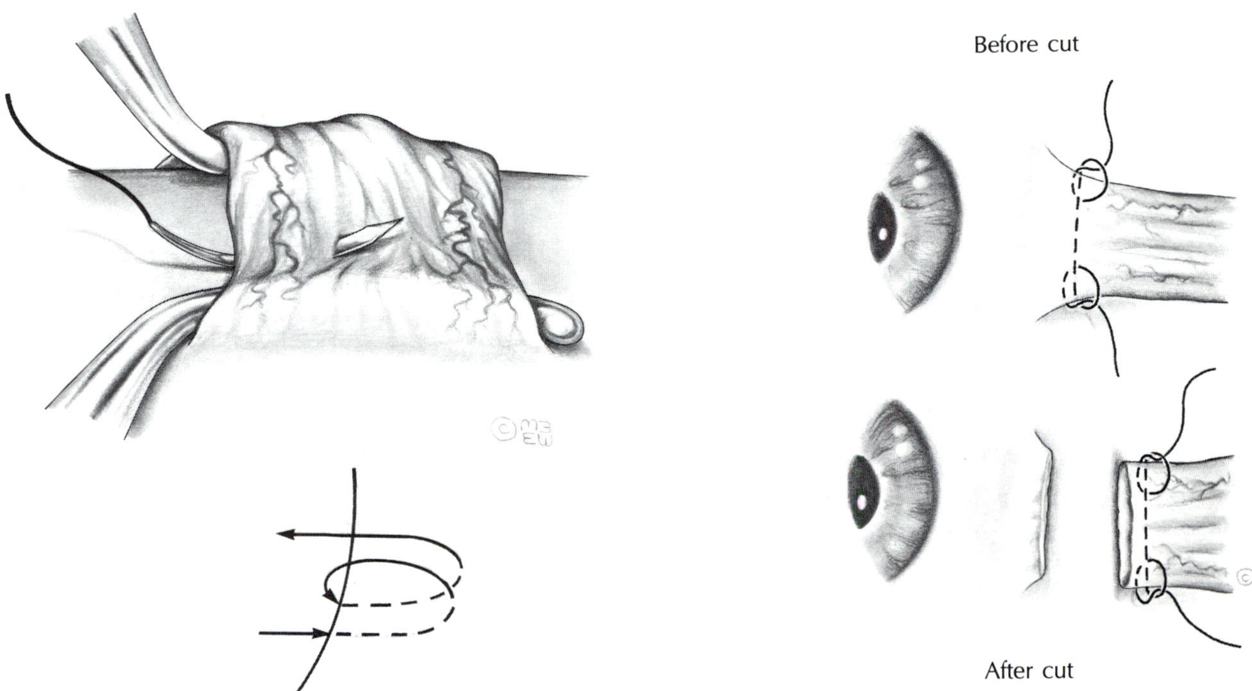

FIGURE 17-7

A double-arm suture reattaching a rectus muscle (Fig. 17-8, *A*) may be anchored with scleral bites that oppose each other but do not cross in a pseudo–crossed swords technique (Fig. 17-8, *B*).

Parks has advocated the "crossed-swords" technique when one is using a double-armed suture (Fig. 17-9). This method secures the muscle at the intended point of recession before the suture is tied.

When two single-arm sutures are used, needles are placed into sclera at approximately the width of the muscle (Fig. 17-10, *A*). The exact direction of needle placement is not crucial. The muscle is brought up to the point of entry of the needle into sclera.

Both sutures are tied securely in front of (Fig. 17-10, *B*) or on the side of the muscle's new insertion (Fig. 17-10, *C*).

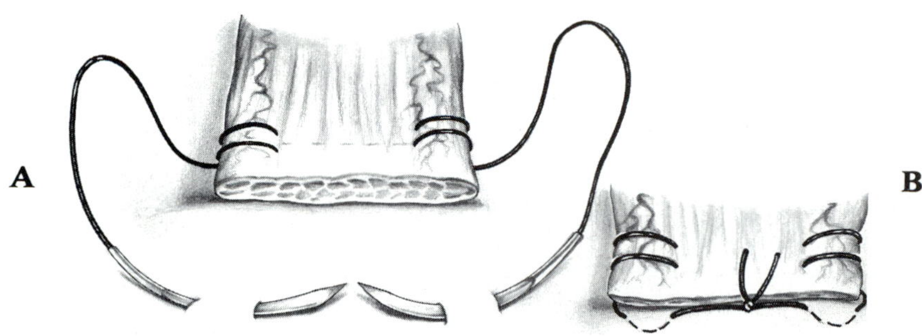

FIGURE 17-8

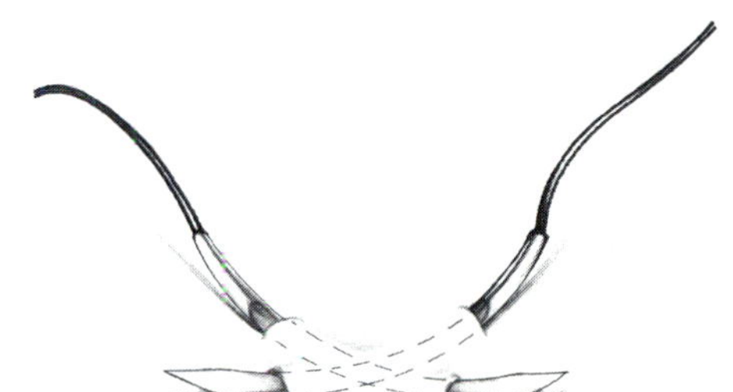

FIGURE 17-9

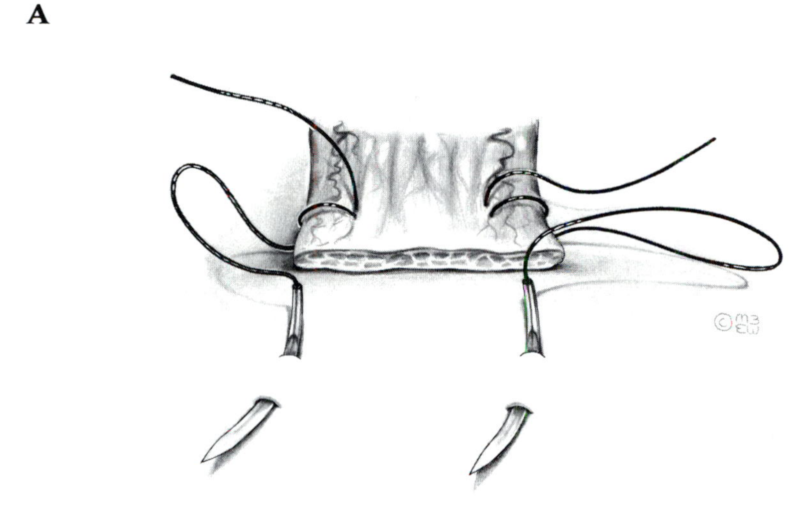

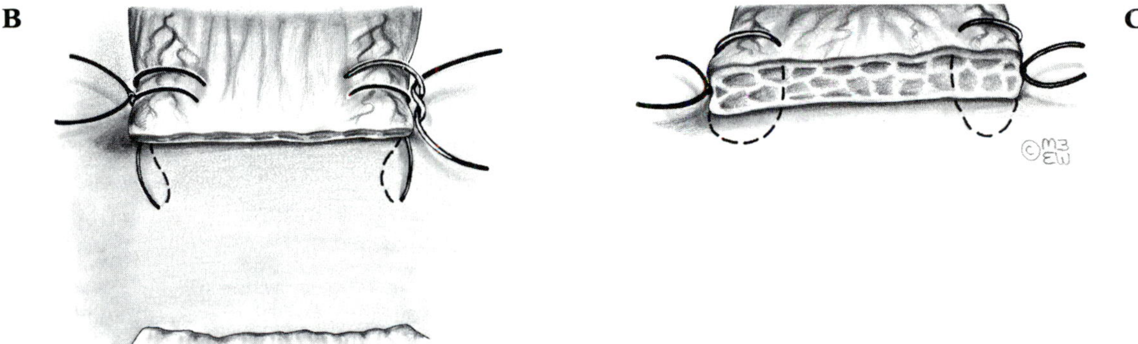

FIGURE 17-10

Weakening Procedures

To determine the length necessary for weakening, calipers are used to measure from the limbus (Fig. 17-11). This actually measures a chord. For measurements up to approximately 11.5 mm the difference between the chord and the surface of the sclera is not significant. A curved caliper that eliminates the chord error may be used. Recession may be measured from the insertion.

My preferred technique for weakening the inferior oblique is myectomy in the inferior temporal quadrant. One begins the procedure by grasping the conjunctiva and Tenon's capsule at the limbus midway between the insertion of the lateral and inferior rectus muscle (Fig. 17-12). The eye is brought into elevation in adduction. A forcep grasps the conjunctiva and Tenon's capsule 8 mm from the limbus halfway between the insertion of the lateral and inferior rectus muscle. A snip incision is carried down to bare sclera.

Muscle hooks are placed behind the lateral and inferior rectus muscle, and the incision is spread (Fig. 17-13). A small muscle hook is then used to triangulate the incision so that conjunctiva and anterior and posterior Tenon's capsule are pulled inferolaterally.

A second small hook is placed with the tip against bare sclera and is guided gently posteriorly until the tip is behind the posterior belly of the inferior oblique muscle. The inferior oblique muscle is brought out into the incision (Fig. 17-14).

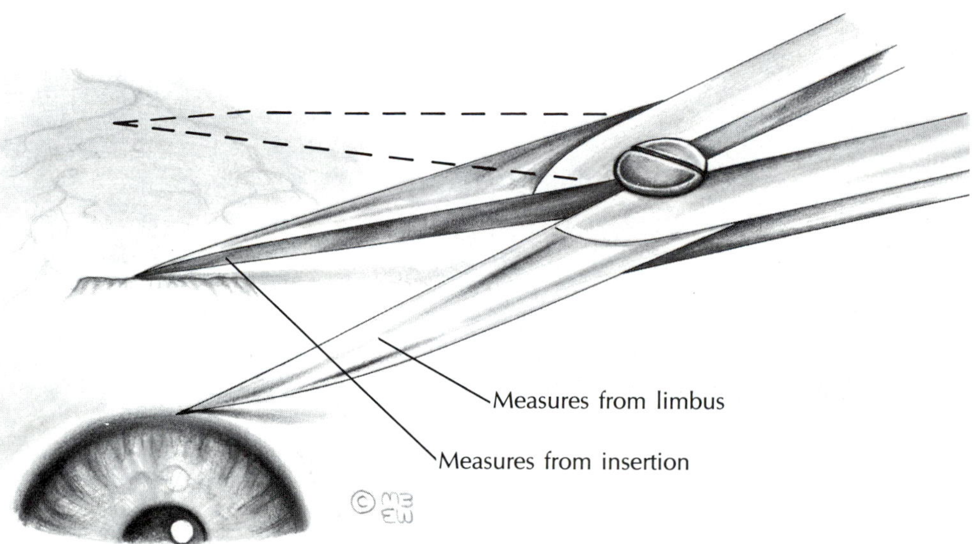

FIGURE 17-11

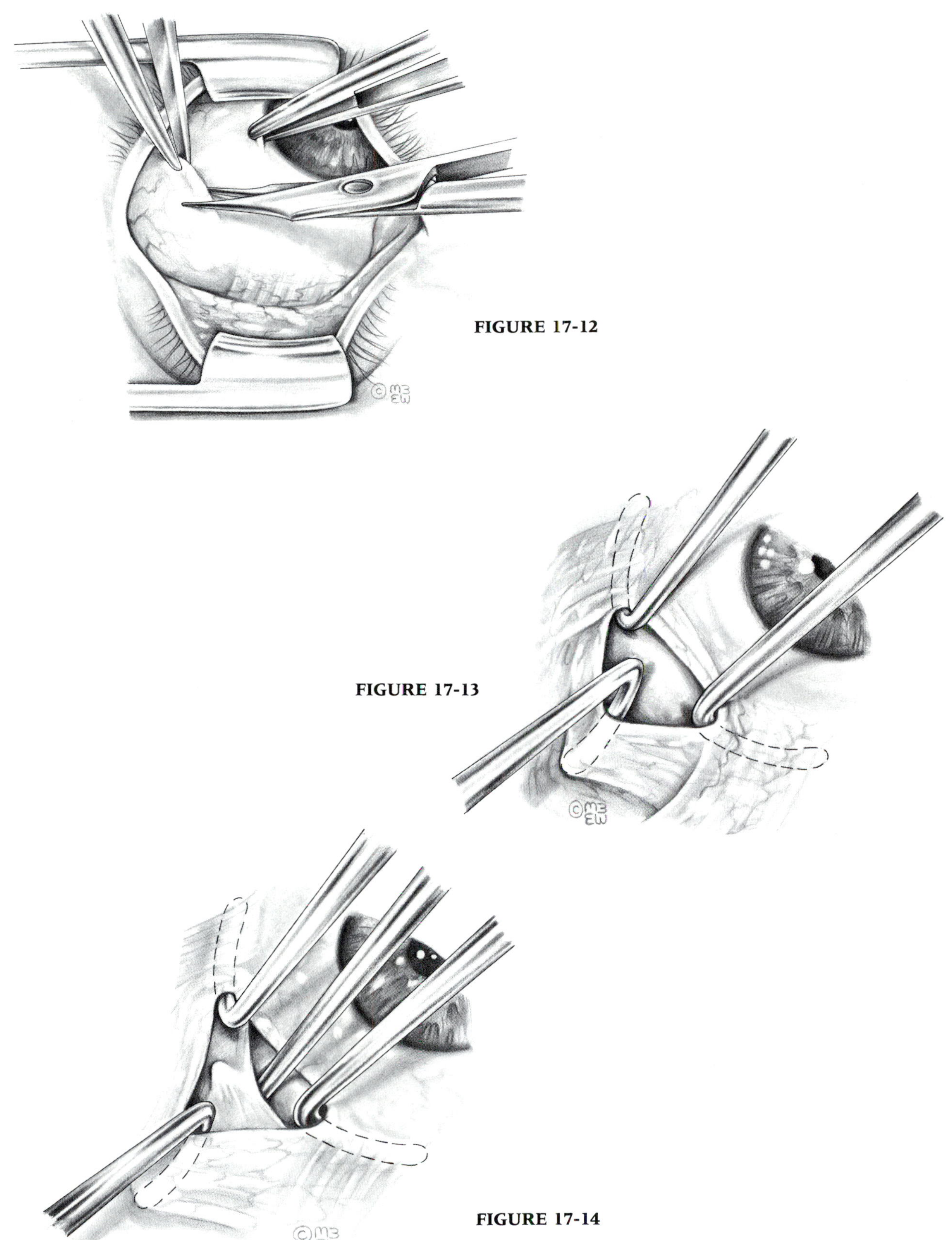

FIGURE 17-12

FIGURE 17-13

FIGURE 17-14

A second small muscle hook is placed under the inferior oblique muscle (Fig. 17-15).

A 5 to 8 mm section of the inferior oblique muscle is cut between two hemostats, which have replaced the two small muscle hooks (Fig. 17-16).

The cut ends of the inferior oblique muscle are cauterized heavily to control bleeding (Fig. 17-17).

The muscle is allowed to retract (Fig. 17-18).

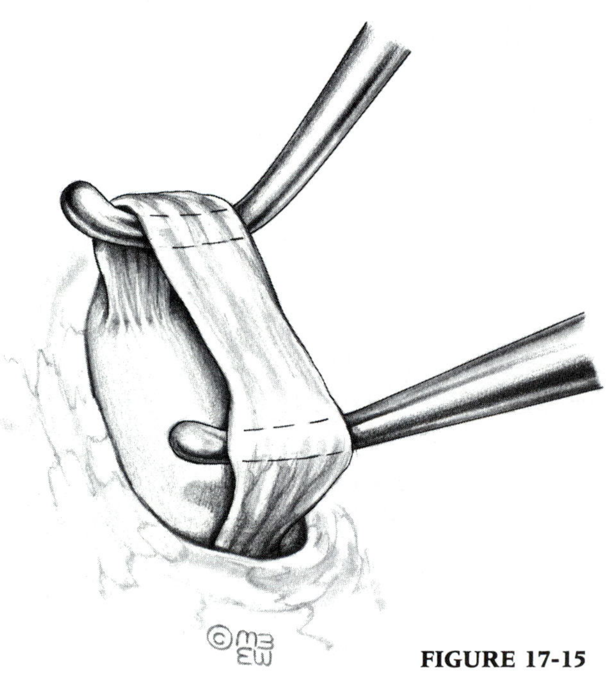

FIGURE 17-15

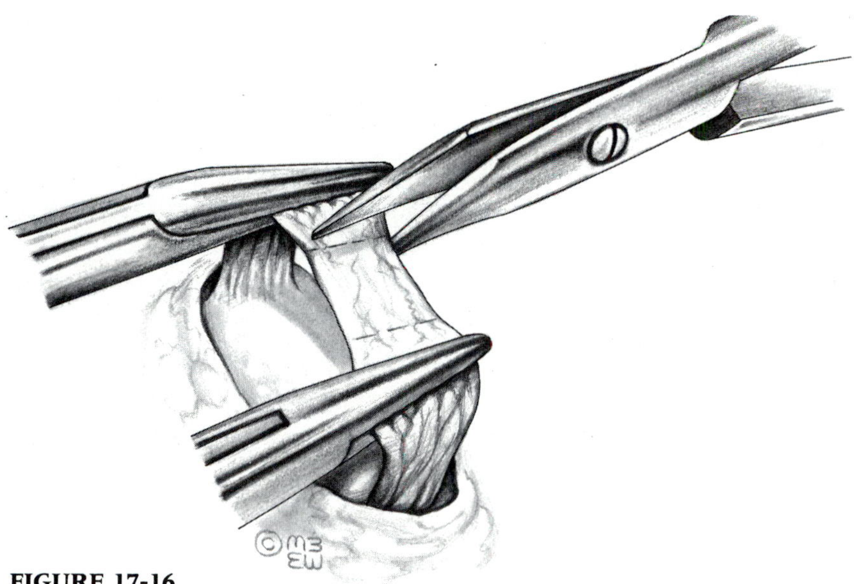

FIGURE 17-16

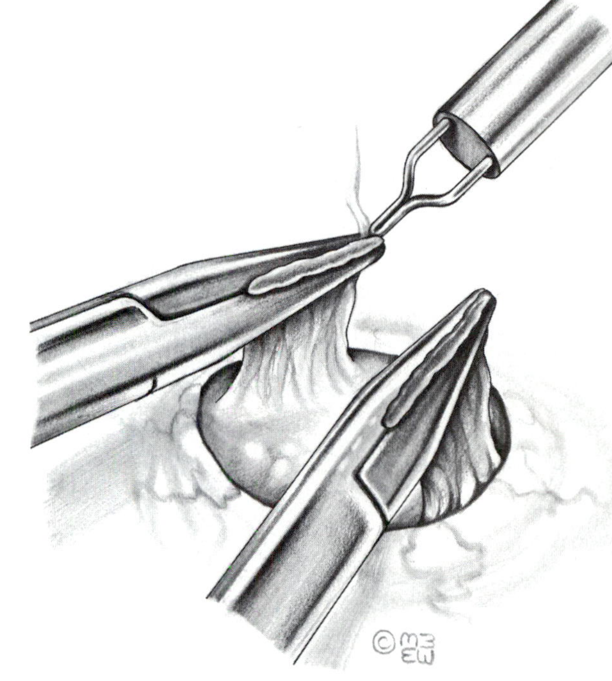

FIGURE 17-17

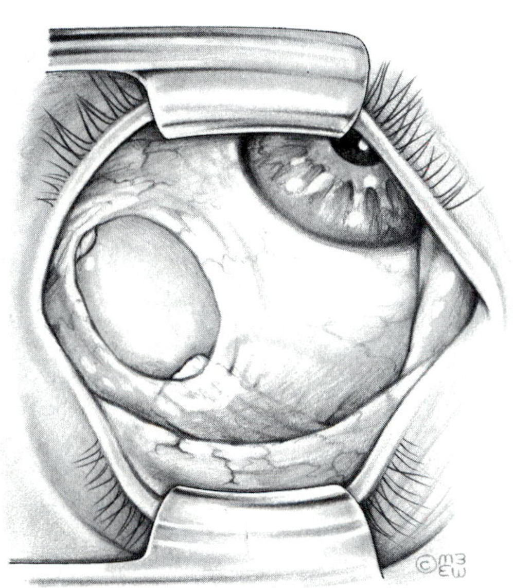

FIGURE 17-18

The incision may be closed with one or two 8-0 Vicryl sutures, or the incision may be left unsutured (Fig. 17-19).

If a hole is made in the posterior Tenon's capsule so that fat is allowed to protrude, this should be closed carefully with interrupted sutures. Careful attention to detail in inferior oblique surgery is extremely important. Fat prolapse with excessive bleeding and so on will lead to the inferior oblique adherence syndrome with a mechanically induced vertical deviation (Fig. 17-20).

One may weaken the superior oblique muscle by simply disinserting and allowing it to retract under the superior rectus muscle (Fig. 17-21).

The superior oblique tendon may be weakened by a type of "hang-loose" recession (Fig. 17-22).

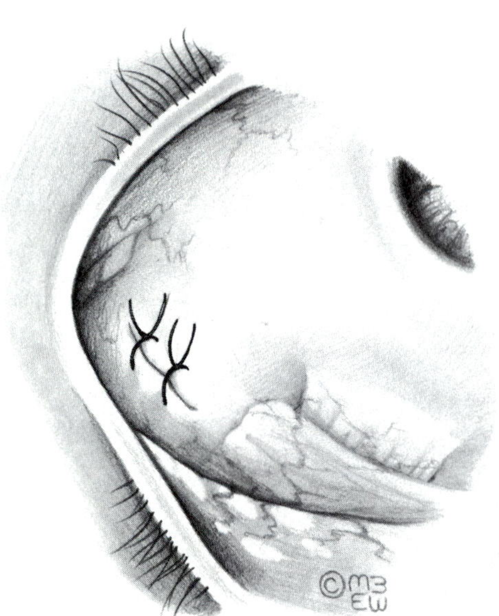

FIGURE 17-19

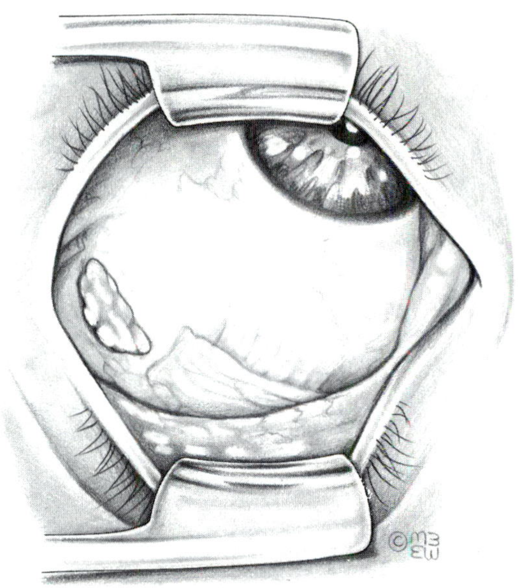

FIGURE 17-20

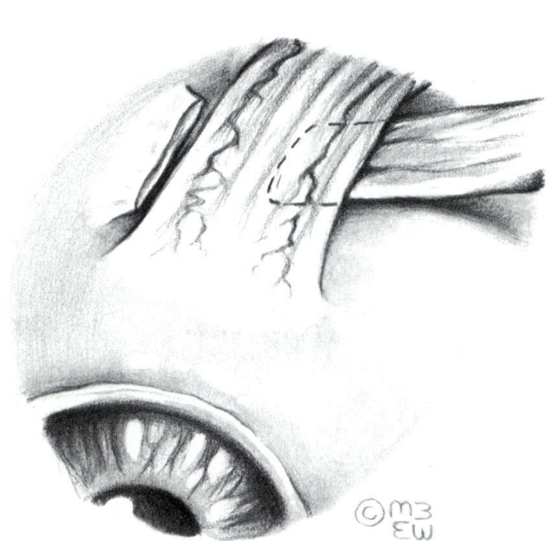

FIGURE 17-21

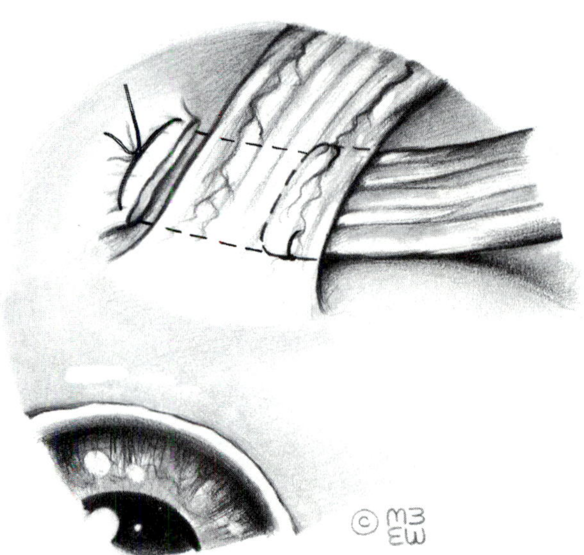

FIGURE 17-22

The anterior fibers of the superior oblique tendon may be cut to weaken intorsion while the depression effect is maintained (Fig. 17-23).

The posterior fibers of the superior oblique tendon may be disinserted to weaken the depression affect while intorsion is maintained (Fig. 17-24).

Some prefer to transect the superior oblique tendon nasal to the superior rectus (Fig. 17-25).

As a rule, the closer to the trochlea that tendon transection occurs and the more extensive the dissection of adjacent Tenon's capsule, the more the effect will be obtained from superior oblique weakening procedures.

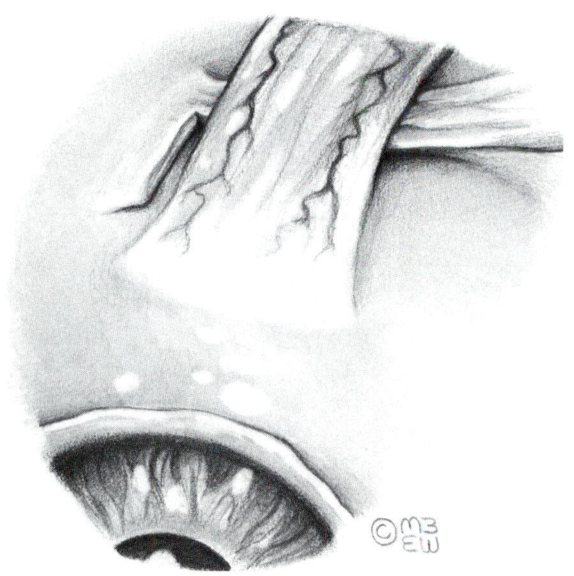

FIGURE 17-23

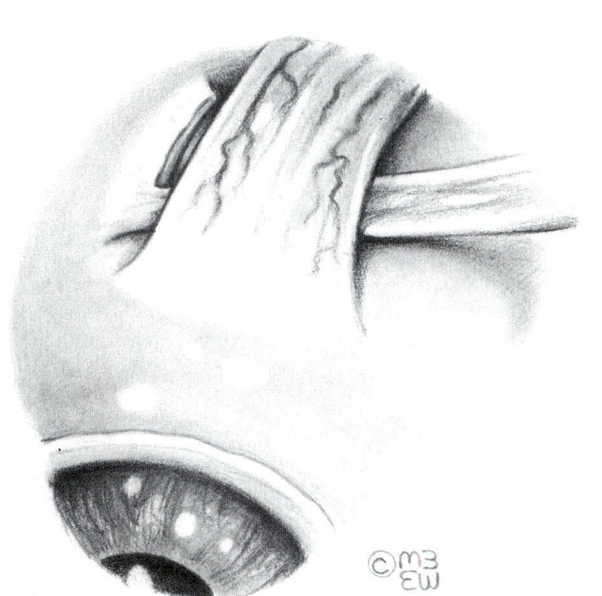

FIGURE 17-24

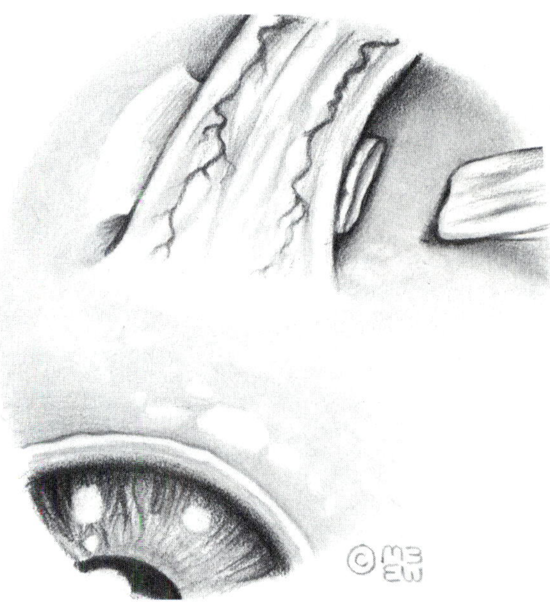

FIGURE 17-25

CHAPTER 18

Muscle Resection and Strengthening Procedures

Eye muscle resection procedures are commonly called "strengthening procedures." In fact, the muscles have a segment removed and are plicated, or advanced, so that a sort of tether is placed on the globe. The muscles are not strengthened in that no more grams of force are created. It is widely held that the principal value of an eye muscle resection procedure is accomplished by enhancement of the recession effect of the antagonist. Resection procedures may be done alone for specific indications such as unilaterally for mild vertical rectus underaction or bilaterally for convergence insufficiency. However, in most instances extraocular muscle resection (strengthening) is done with recession of the antagonist.

Muscle Resection

The essence of resection is removal of a distal segment of a muscle (tendon) and reattachment of the shortened muscle (Fig. 18-1).

For resection of a rectus muscle, a muscle clamp is placed posteriorly along the rectus muscle just anterior to the intended point of resection. This distance may be measured with a caliper according to the preference of the surgeon. After placement of the resection clamp and measurement, the muscle is detached from the globe leaving a 1 mm tendon stump (Fig. 18-2).

Double-arm sutures are placed backhand through the stump and brought out posterior to the muscle clamp (Fig. 18-3).

The muscle clamp is advanced to the cut end of the muscle. The sutures are tied while the clamp advances the muscle (Fig. 18-4).

When the shortened muscle is secured (Fig.18-5, *A*), the excess tendon-muscle is cut off (Fig. 18-5, *B*).

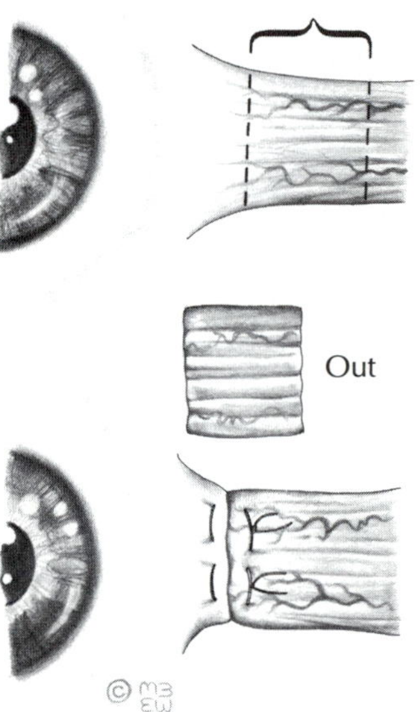

FIGURE 18-1

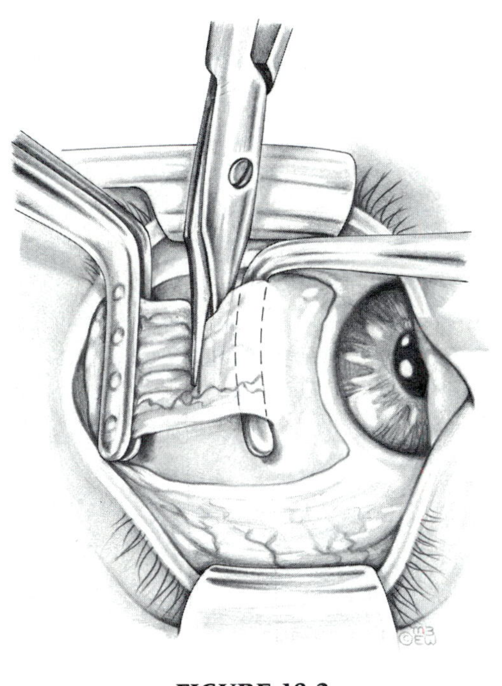

FIGURE 18-2

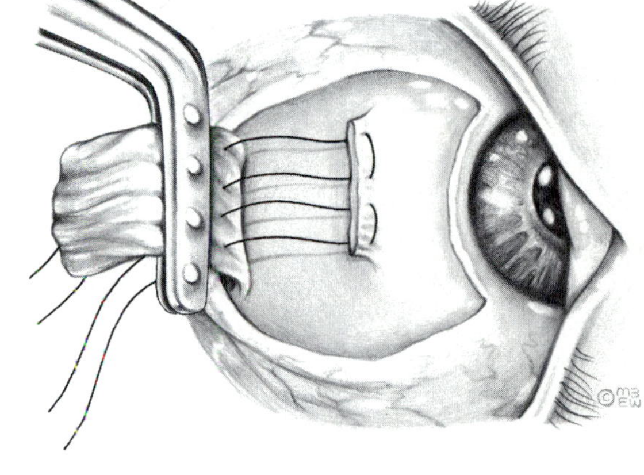

FIGURE 18-3

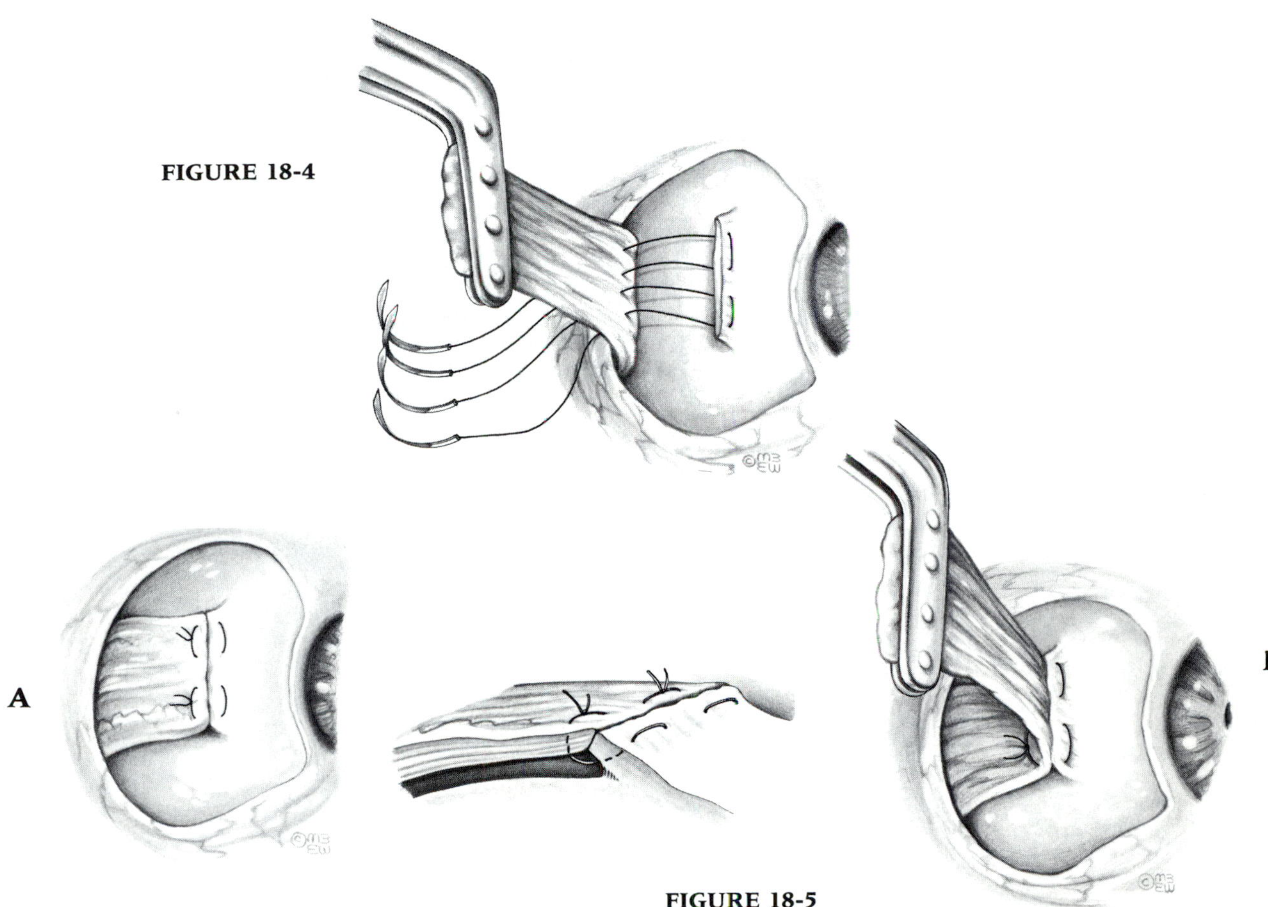

FIGURE 18-4

FIGURE 18-5

A simpler technique for resection is the use of a single double-arm suture placed posteriorly to the intended point of resection (Fig. 18-6). For added security a second suture may be placed immediately behind the first and in a similar manner.

The muscle after being cauterized is transected just anteriorly to the suture placement (Fig. 18-7).

After the tendon has been cut free from the insertion leaving a 1 mm stump, the sutures are brought through the muscle stump (Fig. 18-8).

The sutures may be tied at this point (Fig. 18-9). If two sutures are used, the anterior and posterior arms may be tied to each other at the muscle borders.

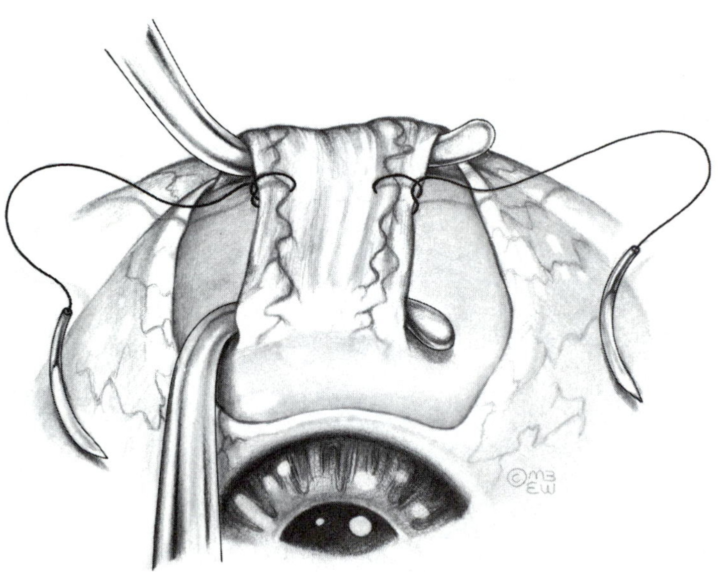

FIGURE 18-6

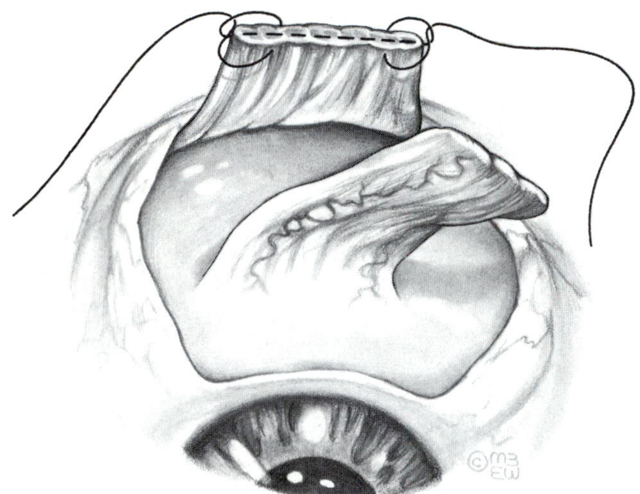

FIGURE 18-7

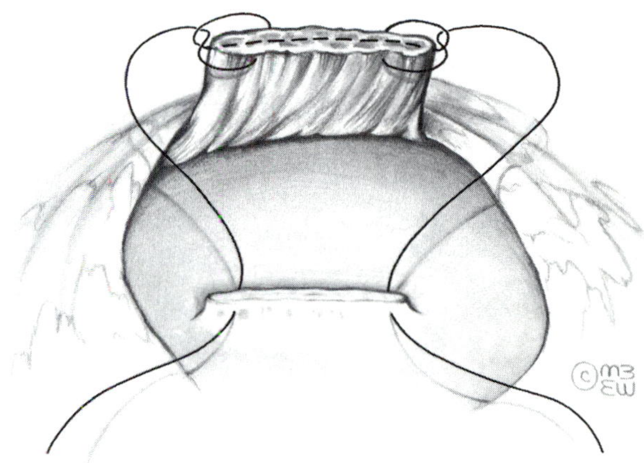

FIGURE 18-8

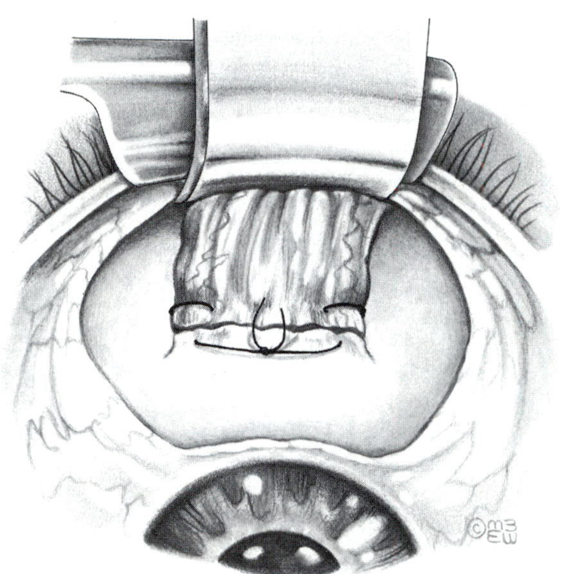

FIGURE 18-9

When a single double-arm suture is used, if the surgeon wishes, he may place the needles back through the muscle stump and out through the muscle posterior to the suture line (Fig. 18-10, *A* and *B*).

A

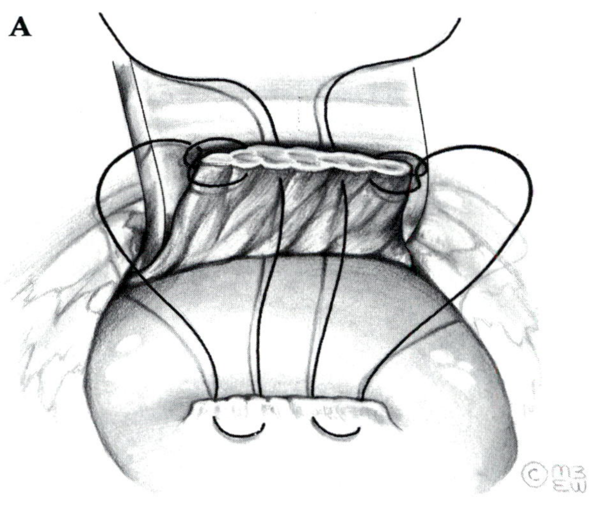

B

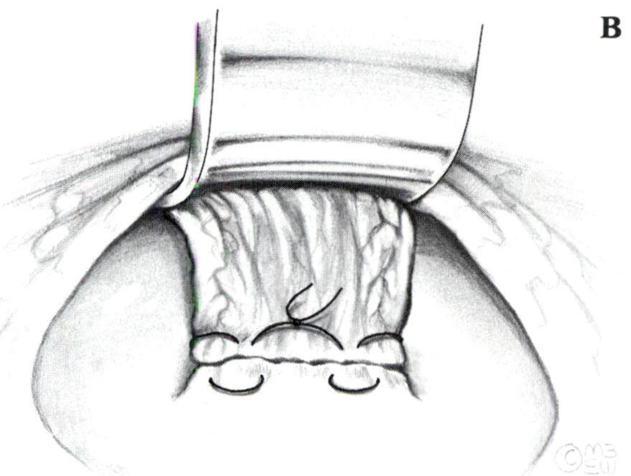

FIGURE 18-10

Strengthening Procedures

Superior oblique strengthening may be carried out in a variety of ways. One of these is a tuck at the insertion. The muscle is brought upward on a muscle hook or tendon tucker, which takes up the redundant or loose tendon (Fig. 18-11). The base of the tuck is secured with a nonabsorbable suture. The loop of tendon may be secured to sclera temporal to the base of the tuck. The amount of tuck depends on the laxity of the tendon, *not* on the amount of vertical deviation being treated. An excessive tuck will cause a postoperative Brown's superior oblique tendon sheath syndrome with limited elevation of the globe. An effective tuck may be as small as 6 mm or less or as large as 20 mm.

As an alternative, the superior oblique tendon can be resected with the proximal superior oblique tendon being resecured to the insertion (Fig. 18-12).

The excess superior oblique tendon is cut off (Fig. 18-13). The effect of this procedure can be altered by the point of superior oblique tendon reattachment. More torsional effect is obtained if the superior oblique tendon is reattached anteriorly and more vertical effect is obtained if the superior oblique tendon is reattached more posteriorly.

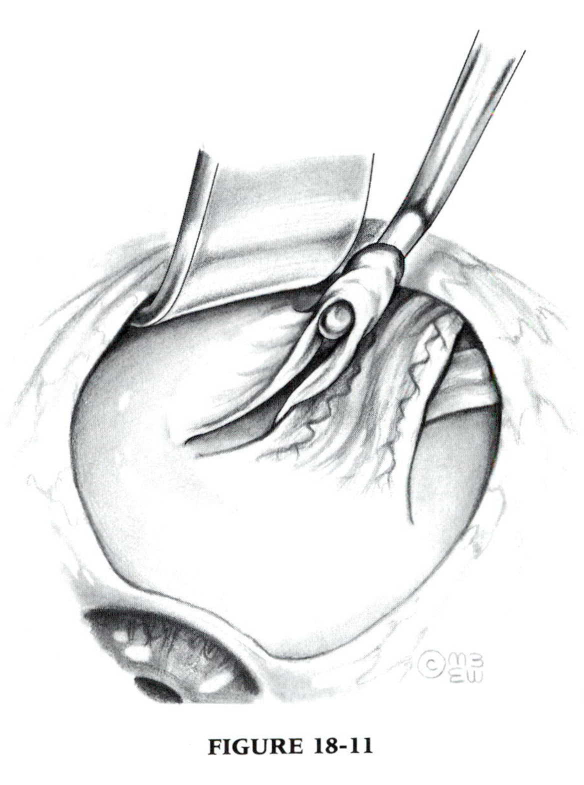

FIGURE 18-11

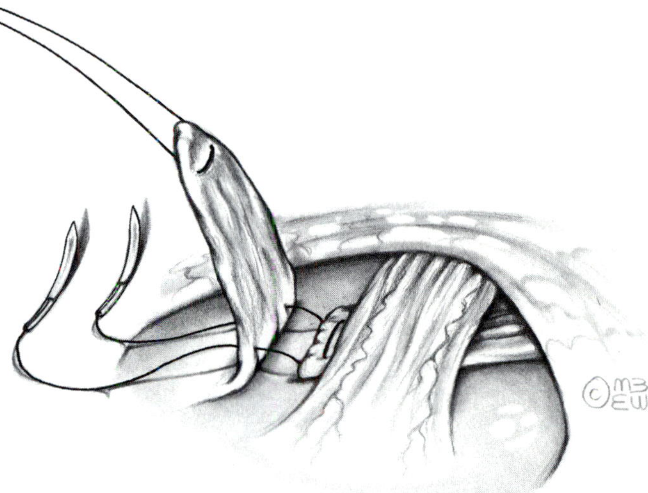

FIGURE 18-12

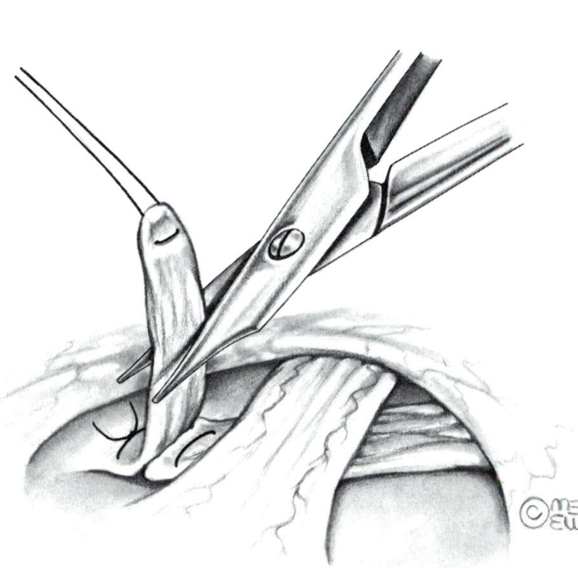

FIGURE 18-13

Increased torsional effect can be obtained if the superior oblique tendon is merely redirected more anteriorly (Fig. 18-14).

The superior oblique tendon may be strengthened by advancement of the tendon with or without detachment (Fig. 18-15).

The torsional effect of the superior oblique tendon can be increased by detachment and reattachment of it anteriorly as originally described by Harada-Ito procedure (Fig. 18-16). Although inferior oblique strengthening procedures have been described, they are of questionable value and are rarely done.

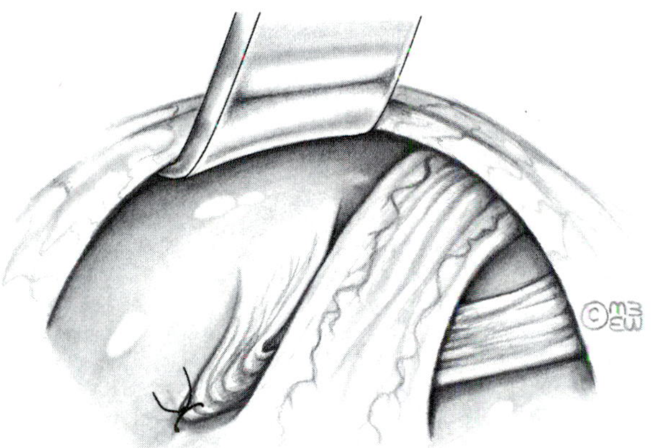

FIGURE 18-14

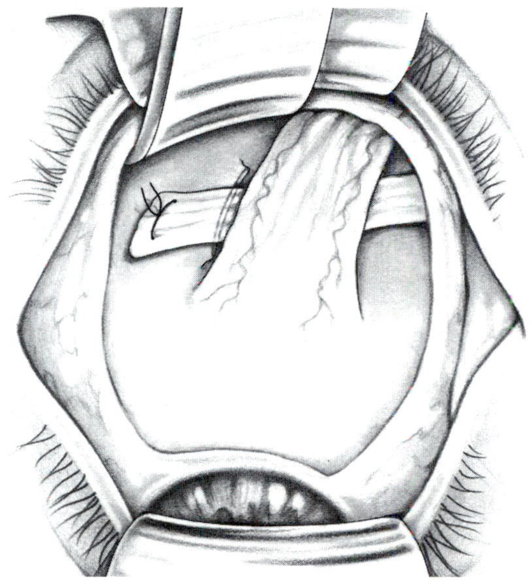

FIGURE 18-15

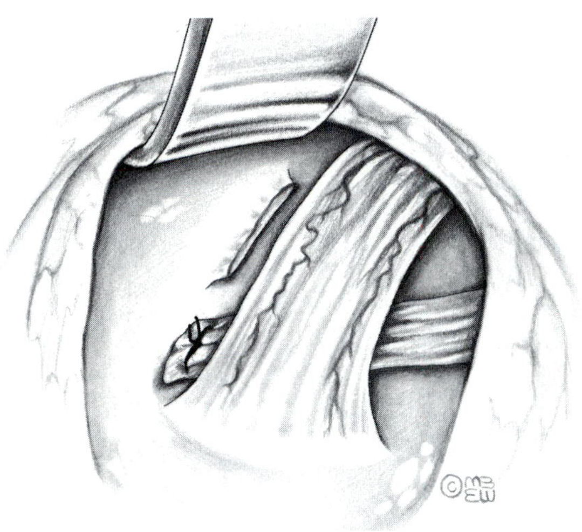

FIGURE 18-16

CHAPTER 19

Muscle Transfer Procedures

Eye muscle transfer procedures are indicated when strabismus is caused by paralysis of one or more rectus muscles. The most commonly employed eye muscle transfer procedure is done by shifting opposing rectus muscles to a point adjacent to the paretic rectus muscle between. For example, the vertical recti may be transposed to either the medial or lateral rectus or the horizontal recti may be transferred to the superior or inferior rectus. The antagonist of the paretic muscle is routinely weakened either by recession or by chemodenervation, botulinum toxin A injection during the course of extraocular muscle transfer to the paretic agonist.

Full Tendon Transfer

One may carry out a full tendon transfer of rectus muscles by shifting antagonist rectus muscles to the sclera adjacent to the insertion of the paretic rectus muscle between them (Fig. 19-1). The procedure is shown with shifting of the medial and lateral rectus muscles adjacent to the superior rectus.

The superior and inferior rectus are reattached adjacent to the medial rectus muscle (Fig. 19-2).

The inferior and superior rectus are reattached adjacent to the lateral rectus (Fig. 19-3).

The medial and lateral rectus are reattached adjacent to the inferior rectus (Fig. 19-4).

In certain cases of third-nerve palsy, the superior oblique tendon may be freed from the trochlea and reattached after shortening to the sclera just above the medial rectus insertion (Fig. 19-5). This step is usually accompanied by recession of the lateral rectus. Botulinum toxin A may be injected into the sound antagonist of the paretic muscle instead of recession of this muscle, or in any case where a transfer is done. From 5 to 7 units of botulinum toxin A are used.

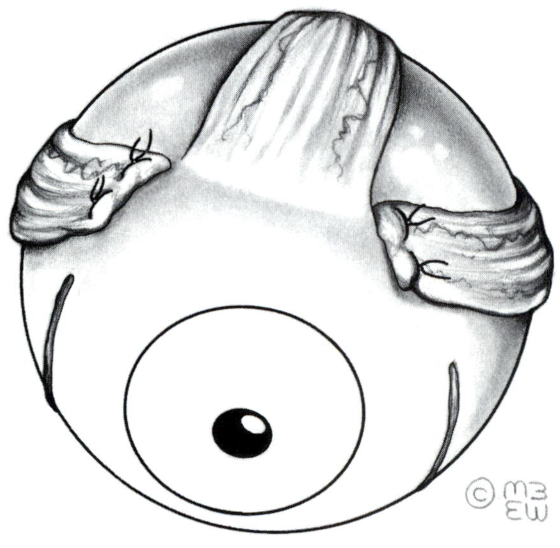

FIGURE 19-1

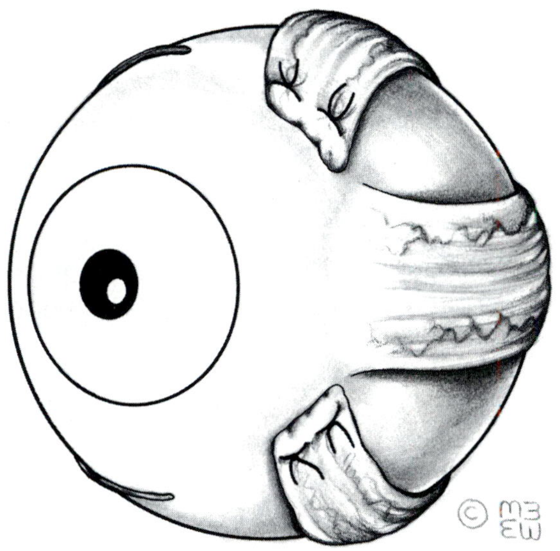

FIGURE 19-2

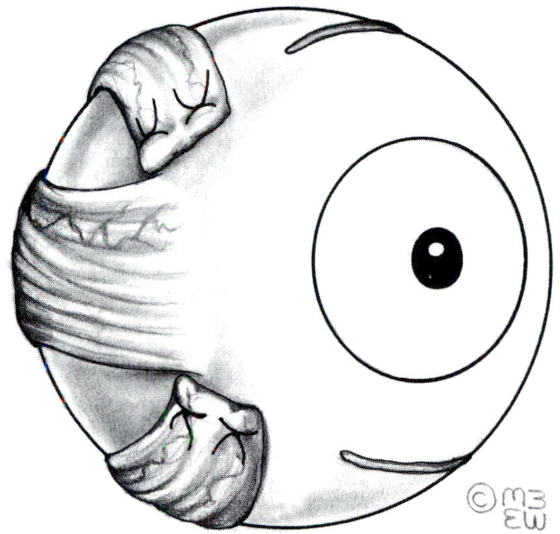

FIGURE 19-3

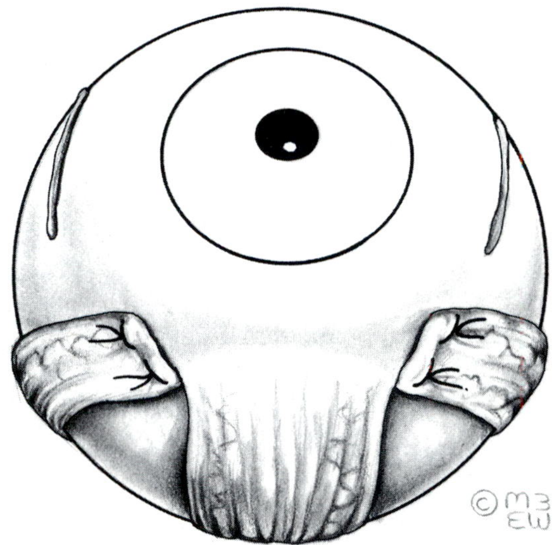

FIGURE 19-4

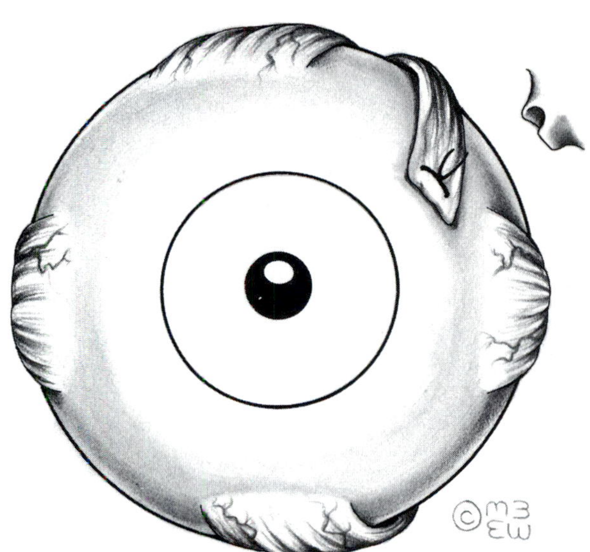

FIGURE 19-5

Jensen Procedure

The Jensen procedure has been largely replaced by full tendon transfer with botulinum toxin A injection of the sound antagonist. However, if the Jensen rectus muscle union is done, one carries out the procedure by joining the temporal half of opposing rectus muscles with the adjacent half of the paralyzed rectus muscle lying between them (Fig. 19-6). This union is carried out by use of nonabsorbable suture joining the muscles approximately at the equator. In most cases the antagonist muscle is recessed. It may also be treated with botulinum toxin A.

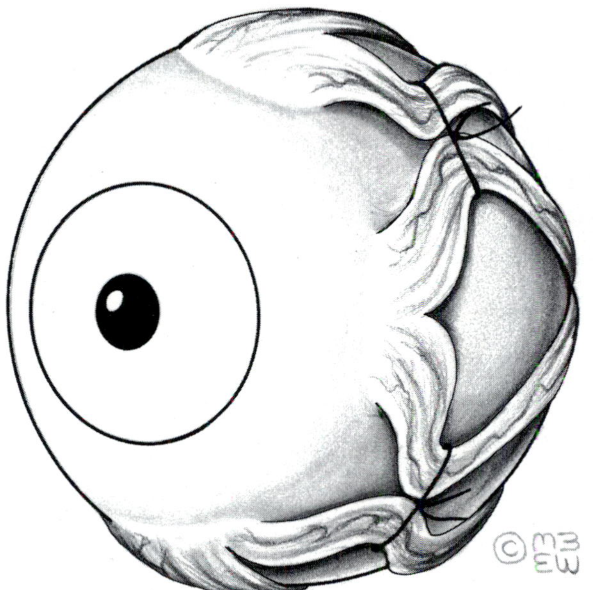

FIGURE 19-6

Scleral Strap Union

In cases of an absent rectus muscle either iatrogenicly, from trauma, or congenitally, the antagonist rectus muscles may have the half of each muscle adjacent to the absent muscle joined by a band of bank sclera (Fig. 19-7, *A* and *B*). Like the Jensen procedure, this is usually associated with recession of the antagonist muscle (Fig. 19-7, *C*). The principal reason for doing the Jensen procedure or scleral strap union is to maintain circulation in at least two rectus muscles. This avoids the complication of anterior segment ischemia. Since a muscle can be weakened at least temporarily with botulinum toxin A while still maintaining circulation, the need for a Jensen procedure or the scleral strap union has been lessened.

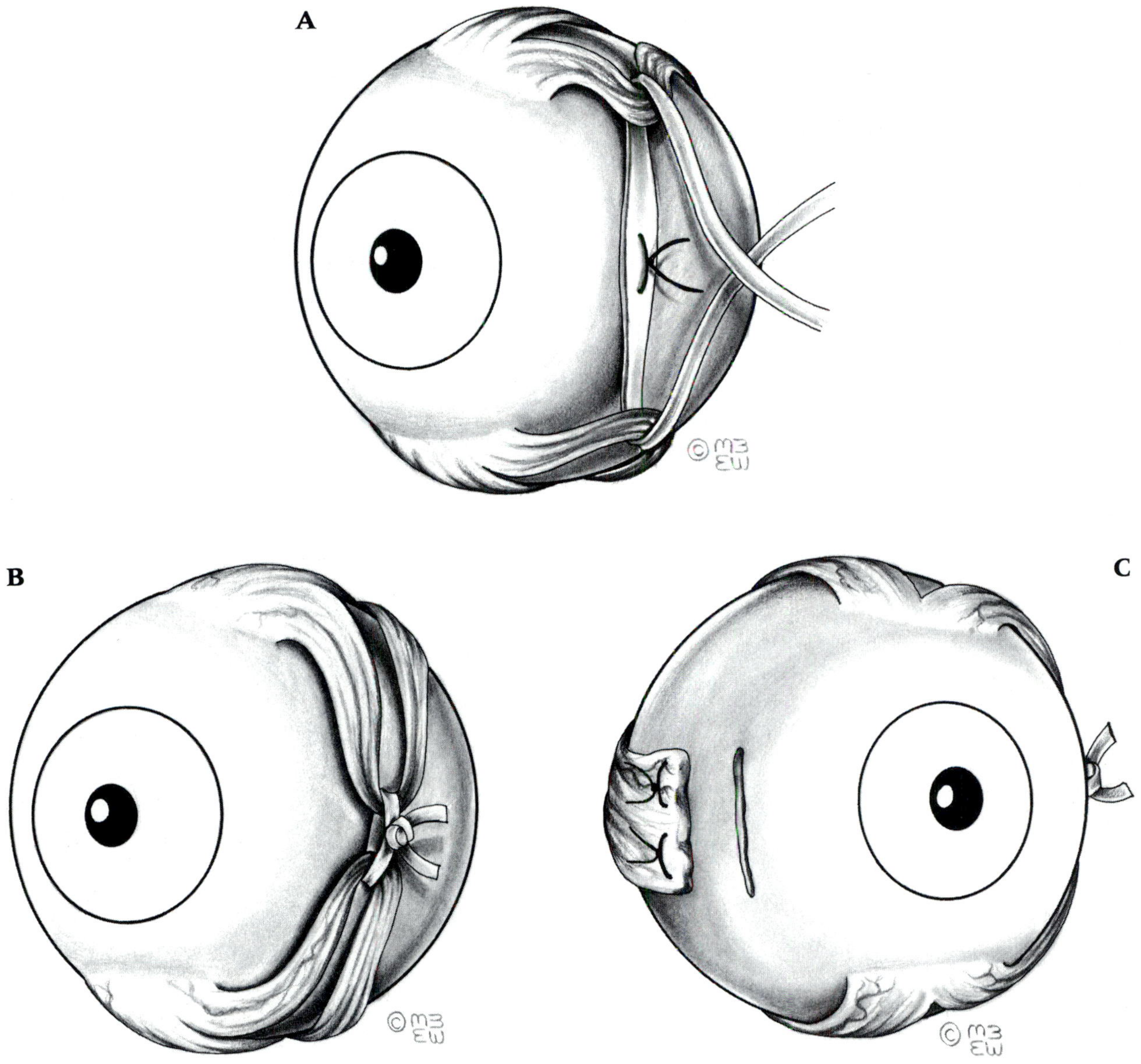

FIGURE 19-7

Other Procedures

To combine horizontal rectus surgery with a vertical effect, both horizontal recti may be shifted upward to relieve a hypodeviation (Fig. 19-8, *A*).

To relieve a hyperdeviation, both recti may be shifted downward (Fig. 19-8, *B*).

For vertically incomitant strabismus, the medial recti are shifted toward the closed end of the A (Fig. 19-8, *C, upper pair*) or V (Fig. 19-8, *C, lower pair*) with or without recession or resection depending on the primary-position deviation.

For A (Fig. 19-8, *D, upper pair*) or V (Fig. 19-8, *D, lower pair*) patterns, the lateral recti are moved toward the open end of the pattern with or without recession, or resection depending on the primary-position deviation.

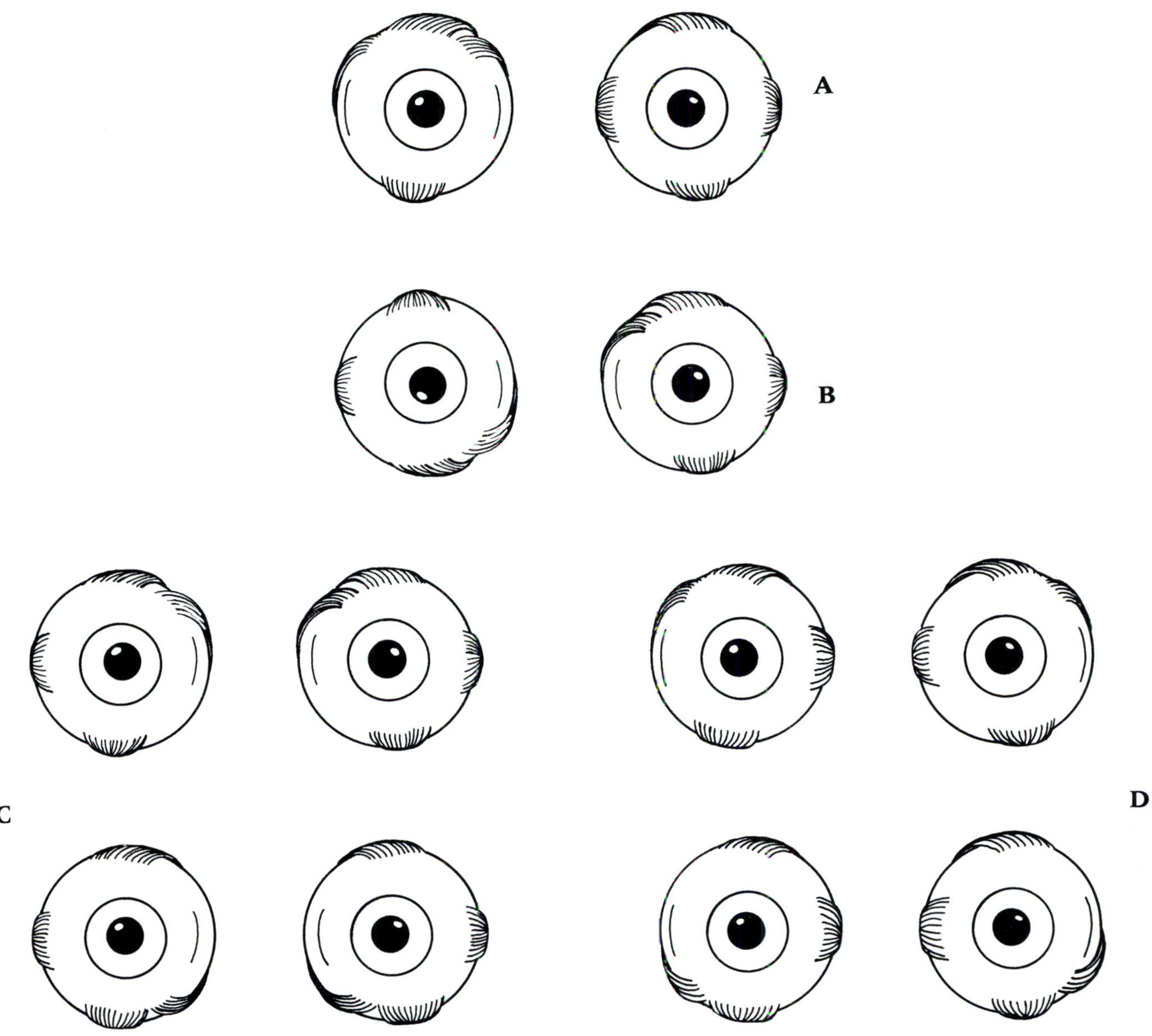

FIGURE 19-8

CHAPTER 20

Adjustable Sutures, Faden Procedure, and Conjunctival Recession

Adjustable sutures are a widely accepted and useful addition to the strabismus surgeon's armamentarium. Since the patient's cooperation is required when this surgery is performed, this technique is most applicable in older teenagers and adults. The ideal candidate can recognize diplopia to assist in the postoperative adjustment or cooperate for cover testing during and immediately after the surgical procedure. Either local or general anesthesia can be used, with local being preferred. All the rectus muscles are suitable for the adjustable suture technique; in this chapter the technique for recession and resection of the superior oblique tendon is described. Various suture placement configurations can be used with adjustable recession and resection, but in each the suture ends are secured temporarily but left available for loosening and tightening depending on the patient's alignment. Even after achieving entirely satisfactory alignment with an adjustable suture, postoperative drift can occur.

The Faden operation, posterior fixation suture, or retroequatorial myopexy, was introduced by Cuppers. It was at first widely heralded but is now used very selectively. The principle of this operation is to move the arc of contact for a rectus muscle to a point slightly behind the equator and reduce the muscle's effect in its field of action by reducing its lever arm. The procedure may be done alone or combined with recession. No effect is produced on alignment in the primary position if no recession is done. A Faden procedure done on a sound muscle produces a "laudable" secondary deviation in an underacting yoke muscle. One may use this technique to improve the alignment of an eye without operating on it and without adversely affecting the alignment of the fellow eye. When an eye muscle is "crippled" in its field of action, more innervation is required, and according to Hering this innervation is sent to the yoke muscle.

Conjunctival recession is useful when the conjunctiva is tight and inelastic, causing restricted movement, or when the conjunctiva is reddened, rough, and unsightly. The conjunctiva may be recessed and reattached to sclera at or near the point of rectus muscle insertion.

Adjustable Sutures

Adjustable sutures of the rectus muscles are employed in the form of a simple double-arm suture (Fig. 20-1, *A*). After the suture is placed near the muscle's insertion, the muscle is detached. Sutures are brought through the original insertional stump and tied with the muscle recessed.

The conjunctiva may be recessed if it is tight, scarred, or restrictive (Fig. 20-1, *B*). The surgeon may employ a slip knot or a bow knot to temporarily secure the muscle. Adjustment is carried out on the table, on the afternoon of surgery, or 24 hours later. Resection of the muscle can be done by placement of the suture in the muscle at the approximate point of intended resection. The suture may be tied under conjunctiva or on top of conjunctiva.

A small plastic band may serve as a bolster after the suture is brought through the conjunctiva with or without recession (Fig. 20-2). 6-0 Vicryl suture is of adequate tensile strength for this procedure. The bolster is removed at the time of adjustment, and the suture may be tied externally over conjunctiva. Several variations on the adjustable suture are used. These include reaching under the conjunctiva to assist in further recession of the rectus muscle, closing the conjunctiva at surgery, and lifting it at adjustment.

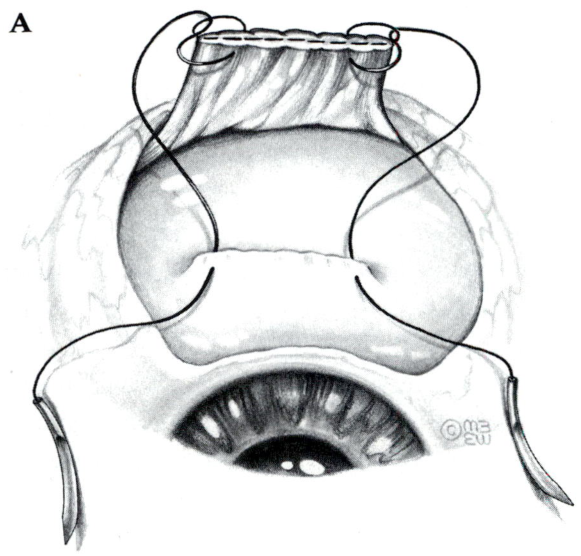

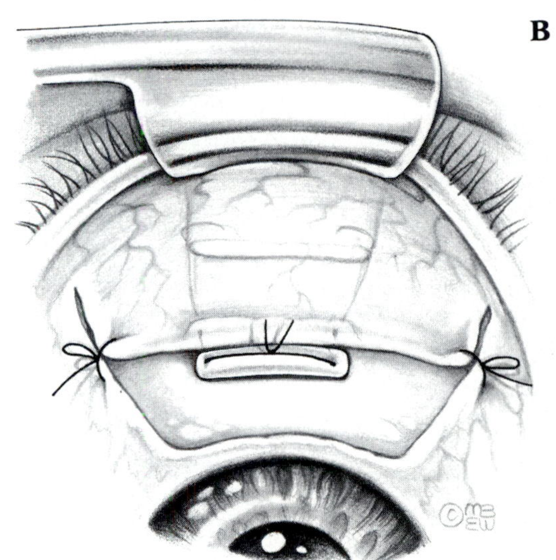

FIGURE 20-1

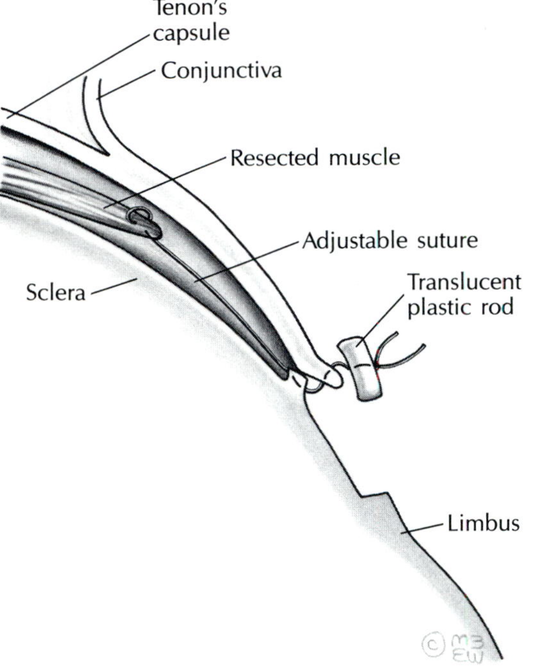

FIGURE 20-2

Faden Procedure

The principle of the Faden operation or posterior fixation suture is to weaken the muscle in its field of action without altering the primary position alignment (Fig. 20-3). One does this by reducing the lever arm of the rectus muscle. This reduced lever arm with reduced torque weakens the muscle in its field of action. It is also useful in producing a laudible secondary deviation. That is, the yoke muscle of the Faden-treated muscle will react to an increased innervation. The rectus muscle body is attached to sclera at the equator. The sutures are placed, for example, 12 mm posterior to the insertion of the superior or medial rectus muscle (when one considers functional insertion).

The Faden operation may be done with recession (Fig. 20-4). Two sutures may be used at the muscle's border. These should be nonabsorbable, usually 5-0 or 6-0. For the Faden operation a single suture securing the center of the muscle to underlying sclera may be used.

The Faden operation may also be carried out without detachment of the muscle (Fig. 20-5).

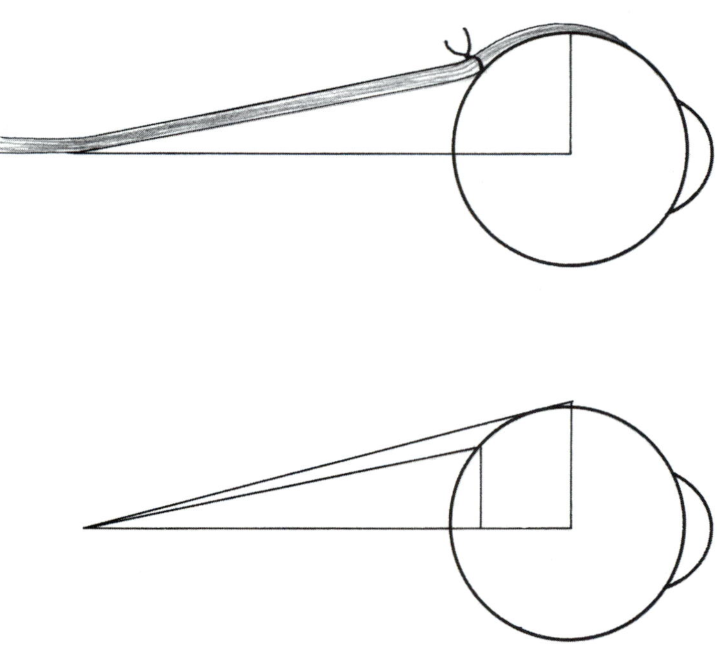

FIGURE 20-3

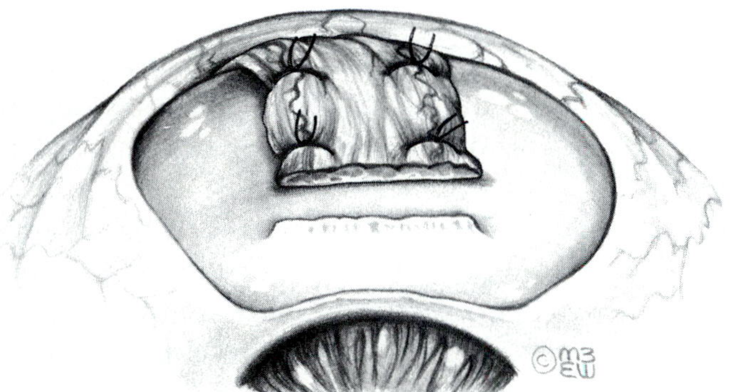

FIGURE 20-4

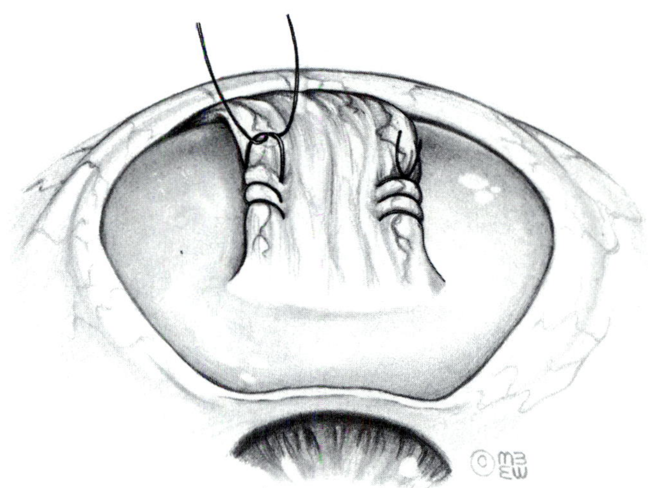

FIGURE 20-5

Conjunctival Closure

The limbal incision may be closed with 8-0 Vicryl sutures at the limbal corners by use of a conventional or buried knot. The radial relaxing wings may be sutured or left unsutured (Fig. 20-6).

One carries out conjunctival recession with a limbal incision by securing conjunctiva and anterior Tenon's capsule at the center of the previous insertion of the recessed muscle and the corners of the recessed flap of conjunctiva to adjacent conjunctiva (Fig. 20-7).

Proper management of the conjunctiva is essential to the successful management of the strabismus operation. Proper alignment of the eyes in the presence of red, scarred, and irregular conjuctiva is no success at all. Careful dissection and repair of conjuctiva and Tenon's capsule is as important as proper management of muscle placement in the overall management of strabismus.

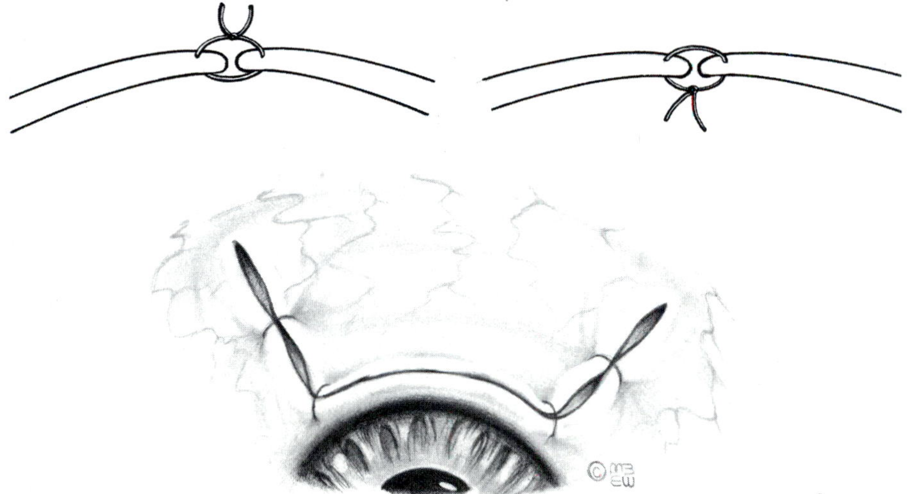

FIGURE 20-6

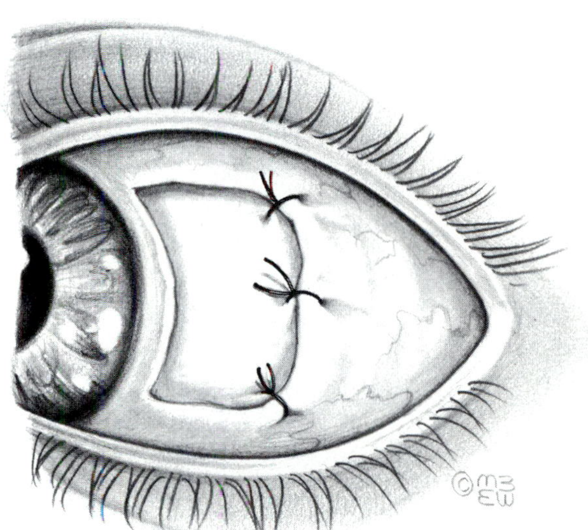

FIGURE 20-7

PART FIVE

VITREOUS SURGERY

Steve T. Charles

CHAPTER 21

Essentials of Vitreous Surgery

Vitreoretinal surgery blends high technology microsurgery with a complex pathobiologic system and presents the surgeon with a significant challenge. The team that undertakes this challenge must be well trained, efficient, and competent technologically. The complex equipment that is required must be well maintained and updated with meaningful modifications as they are developed.

PATIENT EVALUATION AND PREPARATION

Patients requiring vitreoretinal surgery range from premature babies to the elderly and from the healthy athlete to those with advanced systemic complications of diabetes. As in all of clinical medicine, decision making is a multiparametric process utilizing social, scientific, and statistical principles, with the patient's overall welfare being the primary concern.

Clinical evaluation must begin with visual acuity testing. Patients must have light perception to be eligible, and those with acuities of 20/400 or better must undergo refraction. Other psychophysical testing such as two-point discrimination, Maddox rod orientation, entoptic phenomena, photostress, color vision testing, and light projection have not been found to be of value.

Ultrasound testing using contact real-time gray scale B-scan or volumetric imagery must be performed in any case in which the retina cannot be visualized. It is preferable that this be performed by the surgeon.

Bright flash electroretinogram testing is dangerous to patients with clear media and produces many false-negative results because of proliferative retinopathy and vascular disease, largely negating its value.

Clinical examination requires slitlamp examination with special emphasis on iris neovascularization, lens clarity, retrolenticular neovascularization, and fundus examination with the +90D lens. Indirect ophthalmoscopy is crucial and is best performed with the brightest light and +20D lenses.

Careful discussion with the patient and family of the success rates, complications, and patient-positioning requirements must precede surgery.

The majority of the illustrations in this chapter have been modified and redrawn from Charles ST: Vitreous microsurgery, ed 2, Baltimore, 1987, Williams & Wilkins.

SURGICAL ANATOMY

The vitreous can be viewed as a three-dimensional matrix of collagen fibers and hyaluronic acid gel. Normally the outer surface of the vitreous contacts the retina, pars plana, and ciliary body in a roughly spherical shape with a facet anteriorly for the lens. Disease can produce a modest cellular infiltration, and this, along with changes that are induced in the aging process, causes the collagen matrix to contract. Most of the resulting alterations occur along the continuous outer surface. The anterior hyaloid face is continuous with the posterior hyaloid face and is generally nonfenestrated.

Cells that are abnormal migrate along the front and back surfaces of the retina and vitreous. Many of these cells have coated pits that contain fibronectin, which allows them to attach to and produce contraction of the collagen matrix. Since the retina normally does not contract or contain intraretinal proliferation, any changes that occur in contour are the result of perpendicular vitreous traction (which produces funnel-, plateau-, or ridge-like elevations) or tangential periretinal membrane traction (producing starfolds).

The epiretinal membranes are white with a matte finish, and the retina appears pale yellow with a surface luster. Unless a complete posterior vitreous detachment has occurred, the areas of epiretinal membrane and adjacent detached posterior hyaloid face are continuous.

A relative decrease or loss of normal transretinal pressure gradient results from retinal breaks. The flow through the break is related to intraocular pressure, health of the retinal pigment epithelium, viscosity of the fluid, and the size of the break.

MECHANICS OF VITREOUS SURGERY

Cutter frequency. Moving the cutter along at high speed makes use of tissue inertia to provide cleaner cutting and less traction. If a constant flow rate is assumed, Fig. 21-1 shows the effect of cutter velocity. It should be noted that high-frequency cutter use allows less vitreous fiber travel before cutting, therefore reducing traction.

Moving mass. A cutter mechanism with small moving mass allows for (1) reduced vibration, (2) reduced motor size and weight of the cutter, and (3) use of high-speed inertial cutting (Fig. 21-2).

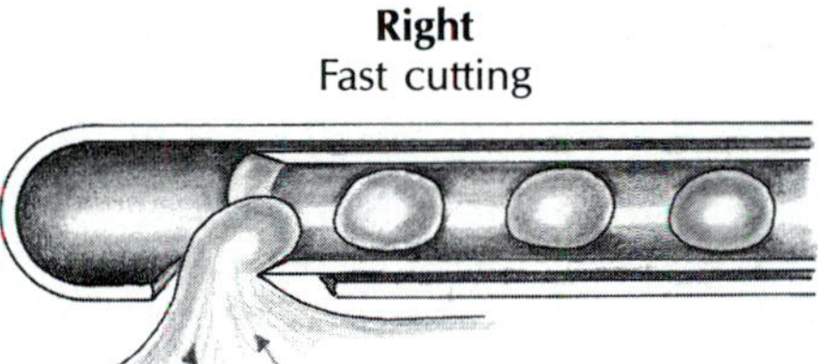

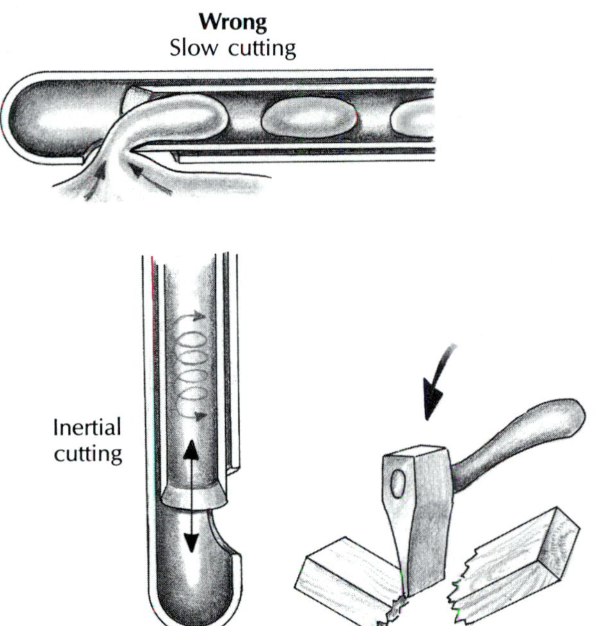

FIGURE 21-1. Effect of cutter velocity.

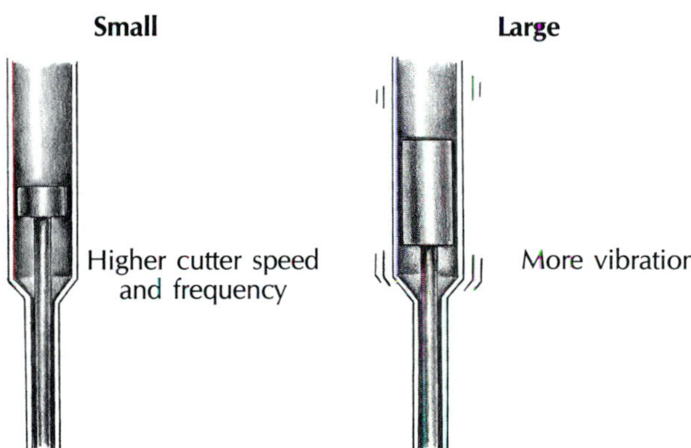

FIGURE 21-2. Cutter mechanism.

Direction of cutting. One should cut while advancing the cutter port (Fig. 21-3, *A*). The cutter port should be placed directly on the tissue to be removed, so that excessive vitreous fiber travel and retinal traction are eliminated. If cutting is performed while the cutter is being withdrawn and suction is being applied, undue traction results (Fig. 21-3, *B*).

Cutting methods. The correct cutting method employs proportional suction force (Fig. 21-4, *A*). With this method suction may be applied at a low level, which will reduce vitreoretinal traction. If tissue is inadvertently caught in the port, the surgeon should delay slightly, to allow the pressure to equalize through the porous tissues or through use of a small-volume back flush. Along with the high-speed cutter movement, this method reduces vitreoretinal traction and allows better cutting to be achieved.

If tissue is entrapped in the port, the surgeon must avoid jerking the hand away (Fig. 21-4, *B*).

Infusion options. As outlined in Fig. 21-5, various options are available with regard to infusion tools. When visualization of the pars plana is not possible, hand-held infusion cannulas are used.

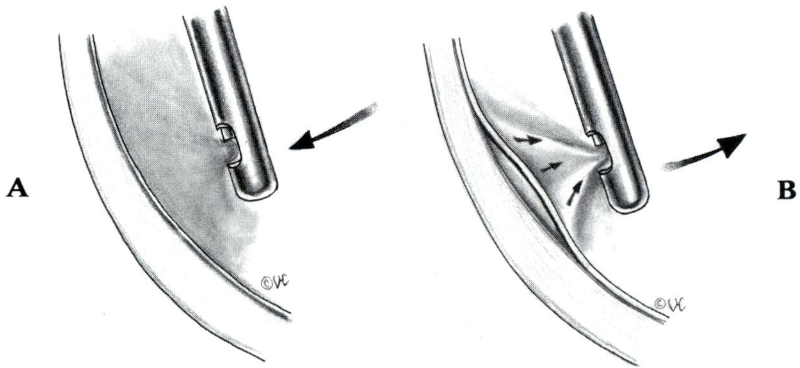

FIGURE 21-3. **A,** Correct position for cutting while advancing. **B,** Cutting while pulling creates undue traction.

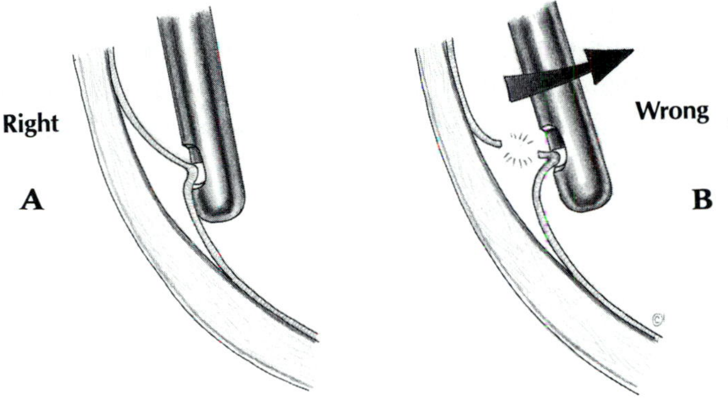

FIGURE 21-4. Cutting methods. **A,** Correct method. **B,** Sudden movement may cause entrapment of retina or iris.

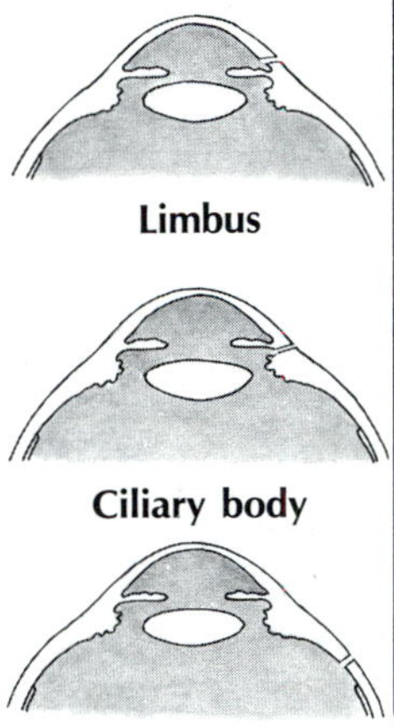

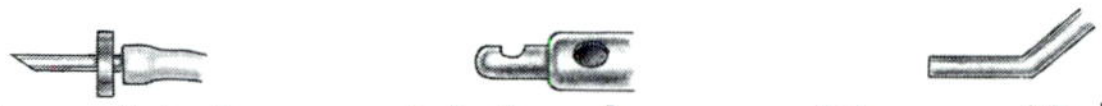

	4 mm infusion cannula	Infusion sleeve	20-gauge 30-degree blunt cannula
Limbus	No	VITREOUS LOSS PREEXISTING WOUNDS Phacoemulsification Aphakic trabeculectomy Extracapsular cataract extraction (ECCE)	Traumatic cataract Hyphema ECCE with fragmenter
Ciliary body	No	No	Persistent hyperplastic primary vitreous Retinopathy of prematurity Choroidal edema or hemorrhage
Pars plana	Best method for all anterior and posterior approaches except as noted	No	Retro-intraocular lens membrane Opaque pupillary membrane

FIGURE 21-5. Infusion options.

Handpieces. Instruments should be held in the surgeon's fingertips (Fig. 21-6). Three fingertips should be used to allow sufficient sensitivity and stability. Contouring of the instruments reduces holding-pressure requirements. The contour should be axially symmetric to permit rotation.

Spherical coordinates (Fig. 21-7). The surgeon must mentally separate the spherical coordinates of the tissue-access port from the tool-tip location. The sclerotomies are used to rotate the eye, but the eye should be stable if the intent is to move only the instruments to a new location.

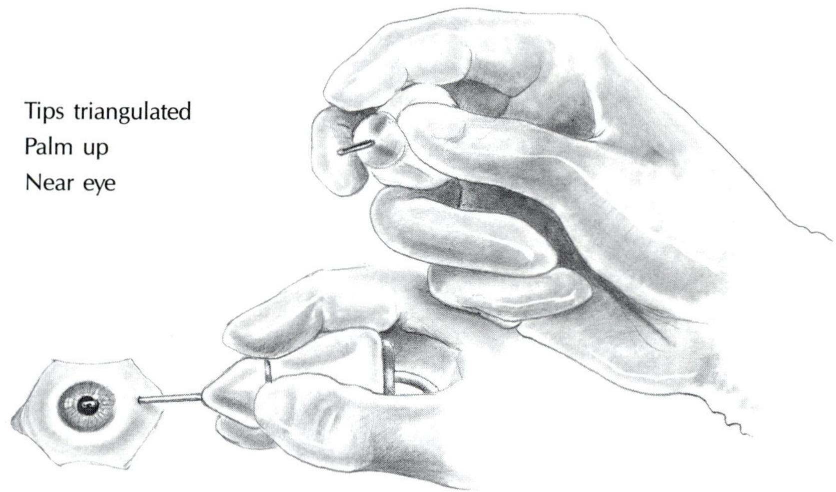

FIGURE 21-6. Finger position.

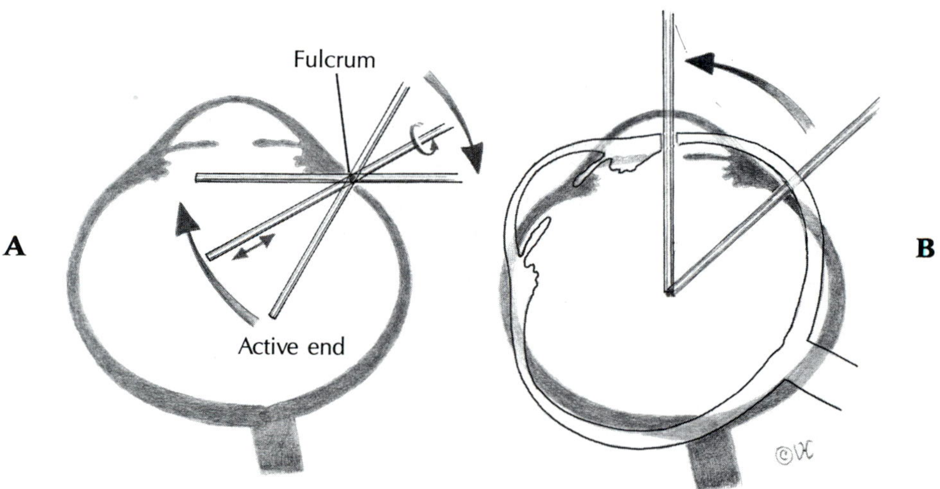

FIGURE 21-7. Two sets of spherical coordinates. **A,** Move tip to pathologic area. **B,** Use instruments to rotate eye.

CHAPTER 22

Anterior Segment Procedures

Instrumentation developed for posterior segment vitreous surgery is useful to cut and remove a wide variety of tissues from the anterior segment. Vitrectomy, lensectomy, iridectomy, and removal of hemorrhage and fibrous tissue can all be accomplished with standard vitreous cutters. Two-port systems allow infusion to be maintained while a wide variety of cutters, scissors, and fragmenters are utilized. A third port allows visibility of access under the iris plane, and the endoilluminator improves visualization. The sleeve over 20-gauge cutters is used only when a larger procedure opening, such as a trabeculectomy site or phacoemulsification wound, is present because it causes more turbulence and endothelial damage. The infusion handle is used in lieu of the sew-on cannula when the pars plana cannot be visualized. The anterior pars plana is an appropriate access site for all anterior segment microsurgery with vitreous problems. Compared to limbal views, it reduces corneal damage and iris damage and permits more complete removal of lens material and vitreous.

The majority of the illustrations in this chapter have been modified and redrawn from Charles ST: Vitreous microsurgery, ed 2, Baltimore, 1987, Williams & Wilkins.

Vitrectomy

The use of vitrectomy in *penetrating keratoplasty* (Fig. 22-1) involves the simplest and most frequently performed type of anterior vitrectomy—open-sky vitrectomy. No infusion is required, and neither cellulose sponges nor vitreous aspiration should be used. The instrument is placed in the central anterior vitreous space and moved only minimally. The vitreous base must be avoided to reduce vitreoretinal traction. More suction is required than with closed vitrectomy because of the absence of a closed system with infusion pressure. The port should be maintained within the vitreous, moving and cutting while advancing. Penetrating keratoplasty necessitates a more extensive vitrectomy than with the basic aphakic technique to prevent adhesion between the vitreous and the donor cornea (see also p. 36). Closure over an air bubble is recommended to avoid creation of residual strands to the wound (see also p. 220).

In the presence of large wounds, such as a trabeculectomy incision or planned extracapsular extraction, use of a combined infusion and suction probe is appropriate (Fig. 22-2), though this combination is now obsolete in other anterior and posterior vitrectomies.

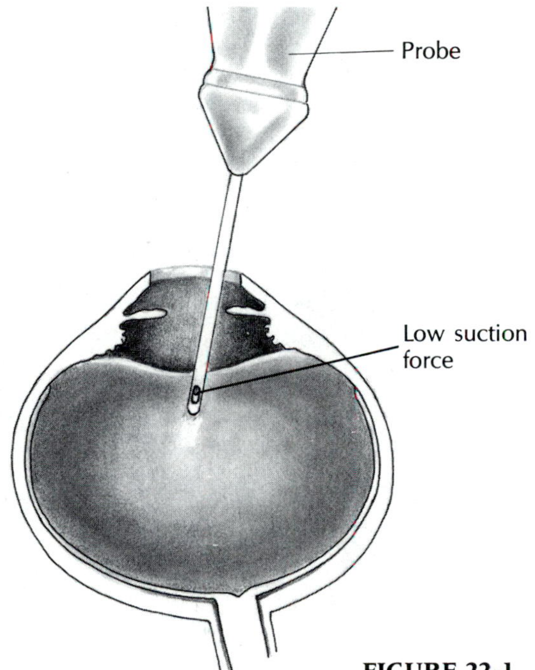

FIGURE 22-1. Vitrectomy in penetrating keratoplasty.

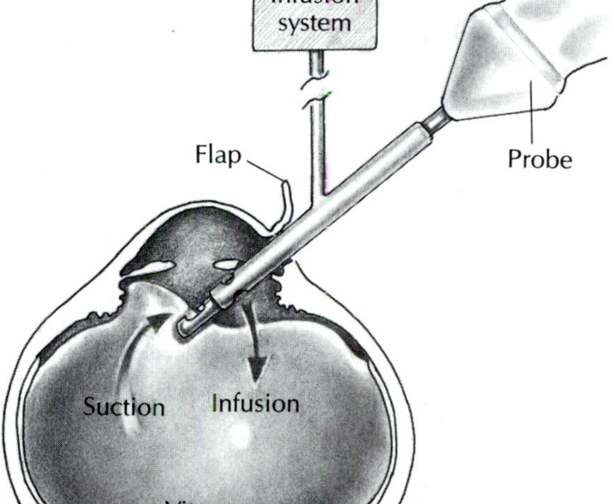

FIGURE 22-2. Anterior vitrectomy in aphakic trabeculectomy.

Lensectomy

Bimanual translimbal or pars plana lensectomy (Fig. 22-3) is useful for pediatric, persistent hyperplastic primary vitreous, retinopathy of prematurity, and some trauma cases. Use of 20-gauge infusion allows the instruments to be interchanged to permit more complete removal of the lens material.

The indications and contraindications for lensectomy are as follows:

Indications	Contraindications
Indicated vitrectomy and cataract	Routine cataract extraction in adults
Giant breaks	
Proliferative vitreoretinopathy	Most diabetic vitrectomies
Stage 5 retinopathy of prematurity	
Most trauma cases	

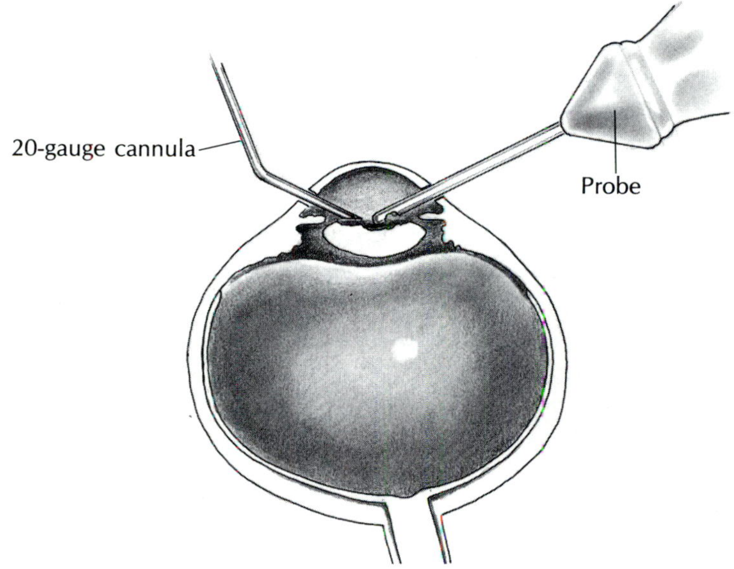

FIGURE 22-3. Translimbal lensectomy.

Trans–pars plana lensectomy with fragmentation (Figs. 22-4 and 22-5)

Continuous and simultaneous aspiration and sonification allow safe, rapid, "in-the-bag" lensectomy. Proportional vacuum should be used with a high flow rate and a "sew-on" 20-gauge infusion system to maintain normal intraocular pressure. The lancet blade should enter only the equatorial capsule to reduce zonule rupture.

Points to remember include the following:

- Stay in a horizontal plane.
- Avoid anterior and posterior capsules.
- Empty the capsular bag.
- Do not dislocate.

Problematic situations arise with lensectomy, including (1) opening the anterior capsule, (2) damaging the iris, (3) creating a shallow chamber, (4) producing vitreous traction, and (5) posteriorly dislocating the lens material. To avoid these, the surgeon must keep the instrument in a horizontal plane (eliminates situations 1 to 3) and avoid the posterior capsule (eliminates situations 4 and 5). The "coal-mining approach" is recommended (Fig. 22-5).

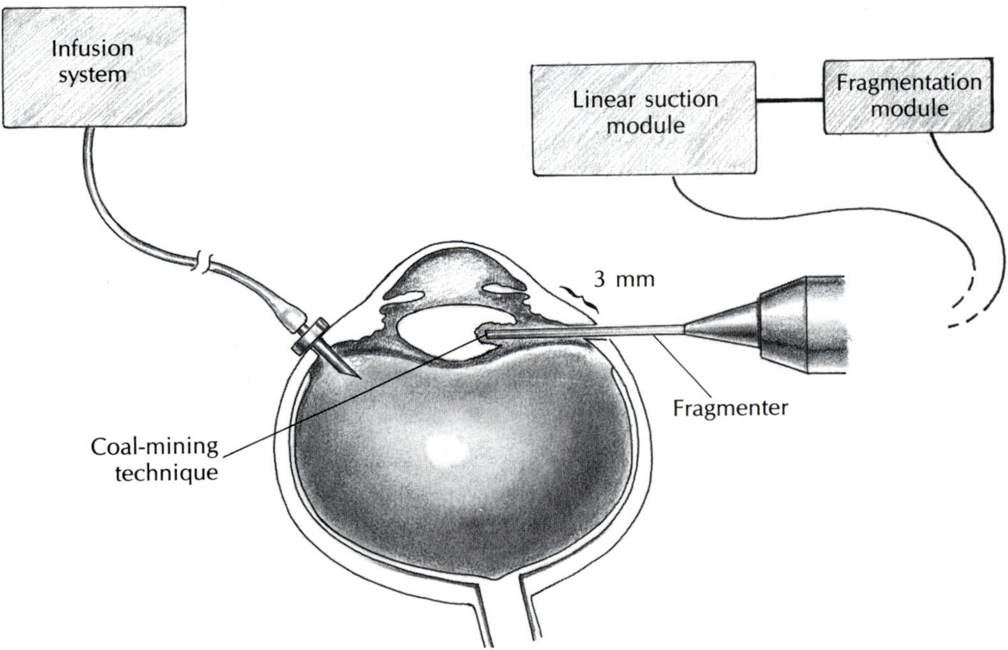

FIGURE 22-4. Trans–pars plana lensectomy with fragmentation.

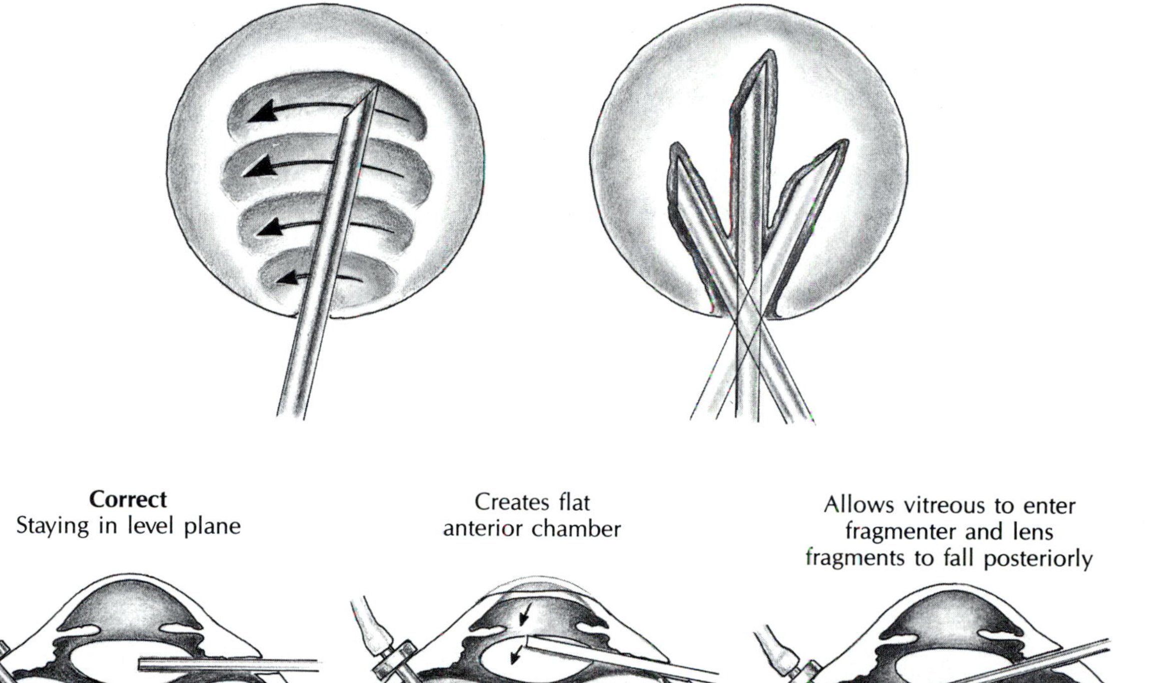

FIGURE 22-5. Problems in lensectomy.

Scleral depression

To see the peripheral lens, one should remove all cortex and capsule should be removed by using scleral depression (Fig. 22-6). To accomplish this, either the surgeon or an assistant applies and holds the scleral depressor. Complete removal prevents lens-induced inflammation, iridovitreocapsular membranes and secondary vitreoretinal traction.

Infusion system (Fig. 22-7)

Sew-on cannulas are preferred for all anterior and posterior lensectomies to provide flexibility and reduce turbulence. Sleeves are used only with preexisting large wounds. Irrigation handles are used initially if the pars plana cannot be seen and for bimanual lensectomy. Prior discission of the anterior capsule is accomplished with a fragmenter or lancet blade. The surgeon must remember to hold the port down to avoid contact with the iris.

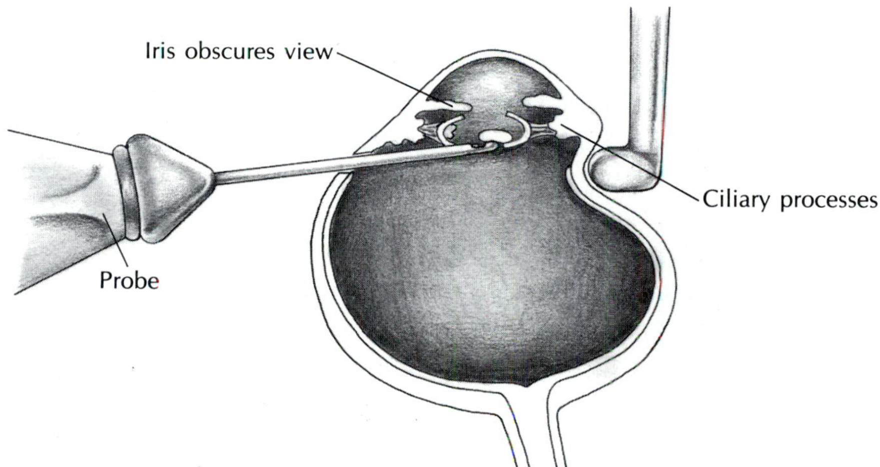

FIGURE 22-6. Scleral depression to see peripheral lens.

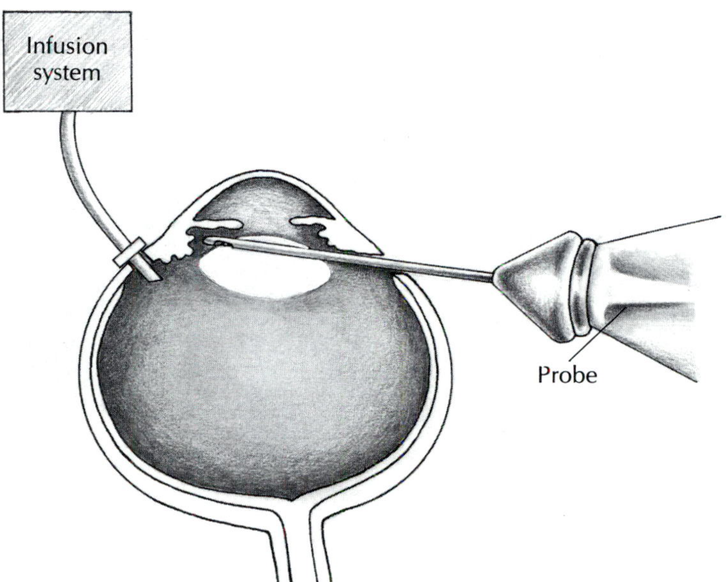

FIGURE 22-7. Capsulectomy after lensectomy.

Dislocated lens procedures

A total vitrectomy with conventional posterior methods should precede aspiration pickup of lens, nucleus, or fragments (Fig. 22-8). Sonification should be initiated after the lens material is lifted away from the retina. The surgeon must never touch the fragmenter to the vitreous.

Moderately dense nuclei or nuclear fragments can be crushed between the endoilluminator and the fragmenter or vitreous cutter (Fig. 22-9). Total vitrectomy should also precede this maneuver. Aspiration pickup of the crushed fragments is accomplished, and the fragments are moved away from the retina before sonification.

Occasionally translimbal removal of dislocated hard lens (nucleus) (Fig. 22-10) is required. A total vitrectomy should precede any manipulation of the posterior lens, nucleus, or fragments. If the material is too dense for crush aspiration, fluid-air exchange with the air pump and proportional suction should be performed. A limbal cataract section of appropriate size permits a straight suction cannula or a 1 mm cryoprobe access to extract the lens under air. This topic is also discussed on p. 222.

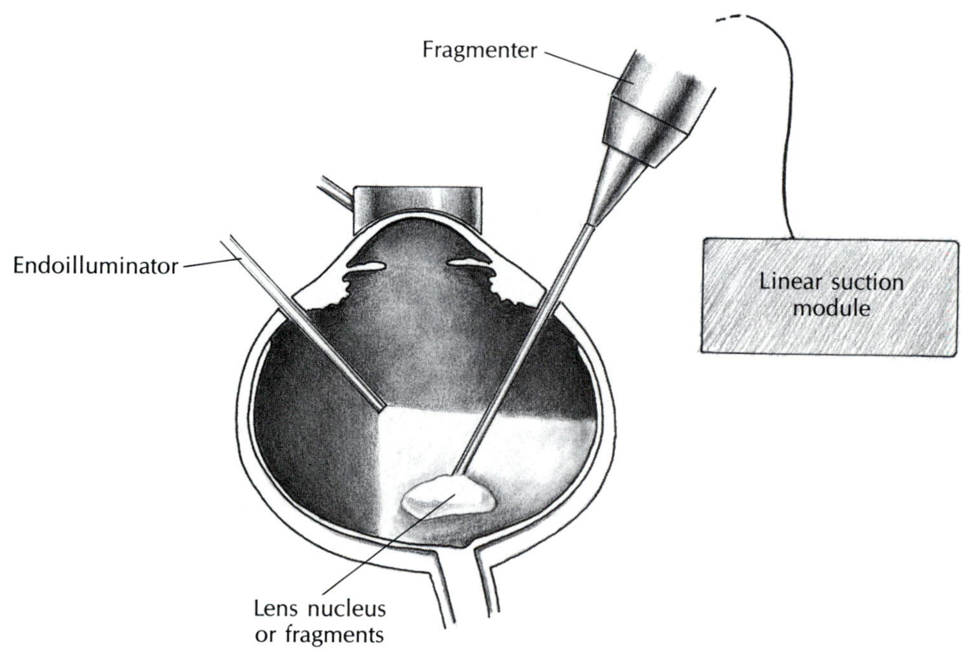

FIGURE 22-8. Fragmentation aspiration of dislocated material lens.

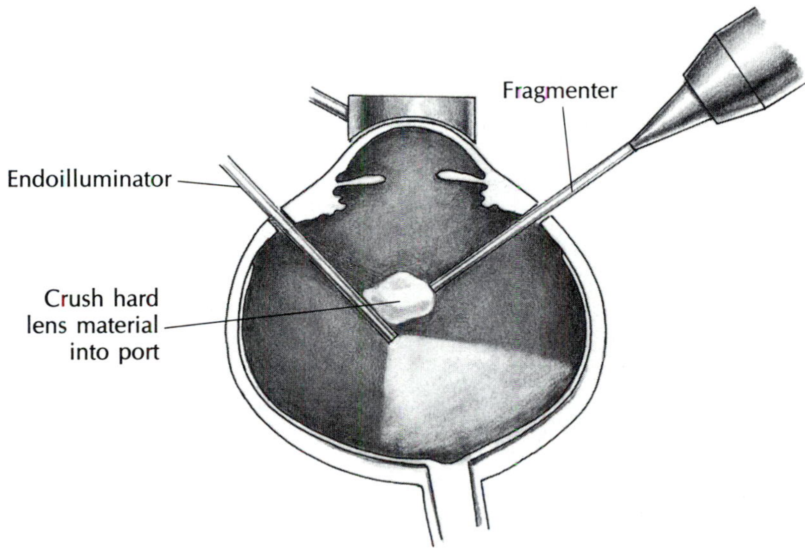

FIGURE 22-9. Crush-aspiration of dislocated crystalline lens.

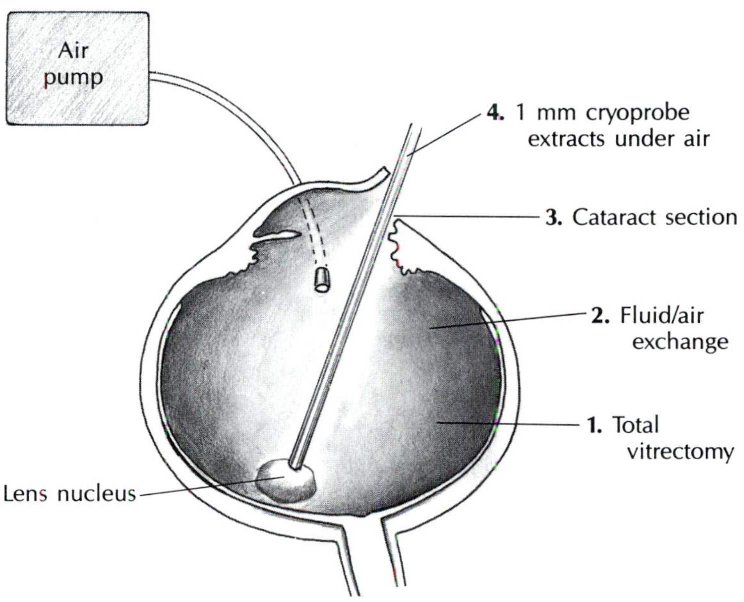

FIGURE 22-10. Translimbal removal of dislocated hard lens (nucleus).

Retrointraocular lens pupillary membrane management

The wide variety of materials causing retrointraocular pupillary membrane leads to a variety of management schemas:

Type	Neodymium-YAG laser	Scissors-TPPV*, 1 MHz bipolar radio frequency cautery
Thin	×	
Moderate	×	
Thick, calcium		×
Vascular		×

*TPPV, Trans–pars plana vitrectomy.

A blunt 30-degree 20-gauge infusion handle is used for infusion if the pars plana cannot be seen while the sew-on cannula is used after removal of dense or semiopaque pupillary membranes (Fig. 22-11). A prior lancet blade or scissors discission creates an edge for the vitreous cutter. Scleral depression allows complete removal of the membrane.

For moderately dense pupillary membranes, a straight 20-gauge scissors or shears can be used to accomplish sectioning (Fig. 22-12) after prior discission with a lancet blade or scissors. The membrane can be completely detached from other tissue with the scissors and sectored to permit its removal with the vitreous cutter, avoiding traction and high suction force.

In retrointraocular lens membrane removal (Fig. 22-13), a blunt 30-degree 20-gauge infusion handle is once again used if the pars plana cannot be seen. The sew-on cannula is used if the sew-on cannula can be visualized. A lancet blade or straight scissors should be applied to create an edge for the vitreous cutter and to section the membrane so that suction force is reduced.

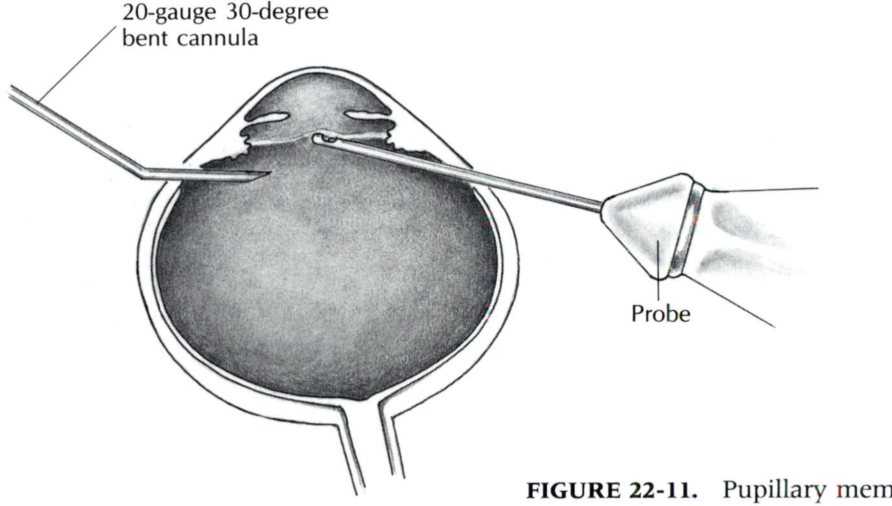

FIGURE 22-11. Pupillary membrane management.

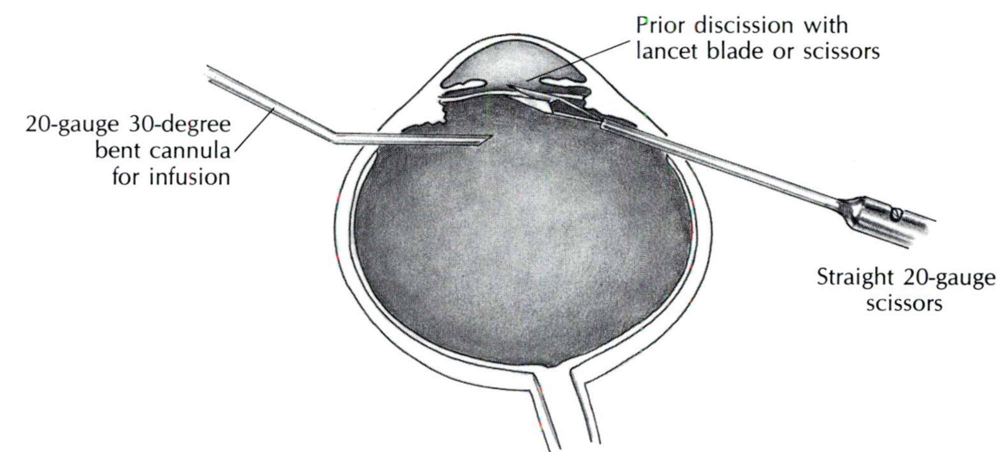

FIGURE 22-12. Dense pupillary membranes.

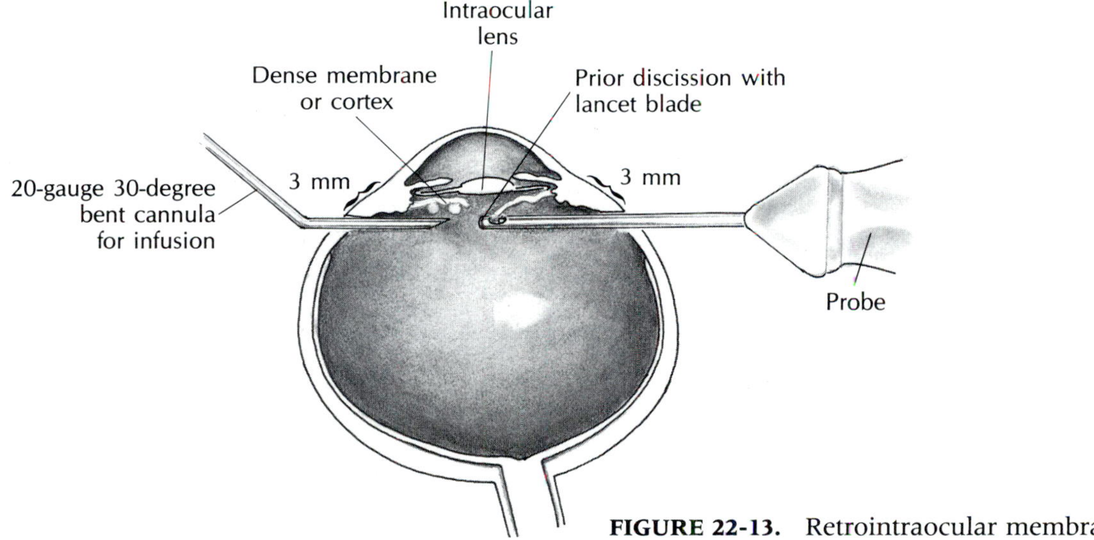

FIGURE 22-13. Retrointraocular membrane removal.

Pars Plana Vitrectomy

The applications of pars plana vitrectomy include use in pupillary block, vitreous touch, repositioning of the intraocular lens, uveitis, and cystoid macular edema.

If neodymium–yttrium-aluminum-garnet (Nd:YAG) laser iridotomy cannot relieve phakic or aphakic *pupillary block,* a pars plana vitrectomy is preferred over slashing the anterior hyaloid face or vitreous aspiration (Fig. 22-14) (see also p. 332).

If the cornea was initially clear after cataract extraction and a recent *vitreous touch* and corneal edema occur, an aphakic or pseudophakic pars plana vitrectomy is preferred to a limbal approach (Fig. 22-15).

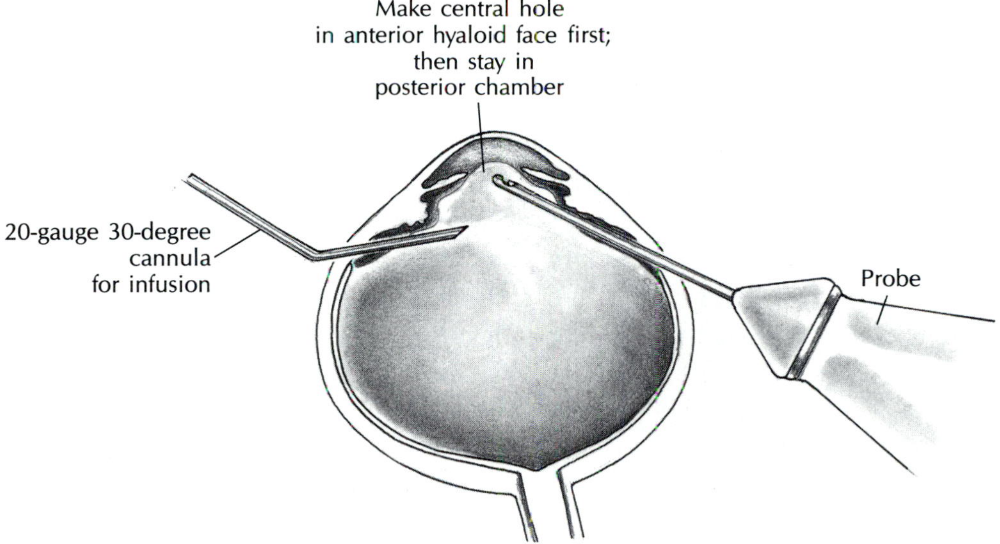

FIGURE 22-14. Trans–pars plana vitrectomy in phakic pupillary block.

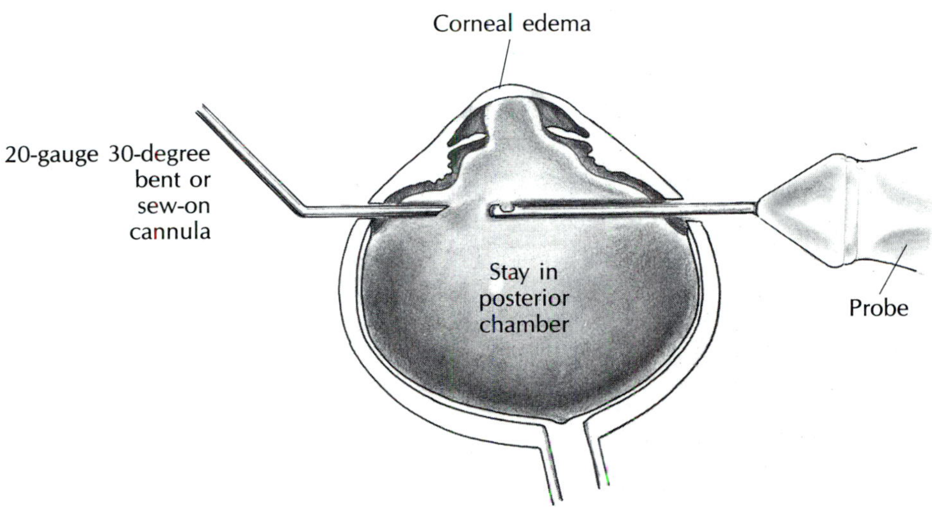

FIGURE 22-15. Trans–pars plana vitrectomy in vitreous touch.

In dealing with *repositioning of the intraocular lens* (Fig. 22-16), total pars plana vitrectomy *(1)* with a sew-on infusion cannula, proportional suction, and an endoilluminator should precede manipulation of the implant. Care should be taken to avoid haptic damage. Twenty-gauge forceps *(2)* are used to pick up the implant, with care being taken not to force the intraocular lens against the retina. The intraocular lens is moved anteriorly, and a second pair of forceps is used to reposition the lens. The loops are rotated into preplaced 10-0 polypropylene sutures *(3)*. Although the lens can be placed in the anterior chamber, it is preferable to use ciliary sulcus suturing after total capsulectomy. This suturing (Fig. 22-17) is accomplished as follows: Sutures (10-0 polypropylene) can be passed through implant-positioning holes and sutured inside sclerotomies 180 degrees apart and just posterior to the iris. If positioning holes are not present, a transscleral suture bite after positioning can be used for ciliary sulcus suturing. Suturing to the iris is not recommended. (See also p. 244.)

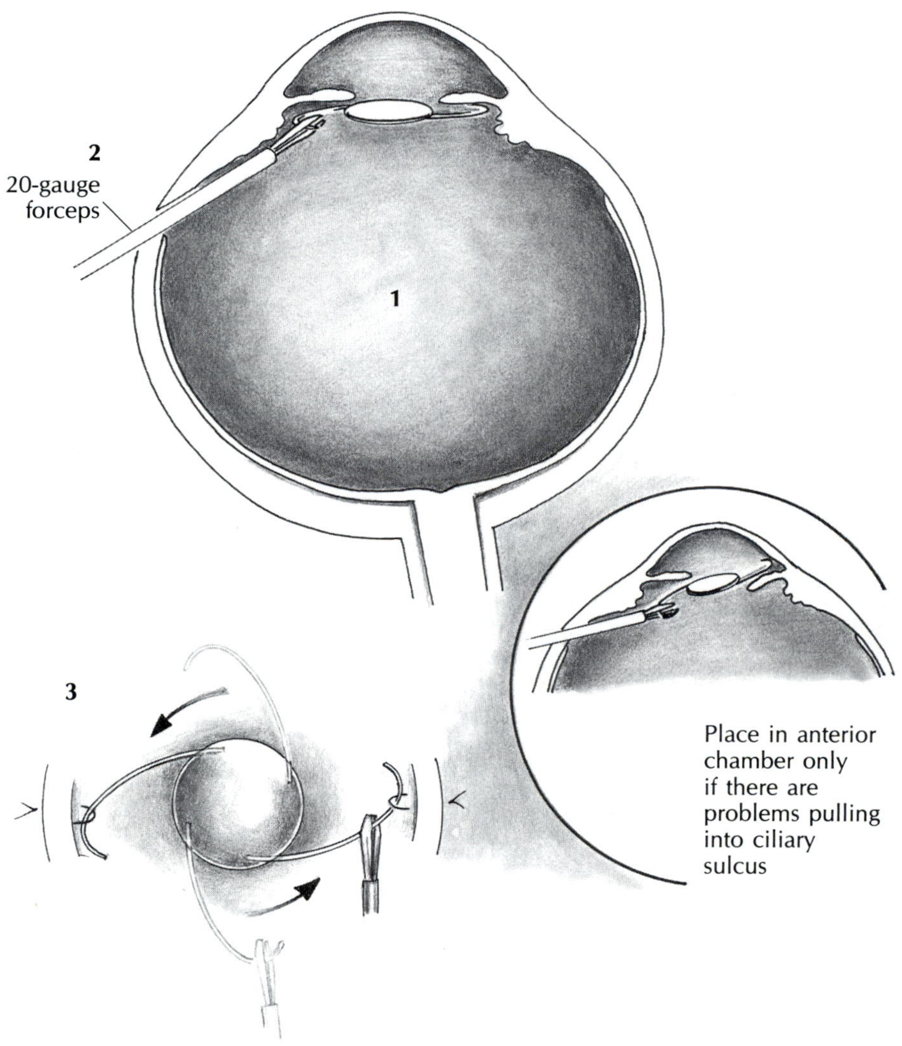

FIGURE 22-16. Repositioning of intraocular lens.

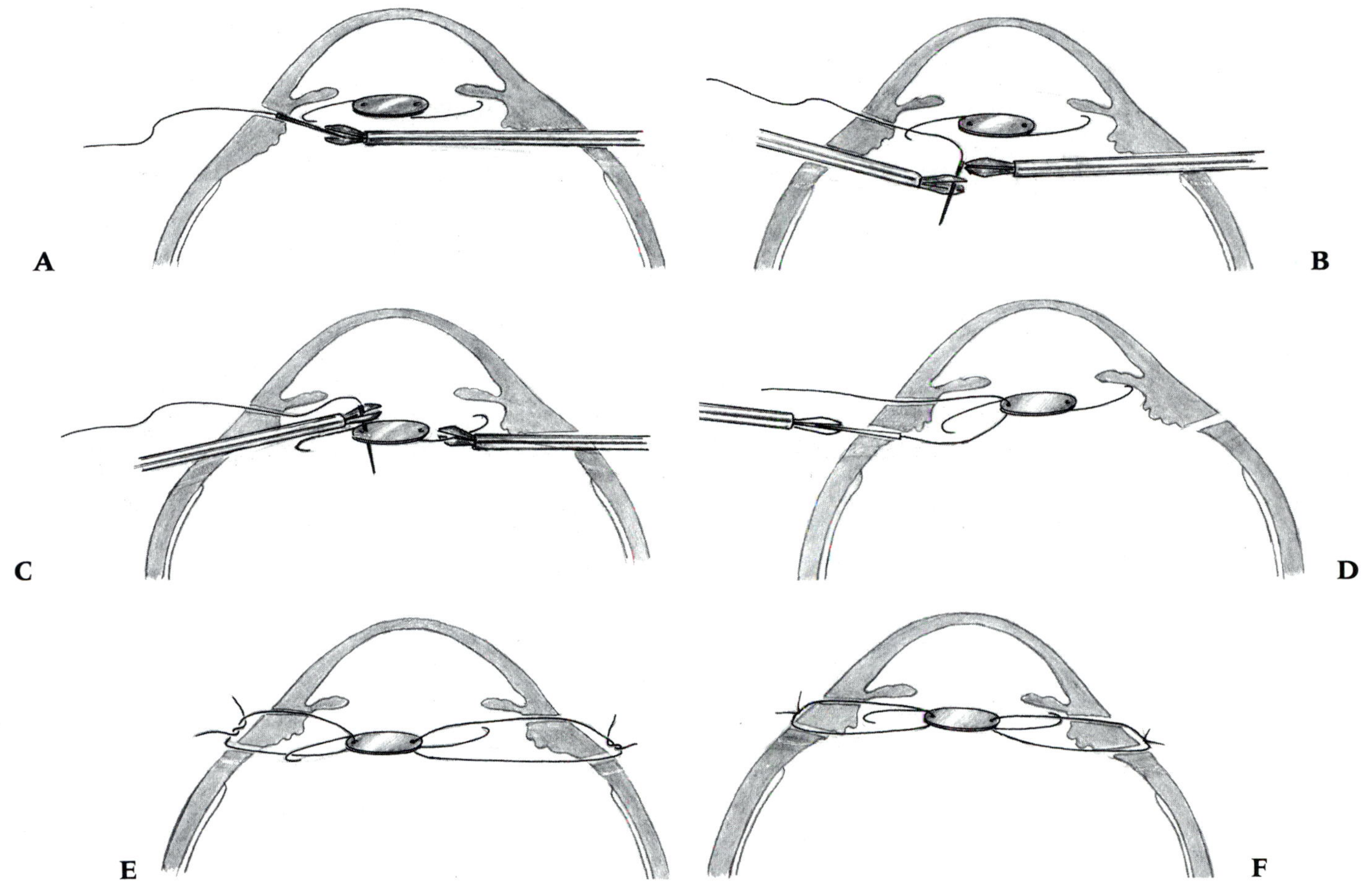

FIGURE 22-17. Suturing of intraocular lens.

If the intraocular lens is dislocated and must be removed, the following summary should be applied:

Leave	Remove
Cystoid macular edema	Epithelial ingrowth
Endophthalmitis	Cyclitic membrane–vascular, nonvascular
Dislocation	Giant break Proliferative vitreoretinopathy

One should remember that an intraocular lens should be removed only if the haptics are bent or broken, preventing ciliary sulcus suturing. A total vitrectomy and use of an air pump with proportional-suction fluid-air exchange should precede limbal section and forceps removal of the damaged intraocular lens (Fig. 22-18). However, *repositioning and suturing in the ciliary sulcus is usually preferable to complete removal.* (See also p. 250.)

Lensectomy should be performed in all *uveitis* vitrectomies. Indications and strategies may be summarized as follows:

Indications	Rationale
Pars planitis and cataract	Decompartmentalize: reduce cells, reduce factors
Uveitis and cataract	Remove substrate for cyclitic membrane, retinal traction
Cystoid macular edema	Remove vitreous opacities

Avoiding the iris reduces postoperative inflammation. Scleral depression to remove all lens material is advised. Prophylactic buckling without retinopexy greatly reduces postoperative retinal detachment.

Trans–pars plana vitrectomy reduces *cystoid macular edema* in many cases that do not respond to the 4- to 6-month wait usually imposed and to the subconjunctival corticosteroids as well as oral and topical antiprostaglandins (Fig. 22-19). This is particularly useful when the Nd:YAG laser has dispersed lens cortex posteriorly and vitritis is present.

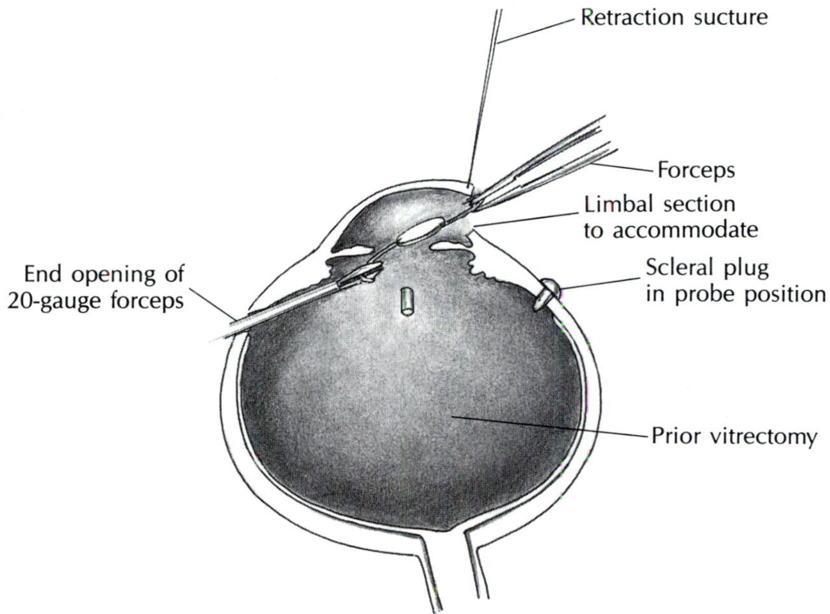

FIGURE 22-18. Removal of dislocated intraocular lens.

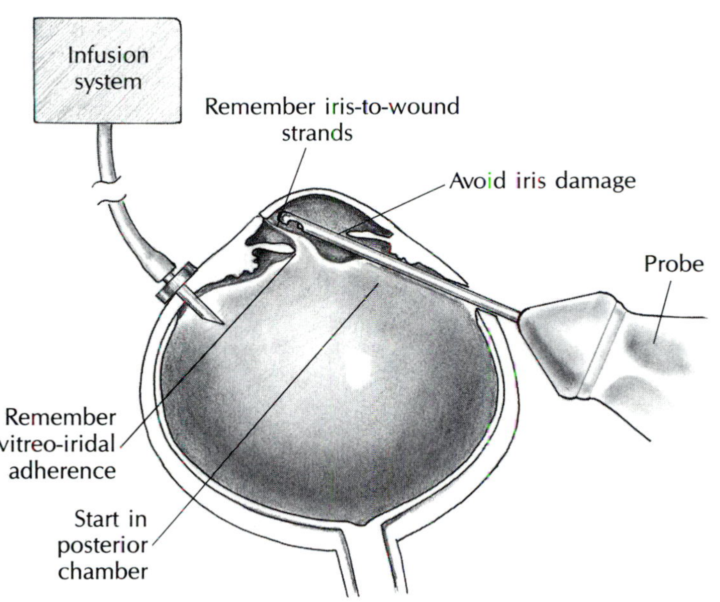

FIGURE 22-19. Total pars plana vitrectomy in cystoid macular edema.

COMPLICATIONS

Endophthalmitis

Care must be taken not to disrupt the cataract wound in vitrectomy for endophthalmitis (Fig. 22-20). The first 5 ml of fluid should be retained for culture and sensitivity testing. One applies the probe using low suction force and avoiding the iris. If a wound leak does occur, the wound should be oversewn. The implant should never be removed, but the capsular bag must be opened. However, there are entities where the infectious material is sequestered in the capsular bag, which has to be removed to effect a cure. This necessitates opening of the capsular bag with the vitreous cutter. The use of low suction force and avoidance of the retina reduce retinal breaks and detachment.

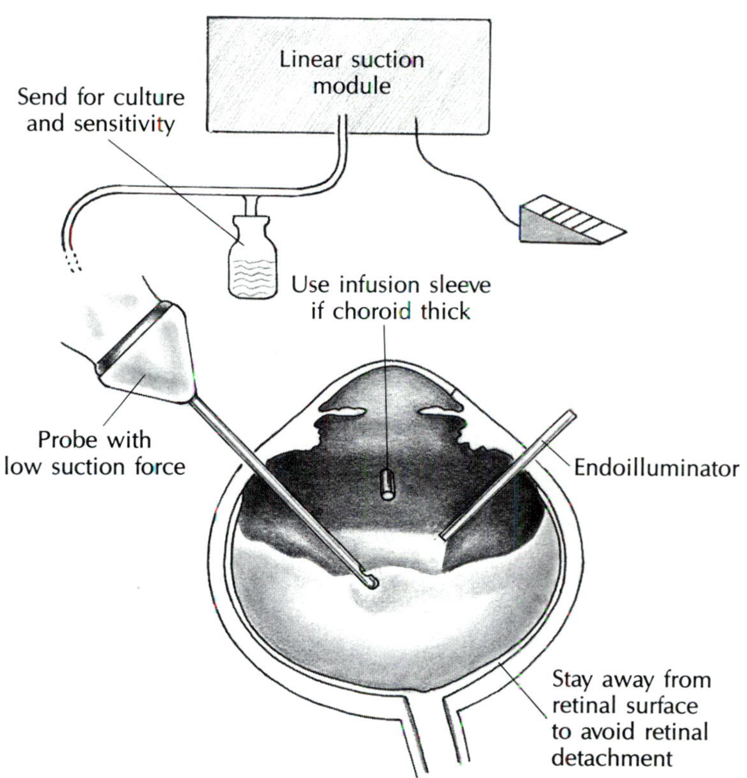

FIGURE 22-20. Endophthalmitis.

Epithelial ingrowth

Fibrous or epithelial tissue covering iris, vitreous, ciliary body, or implant can be removed with 20-gauge scissors and the vitreous cutter. As shown in Fig. 22-21, *A*, the wound is reopened and a lamellar sclerotomy and fistulectomy are performed. The involved iris is elevated with forceps to achieve a 2 mm margin, and Vannas scissors are used to perform a basal iridectomy (Fig. 22-21, *B*). The wound is closed (Fig. 22-21, *C*) with an 8-0 nylon running shoelace suture. An anterior vitrectomy is performed, and the epithelium or anterior hyaloid face is removed if present, while infusion is maintained on the opposite side. Using a probe the surgeon removes fluid during internal fluid and air exchange (Fig. 22-21, *D*). The cryoprobe is applied to freeze the area (−80° C for 1 minute) and obtain a good margin. Then all involved ciliary body is frozen against an air bubble, allowing a 2 mm margin. Implants should be removed, and a total vitrectomy performed. Scleral depression allows dissection along the ciliary body. Fluid-air exchange allows the transcorneal cryoprobe to eliminate the retrocorneal epithelium.

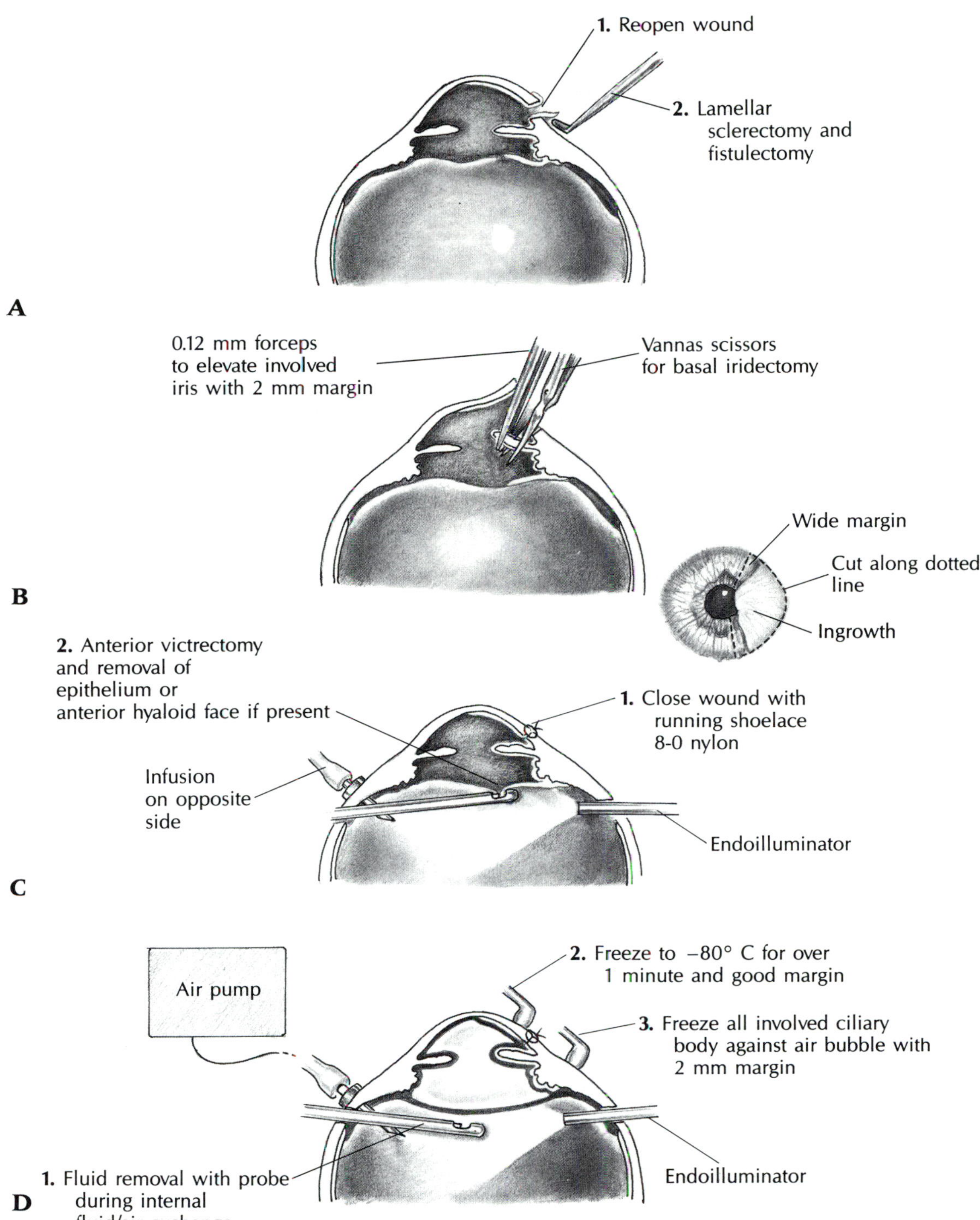

FIGURE 22-21. Epithelial ingrowth.

CHAPTER 23

General Posterior Segment Procedures

This chapter presents the steps to be followed in performing posterior segment surgery. The procedures are discussed as the surgeon would encounter them within the standard operating sequence, as follows:

Conjunctival incision and retromuscle sutures (if required for scleral buckling)
Sclerotomies
Infusion cannula basics
Entering the posterior hyaloid face
End-opening suction
Epiretinal membrane management
Exchange procedures
Sequential fluid-gas exchange
Subretinal fluid drainage
Internal fluid-air exchange
Internal drainage of subretinal fluid
Retinoplexy
Cryopexy versus diathermy
Use of silicone
Wound and conjunctival closure

The majority of the illustrations in this chapter have been modified and redrawn from Charles ST: Vitreous microsurgery, ed 2, Baltimore, 1987, Williams & Wilkins.

Conjunctival Incision and Retromuscle Sutures

Because most posterior segment surgery involves access through the pars plana, one or more conjunctival incisions are usually required. When scleral buckling is not required, two incisions are needed: one for temporal instruments and one for nasal instruments. The first one should extend for 120 degrees centered on the lateral rectus muscle and be parallel and 2 mm posterior to the limbus. The second one should begin at the upper border of the medial rectus muscle, extend for 60 degrees, and be parallel and 2 mm posterior to the limbus. When scleral buckling is required, a single 360-degree incision should be made 2 mm posterior to the limbus.

Making a small (2 mm) limbal flap permits running single-layer closure of Tenon's capsule and the conjunctiva; thus one avoids bleeding under the surgical contact lens, as well as eliminates postoperative redundancy. Retromuscle traction sutures are placed with a short fenestrated muscle hook only if scleral buckling is anticipated. Use of 2-0 black silk creates less trauma to the muscle and gives a better grip (Fig. 23-1).

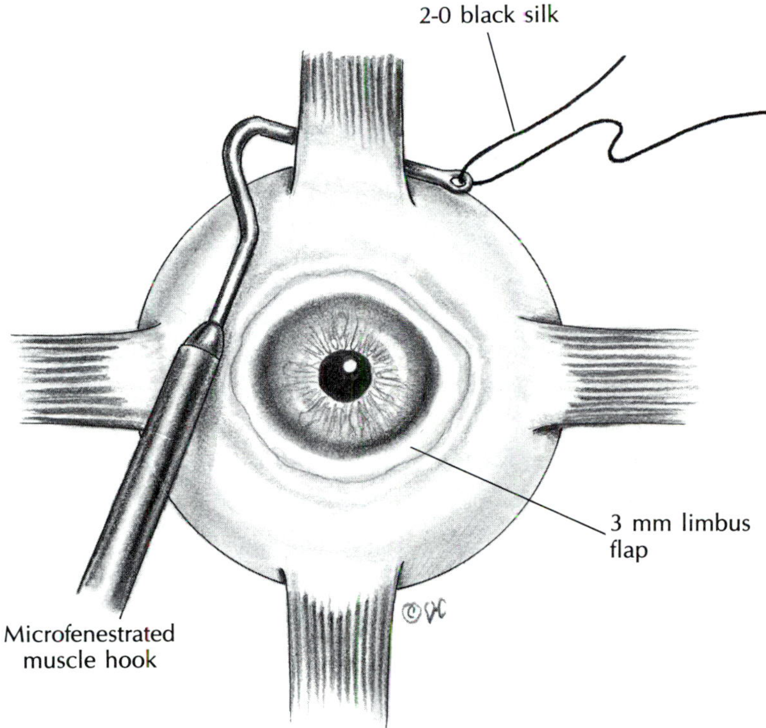

FIGURE 23-1. Conjunctival incision and retromuscle sutures.

Sclerotomies

The scleral suture to affix the infusion cannula must be correctly placed so that one can avoid negatively influencing the rest of the operation. The first limbus-parallel bite is placed from superior to inferior while one holds the sclerotomy edge with forceps (Fig. 23-2). The second bite is placed in the opposite direction.

Next the cannula is placed into the sclerotomy site. To achieve this, the infusion cannula is rotated back and forth to penetrate the elastic choroid and ciliary epithelium (Fig. 23-3). Before the cannula is turned on, the tip must be inspected for proper placement with the operating microscope when the operated eyes lack a lens or when the lens is to be removed. The indirect ophthalmoscope should be used for inspection if the lens is to be retained. In all phakic or aphakic eyes, 4 mm cannulas should be used unless a thickened choroid dictates use of a 6 mm cannula (Fig. 23-4). The incision should be placed 4 mm from the limbus if the lens is to be retained; otherwise, an incision at 3 mm should be used. The silver tip must be clear of the retina and uvea as observed under the microscope or through indirect methods. The suture must be tied tightly.

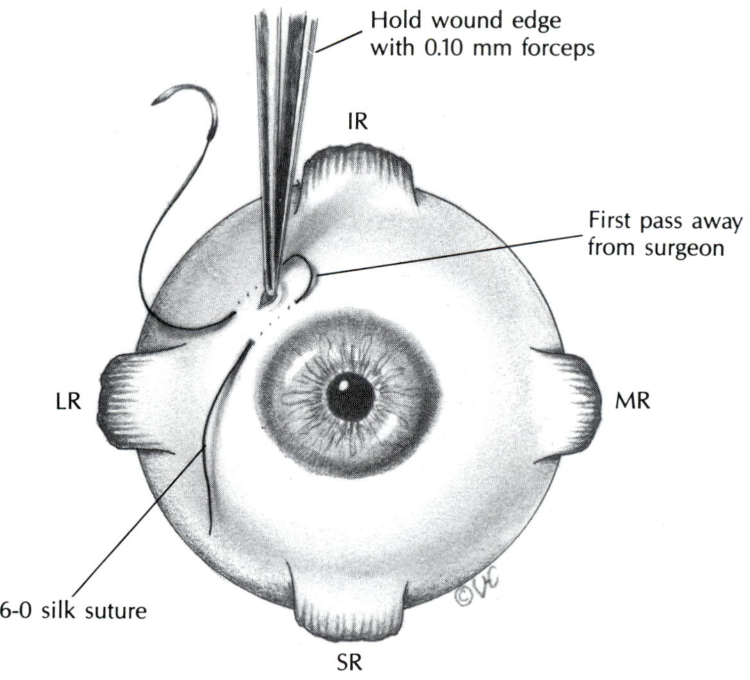

FIGURE 23-2. Scleral suture to affix infusion cannula.

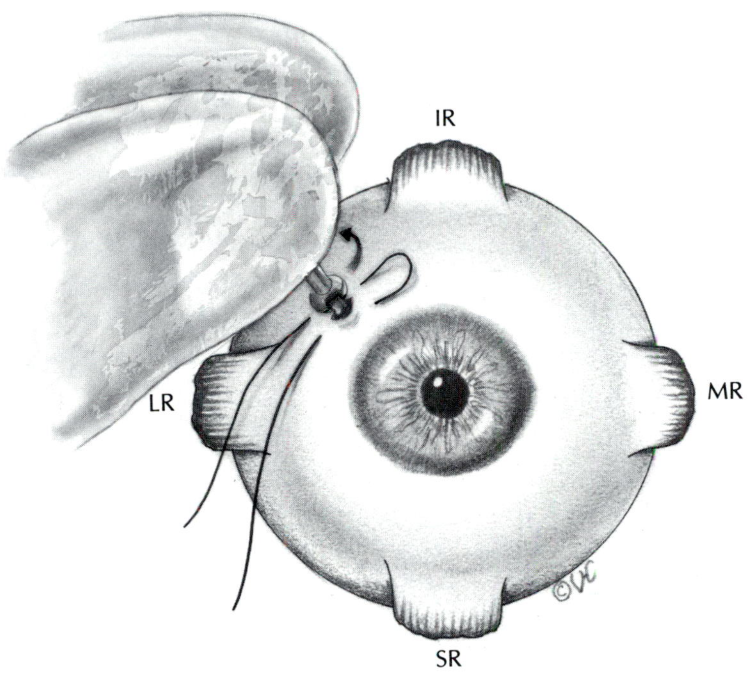

FIGURE 23-3. Placing cannula into sclerotomy site.

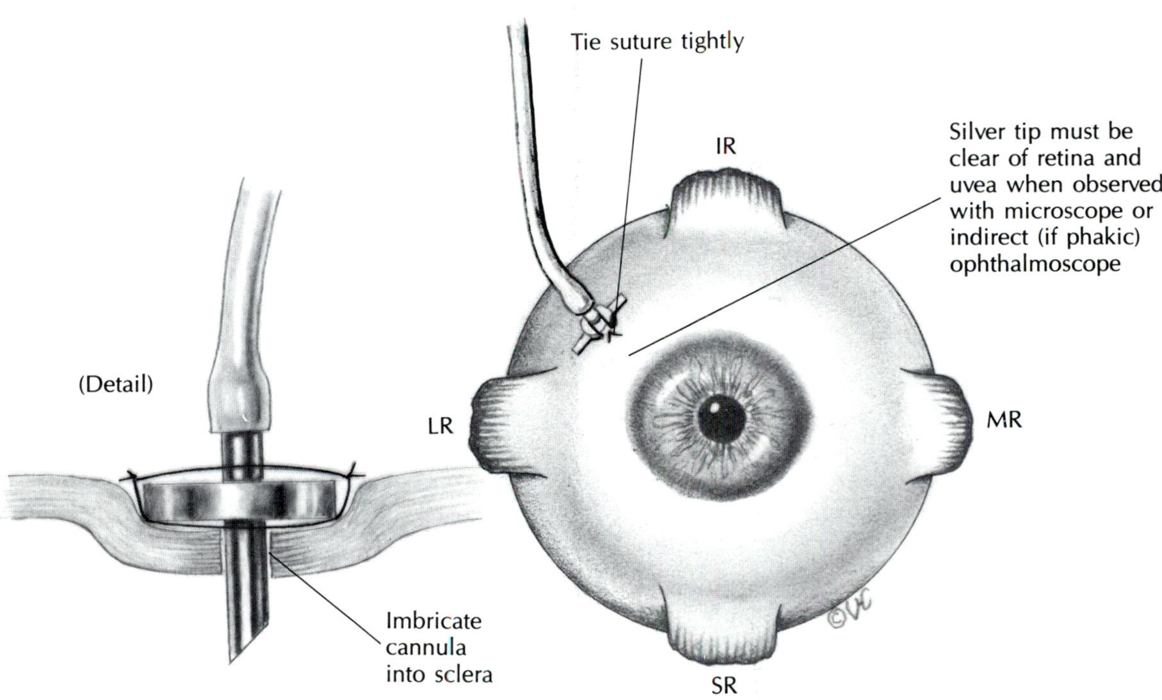

FIGURE 23-4. Correct placement of infusion cannula.

The second incision (Fig. 23-5, *1,* supranasal) should be placed just above the 3 or 9 o'clock position supranasally at the same distance from the limbus as the first. The endoilluminator is inserted into this sclerotomy incision. The third incision (supratemporally) will be placed just above the 3 or 9 o'clock position (*2* or *3*). This will pass into the lens equator if the lens is to be removed. Previous wounds should be avoided.

Most bleeding from these incisions will be controlled by instrument placement into the wound. Bipolar diathermy can be used for severe bleeding (Fig. 23-6). The diathermy forceps is rotated 360 degrees around a scleral plug, and the energy flows between the plug and the forceps touching the sclera. Scleral damage should be minimal.

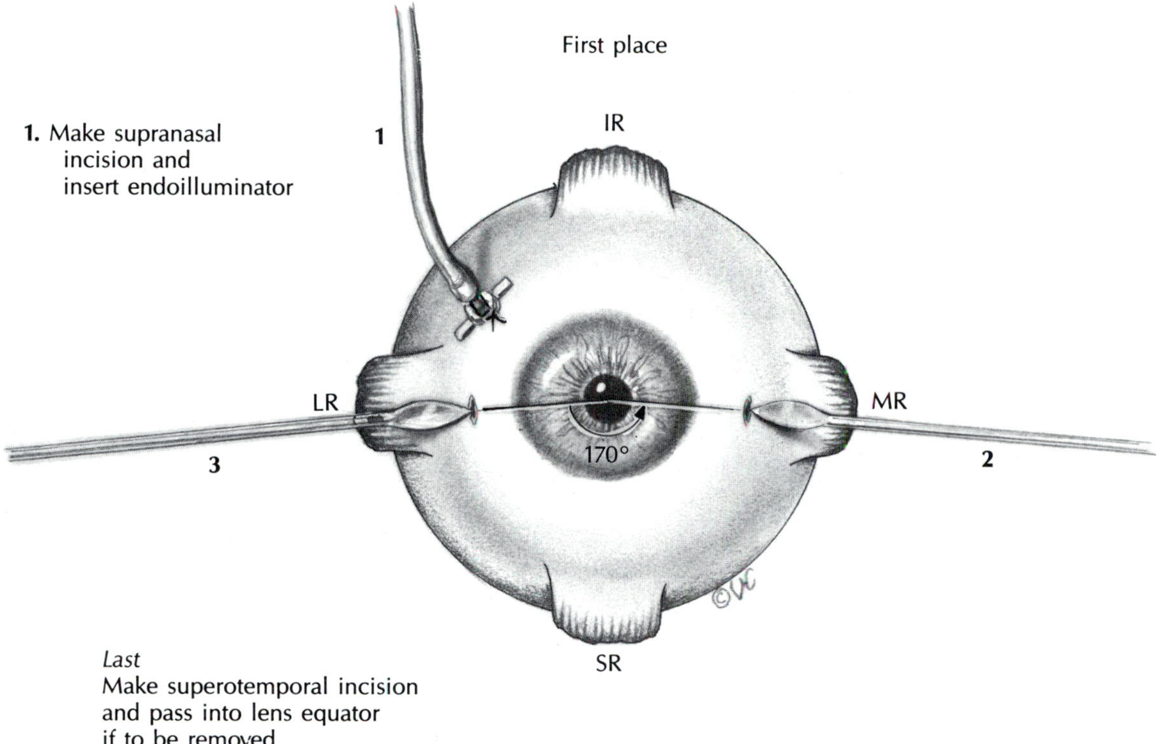

FIGURE 23-5. Second incision.

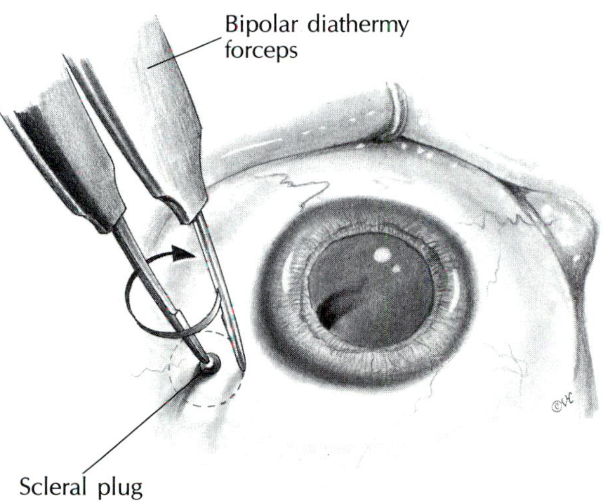

FIGURE 23-6. Bipolar diathermy for bleeding from sclerotomy.

Infusion Cannula Basics

Placement of the infusion cannula is always the first step to prevent hypotony and miosis, bleeding, and striate keratopathy (Fig. 23-7). As already stated, its placement is checked with magnification, and then it is turned on and left on unless there is iris or retinal prolapse, or suprachoroidal or subretinal infusion. An important precaution to be taken is to infuse only with a cannula that can be seen (Fig. 23-7). In this way, subretinal and choroidal infusion is avoided.

If inadvertent suprachoroidal or subretinal infusion occurs, management involves cutting the tissue internally with the lancet blade *if the lens is not to be retained* (Fig. 23-8). Prefirming the globe with a 20-gauge needle followed by replacement of the infusion cannula is done in phakic eyes.

If hyphema or cataract prevents visualization of the pars plana, a blunt 20-gauge 30-degree infusion cannula should be used until a sew-on cannula can be seen (Fig. 23-9).

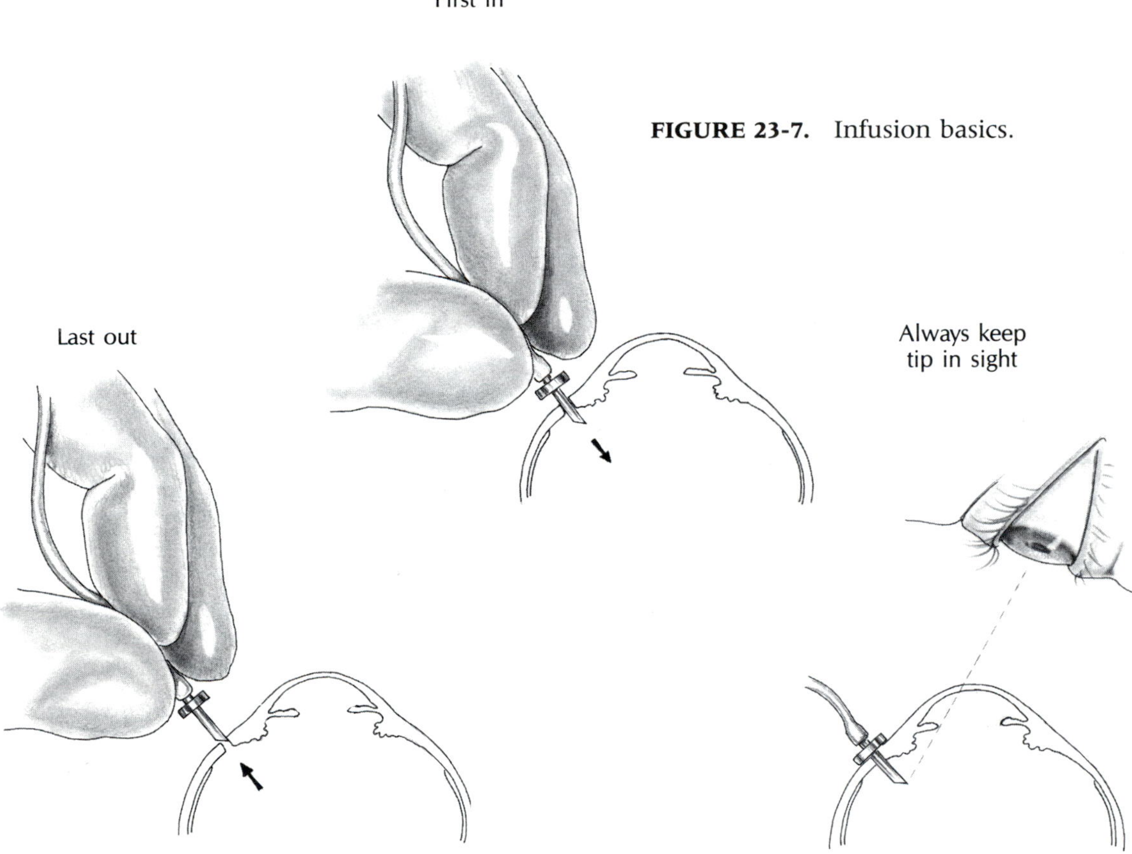

FIGURE 23-7. Infusion basics.

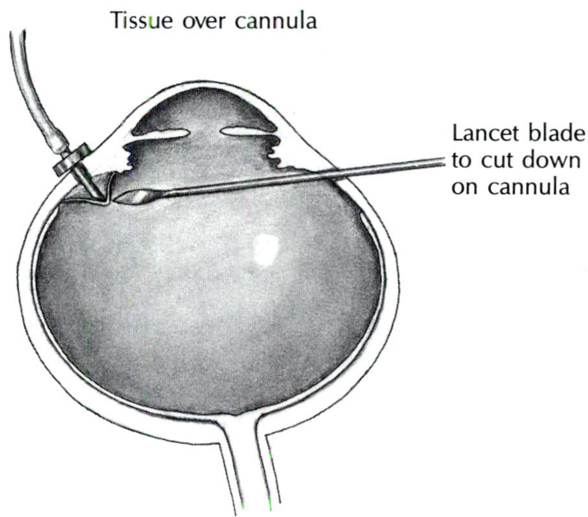

FIGURE 23-8. Management of infusion cannula problems, tissue over cannula.

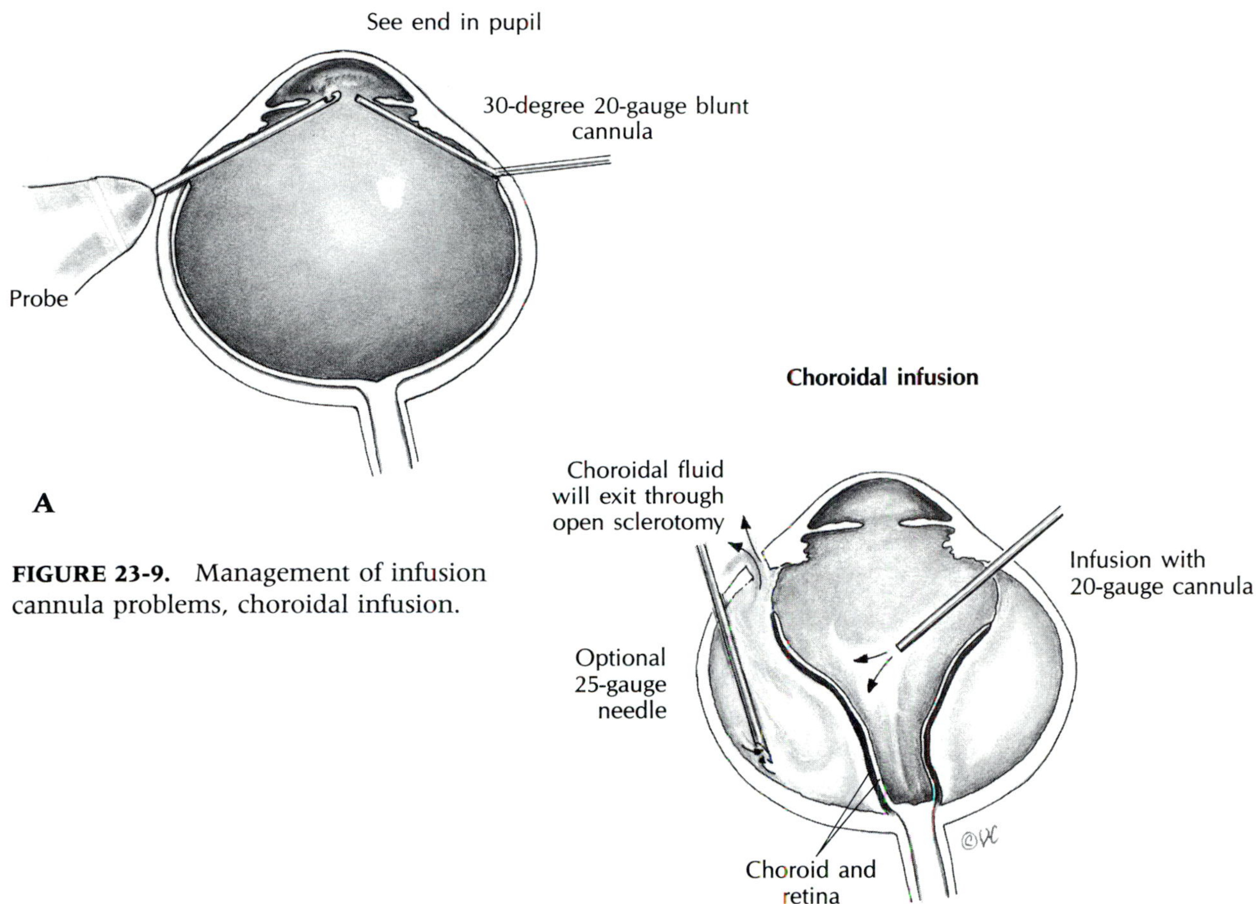

FIGURE 23-9. Management of infusion cannula problems, choroidal infusion.

Entering the Posterior Hyaloid Face

The posterior hyaloid face should be entered after removal of the opaque or taut anterior face (Fig. 23-10). No "core" vitrectomy is required except in very young patients with recent disease. The opening in the posterior hyaloid face should be made in a place determined to be away from the retina, and a 360-degree extension of this opening must be accomplished. The opening is generally made on the nasal side unless another area is confirmed as safe by either ultrasonography or direct observation of the retina. A taut posterior hyaloid face can cause anterior and posterior retinal breaks as it is imbricated into the vitrectomy port. It should not be removed in sequential layers because this requires repeated searching for the vitreoretinal interface (Fig. 23-11, *A*). Prior inside-out delamination of the posterior hyaloid face from the retina allows removal of the epiretinal membrane/posterior hyaloid face in a single sheet if a posterior vitreous detachment is not present. One safe place is identified, and dissection is achieved along a single plane (Fig. 23-11, *B*).

End-opening suction

If blood products are in the subposterior vitreous detachment space, low proportional suction with a blunt 20-gauge cannula through the posterior hyaloid face opening should be used until the fluid is clear (Fig. 23-12, *A*). Constant, very low (20 to 40 mm Hg), nonpulsatile suction with a straight, blunt, 20-gauge cannula or a soft rubber tip should be used for preretinal blood products (Fig. 23-12, *B*). Complete removal allows safer dissection and photocoagulation and reduces postoperative residual blood and erythroclastic glaucoma.

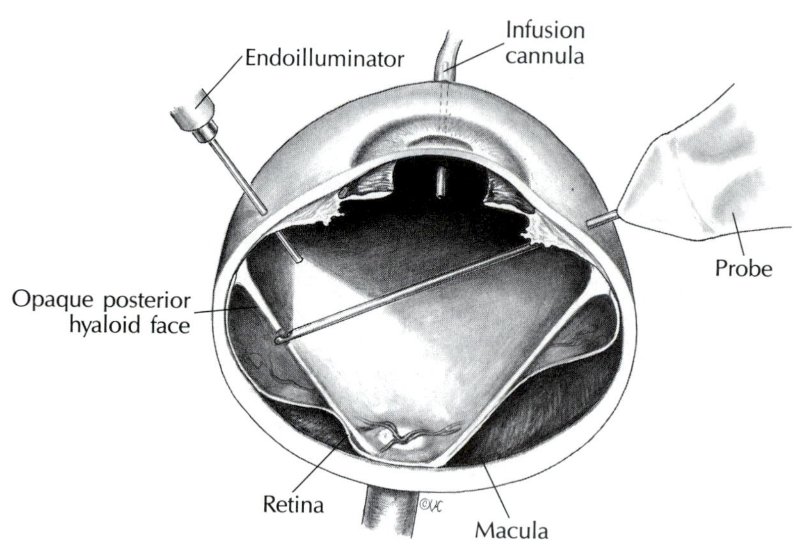

FIGURE 23-10. Entering of posterior hyaloid face.

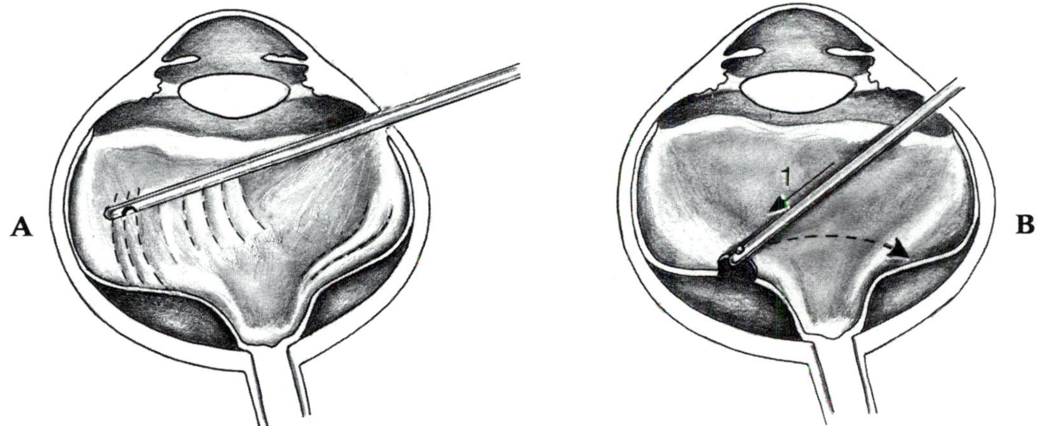

FIGURE 23-11. A, Do not remove in sequential layers. **B,** Dissect along plane.

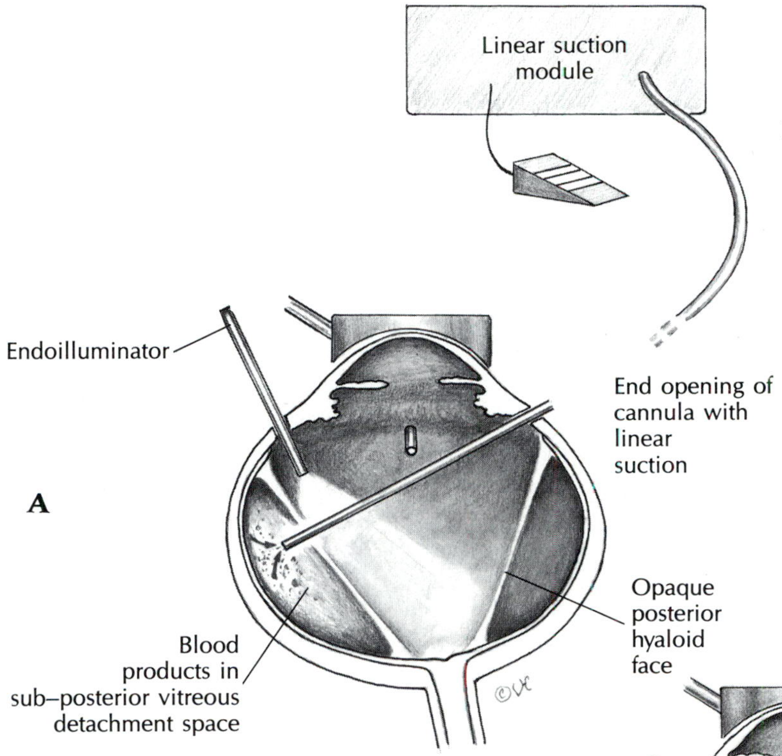

Linear suction module

End opening of cannula with linear suction

Endoilluminator

A

Opaque posterior hyaloid face

Blood products in sub–posterior vitreous detachment space

Linear suction module

Endoilluminator

End opening of cannula with linear suction

Low-pressure infusion

Blood products

B

FIGURE 23-12. A, End opening suction in subposterior vitreous detachment space. **B,** End opening of preretinal hemorrhage.

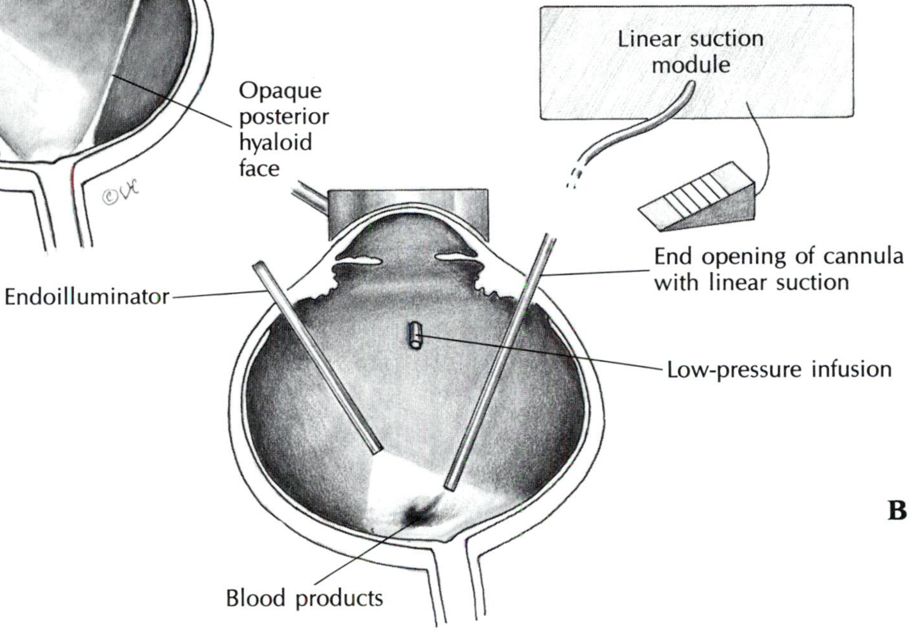

Epiretinal Membrane Management

Fig. 23-13 presents an algorithm to be applied in the management of the epiretinal membranes.

Exchange Procedures

The recognized methods of fluid-air (gas) exchange fall into two general categories: sequential and internal (or simultaneous). Sequential exchange is performed only in the office and can be associated with several disadvantages:

Incomplete exchange
Hypotony
Bubbles
Poor visualization during injection
Ocular collapse combined with an intraocular sharp needle

Internal exchange involves the injection of air through one opening in the eye while fluid is removed through another opening. Hypotony with ocular collapse and bleeding can be avoided; thus this method is safer and permits better visualization than sequential exchange can.

Sequential fluid-gas exchange (office procedure)

Translimbal fluid-air (gas) exchange is used in the aphakic vitrectomized eye, whereas exchange in the pars plana is used for the phakic vitrectomized eye. *Vitreous aspiration is dangerous and should be avoided.* The patient's head should be moved forward to aspirate fluid and backward to inject air into the first bubble placed; this will avoid multiple small bubbles (Fig. 23-14). A small initial aspiration of air just before injection clears the needle of fluid. The correct sequence is thus:

Inject → Aspirate → Inject into bubble → Aspirate

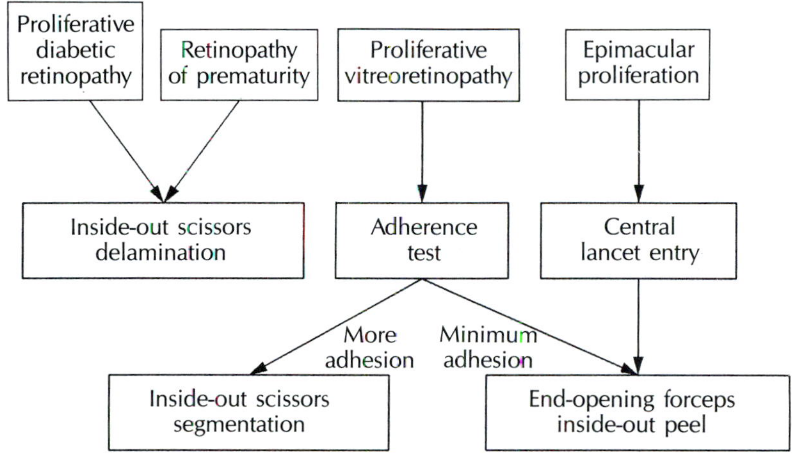

FIGURE 23-13. Algorithm of management of the epiretinal membrane.

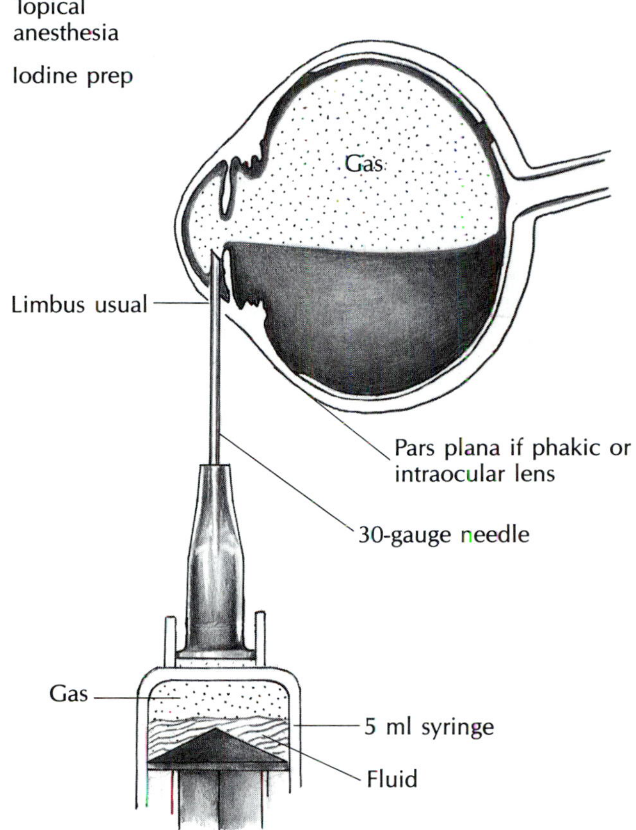

FIGURE 23-14. Sequential fluid-gas exchange.

Subretinal fluid drainage

The indications for use of needle drainage are as follows:

Use of scleral buckle without vitrectomy but with retinal detachment
Vitrectomy with retinal detachment and no retinal breaks
Choroidal infusion with hemorrhage
Subretinal infusion

If no break is present, needle drainage of subretinal fluid is used (Fig. 23-15). A clear hub, disposable 25- to 27-gauge needle on a tuberculin syringe without a plunger or a proportional suction handle should be used. The bevel is directed away from the retina. This permits controlled fluid removal without incarceration under direct visualization.

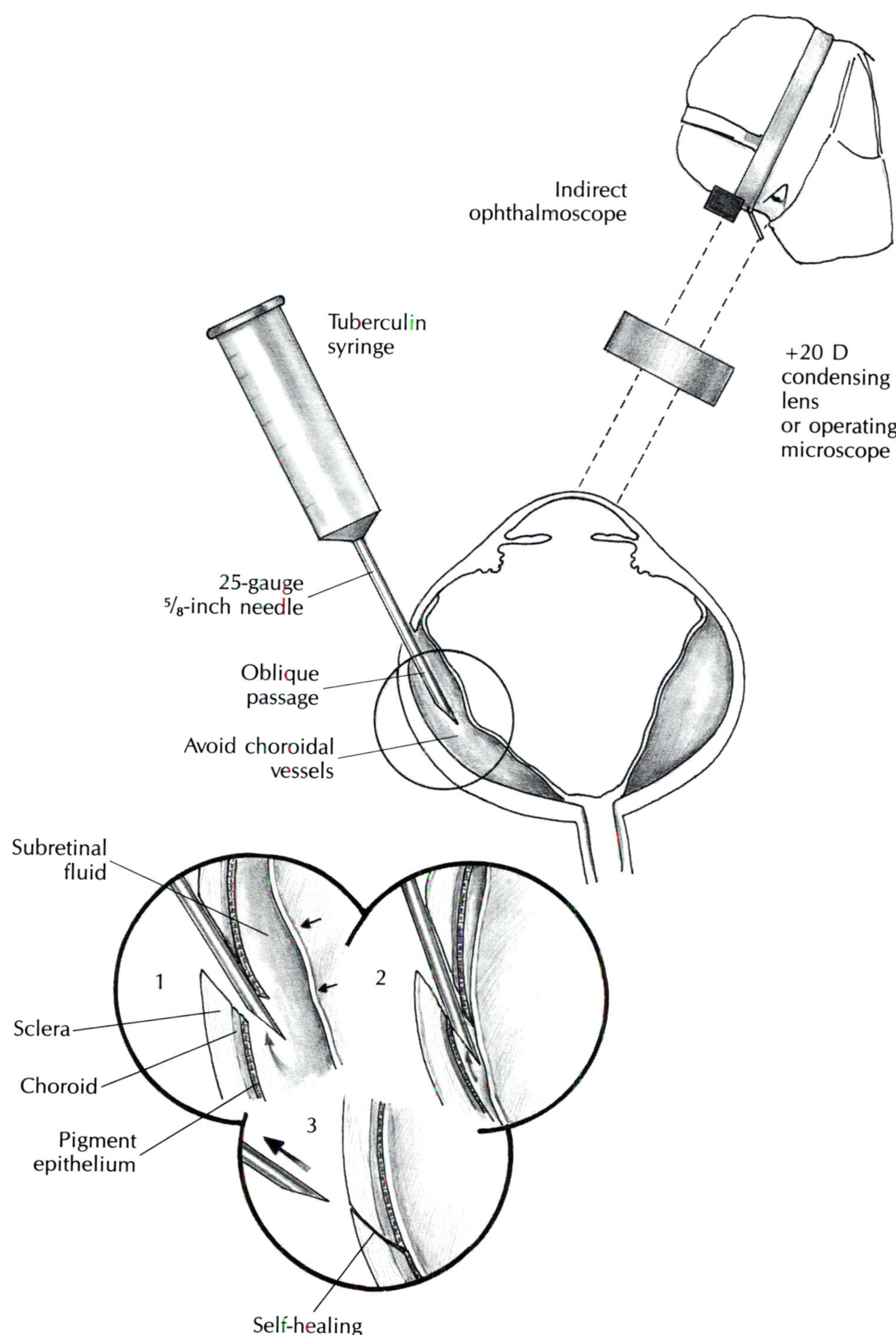

FIGURE 23-15. Needle drainage of subretinal or suprachoroidal fluid.

Internal fluid-air exchange

A pressure-controlled air pump that provides air to the sew-on infusion cannula is combined with proportional suction through a bent, tapered 20-gauge cannula (Fig. 23-16). No contact lens is used in the aphakic eye. In the phakic or pseudophakic eye, a high minus contact lens is used for fluid-air (gas) exchange (Fig. 23-17). Exchange stops when air egress begins.

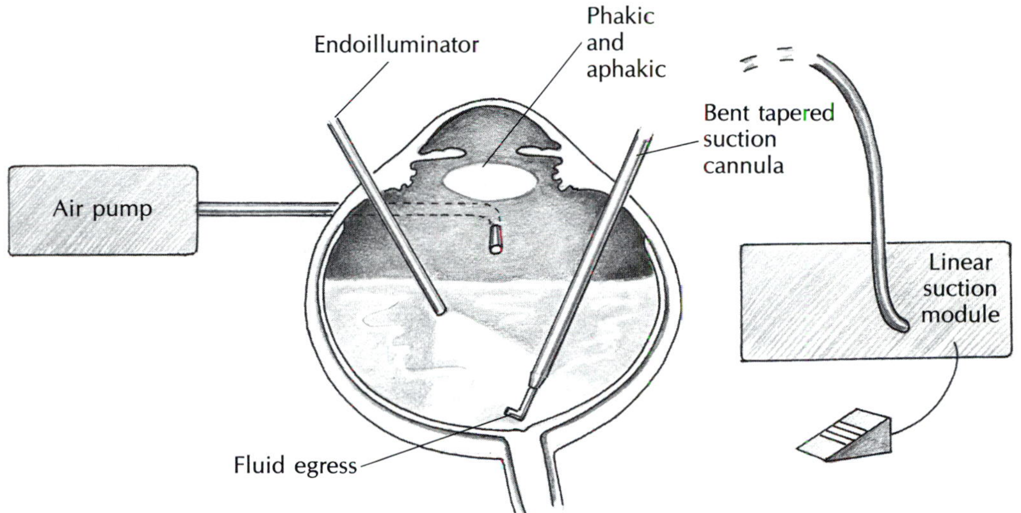

FIGURE 23-16. Internal fluid-air exchange.

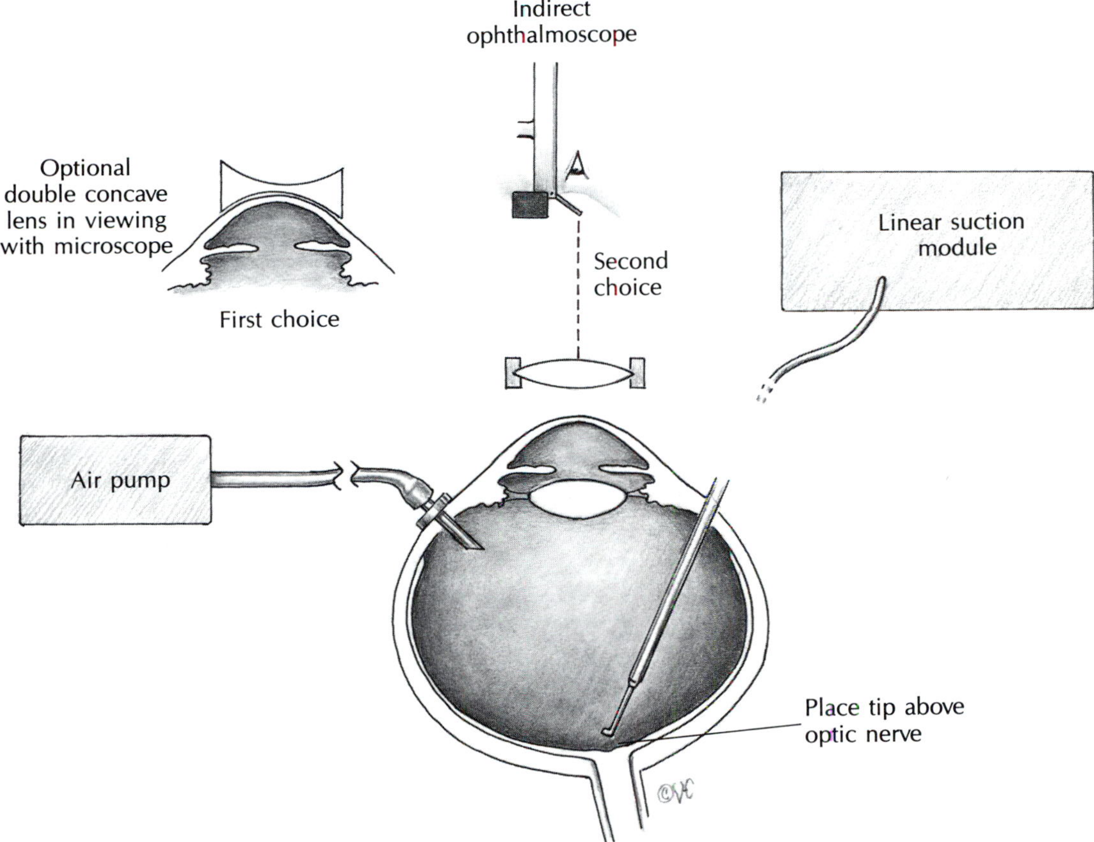

FIGURE 23-17. Fluid-air exchange in the phakic eye.

Direct injection of gas into an air-filled eye is to be avoided because the volume and therefore the concentration is highly variable. Air-gas exchange with a volumetric or automatic gas mixer permits total filling with a nonexpansile concentration (25% sulfur hexafluoride, 15% perfluropropane) (Fig. 23-18).

Internal drainage of subretinal fluid

A tapered, bent, 20-gauge, proportional, suction-controlled cannula is placed through the retinal break near the retinal pigment epithelium to drain subretinal fluid (Fig. 23-19). Retinotomy procedures should not be performed for this purpose. The sequence to be followed is drain, perform fluid-air exchange, and completely drain the subretinal fluid.

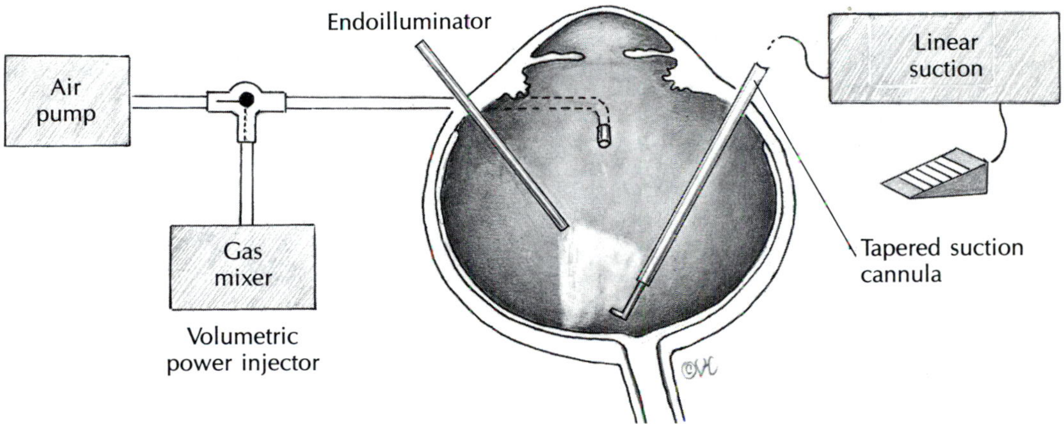

FIGURE 23-18. Air-gas exchange.

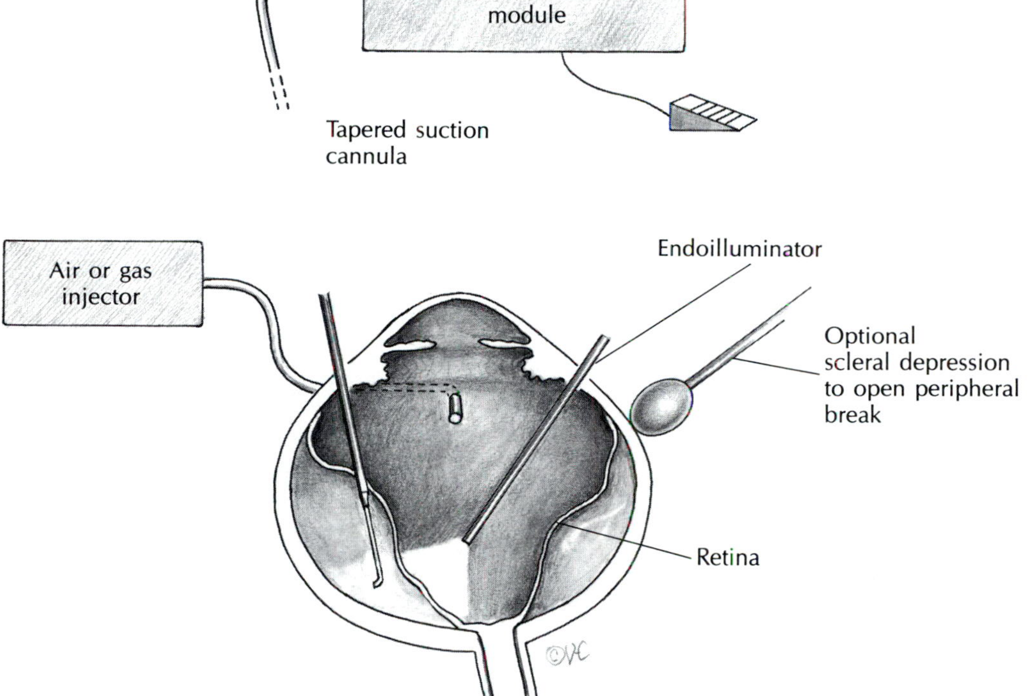

FIGURE 23-19. Internal drainage of subretinal fluid.

Retinopexy and Endophotocoagulation

Although neovascularization frequently occurs in vitreous surgery, significant intraoperative bleeding seldom occurs. However, every attempt should be made to prevent and control bleeding because blood can form a substrate and stimulate postoperative cellular proliferation. The primary methods available to control bleeding are endodiathermy and endophotocoagulation.

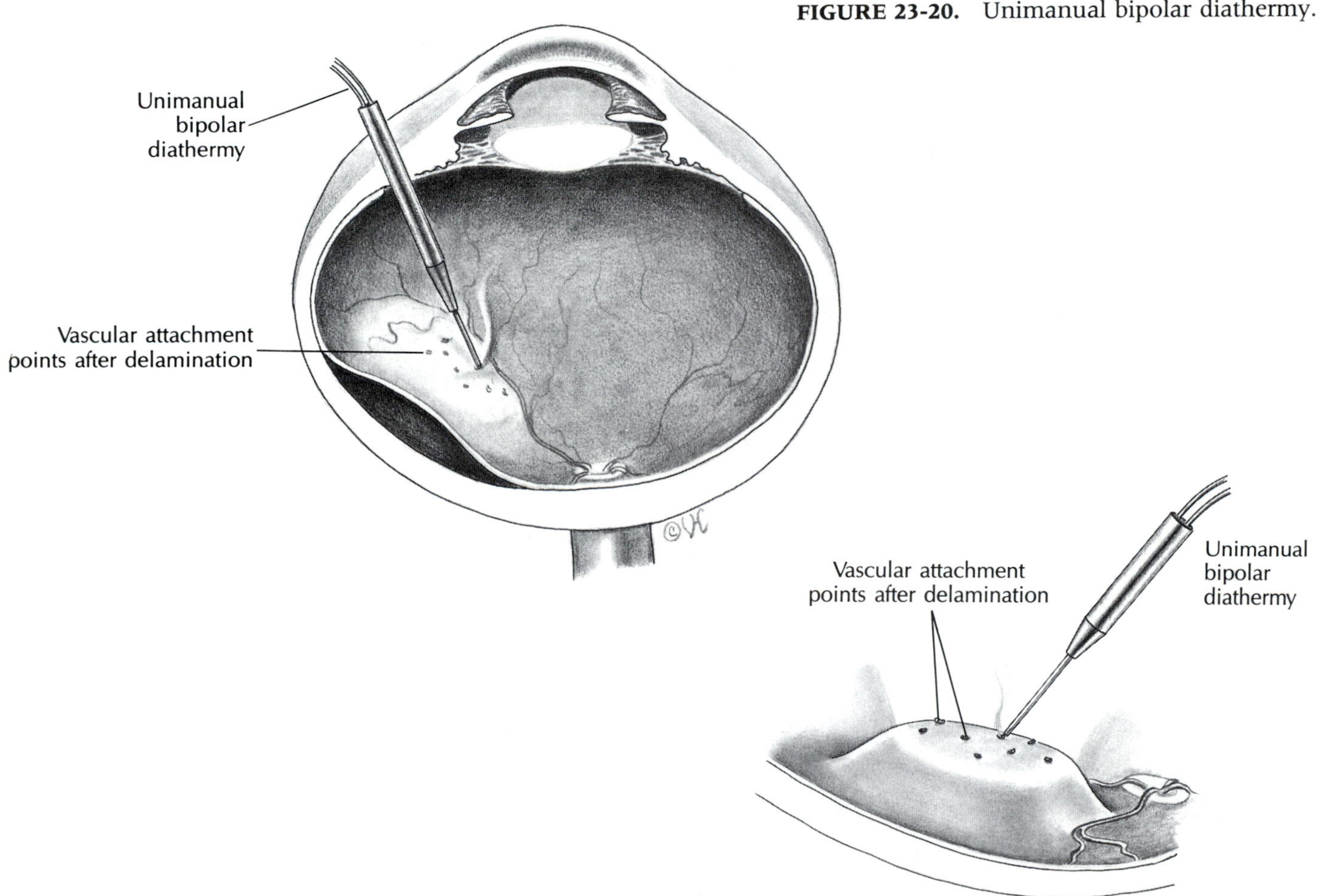

FIGURE 23-20. Unimanual bipolar diathermy.

Unimanual bipolar diathermy can be combined with supplemental infusion, endoillumination and endophotocoagulation, or a monofunctional 1 MHz bipolar radio-frequency (RF) probe may be used for elevated bleeding vessels (Fig. 23-20). Predelamination diathermy can lead to retinal necrosis, however. *Bipolar bimanual diathermy* can also be used by attachment of cables from the 1 MHz RF source to any two metallic intraocular instruments to permit flexibility in the control of bleeding (Fig. 23-21). Simultaneous linear suction permits excellent visualization. The tissue is placed between the tips of the endoilluminator and the linear suction cannula. Bipolar diathermy prevents inadvertent damage to the optic nerve. Diathermy should never be used within 1 mm of the optic nerve.

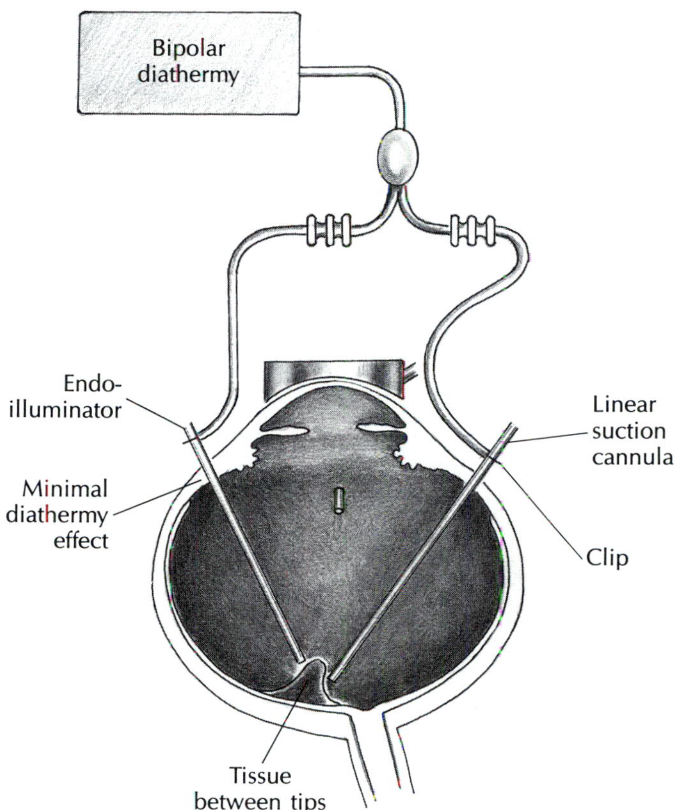

FIGURE 23-21. Bipolar bimanual diathermy.

The indications for *endophotocoagulation* are as follows:

Endo-panretinal photocoagulation	Proliferative diabetic retinopathy and indicated trans–pars plana vitrectomy Trans–pars plana revision for iris neovascularization or retrolental neovascularization
Focal photocoagulation	Macular hole or peripapillary break Break over previous buckle Break without retinal detachment

Endophotocoagulation can be accomplished with an argon, krypton, or diode laser. Xenon is less useful. Illumination is provided by a coaxial white light or a separate endoilluminator (for diffuse illumination). The assistant should wear protective goggles and the microscope requires a laser filter. Endophotocoagulation is used for all retinopexy procedures unless the sclera is exposed, for panretinal photocoagulation, for flat bleeding vessels, and for cyclophotocoagulation (Fig. 23-22).

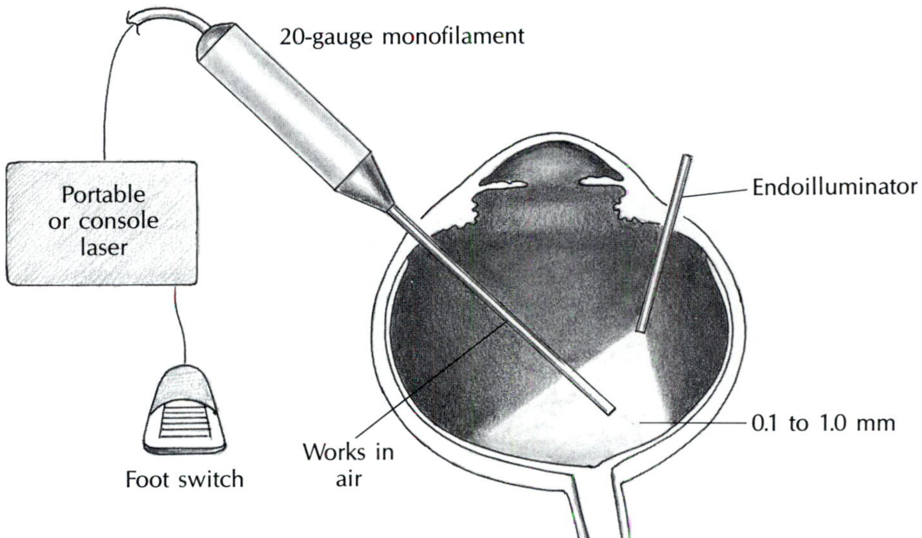

FIGURE 23-22. Endophotocoagulation.

Cryopexy versus diathermy (Fig. 23-23)

Cryopexy causes more dispersion of viable retinal pigment epithelial cells, proliferation, and inflammation than diathermy does. Diathermy causes minimal scleral damage and is also preferred for its small-diameter probe with fiberoptic illumination. Scleral damage can be minimized by retinopexy after reattachment, utilizing low-energy long-duration treatment, and instillation of air or gas into the eye to create a thermal and electrical insulation. The small conical fiberoptic tip of the transscleral diathermy probe (13.56 MHz RF) is used to perform postattachment retinopexy in the air-filled eye in cases involving giant breaks and proliferative vitreoretinopathy combined with scleral buckling (Fig. 23-24).

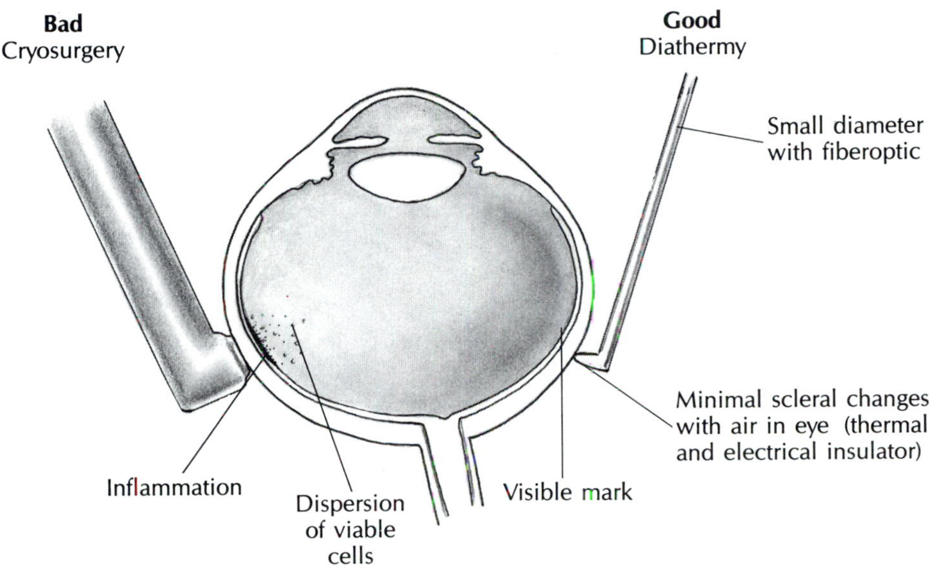

FIGURE 23-23. Cryopexy versus diathermy.

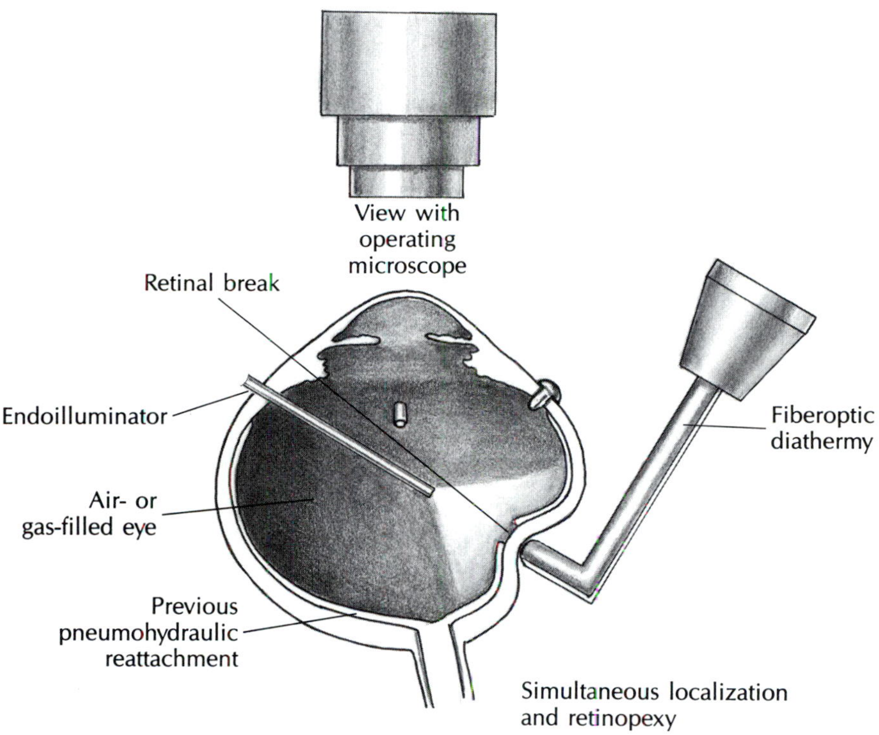

FIGURE 23-24. Transscleral diathermy.

Use of Silicone

Silicone is used for permanent or long (as compared to gas)–duration surface-tension management (tamponade). It is used to avoid retinopexy in cases of extensive retinal breaks or retinotomy to reduce reproliferation. Its other purpose is rhegmatogenous confinement for missed or new breaks or those that cannot be reapproximated to the retinal pigment epithelium. Silicone like gas causes recompartmentalization and is a factor in reproliferation.

Fluid-air exchange should always precede air-silicone exchange because a fluid-air interface has 50% more surface tension than a fluid-silicone exchange has (Fig. 23-25). Also, the retina should be reattached under air before the power silicone injector is used for air-silicone exchange.

A large silicone instillation is more likely to lead to the attachment of the inferior retina but causes corneal contact and endothelial damage. An inferior peripheral iridectomy allows aqueous humor access to the endothelium and reduces silicone keratopathy and subacute angle closure glaucoma (Fig. 23-26).

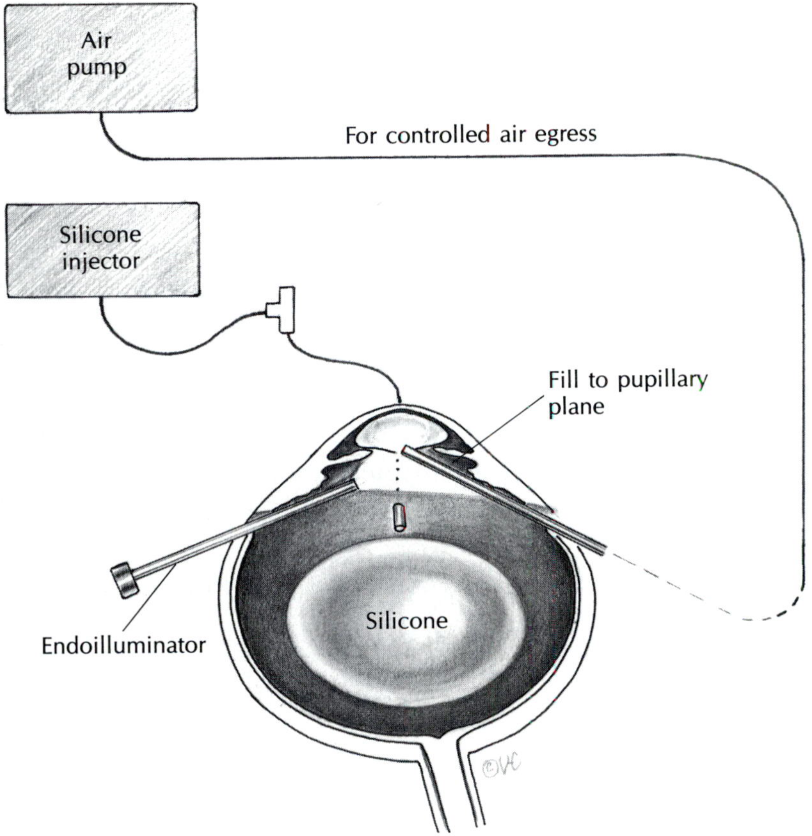

FIGURE 23-25. Air-silicone exchange.

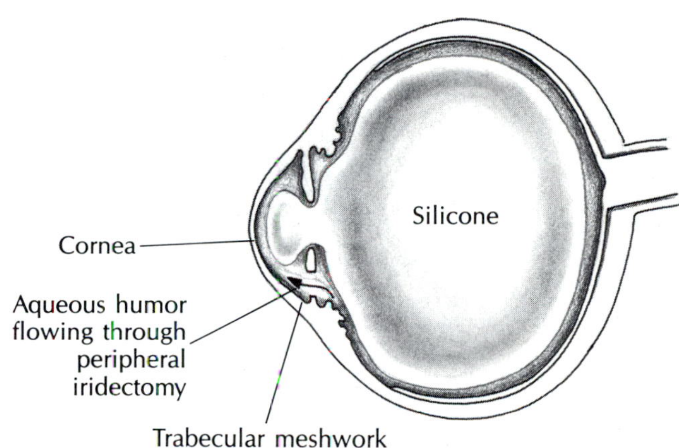

FIGURE 23-26. Prevention of silicone keratopathy.

Closing Procedures

Positioning of air (gas) bubble

The patient must be instructed to position the head in order to position the bubble on the retinal break and away from lens, cornea, and iris diaphragm to prevent cataract, corneal damage, and creation of a flat chamber (Fig. 23-27).

Wound closure

Fig. 23-28 shows the steps in wound closure:

1. Cut off the vitreous with Vannas scissors while squirting the area with balanced saline solution. *Never use cellulose sponges or forceps on the vitreous.*
2. Use a running shoelace suture with three or more bites of an 8-0 elastic monofilament suture with the knot set flat and the ends cut flush with a blade. Do not use absorbable sutures because leakage may occur in the postoperative period. Retinopexy and cautery should also be avoided.
3. Pull the wound very tight with a pair of needle holders and set the suture ends parallel to the sclera.
4. Trim the ends flush with a razor blade, without lifting, to avoid subsequent conjunctival erosion.

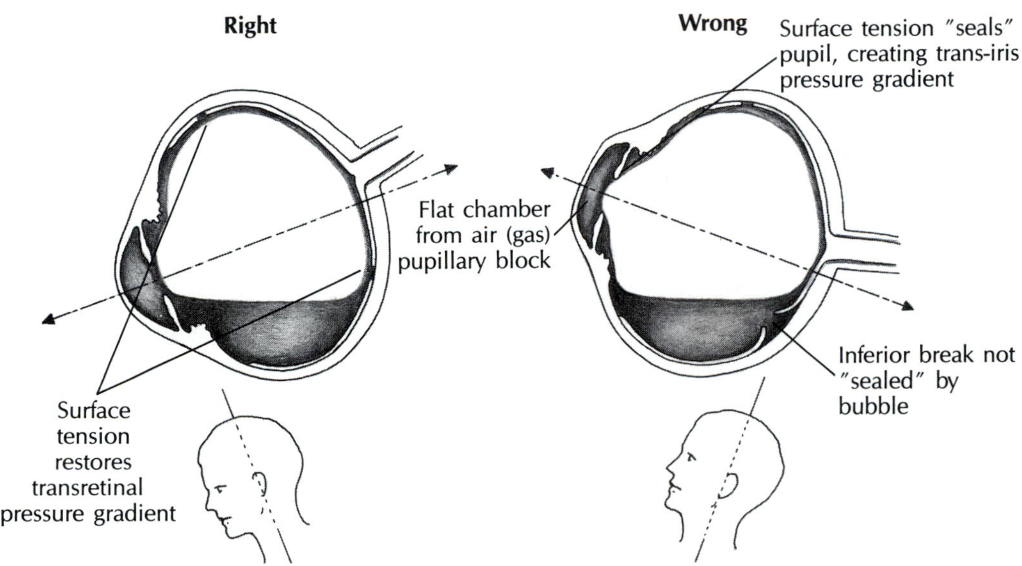

FIGURE 23-27. Positioning with air (gas) bubbles.

Closure of conjunctiva

The conjunctiva should never be sewed to the sclera or advanced (Fig. 23-29). A running 6-0 plain single-layer closure of Tenon's capsule and the conjunctiva provides the safest and most cosmetic closure. Irrigation with gentamicin and bacitracin should be carried out near the buckle in each quadrant before closure. Sutures at 3 and 9 o'clock bunch up the conjunctiva, and fornix flaps heal in unpredictable locations with conjunctival redundancy, ptosis, and symblepharon.

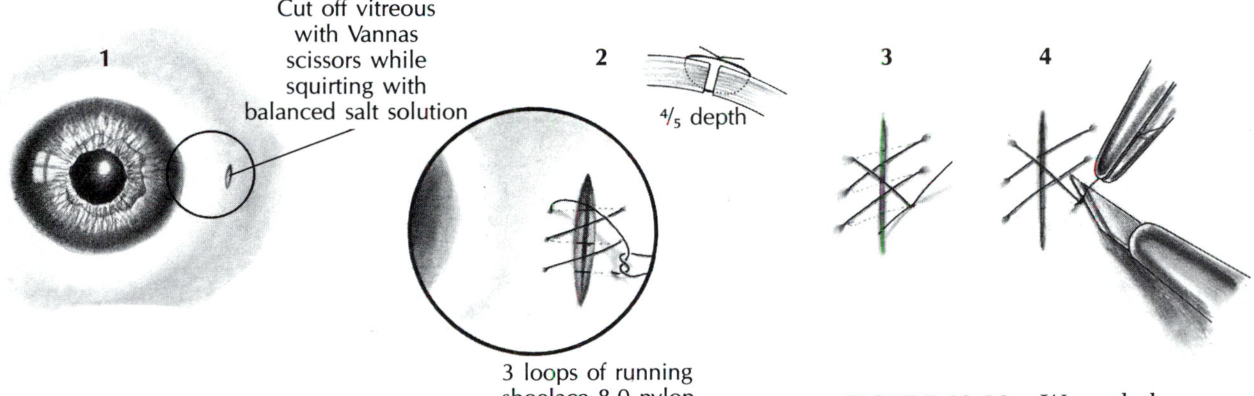

FIGURE 23-28. Wound closure.

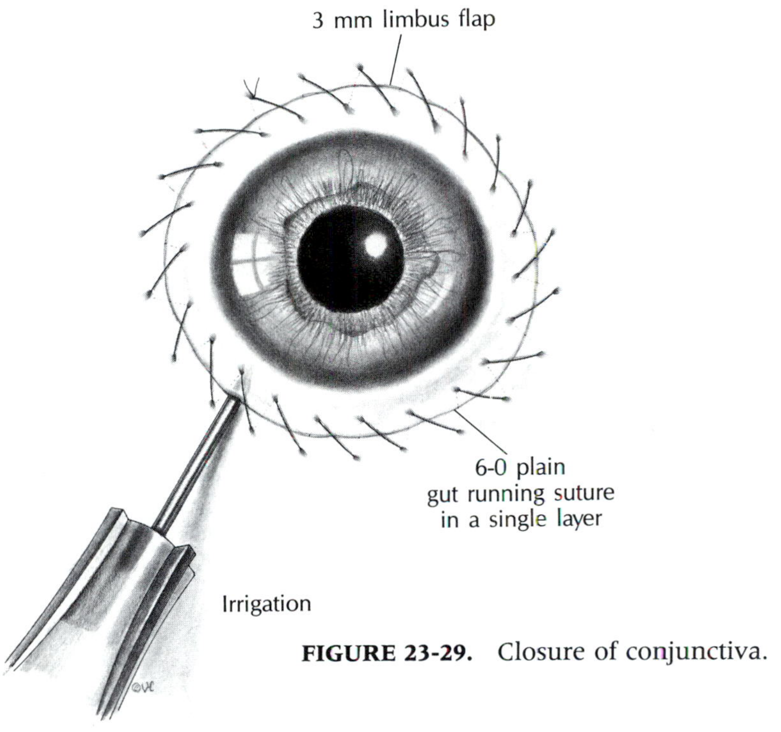

FIGURE 23-29. Closure of conjunctiva.

CHAPTER 24

Proliferative Diabetic Retinopathy

Proliferative diabetic retinopathy is among the leading causes of blindness in the United States today. Complications related to this disorder are the most common indications for vitreous surgery. Severe visual loss is associated with proliferative retinopathy caused by diabetes, and the search for better ways of treating this disorder is ongoing. Advances have been made both in focal photocoagulation and in the understanding of the mechanisms of panretinal photocoagulation.

The majority of the illustrations in this chapter have been modified and redrawn from Charles ST: Vitreous microsurgery, ed 2, Baltimore, 1987, Williams & Wilkins.

The indications for surgery in proliferative diabetic retinopathy are as follows:

1. Presence of nonabsorbing vitreous hemorrhage if bilateral or in only eye
2. Traction retinal detachment with recent macular involvement
3. Combined traction and rhegmatogenous retinal detachment with retinal breaks not amenable to closure by conventional scleral buckling
4. Continued growth of preretinal or epiretinal membrane resulting in visual loss by covering, dragging, or distorting the posterior retina
5. Early iris neovascularization and vitreous hemorrhage

All of these are discussed, and treatment alternatives are outlined (Fig. 24-1).

The indications for considering surgery in vitreous hemorrhage include the following:

Macular traction retinal detachment
Recent traction retinal detachment
Bilateral hemorrhage
Dense clot
Good health of the patient generally
Hemorrhage of long duration
Poor vision in the other eye

Bilateral visual loss or irreversible conditions such as macular detachment, neovascular glaucoma, or retrolental neovascularization are the only safe indications for trans–pars plana vitrectomy in the diabetic because of the high rate of biologic complications and medical risk factors.

Surgery should in general not be performed in the following situations:

Extramacular traction retinal detachment
Old traction retinal detachment
Unilateral hemorrhage
Subposterior vitreous detachment hemorrhage
Dialysis or other long-term health problems
Short-duration hemorrhage
Good vision in the other eye

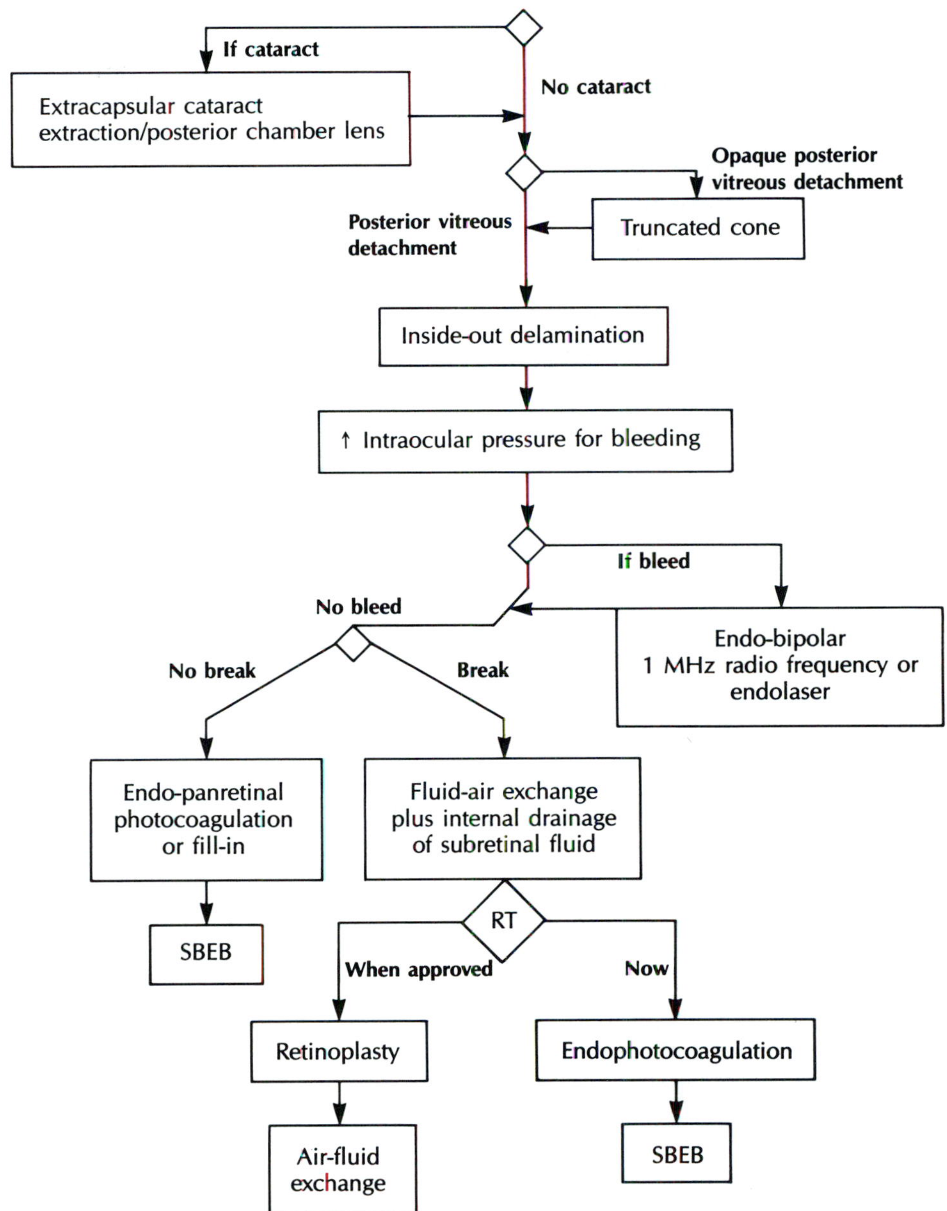

FIGURE 24-1. Proliferative diabetic retinopathy algorithm. *RT,* Retinal tear; *SBEB,* scleral buckle with encircling band.

Procedure

The first step to take requires ophthalmoscopic and ultrasonic evaluation of the eye to determine if a traction retinal detachment is present. Fig. 24-2 shows how the posterior hyaloid face and epiretinal membrane appear in cases involving traction retinal detachment. If the posterior hyaloid face is opaque or semiopaque, it must be entered in a safe area and incised at full thickness, and the opening must be extended 360 degrees to accomplish truncation (Fig. 24-3).

Inside-out delamination with right-angled scissors and a few segmentation cuts for the delamination scissors shank is the preferred method of epiretinal membrane management (Fig. 24-4). Peeling applies too much traction to the retina, and segmentation leaves tissue behind.

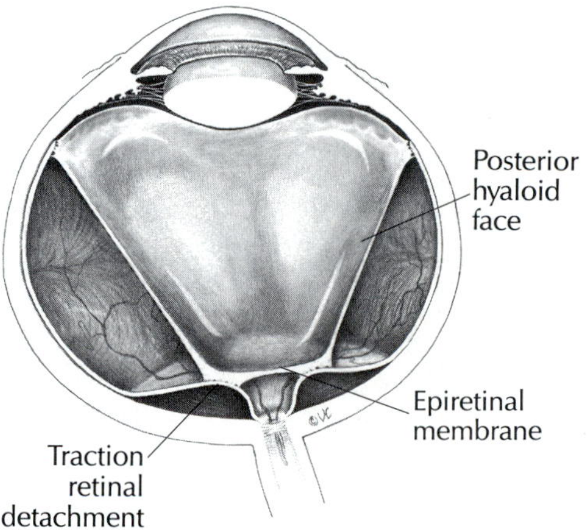

FIGURE 24-2. Posterior hyaloid face in cases involving traction retinal detachment.

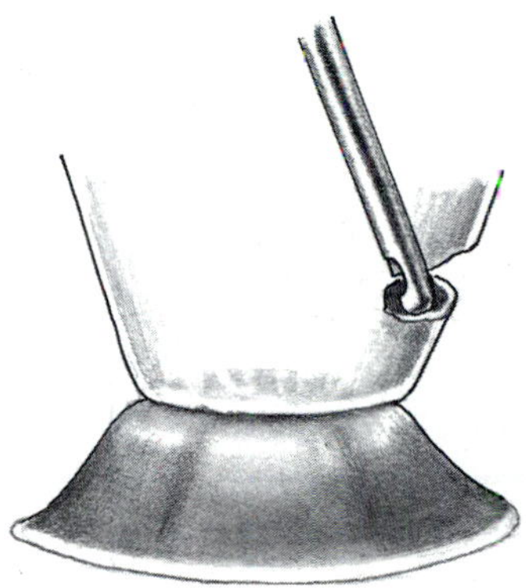

FIGURE 24-3. Opaque posterior hyaloid face.

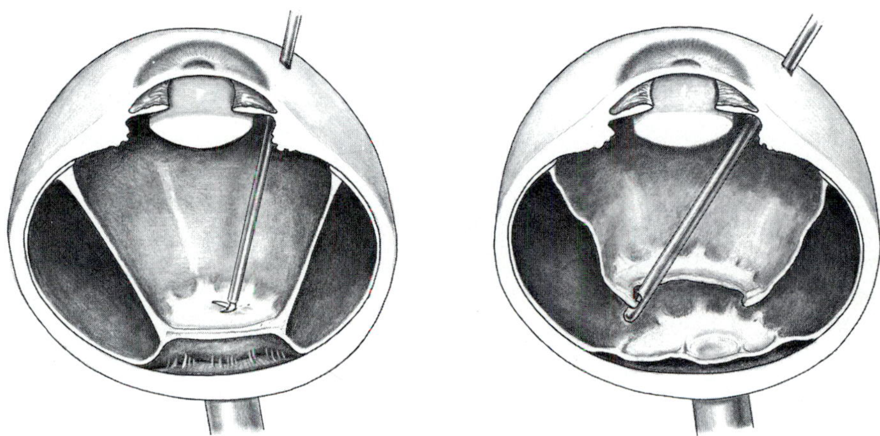

FIGURE 24-4. Inside-out delamination.

Bleeding is controlled by transient elevation of intraocular pressure. Endo-bipolar diathermy to elevated vessels or endophotocoagulation may be used if bleeding continues. This is summarized as follows:

Control of bleeding for proliferative diabetic retinopathy and retinopathy of prematurity

Method of control	Problem	Solution
Increase the intraocular pressure	Vascular occlusion, corneal edema	Brief use
Diathermy, laser	Tissue damage, reproliferation	Minimize use

A full vitrectomy setup to permit delamination of recurrent membranes should be used instead of the washout technique (Fig. 24-5). Endopanretinal photocoagulation fill-in should always be used in reoperation (Fig. 24-6).

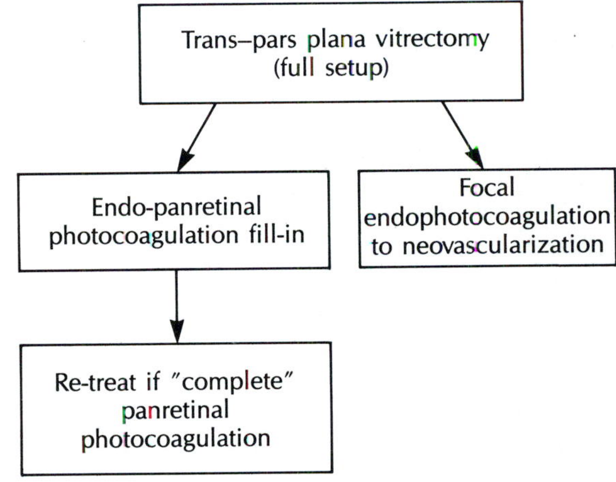

FIGURE 24-5. Postvitrectomy rebleeding algorithm.

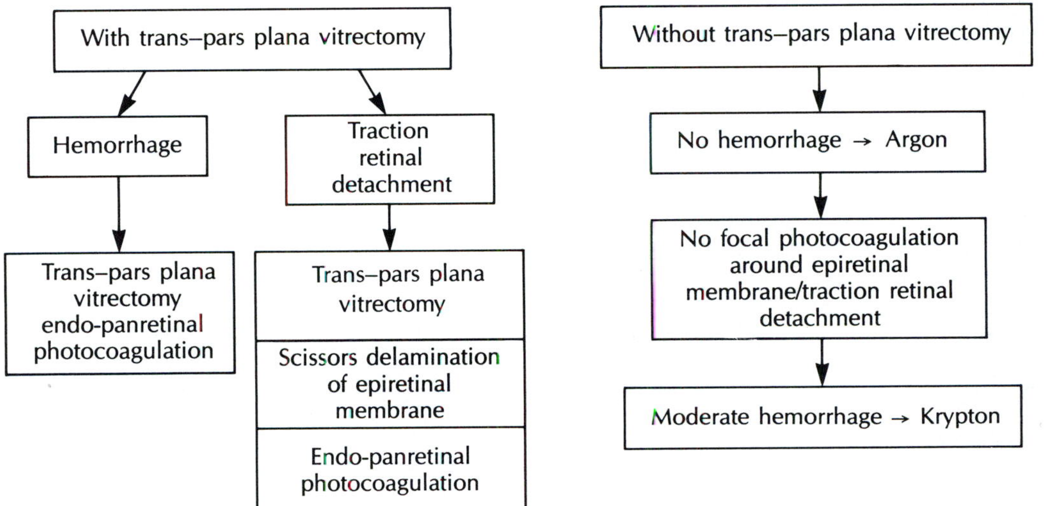

FIGURE 24-6. Indications for panretinal photocoagulation.

Neovascular Complications—Vasoproliferative Factor (VPF) Concepts

A diffusible factor causing endothelial cell mitosis and neovascularization is released by hypoxic retina. Detached retina releases more vasoproliferative factor because of increased hypoxia (Fig. 24-7). The key to management is titrated, extensive panretinal photocoagulation with light small lesions and no focal treatment (Fig. 24-8). This, along with judicious use of vitrectromy, carries the best results.

The posterior and anterior hyaloid face, lens, and trabecular meshwork are natural barriers to vasoproliferative factor diffusion and are substrates for neovascularization (Fig. 24-9). Intraocular lens and silicone oil create similar barriers.

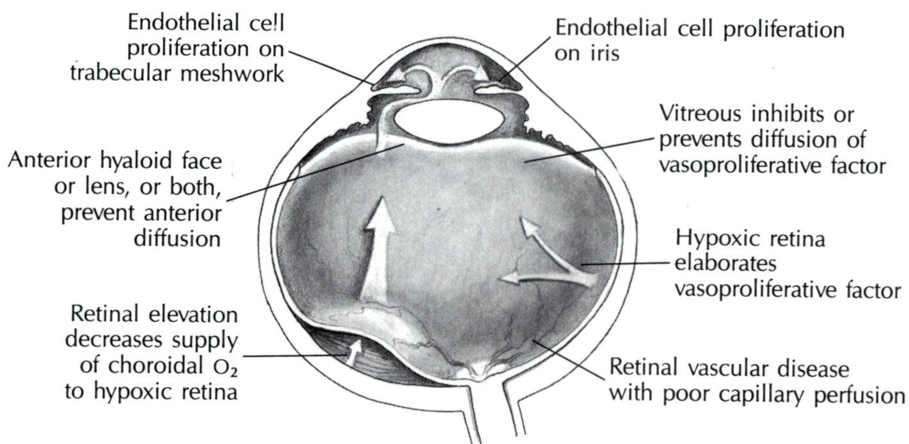

FIGURE 24-7. Vasoproliferative factor concepts.

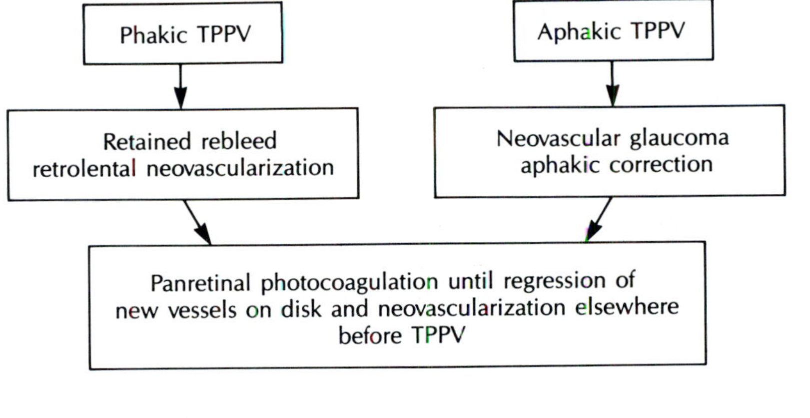

FIGURE 24-8. Neovascularization algorithm.

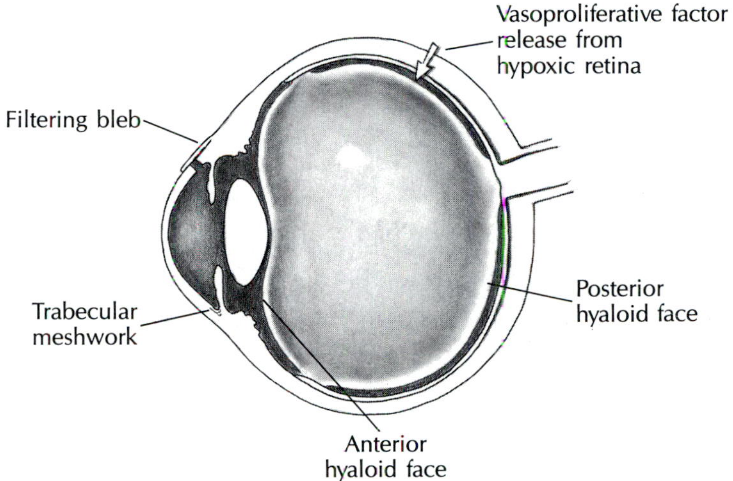

FIGURE 24-9. Barriers to vasoproliferative factor.

Neovascular Complication—Retrolenticular Neovascularization

Retrolenticular or retrointraocular lens neovascularization is caused by vasoproliferative factor and is followed by glial proliferation and contraction with a secondary equatorial ring–like traction detachment (Fig. 24-10). Retrolenticular neovascularization is similar to stage 5 retinopathy of prematurity (Fig. 24-11).

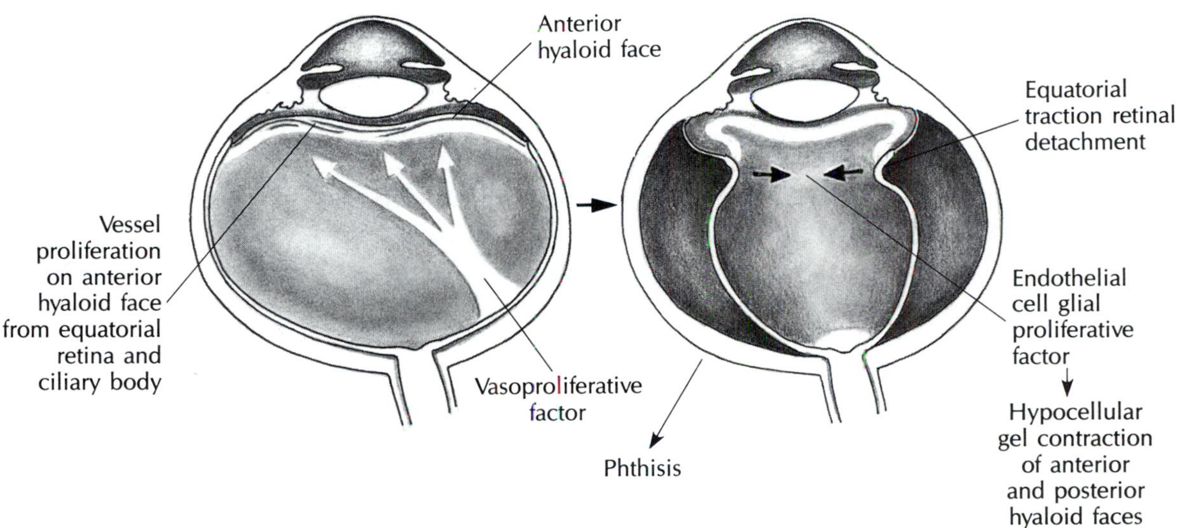

FIGURE 24-10. Retrolenticular neovascularization.

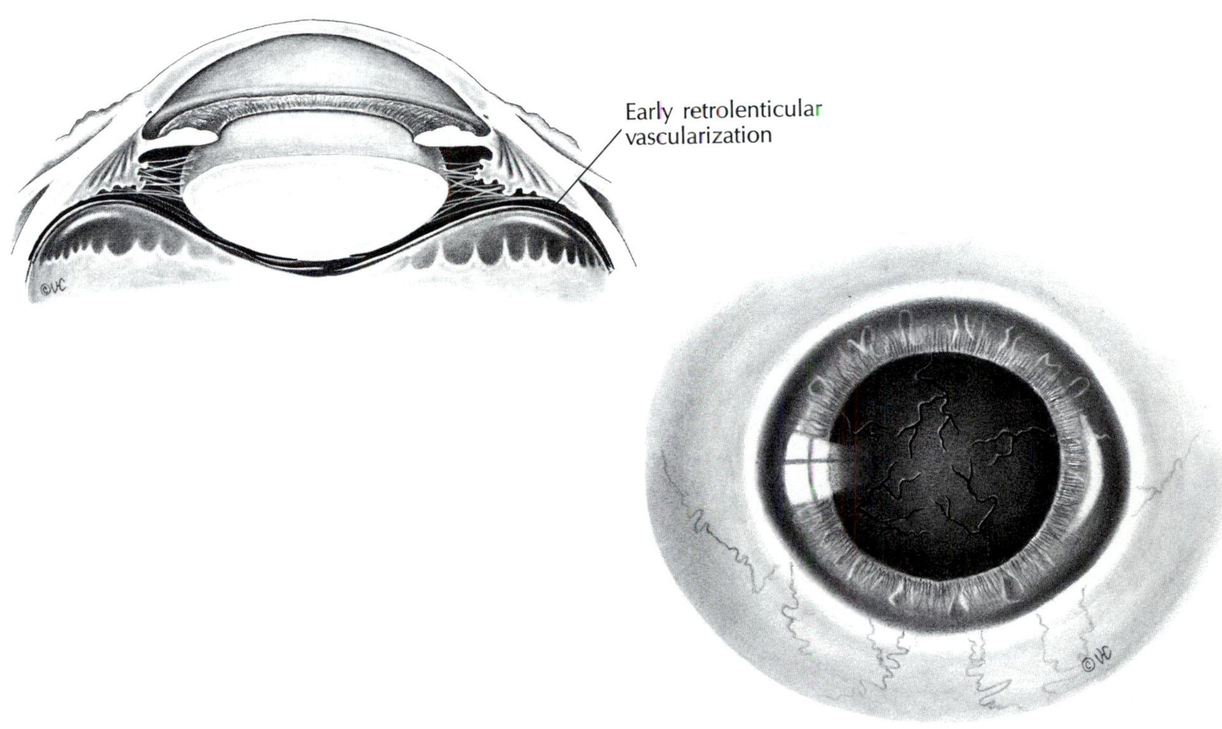

FIGURE 24-11. Retrolenticular neovascularization is similar to stage 5 retinopathy of prematurity (see p. 496).

Retrolenticular neovascularization has the same configuration as proliferative vitreoretinopathy seen in anterior loop traction and severe trauma or uveitis cases (Fig. 24-12). If untreated, it leads first to retinal detachment and then to phthisis in most cases. The eye must be rotated at the slitlamp for early diagnosis of retroventricular vascularization (Fig. 24-13).

An eye with retrolenticular neovascularization must be decompartmentalized, and endo-panretinal photocoagulation must be performed to save the eye (Fig. 24-14).

• • •

It is hoped that retinoplasty (cyanoacrylate retinopexy) will replace gas, silicone, and all forms of retinopexy in future years for the management of retinal breaks. Extensive panretinal photocoagulation is essential. Eyes may have fewer postoperative complications if they are made aphakic in conjunction with extensive endo-panretinal photocoagulation.

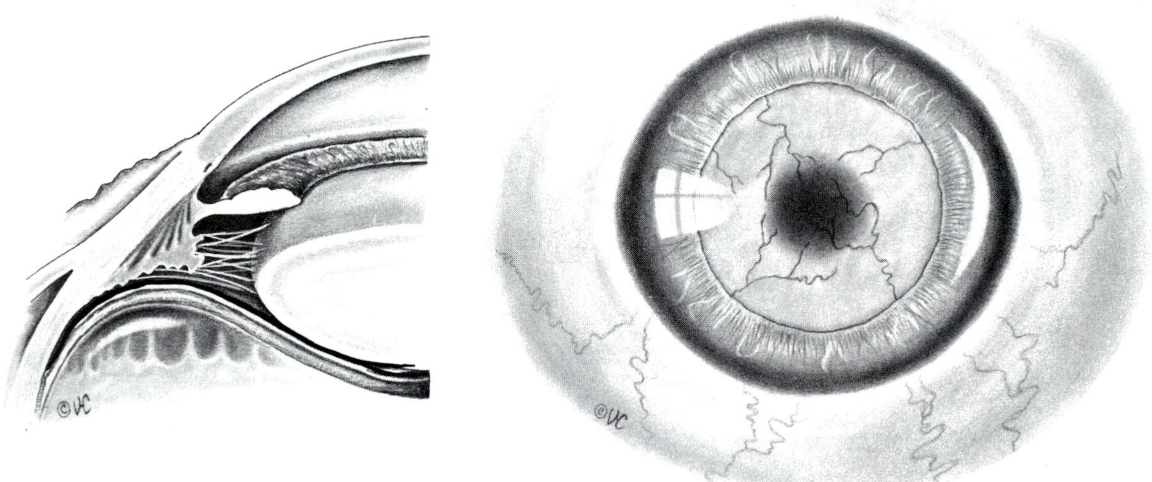

FIGURE 24-12. Retrolenticular neovascularization has same configuration as proliferative vitreoretinopathy seen in anterior loop traction.

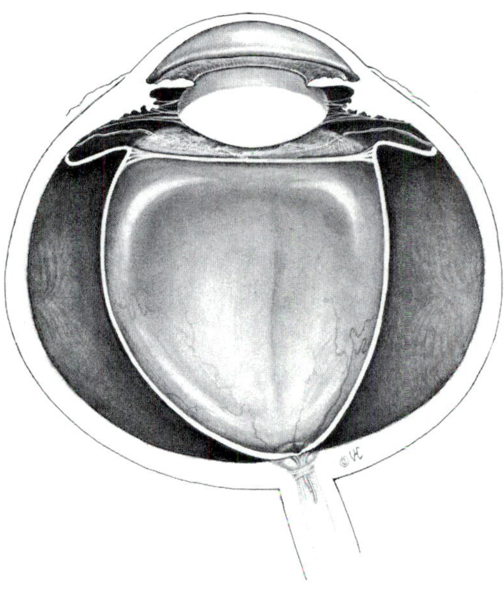

FIGURE 24-13. Rotation at slitlamp.

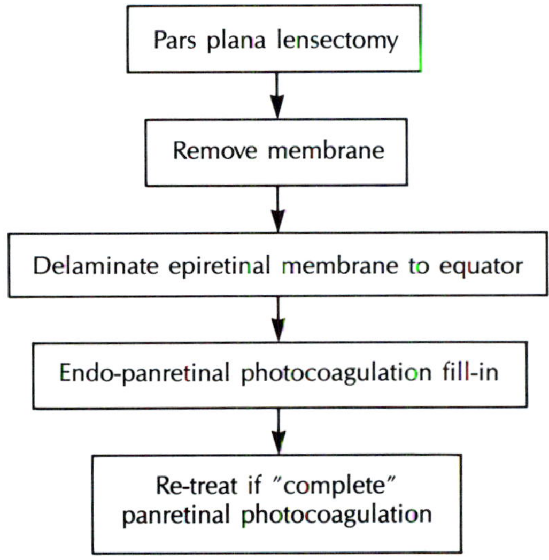

FIGURE 24-14. Retrolenticular neovascularization algorithm.

CHAPTER 25

Epimacular Proliferation

Epimacular proliferation has also been called macular pucker, premacular fibrosis, and surface wrinkling retinopathy. It involves the presence of hypocellular membranes on the macular surface and can result from a variety of conditions, as follows:

Cause	Type
Retinal break	Glial Retinal pigment epithelium
Posterior vitreous detachment with internal limiting membrane defect	"Idiopathic"
Retinopexy	Cryopexy Argon Xenon
Inflammation	Inflammatory

The majority of the illustrations in this chapter have been modified and redrawn from Charles ST: Vitreous microsurgery, ed 2, Baltimore, 1987, Williams & Wilkins.

The typical configuration of epimacular proliferation includes retinal elevation, whiteness from axoplasmic stasis, and retinal edema; this generally involves a single large membrane on the macular surface (Fig. 25-1).

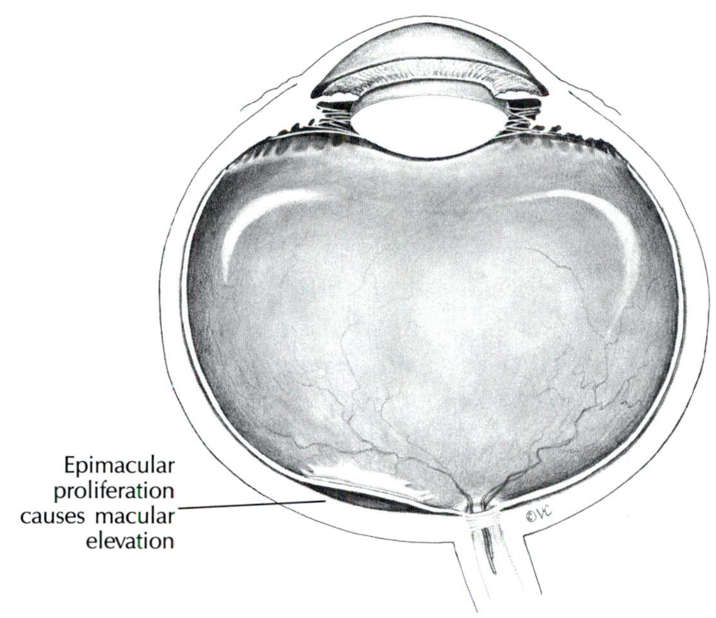

FIGURE 25-1. Typical configuration of epimacular proliferation.

Procedure

The steps to be taken in repairing this problem are outlined in Fig. 25-2. Each step is described and illustrated in this chapter.

As shown in Fig. 25-2, vitrectomy is performed only if the vitreous is abnormal, that is, under traction or partially opaque. Complications associated with vitrectomy include increased incidence of phakic-like, rhegmatogenous retinal detachment as a result of the intraoperative suction-induced traction and increased posterior subcapsular cataract.

The procedure is initiated by central entry with a sharp lancet blade (Figs. 25-3 and 25-4, *A*), and an edge is created when the membrane is thickest (Fig. 25-4, *B*). Inside-out peeling can then be performed with end-opening forceps (Fig. 25-5). The retina should be avoided during this procedure, and the fovea observed so that a macular cyst is not inadvertently unroofed.

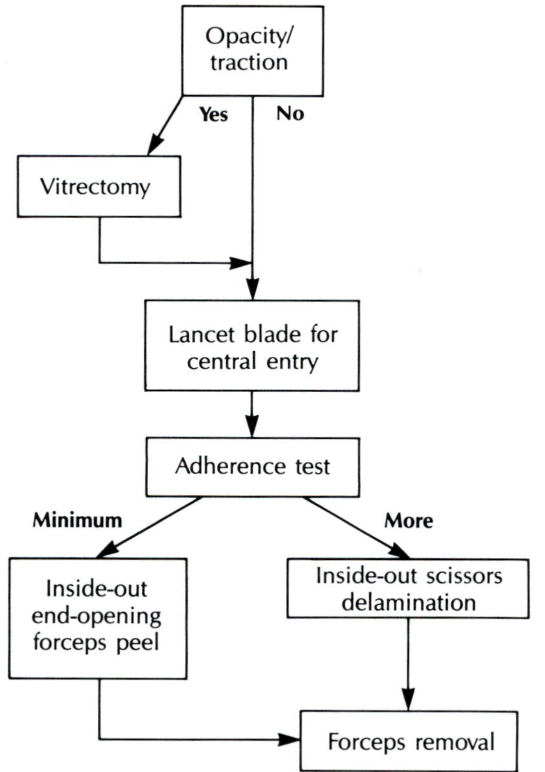

FIGURE 25-2. Epimacular proliferation algorithm.

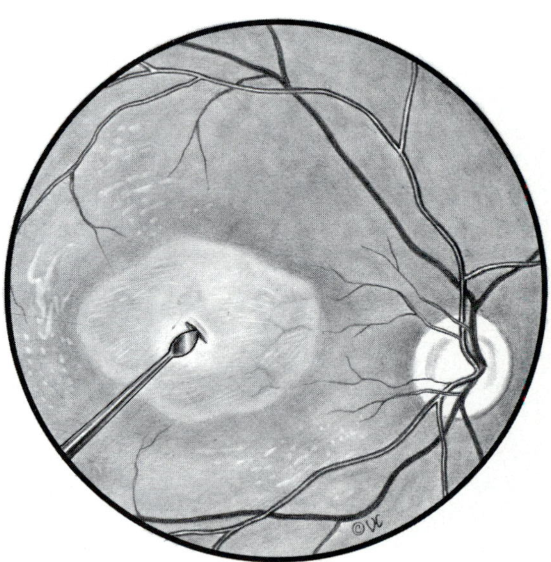

FIGURE 25-3. Central entry, fundic view. See Fig. 25-4, *A*.

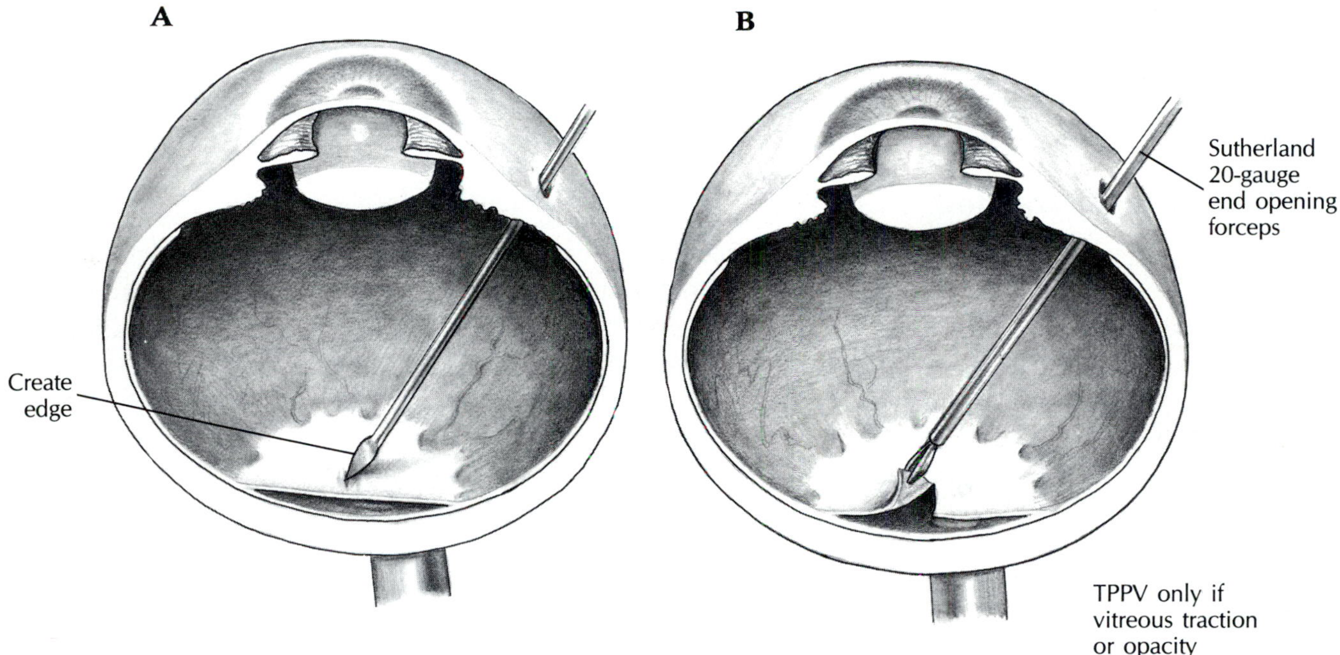

FIGURE 25-4. A, Central entry with a sharp lancet blade. **B,** Edge is created.

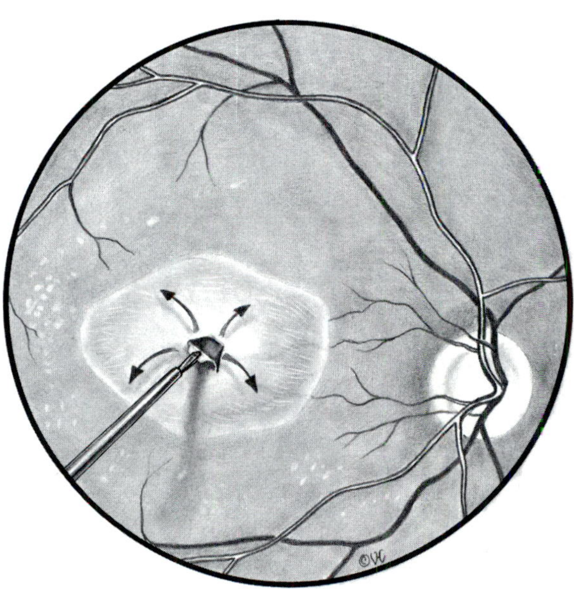

FIGURE 25-5. Peeling off membrane.

If the membrane is dense and more adherent, delamination may be required (Fig. 25-6). The forceps or vitrectomy probe is then used to remove the membrane from the eye.

Vitreomacular traction

Macular elevation and macular holes can be created by traction forces from the posterior hyaloid face and partial posterior vitreous detachment. Taking care not to pull on the fovea, the surgeon can perform vitrectomy and thereby allow reattachment and possibly prevent macular holes in some cases (Fig. 25-7).

COMPLICATIONS

The principal complications are rhegmatogenous retinal detachment, proliferative vitreoretinopathy, recurrence of epimacular proliferation, retinal whitening, and cataract. These can for the most part be reduced if the following general principles are remembered:

1. Avoid damaging the retinal surface, and perform vitrectomy only if the vitreous is abnormal.
2. Retinal whitening results from axoplasmic stasis and usually disappears spontaneously in several days. It should not be interpreted as a second layer.
3. The epiretinal membrane should always be removed in a single layer.
4. No edge is necessary for surgery to be successful.
5. Visual acuity loss is generally secondary to subretinal fluid.
6. Cystoid macular edema is secondary to retinal elevation.
7. Trans–pars plana vitrectomy causes posterior subcapsular cataracts and aphakic-like retinal detachment.
8. If possible, general anesthesia should be used.
9. Ultraviolet radiation probably accelerates nuclear sclerosis and should be avoided.

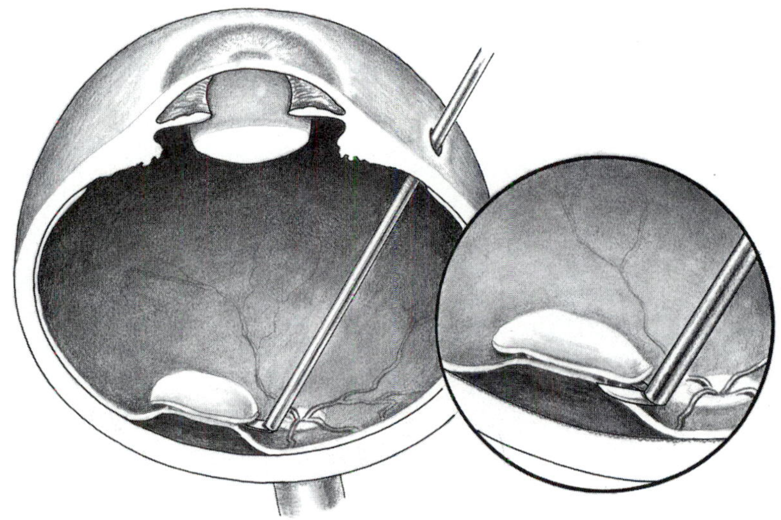

FIGURE 25-6. Delamination of epimacular membrane.

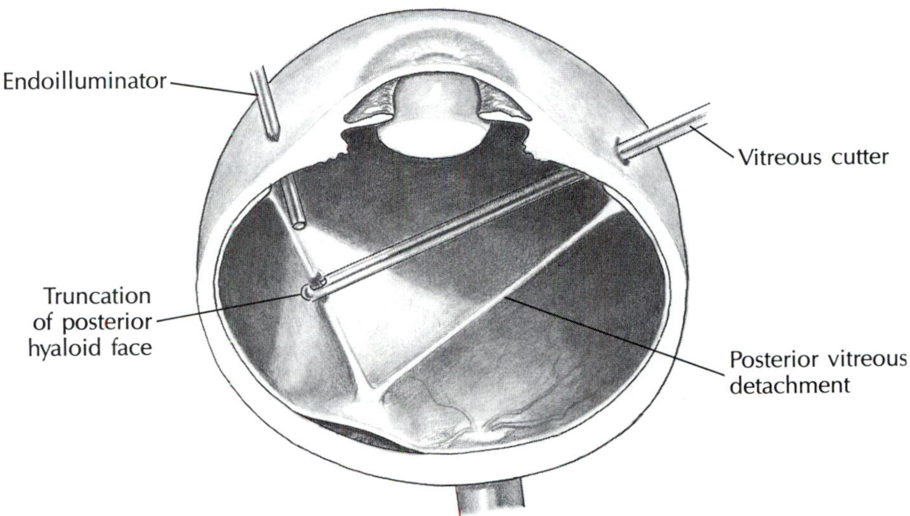

FIGURE 25-7. Vitreomacular traction.

CHAPTER 26

Retinopathy of Prematurity

Retinopathy of prematurity involves glial proliferation at the interface of the posterior hyaloid face and the retina. Both adherence and curved planar contraction result, causing traction retinal detachment and a concave retina preequatorially. Hypocellular gel contraction of the anterior hyaloid face occurs as well. This layer combines with the posterior hyaloid face–retinal interface and develops into a four-layer complex known as the "retrolental membrane complex."

Optimally the patient is examined while being held by the parent. Sedation should never be used in the office. If anesthesia must be used for examination, it should be combined with surgery at the same time. Electroretinography and visual evoked response are of no value. Ultrasonography is of nominal value because the retina can usually be visualized in these cases.

The majority of the illustrations in this chapter have been modified and redrawn from Charles ST: Vitreous microsurgery, ed 2, Baltimore, 1987, Williams & Wilkins.

The indications for treatment are shown in Fig. 26-1. They may be summarized as follows:

Extensive macular detachment (stage 4B) or preferably total retinal detachment (stage 5)
Inactive iris and retinal vessels
Medically stable

Fig. 26-2 is an algorithm outlining treatment modalities.

EARLY INTERVENTIONS

Premature infants with active iridal or retinal vessels or medical instability require lensectomy and chamber deepening without vitrectomy to manage the pupillary block glaucoma and corneal edema that may occur at 3 to 4 months of age—too early for definitive treatment. Early recognition of a change in corneal luster and lid edema by the parents and frequent physician monitoring are essential for early diagnosis and treatment (Fig. 26-3).

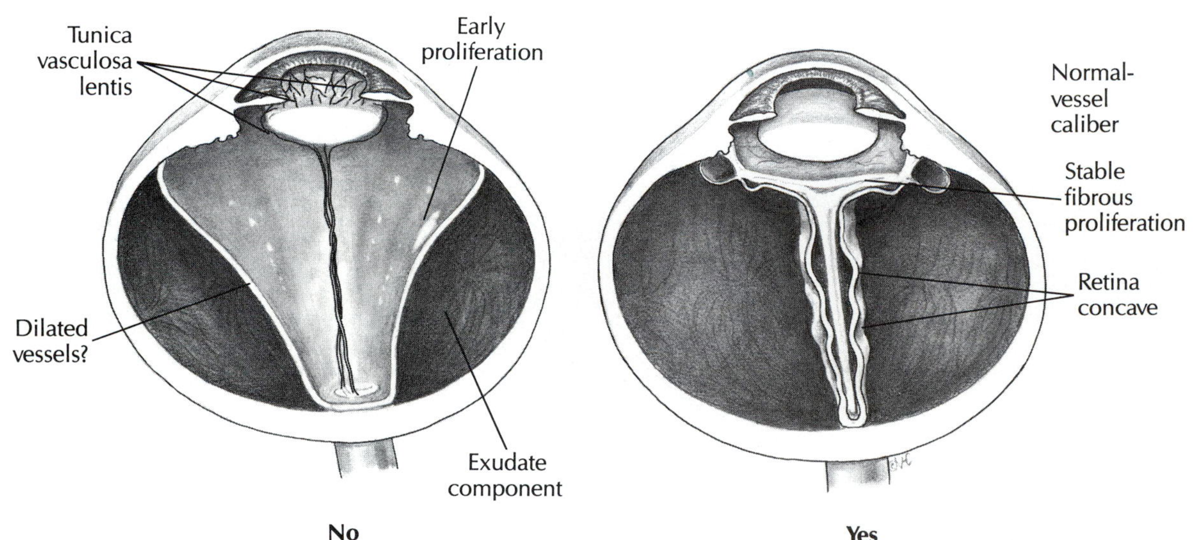

FIGURE 26-1. Indications of retinopathy of prematurity.

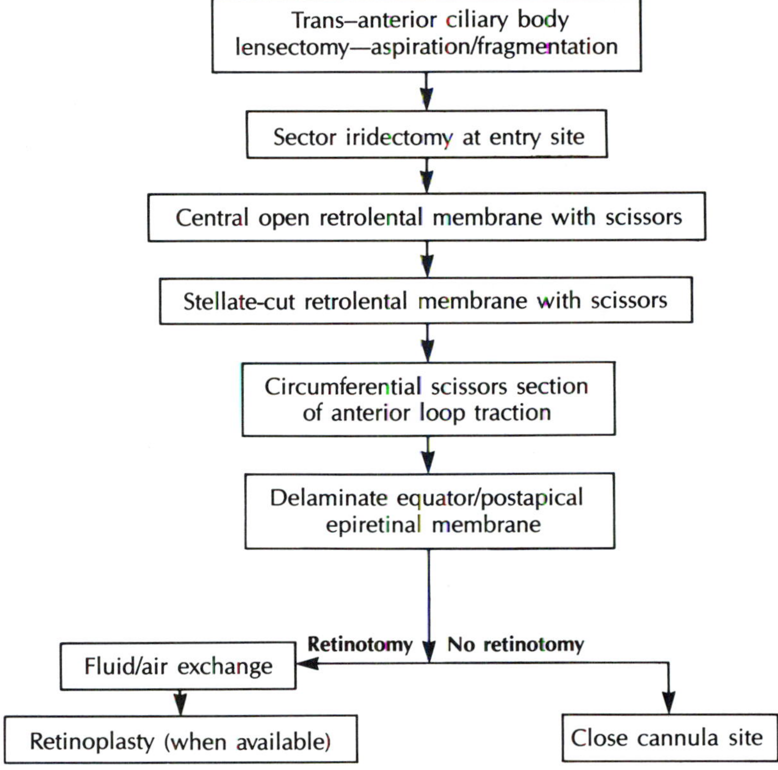

FIGURE 26-2. Algorithm for retinopathy of prematurity.

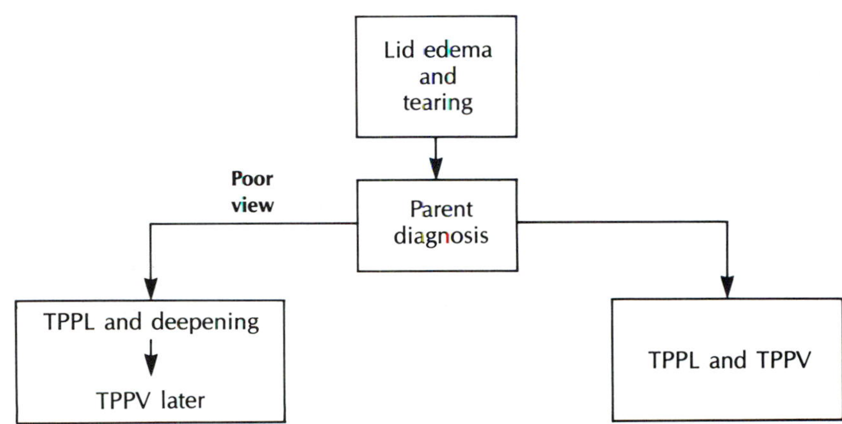

FIGURE 26-3. Algorithm for management of retinopathy of prematurity with flat chamber.

STAGES OF DISEASE

The stage 5 *wide funnel configuration* (Fig. 26-4) has a better prognosis than the narrow funnel configuration does. Presence of macular folds in stages 4A and 4B disease does not require vitrectomy. The *narrow configuration* is always initially mechanically operable, but surgery also depends on the infant's medical status and the visual potential in the other eye (Fig. 26-5). See Table 26-1.

TABLE 26-1
Stages of Retinopathy of Prematurity

Stage	Characteristic		
1	Demarcation line		
2	Ridge		
3	Ridge with extraretinal fibrovascular proliferation		
4	Subtotal retinal detachment		
	A. Extrafoveal		
	B. Retinal detachment including fovea		
5	Total retinal detachment		
	Funnel:	*Anterior*	*Posterior*
		Open	Open
		Narrow	Narrow
		Open	Narrow
		Narrow	Open

From International Committee for Classification of the Late Stages of Retinopathy of Prematurity, Arch Opthalmol 105:906, 1987.

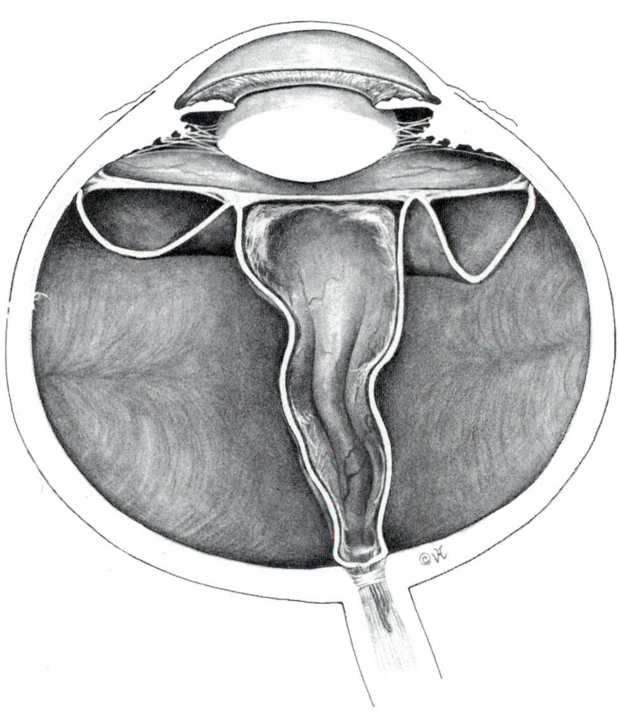

FIGURE 26-4. Wide funnel configuration.

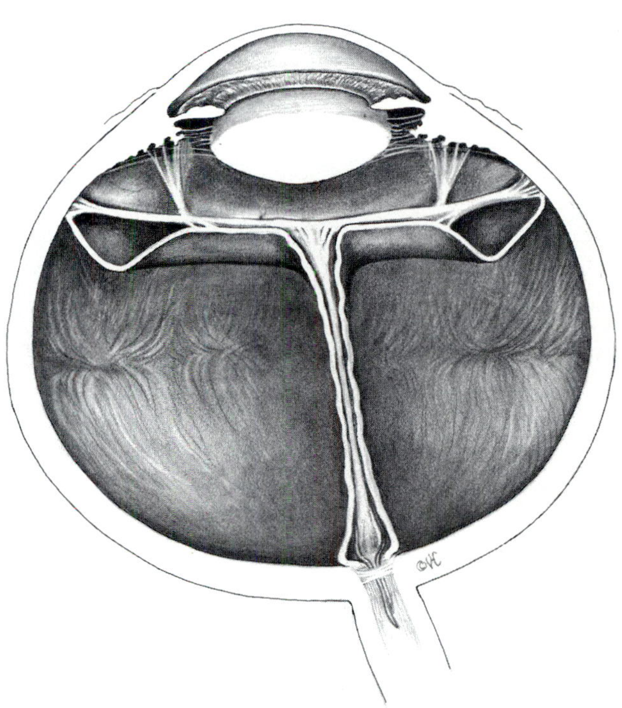

FIGURE 26-5. Narrow configuration.

Surgical Sequence

Lensectomy and capsulectomy

The three possible sites of entry are limbal, pars plana, and ciliary body, which create the following situations:

1. *Limbal:* striate keratopathy, regional corneal edema, wound leaks, poor access to the area of preequatorial traction
2. *Pars plana:* instruments brought into subretinal space, resulting in inoperable retinal dialysis and detachment
3. *Ciliary body:* frequently requires sector iridotomy or passage anterior to the iris

Overall the ciliary body entry is safest.

Aspirating, bimanual fragmenter lensectomy is faster than using vitrectomy probes for lensectomy (Fig. 26-6). All peripheral cortex should be removed (Fig. 26-7), with scleral depression employed to visualize the periphery (Fig. 26-8). Luminal fluid flow cools the sclera better than pulsed ultrasound, and so continuous and simultaneous aspiration and fragmentation should be used.

All this is done to reduce postoperative iris-retinal adherence. The scleral depression must be done carefully to avoid rupturing the nonpigmented ciliary epithelium. Less iris surgery results in decreased bleeding and inflammation.

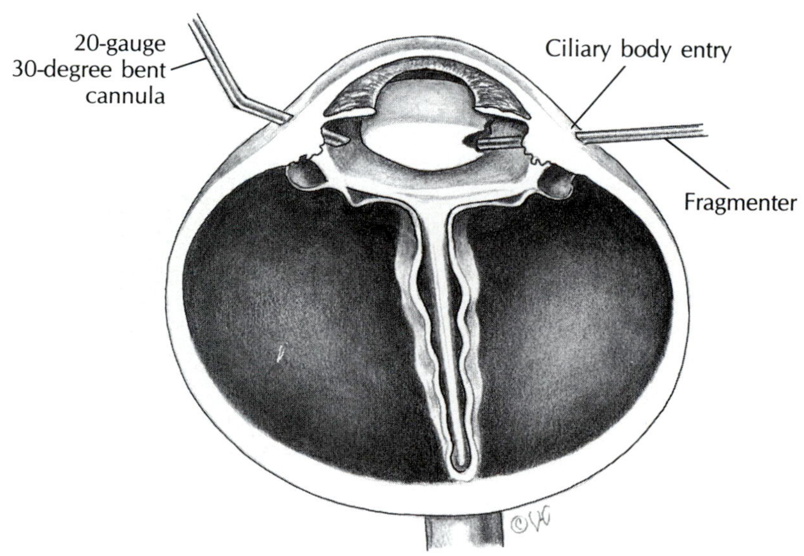

FIGURE 26-6. Lensectomy.

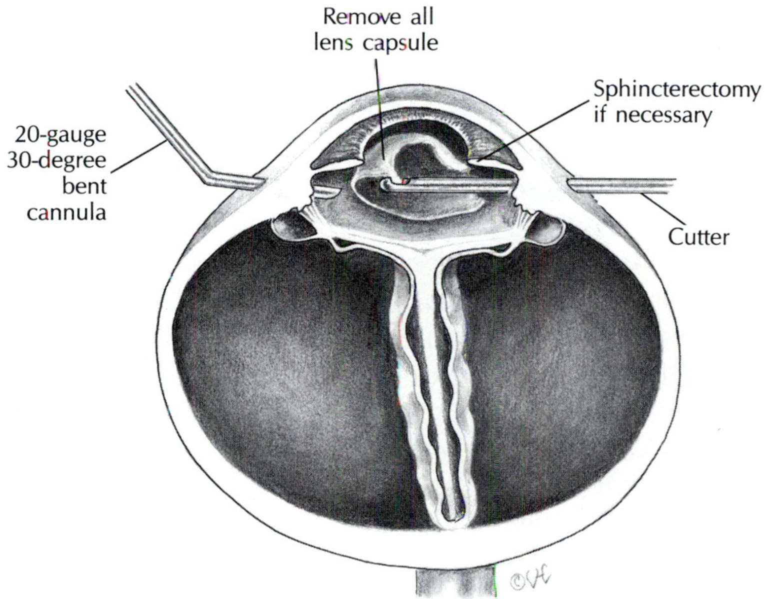

FIGURE 26-7. Capsulectomy.

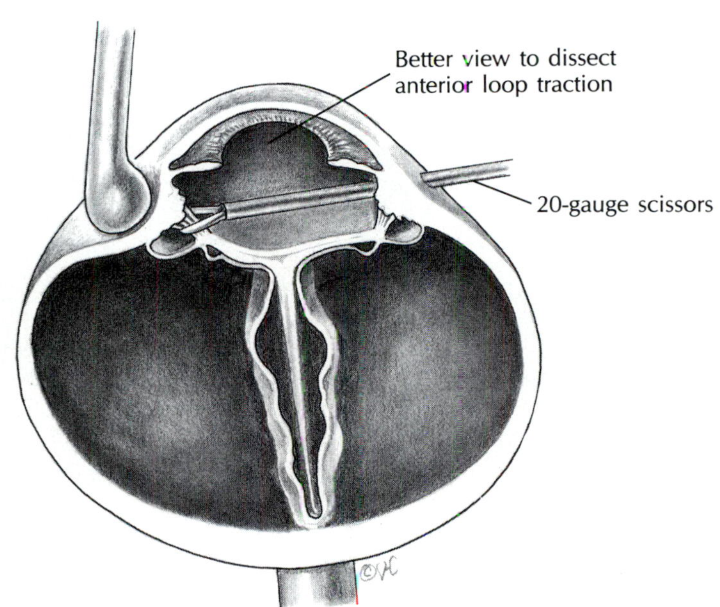

FIGURE 26-8. Scleral depression in retinopathy of prematurity.

Epiretinal membrane

The retrolental complex referred to earlier usually extends from equator to equator. Generally the retina is not in contact in the central area. Therefore central stellate scissors incisions are made in the retrolental membrane and carried to the periphery, with careful avoidance of displacement of the membrane (Fig. 26-9). These should be full-thickness cuts to allow visualization of the retinal surface.

In most instances, total 360-degree circumferential segmentation of the anterior loop traction is essential (Fig. 26-10), even if it is difficult. Then the segments of epiretinal membrane should be carefuly delaminated from the retinal surface and removed from the eye with the vitreous cutter (Fig. 26-11).

With excellent pupillary dilatation all retrolental membranes can be delaminated away from the ciliary body. It should be noted that internal fluid-air exchange or fluid-gas exchange with an air pump or gas injection and proportional suction is used if a retinal break is seen or suspected during these procedures (Fig. 26-12). Frequently the break cannot reach the retinal pigment epithelium, and retinoplasty if available would be indicated.

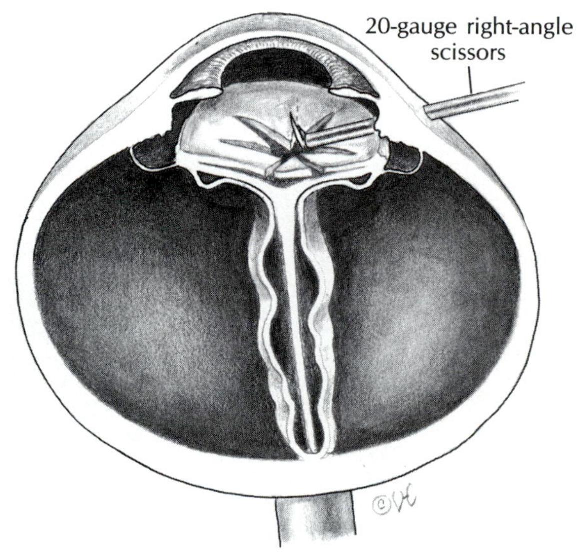

FIGURE 26-9. Stellate incisions in epiretinal membrane.

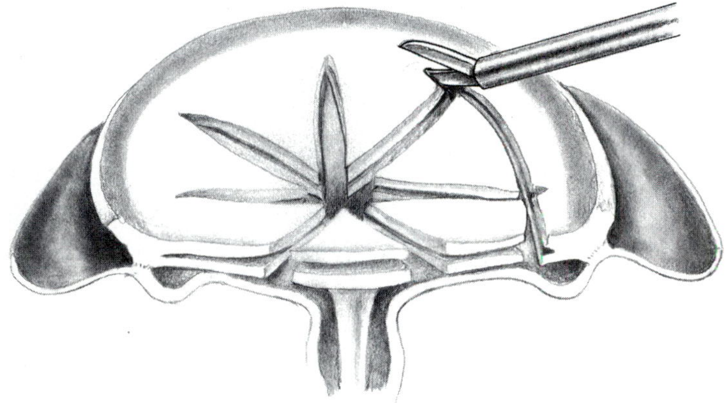

FIGURE 26-10. Anterior loop dissection.

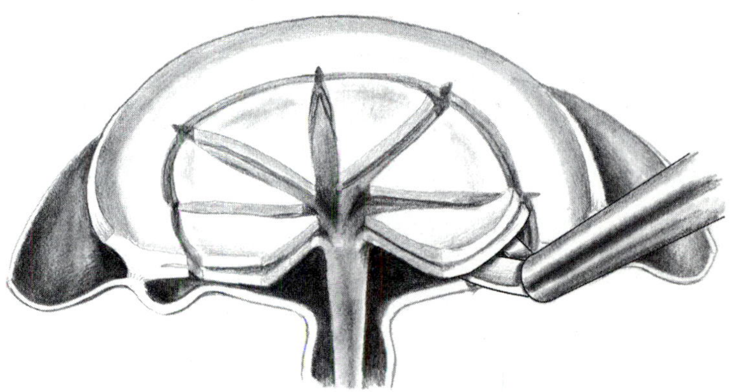

FIGURE 26-11. Epiretinal membrane delamination.

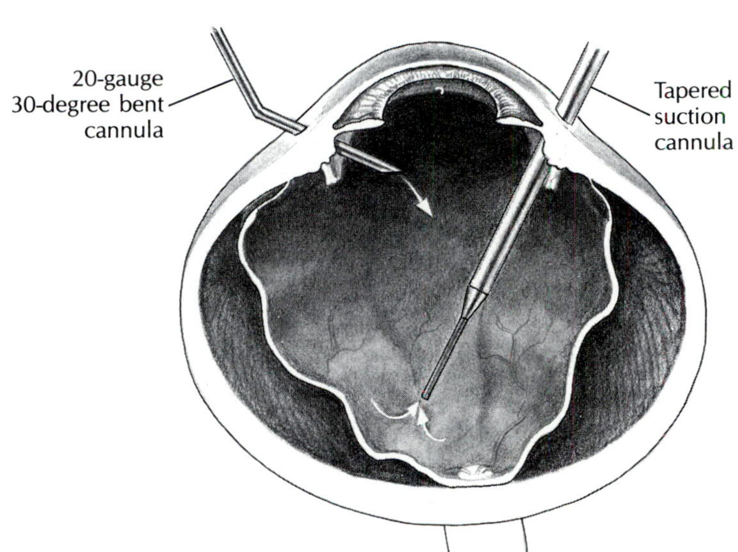

FIGURE 26-12. Internal fluid-air exchange.

Proliferation

Iris-retinal adherence

Iris-retinal adherence is a common form of the reproliferation that frequently occurs after vitrectomy (Fig. 26-13). Total removal of lens material (thus avoiding hemorrhage, avoiding retinopexy, and avoiding scleral buckling) helps to reduce iris-retinal adherence forms of reproliferation.

• • •

Small-displacement inertial inclusive shears will also improve the dissection procedure when these are available. Until prevention can be accomplished, it is hoped that antireproliferation peptides will be developed to prevent the reproliferation that occurs in about 50% of these cases.

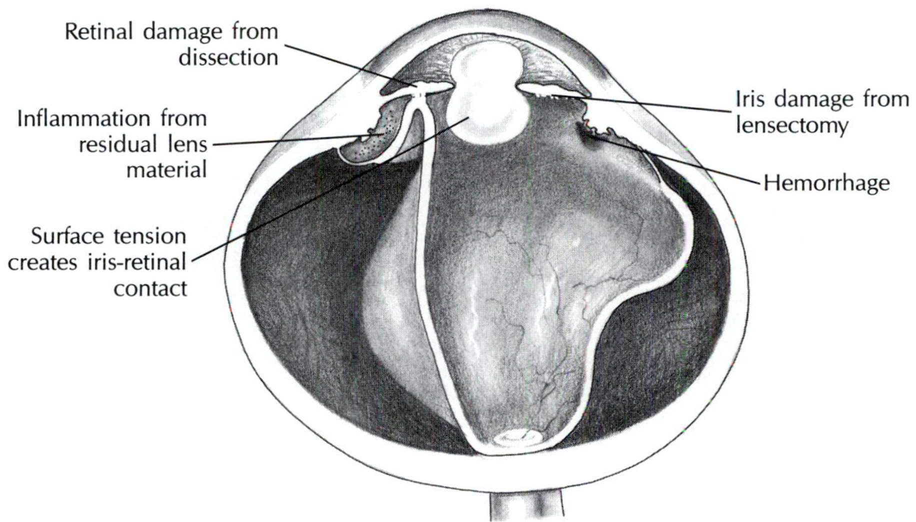

FIGURE 26-13. Iris retinal adherence.

CHAPTER 27

Trauma

Injuries caused by steel, copper, and biologic materials require immediate vitrectomy to reduce retinal toxic damage and infection (Fig. 27-1). In contrast, double penetrating injuries and nontoxic foreign bodies are best managed by a 5- to 10-day delay to allow posterior vitreous detachment and to reduce bleeding and choroidal edema. Primary repair of entry sites and corneal lacerations should usually precede vitrectomy instead of using a combined approach. Better visualization through the cornea usually results from this approach.

The majority of the illustrations in this chapter have been modified and redrawn from Charles ST: Vitreous microsurgery, ed 2, Baltimore, 1987, Williams & Wilkins.

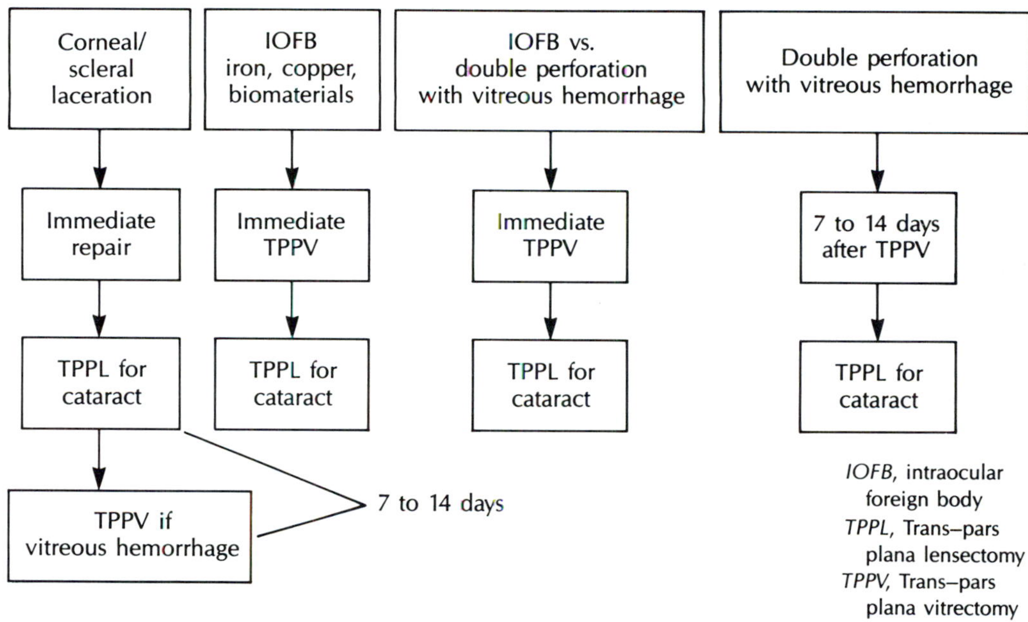

FIGURE 27-1. Trauma algorithm.

Procedure for Corneal-Scleral Lacerations

Repair involves closing the laceration with running-shoelace 8-0 to 10-0 elastic monofilament sutures. These leak less, cause less striation, and can be placed quickly (Fig. 27-2). Absorbable sutures should never be used in either the sclera or the cornea. Scleral lacerations should not require grafting unless large pieces of sclera are missing.

Recently prolapsed iris that does not appear necrotic can be reposited. Lensectomy for traumatic cataract is usually best delayed to allow corneal sealing to occur. Posterior vitrectomy should be performed if a retinal detachment is seen on ultrasonography, if erythroclastic glaucoma occurs, if foreign body is present, or if vitreous mobility decreases, indicating hypocellular gel contraction. Posterior wounds should be sutured only if such suturing can be done without prolapsing tissue. Cellulose sponges should never be used because the retina can be pulled out of the wound. No cryopexy should be applied to wounds because this increases proliferation.

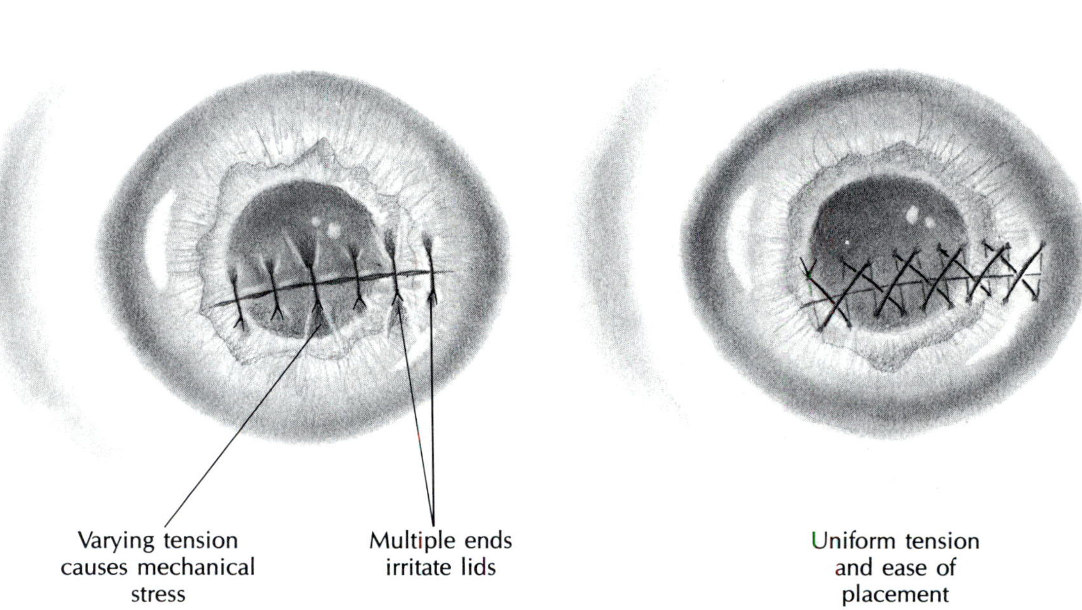

FIGURE 27-2. Wound suturing for corneal lacerations.

Intraocular Foreign-Body and Double Penetrating Injury Management

Before vitrectomy, any visible corneal or scleral wound should be sutured by use of the running-shoelace sutures recommended for corneal repair. Small sutures (10-0) are used for central cornea, 9-0 for the midcornea region, and 8-0 for the peripheral cornea or sclera.

Evaluation of prolapsed tissue is undertaken next. In recent injuries wherein the iris or ciliary body appears viable, it can be irrigated and repositioned. If there is evidence of infection or tissue destruction, excision is recommended. Retinopexy should be reserved for use only in retinal breaks. It should be performed after vitrectomy so that the risk of choroidal hemorrhage is decreased and better visualization is achieved.

If pressure on the globe can be avoided, the posterior wound can be explored if needed. However, there is a risk of prolapse of the vitreous and retina in response to surgical manipulation in this area, and so caution should be exercised. After vitrectomy is completed, the wound can be well localized and the eye softened and filled with air (or gas) before posterior wound repair. It should be noted that most posterior wounds seal themselves and do not require repair.

The vitrectomy instrument, infusion cannula, and endoilluminator enter the wound through an incision in the usual position, 3 mm posterior to the limbus if the lens is to be removed or 4 mm posterior if not. Hypotony and choroidal edema are frequently present in trauma cases, and so care should be taken when one is making this incision.

In cases where the lens is clear, it should remain; one exception to this would involve a very large foreign body that is to be removed translimbally. The aspirating fragmenter is faster in lensectomy, but it should never be used on the vitreous.

In acute cases involving an intraocular foreign body, the vitreous should be removed entirely, whether or not it contains blood. A relatively complete vitrectomy should be done before the foreign body is removed, even though the foreign body may be seen earlier on. Doing so avoids undue traction.

After vitrectomy has been performed, diamond forceps can be used to remove virtually all types of foreign bodies without creating torsion against the retina (Fig. 27-3). Their use has basically eliminated the need for magnets.

For large intraocular foreign bodies, one can enlarge the sclerotomy incision after picking up the foreign body to prevent wound leakage during the pick-up process (Fig. 27-4). Very large intraocular foreign bodies should be removed translimbally after vitrectomy, lensectomy, and fluid-air exchange have been completed. The proper technique is illustrated in Fig. 27-5.

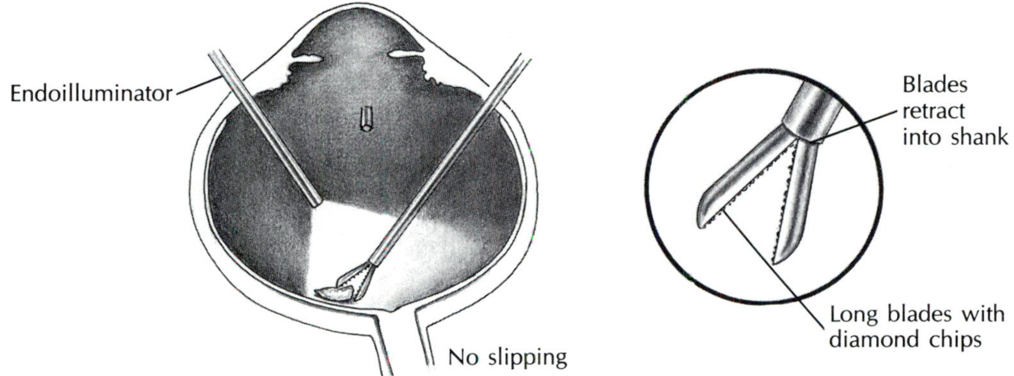

FIGURE 27-3. Diamond intraocular foreign-body forceps.

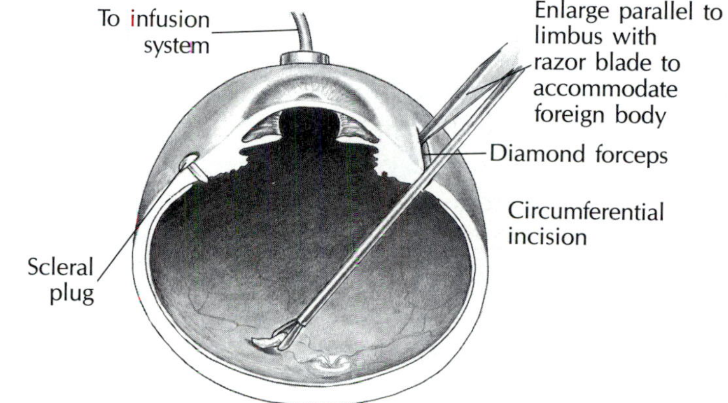

FIGURE 27-4. Enlarging wound for foreign-body removal.

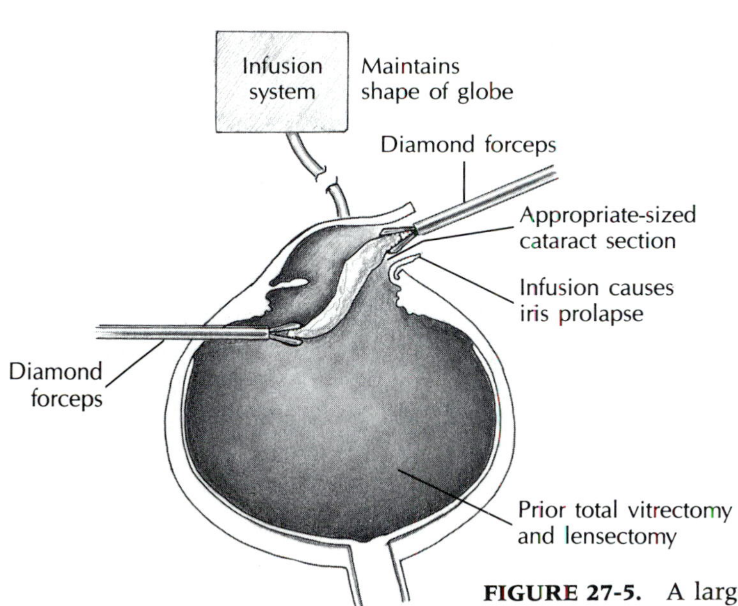

FIGURE 27-5. A large intraocular foreign body (IOFB) should be removed translimbally via a cataract section after vitrectomy and lensectomy.

Long intraocular foreign bodies, such as wire, are usually picked up at right angles to the forceps and require a second pair of forceps to grasp the end and facilitate removal (bimanual transfer, Fig. 27-6). Encapsulated foreign bodies should be excised from the capsule with scissors to prevent retinal traction caused by pulling on the capsule (Fig. 27-7).

Finally, all subretinal foreign bodies can be removed through the original retinal break, or a retinotomy if the foreign body has migrated away from the retinal break (Fig. 27-8). Transscleral removal causes incarceration of the retina and choroidal bleeding.

Once the foreign body is removed, sclerotomy closure can proceed with a running-shoelace 8-0 nylon suture, with care being taken to leave a 20-gauge size opening around a scleral plug. If any material remains, vitrectomy should be completed.

If a definite retinal break is seen, retinopexy should be performed. An exception to this exists if the break is next to the optic nerve, the papillomacular bundle, or the macula, which can lead to detachment and decreased central vision. If the 360-degree conjunctival incision was made, transscleral diathermy in the air-filled eye is a safe method for retinopexy. Internal fluid-air exchange and air-gas exchange should be used for definite retinal breaks. Then any subretinal fluid is drained internally if there is detachment. Finally, diathermy can be performed after the reattachment is completed. Encircling scleral buckles should be used if retinal detachment or peripheral breaks are present.

Antibiotics against both gram-positive and gram-negative organisms should be instilled subconjunctivally as in all vitrectomies. In addition, steroids must be reposited subconjunctivally to decrease fibrin formation and choroidal effusion postoperatively.

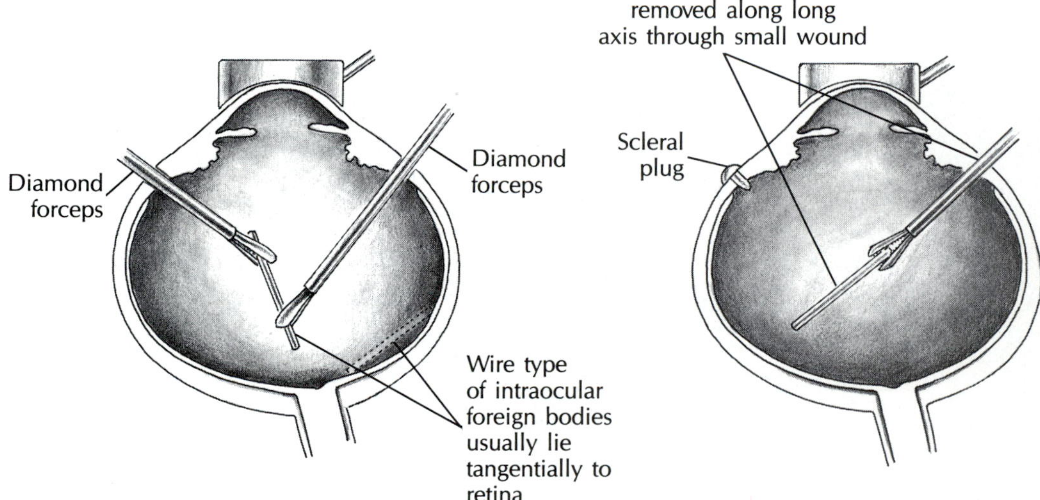

FIGURE 27-6. Bimanual transfer of long intraocular foreign bodies.

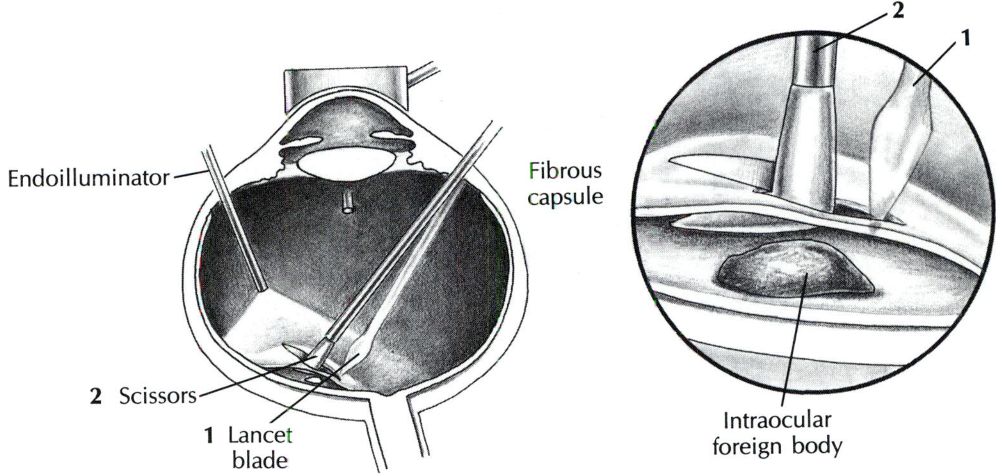

FIGURE 27-7. Opening capsule for encapsulated intraocular foreign bodies.

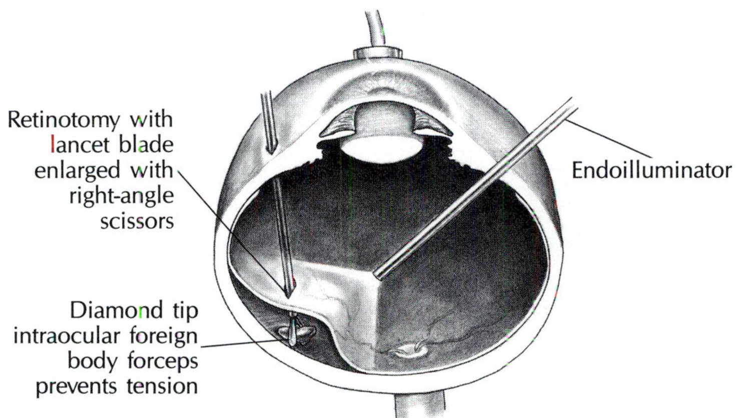

FIGURE 27-8. Subretinal removal of intraocular foreign bodies.

CHAPTER 28

Proliferative Vitreoretinopathy

Proliferative vitreoretinopathy (PVR) is aberrant repair in response to tissue destruction such as retinal break formation, epiretinal membrane dissection, retinotomy, retinal tacks, and all forms of retinopexy (especially cryopexy) (Fig. 28-1). Blood components and inflammation play a role in this process. Because it is indicated by cells and factors, natural and man-made barriers such as the lens, silicone, and gas bubbles cause compartmentalization with an increase in the process of reproliferation.

The majority of the illustrations in this chapter have been modified and redrawn from Charles ST: Vitreous microsurgery, ed 2, Baltimore, 1987, Williams & Wilkins.

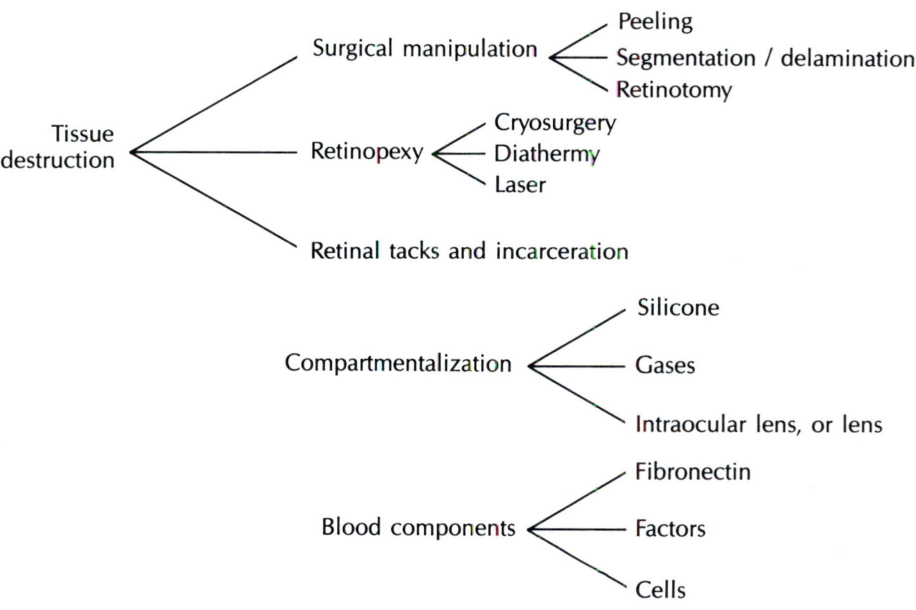

FIGURE 28-1. Factors causing aberrant healing.

The locomotion and contraction mechanism is one and the same. To understand the mechanics of this disease is to understand the role of cellular interactions with the extracellular matrix. The process is hypocellular and has little mitotic activity. In a process known as recruitment the initial cells are joined by other cells resulting in a combination of retinal pigment epithelial, glial, monocytic, and other cells. The process is analogous to keloids and other aberrant processes observed in the body. Complete removal plays a role in recurrent proliferation in contrast to neoplastic diseases.

CLINICAL APPEARANCE

Starfold configuration

Retinal pigment epithelial, glial, and monocytic cells proliferate on the retina and attach with coated pits and fibronectin to the retinal–internal limiting lamina collagen. Pulling on the retina causes the star-fold configuration (Fig. 28-2). Collagen is produced after the star fold is formed. Moderately extensive star folds cause retinal foreshortening and the picture of moderate proliferative vitreoretinopathy (Fig. 28-3). Further star-fold production, creation of the frontal plane by the confluence of the anterior hyaloid and posterior hyaloid faces, anterior loop traction, and circumferential traction lead to the closed-funnel appearance (PVR D3). Annular subretinal proliferation also produces this picture (Fig. 28-4).

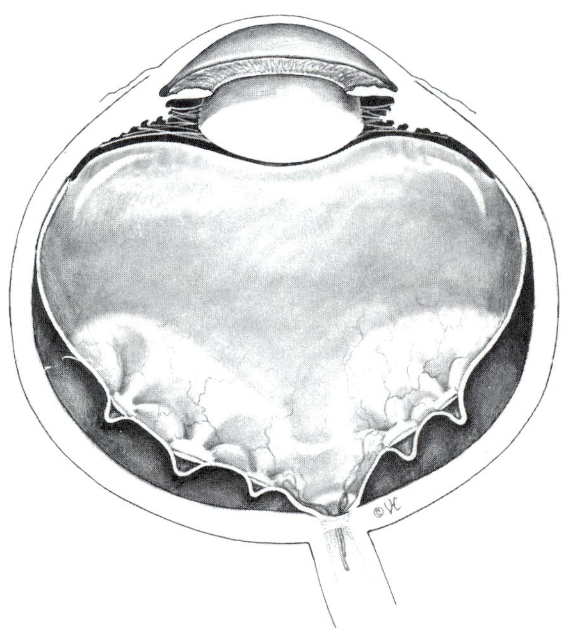

FIGURE 28-2. Pulling on retina causes star-fold configuration.

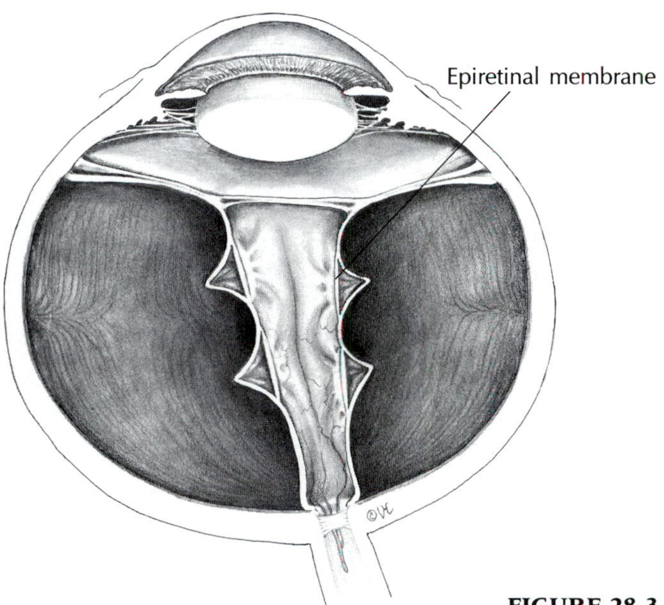

FIGURE 28-3. Moderately extensive star folds.

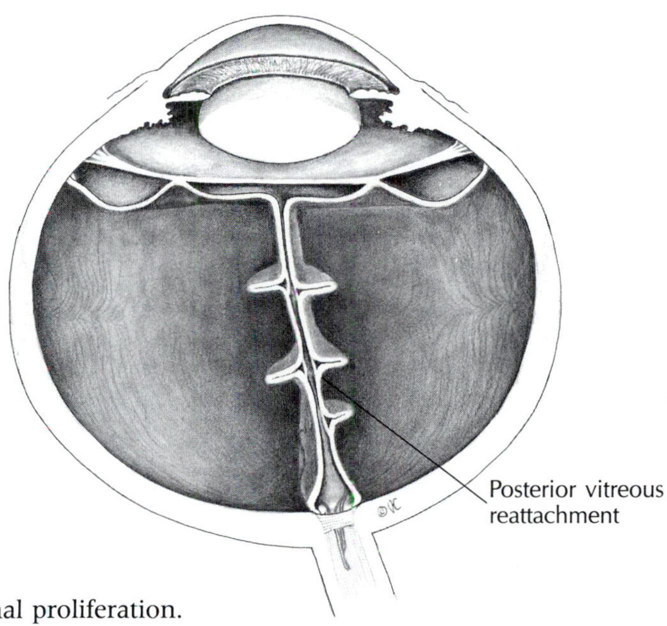

FIGURE 28-4. Annular subretinal proliferation.

Anterior loop traction

Anteroposterior hypocellular gel contraction of preequatorial vitreous cortex results in anterior loop traction (Fig. 28-5). This pulls the equatorial retina anteriorly. Contraction of the anterior hyaloid and posterior hyaloid faces pulls the retina centrally while equatorial fiber contraction accomplishes the same result.

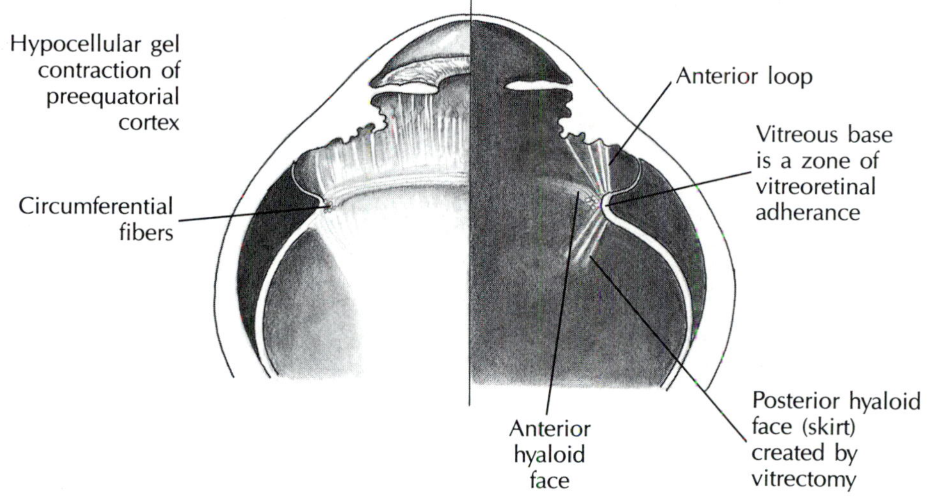

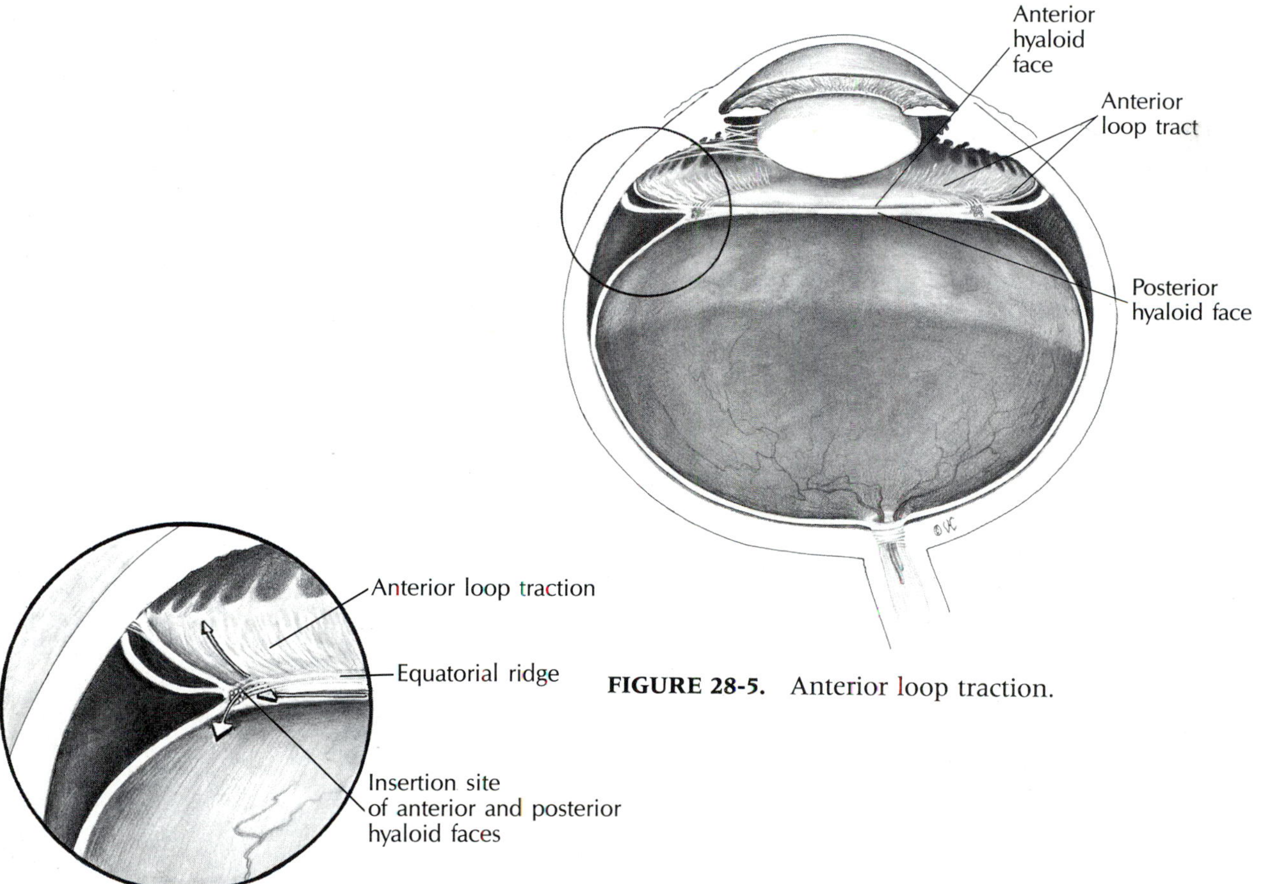

FIGURE 28-5. Anterior loop traction.

Surgical Steps

As outlined in Fig. 28-6, the first step to be taken is decompartmentalization, which involves removing the lens or intraocular lens. This is done to permit cells and factors from the posterior compartments to egress through the trabecular meshwork and to permit the dissection or anterior loop traction. Unless there is extremely dense nuclear sclerosis, an aspirating fragmenter should be used through a pars plana approach.

Next the anterior hyaloid face is removed along with all vitreous attachments to cataract wounds, traumas, and the iris. The posterior hyaloid face is frequently contiguous with the anterior hyaloid face and should be removed in a single step. A configuration typical of proliferative vitreoretinopathy is formed by the hypocellular gel contraction, causing the posterior and anterior hyaloid faces to join and form the "frontal plane."

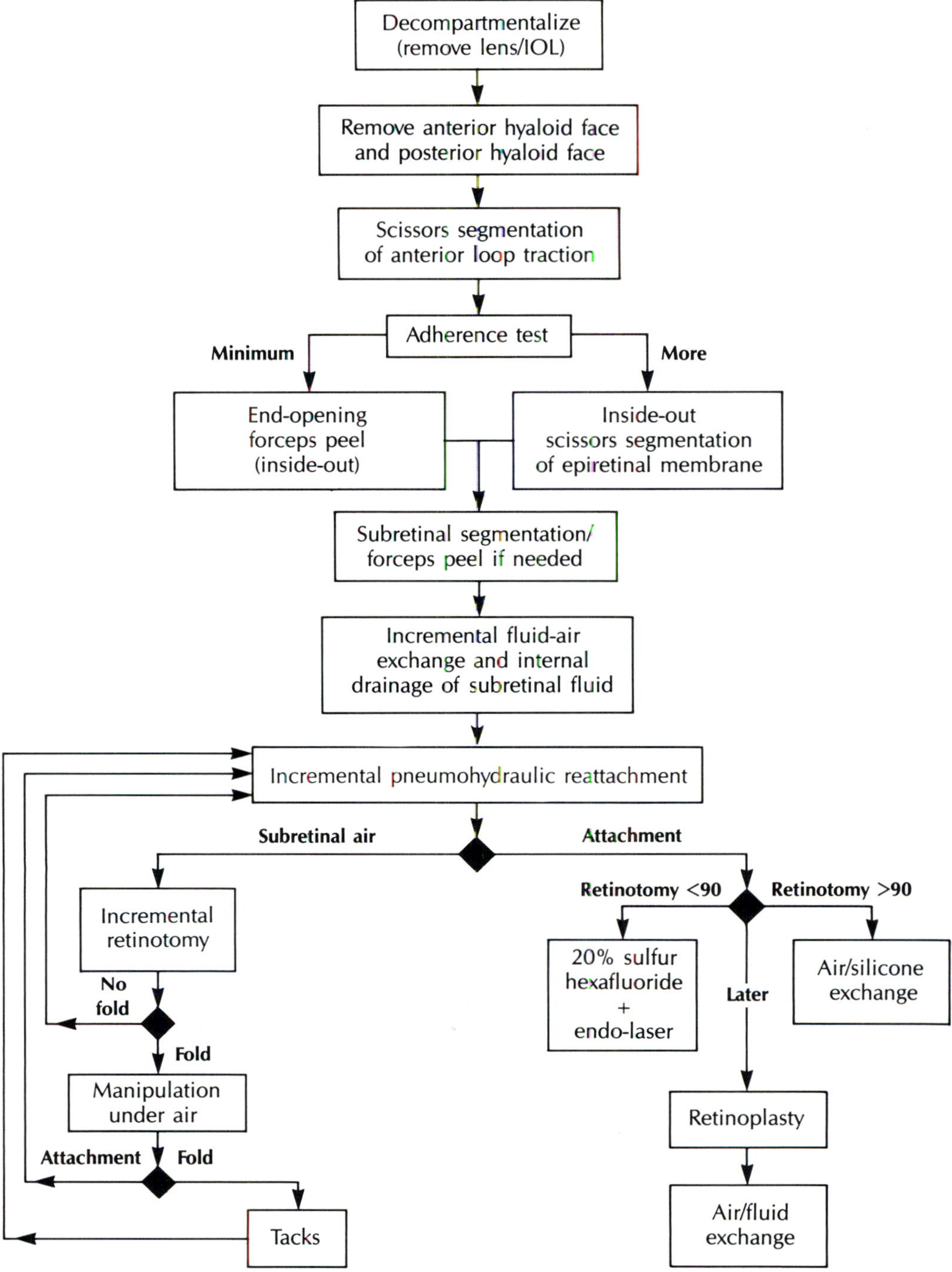

FIGURE 28-6. Algorithm of proliferative vitreoretinopathy.

In the next step, the anterior loop traction is released by dissection. Scleral depression is better than special contact lenses to view the periphery in this procedure (Fig. 28-7). Circumferential cutting with scissors is the preferred method of dissection. Peeling is particularly unsafe, and the vitreous cutter is used only if the anterior loop traction area is wide.

If attempted peeling of epiretinal membrane reveals fibers of retina, segmentation or delamination should then be used. Immature, thinner, and less adherent membranes are removed with end-opening forceps, whereas mature, denser, and more adherent membranes should be segmented before removal (Fig. 28-8).

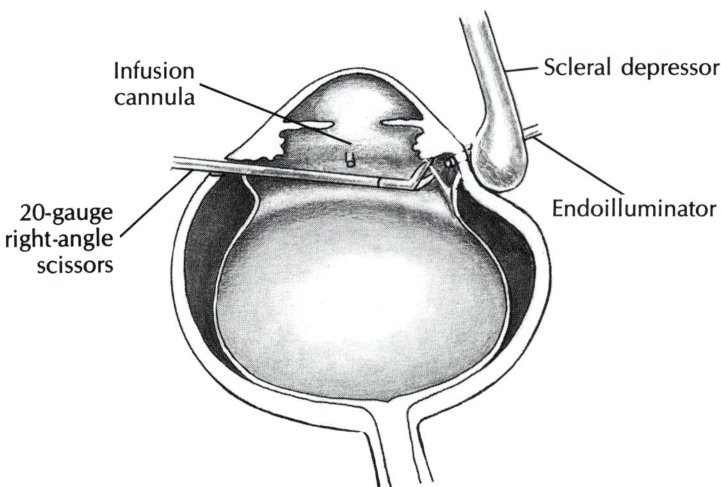

FIGURE 28-7. Anterior loop dissection.

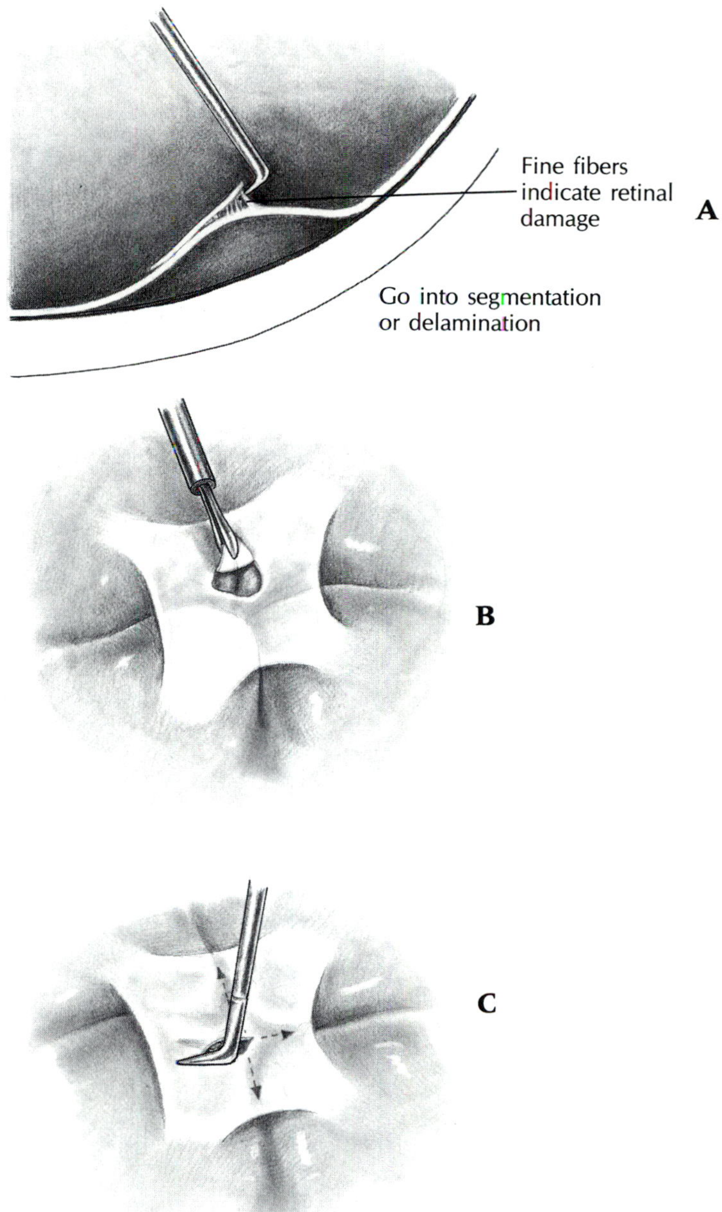

FIGURE 28-8. **A,** Adherence test. **B,** Forceps peel membranes. **C,** Scissors segmentation for star folds.

If there is annular subretinal proliferation, 20-gauge right-angled scissors can be passed through preexisting retinal breaks or a scissors retinotomy can be made to permit section (Fig. 28-9). Many annular, placoid, and extended dendritic subretinal types of subproliferation can be removed with a long, 20-gauge subretinal forceps (Fig. 28-10).

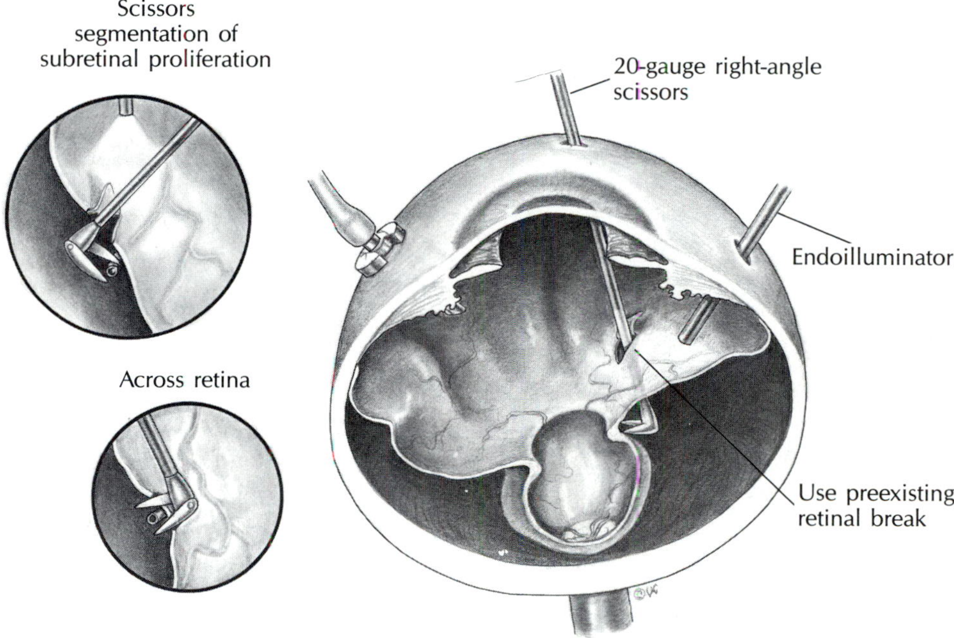

FIGURE 28-9. Scissors segmentations of subretinal tissue.

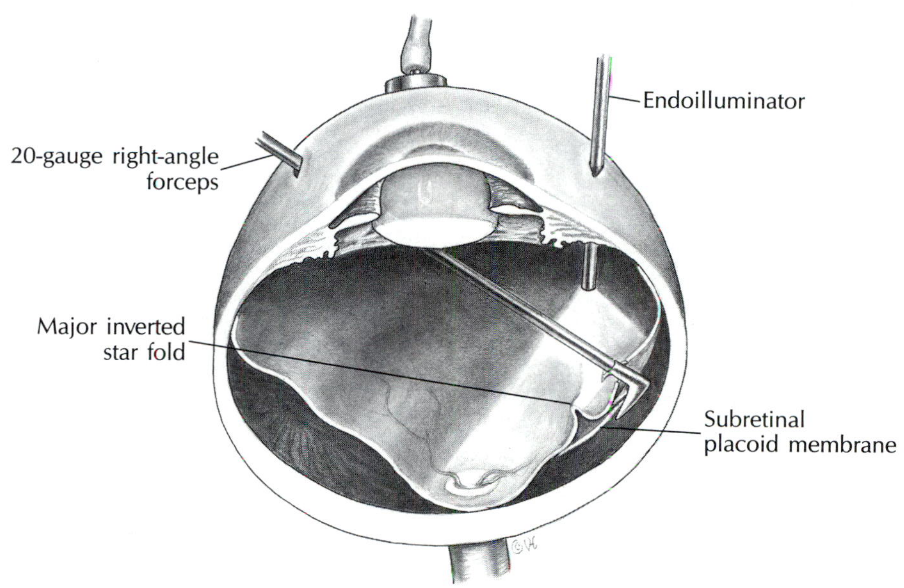

FIGURE 28-10. Subretinal membrane peeling.

Retinotomy

All retinotomies should be performed under air after an initial attempt has been made at reattachment by use of subretinal fluid drainage (Fig. 28-11). Only large vessels require endodiathermy. The retinotomy is managed with endophotocoagulation and gas or silicone.

The implication of incremental retinotomy is to perform as little retinotomy as possible to reduce reproliferation and exposed retinal pigment epithelium (Fig. 28-12). Retinotomy should always follow fluid-air exchange procedures and use of internal drainage of subretinal fluid (see pp. 452 to 459).

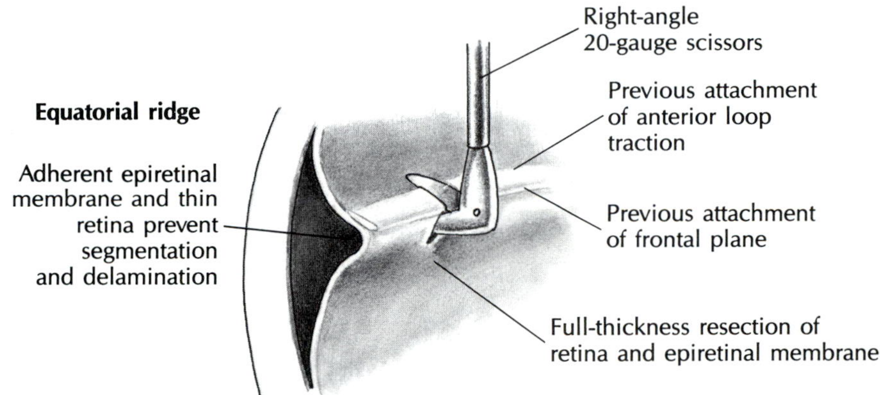

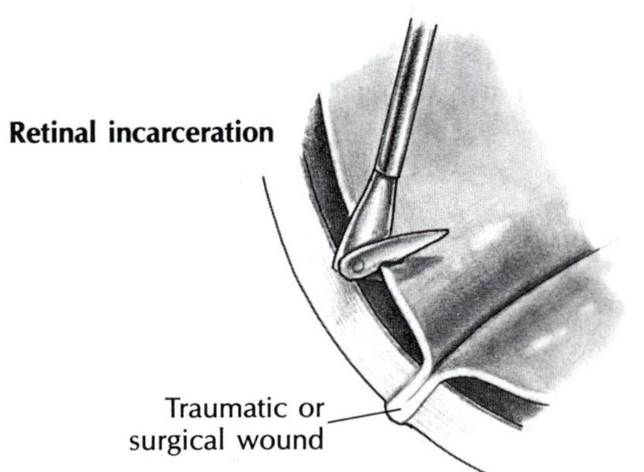

FIGURE 28-11. Retinotomy.

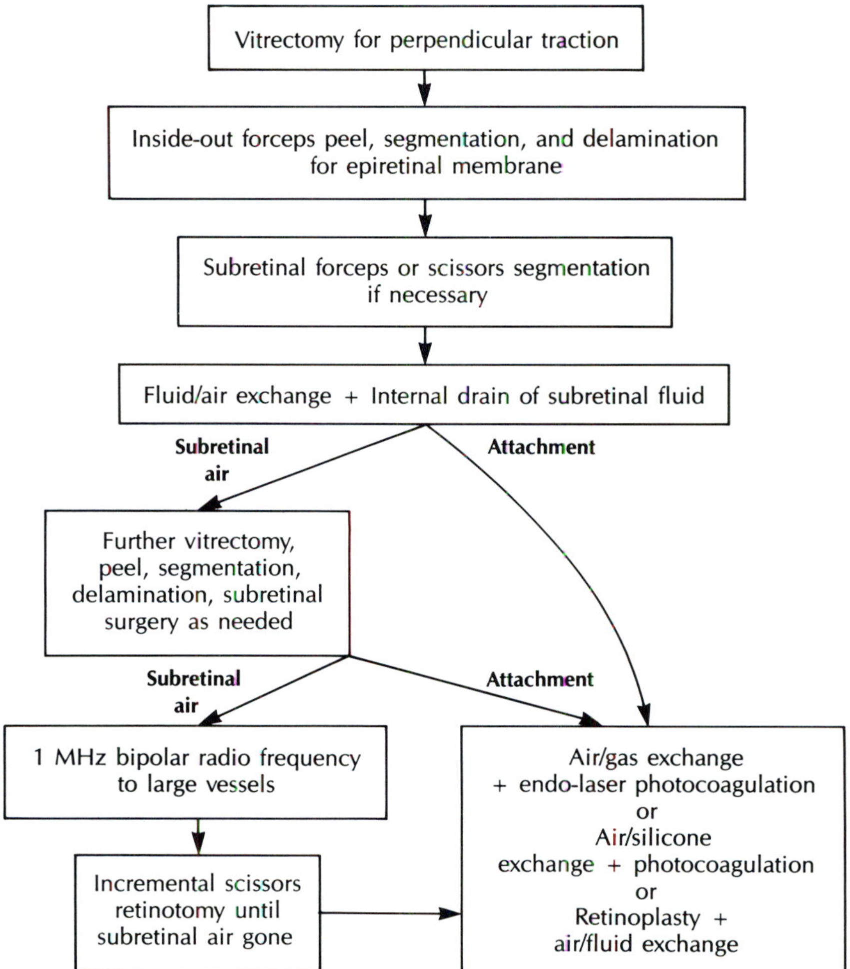

FIGURE 28-12. Algorithm of retinotomy.

Small circumferential retinotomy cuts under air are the safest retinotomy method. When surface tension and molecular adhesion forces exceed the level of traction on the retina, it will reattach (Fig. 28-13).

Radial folds through the macula or causing fluid leakage can be managed with circumferential incremental retinotomy (Fig. 28-14). Circumferential folds can be managed with radial retinotomy, fluid-gas exchange, internal drainage of subretinal fluid, and endophotocoagulation.

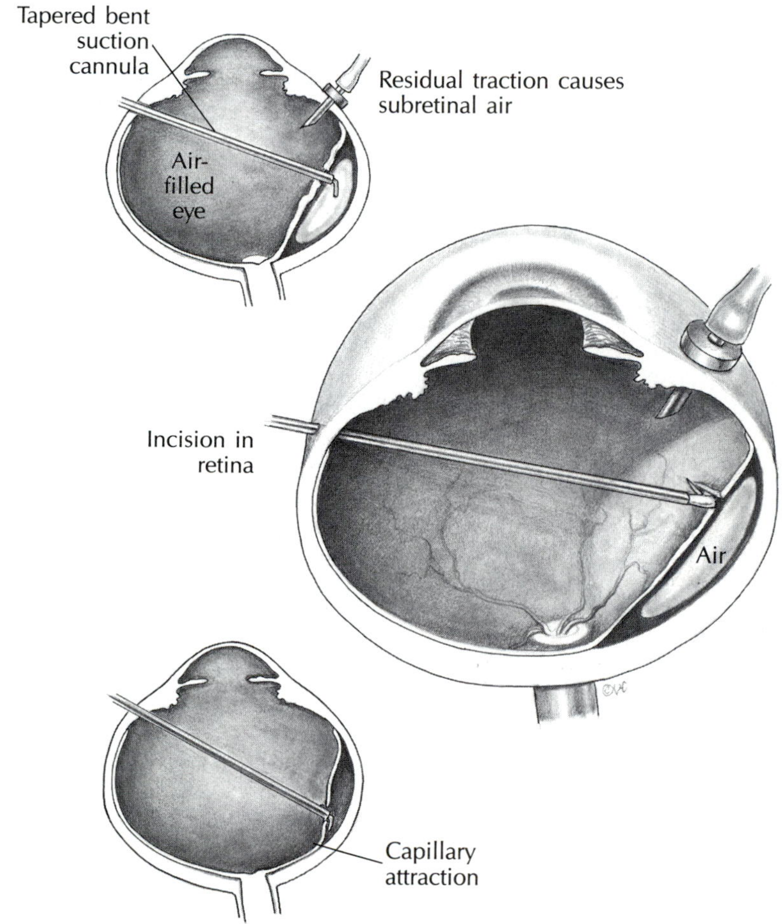

FIGURE 28-13. Incremental retinotomy pneumohydraulic reattachment.

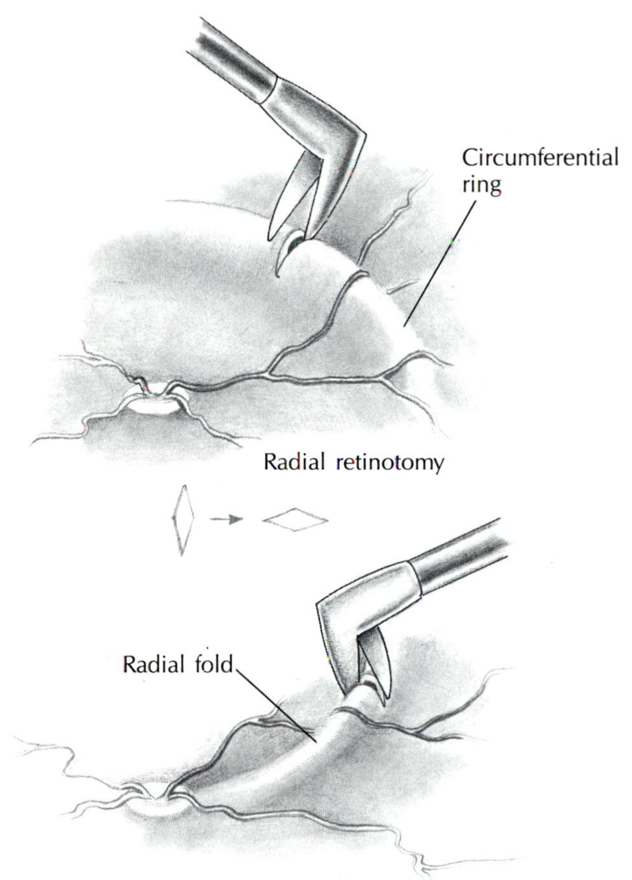

FIGURE 28-14. Retinotomy for folds.

Scissors segmentation, delamination, and retinotomy under air

If the initial fluid-air exchange and internal drainage procedures reveal residual elevation or subretinal air, the retinal surfaces should be inspected and further vitrectomy, delamination, and subretinal surgery performed until the retina flattens (Fig. 28-15). Retinotomy may again be required at this point. Retinoplasty, when available, will be the best management.

Surface tension effect

Air (gas)–fluid interfaces have a surface tension of about 70 dynes/cm, whereas silicone at best has only 42 dynes/cm of surface tension (Fig. 28-16). Hyaluronic acid, blood, and inflammation greatly reduce the surface tension of silicone, leading to emulsification, glaucoma, and incorporation into tissue.

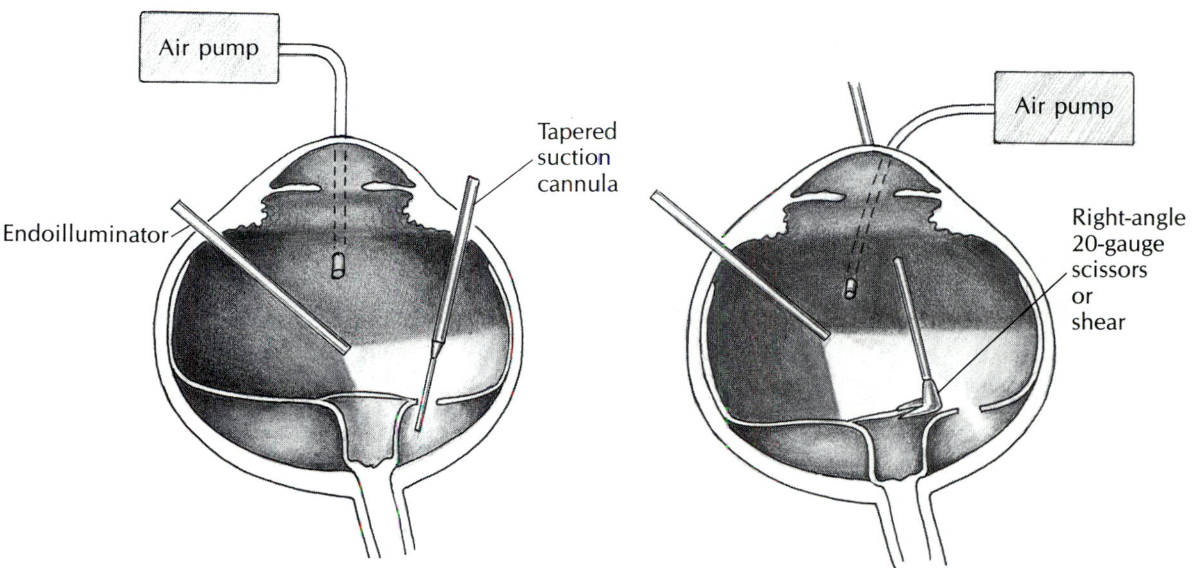

FIGURE 28-15. Scissors segmentation, delamination, and retinotomy under air.

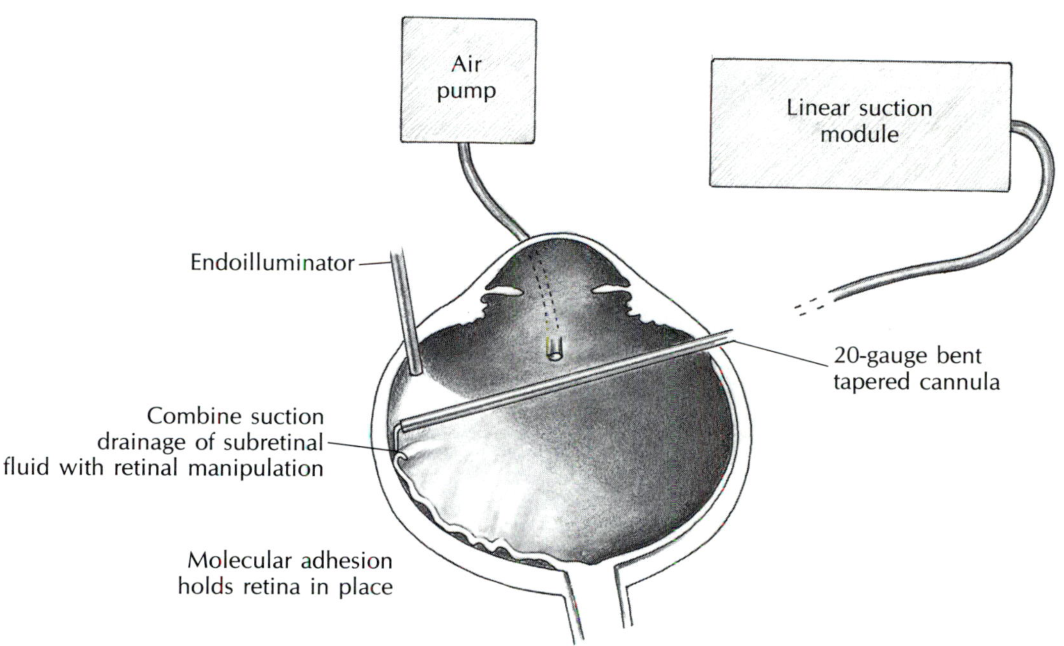

FIGURE 28-16. Retinal manipulation under air.

Silicone and gas

Silicone and gas cause cells and factors (including oxygen and metabolites) to be sequestered at the retinal surface and enhance reproliferation (Figs. 28-17 and 28-18). They also prevent aqueous-phase pharmacologic agents from reaching the retina. Silicone removal in the early postoperative period is the same as for gas (Fig. 28-19). Removal later will produce many corneal-decompensation and permanent-glaucoma cases. Many patients refuse removal, and many retinas redetach when the silicone is removed. Many types of silicone exist, and it is essential to choose that with the highest resistivity and the lowest vapor pressure. A purified silicone with a viscosity of 5000 centistokes has the least monomer and contaminants, thus reducing the emulsification toxicity, inflammation, and corneal problems.

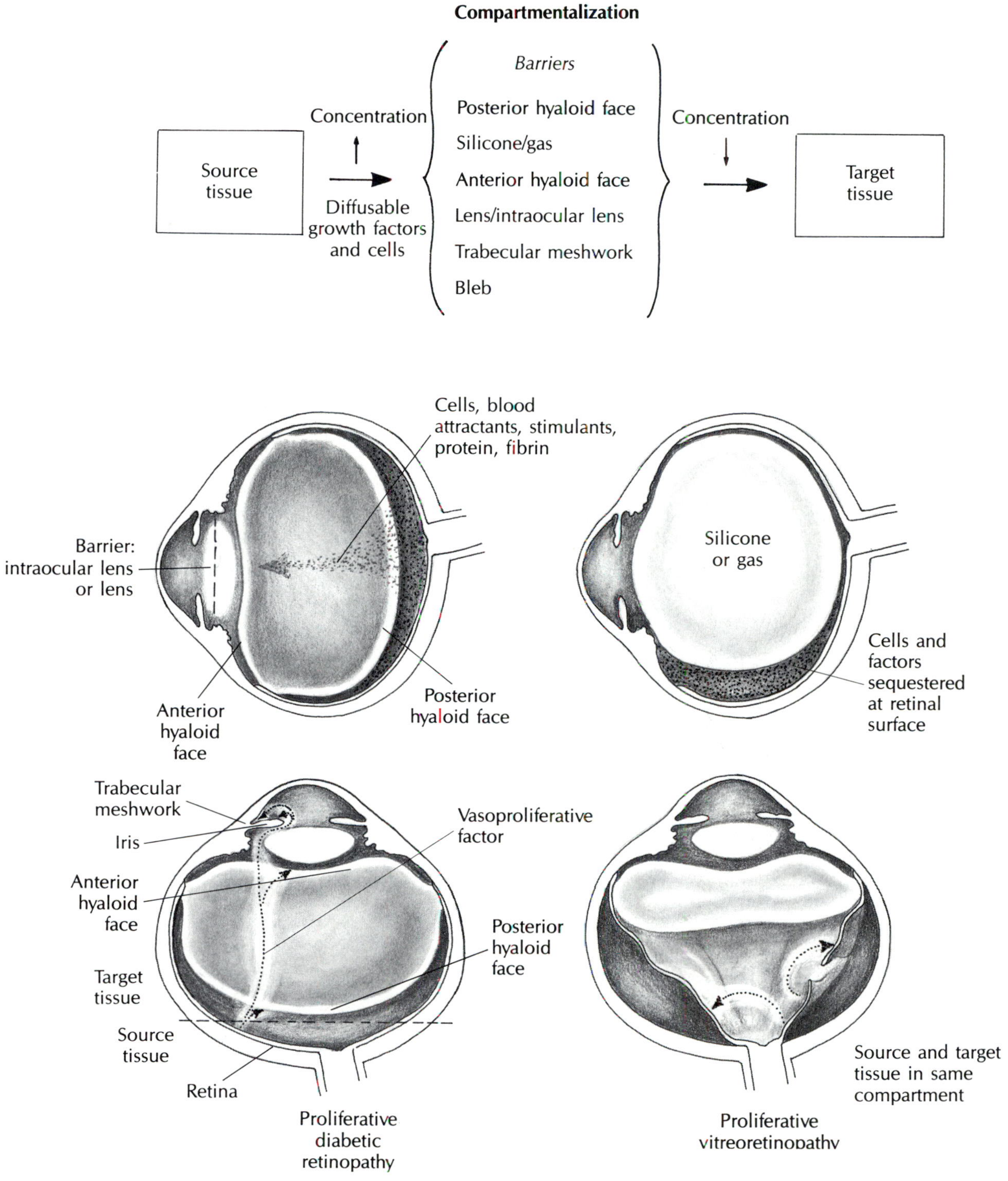

Compartmentalization

Source tissue

Concentration

Diffusable growth factors and cells

Barriers

Posterior hyaloid face

Silicone/gas

Anterior hyaloid face

Lens/intraocular lens

Trabecular meshwork

Bleb

Concentration

Target tissue

Cells, blood attractants, stimulants, protein, fibrin

Barrier: intraocular lens or lens

Anterior hyaloid face

Posterior hyaloid face

Silicone or gas

Cells and factors sequestered at retinal surface

Trabecular meshwork

Iris

Anterior hyaloid face

Target tissue

Source tissue

Retina

Vasoproliferative factor

Posterior hyaloid face

Proliferative diabetic retinopathy

Source and target tissue in same compartment

Proliferative vitreoretinopathy

FIGURE 28-17. Effects of silicone or gas.

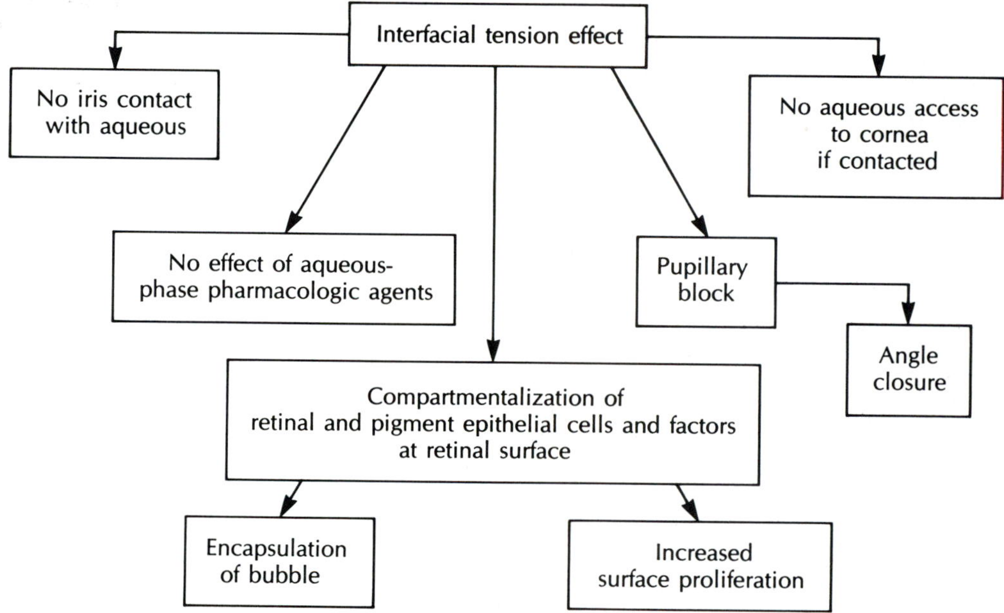

FIGURE 28-18. Algorithm of effects of silicone or gas.

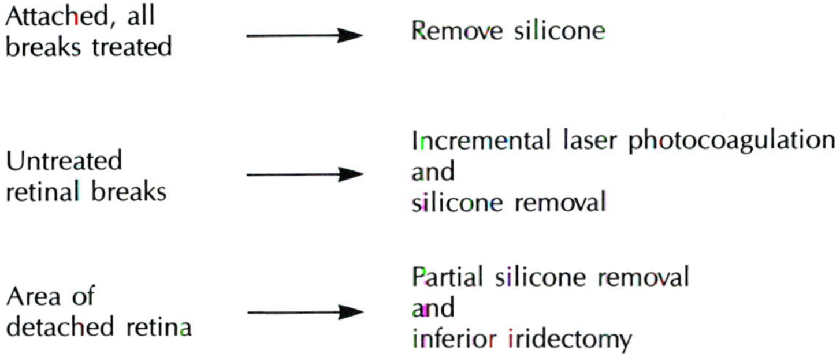

FIGURE 28-19. Silicone postoperative management.

Retinal tacks

Retinal tacks are occasionally needed if retinal manipulation under air cannot correctly reposition giant breaks or large retinotomies (Fig. 28-20). Because of the bleeding, retinal, retinal pigment epithelial, and choroidal damage they produce, their use should be avoided if possible.

Scleral buckling with foreshortened retina

Buckles should be moderately high, uniform in contour, and circumferential in orientation. High localized, especially radial, buckles frequently push the rigid retina away from the retinal pigment epithelium (Fig. 28-21).

POSTOPERATIVE RESULTS

Compulsive decompartmentalization and avoidance of retinal damage reduces postoperative recurrences of proliferative vitreoretinopathy. Minimizing the use of retinopexy and silicone until retinoplasty is available will also reduce reproliferation.

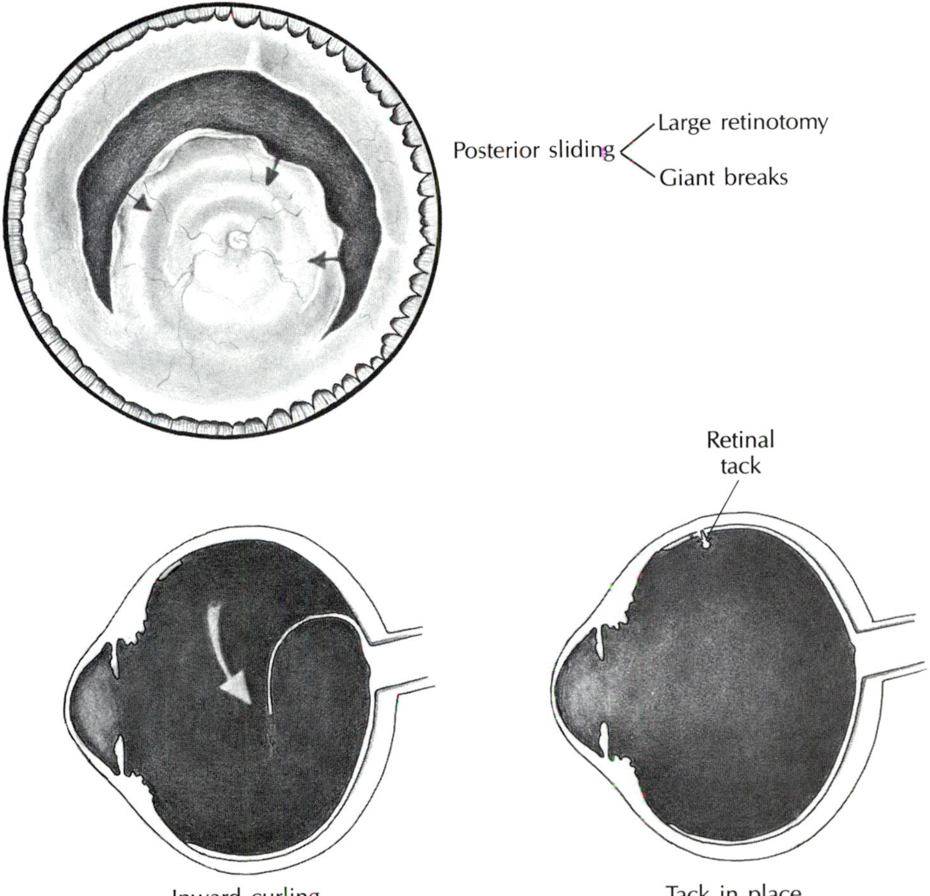

FIGURE 28-20. Purpose of retinal tacks.

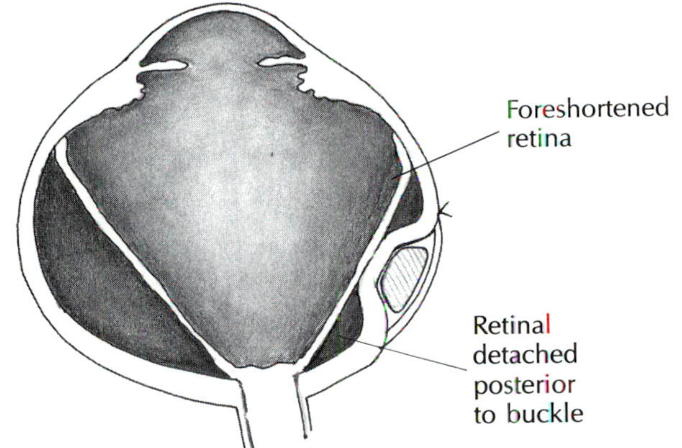

FIGURE 28-21. High buckles with foreshortened retina.

PART SIX

RETINAL SURGERY

Jesse L. Sigelman

CHAPTER 29

Essentials of Retinal Surgery

This chapter encompasses the two major areas of retinal surgery retinal detachment and retinal vascular disease. Both these categories are constituted by individual diseases that by themselves are relatively rare but as a group are epidemiologically significant in the increasing aged population. Large retinal detachment requiring scleral buckling has become a relatively less common disease because of improvements in cataract surgery, whereas small retinal detachments now have a higher incidence because they are being detected even before detachment of the posterior retina. Retinal vascular disease is becoming very common because of the aging of the general population.

The two major groups of retinal surgery have fundamentally different causes. Retinal detachment originates predominantly from a developmental vitreoretinal disorder that predisposes toward tearing of the retina in adulthood. Retinal vascular disease is usually secondary to systemic medical disorders, including diabetes mellitus, hypertension, and arteriosclerosis. The great strides in the treatment of retinal diseases have increased their clinical identification. The advanced techniques described in this chapter most effectively minimize vision loss when the diseases are detected and treated in their early stages.

In retinal detachment, laser photocoagulation and local scleral buckling are among the most significant developments for the treatment of retinal breaks and small retinal detachments. The application of mixed types of scleral buckling using both circumferential and meridional components has provided a tremendous advance in the outcome of surgery for large retinal detachments.

The prognosis of retinal vascular disease has been sharply improved by the use of detailed fluorescein angiography and high magnification biomicroscopy for early and precise diagnosis. For example, senile macular degeneration can only be treated if detected in its extrafoveal stage. Diabetic maculopathy is best treated before the onset of cystic macular degeneration. The recent introduction of new laser wavelengths in the 577 and 640 nanometer ranges has increased the treatment modalities for macular diseases beyond the traditional argon green laser.

PATIENT EVALUATION AND PREPARATION

Patient evaluation for retinal detachment must include complete mapping of the retina with emphasis on preequatorial periphery. Indirect ophthalmoscopy with scleral depression should be augmented by biomicroscopy either by the slitlamp or by the slitbeam indirect ophthalmoscope to obtain full understanding of the vitreoretinal relationship as well as the identification of all retinal breaks. In cases where the patient will require surgery rather than laser treatment, complete surgical preparation must include attention to possible endogenous sources of infection and to possible blood-coagulation abnormalities.

The evaluation for retinal vascular disease necessitates a detailed study of the retina with biomicroscopy, with special attention being paid to the topography of the retina and the pigment epithelium. The relationship between abnormal retinal vasculature and the retina necessitates a geographic analysis of the relationship of the vascular disease to the retina. For example, the relationship between macular edema and a zone of microaneurysms in either diabetic maculopathy or branch vein occlusion is essential to prove the cause-and-effect relationship between them. Retinal vascular diseases also warrant a detailed medical evaluation as part of the diagnostic work-up. The poor control of diabetes can be responsible for worsening maculopathy, and systemic hypertension can be the underlying cause for a retinal vein occlusion. A full ocular examination is also necessary because of the relationship of other ocular conditions and retinal diseases, such as glaucoma and central retinal vein occlusion.

SURGICAL ANATOMY

The surgical anatomy most important for retinal detachment is the retinal periphery anterior to the equator and its relationship to the vitreous base as it inserts approximatey 3 mm posterior to the ora serrata. In retinal vascular disease, the essential surgical anatomy includes not only all the retinal vasculature with particular attention to the retinal capillary bed but also the status of the pigment epithelium, Bruch's membrane, and the choroid. Biomicroscopic analysis of these anatomic components, along with their topographic irregularities and their relationships, is the most important diagnostic step in the diagnosis of retinal vascular disease. Although fluorescein angiography is critically important, it can only augment the conception of the disease as suggested by the biomicroscopic findings.

CHAPTER 30

Diabetic Maculopathy

Diabetic maculopathy refers to the set of changes unique to the macula in diabetic patients. The components of diabetic maculopathy are microaneurysms, cotton-wool exudates, hemorrhages, lipid deposits, and serous fluid. These components are all found in other maculopathies associated with decreased capillary circulation—Coats's disease, branch retinal vein occlusion, and hypertensive retinopathy. The distinctive feature of diabetic maculopathy is its bilaterality, symmetry in both eyes, and inexorable progression. Diabetic maculopathy results from incompetent retinal vasculature with leakage. This differs from proliferative diabetic retinopathy wherein the major problem is neovascularization secondary to ischemia.

ETIOLOGY

The fundamental cause for the changes associated with diabetic maculopathy is abnormal hyperpermeability of the retinal capillary network of the macula. The earliest detectable change is the breakdown of the blood-retinal barrier; this breakdown is observable by vitreous fluorophotometry as soon as 1 year after the onset of diabetes. The other changes of diabetic maculopathy do not appear until more than 10 years after diabetic onset.

The first ophthalmoscopically observable sign of diabetic maculopathy is the appearance of microaneurysms, which occur when macular function remains normal. The microaneurysms are most common at the temporal raphe, which is a watershed zone of circulation. The capillary bed in the region of the microaneurysms shows zones of nonperfusion with the surrounding capillaries acting as shunt vessels around the blocked circulation. The nonperfused retinal areas form discrete units called "ischemic foci." Leakage from the margins of the ischemic foci produces the subsequent exudative maculopathy.

Swelling occurs at the site of ischemic foci because of accumulation of exudate from the diseased capillary system and from cellular edema in reaction to the ischemia.

HISTOLOGY

Histologic examination and angiography show that leakage occurs from microaneurysms and from the shunt capillaries at the margins of ischemic foci. Intraretinal neovascularization lacking tight junctions between endothelial cells is an additional source of edema fluid. Leakage tends to increase as the ischemic foci enlarge because of the increased number of diseased vessels and the progression in breakdown of the endothelial tight junctions.

Plasma leakage and retinal ischemia produce the ophthalmoscopically observable findings. The yellow exudates are composed of both lipid and mucopolysaccharides and accumulate in the outer plexiform layer of the retina because of the large potential interstitial space between the cells in that layer. Albuminous material fills the early deposits. Gradually the inner retinal layers become increasingly involved. This involvement changes the exudate's color from dark yellow to lighter yellow. The presence of serous fluid causes diminished visual acuity because of distortion of the photoreceptors. The deposition of lipid exacerbates the distortion and blocks light transmission to the photoreceptors. Eventually, cellular degeneration produces the final, irreversible loss of macular function as cysts form in the macula.

DIAGNOSIS

The diagnosis of diabetic maculopathy should be made before the onset of symptoms. Stereoscopic biomicroscopy (slitlamp) shows a degree of edematous fluid separating the inner retinal layers from the outer retinal layer. Biomicroscopy also shows the presence of cystoid edema or massive cystic cellular degeneration.

Fluorescein angiography is the most accurate method of determining the status of the macular capillary bed, including the full extent of ischemic foci. Cystoid macular edema is best diagnosed in the late phase of angiography, approximately 45 minutes after the fluorescein injection in comparison to the early phase of angiography, which shows the capillary details. Angiography is crucial in allowing delineation of the degree and location of leakage from ischemic foci surrounding the macula. Ischemic foci are delineated in the arterial venous phase when the leakage is not so copious that it blurs the capillary margins. The degree of fluorescein leakage in the later phases of angiography is variable: one area may show extensive leakage, whereas another ischemic area may show only minor leakage.

NATURAL HISTORY AND CLASSIFICATION

Background maculopathy is the early stage when ischemic foci are sparse, small, and only slightly leaky. Edema of the macula is minimal at this stage, and there is only a small degree of capillary closure. Cases with background maculopathy can show cystoid macular edema from ischemia. In background maculopathy, the macula shows little serous fluid or lipid exudate. In cases of advanced ischemia, cotton-wool spots are prevalent. Background maculopathy does not warrant treatment by photocoagulation.

Focal leakage is the second stage of diabetic maculopathy and shows ischemic foci that are large and more numerous than those of background maculopathy. By this stage, the ischemic foci demonstrate fluorescein leakage and produce retinal thickening. It is at this stage that the diabetic maculopathy can first interfere with macular function. Vision can also be normal at this stage. The focal leakage stage has the best potential response to photocoagulation treatment of any stage of diabetic maculopathy. Treatment is indicated for cases where there is a swollen ischemic focus within 500 μm of the fovea.

In diffuse leakage maculopathy, the next stage, the macula is diffusely swollen from capillary leakage and ischemic foci scattered throughout the macula. The accumulation often is associated with severe metamorphopsia and decreased visual acuity. At this stage, the cellular elements of the retina are beginning to undergo degeneration as the result of nutritional deprivation from microcystic edema. Photocoagulation is indicated in a grid pattern in an attempt to stabilize or improve the macular edema.

At the stage of cystic degeneration, the cellular elements of the macula are so far degenerated that no treatment is possible. The extensive accumulation of edema fluid along with lipid exudate and necrosis of the Müller cells, the supporting cells of the retina, give a poor functional or anatomic prognosis.

The degree of ischemia can play a significant role in maculopathy. In cases where there is extensive closure of the macular capillary bed, laser photocoagulation is of no use. In addition, laser photocoagulation of the withdrawn perifoveal capillary network can produce chronic edema where none existed before. Destruction of a significant percentage of the macular capillary bed by photocoagulation can produce a permanent devastating result.

Photocoagulation Technique

Argon green is the most effective wavelength for treatment of diabetic maculopathy because of its absorption by the pigment epithelium and possible absorption by the retinal vasculature. Krypton red can be used in cases where hemorrhage or cataract prevents passage of the green wavelength.

For treatment of focal leakage maculopathy, photocoagulation aims to seal the ischemic focus, which is causing the accumulation of edema fluid and exudate in the macula. A recent fluorescein angiogram is necessary to localize the full extent of the ischemic zone, which appears in the fundus as a swollen retinal area demarcated by exudate primarily on its macular side (Fig. 30-1, *A*).

With the argon green laser, use a spot size as small as 100 μm. Starting with a power setting of 100 milliwatts and a duration of 0.5 seconds, gradually increase the power until a faint gray burn appears. A small increment in power should then produce a gray-white reaction. A dense white reaction is unnecessarily severe and worsens postoperative symptoms by producing destruction of the overlying nerve fiber layer. Place the burns to overlap so that the entire area of the ischemic focus and its margins are coagulated.

For the krypton red laser, set the laser for a 200 μm spot size and 0.5 second duration. Gradually increase the power setting until a yellow-white reaction results. A more intense reaction is unnecessary. Cover the entire area of the ischemic focus with contiguous and even overlapping coagulations. There is no need to re-treat already treated zones (Fig. 30-1, *B*).

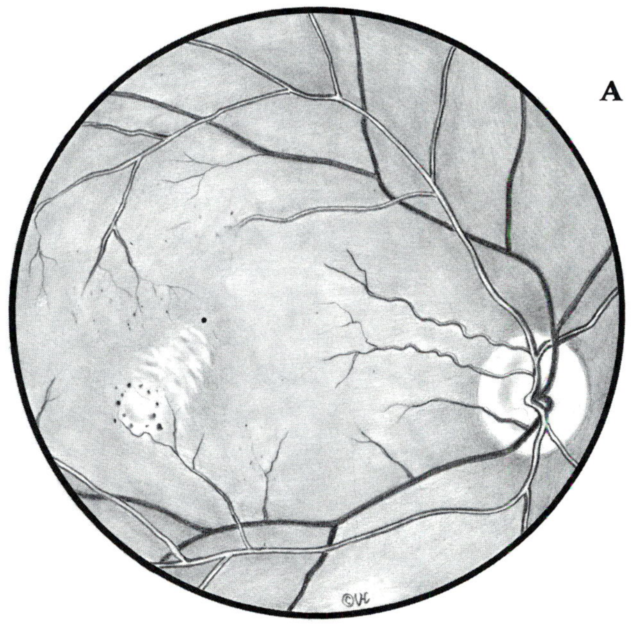

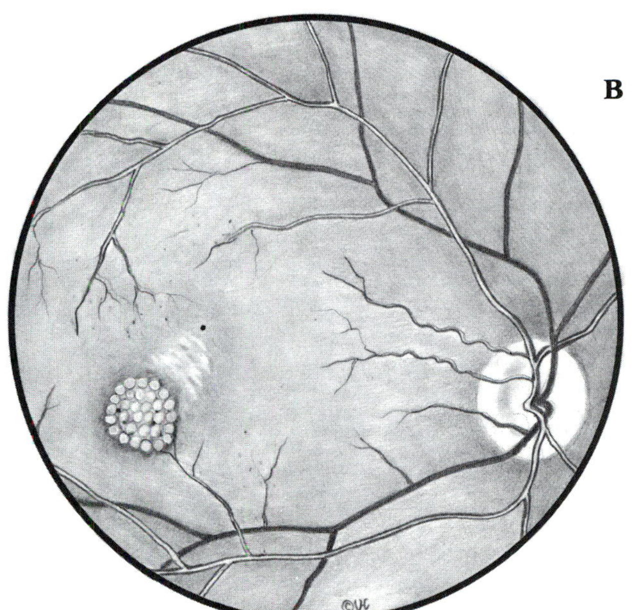

FIGURE 30-1. **A,** Focal leakage before laser treatment. **B,** Laser photocoagulation.

Follow-up study for focal leakage photocoagulation

By 4 weeks after photocoagulation the treated areas should show pigmented scars, and by 8 weeks after treatment the scars should be mature, the ischemic focus closed, and the exudate diminished. Fluorescein angiography should show no retinal perfusion and no late leakage from the treated zone (Fig. 30-2). The macula should show resolution of exudate and edema. Failure of this type of resolution by 8 weeks after treatment warrants repeat photocoagulation. It is unnecessary to repeat the photocoagulation sooner than that.

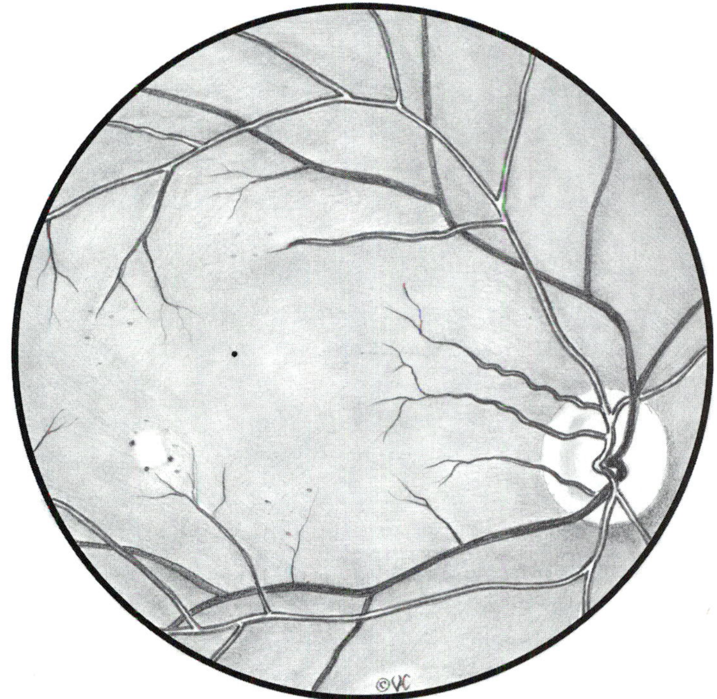

FIGURE 30-2. After treatment.

Laser Photocoagulation of Diffuse Maculopathy

In diffuse leakage maculopathy, the aim of photocoagulation is to diminish edema. The photocoagulation is unable to diminish retinal leakage because of the density of ischemic foci (Fig. 30-3, *A*). Destruction of all the foci would leave the posterior pole without adequate circulation. The aim of photocoagulation for diffuse maculopathy is to diminish macular edema by increasing the ability of the pigment epithelium to pass the edema fluid into the choriocapillaris. The edema accumulation that diminishes vision by distorting the retina (Fig. 30-3, *B*) can pass to the choriocapillaris and allow the macula to reapproach its normal configuration and improve photoreceptor and retinal function.

Grid-pattern laser photocoagulation consists in creating an approximately even grid of 50 or 100 μm argon green or 200 μm krypton red photocoagulation spots throughout the posterior pole so that the perifoveal capillary network is spared. The large krypton spot is necessary to diminish the risk of choroidal rupture and hemorrhage. The smaller spot size with argon has the advantage of diminishing postoperative complication of symptomatic positive scotomas.

The intensity of the laser burns for grid pattern should be low. The ultimate coagulation should produce only a faint gray reaction in the case of argon green and faint yellow reaction in the case of krypton. A more intense photocoagulation is unnecessary. The coagulation should not be contiguous (Fig. 30-3, *C*). Be certain that the photocoagulation burns do not extend closer than 250 μm from the perimeter of the perifoveal capillary net.

A

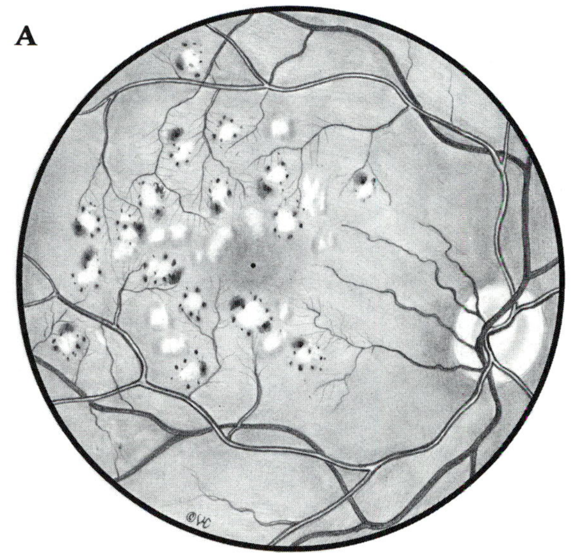

B

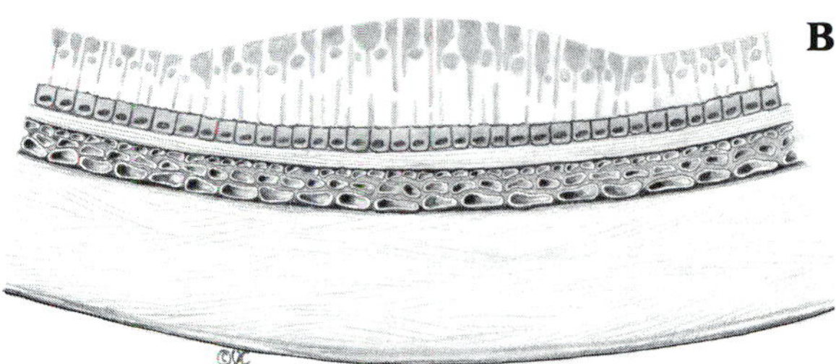

C

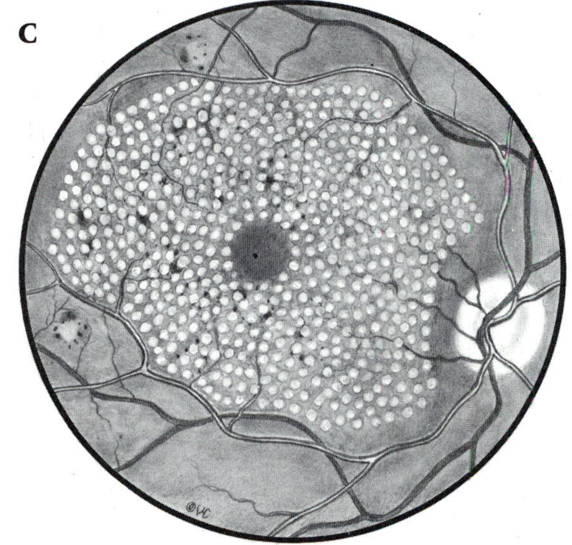

FIGURE 30-3. **A,** Diffuse leakage. **B,** Distortion of retina by edema. **C,** Treatment area.

FOLLOW-UP STUDY

Alert the patient before treatment that visual acuity is likely to worsen after grid-pattern laser for a period of up to 6 weeks, when the vision will begin to resolve. The resolution tends to be maximal at 3 months after laser, but the grid-pattern laser treatment should not be repeated until at least 3 to 4 months after the initial treatment. A satisfactory result shows partial resolution of the edema (Fig. 30-4, *A*) with only faintly visible laser scars (Fig. 30-4, *B*). Failure to observe any resolution of the edema or diminution of lipid exudate warrants repeat grid-pattern treatment. After an initially good result with the grid pattern, the macular edema can begin to worsen again at 6 months to 1 year after the initial treatment. The grid-pattern laser should be repeated then.

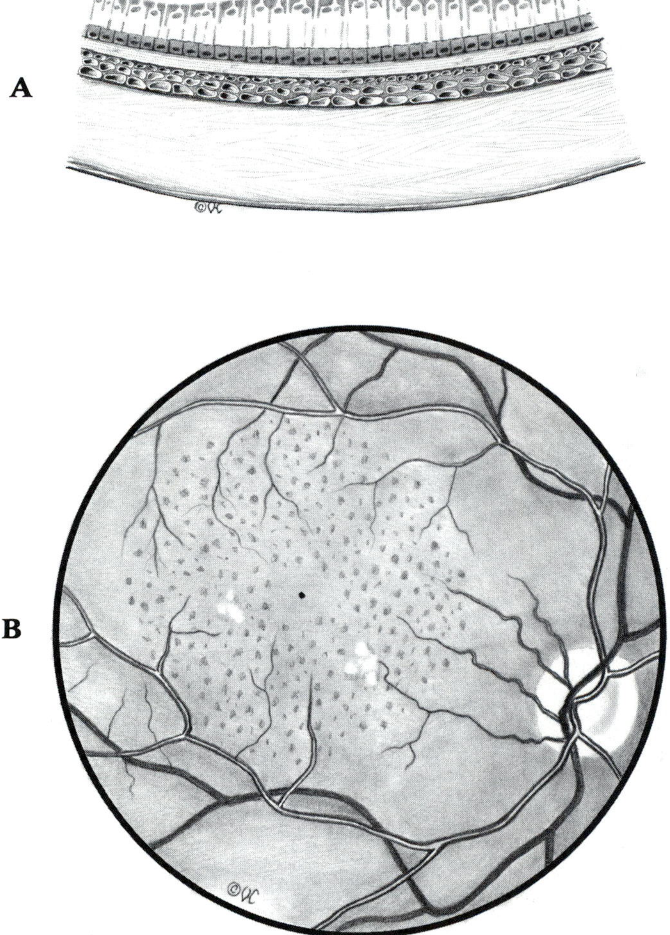

FIGURE 30-4. A, Reduced retinal swelling after treatment. **B,** Grid laser of diffuse leakage.

COMPLICATIONS

The major complication is photocoagulation within the area of the retracted perifoveal capillary zone. In diabetic maculopathy, the extension of the capillary zone and sparsity of capillaries around the fovea make the circulation precarious (Fig. 30-5). If the photocoagulation extends into the perifoveal zone, destroying the residual capillary net, chronic edema will result. In addition, photocoagulation should not extend heavily through areas where there is no extensive leakage as shown on angiography in order to diminish the reactive edema after treatment and the ultimate scotoma.

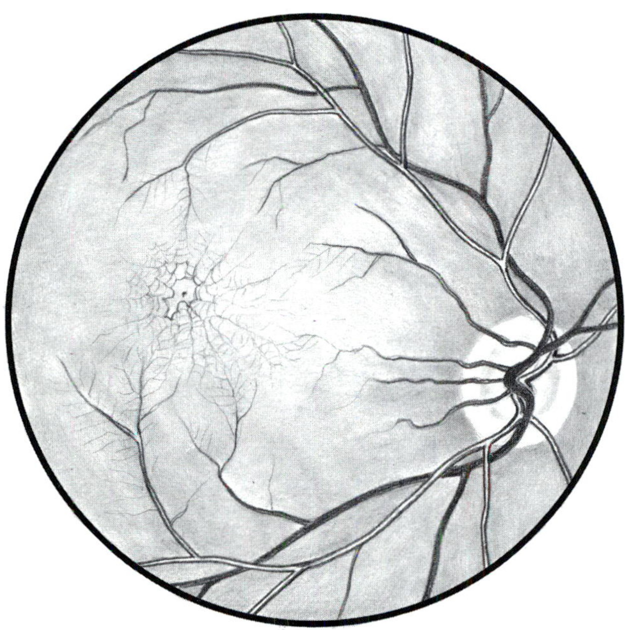

FIGURE 30-5. Excessive laser photocoagulation destroying residual perifoveal capillary net.

CHAPTER 31

Macroaneurysm

A retinal macroaneurysm is an isolated dilatation of a major retinal arterial branch. It is a unique retinal angiopathy because of its association with systemic hypertension, arteriosclerosis, and retinal embolization. Unlike the multiple aneurysms of Coats's disease, cavernous hemiangioma of the retina, or Leber's multiple miliary aneurysms, a retinal macroaneurysm is a primary isolated arterial dilatation that is the fundamental cause for the surrounding microangiopathy and vascular incompetence. The macroaneurysm is, of course, larger than a microaneurysm. The macroaneurysm is an isolated abnormality in an otherwise normally perfused but arteriosclerotic vasculature. The macroaneurysm occurs without association with diabetes or ischemia.

ETIOLOGY

Old age, hypertension, arteriosclerosis, and focal damage to the arterial wall cause the formation of the macroaneurysm. The focal damage can result from retinal arterial emboli, which cause incomplete arterial occlusions and zones of retinal arterial infarction.

The average age of patients with macroaneurysms is 66 years, with a range from 49 to 83 years. As with intracranial aneurysms, macroaneurysms show a predominance in women over 50 years of age. Approximately 25% of patients with macroaneurysm show the effects of systemic vasculopathy (myocardial infarction, stroke, and abdominal aortic aneurysm) within 5 years of the retinal diagnosis. They have a high mortality. Ophthalmodynamometry is unremarkable in this patient group.

DIAGNOSIS

A macroaneurysm can be detected as an isolated phenomenon or it can be the cause for decreased visual acuity from macular edema, circinate maculopathy, or vitreous hemorrhage. When little exudation or hemorrhage is present, the balloon-shaped appearance of the macroaneurysm is evident. The macroaneurysms usually are single and located at the first or second branch of the temporal arteries, often at a bifurcation. The macroaneurysms can be multiple and located on any arterial branch. Their size ranges from a subtle expansion of the artery up to three times the normal arterial width. Systolic pulsations are evident in cases where the vessel wall is thin.

Yellow lipid deposition in the intraretinal and subretinal space can accumulate sufficiently around the macroaneurysm to obscure the aneurysm's detection. Most commonly the exudate and edema surround the macroaneurysm. Only occasionally do macular edema and exudate show no obvious geographic connection to the macroaneurysm (in contrast to the common geographic separation in angiomatosis retinae).

The hemorrhage from a macroaneurysm collects in the preretinal and subretinal spaces and in the retina itself. The hemorrhage can break through the hyaloid to produce a dense intravitreal hemorrhage. Vitreous haze can develop solely from exudation.

Fluorescein angiography demonstrates the full size of the macroaneurysm despite the enormity of circinate retinopathy. During angiography, the aneurysmal wall stains and dye leaks eventually into the surrounding retina. Intraretinal microvascular abnormalities surrounding the macroaneurysm are an additional source of leakage. The structure resembles the ischemic zone in diabetic maculopathy with widening of the periarterial capillary-free zone, dilatation of the adjacent capillary bed with small zones of capillary nonperfusion, capillary microaneurysms rimming the avascular zone around the aneurysm, and fine-caliber intraretinal collateral vessels.

INDICATIONS FOR TREATMENT

The indication for treatment of macroaneurysm is exudation or hemorrhage, or both. A macroaneurysm without these complications carries a good prognosis and requires no treatment. An asymptomatic macroaneurysm should be observed at regular intervals (approximately every 6 months) and considered for photocoagulation treatment only if it causes maculopathy or threatens a massive hemorrhage.

A macroaneurysm that produces only local edema and exudate does not warrant photocoagulation if the macula is uninvolved. The edema and exudation can remain localized for months or years without macular involvement. Eventually the exudate is resorbed after thrombosis, whose immediate effect is a small, local hemorrhage that seals the macroaneurysm. Hemorrhage of the retina alone is not an indication for photocoagulation. If hemorrhage dissects into the macula, it usually does so quickly and resorbs spontaneously. Photocoagulation is of no benefit for those cases in which the macula suffers morphologic change from subretinal hemorrhage or from dissection of blood into the subpigment epithelial space where it can produce a clinical picture that mimics senile macular degeneration.

The principal indication for photocoagulation of a macroaneurysm is the persistence by the macular edema or circinate retinopathy without spontaneous improvement in visual acuity after 3 months of observation. Enlargement of the macroaneurysm or extension of exudation into the macula during sequential observation is another indication for photocoagulation. Pulsatile movement of a macroaneurysm's wall is a third indication because the pulsatility indicates that the wall is so thin that it could rupture and produce a vitreous hemorrhage.

Photocoagulation Technique

The aim of photocoagulation is to stimulate fibrosis of the wall of the macroaneurysm and to coagulate its surrounding leaking capillaries. In cases with multiple macroaneurysms, photocoagulation should be directed to the leaking macroaneurysm as demonstrated on fluorescein angiography or as shown by the collection of circinate retinopathy (Fig. 31-1, *A*). Do not photocoagulate macroaneurysms unassociated with leakage.

Use the argon green laser with a 100 or 200 μm spot size for a duration of 0.2 or 0.5 seconds with a power setting of 200 milliwatts or higher in order to obtain a gray-white reaction on the surface of the macroaneurysm. Do not attempt to produce a dense white reaction, which could produce rupture of the macroaneurysm and hemorrhage. Usually, between 50 and 75 photocoagulation spots suffice to produce a moderate coagulative reaction in the macroaneurysm and the surrounding retina (Fig. 31-1, *B*). Do not photocoagulate the macula where exudate has accumulated. For treating a large, pulsatile microaneurysm, increase the spot size to 200 or 500 μm in order to decrease the risk of rupturing the wall of the macroaneurysm during photocoagulation.

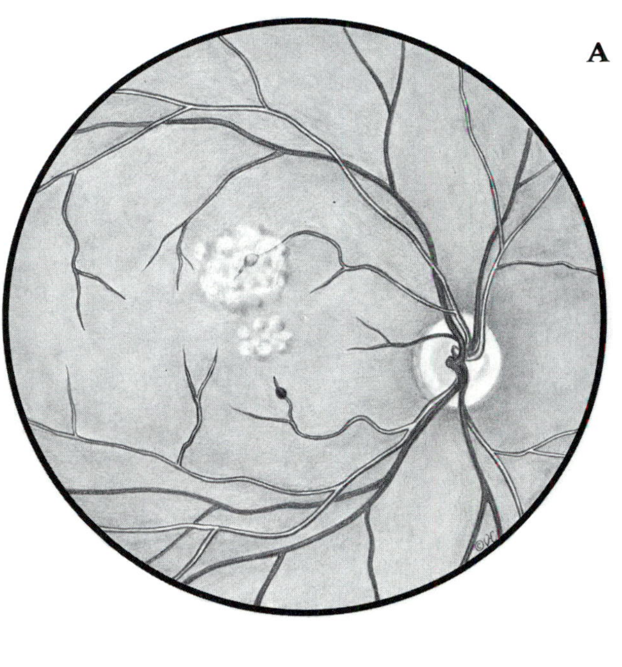

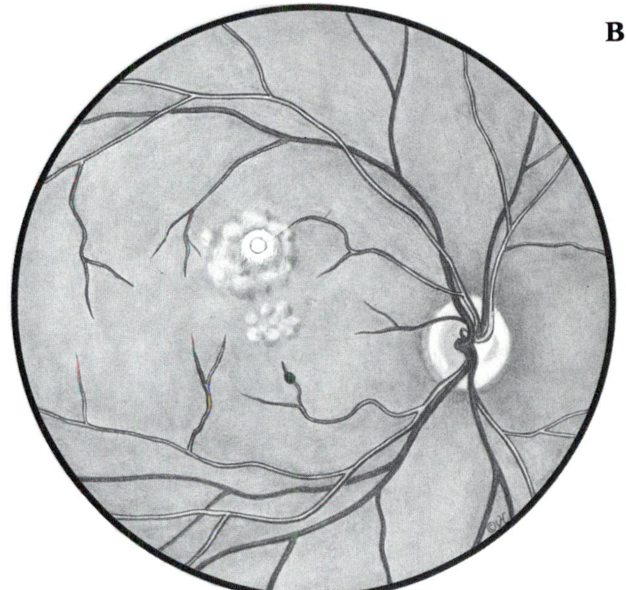

FIGURE 31-1. Photocoagulation technique.

FOLLOW-UP STUDY

The ideal response to treatment is fibrosis of the wall of the macroaneurysm. By approximately 3 to 6 months after treatment, a pigmented scar develops at the treatment site and there is at least partial restoration of macular anatomy with the improvement of macular function depending on the degree of degeneration of retinal cells during the pretreatment exudative phase. The exudate should undergo resorption within 3 to 6 months (Fig. 31-2). By 6 weeks after photocoagulation, fluorescein angiography should show staining but no leakage at the macroaneurysm site.

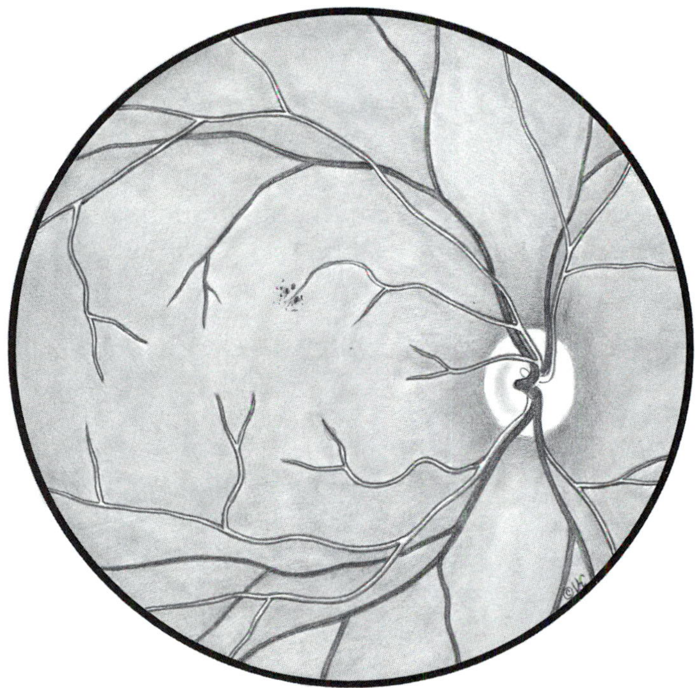

FIGURE 31-2. Result of treatment.

COMPLICATIONS

Closure of the treated artery and macular pucker are the major potential complications of photocoagulation. To avoid closure of the artery, keep in mind that photocoagulation does not have to produce an intense response to achieve fibrosis of the macroaneurysm wall. The ideal outcome of photocoagulation is to thicken the tissue surrounding the macroaneurysm so that leakage or hemorrhage will not result (Fig. 31-3, *A*). Excessive photocoagulation can produce complete closure of the treated artery (Fig. 31-3, *B*). This outcome produces chronic cystoid edema by destroying a portion of the perifoveal capillary network (Fig. 31-3, *C*). No treatment helps this complication.

The risk of macular pucker can be diminished by avoidance of full-thickness retinal photocoagulation. Preventing absorption of the photocoagulation energy by the innermost retinal layers and internal limiting membrane surrounding the macroaneurysm diminishes the risk of pucker.

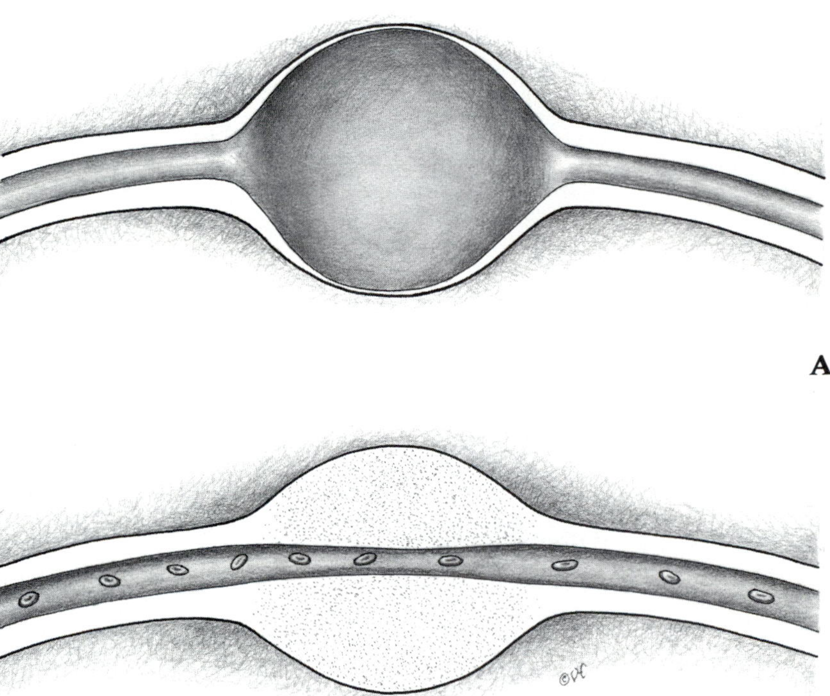

FIGURE 31-3. Complications of technique.

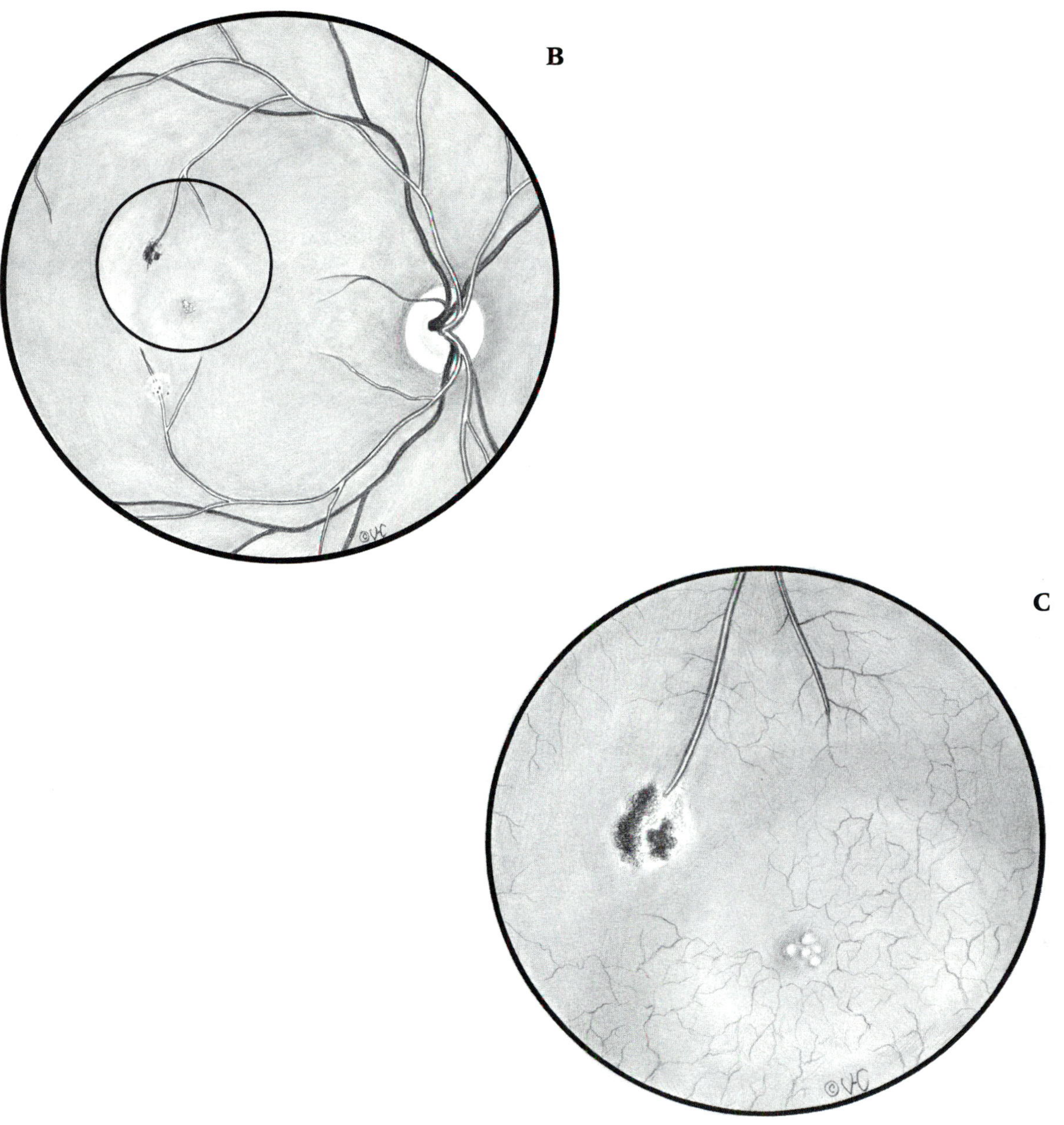
B
C

CHAPTER 32

Coats's Disease

Coats's disease is a specific exudative retinopathy produced by telangiectasis of the retinal vessels. Synonymous terms are "Leber's disease," "retinal telangiectasis," and "Leber's miliary aneurysms," which is the term used when the telangiectasis is evident without extensive exudation.

Coats's disease is unassociated with genetic inheritance and has only rare systemic associations in comparison to exudative retinopathy resulting from angiomatosis retinae, which has genetic association and systemic involvement and can be confused with the advanced exudative stage of Coats's disease.

Coats's disease can be divided into types on the basis of the patient's age at onset. Juvenile Coats's disease includes patients with onset under 30 years of age. These patients form the vast majority of all cases and have no association with systemic disease. Patients with adult Coats's disease, with onset at age over 30 years, frequently have elevated serum cholesterol levels, a history of uveitis, or both. Some adult cases show no distinguishing characteristics from patients with juvenile Coats's disease. The two groups share much in common: predominant unilaterality of ocular involvement, retinal telangiectasis as the primary problem, and gradual accumulation of exudation secondary to leakage from the telangiectasis.

ETIOLOGY

The fundamental problem in Coats's disease is the formation of a retinal telangiectasis and the breakdown in the blood-retinal barrier at the telangiectasis. The breakdown results in all the progressive developments in Coats's disease: intraretinal and subretinal exudation, hemorrhages, lipid and fibrin deposition, phagocytic proliferation, and ultimately glial and fibrous tissue organization of the retina. Telangiectasis of the internal retinal circulation produces intraretinal exudation in comparison to telangiectasis of the external retina, which is more likely to produce subretinal exudation leading to retinal detachment without obscuration of the causative telangiectasis. Intraretinal exudation can obscure the visualization of the telangiectasis. Both types of telangiectasis produce serous leakage that migrates to the retina to cause cystoid macular edema, reducing visual acuity even before intraretinal lipid or exudative retinal detachment is sufficiently extensive to involve the macula.

The primary cause for the formation of the telangiectasis remains unknown. Probably the telangiectasis results from a developmental abnormality in a sector of the retinal capillary bed. The time gap between the formation of the telangiectasis and the accumulation of exudative material sufficient to produce visual symptoms is approximately 8 years in juvenile cases and longer in adult cases of Coats's disease.

HISTOPATHOLOGY

Patients with Coats's disease who have not yet developed subretinal organization or cholesterol deposition show the retinal vascular abnormalities at the telangiectasis to consist in gross thickening of the walls of the smaller vessels with relatively normal or slightly dilated lumens and continuous endothelium to a gross thinning of these walls with irregular and dilated lumens and a total absence of the endothelial lining. The absence of the endothelium would explain the exudation. The lumens present impacted circulatory products including red blood cells, plasma, thrombi, and platelet aggregation. The thickening of the capillary wall results from insudated lipid, plasma, and fibrin in an amalgam with basement membrane–like material and leukocyte and macrophage infiltration. Abnormal permeability through the endothelium appears to be an early event in Coats's disease. What is unknown is whether the permeability increases because of a deficiency in the structure of the vessels or a deficiency in the function of the vacuolated endothelial cells. Regardless of the fundamental mechanism, the formation of the telangiectasis and leakage of fluid into the intraretinal space and eventually into the subretinal space are sequelae of the abnormality of the vascular permeability at the telangiectasis. Necrosis of the endothelial cells in the area of the diseased capillaries is the most likely mechanism for the formation of the irregular dilatation with microaneurysm formation and capillary closure.

Retinal ischemia secondary to the telangiectasis can result in retinal neovascularization, hemorrhage, and even vitreous hemorrhage. The area surrounding the telangiectasis shows irregular shunt vessels and microaneurysms similar to the pattern found surrounding the ischemic focus in diabetes.

NATURAL HISTORY AND CLASSIFICATION

The natural progression of Coats's disease leads to the classification of the following stages, which are used for treatment indications.

Clinical stages of Coats's disease

1. Retinal telangiectasis
2. Focal intraretinal exudates (yellow or white)
3. Partial retinal detachment (yellow or green subretinal mass)
4. Total retinal detachment
5. Chronic retinal detachment
   A. Subretinal membrane
   B. Uveitis
   C. Glaucoma
   D. Cataract

The rate of progression of Coats's disease is unpredictable but a small telangiectasia involving only one quadrant of the retina augers a slower rate of accumulation of exudate than the rate when the vascular malformation is present in two quadrants. With involvement in three or four quadrants, exudation is rapid and prognosis is poor. Approximately two thirds of all cases of Coats's show telangiectasis involving only one quadrant of the retina with almost all the additional cases involving only two quadrants. It is very rare to involve three or four quadrants. Involvement of the optic nerve head or at the macula by telangiectasis shows a rate of exudative accumulation corresponding, in general, to the extent of the telangiectasis.

Spontaneous regression is rare in any of the stages in Coats's disease earlier than stage 4 or 5, when the massive exudation and uveitis can regress, though retinal function shows no subsequent improvement because of the irreversible degeneration of the neural elements. Stage 4 or 5 can involve such severe exudation that exudate drains into the orbit and causes an inflammatory reaction.

DIAGNOSIS

The telangiectasis of Coats's disease is best observed in the early stages before cholesterol exudate obscures the vascular malformation, which can then only be identified on fluorescein angiography. In the earliest stage, the affected vessels show enlargement and distension in the form of sausage-like intermittent dilatations. Balloon-shaped structures resembling microaneurysms appear on both the arteriole and venule surrounding the distorted capillary bed. An intraretinal hemorrhage can result from the rupture of these aneurysmal dilatations. Aneurysmal pulsations do not occur in Coats's disease. The beading and tortuosity of the feeder vessels common in angiomatosis retinae usually are not found. Small, localized telangiectases surrounded by exudate may be present away from the initially discovered large telangiectasis. By the time one full quadrant of the retina is involved with telangiectasis, the exudate usually causes a localized retinal detachment of that quadrant.

In the posterior pole, the presenting sign of telangiectasis is a cluster of tiny, balloonlike dilatations caused by the miliary aneurysms on the terminal vessels. The dilatations may involve any portion of the perimacular capillary bed to the entire macular vasculature. Lesions at the macula are most likely to be observed at their early stage without exudation, hemorrhage, or detachment because of the direct effect of the telangiectasia on foveal function.

Peripheral telangiectases show closure of the retinal vessels peripheral to the lesion. The main retinal draining veins show dilatation in proportion to the extent of the telangiectasis. Cholesterol sheathing may accumulate along the veins and arteries along the telangiectasis. Angiomas smaller than one-half disc diameter can develop on the retinal surface overlying the telangiectasis. These lesions are smaller than the ones found in angiomatosis retinae.

The exudation of Coats's disease can produce tumorlike, cholesterol masses in the subretinal space. The mass usually appears as a gray–yellow green or yellow-white mound with its central portion showing a moderate retinal hemorrhage at the peak. The mounds can be multiple or located anywhere in the fundus with telangiectatic vessels coursing over them. Yellow crystals develop in long-standing masses.

The exudation of Coats's disease occurs as fragmented material of light yellow in the outer retina in the vicinity of the telangiectasis but separated from the telangiectasis by a clear interval. These accumulations often have a stellate appearance and can occur at the macula secondary to a peripheral telangiectasis. This occurrence can result from migration of lipid through the retina or deprivation of the macular circulation.

The second type of exudate occurs as broad sheets that appear predominantly in the posterior pole. After successful treatment of the telangiectasis, the broad sheets of exudation gradually resorb over the ensuing months.

INDICATIONS FOR PHOTOCOAGULATION

Photocoagulation should be applied to all cases of Coats's disease in stages 1 and 2. In stage 3, photocoagulation should be applied to cases where there is only a shallow retinal detachment so that heat can be transferred through the pigment epithelium to the retinal vessels or where there is sufficient intraretinal opacification secondary to exudation to provide a basis for light absorption directly by the retina; the retinal vasculature itself usually cannot absorb adequate amounts of laser photocoagulation light to produce closure without augmented heating by the surrounding tissues. Advanced cases of stage 3, not amenable to photocoagulation, and all cases of stage 4 require cryocoagulation, with scleral buckling in cases of stage 4 or 5.

Laser Technique

For photocoagulation of stage 1, first delineate the full extent of the telangiectasis either by direct observation or by fluorescein angiography or angioscopy (Fig. 32-1, *A*). Use argon green laser with a spot size of 200 or 500 μm and a time duration of 0.5 seconds with a power setting adjusted upward from 100 milliwatts until a white spot results. Place laser burns in an almost contiguous pattern throughout the bed of the telangiectasis and also in the normal retina at the margin of the telangiectasis in order to destroy vessels that may be partially involved and produce future leakage (Fig. 32-1, *B*).

FOLLOW-UP STUDY

Approximately 6 weeks after laser photocoagulation, pigment will appear in the areas of treatment and the telangiectasis should appear atrophic. In cases where exudate has been present, exudation should show a resorption pattern. Failure of either the appearance of atrophy or of resorption of exudate warrants repeat photocoagulation. The energy setting for repeat photocoagulation must be greatly reduced because of improved light absorption by the newly pigmented fundus in the area of treatment.

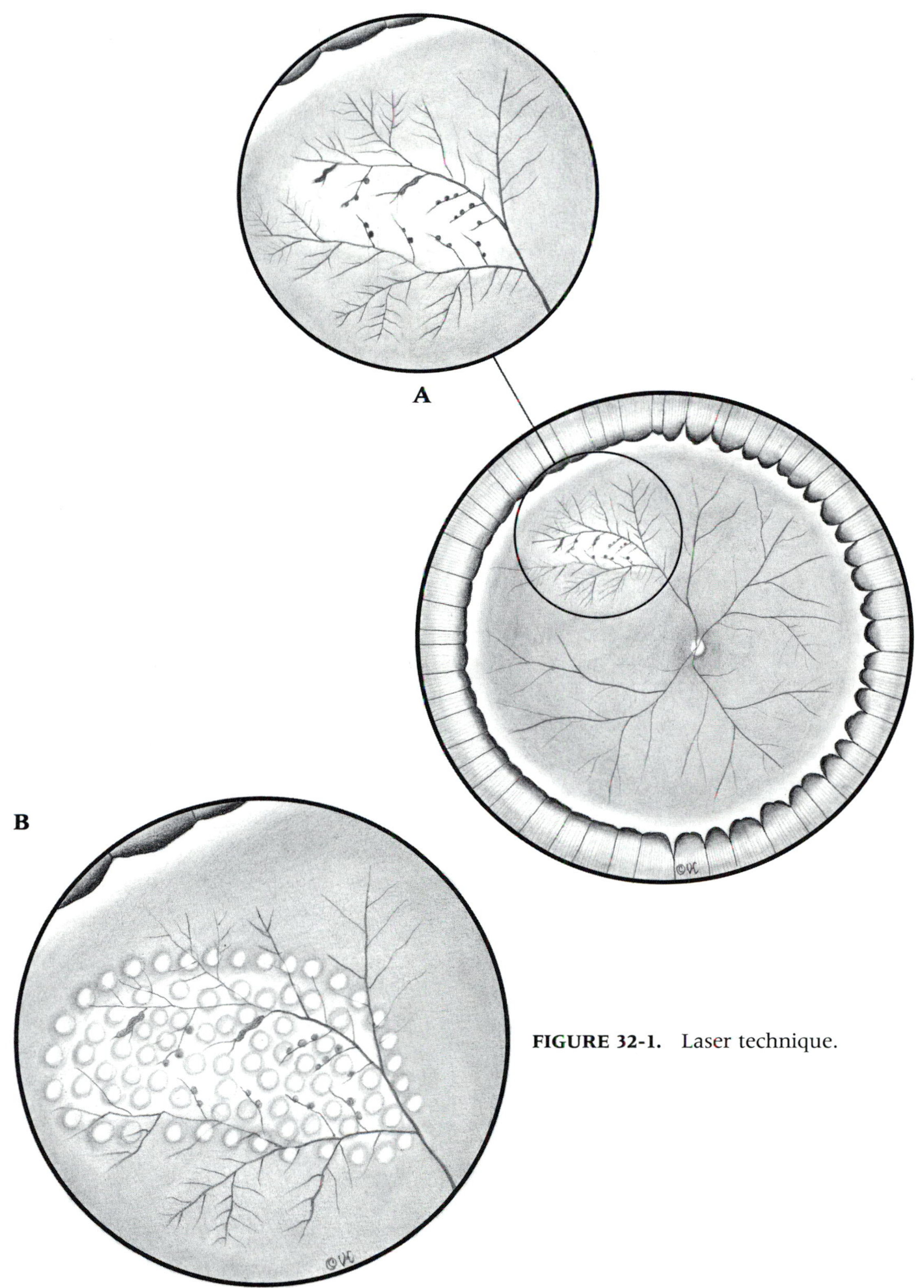

FIGURE 32-1. Laser technique.

TREATMENT OF STAGE 3

In stage 3, with partial retinal detachment resulting from exudation from the telangiectasis (Fig. 32-2, *A*), photocoagulation with laser can be attempted. If argon green laser photocoagulation cannot produce whitening of the area of telangiectasis, cryocoagulation must be applied.

If the lesion is sufficiently anterior, the cryocoagulation can be performed transconjunctivally. If the lesion is more posterior, a sterile surgical procedure must be performed with removal of the conjunctiva and Tenon's capsule. Apply cryocoagulation with a direct view with a binocular indirect ophthalmoscope. Applications should cover all areas of the telangiectasis so that the ice ball penetrates through to the surface of the retina and causes intense whitening. In order for this to be done, indentation of the sclera with the cryoprobe is necessary (Fig. 32-2, *B*). Best results are achieved with three cycles of freeze and thaw to destroy the telangiectatic vessels. If the retina is too highly elevated, the ice ball will be unable to reach the retina even with scleral depression. Failure of the procedure will appear as the inability to whiten the inner surface of the retina with extension of the ice ball from the wall of the eye (Fig. 32-2, *C*). In such a case, drain subretinal fluid to bring the retina nearer to the wall of the eye.

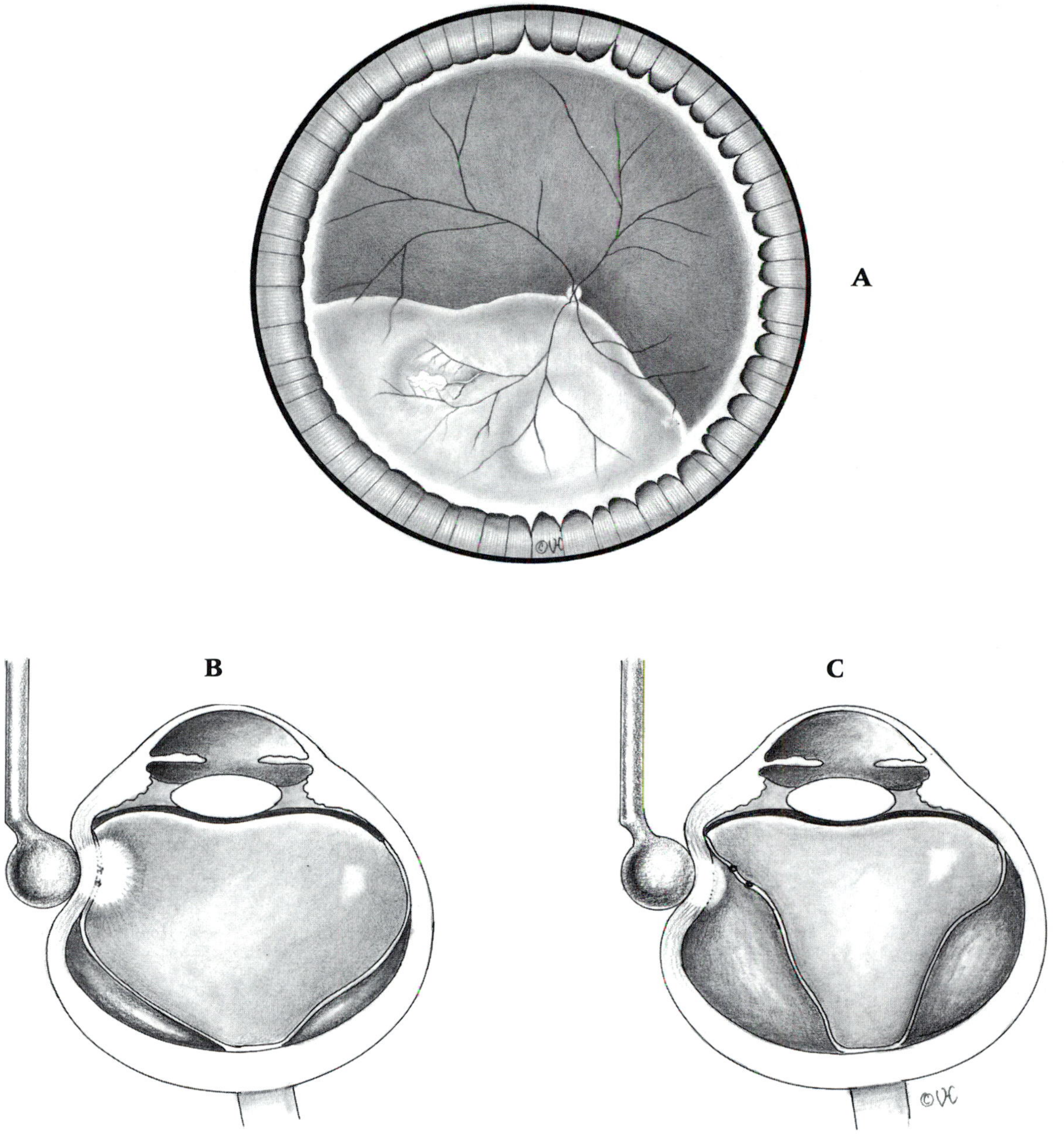

FIGURE 32-2. Treatment of stage 3.

TREATMENT OF STAGE 4

In stage 4, where the retina is totally detached and there is extensive hard exudation in the subretinal space (Fig. 32-3, *A*) scleral buckling with cryosurgery is indicated. Expose and prepare the scleral surface as for a scleral buckling procedure for retinal detachment. Mark the area on the sclera corresponding to the telangiectasis. Prepare the sutures for placement of a scleral buckle to support the peripheral retina at the vitreous base and posterior to it or at any point where there is obvious vitreoretinal traction. After drainage of subretinal fluid, perform cryocoagulation to freeze through the thickness of the retina and telangiectasis. Then tie the broad scleral buckle supported by an encircling band as an explant to indent the entire vitreous base region of the retina (Fig. 32-3, *B*).

COMPLICATIONS

The major complication of the cryoprocedures for telangiectasis is recurrence of the exudation because of failure to close the telangiectasis. Repeated attempts at cryosurgery with or without augmentation of photocoagulation should be done. The resorption of some of the exudate should occur within 10 weeks after successful surgery, but the hard exudates that have accumulated over months or years can take many months to show even partial resorption. If the retina remains in as good a position to the scleral buckle as it was at the end of surgery, the operation should be considered a success until the retina is seen to become more detached by the reaccumulation of fluid.

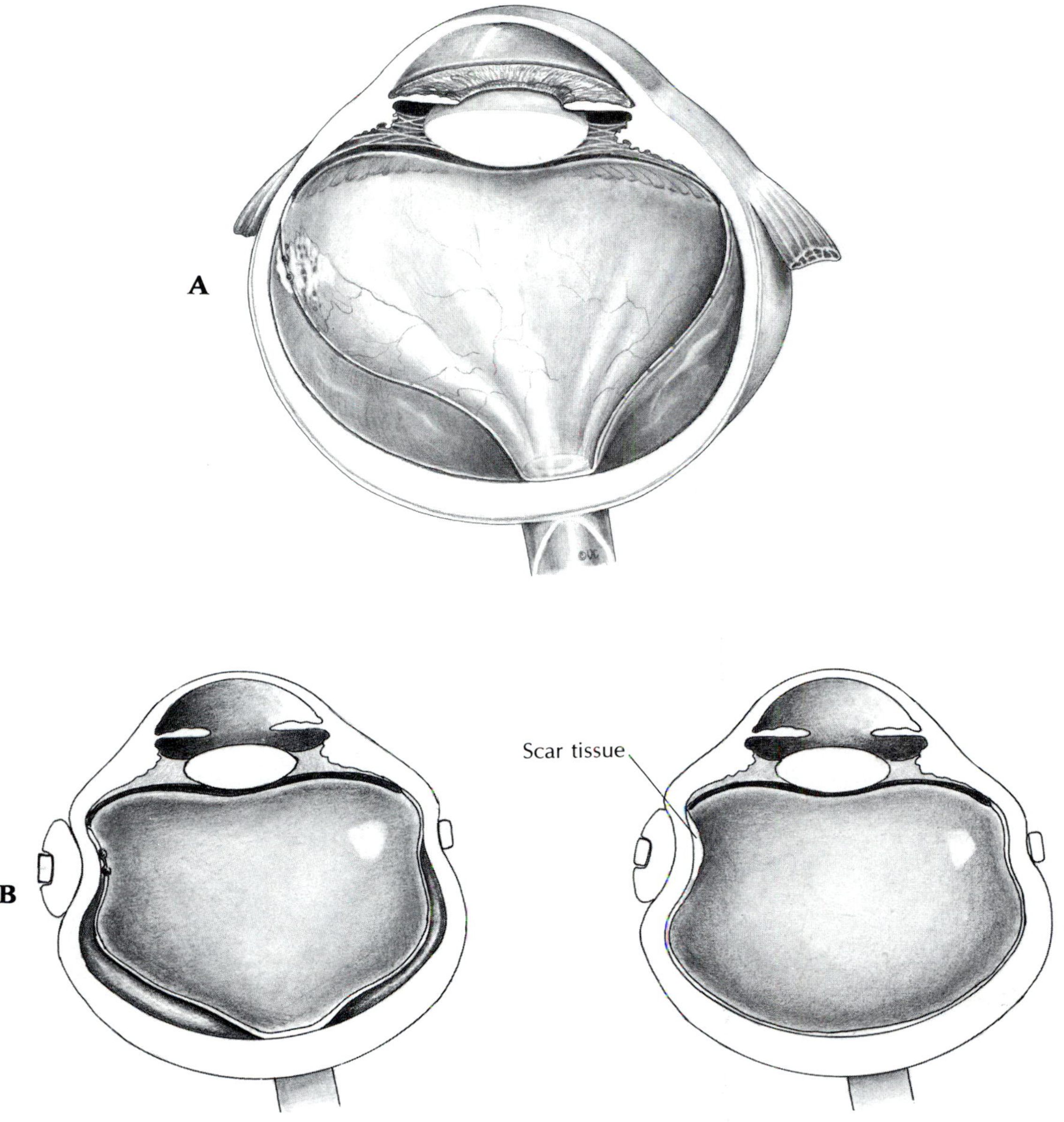

FIGURE 32-3. Treatment of stage 4.

CHAPTER 33

Central Serous Retinopathy

Central serous retinopathy (CSR) is the syndrome consisting of transient episodes of serous detachment of the retina and the pigment epithelium in eyes of patients under 50 years of age with no obvious predisposing pathologic changes at the macula such as drusen, subretinal neovascularization, angioid streaks, optic pit, myopic degeneration, retinal break, retinal angiomatosis, choroidal tumor, or uveitis. An alternative name for this syndrome is *idiopathic central serous chorioretinopathy*.

ETIOLOGY

Dysfunction of the pigment epithelium appears as the primary observable cause of CSR. The dysfunction consists of a breakdown in the tight junctions between pigment epithelial cells allowing serous fluid to pass from the choroid through the pigment epithelium into the subretinal space. The serous fluid separates the retina from the pigment epithelium. Frequently the group of diseased pigment epithelial cells shows detachment from the underlying Bruch's membrane. The ultimate cause for this pigment epithelial defect is unknown and may involve a relationship to vasomotor stress.

CLINICAL HISTORY

Patients with CSR show an average 34 years of age at onset of the disease, with a range from 27 to 58 years. Eighty percent of patients range from 35 to 45 years of age with a strong predisposition for males. CSR occurs infrequently in black patients but is seen in all other groups.

The accumulation of serous fluid beneath the retina produces a sudden onset of mild, unilateral distortion of central vision with central metamorphopsia or micropsia or a positive scotoma. Visual acuity with the patient's usual optical correction is diminished but frequently can be improved to normal with refraction by use of convex lenses that compensate for the macula's convex elevation. The accumulation of proteinaceous yellow material on the subretinal surface in protracted cases correlates with diminution in best corrected visual acuity.

CLINICAL COURSE

CSR differs from senile macular degeneration because it shows as many as 90% of affected patients having a spontaneous resolution with the return of visual acuity to at least 20/40 within 1 to 6 months after the onset of symptoms. Between 50% and 60% of patients wtih CSR recover visual acuity of 20/20. In pregnancy, CSR resolves by the third trimester, with complete resolution of symptoms in the postpartum weeks. Fluid recurs in about 50% of patients, with multiple recurrences in many patients. The number of recurrences, however, usually has no harmful effect on the ultimate recovery of visual acuity. Over 60% of the recurrences result from reopening of the original leakage site as seen on fluorescein angiography. Only a small group of patients with recurrence (approximately 9%) develops pigment epithelial atrophy and ultimately suffers a diminution in visual acuity. Although pigment epithelial atrophy can follow a recurrent CSR episode by as much as 5 years, the benignity of even recurrent CSR is confirmed by the finding that only 5% to 10% of patients experience permanent loss of acuity worse than 20/40.

Even with complete resolution of the serous detachment of the retina, at least 80% of patients will show some degree of permanent visual deficit resulting from pigmentary disturbance at the macula, small foveal cysts, or irregularity in the alignment of the photoreceptor outer segments. Metamorphopsia and micropsia are the most common symptoms after disease resolution, with approximately 40% of all patients being unaware of the residual deficit.

CSR occurs in the opposite eye in approximately 10% to 25% of cases. The second eye tends to become involved after a delay of weeks after onset in the first eye. Often, the second eye is uninvolved until long after complete healing in the first eye.

DIAGNOSIS

The diagnosis of CSR is confirmed by biomicroscopy showing elevation of the retina by serous fluid. Pigment epithelial detachments ranging in size from 0.25 up to 1 disc diameter may be single or multiple. CSR can occur eccentrically in the peripheral fundus sometimes showing a long, narrow track extending from the peripheral fundus to the macula.

Fluorescein angiography shows a variety of patterns of leakage ranging from the most common, a discrete punctate stain appearing in the venous phase with gradual enlargement, to a faintly staining circular mass beneath the retina, to a point source of leakage that develops a "smokestack" appearance in late angiography and the fluorescein leaks superiorly into the subretinal space.

INDICATIONS FOR PHOTOCOAGULATION

Most cases of CSR should not be photocoagulated because of the strong proclivity of CSR for spontaneous, favorable resolution. Although the risks of photocoagulation treatment are less than 5%, even the most satisfactory treatment is likely to leave a visual deficit. At worst, photocoagulation can cause foveal scarring, macular striae, or subretinal hemorrhage with severe, irreversible loss of macular function.

The most common indication for photocoagulation treatment is the patient's desire for alleviation of the annoying symptoms. Although photocoagulation can speed recovery, it will not improve the acuity, metamorphopsia, or the relative central scotoma more than the natural healing will. Therefore photocoagulation should be delayed as long as the patient can tolerate the symptoms. Only in rare cases will delay cause irreversible degeneration of the macula. Such cases are heralded by the failure of refraction to bring visual acuity to its pre-CSR level and by the accumulation of turbid subretinal fluid.

It is uncertain whether a past episode of CSR is an indication for treatment of a new episode. A subjective impression is that there is a lower rate of recurrence in treated than in untreated patients though photocoagulation does not guarantee against recurrence. If leakage recurs in a previously photocoagulated case, the fluid originates from a new site. In spontaneously healed cases, fluid frequently originates from an old site. Predegenerative cases of CSR usually show persistent fluid without improvement for more than 4 months. In order to be considered for photocoagulation, the leakage point should lie outside the foveal avascular zone. Location within the papillomacular bundle is not a contraindication to treatment. Photocoagulation should also be considered for the predegenerative phases of cases that represent a recurrence in an eye that has suffered a permanent visual deficit from a previous CSR attack. A residual visual deficit from CSR in the opposite eye also is an indication for treatment.

Photocoagulation Technique

Photocoagulation requires the use of a fluorescein angiogram no more than 1 week old in order to ensure proper localization of the leakage site. If the leakage site is farther than 250 μm from the foveal perimeter, the direct treatment technique is best. If the leak is closer to the fovea, indirect laser treatment is safest: the placement of laser burns far from the fovea can eliminate the subretinal fluid even though the treatments are not administered to the leakage site.

Krypton red laser photocoagulation is ideal because it spares the neurosensory retina. Argon green can also be used. The laser burns for krypton red should be 200 μm or wider with a time duration of 0.5 seconds and a very low power setting started at 100 milliwatts and worked upward until a faint reaction results. Intense reaction is unnecessarily destructive. With argon green, a smaller spot size, 100 μm, is adequate for treatment and safe compared to krypton red where the small spot size risks producing a choroidal hemorrhage. An argon green laser should also be used with a low power setting to produce only a faint gray-white reaction. The entire area of leakage should be covered by either laser technique.

The direct treatment method places the laser burns directly on the pigment epithelial detachment; the treatment need extend no further (Fig. 33-1, *A*). If the total energy input is kept weak, there is no reason for the retina overlying the pigment epithelial detachment to be involved by the laser burn. The presence of subretinal fluid provides a thermal barrier (Fig. 33-1, *B*). Only if the laser burn is excessive will the overlying retina be coagulated. Laser photocoagulation should be limited to the primary leakage spot of the angiogram rather than to the area where fluorescein may flow in the later phase of the angiogram, as in the classic mushroom appearance wherein only the base of the mushroom should be coagulated and the remaining area should be left untreated (Fig. 33-1, *C*).

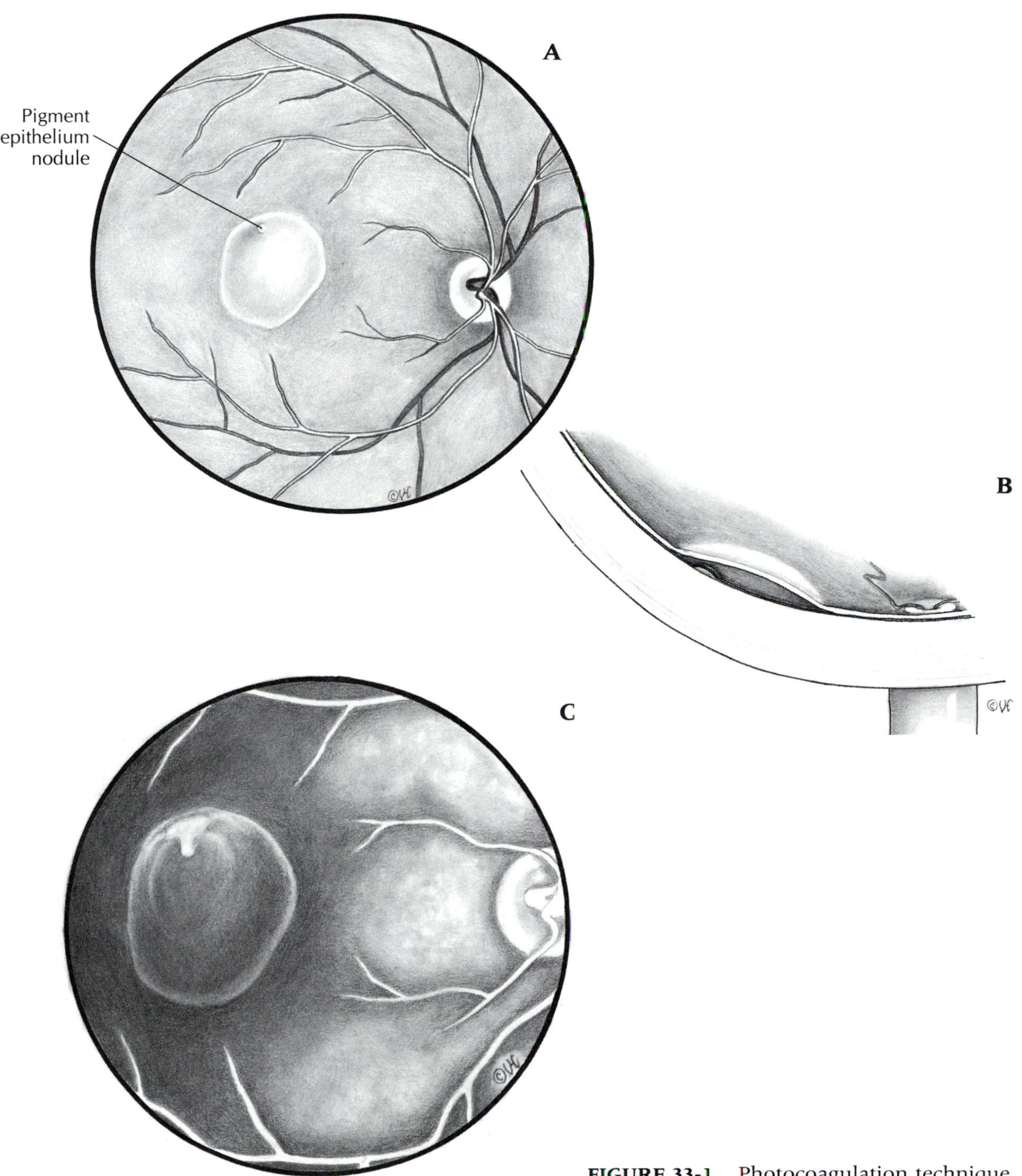

FIGURE 33-1. Photocoagulation technique.

Indirect Photocoagulation Technique

If leakage is too close to the fovea, laser burns can be placed farther away from the fovea in an area where there is subretinal fluid but no leakage site. The spots are best placed toward the inferior aspect of the serous detachment because of the effect of gravity to move the subretinal fluid toward the treatment zone where the fluid can be resorbed through the treated pigment epithelium (Fig. 33-2, *A*).

Using argon green or krypton red, place small laser burns, usually three or four burns (near each other and almost contiguous). The burns should be of low intensity, producing only a faint reaction of the pigment epithelium. If successful, resorption of the subretinal fluid will gradually occur over the ensuing 3 weeks.

The major risk of this treatment is excessive photocoagulation, which can produce a scotoma if the retina is involved or a hemorrhage if the choroid is involved. Retreatment should be considered if there is no appropriate response within approximately 6 weeks. The accumulation of pigment at the site of treatment or at the fovea is a normal response in this treatment and should not be viewed as a complication (Fig. 33-2, *B*).

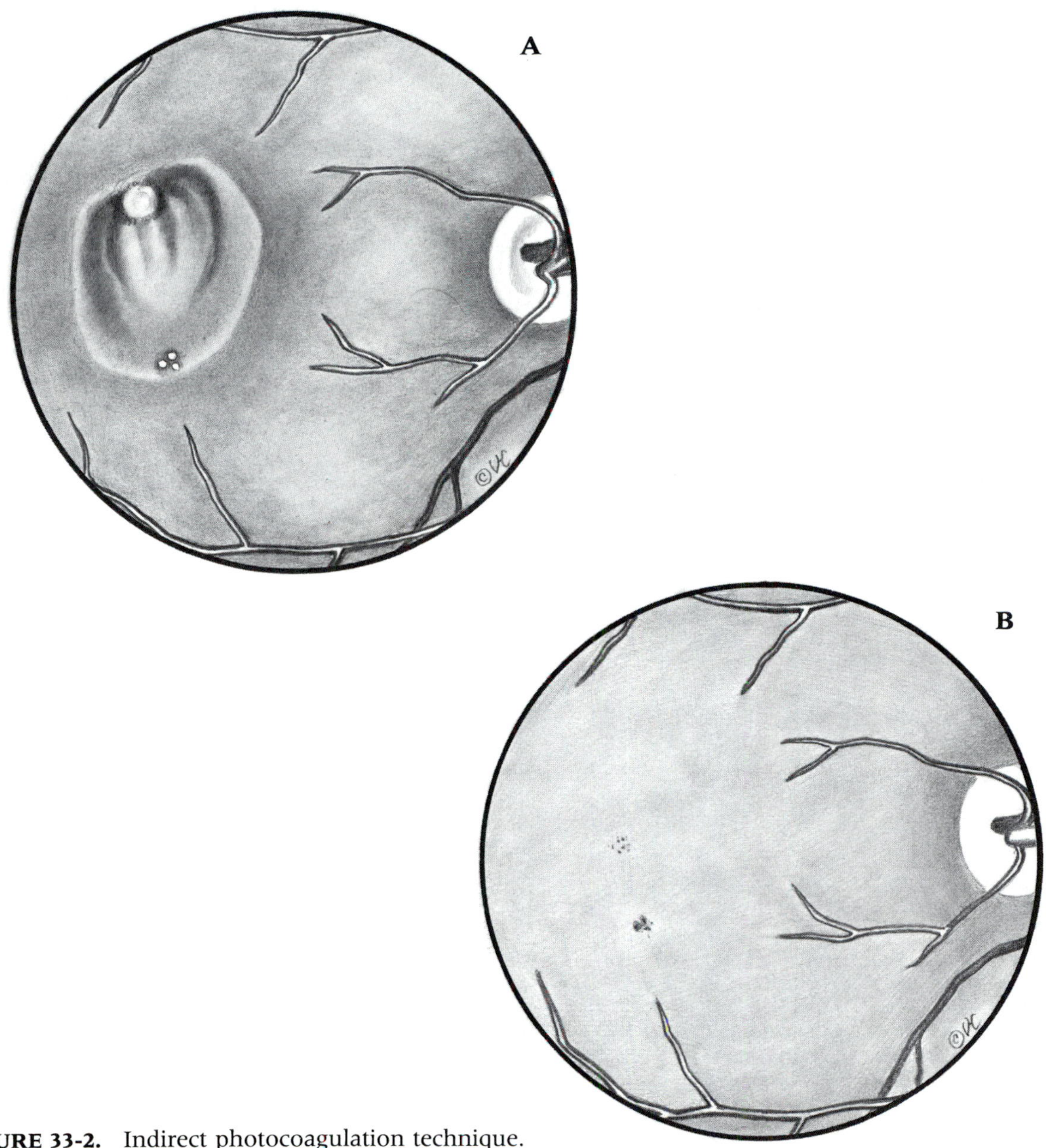

FIGURE 33-2. Indirect photocoagulation technique.

FOLLOW-UP STUDY AND COMPLICATIONS

Successful treatment is not obvious immediately. At first, the subretinal fluid may persist despite successful photocoagulation of the leakage spot (Fig. 33-3, *A*). Over the ensuing 3 weeks, the subretinal fluid should show resorption with pigmentation of the laser spots (Fig. 33-3, *B*). The accumulation of pigment at the fovea is not a complication but is the result of the previous serous separation of the retina.

The major complication risk is production of hemorrhage by excessive photocoagulation. The other risk is the failure to identify a choroidal neovascular network that can hemorrhage during the photocoagulation or subsequently. Rapid identification of any neovascularization either during or after treatment warrants immediate photocoagulation in an attempt to destroy the entirety of the membrane before the fovea is involved.

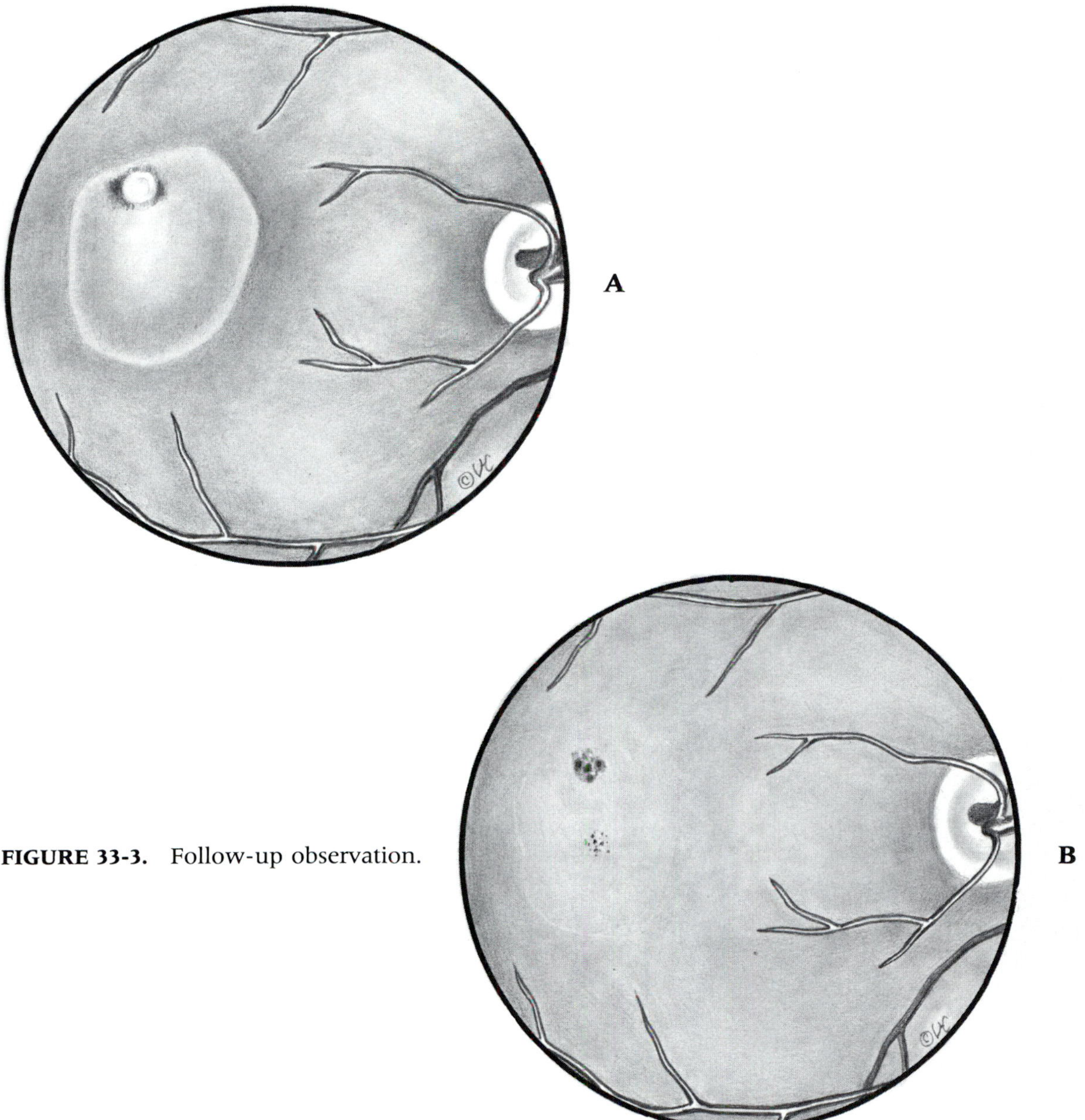

FIGURE 33-3. Follow-up observation.

CHAPTER 34

Senile Macular Degeneration

Senile macular degeneration (SMD) refers to the exudative degeneration that occurs primarily after 50 years of age at the macula. For purposes of this discussion, atrophic or "dry" macular degeneration is not included because of the absence of any therapeutic modality. SMD consists of two entities: (1) serous pigment epithelial detachment with secondary serous retinal detachment and (2) sub–pigment epithelial neovascularization with secondary serous and hemorrhagic detachment of the pigment epithelium and retina.

ETIOLOGY AND HISTOPATHOLOGY

The first change at the macula in SMD is hyalinization and thickening of Bruch's membrane. Bruch's membrane shows thickening as early as 20 years of age, with the first thickening being noticeable in the inner collagenous zone and resulting from the accumulation of vesicular, granular, and filamentous material. By 40 years of age, the material includes residual bodies, undigested outer segments, debris from the pigment epithelium, collagen (both round and intermediate spacing), long-spacing collagen, and elastic fibers that are dense and calcified. During these years, drusen accumulate, either as the result of aberrant biochemical activity by the pigment epithelium or from the pathologic autolysis of pigment epithelial cells caused by the breakdown of cellular lysozymes. The drusen take two forms—globular or granular—with globular drusen appearing first and associated with ophthalmoscopically observable irregular drusen combined with pigment irregularities in the pigment epithelium. Granular drusen may represent a more advanced stage in the degeneration of the pigment epithelial cells. The final aging change in Bruch's membrane is the accumulation of a fine granular deposit between the pigment cells and the inner layer of Bruch's membrane. This deposit consists of spindle-shaped collagen embedded in a granular material. The basal linear deposit between the basal plasma infoldings and the basement cells collates not only with diffuse pigmentary degeneration overlying the region of formation of the deposit but also with a tendency toward the growth of choroidal neovascularization into the sub–pigment epithelial space at the site of the deposit. The deposit seems to act as an entrance path for neovascular ingrowth and a site for breakdown of adhesion between the pigment epithelium and Bruch's membrane to form a pigment epithelial detachment. The accumulation of material between the degenerated pigment epithelium and Bruch's membrane encourages spontaneous detachment of the sheet of pigment epithelial cells from Bruch's membrane and the subsequent ingrowth of choroidal neovascularization into the subpigment epithelial space whether the pigment epithelium is detached. If the pigment epithelium becomes detached without neovascularization or hemorrhage, the serous fluid that accumulates in the subpigment space eventually migrates into the subretinal space through the degenerated pigment epithelial tight junctions. Initially, this fluid accumulation causes metamorphopsia. Subsequently, it diminishes visual acuity because of interference with metabolism in the photoreceptors.

The growth of neovascularization from the choriocapillaris through the brittle-hyalinized Bruch's membrane invades the basal linear deposit between the pigment epithelial cell membranes. In the presence of neovascularization, leakage of subretinal fluid separates the pigment epithelial cells further from Bruch's membrane. The fluid also seeps into the subretinal space. Eventually, hemorrhage can occur, first limited to the subpigment epithelial space and later spreading into the subretinal space and even into the vitreous. In the end, an organized fibrous scar results.

DIAGNOSIS

Pigment epithelial detachment occurs as both a serous detachment of the pigment epithelium and (in 95% of cases) a serous separation between the retina and the pigment epithelium. The diagnosis of pigment epithelial detachment requires stereoscopic biomicroscopy, which shows the detachment best in retroillumination. Fluorescein angiography shows the accumulation of fluorescein under the entire bed of the detached pigment epithelium. In some cases, the fluorescein accumulation is even, whereas in others it is scattered by pigment accumulation. The absence of choroidal neovascularization can be judged by the failure of fluorescein to spread beyond the margins of the pigment epithelial detachment in the late phase of angiography.

In its early stages, choroidal neovascularization can be detected by discoloration of the overlying pigment epithelium, which changes from its natural yellow to a dark gray. Fluorescein angiography shows a network of vessels in the early phase with gradual leakage. In rare cases, a bicycle-wheel pattern of vessels can be seen to originate from a central single vessel. The hallmark of sub–pigment epithelial neovascularization is extravasation of fluorescein within and at the margins of the lesion throughout the fluorescein study. At 30 minutes after injection, the lesion looks larger than it did during the arteriovenous phase and its borders are fuzzy compared to the usually neat borders of a pigment epithelial detachment without neovascularization. In more advanced cases of neovascularization, hemorrhage appears beneath the pigment epithelium as a dark gray mound that can extravasate into the subretinal or preretinal space as red blood. In advanced cases, fibrous tissue accumulates both in the subretinal and sub–pigment epithelial space to produce a disciform scar, which cannot be treated.

INDICATIONS

Laser photocoagulation is indicated for all cases of exudative macular degeneration that show signs of exudation or hemorrhage if the responsible choroidal neovascularization does not extend closer than 200 μm to the center of the fovea. Nonexudative, or "dry," degeneration consisting of atrophy of the pigment epithelium or choroid, drusen, or small avascular pigment epithelial detachments are not currently indices for laser photocoagulation.

Photocoagulation Technique

Krypton red laser is the best means currently available for treating choroidal neovascularization as the cause of senile macular degeneration. The deep penetration of the red wavelength spares the neurosensory retina and produces maximum coagulation at the choroid and pigment epithelium. The only potential advantage of argon green is its absorption by hemoglobin at the site of the neovascularization. Green has the disadvantage of absorption by the retina and its vasculature, however, and substantial absorption by the pigment epithelium thereby blocking penetration to the choroid.

Photocoagulation treatment requires determination of the focus of the choroidal neovascularization and accompanying pigment epithelial detachment. The combination of fundus examination and fluorescein angiography shows the neovascular area (Fig. 34-1, *A*) to lie beneath the shallow pigment epithelial detachment often surrounded by exudation. The choroidal neovascularization lies beneath both the retina and the pigment epithelium (Fig. 34-1, *B*). The ideal laser treatment will produce coagulation of the neovascularization along with the superficial choroid and the pigment epithelium. The treatment would leave the retina spared (Fig. 34-1, *C*). Drusen or shallow pigment epithelial detachment without neovascularization should not be included in the treatment.

Once the neovascular zone is determined, direct full attention toward this zone in comparison to distracting landmarks of exudation and hemorrhage (Fig. 34-1, *D*), particularly if hemorrhage is present at the margin of the pigment epithelial detachment, begin photocoagulation treatments at the margin of the pigment epithelial detachment facing the macula. The purpose of locating the initial treatments in this position is to create a relative barrier to diminish the risk of spread of hemorrhage toward the fovea (Fig. 34-1, *E*). Using krypton red with a 200 μm spot size and a 0.5 second duration, gradually increase the power until a yellow-white scar results. A dense white scar is unnecessary. With argon green, follow the same procedure using a 100 μm spot size until a gray-white reaction results.

Continue the initial photocoagulations to surround the pigment epithelial detachment and choroidal neovascularization (Fig. 34-1, *F*). Then continue the photocoagulation through the center of the lesion with overlapping spots. Gradually increase the power until an almost white reaction results (Fig. 34-1, *G*).

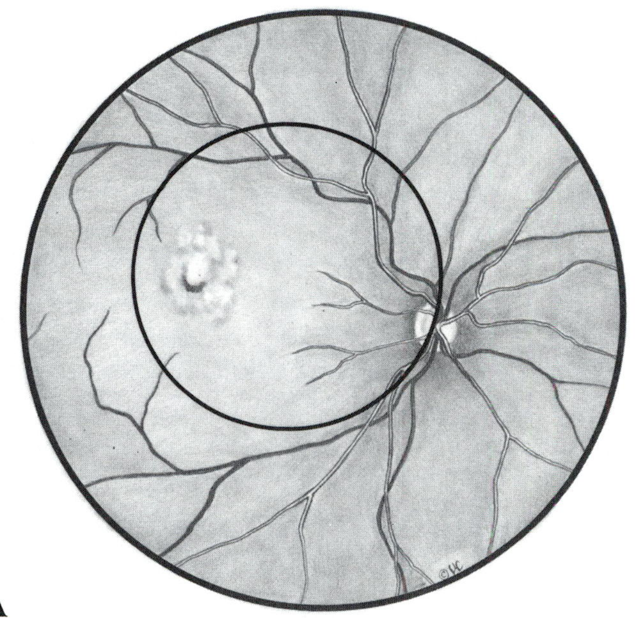

FIGURE 34-1. Photocoagulation technique.

A

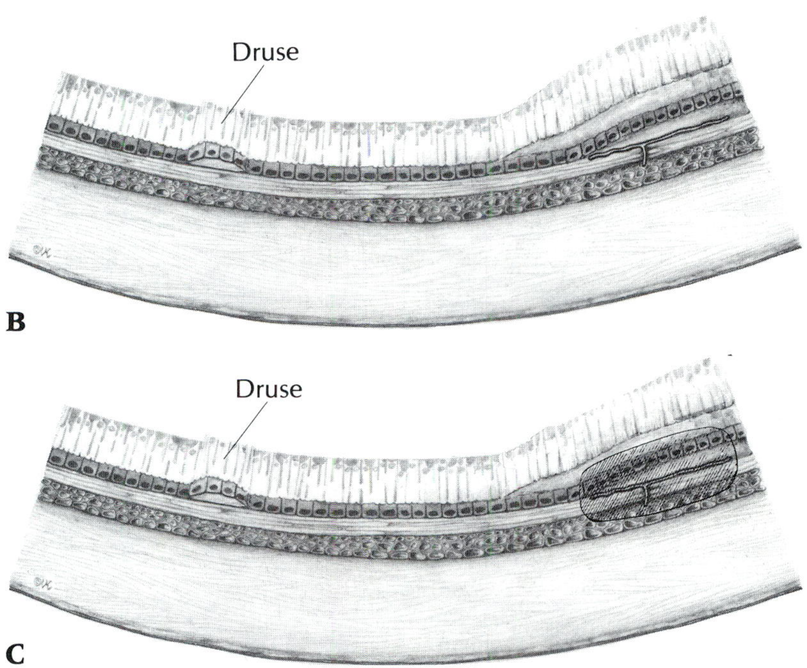

B

C

Continued.

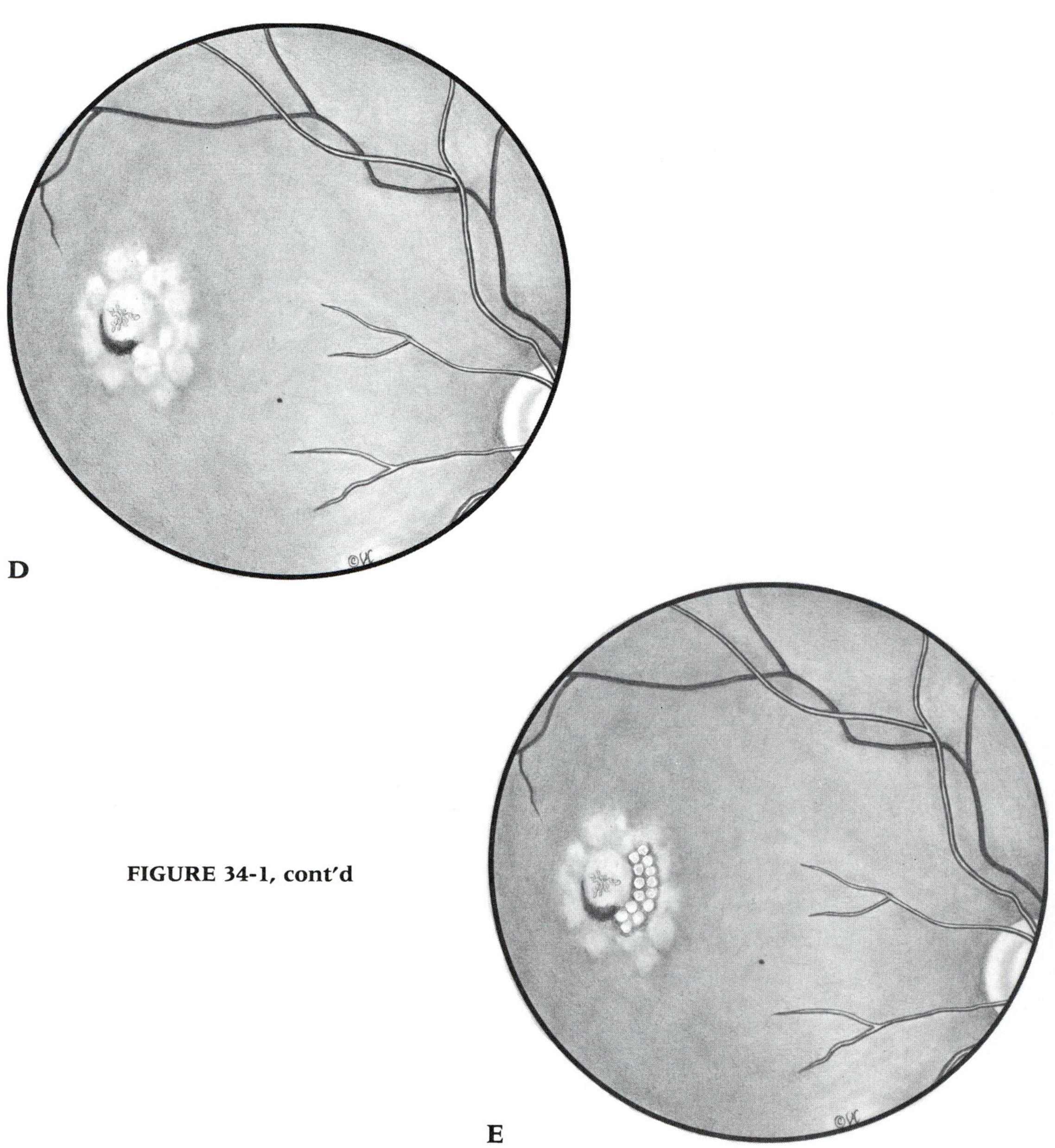

FIGURE 34-1, cont'd

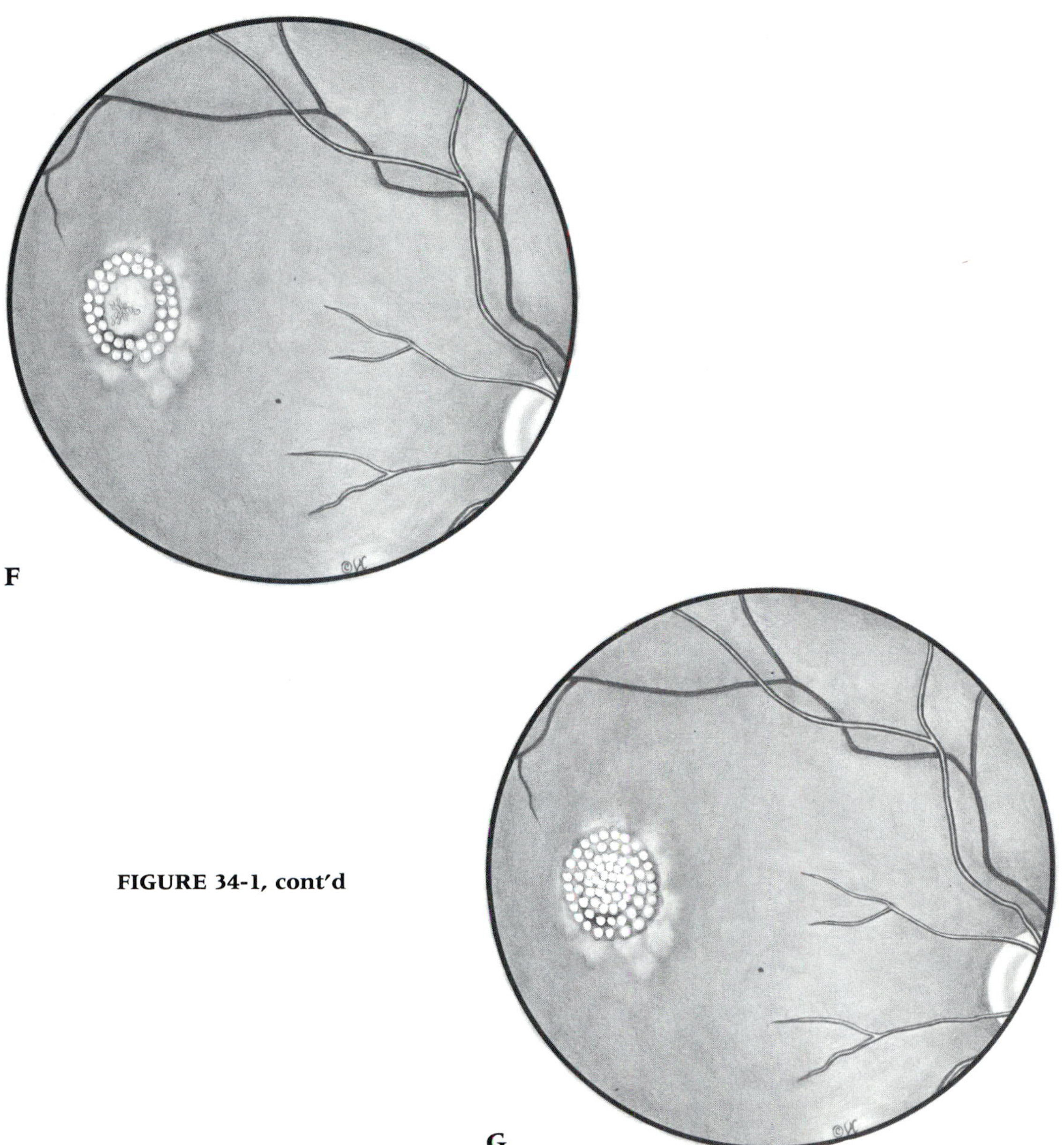

F

G

FIGURE 34-1, cont'd

Photocoagulation of Juxtapapillary Neovascularization

Photocoagulation of juxtapapillary neovascularization should be aimed at the neovascularization as delineated by fluorescein angiography rather than at the exudate, which tends to accumulate through the macula (Fig. 34-2, *A*).

Krypton red laser photocoagulation is the safest means for destroying juxtapapillary neovascularization. The deep absorption of the krypton red wavelength relatively spares the nerve fiber layer and diminishes the risk of producing a dense centrocecal scotoma.

Begin the laser treatment at the perimeter of the neovascular network and outside it, creating 200 μm spots that are contiguous and are yellow-white in appearance rather than dense white. Then proceed to fill in the interior of the demarcated space up to the margin of the optic nerve. After initial treatment with 200 μm spot size to produce a yellow reaction, re-treat to produce a yellow-white reaction (Fig. 34-2, *B* and *C*).

Initial photocoagulation of the neovascularization with low energy level presents less of a risk of hemorrhage than initial coagulation with high energy input does.

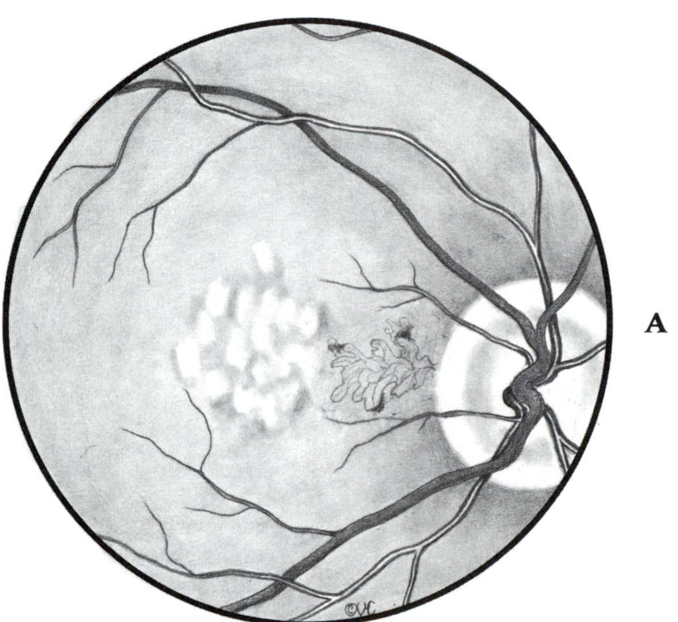

FIGURE 34-2. Photocoagulation of juxtapapillary neovascularization.

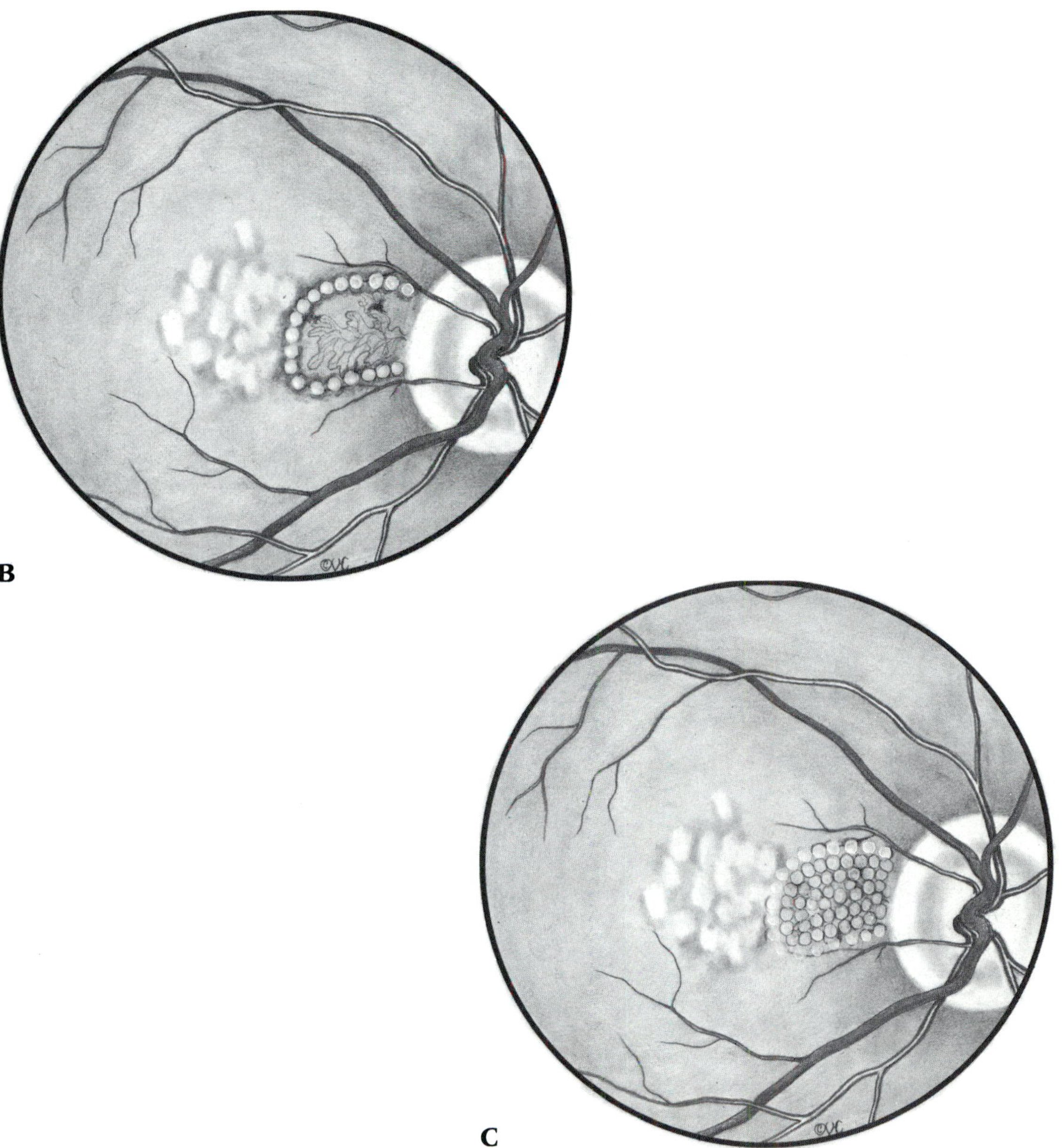
B
C

Neovascularization from angioid streaks

The aim of laser photocoagulation for choroidal neovascularization stemming from angioid streaks must be at the entire neovascular network and its origin in the angioid streak. The angioid streaks themselves do not warrant photocoagulation (Fig. 34-3, *A*). The area for photocoagulation must be delineated by fluorescein angiography to show the extent to the neovascular network in the midst of the exudate (Fig. 34-3, *B*).

Using krypton red with a 200 or 500 μm spot size and a duration of 0.5 seconds with a power setting to produce a yellow-white reaction, coagulate the entirety of the neovascular membrane up to and including the angioid streak. There is no need to extend the photocoagulation along the angioid streak where there is no neovascularization: photocoagulation of the angioid streak carries risks of producing further rupture in Bruch's membrane (Fig. 34-3, *C*). After initial treatment, re-treat the neovascular zone more intensely to produce an almost dense white reaction.

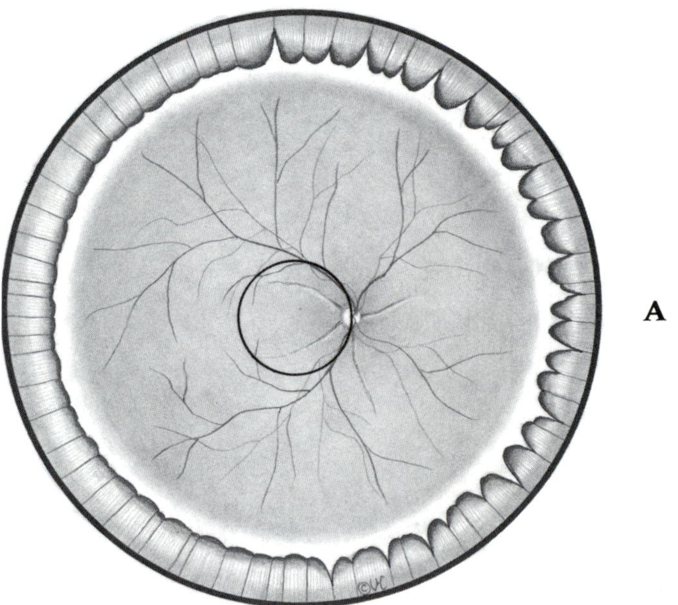

FIGURE 34-3. Photocoagulation for neovascularization from angioid streaks.

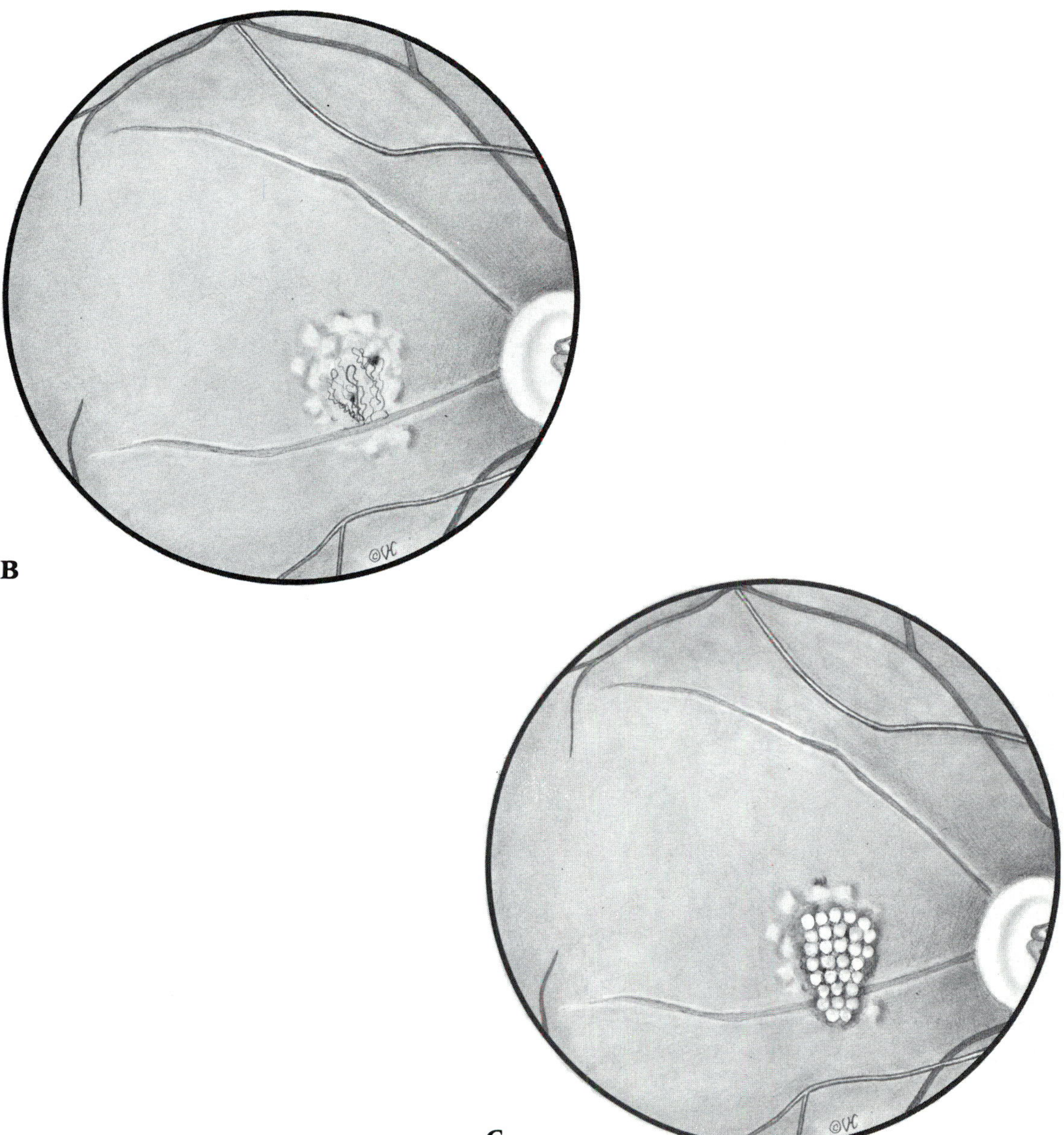
©VC
B
©VC
C

Pigment epithelial detachment

The aim of photocoagulation of a pigment epithelial detachment should be at the pigment epithelial detachment alone and the area of accompanying subretinal fluid being left untouched (Fig. 34-4, *A*). Fluorescein angiography and biomicroscopy show the full extent of the pigment epithelial detachment.

Using either krypton red or argon green laser, surround the margins of the pigment epithelial detachment but remain at least 250 μm from the fovea (Fig. 34-4, *B*). Then continue the laser photocoagulation to cover the entirety of the pigment epithelial detachment. Initially, use a reaction that produces only faint yellow with krypton or faint gray with argon. Gradually increase the power on re-treatment to produce a moderate reaction of yellow with krypton or gray-white with argon. Do not overtreat because of the risk of producing a tear of the pigment epithelium. Use the moderate intensity to treat the entire pigment epithelial detachment and its margins (Fig. 34-4, *C*).

Photocoagulation can also be aimed at "notches" in the margin of the pigment detachment because of possible occult neovascularization in the notch.

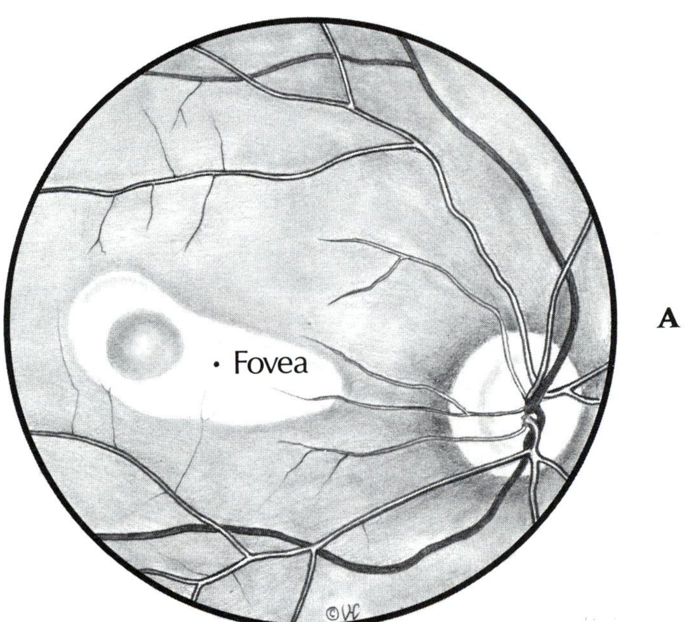

FIGURE 34-4. Photocoagulation of pigment epithelial detachment.

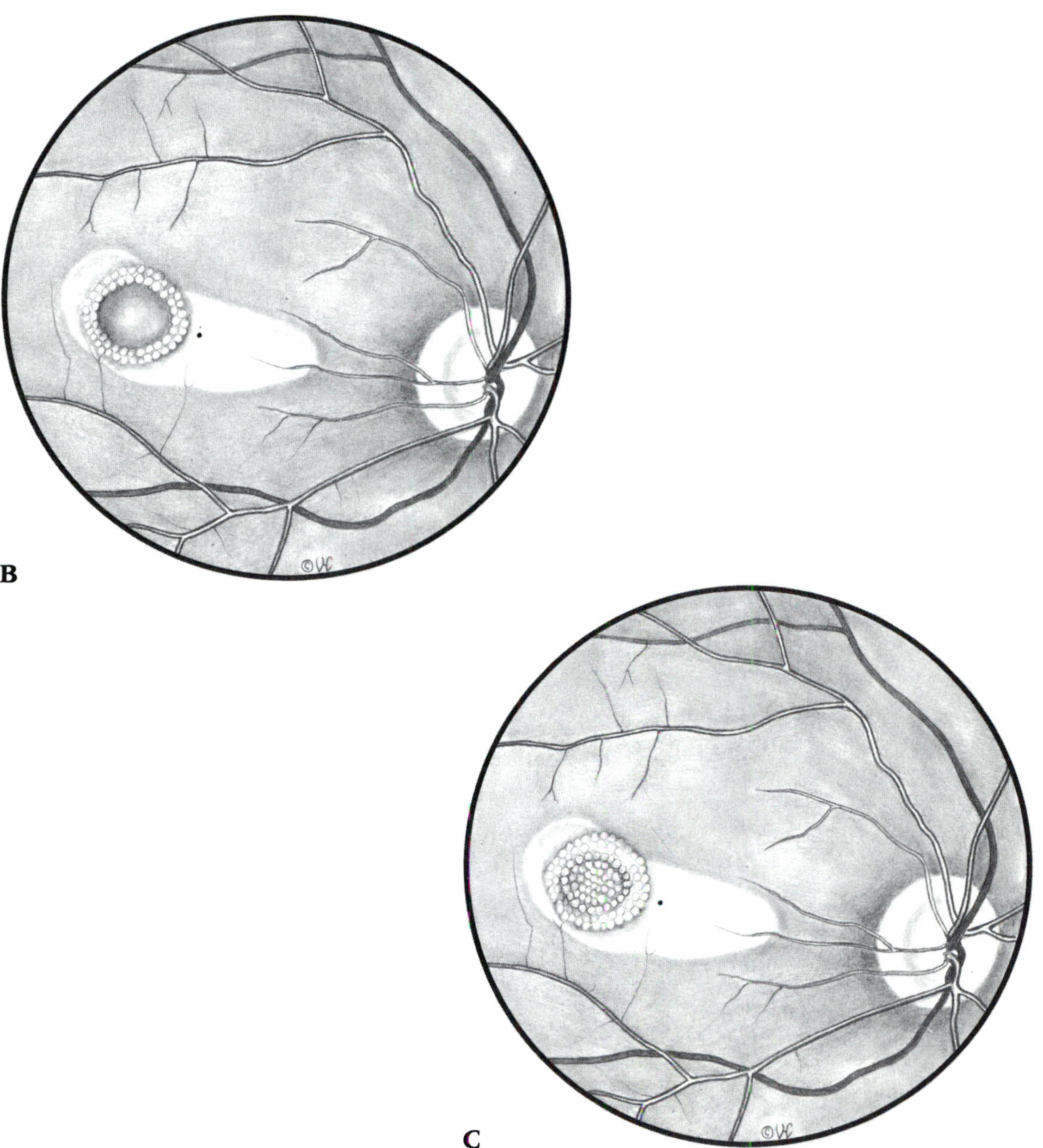
©VC
B
©VC
C

FOLLOW-UP STUDY

For choroidal neovascularization, the appearance of a well-pigmented scar with atrophy of the pigment epithelium and choroid at the treatment zone is the ideal result (Fig. 34-5, *A*). Gradually, subretinal fluid should resorb over the ensuing weeks and fluorescein angiography should confirm the absence of residual neovascularization. The lesion should not be considered successfully treated until 2 months after the most recent treatment for leakage.

For juxtapapillary neovascularization, a pigmented scar at the margin of the disc with atrophy of the underlying layers is the desired outcome (Fig. 34-5, *B*). Any change in morphology and subsequent examinations would indicate the possible regrowth of neovascularization from either the disc margin or the margins of treatment. Retreatment should be undertaken if there is any change in morphology. Similarly the treatment of angioid streak neovascularization should also result in a pigmented and partially atrophic scar with gradual drying of the subretinal fluid. The remainder of the angioid streaks should appear unchanged (Fig. 34-5, *C*). Any change in the surrounding angioid streak could indicate further breakdown with new neovascularization, which would require immediate treatment.

A successfully treated pigment epithelial detachment can show one of two appearances. The most common is for persistence of a shallow pigment epithelial detachment surrounded by a margin of scarred tissue that is flat (Fig. 34-5, *D*). The alternative successful appearance is flattening of the pigment epithelial detachment in its entirety with atrophy of the pigment and choroidal layers. Failure of the central pigment epithelial detachment to flatten is not an indication for retreatment. Extension of the pigment epithelial detachment through the margins of treatment or the appearance of choroidal neovascularization with fresh extravasation is an indication for reevaluation for treatment. A successfully treated pigment epithelial detachment should show resolution of the accompanying subretinal fluid.

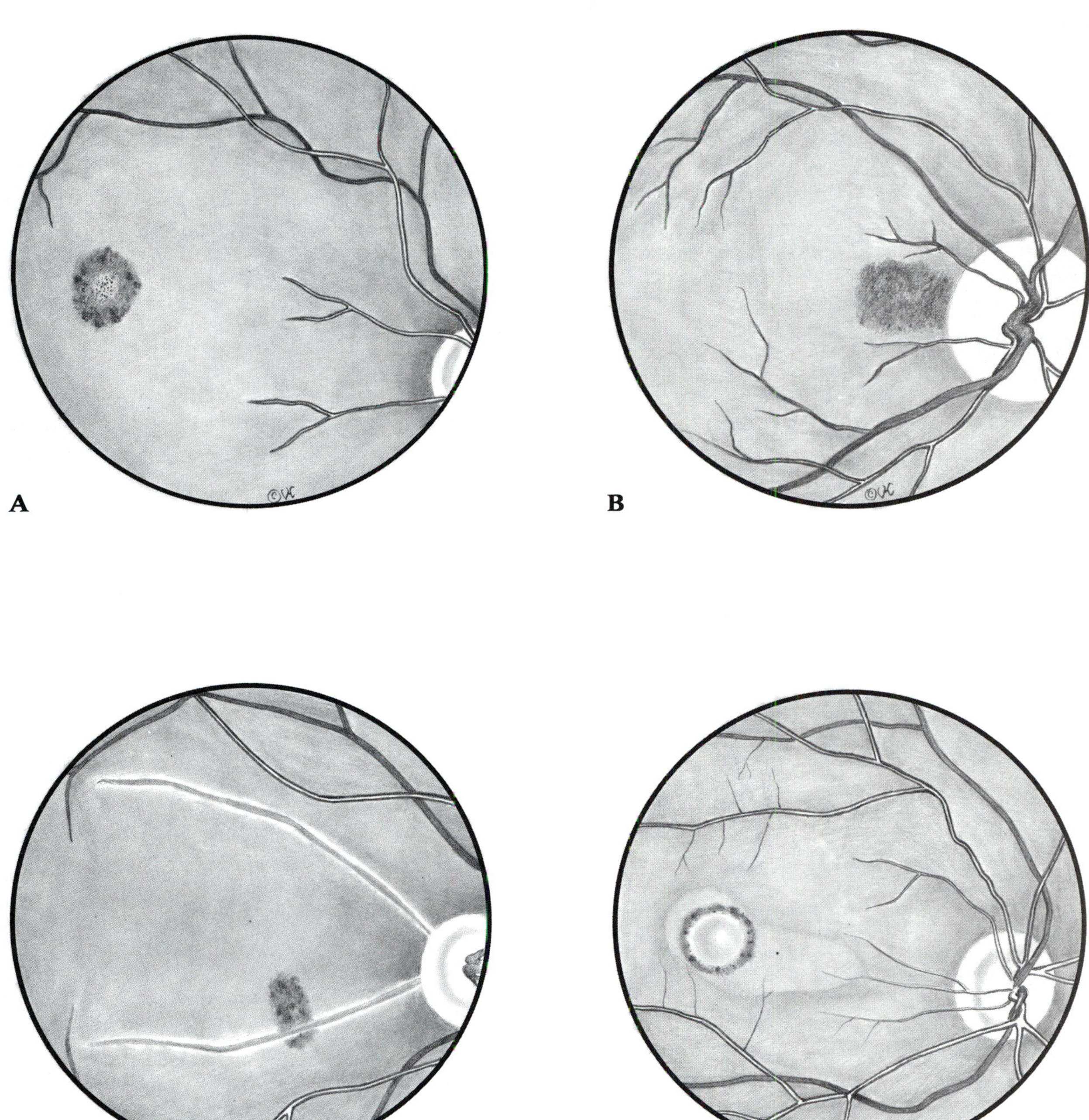

FIGURE 34-5. Follow-up observation.

POSTOPERATIVE INSTRUCTIONS

All patients treated for macular degeneration with laser should be instructed to avoid any form of anticoagulation or Valsalva maneuver in the postoperative 2 weeks until the lesion is stable. They must be warned that their vision will be worse immediately after laser and will begin to stabilize or improve starting only at approximately 4 to 7 days after treatment. Reevaluation as early as 2 days after treatment should be done for cases where the lesion is juxtafoveal. Failure to produce sealing in a juxtafoveal lesion requires frequent retreatment at short intervals to increase the poor chance for successful closure.

COMPLICATIONS

The most common complication of photocoagulation for macular degeneration is failure to seal the choroidal neovascular membrane in its entirety. The failure can occur either because photocoagulation did not extend to the entire neovascular membrane or because part of the photocoagulation is not sufficiently intense to produce total destruction.

This complication is avoided by careful postoperative checkups involving biomicroscopy and fluorescein angiography at no more than 2 weeks after the initial treatment. If the leakage persists, photocoagulation should be repeated immediately. Differentiation must be made between staining, which does not require retreatment, and leakage, which does require retreatment.

Choroidal hemorrhage, tear of the pigment epithelium, and macular pucker can be avoided through use of moderate laser energy for treatment.

CHAPTER 35

Toxoplasmic Retinitis and Presumed Ocular Histoplasmosis Syndrome

TOXOPLASMIC RETINITIS

The retinitis produced by *Toxoplasma gondii* is treatable by surgical means in cases where medical management is inappropriate or inadequate. The retinitis can occur as part of acquired systemic toxoplasmosis but more commonly results from reactivation of congenital toxoplasmosis, which is difficult to detect because of the absence of ophthalmoscopic evidence in areas of the retina harboring dormant congenital toxoplasmosis.

Etiology

Toxoplasma gondii has a strong proclivity for the nerve fiber layer of the retina. As an obligate intracellular parasite, the protozoa move easily in tissues, can multiply in any nucleated cell, and can infect adjacent healthy cells when each infected cell bursts. If the *Toxoplasma* is of low virulence or the host is highly resistant, the infected cell may fail to burst but, instead, will form a membranous cyst harboring thousands of *Toxoplasma* organisms. These organisms can remain viable in the congenital cyst for 25 years or more. Infection can occur from the ingestion of cat feces or the intake of insufficiently cooked beef or lamb as well as by inhalation of *Toxoplasma*-bearing fomites.

Natural history

Primary toxoplasmic retinitis can occur in apparently healthy persons after the ingestion of infected material (frequent uncooked or partially cooked meat). The retinitis also occurs as part of a primary infection in patients with immunodeficiency. The initial recurrent attack of congenital retinal toxoplasmosis occurs at any age between 50 and 60 years, with the average age of the first attack being approximately 25 years. The average duration of a toxoplasmic retinochoroiditis attack is 4.2 months with a range from 1 week to 2 years. The majority of patients (62%) have more than one recurrence. The average number of recurrences is 2.7.

After each recurrence, the area that has been inflamed shows a pigmented chorioretinal scar. The area of inflammation usually is contiguous with a pigmented site of previous scarring though the site of recurrence can be removed from the original. Each inflammatory episode can diminish visual acuity by either direct scarring of the macula or by the formation of preretinal membranes. Severe inflammation can cause vitreous fibrosis and lead to retinal tearing and detachment. Neovascularization of the disc or retina can follow an inflammatory episode. Choroidal neovascularization may grow into the sub–pigment epithelial space at the margin of a toxoplasmosis scar and produce hemorrhagic macular degeneration.

Diagnosis

White blood cells emanating from a focus of white inflamed retina adjacent to a pigmented chorioretinal scar extravasate into the overlying vitreous and produce the most common sign of toxoplasmic retinitis. There may be no pigmented scar, or the areas of retinal inflammation may be multiple and scattered throughout the fundus. The active white lesion in the retina can vary in size from less than one to more than four disc diameters.

When the nidus of retinitis is larger than approximately two disc diameters, the entire retinal thickness is inflamed. The panretinal inflammation can produce inflammation of the choroid and the vitreous with secondary iridocyclitis. Retinitis lesions larger than four disc diameters can produce chronic iridocyclitis that lasts for months, clouding the vitreous enough to obscure the entire fundus. Mutton-fat keratoprecipitates can accumulate and produce corneal edema and secondary glaucoma.

Blood testing using the Sabin-Feldman technique measures the antitoxoplasmosis antibody titer in serum with the titer starting to rise approximately 1 week after the original infection and reaching a maximum 1 to 2 months after infection and remaining weakly positive throughout life. It is a pattern rather than the magnitude of the titer level that is important for diagnosis. Fluorescent antibody testing provides the ultimate diagnosis in cases where the Sabin-Feldman test is negative.

Medical treatment

All but the mildest cases of toxoplasmosis require treatment. Corticosteroids are used for suppression of the inflammation. A combination of pyrimethamine and sulfadiazine is the traditional antimicrobial therapy. Clindamycin and sulfadiazine can be used simultaneously because of their synergistic effect. The risk of complications from the use of systemic corticosteroids, pyrimethamine (from platelet suppression), and clindamycin (from colitis) make medical therapy hazardous.

Photocoagulation

The photocoagulation of toxoplasmosis retinitis requires full-thickness retinal destruction because of the location of the organisms in the nerve fiber layer. Photocoagulation must destroy the entire region of inflamed retina to bring the inflammation under control. Leaving a margin of the inflamed area untreated leads to prolonged inflammation and invites recurrent fulminant inflammation after months of smoldering inflammation. It is unnecessary, however, to coagulate beyond the margins of the inflammatory focus. Pigmented areas adjacent to this focus should not be treated.

Krypton red laser photocoagulation provides the better means of coagulating the inflamed retina because of its relatively better penetration of the overlying inflammatory debris compared to the greater scattering of the shorter one, the green argon wavelength.

Aim the photocoagulation through the inflammatory debris overlying the nidus of retinitis (Fig. 35-1, *A*). Using 200 or 500 μm spot size with a duration of 0.5 seconds, calibrate the power level until a dense white reaction results. The 500 μm size is preferable because of its lesser risk of producing choroidal hemorrhage. Place contiguous laser burns over the entire nidus of inflammation (Fig. 35-1, *B*).

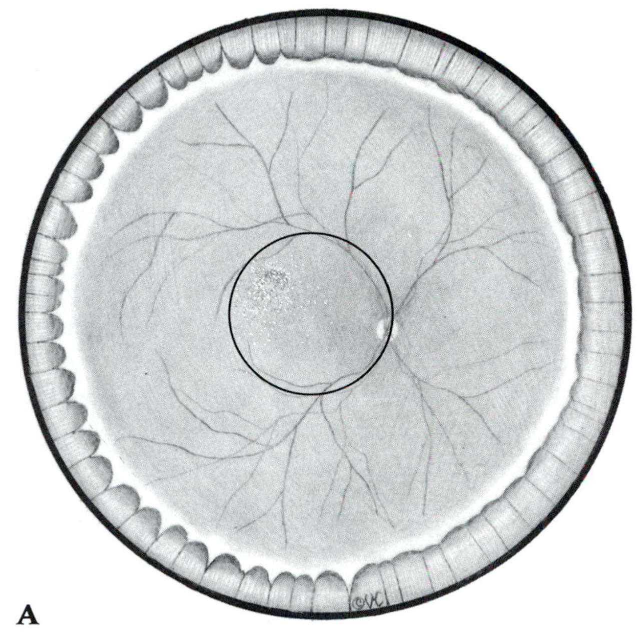

FIGURE 35-1. Photocoagulation technique of toxoplasmic retinitis.

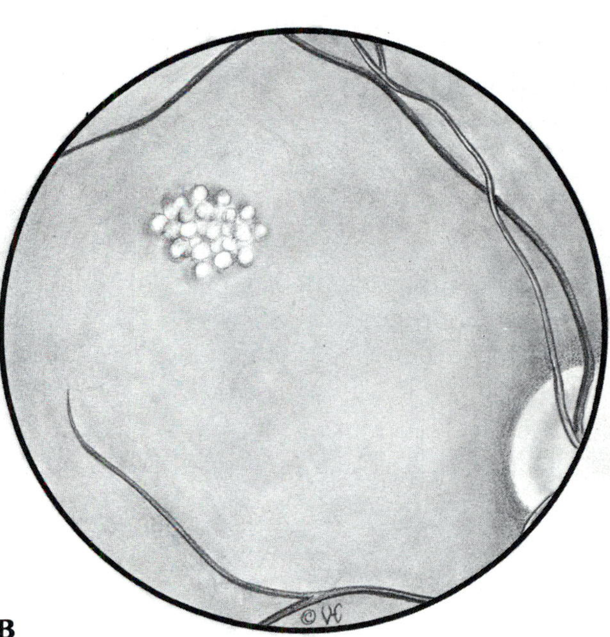

Cryosurgery

For lesions that are excessively obscured by overlying inflammation so that laser photocoagulation cannot penetrate, use cryocoagulation along with binocular indirect ophthalmoscopy. For peripheral lesions, the cryocoagulation can be used transconjunctivally, whereas a conjunctival and Tenon's incision is necessary for more posterior lesions. Because thermal sensitivity of the toxoplasmosis organisms is the basis of cryotreatment, it is necessary that the cryotherapy freeze-penetrate the entire retinal thickness to ensure destruction of the organisms. When freezing has penetrated sufficiently, it produces frozen whitening of the inner retinal layer whereupon the treatment should cease. As with photocoagulation, cryocoagulation must treat the entire nidus of inflammation without unnecessary damage to the surrounding retina. The freeze-thaw process should be repeated two times after the initial treatment during one single treatment session in order to maximize the damage to the organisms (Fig. 35-2).

Because cryocoagulation can cause a temporary exacerbation of the retina's inflammatory reaction, the use of systemic prednisone should be considered for severe cases for several days postoperatively to minimize the accumulation of visually disabling vitreous debris.

Follow-up study

The initial response to any treatment is edema of the retina, pigment epithelium, and choroid. The original whitening of the retina can be more intense and vitreous debris worse on the day after surgery. Four to 6 weeks after treatment, pigmentation should appear at the treatment site. Usually, debris begins to show improvement within 1 week after treatment. Failure of all retinal whitening to disappear by 6 weeks after surgery is an indication that surgery should be repeated. A pigmented area without any residual retinal whitening and clearing of overlying debris indicates a successful outcome (Fig. 35-3).

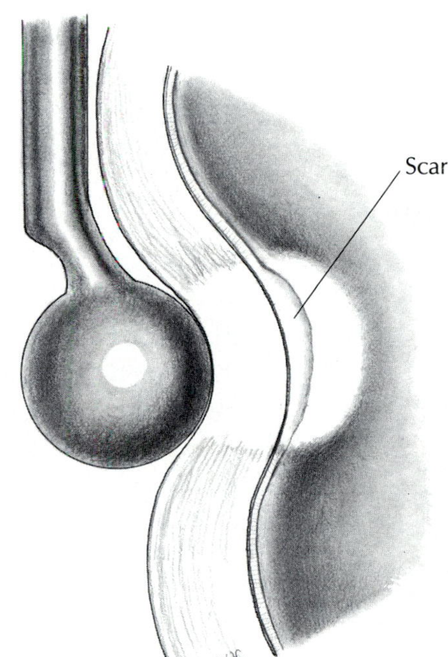

FIGURE 35-2. Cryosurgery.

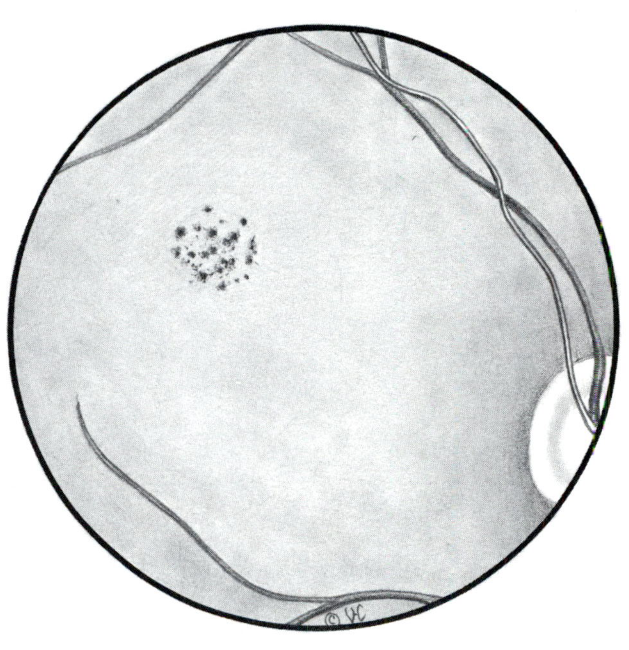

FIGURE 35-3. Follow-up observation.

PRESUMED OCULAR HISTOPLASMOSIS SYNDROME

The *presumed ocular histoplasmosis* (POH) syndrome consists in a triad of clinical findings: (1) serous or hemorrhagic macular degeneration, (2) yellow choroidal spots, and (3) peripapillary scars. The most important clinical component of POH is its hemorrhagic macular degeneration, which occurs at a young age. POH carries the term "presumed" because histologic or immunologic proof of the cause-and-effect relationship of the *Histoplasma capsulatum* organism is lacking.

Clinical findings

The patient with presumed ocular histoplasmosis presents because of diminished visual acuity from macular involvement. The growth of neovascularization from the choroid into the sub–pigment epithelial space produces a pigment ring at the site of an old, atrophic yellow scar at the level of the choroid. The neovascular network gives rise to serous detachment separating the pigment epithelium and retina and, eventually, to hemorrhagic detachment of both layers. Unlike senile macular degeneration, POH is unassociated with drusen or the accumulation of yellow basal linear deposits on Bruch's membrane.

The inactive POH spots appear at both the macula and the peripheral fundus as yellow-orange, with pigment loss in the overlying pigment epithelium and with hyperpigmentation surrounding the spots, which range in size from 0.1 to 0.7 disc diameter. As many as 70 spots can fill one fundus.

At the optic disc, the choroidal lesion produces a depigmented halo separating the margin of the disc from a thin ring of surrounding hyperpigmentation. An alternative pattern produces nodular involvement of the choroid and the pigment epithelium surrounding the disc, with normal peripapillary choroid and pigment epithelium surrounded by discreet areas of patchy loss of both the choriocapillaris and the pigment epithelium. The choroidal neovascularization grows from the nodules toward the macula where it produces hemorrhage. POH lesions cause vision loss only if there is macular involvement.

Patients with POH range in age from 7 to 77 years with rare occurrence below age 20 or over age 50. POH is evenly distributed between the sexes but is far more frequent in whites than in blacks. Both inactive and active POH are unaccompanied by any other ocular inflammatory or vascular disease: the absence of inflammatory debris overlying the active lesion differentiates it from infectious lesions. POH is associated with the HLA-B7 cell surface antigen.

Etiology

The POH choroidal nodules most likely result from episodes of disseminated blood-borne histoplasmosis during mild dissemination. A self-limited choroiditis destroys the fungi and forms the choroidal granuloma. With damage to Bruch's membrane in the final scar, choroidal vessels are able to penetrate the sub–pigment epithelial space where they present the same risks as in senile macular degeneration.

Categorization

The categorization of presumed ocular histoplasmosis according to the degree of macular involvement is the basis for selecting cases for treatment. In stage I of macular involvement, a yellow-white spot similar to the peripheral spot is the only abnormality. Usually, there is only one spot, but occasionally two or three spots are present in the macula. The yellow spots can remain quiescent or progress to stage II activity. The stage I lesion results from a granulomatous elevation of the pigment epithelium extending from the choriocapillaris through Bruch's membrane to the base of the overlying pigment epithelium (Fig. 35-4, *A*). The absence of leakage as shown by no fluorescein leakage and the absence of subretinal fluid result from the dearth of choroidal vessels within the lesion or at its margins. In stage I, the patient is usually asymptomatic but can notice metamorphopsia caused directly by distortion of the pigment epithelium at the site of the lesion.

Stage II lesions result from the growth of choroidal neovascularization into the sub–pigment epithelial space producing serous elevation of both pigment epithelium and the retina and reactive hyperpigmentation surrounding the neovascularization (Fig. 35-4, *B*). The neovascular network first is confined by the pigment ring but later extends beyond it. Stage II most commonly appears as a cluster of gray nodules caused by small, localized detachments of the pigment epithelium. Eventually the nodules coalesce to form pigment rings approximately 0.5 disc diameter wide. A partial central scotoma results from the retinal serous detachment, which is far larger than the pigment epithelial detachment. This stage can undergo spontaneous resolution but can progress to stage III.

The stage III lesion is the most common to lead a patient to seek ophthalmic consultation. The lesion shows a dark, greenish gray circular or oval area caused by sub–pigment epithelial hemorrhage from neovascularization. If blood dissects through the pigment epithelium, a bright red color appears surrounding the lesion. Fluorescein angiography shows choroidal neovascularization originating from a central vascular spoke.

The stage IV lesion results from hemorrhages that have been recurrent for a period of approximately 2 years. The chronic hemorrhagic process produces a fibrous scar and atrophy. The pigment epithelium and the retina are chronically detached at the macula.

The circumpapillary lesions of POH produce the same changes as those at the macula but with a more obvious appearance because of the lower density of pigment epithelial cells. Although POH lesions at the disc are less dangerous than those nearer to the fovea, fully 10% of them develop hemorrhage. Of the hemorrhagic group, 50% of cases lead to legal blindness.

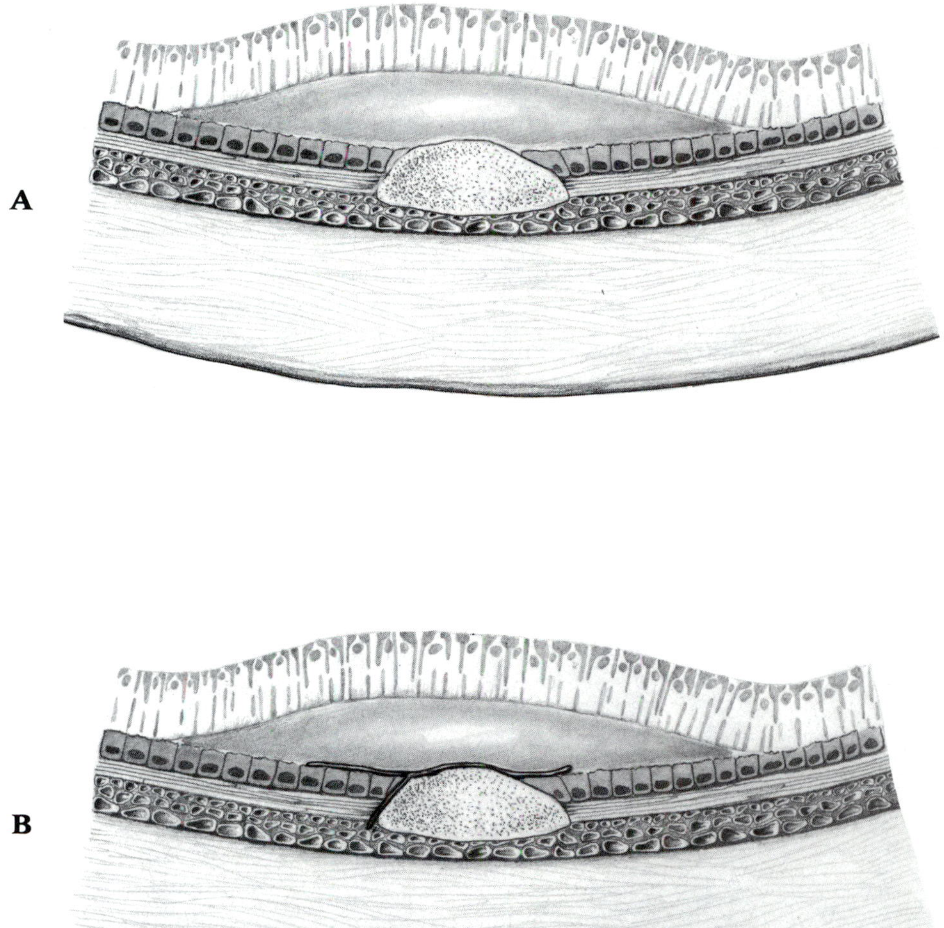

FIGURE 35-4. Categorization of presumed ocular histoplasmosis syndrome.

Photocoagulation Technique

Krypton red is the ideal wavelength for photocoagulation of avascular or vascular histoplasmosis lesions. With avascular histoplasmotic lesions with leakage the laser must reach to the primary focus of the lesion at Bruch's membrane, the choroid, and the pigment epithelium (Fig. 35-5, *A*). There is no need for photocoagulation to involve the neurosensory retina. Similarly for vascular lesions of histoplasmosis with leakage where a choroidal neovascular membrane penetrates into the subretinal space, krypton red is ideal for coagulating the layers from the choroid through the pigment epithelium and sparing the overlying retina (Fig. 35-5, *B*). Argon green wavelength can be used but presents the combined disadvantages of coagulating primarily the pigment epithelium and only secondarily coagulating the choroid. The argon laser also risks coagulation of the neurosensory retina because of absorption by hemoglobin.

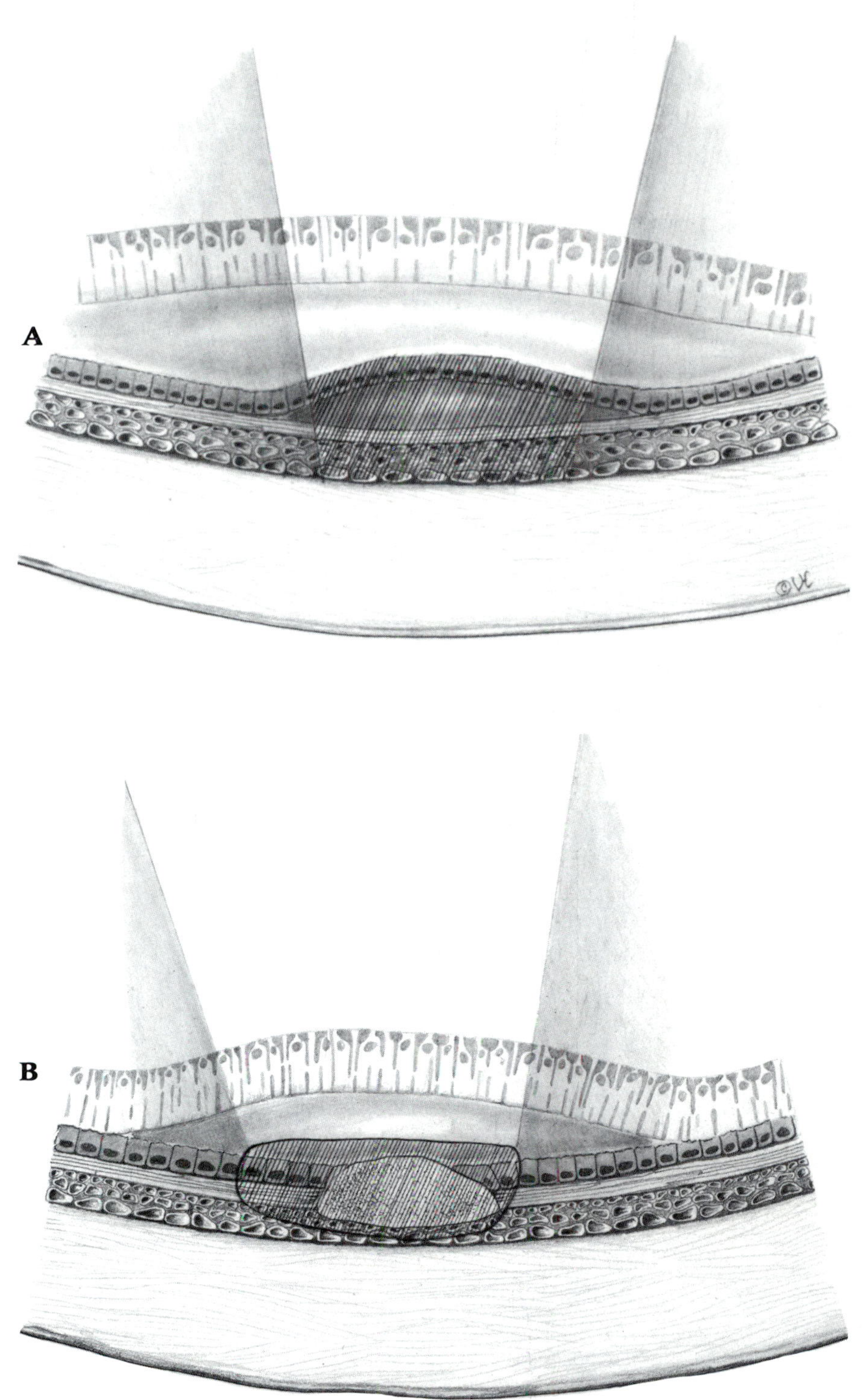

FIGURE 35-5. Photocoagulation of avascular or vascular histoplasmotic lesions.

Continued.

Place the intital photocoagulations to surround the pigment epithelial detachment and choroidal focus rather than through the area of exudation (Fig. 35-5, *C*). Then fill the entire leakage zone with krypton red 200 μm spot size with a duration of 0.5 seconds and a power sufficient to produce a yellow-white reaction (Fig. 35-5, *D*). Then return to the treated zone and introduce more intense treatment to bring it to a near white. Intense whitening is unnecessary and risks hemorrhage and macular pucker.

Photocoagulation of a vascular histoplasmotic lesion with hemorrhage differs from photocoagulation of a leaking avascular lesion by the need to limit photocoagulation to the neovascular zone and its perimeter without excessive involvement of the hemorrhage (Fig. 35-5, *E*). Krypton red laser photocoagulation is the best available method for this purpose because of its ability to penetrate shallow layers of blood to reach the vascular zone.

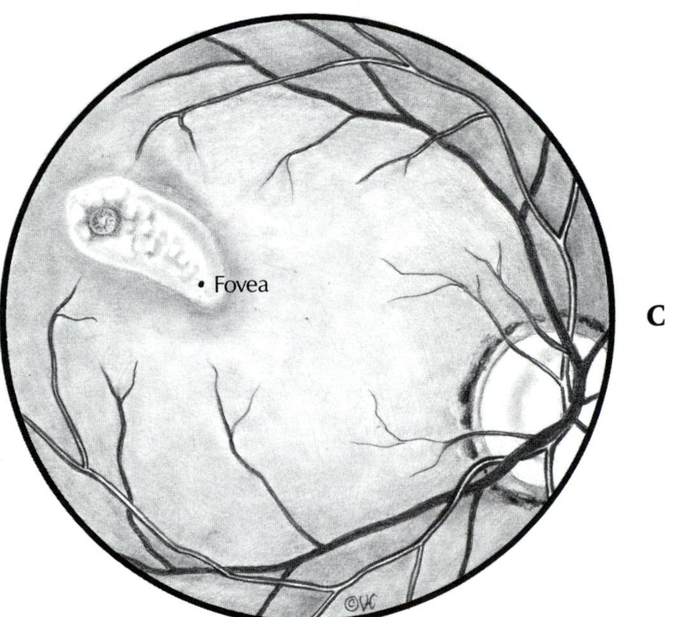

FIGURE 35-5, cont'd

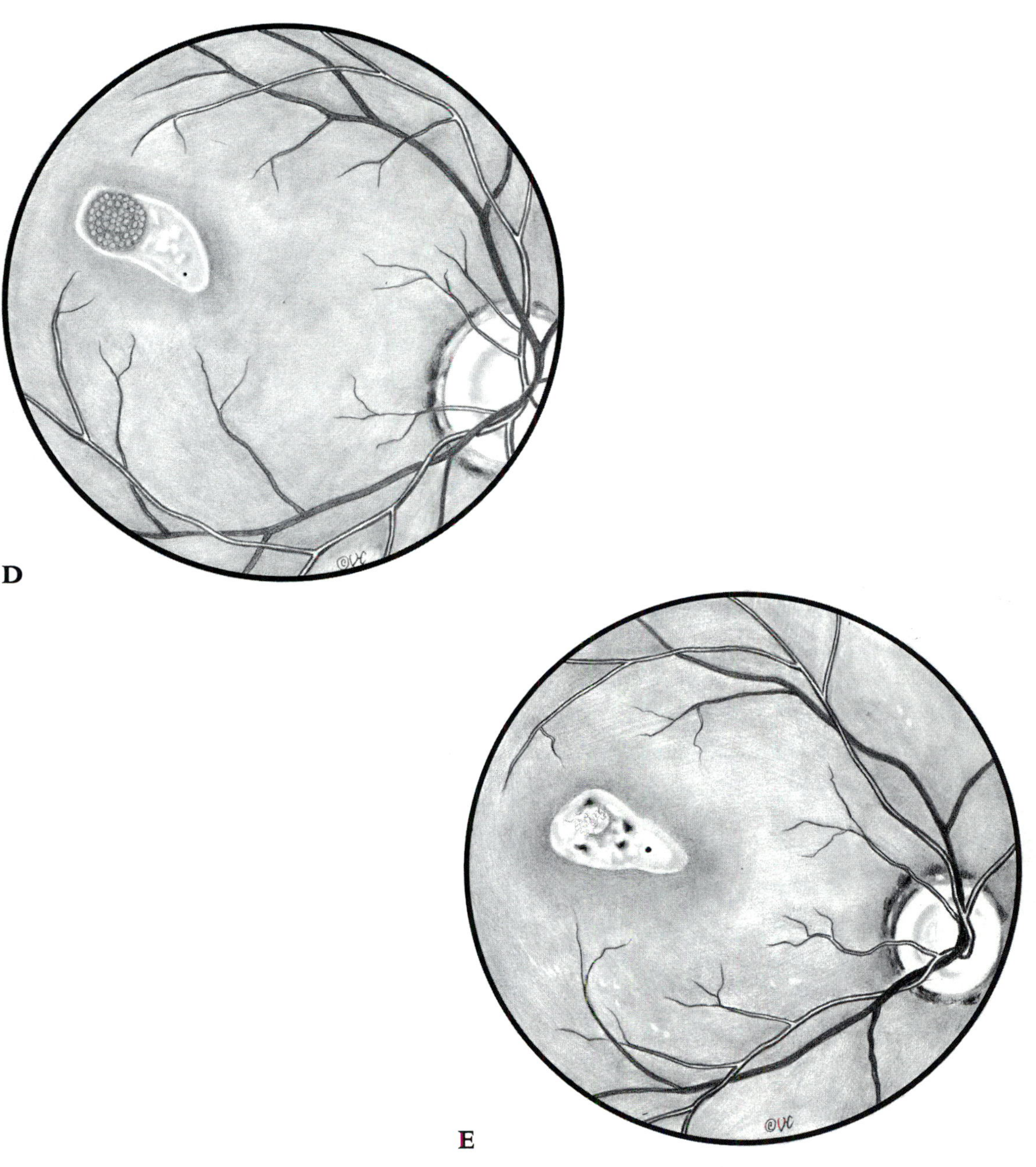

Continued.

After identification of the extent of the neovascularization on a fluorescein angiogram done within 72 hours, use the krypton red wavelength to create yellow-white burns in a contiguous fashion first surrounding the lesion and then covering the entirety of the lesion. Then re-treat the lesion to create a yellow-white reaction, which is more intense than the original treatment (Fig. 35-5, *F*). Err in the direction of treating beyond the limits of the neovascularization rather than risking leaving a portion of the neovascular network untreated.

FOLLOW-UP STUDY

The absorption of subretinal fluid during the period immediately after photocoagulation indicates that the neovascularization has been coagulated. If subretinal fluid persists, fluorescein angiography must be repeated to determine the source of the leakage. If the lesion is close to the fovea, the reexamination should be done within days of the original treatment. If the lesion is far from the fovea, greater than 400 μm, follow-up observation should be done at 10 days to 2 weeks. Photocoagulation must be repeated to any persistent areas of leakage or areas that show new leakage where neovascularization may have spread.

Patients with POH can use the Amsler grid for weekly self-testing and undergo regular fundus examinations so that the activity from either a fresh lesion or an old lesion can be treated during the early stage.

The desired fundus outcome ultimately produces scarring and atrophy in the area of treatment with drying of the edema at the macula (Fig. 35-5, *G*). Atrophic changes at the macula result from the previous insult and the fluid accumulation and do not necessarily indicate the ingrowth of choroidal neovascularization. Any change in the morphology of the scar can indicate regrowth of neovascularization and need for reevaluation for possible treatment.

COMPLICATIONS

The major complication is inadvertent photocoagulation of the fovea or of the perifoveal capillary network. Lower the laser energy input when treating near the fovea because of the lateral spread of the burn toward the fovea and increased absorption by the foveal xanthophyll pigment.

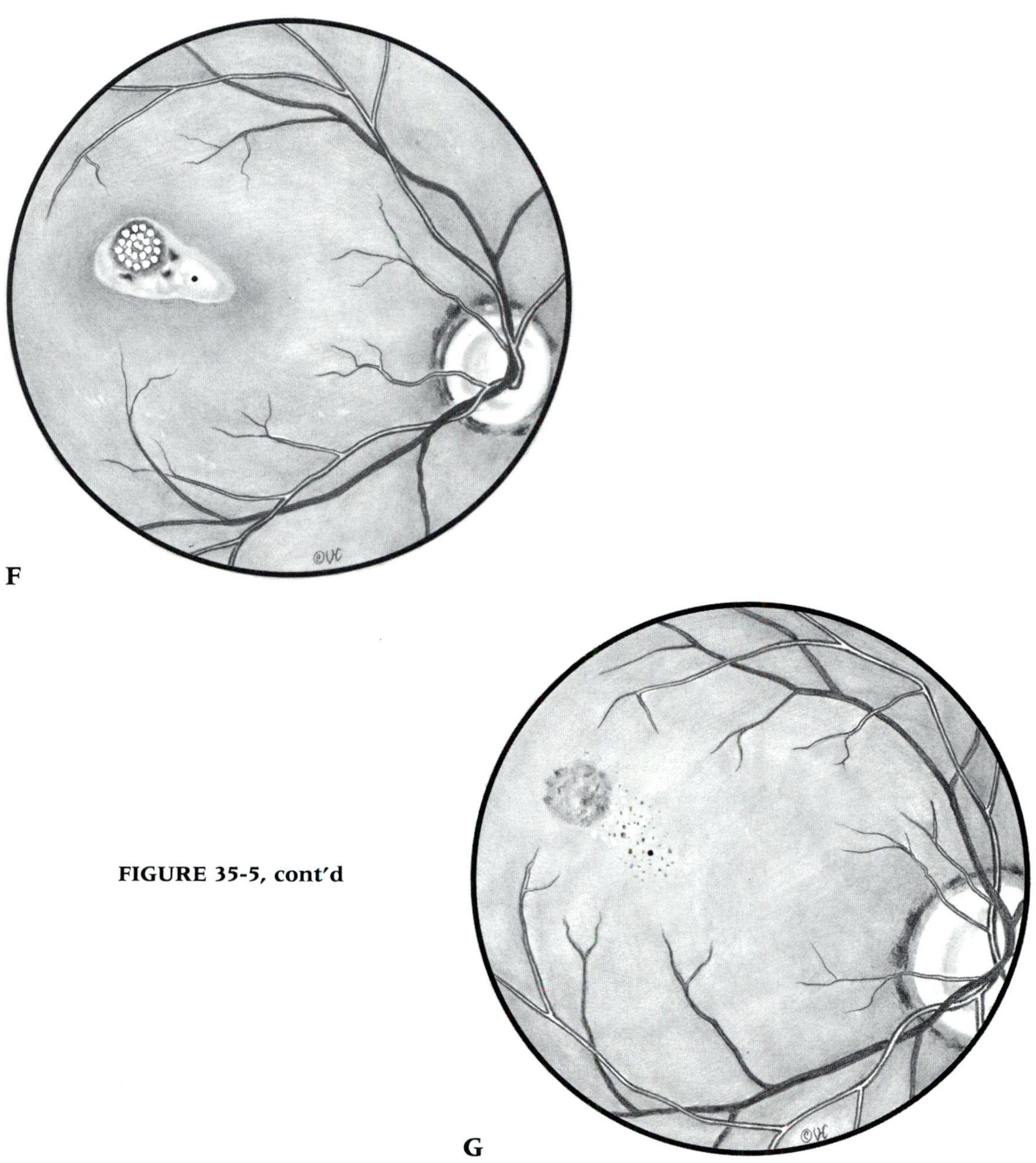

FIGURE 35-5, cont'd

CHAPTER 36

Macular Hole with Retinal Detachment

A macular hole is a full-thickness retinal break occurring at the macula. In comparison to lamellar holes, macular cysts, cystoid macular edema, and serous elevation of the macula, the macular hole is a full-thickness break that permits the accumulation of subretinal fluid and has the potential to lead to rhegmatogenous retinal detachment. Although the loss of central visual acuity caused by a macular hole is irreparable, the repair of the resulting retinal detachment can preserve peripheral vision.

ETIOLOGY

Macular holes result from concussive ocular trauma in approximately 10% of cases and spontaneously without a history of trauma in 90% of cases. The macular hole can result from prolonged macular edema with atrophy of the cellular elements. More commonly, a macular hole can result from vitreous traction from an abnormal adhesion between the posterior hyaloid and the macula. Most macular holes result from cystoid macular edema secondary to a primary vascular abnormality, systemic hypertension, occlusion of the central retinal artery or vein, periphlebitis, syphilitic vasculitis, Behçet's syndrome, Coats's disease, solar retinitis, or nonspecific chorioretinitis. Once cystoid edema progresses to form intraretinal cysts, the tissue atrophy resulting in macular hole formation has begun. The low incidence of bilaterality of macular holes (approximately 10%) has made evaluation of medical vasodilatation or prophylactic vitrectomy in the second eye difficult.

NATURAL PROGRESSION AND INDICATIONS FOR TREATMENT

A macular hole without detachment should not be treated because 80% of such cases remain unchanged or even improve by spontaneous reattachment of the hole's rim. These results are better than the results of photocoagulation, which worsen acuity by enlarging the central scotoma. The only indications for prophylactic laser photocoagulation of the margins of a macular hole without concomitant detachment are myopia greater than 6 diopters and an unequivocal history of truma.

Retinal detachment combined with macular hole progresses from focal detachment surrounding the hole (type I) to retinal detachment extending to the equator and resembling an effusion detachment (type II) to a retinal detachment extending to the ora in a minimum of one quadrant (type III). Type I and type II detachments can be managed by scleral buckling and vitrectomy. In a type III retinal detachment the macular hole is always putative and can be a false-positive diagnosis. Only 0.5% of retinal detachments involving the macula are caused by a macular hole. In eyes with myopia greater than 8 diopters, 2% of detachments are caused by a macular hole. Females have a seven times greater rate of detachment caused by a macular hole than males do. In type III retinal detachment, which extends to the ora serrata, a search should be made for a peripheral retinal break. What appears to be a macular hole can be a cyst or the optical illusion of a full-thickness hole. In cases where there is some question as to whether the detachment results from a peripheral retinal break or a retinal hole, the primary operation should be an attempt to buckle the retinal periphery. Only if the operation fails and subretinal fluid reaccumulates in the postoperative days should a surgical procedure be performed to seal the macular hole.

Pars Plana Vitrectomy

Pars plana vitrectomy seals a macular hole by severing any adhesions of the vitreous to the perimacular retina and lowers the intraocular pressure sufficiently to permit an intraocular gas injection which tampons the retina at the site of the macular hole as the patient lies prone during the postoperative days.

Remove only the posterior half of the vitreous leaving the retrolenticular vitreous intact (Fig. 36-1, *A*). After removal of the vitreous and closure of the vitrectomy sclerotomies, inject a gas bubble into the vitreous cavity without raising the intraocular pressure. To accomplish this, release liquid vitreous through the vitrectomy incision at the pars plana with a needle and syringe. An expansile bubble of long duration is the best means of management. The bubble must last for at least 10 days in order for the retina to seal against the pigment epithelium. During the 10 postoperative days, the patient must lie prone. Initially the gas bubble will be insufficient to tampon the entire area of detachment (Fig. 36-1, *B*). In the postoperative hours the bubble will expand and produce retinal reattachment (Fig. 36-1, *C*). The techniques of posterior segment vitrectomy are discussed in Chapter 23.

Laser photocoagulation provides the safest method of producing a scar with minimal enlargement of the central scotoma. The photocoagulation should be done before vitrectomy surgery if possible. Krypton red is preferable to argon green because it penetrates through the detached retina. The photocoagulation should create a white reaction in the pigment epithelium so that a scar forms between the retina and the pigment epithelium while the gas bubble juxtaposes the two layers. If photocoagulation cannot whiten the pigment epithelium, perform laser coagulation as soon after surgery as inflammation and optical clarity permit.

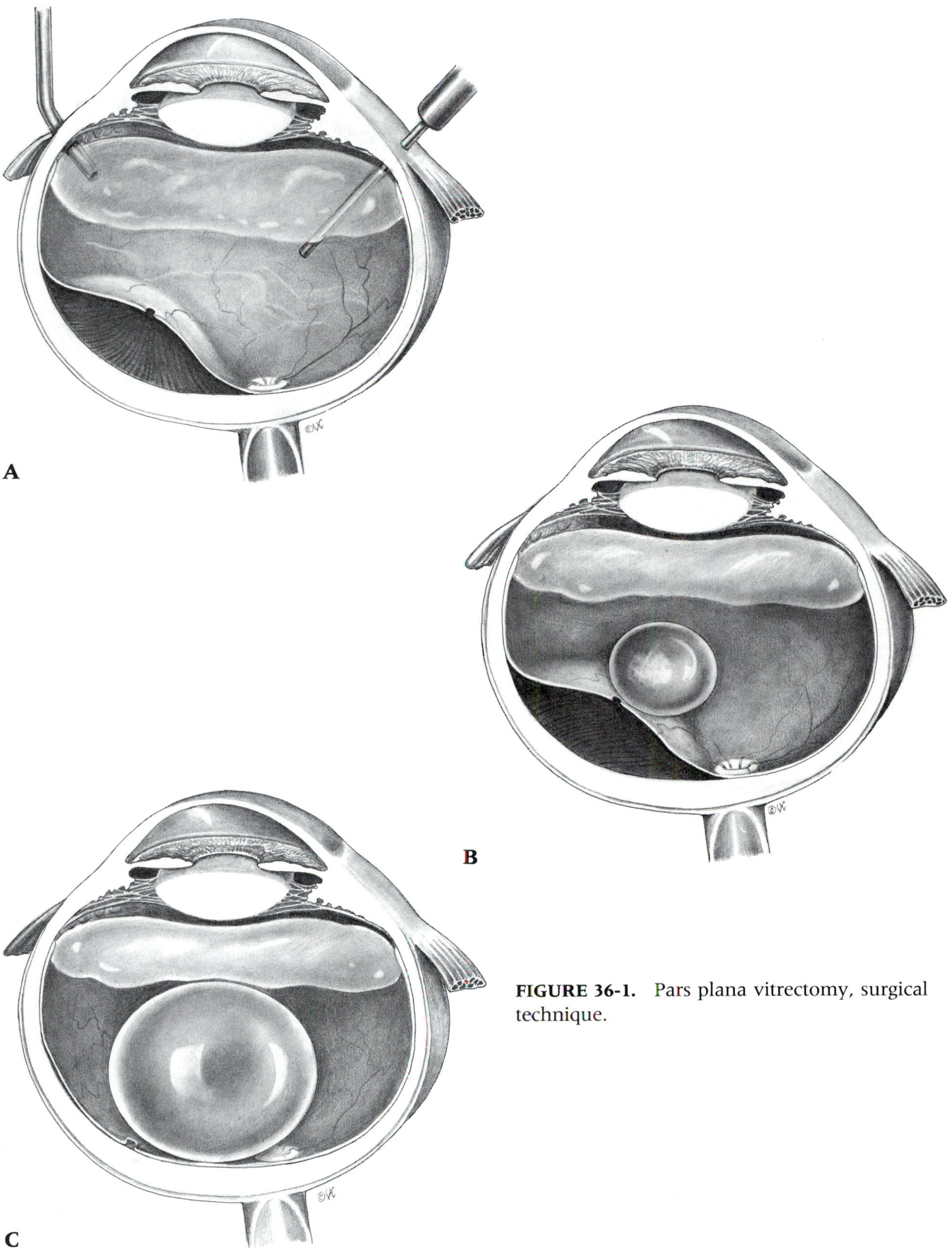

FIGURE 36-1. Pars plana vitrectomy, surgical technique.

Macular Scleral Buckling

The decision to perform scleral buckling surgery can be made before surgery in some cases. When the macula contains a posterior staphyloma, there is less chance of permanent retinal reattachment after the release of vitreous traction by vitrectomy surgery because depth of the staphyloma may prevent the retina from reshaping itself to the wall of the eye. Periretinal proliferation on the surface of the macula is a second preoperative indication for scleral buckling surgery. The membrane shrinks the diameter of the detached retina and prevents retinal reattachment despite the release of vitreous traction. Theoretically, membrane peeling allows the retina to reattach, but this type of surgery carries hazards that are not warranted because of the strong possibility of the success of the alternative buckling procedure. Cases in which the macula does not settle against the pigment epithelium on completion of vitrectomy surgery also requires scleral buckling surgery.

Solid silicone buckling of the macular hole requires the placement of a sling around the posterior segment of the globe. Adequate exposure of the globe requires a deep lateral canthotomy and detachment of the lateral rectus and the inferior oblique muscles. Place traction sutures through the stump of the lateral rectus to allow its use for rotation of the globe. When the globe is rotated, you can determine the position of the macula by finding the midpoint between the medial border of the insertion of the inferior oblique muscle and the optic nerve (Fig. 36-2). Sever the inferior oblique insertion after identifying it. Leave the superior oblique tendon insertion and the vortex veins intact because they do not limit surgical exposure.

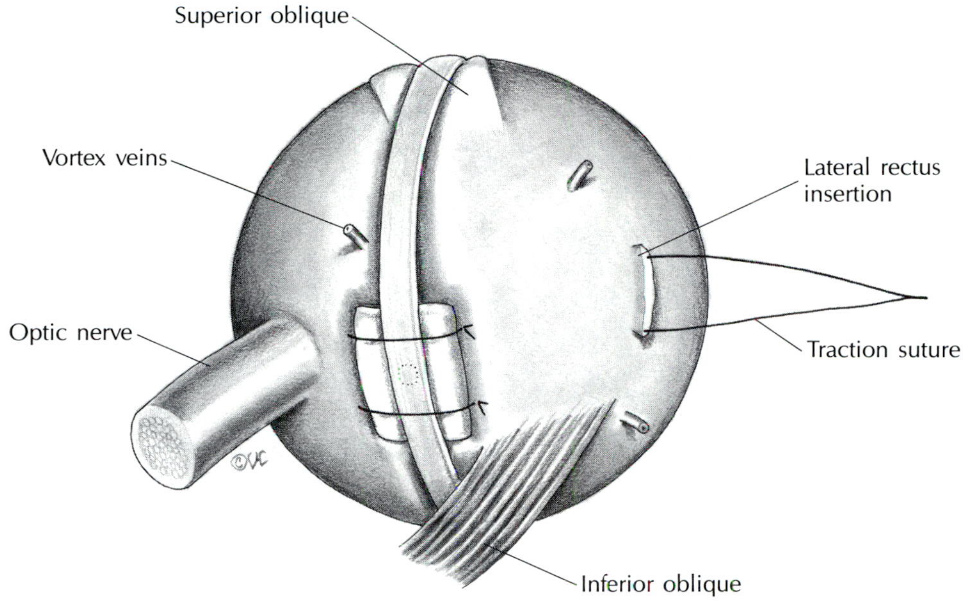

FIGURE 36-2. Macular scleral buckling.

In cases with a deeply set globe, the detachment of the inferior rectus can expedite exposure. Rotate the globe superonasally so that its posterior aspect becomes clearly visible. Examine the posterior aspect for a possible staphyloma or a scleral dehiscence. Do not sharply dissect tissues at the posterior aspect of the globe because of the risk of scleral rupture or excessive bleeding, which will reduce exposure. Remove only the loosely adherent fascia from the posterior aspect of the globe.

To indent the macula, place the silicone band over the posterior half of the globe in the meridian extending from 12 to 6 o'clock positions. The band should be sighted directly over a localization mark. The band should have a solid silicone explant tied to it before the band is placed over the macula. Cut the band so that its ends lie at the equator of the globe, and place it beneath the lateral vortex veins to avoid compressing them. To prevent lateral migration of the band, place it on a great circle route passing through the macula, with the superior end carried through a tunnel cut in the insertion of the superior temporal vortex vein. Place a nonabsorbable, anchoring mattress suture into the medial border of the superior rectus muscle at the globe's equator to anchor the sling. Pass the inferior end of the band beneath the inferotemporal vortex vein to anchor this end of the equator to the globe near the temporal border of the inferior rectus muscle. Tie both equatorial anchoring sutures over the band with a temporary slip knot, and place a wider piece of silicone with a grooved fit under the sling. Attaching this wide silicone piece to the band prior to the band's placement simplifies the attachment of the silicone explant. Drainage of subretinal fluid softens the globe for buckling. Because of the thickness of the sclera at the macula, usually more than 1 mm, perform the draining procedure with a long, fine 2 mm perforating needle pushed through the sclera at the point of previously placed diathermy to decrease the risk of choroidal hemorrhage. This technique drains subretinal fluid slowly because of the small scleral perforation without cutdown. If the retinal detachment is extensive, the scleral perforation can be placed more anteriorly within the area of detachment. This technique decreases the risk of perforation of the long posterior ciliary artery. Subretinal fluid of long-standing macular detachment can be so viscid that only a small amount of fluid escapes with the original single perforation of either technique, and multiple perforations through the original site or through added neighboring sites may be necessary to release enough subretinal fluid to soften the globe and allow buckling. The release of viscid subretinal fluid is important because the fluid's spontaneous resorption is so slow that the retina may not reattach during the 2-week period required for scarring either by diathermy placed at the time of surgery or by postoperative laser.

When the globe is softened, permanently tie one of the mattress sutures over the overlying equatorial sling. Any traction should pull the other end of the sling so that the height and position of the buckle can be evaluated and controlled with examination of the fundus. To prevent slippage, even after the second end of the band is permanently tied, use two additional mattress sutures across the silicone band. Do not place sutures within a scleral staphyloma. At completion of the buckling procedure, the buckle height should be adequate to seal the macular hole. If there is no laser in the operating room, perform photocoagulation to the rim of the hole as soon as the orbital swelling permits.

Sponge Silicone Buckling

Silicone sponge material can be used in place of solid silicone to create a sling for buckling over the macula. The sponge buckling eliminates the necessity to soften the globe to achieve indentation. During the postoperative hours the elasticity of the sponge indents the globe enough to close the macular hole.

Using a procedure similar to the one described for the placement of the solid silicone sling, place a 5 mm wide cylindrical silicone sponge from the superior nasal quadrant across the back of the globe to the inferotemporal quadrant (Fig. 36-3, *A*). Introduce the end of the sponge at the superonasal quadrant of the globe at the margin of the insertion of the superior rectus muscle and on top of the insertion of the superior oblique tendon. Pass the sponge inferiorly. Its distal end should emerge in the inferotemporal quadrant at the lateral margin of the inferior rectus muscle. Fix the superonasal end of the sponge with a permanent mattress suture at the equator. A second mattress suture, posterior to the initial suture, provides further anchoring for this end of the sponge. Before placing the sponge, maneuver its inferotemporal extremity to place it over the scleral area marked by diathermy treatment for treatment of the macular hole. Final positioning requires observation by the indirect ophthalmoscope to create an indentation over the site of the macular hole (Fig. 36-3, *B*). When the sponge is placed properly, increase the tension on it until there is a visible buckling of the macula. Place a permanent suture in the equatorial sclera of the inferotemporal quadrant at the site that anchors the sponge in the correct position. Before tying the suture, determine if globe softening is necessary to produce adequate indentation. Create tension on the sponge by pulling its inferotemporal end while the permanent suture is tied. Tie a second suture in the inferotemporal quadrant into a tight mattress suture only when the tension on the sponge is adequate. Finally, trim the two ends of the sponge to prevent the superficial edge of these ends from causing conjunctival erosion.

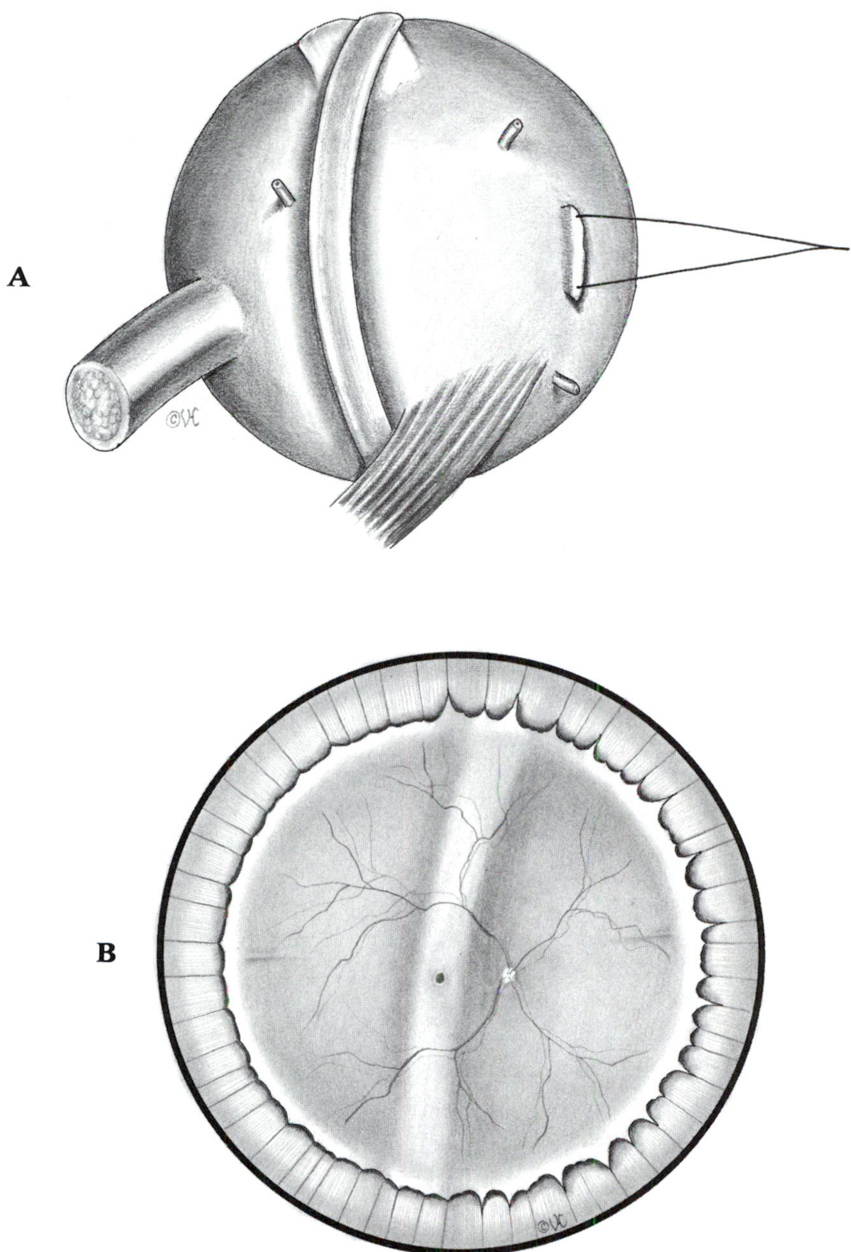

FIGURE 36-3. Sponge silicone buckling.

Y-Shaped Sponge Buckling

A variation of the sponge technique is to divide a wide sponge along its length after its inferotemporal end has been anchored to the sclera and after the position for anchoring the superonasal quadrant has been determined (Fig. 36-4). Dividing the sponge in this manner creates a semi-inverted Y shape with the division of the arms of the Y halfway between the macula and the superotemporal point of suturing. Attach the inferior portion of the Y to the sclera, 3 mm inferior to the equatorial mark, and secure it with a permanent suture temporarily tied with a slipknot. Bring the upper arm of the Y deep to the edge of the insertion of the superior rectus muscle, and secure it at the equator in the superonasal quadrant with a permanent mattress suture tied as a slipknot. If subretinal fluid drainage or paracentesis is to be performed, do it now. It is easiest to drain the subretinal fluid in the inferotemporal quadrant.

After drainage, in order to produce indentation on the scleral surface, manipulate the struts of the Y as the assistant gently draws the two temporal struts taut after the slipknots. Precise localization of the indentation over the diathermy marks at the macula can require several separate repositioning steps. It is often helpful to fix one strut to the sclera temporarily while the other is being manipulated because such fixation permits the sponge to be moved to a more effective great-circle path. When observation of the indentation by binocular indirect ophthalmoscopy shows that the hole is sealed, tie the suture permanently and excise the excess sponge. This surgical procedure has the advantage of placing the sponge precisely, with a minimum of manipulation.

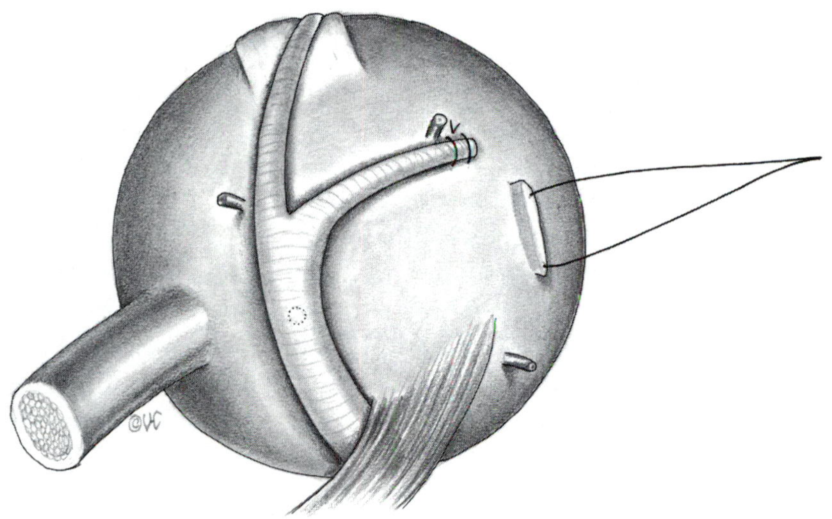

FIGURE 36-4. Y-shaped sponge buckling.

Intrascleral Pouch

The intrascleral pouch technique for macular buckling differs from the previously described techniques in that it requires scleral surgery directly at the macula. While this technique presents obvious hazards to a tyro surgeon, it can be safer and easier for the surgeon who is more experienced in scleral dissection than in the placement of intrascleral sutures. The two essential requirements for dissecting an intrascleral pouch at the macula are adequate surgical exposure and precise localization. Exposure requires the removal of the lateral and inferior recti. External topographic localization is simpler than localization using the binocular indirect ophthalmoscope. The posterior end of the insertion of the inferior oblique muscle lies 3 to 6 mm in front of the optic nerve and 1 mm below and 1 to 2 mm in front of the macula. The temporal long posterior ciliary artery is another landmark; it runs in the horizontal meridian 3 to 4 mm superior to the access of the optic nerve. The use of these landmarks permits localization of the macula within 1 mm without the difficulty of using binocular indirect ophthalmoscopy.

To create the macular scleral pouch, make a scleral incision with the posterior tip of the inferior oblique muscle insertion at the midpoint. Extend the excision 6 to 8 mm on the horizontal meridian. Anterior dissection of this pouch risks rupture of the posterior ciliary artery. Should a rupture occur, cauterize the vessel with diathermy. The complete dissection should result in slight listing of the posterior tip of the inferior oblique muscle insertion. The short ciliary vessels produce hemorrhage, which requires diathermy coagulation to maintain a sufficiently clear view. From a sheet of Gelfilm 0.75 mm thick, cut a 6 by 6 mm piece. Keep this piece at least partially nonhydrated so that it will increase in size during its hydration in the scleral pouch. Tie the two overlying permanent mattress sutures after the Gelfilm is placed in the pouch (Fig. 36-5, *A*). Binocular indirect ophthalmoscopy will show only a slight buckling effect beneath the macular hole, but during the 48 hours after surgery increased hydration of the Gelfilm increases the height of the buckling and seals the tear. As soon as the hydration of the Gelfilm has caused the pigment epithelium to touch the retina at the macula (Fig. 36-5, *B*), during the first few days after surgery, surround the macular hole with either laser or xenon arc photocoagulation. Failure to place these scars can result in redetachment months after surgery when the height of the scleral buckle decreases.

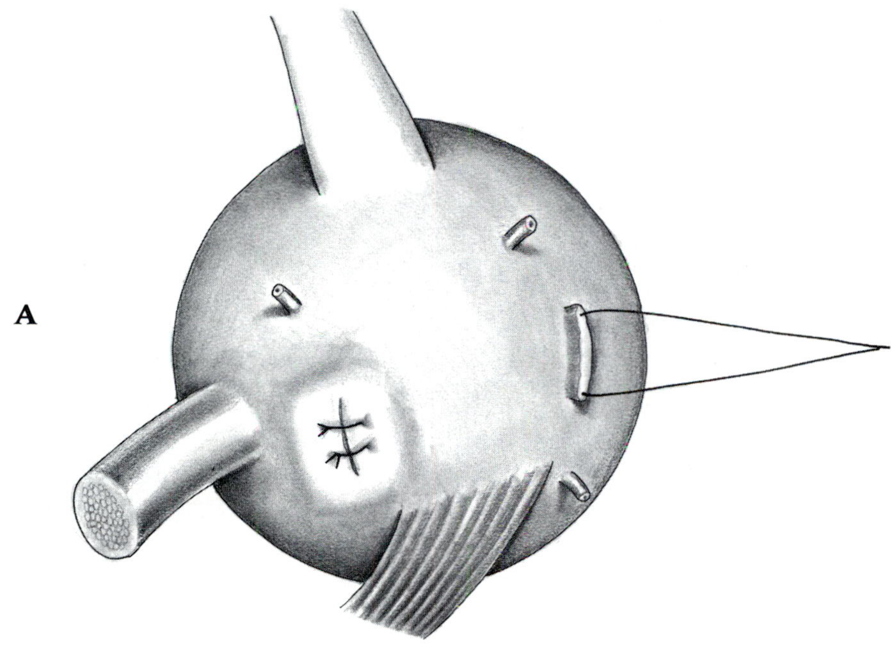

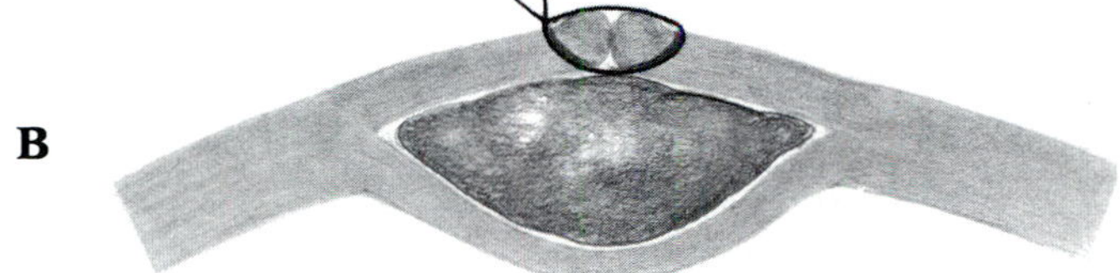

FIGURE 36-5. Intrascleral pouch.

FOLLOW-UP STUDY

Redetachment of the retina after macular hole surgery most frequently indicates that a peripheral retinal break was the cause of the detachment in a type III case. The pattern of accumulation of fluid from the retinal periphery indicates the need for peripheral buckling. Reopening of the macular hole after initially successful surgery can indicate inadequate scarring by laser or other means during surgery. If the margins of the tear are seen to begin to separate again from the pigment epithelium, laser photocoagulation should be performed as an emergency procedure.

COMPLICATIONS OF MACULAR BUCKLING

Macular buckling carries all the complications of scleral buckling surgery. In addition, macular buckling can cause optic nerve compression either by intraoperative maneuver or by postoperative shifting of an external buckle. The compression is evidenced by the appearance of papilledema during the first or second postoperative day and is an indication for emergency surgical readjustment of the sling. Failure to readjust the sling when papilledema appears will result in optic atrophy. The absence of papilledema does not guarantee that the optic disc will not atrophy during the postoperative week.

A type III detachment, wherein the detachment involves both the macula and the peripheral retina out to the ora serrata, carries the complication that treatment of a macular hole may fail to cause permanent retinal reattachment because of the presence of an occult retinal break. In 75% of cases of a type III detachment with a putative macular hole, treatment of the periphery alone, without treatment of the macular hole, produces retinal reattachment. The best indication of the need for macular buckling in addition to peripheral buckling is the pattern of accumulation of subretinal fluid after initially successful peripheral buckling surgery. If there is no recurrence of retinal detachment after closure of a suspected peripheral break, it is inadvisable to treat a putative macular hole with photocoagulation.

CHAPTER 37

Retinal Break Without Retinal Detachment

A retinal break should be considered as a special entity when it is unaccompanied by retinal detachment beyond the immediate margins of the break. Regardless of the degree of elevation of the flap of the break, the absence of more than peripheral retinal detachment makes the treatment of the break a simpler procedure than breaks that are accompanied by significant retinal detachment.

ETIOLOGY

Retinal breaks result from the tractional force exerted by an irregularly positioned vitreous base. In almost all cases the retinal break occurs at the time of posterior vitreous detachment. In rare cases a retinal break can occur at the time of partial vitreous detachment. The absence of significant retinal detachment results from either the short duration of time between the occurrence of the break and its detection or from weak vitreoretinal tractional force or from unusually strong adhesion between the pigment epithelium and the retina surrounding the break. The development of retinal detachment surrounding the break occurs if the break is untreated for days or weeks. During this time lag, vitreoretinal traction exerted on the flap elevates the break and liquid vitreous hydrates the subretinal mucopolysaccharide, destroying the adhesion between the pigment epithelium and the outer retina.

Most retinal breaks do not require treatment because they are not the result of direct vitreoretinal traction. Breaks that occur within the vitreous base, intrabasal breaks, are safe to observe because of the absence of direct traction. Breaks at the ora serrata, oral breaks, require treatment because of tractional force by the vitreous. Juxtabasal breaks, at the posterior margin of the vitreous base, are the most dangerous because of the strong vitreoretinal force at this junction. The juxtabasal break forms the characteristic horseshoe flap tear and requires immediate treatment. Extrabasal breaks, located posterior to the posterior margin of the vitreous base, do not require treatment in almost all cases because they are operculated and relieved of vitreous traction. Only if an extrabasal break remains partially attached to the vitreous should it be treated.

NATURAL HISTORY AND DIAGNOSIS

Retinal breaks occur suddenly. Photopsia and floaters are the most common symptoms and result from tractional force on the retina and dispersion of pigment or blood from torn capillaries at the margin of the break. Visual field will be lost only after the passage of days or weeks as retinal detachment develops.

INDICATIONS FOR TREATMENT

All juxtabasal and oral ('rim') breaks should be treated immediately upon diagnosis. Intrabasal and extrabasal breaks should be observed. Most breaks within lattice degeneration are intrabasal and should not be treated. Only breaks within lattice that are juxtabasal should be treated. Atrophic holes in the intrabasal region should remain under observation and do not require treatment unless change is observed.

Laser Technique

Laser photocoagulation of a horseshoe retinal break begins with the placement of three or more rows of laser coagulation (Fig. 37-1, *A*). For argon green laser, the coagulation size should be either 100 or 200 μm with a duration of approximately 0.2 seconds and a power setting ranging from 150 to 300 milliwatts in order to create a white photocoagulation scar. Argon green is best in cases with a pale fundus coloration. Krypton red should be used with a spot size ranging from 200 to 500 μm with a duration of 0.5 seconds and a power ranging from 150 to 400 mW in order to obtain a photocoagulation that is almost white. Watch each photocoagulation burn, and terminate it prior to 0.5 seconds if necessary in order to prevent the photocoagulation from reaching a dense white coloration, which indicates risk of choroidal rupture. Krypton red laser is desirable in cases complicated by cataract or vitreous hemorrhage. Although argon laser may produce little or no pain, krypton laser often produces pain and warrants a sub-Tenon's anesthetic injection before treatment. Place the photocoagulations so that their perimeters are separated by approximately 100 μm. Unless the retinal break is far posterior to the ora serrata, the optical difficulty of focusing the laser beam will prevent photocoagulation of the anterior margin of the break.

The ideal laser photocoagulation pattern should completely surround the retinal break including the anterior margin (Fig. 37-1, *B*). If the anterior margin of the break is near the ora serrata, extend the photocoagulation scars on the sides of the retinal break up to the ora serrata.

A

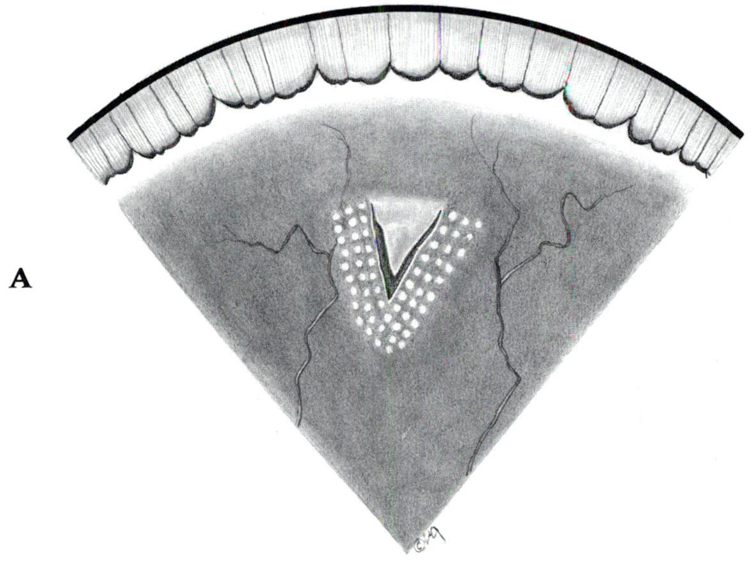

B

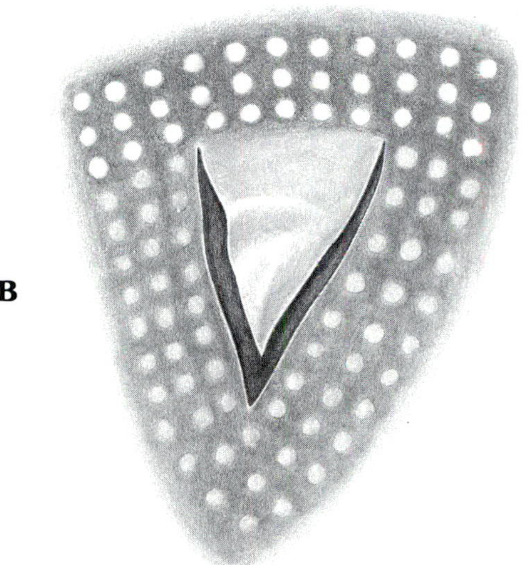

FIGURE 37-1. Laser technique of a horseshoe retinal break.

Continued.

In order to photocoagulate the anterior margin of the retinal break or to extend the photocoagulation to the ora serrata, use an identation funnel with the triple-mirror Goldmann corneal lens (Fig. 37-1, *C*). The photocoagulation treatments to the posterior margin of the retinal break do not require indentation. The optical pathway is able to transmit the laser beam to the preequatorial retina. Photocoagulation of the retina near the ora serrata requires advancing the indentation device on the indentation funnel to move the peripheral retina into the optical pathway of the laser. The Eisner indentation funnel is the ideal instrument for this maneuver because of the flexibility of its indentation probe. The use of the indenter may cause pain, which requires sub-Tenon's anesthesia in addition to topical anesthesia.

Laser photocoagulation within an area of already detached retina is the leading cause for failure in the treatment of a retinal break. The detached area most commonly lies at the anterior margin of the break rather than at the posterior margin (Fig. 37-1, *D*). Although laser photocoagulation can produce a reaction in the area of detachment by whitening the pigment epithelium and choroid, the reaction is less intense in appearance than are the reactions in the more posterior aspect of treatment where the retina is attached. Failure to achieve a white or nearly white reaction indicates that the photocoagulation is likely placed within an area of retinal separation. Stereopsis in the far retinal periphery is difficult. Extend the laser burns farther laterally until they produce a white or near-white reaction with the same energy input that produced a white reaction in the more readily observable attached posterior retina.

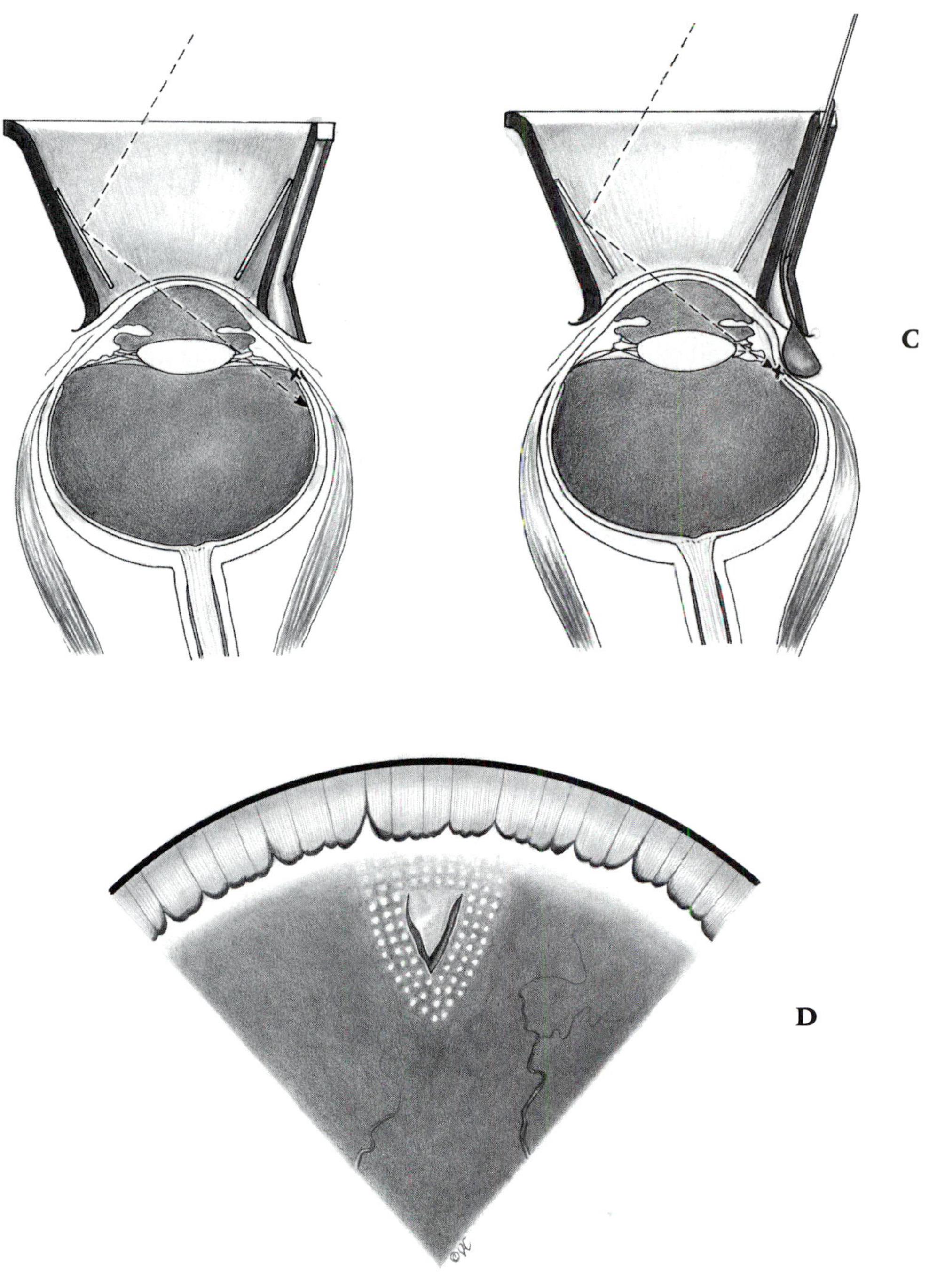

FIGURE 37-1, cont'd

Continued.

The extension of retinal detachment can occur through an area of retina within several days of laser photocoagulation, before an adequate scar has begun to form. Most commonly the extension of detachment occurs because of the failure to extend the laser photocoagulations to the ora serrata or along the anterior margin of the retinal break (Fig. 37-1, *E*). Failure to repair an extension of the retinal detachment results in the progression of the small retinal detachment accompanying the break into a large clinical retinal detachment. Laser photocoagulation should be repeated as soon as the extension of retinal detachment appears.

The repair of the extension of retinal detachment requires laser photocoagulation within the attached retina at the margins of the extension of the detachment (Fig. 37-1, *F*). Laser photocoagulation within the area of detachment is unproductive. The pattern of photocoagulation to circumscribe the extension of detachment is the same as the multiple-row pattern used for the initial treatment. Indentation of the sclera at the time of photocoagulation permits the extension of the laser photocoagulations to the ora serrata. The width of the laser zone for treatment of an extension of detachment should be at least as wide or wider than the initial treatment in order to create scars even if the detachment extends slightly during the approximately 2- to 3-week scarring period.

E

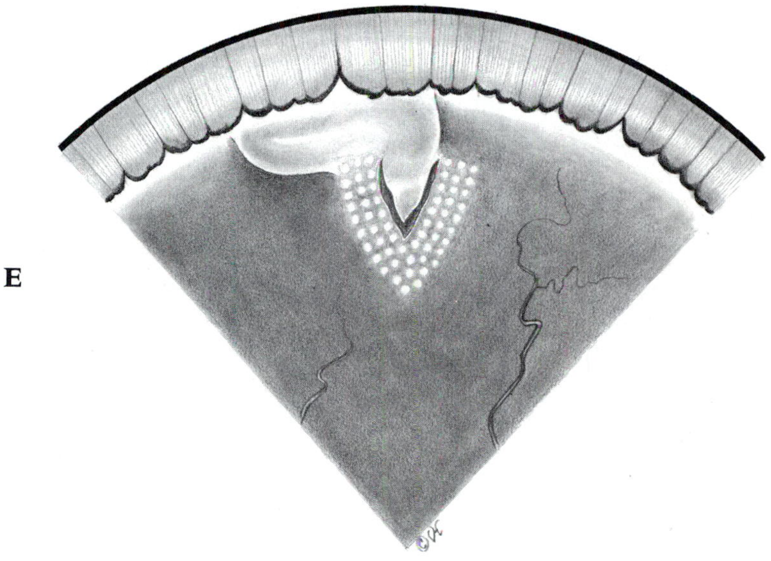

F

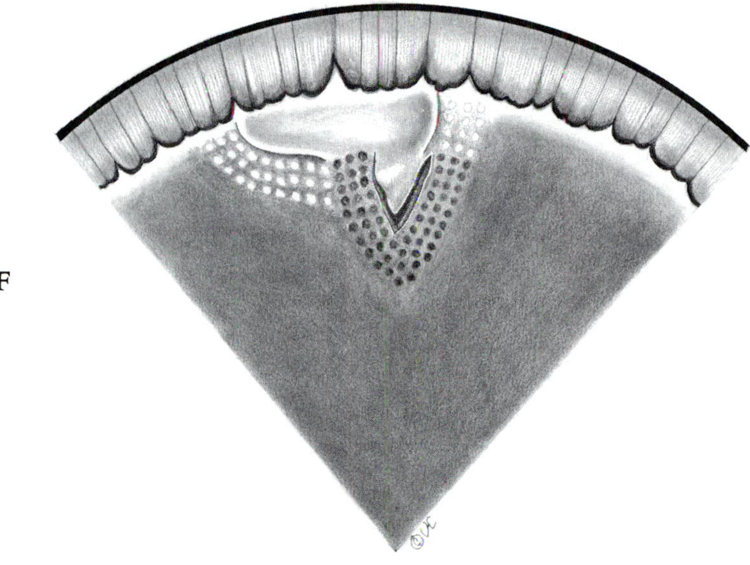

FIGURE 37-1, cont'd

Cryosurgical Technique

Cryosurgery of a retinal break necessitates the passage of the freezing zone through all the eye-wall thickness and through the retina up to the internal limiting membrane of the retina. The treatment must be performed within attached retina at the margins of the detached retina (Fig. 37-2, *A*). Cryosurgery within the area of retinal detachment is contraindicated. Determine the intensity of cryocoagulation by observation using the binocular indirect ophthalmoscope during treatment. Continue freezing until the central portion of the treatment zone becomes white, indicating that the frozen zone has reached to the internal limiting membrane of the retina. Stop the freeze immediately but do not remove the cryoprobe until the white spot is completely returned to normal coloration. Premature removal of the cryoprobe can produce cracking of the frozen retina. Although cryosurgery can sometimes be done with topical anesthetic, sub-Tenon's anesthesia can eliminate almost all pain. Try to avoid placing excessive anesthetic beneath the conjunctiva at the site where cryosurgery will be given because the anesthesia fluid will act as a thermal barrier.

Place the cryocoagulation spots to surround the retinal break at a distance of approximately 500 to 1000 μm from the margins of the retinal break and its accompanying detachment (Fig. 37-2, *B*). The cryocoagulation spots should overlap slightly because the margins of each treatment zone will not form a dense scar. Try to avoid retreatment of each spot because of the risk of producing hemorrhage, retinal tearing, retinal contraction with macular pucker, or severe exudation.

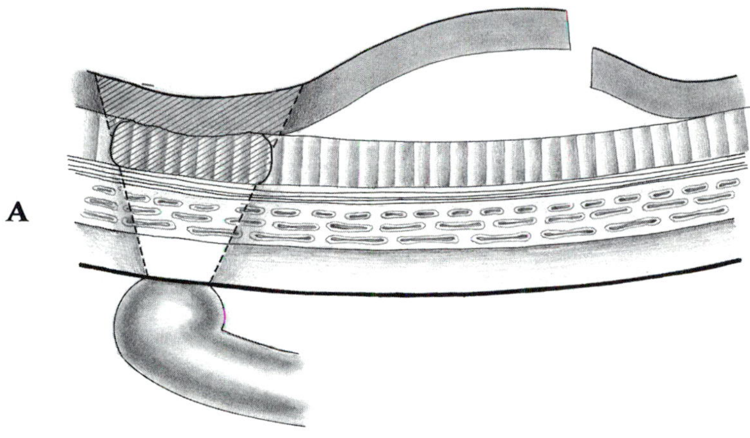

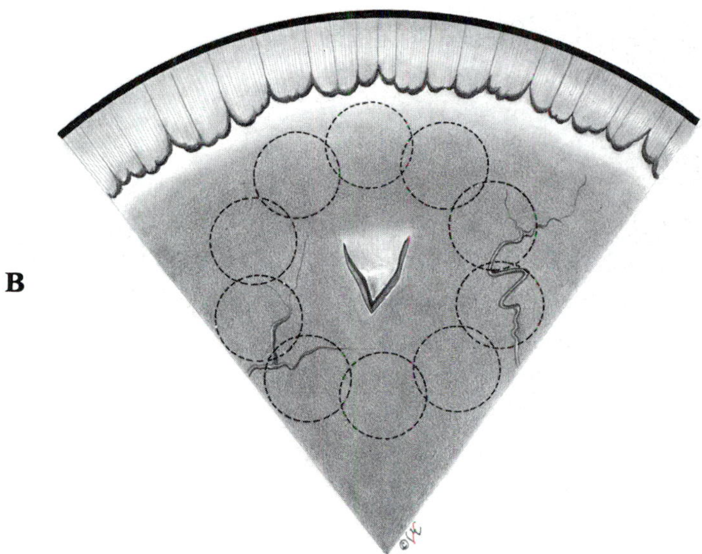

FIGURE 37-2. Cryosurgical technique.

FOLLOW-UP STUDY

The follow-up observation for the treatment of retinal breaks consists in observation using binocular indirect ophthalmoscopy with scleral depression along with contact lens biomicroscopy where necessary for determination of whether retinal detachment develops beyond the margins of the break during the post-treatment weeks. The scars from either the laser or the cryoprobe are not adequately mature and strong until approximately 6 weeks after treatment when one is ensured that detachment will not develop. Any evidence of the beginning of detachment warrants extension of the local treatment or scleral buckling surgery for cases of rapid extension of detachment threatening the macula.

The appearance of continuous pigmentation surrounding the retinal break by 6 weeks after treatment is a sign of success. Any margin of the break that does not show smooth pigmentation should be re-treated.

The chance for development of new retinal breaks in the treated eye, particularly 180 degrees from the location of the original break, necessitates continued observation of the eye over a period of years. The patient must remain alert to symptoms.

COMPLICATIONS

The major complication is development of retinal detachment at the margins of the retinal break. This must be recognized immediately so that an attempt can be made to surround the retinal detachment with either laser photocoagulation or cryocoagulation. Scleral buckling surgery must be considered as an alternative if the detachment extends.

Recurrence of vitreous hemorrhage after successful closure of a retinal break can imply the presence of an avulsed retinal vessel, either at the site of the break or elsewhere. The identification of an avulsed retinal vessel necessitates scleral buckling to relieve traction at the site of the vessel in order to prevent rehemorrhage in cases where the density of the vitreous hemorrhage prevents laser photocoagulation. If the vitreous is clear, laser photocoagulation can be administered to the afferent and efferent aspects of the avulsed vessel at the point where they are adherent to the pigment epithelium. Adequate laser energy must be used to produce narrowing and almost closure of the vessels in order to prevent recurrent hemorrhage. A recurrence of hemorrhage after laser photocoagulation necessitates scleral buckling to relieve traction.

Excessive input of laser photocoagulation energy or the preoperative presence of a premacular membrane can result in premacular fibrosis despite the peripheral location of treatment of the retinal break. Iritis can result from inadvertent photocoagulation of the iris or from intense energy input to the uvea.

CHAPTER 38

Retinal Detachment

Retinal detachment is the separation of the retina from the underlying pigment epithelium. It is an abnormal reformation of the embryologic optic vesicle. The fluid that separates neurosensory retina from the nutrient retinal pigment epithelium causes the loss of retinal function and visual acuity.

Retinal detachment occurs in three types: (1) rhegmatogenous, (2) traction, and (3) exudative. This chapter is devoted to rhegmatogenous retinal detachment, which results from the passage of fluid from the vitreous cavity through a break in the retina into the subretinal space.

ETIOLOGY

The fundamental cause of retinal detachment is the combined presence of a full-thickness retinal break, traction by the vitreous on the break, and inability of the pigment epithelium to dehydrate the subretinal space faster than the accumulation of liquid vitreous in the subretinal space. In a localized retinal detachment, the dehydrational force of the pigment epithelium is stronger than the tractional force on the retina, and so the detachment does not extend far from the margin of the retinal tear. In a large, clinical retinal detachment, the force of traction on the retina overwhelms the dehydrational force of the pigment epithelium. As a result, the mucopolysaccharide glue that normally binds the retina to the pigment epithelium gradually hydrates as the vitreous pulls the retina away from the pigment epithelium. Over a period of days or weeks, the area of hydrated mucopolysaccharide spreads along the route of gravitational extension of the fluid from the tear until all the retina inferior to the tear and, later, the retina superior to the tear detach. Whether the detachment results from an oral dialysis, a horseshoe tear, a small, round hole, or a giant tear, the fundamental cause is the pull at the margin of the break by the vitreous gel that is connected to that margin, and the fundamental approach to treatment is sealing of the retinal break sufficiently so that the traction of the vitreous does not force the break to reopen.

CLINICAL HISTORY

The earliest retinal detachment symptoms are usually photopsia from vitreous traction on the retina and floaters from the scattering of pigment cells or from hemorrhage at the time of retinal tearing. The time interval between initial symptoms and first loss of visual field ranges from hours to months. The process is not painful unless a detachment causes iridocyclitis and glaucoma. A history of trauma to the globe or of intraocular surgery may precede, by days or years, the onset of the symptoms of detachment. A retinal tear or detachment in the opposite eye is part of the history of between 25% and 40% of patients who present with a retinal detachment. The other associated findings are myopia and lattice degeneration.

DIFFERENTIAL DIAGNOSIS

The major differential is between a rhegmatogenous retinal detachment and a serous retinal detachment wherein the source of the subretinal fluid is the choroidal or retinal vasculature. Hallmarks of exudative serous retinal detachment are gravitational shifting of subretinal fluid within minutes or hours of alteration of the patient's position, failure of the retinal detachment to extend to the ora serrata, and choroidal effusions that extend beyond the ora serrata into the pars plana. Although rhegmatogenous detachments undulate, their contours and their geographic extent do not change within minutes, hours, or even days of gravitational change. The serous detachment shows a smooth surface without fibrotic whitening, in contrast to the irregular surface of a rhegmatogenous detachment. Serous detachment is unlikely to present with the extreme elevation of height that can occur in rhegmatogenous detachment. Leakage of choroidal fluid through the pigment epithelium in serous detachment can result from malignant melanoma, metastatic carcinoma, hemangioma of the choroid, and the Vogt-Koyanagi-Harada syndrome. Retinal vascular malformations such as telangiectases or angiomas and pigment epithelial disease such as that found in central serous retinopathy can also produce serous retinal detachment. Surgery must not be performed on serous retinal detachments because the surgery aims to seal retinal breaks in order to resolve the detachment. In serous detachments there are no retinal breaks.

PREOPERATIVE MANAGEMENT

The most important factor in preoperative management is careful mapping of the retina and identification of all retinal breaks by use of binocular indirect ophthalmoscopy with scleral depression combined with biomicroscopy when necessary for a high magnification view. The details of examination should be recorded on a retinal drawing sheet with systematic mapping of each retinal area from the disc to the ora serrata indicating whether subretinal fluid is present and, if so, to what extent so that planning can be made for drainage of subretinal fluid in a safe area where the retina is highly elevated. The failure to identify all retinal breaks is a leading cause for redetachment of the retina postoperatively. A clue that can be helpful in the identification of the retinal break is to look for one near the superior margin of an inferior detachment or near the 12 o'clock meridian in a total detachment. The presence of multiple retinal breaks in approximately 40% of detachments necessitates meticulous examination.

Preoperative management should also include administration of an antibiotic topically to diminish the risk of infection at surgery. Intraocular inflammation should be brought under control before surgery. If a cataract blocks the view of the retina, combined scleral buckling with lensectomy and vitrectomy can be considered or the cataract can be removed as a primary procedure with the scleral buckling several days later. Similarly, if vitreous hemorrhage does not clear spontaneously within approximately 1 week of the diagnosis of retinal detachment, vitrectomy surgery should be considered.

Despite the improved management provided by modern vitrectomy technique, simple scleral buckling should be the primary surgical attempt in all cases of rhegmatogenous retinal detachment except those with dense vitreous hemorrhage, dense cataract, or extensive periretinal proliferation. Vitrectomy surgery carries greater risks than scleral buckling without vitrectomy in the appropriate cases.

Retinal Detachment with Multiple Tears

The retinal detachment with multiple tears (Fig. 38-1, *A*) presents the problem of sealing all the breaks to produce permanent retinal reattachment. One procedure for breaks that are far removed from each other is the placement of meridional sponge buckles with an overlying encircling band (Fig. 38-1, *B*). The meridional sponge buckles seal the breaks and prevent fish-mouthing; the encircling band both exaggerates the indentation of the meridional buckles and provides a permanent indentational effect after the erosion of the scleral sutures holding the sponge (Fig. 38-1, *C*). Placement of the meridional sponges should be done while the surgeon imagines a set of lines surrounding the retinal breaks (Fig. 38-1, *D*). The lines should be evenly spaced laterally from the margins of the breaks with an additional imaginary line connecting the posterior margins of the breaks. The meridional lines should be used to orient the position of the meridional buckle under each break. The imaginary circumferential line is the basis for orientation of the circumferential band.

Place the meridional buckles so that the breaks are centered on the buckles with adequate distance both anteriorly and posteriorly from the margins of the buckle. If possible, place the encircling band to lie over the posterior margin of the retinal breaks where maximal indentation is beneficial. Cryocoagulation can be done before placement of the buckle, or laser can be used at approximately 4 weeks postoperatively.

A

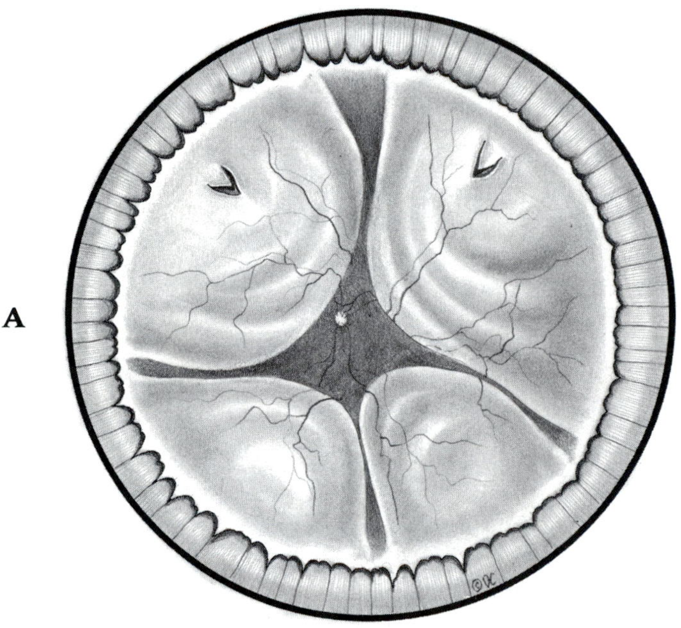

FIGURE 38-1. Retinal detachment with multiple tears.

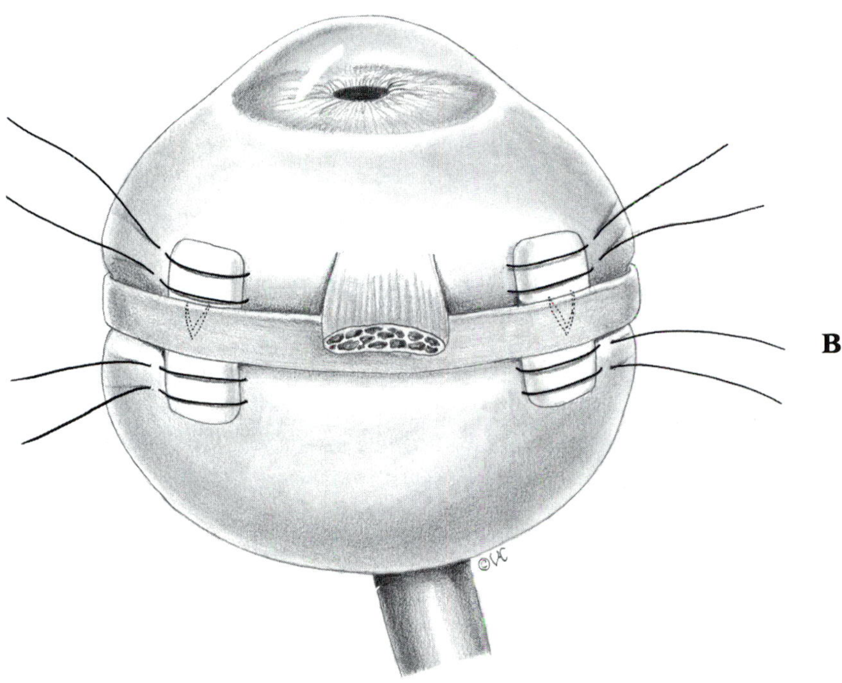

B

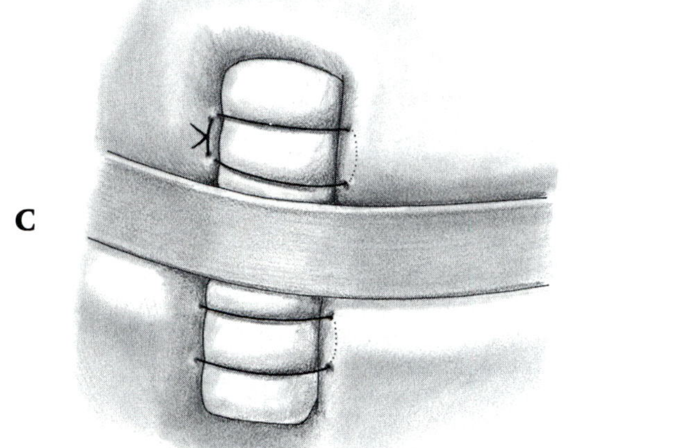

C

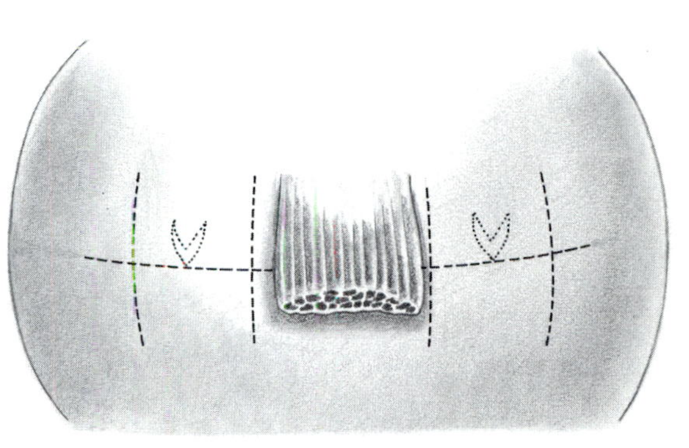

D

Continued.

An alternative approach to the buckling of multiple retinal breaks is the placement of a solid silicone explant beneath an encircling band. The explant extends to include all definite and putative retinal breaks (Fig. 38-1, *E*). Place the explant so that its posterior margin lies at least 2 mm posterior to the posterior margin of the most posterior break. The explant should also extend anteriorly to the anterior margin of the most anterior break by at least 1 to 2 mm or up to the ora serrata, whichever is more posterior. Place the intrascleral imbricating sutures with the anterior intrascleral placement at the point where you want the anterior margin of the explant. When the suture is tied, the explant will migrate up to the anterior suture. The posterior suture should lie approximately 3 mm posterior to the explant in order to create an indentation when the suture is tied.

After the drainage of subretinal fluid, the intraocular pressure is sufficiently soft to permit tying of the buckle. The indentation produced by the buckle need only effect relative sealing of the breaks (Fig. 38-1, *F*). It is unnecessary to redrain subretinal fluid for further flattening (Fig. 38-1, *G*). The relative sealing of the breaks will permit spontaneous resorption of subretinal fluid in the postoperative days (Fig. 38-1, *H*).

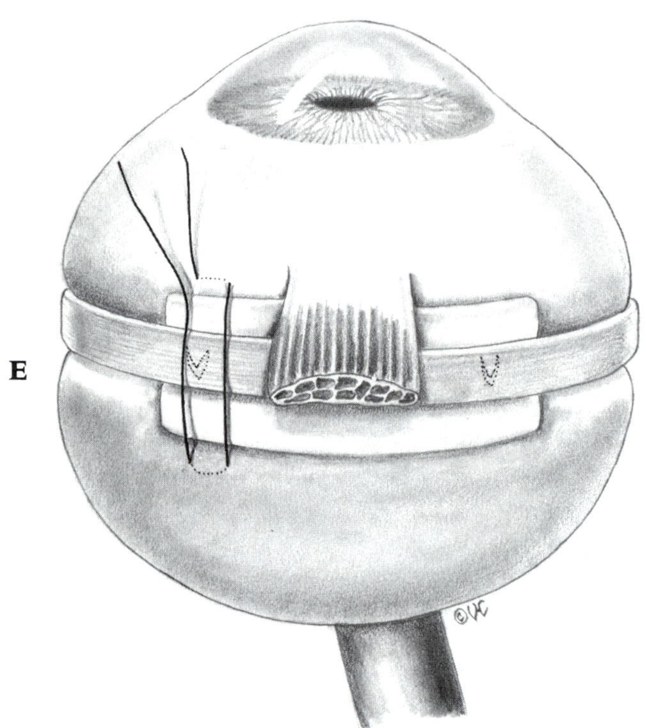

FIGURE 38-1, cont'd

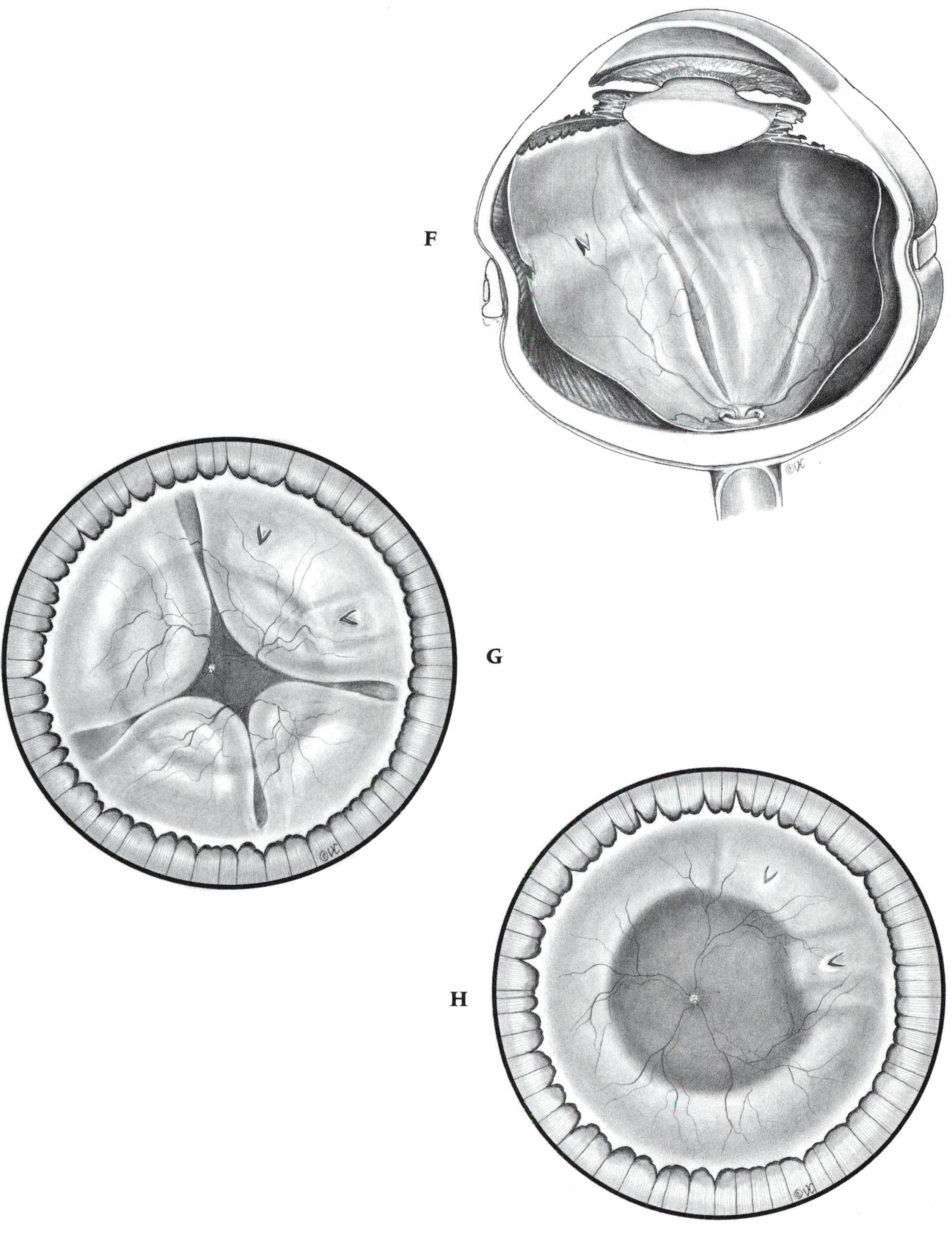
F
G
H

Complications

The leading complication of encircling buckling is the creation of a "fish-mouth" fold at the posterior margin of one of the retinal breaks. This occurs because of the reduction of globe diameter by the encircling buckle. The fish mouth appears as an elevation of the posterior lip of a meriodionally oriented break (Fig. 38-2, *A*). The elevation of the posterior margin of the break permits the accumulation of subretinal fluid. Whether it is observed during surgery or postoperatively, the repair of a fish mouth consists of the placement of a meridional buckle beneath the encircling buckle (Fig. 38-2, *B*). This correction should be taken intraoperatively as soon as fish-mouthing is noticed. Postoperatively, the correction is necessary only if subretinal fluid appears to accumulate and the retinal fails to flatten.

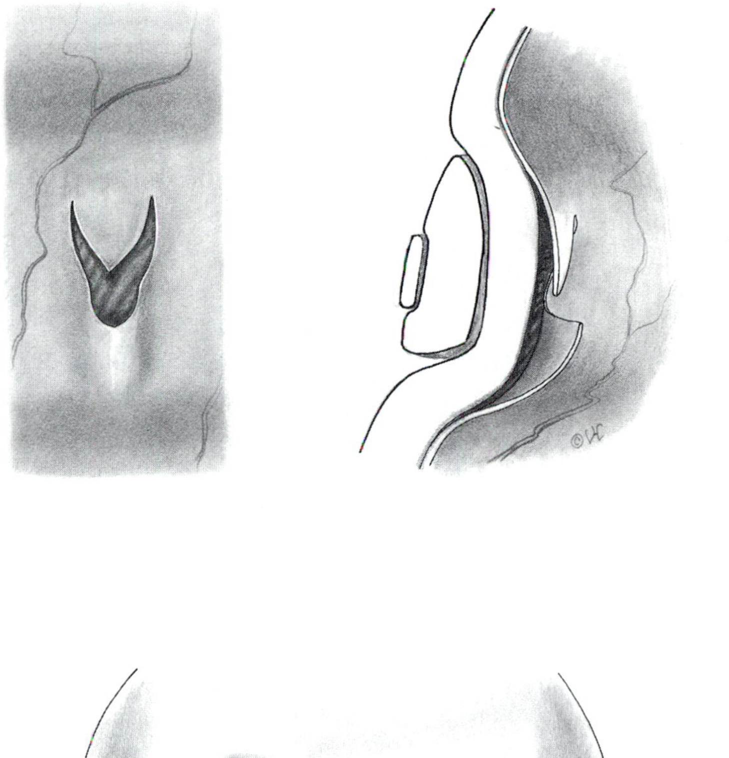

A

B

FIGURE 38-2. Postoperative complications.

Scleral Dissection and Diathermy

This procedure is useful for the placement of large circumferential buckles. Its advantage over the explant technique is that the diathermy has the potential advantage of diminishing scatter of pigment epithelial cells and the concomitant risk of inducing massive periretinal proliferation. In order for diathermy to be performed, scleral flaps must be dissected at approximately one half the scleral thickness (Fig. 38-3, *A*). The flap must extend 3 mm posterior to the intended location of the posterior margin of the buckle to provide sufficient intrascleral space for indentation of the implanted silicone. Apply diathermy only to the portion of the scleral bed underlying the break and where the silicone implant will lie. For example, a 9 mm wide silicone explant extending to the posterior margin of the break should be accompanied by a 9 mm wide bed of diathermy treatments (Fig. 38-3, *B*). The posterior 3 mm of the scleral bed does not require diathermy. The diathermy treatments should be spaced as shown with a blunt-tipped diathermy used for deep diathermy penetration with minimal scleral necrosis. Once the silicone implant is placed with its encircling band to anchor it, the scleral flaps are sutured to each other and pulled tight (Fig. 38-3, *C*). The closing of the scleral pouch produces the indentation for sealing the break. As with explant surgery, subretinal fluid can be left at the end of implant surgery if the retinal breaks are all relatively sealed. Postoperatively, the residual subretinal fluid will be resorbed. The drainage of subretinal fluid should be performed after the diathermy treatment to the sclera and immediately before closing of the scleral flaps. A long time gap between drainage of subretinal fluid and closing of the scleral flaps risks the formation of choroidal hemorrhages from hypotony.

Complications

The major complication of scleral dissection and diathermy is scleral rupture from excessively deep scleral dissection and excessive diathermy coagulation with rupture of the retina. One can avoid the first complication by maintaining a constant plane of scleral dissection with the surgical knife dissecting the fibers that are exposed as the scleral lamella is retracted from the globe. The knife should be held at an approximately 45-degree angle to the scleral surface for the dissection. Never use the knife at an approximately parallel position to the scleral surface because of the risk of moving the scleral dissection plane toward the choroid. At the first sign of dark sclera where black appears through excessively thin sclera, change to a more superficial plane of dissection to avoid choroidal rupture. Diathermy treatment should be administered gently with a low power setting and gradual elevation of the power until an initial diathermy reaction can be seen with the binocular indirect ophthalmoscope. The appropriate retinal reaction is gray-white and not dense white, which indicates an excessive reaction. The scleral surface must be kept as dry as possible for the diathermy current to pass into the globe. Fluid on the surface of the scleral will cause the diathermy current to pass laterally and diminish its retinal effect.

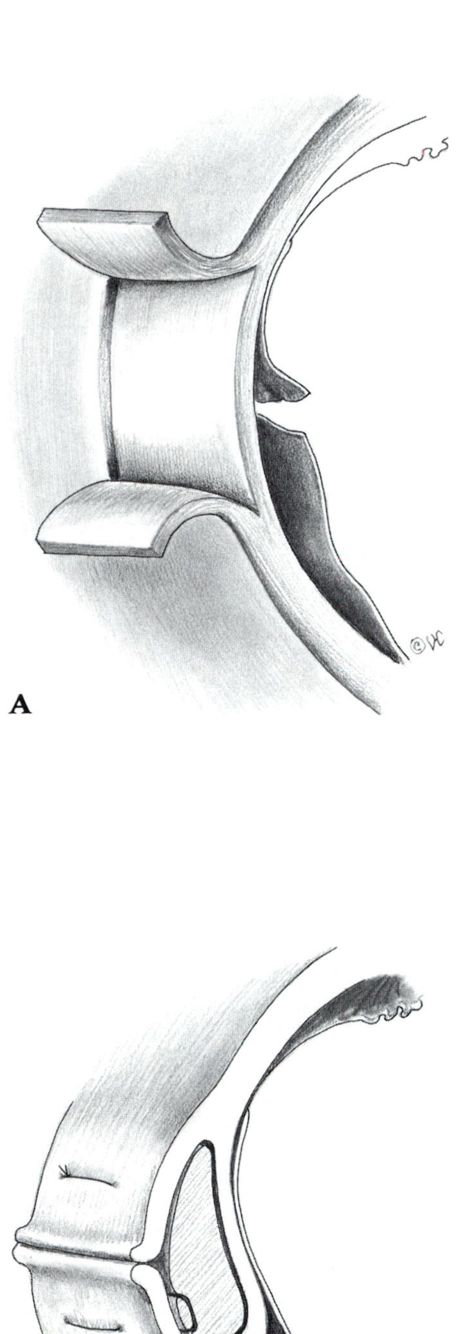

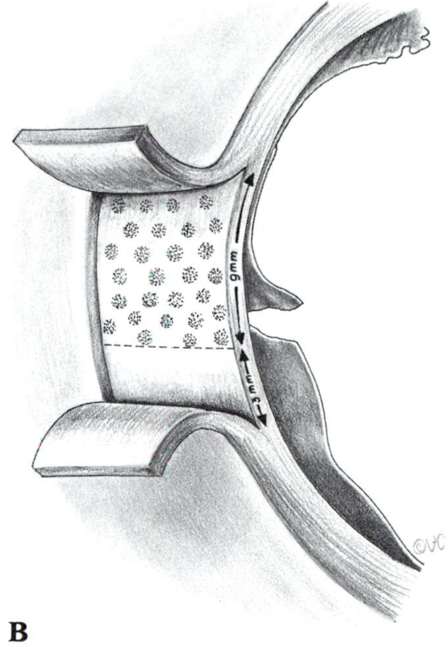

FIGURE 38-3. Scleral dissection and diathermy.

Surgical Management of Retinal Detachment Produced by Oral Dialysis

An oral dialysis usually shows slight eversion of the posterior lip of the tear (Fig. 38-4, *A*). A circumferential sponge buckle is the best technique for sealing a dialysis. Place the buckle so that the apex of the posterior margin of the break lies immediately anterior to the apex of the buckle (Fig. 38-4, *B*). The buckle should be selected so that the width of the buckle is approximately three times the width of the tear.

When the overlying sutures are tied, the buckle should indent the eye wall with the apex of the buckle immediately posterior to the anterior margin of the posterior flap. Cryocoagulation can be performed around the margins of the break before buckling, or laser can be performed at approximately two weeks postoperatively (Fig. 38-4, *C*). The excellent success of buckling for oral dialyses makes the postoperative laser management attractive.

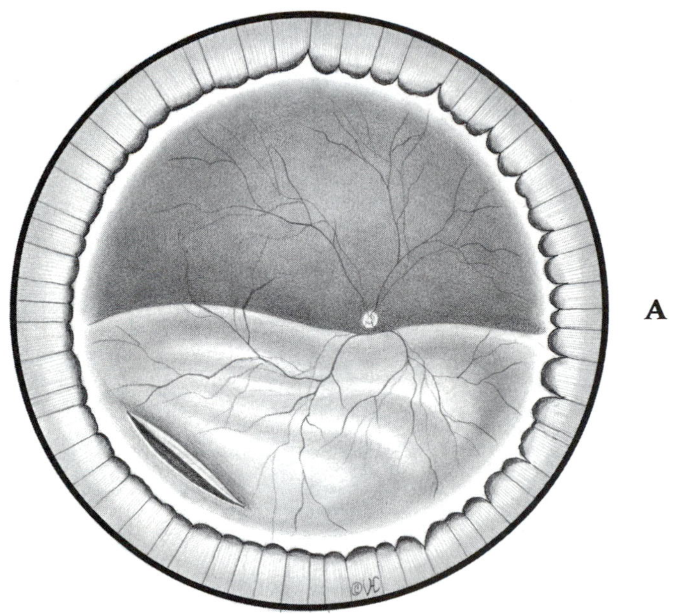

FIGURE 38-4. Surgical management of retinal detachment.

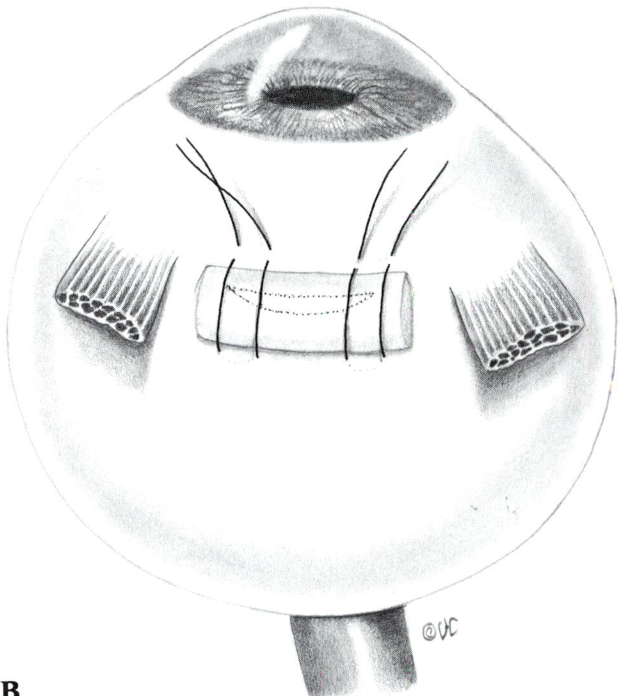

B

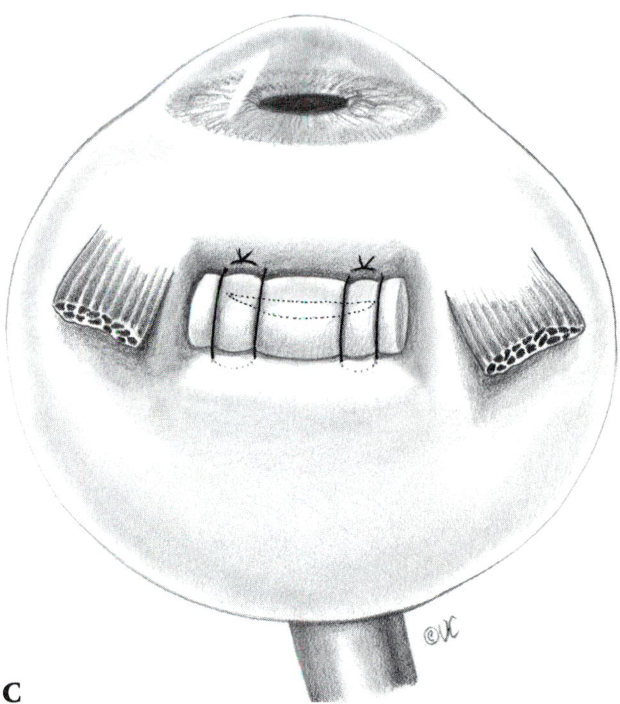

C

FOLLOW-UP STUDY

Reopening of an oral dialysis postoperatively is rare. It can occur because of a "fish-mouth" fold, which forms from excessive indentation of the buckle. In such a case, reoperation must extend the buckling posteriorly. One way this can be done is to include an encircling element posterior to the sponge buckle (Fig. 38-5). The extra indentation by the encircling element will produce adequate indentation to seal the fish-mouth fold at its most posterior aspect.

In all operations for oral dialysis, laser photocoagulation can be used at approximately 2 to 3 weeks after surgery to create a permanent seal.

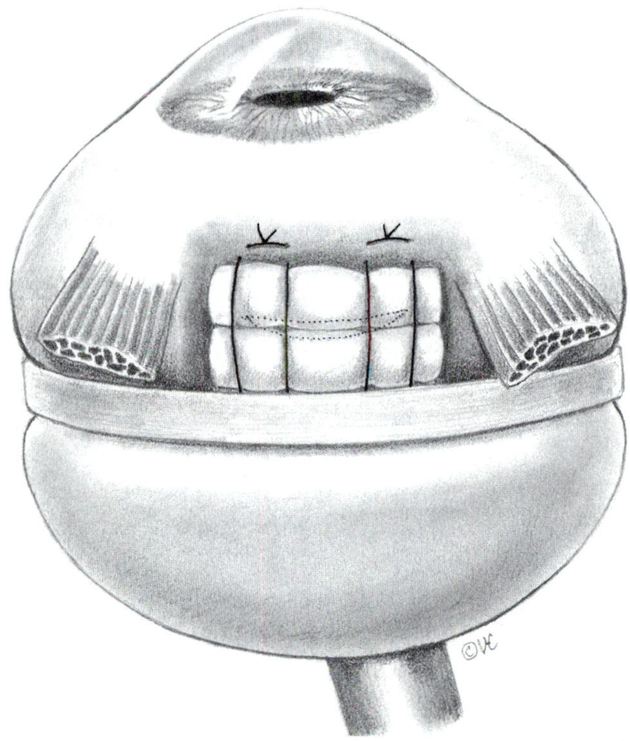

FIGURE 38-5. Follow-up observation.

COMPLICATIONS

The most common complication in the oral dialysis procedure is for the scleral buckle to be excessively narrow and fail to seal the anterior margin of the break (Fig. 38-6, *A*). Following nondrainage procedure, subretinal fluid will continue to accumulate through the anterior margin and the detachment will not improve in the postoperative days. To avoid this complication, or to correct it, broaden the scleral buckle either by the use of a single broad buckle or by the concurrent use of two sponges placed under one set of overlying sutures (Fig. 38-6, *B*). With these sponges the placement should be such that the posterior margin of the break lies at the apex of the buckle or slightly anterior to it. The buckle must extend well anterior (approximately 2 mm) to the anterior margin of the break. No drainage of subretinal fluid is required in the treating of an oral dialysis in most cases. After cryocoagulation or without it, the sutures are gradually tied until the double sponge buckle indents the eye wall (Fig. 38-6, *C*). Ascertain that the buckle produces a significant indentation of the eye wall. Continue to tighten the sutures with a series of slipknots until the indentation is achieved without excessive elevation of the intraocular pressure. If the sutures are tied with pressure on the sponges, the indentation in the postoperative day will be greater than it is at the end of surgery. During the surgery the buckle need be elevated only to the point to produce appositional closure of the break without complete retinal flattening (Fig. 38-6, *D*). In the postoperative 48 hours, the subretinal fluid should be absorbed, and the retinal tear will seal tightly to the buckle.

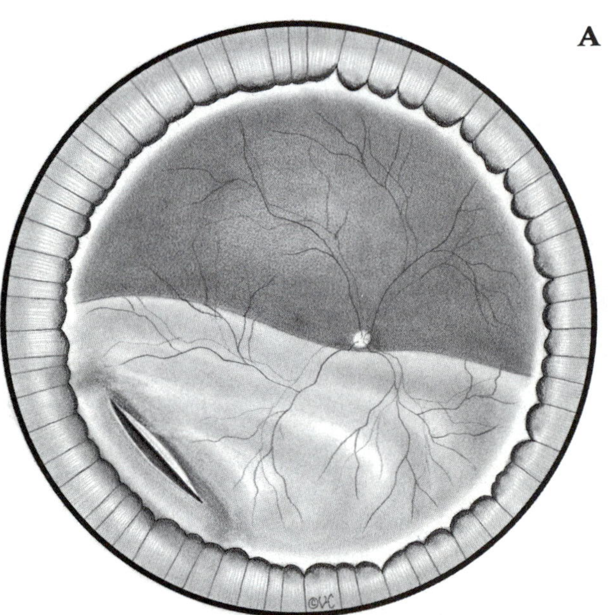

FIGURE 38-6. Postoperative complications.

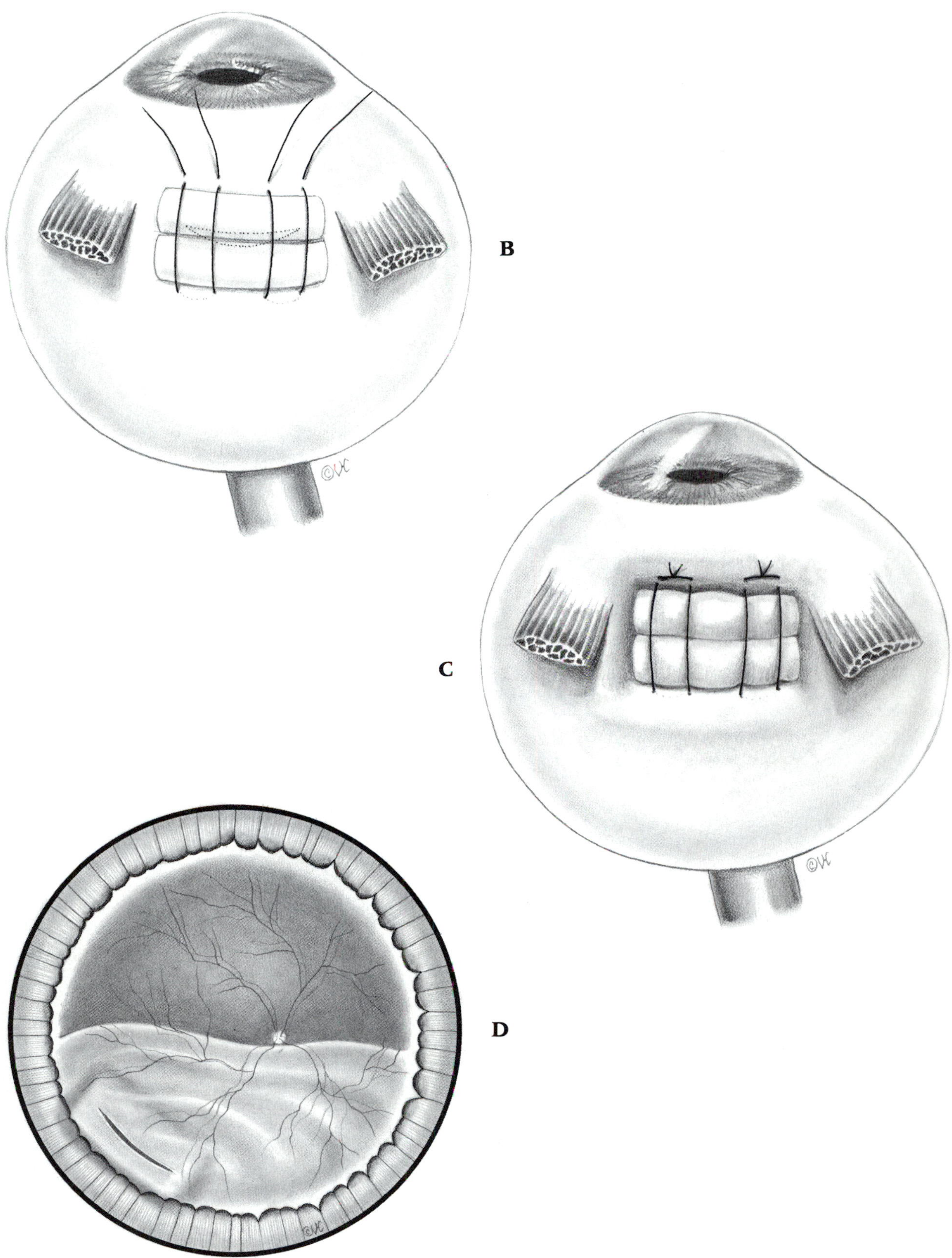
B
C
D

CHAPTER 39

Subclinical Retinal Detachment

Subclinical retinal detachment involves only the preequatorial, nonpercipient retina and does not cause a peripheral visual field defect. Visual acuity suffers only from vitreous hemorrhage, uveitis, or floaters and not directly from detachment.

ETIOLOGY

The cause of subclinical retinal detachment is the same as that for all retinal detachments: the formation of a retinal break by vitreous traction on an area of retina with abnormal vitreoretinal adhesion. The degree of subretinal fluid surrounding the break determines whether the detachment is subclinical, limited to the retinal periphery, or clinical, extending into the percipient retina.

INDICATIONS FOR TREATMENT

Retinal breaks with little or no accompanying retinal detachment are present in approximately 4% to 18% of the adult population. The risk of clinical retinal detachment from any given retinal break is less than 1 in 70. The risk factors for the extension of a retinal break into a large retinal detachment are history of retinal detachment in the opposite eye, impending cataract surgery, or the impending use of miotic therapy for glaucoma. Possibly, high myopia increases the risk of retinal detachment from an existing retinal break.

The most accurate method for determining the prognosis of a retinal break is the classification of the retinal break according to its relationship to the vitreous base. Juxtabasal breaks, lying at the posterior margin of the vitreous base, carry the worst prognosis because they receive the force of vitreous contraction at the time of posterior vitreous detachment. Extrabasal breaks, lying posterior to the vitreous base, usually form operculated holes wherein the traction from the vitreous is completely separated from the margins of the break and no extension of detachment is likely. Intrabasal breaks, lying within the vitreous base, also carry a low-risk of retinal detachment because the vitreous base spreads its traction broadly and does not exert great force at the margin of the break. Oral breaks, occurring at the ora serrata, usually cause slow progression to retinal detachment because they are protected from severe vitreous traction by continued attachment of the vitreous to the posterior lip of the break. The two categories of breaks that warrant prophylactic treatment are juxtabasal and oral breaks. Intrabasal and extrabasal breaks warrant observation.

Photocoagulation

The advantage of laser photocoagulation over cryocoagulation is the precision of energy input and treatment localization provided by laser. Although histologic evidence is controversial, it is my opinion that laser scars are stickier from the onset of treatment and the ultimate scar more long lasting than a cryoscar, which tends to become remodeled and loosen after years.

A partial retinal detachment can sometimes be managed with laser photocoagulation. If a pigment line already surrounds the detachment, photocoagulation can be used to augment the line, which is a sign of the long-standing duration of the detachment and the likelihood that the detachment will not extend by the time the laser scars mature 3 weeks after treatment. In cases of fresh detachment, a laser attempt can be made with the warning that extension of the detachment through the laser scar warrants either immediate reuse of the laser or scleral buckling surgery.

The margins of the detachment must be carefully determined so that the laser scars are placed outside of the detachment into the attached area (Fig. 39-1). Using either argon green or krypton red, place 500 μm wide laser burns in the attached retina surrounding the localized detachment. The photocoagulation spots reach within approximately 200 μm of the ora serrata. Indentation with the Eisner or other indenting funnels provides the best means for performing with this anterior laser. Sub-Tenon's anesthesia is necessary for the anterior photocoagulation with indentation.

Cryosurgery

Cryosurgery can also be used for a local retinal detachment. It is most likely to be effective if there already is a pigment demarcation line at the margin of the detachment. In a rapidly progressive detachment, cryosurgery not only delays the need for the ultimate scleral buckling surgery but also risks involvement of the macula by producing an increase of the volume of subretinal fluid from the exudative reaction to cryocoagulation. In the cryosurgery technique, surround the detachment with contiguous cryotreatments, which are done until there is whitening of the retina at each treatment site. Treat each region only once. The most important point about the cryotreatments is that they be performed in the attached retina surrounding the detachment and not in the detached retina.

If the retinal detachment is seen to extend into the cryocoagulated area in the postoperative period of observation, scleral buckling surgery should be undertaken immediately.

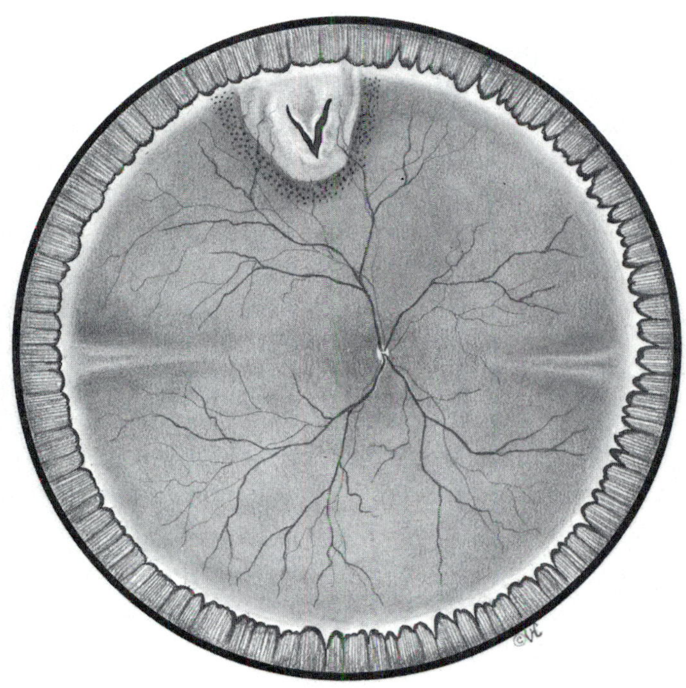

FIGURE 39-1. Laser treatment.

Meridional Sponge Buckling

A meridional buckle must be placed precisely beneath the break in order to produce closure at surgery. Using binocular indirect ophthalmoscopy, mark the sclera so that the meridional buckle will lie directly beneath the retinal break with approximately the orientation of the break (Fig. 39-2, *A*). Place two sutures of 5-0 Mersilene to lie over the sponge. The sutures should pass through half the scleral thickness. Arrange the sutures so that they are evenly spaced and symmetric around the lateral margins of the break. The sutures should be placed to be slightly farther apart circumferentially than the anatomic width of the sponge. Select the sponge buckle to be at least 1 or 2 mm wider than the break on either side (Fig. 39-2, *B*).

Cryosurgery can be performed before placement of either the sutures or the sponge in order to have maximum access to the sclera. If the ocular media are clear, cryosurgery can be eliminated and laser photocoagulation can be performed 4 to 6 weeks postoperatively to the margins of the break (Fig. 39-2, *C*).

After the sponge buckle is in place, gradually tighten the sutures and tie them after the sponge has been indented into the wall of the eye. Tying the sponge buckle loosely against the sclera will not produce buckling.

Successful indentation by the buckle will not necessarily produce complete closure of the break (Fig. 39-2, *D*). Relative closure of the break with indentation of the wall near the retina with relative flattening of the flap of the tear and a change in the shape of the retina is adequate to produce ultimate closure in the postoperative hours. Further tightening of the buckle is contraindicated because of the risks from excess elevation of intraocular pressure and potential for rupture of the sclera from the sutures.

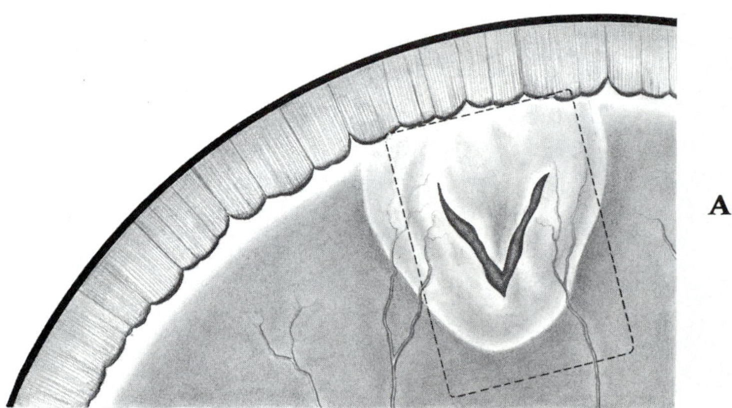

FIGURE 39-2. Meridional sponge buckling.

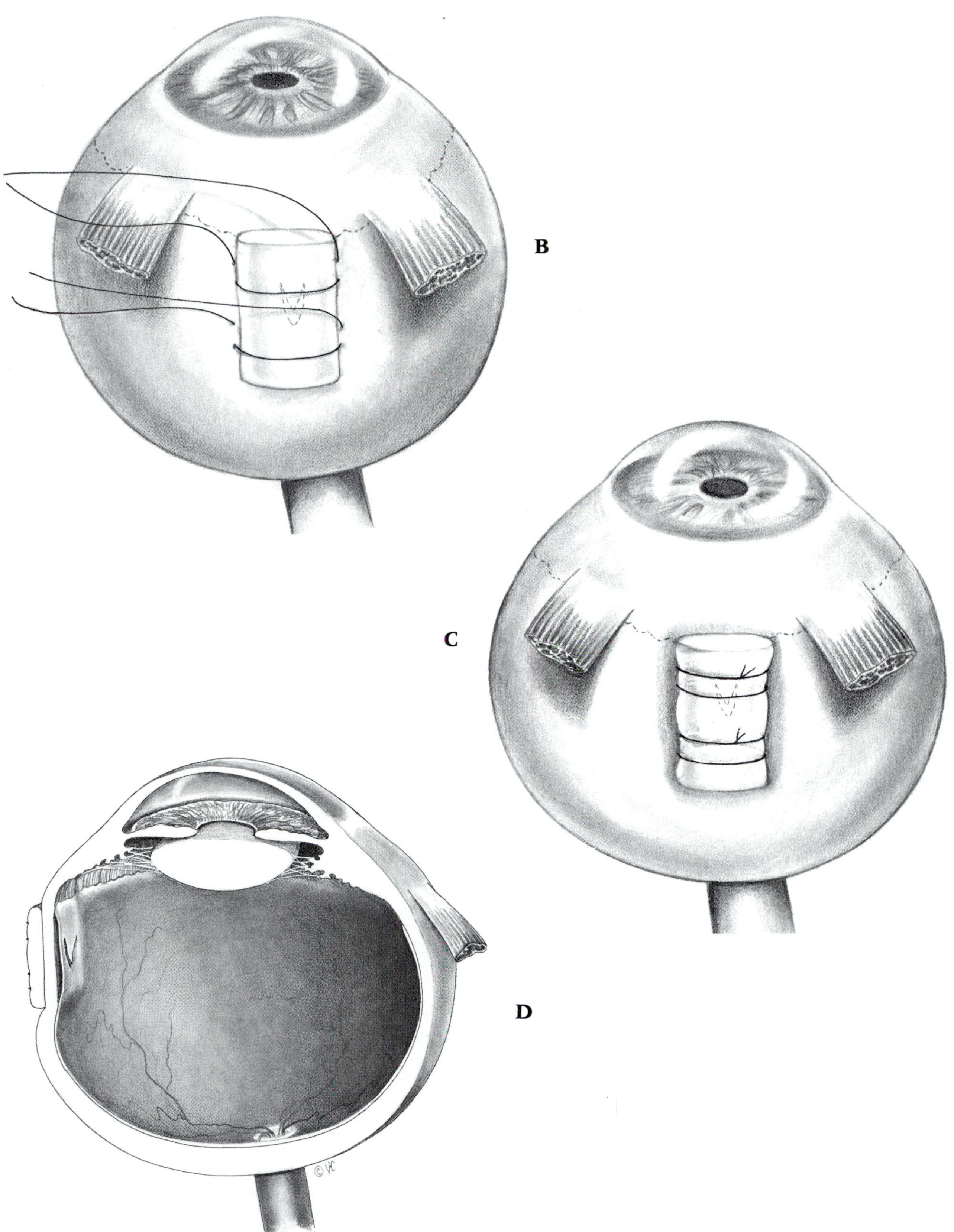
B
C
D
© VC

Postoperative care

On the day after surgery, the retina should be seen to be flattened against the indentation buckle with less subretinal fluid than before surgery (Fig. 39-3, *A*). In the ensuing days, the subretinal fluid should continue to lessen and the tear flatten against the buckle. By 2 weeks after surgery the retina should be completely flattened against the buckle and the tear sealed. If cryocoagulation was used at surgery, pigmentation should appear at the cryosites with the retina sealed flatly down at the cryotreatment areas (Fig. 39-3, *B*).

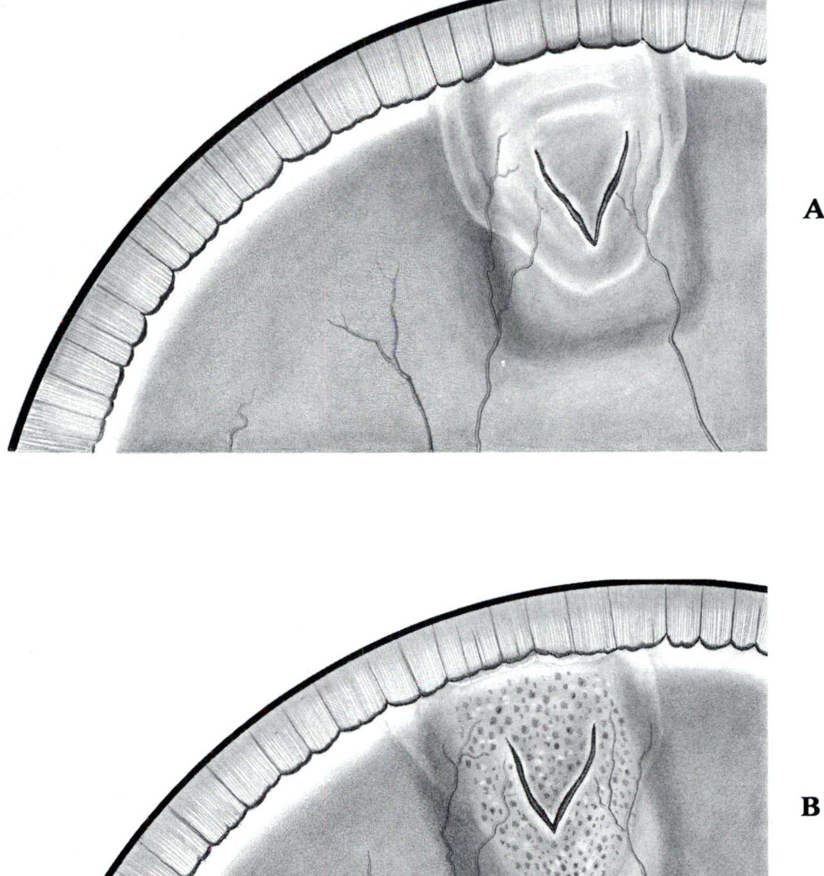

FIGURE 39-3. Postoperative care.

Complications

The most significant complication of meridional buckling is the continued accumulation of subretinal fluid because of failure to seal the tear. The most common cause for this problem is misplacement of the buckle. With the tear mounted toward the side of the buckle (Fig. 39-4, *A*), the lateral aspect of the tear remains unsealed (Fig. 39-4, *B*), and subretinal fluid accumulates despite indentation of the retina at the other aspects of the tear. If this problem is identified at surgery, the buckle should be moved to lie directly under the meridian of the tear. If it is recognized postoperatively, reoperation must be undertaken immediately.

Insufficient extension of the buckle posterior to the tear is another well recognized cause for failure. Although the buckle may extend up to the ora serrata (Fig. 39-4, *C*), it will not produce retinal reattachment of the posterior margin of the tear, and so the tear remains unsealed (Fig. 39-4, *D*).

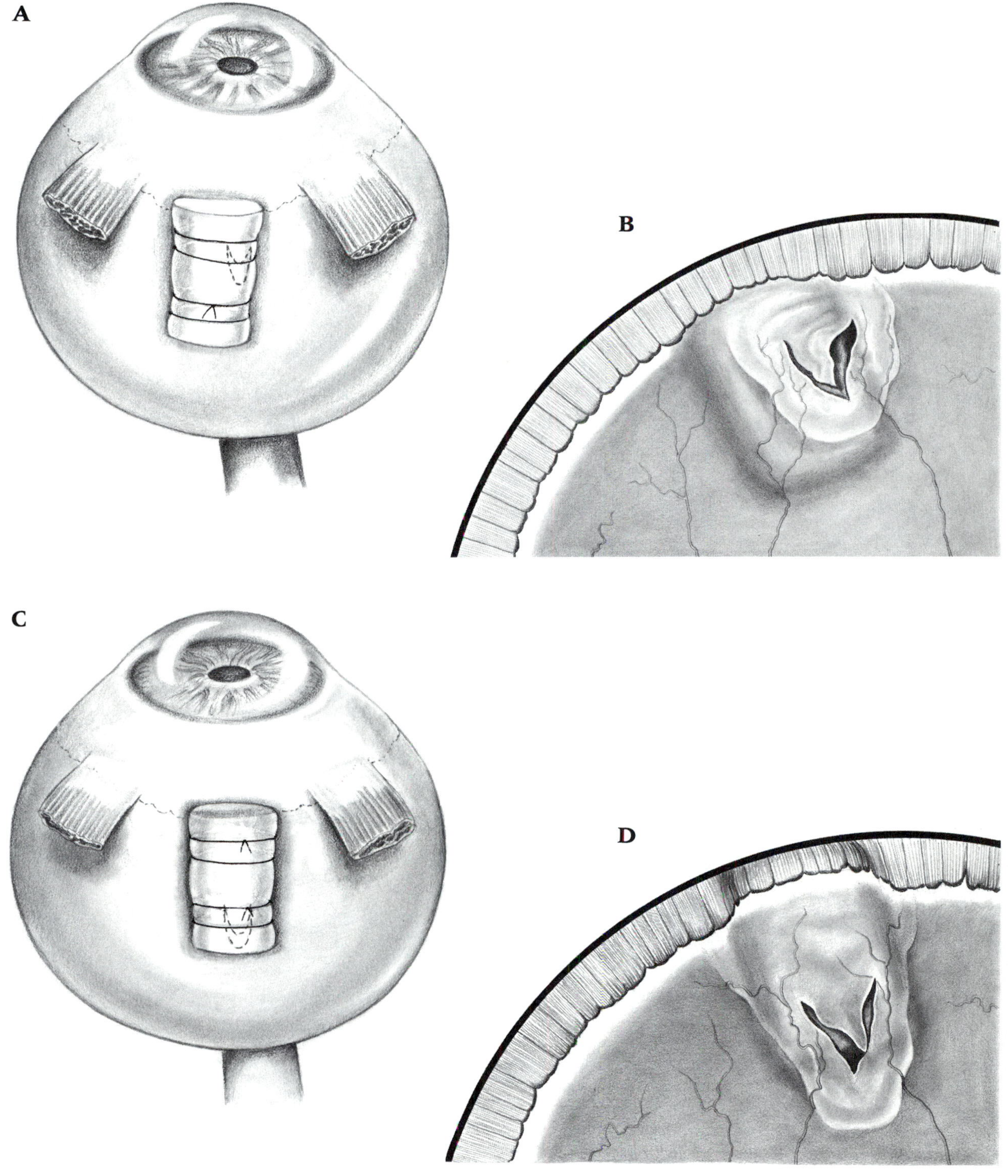

FIGURE 39-4. Complications. *Continued.*

Similarly, insufficient buckling anterior to the tear (Fig. 39-4, *E*) will also cause failure by permitting fluid to pass into the subretinal space through the anterior margin of the tear (Fig. 39-4, *F*). Movement of the buckle more anteriorly is the only correction.

Another complication of the meridional buckle is inadequate closure of the lateral margins of a circumferentially oriented retinal tear (Fig. 39-4, *G*). Despite indentation by the buckle, both lateral ends of the break remain unsealed and subretinal fluid will continue to accumulate at the lateral margins (Fig. 39-4, *H*). One possible method for fixing this situation is the placement of two meridional buckles under one set of imbricating sutures.

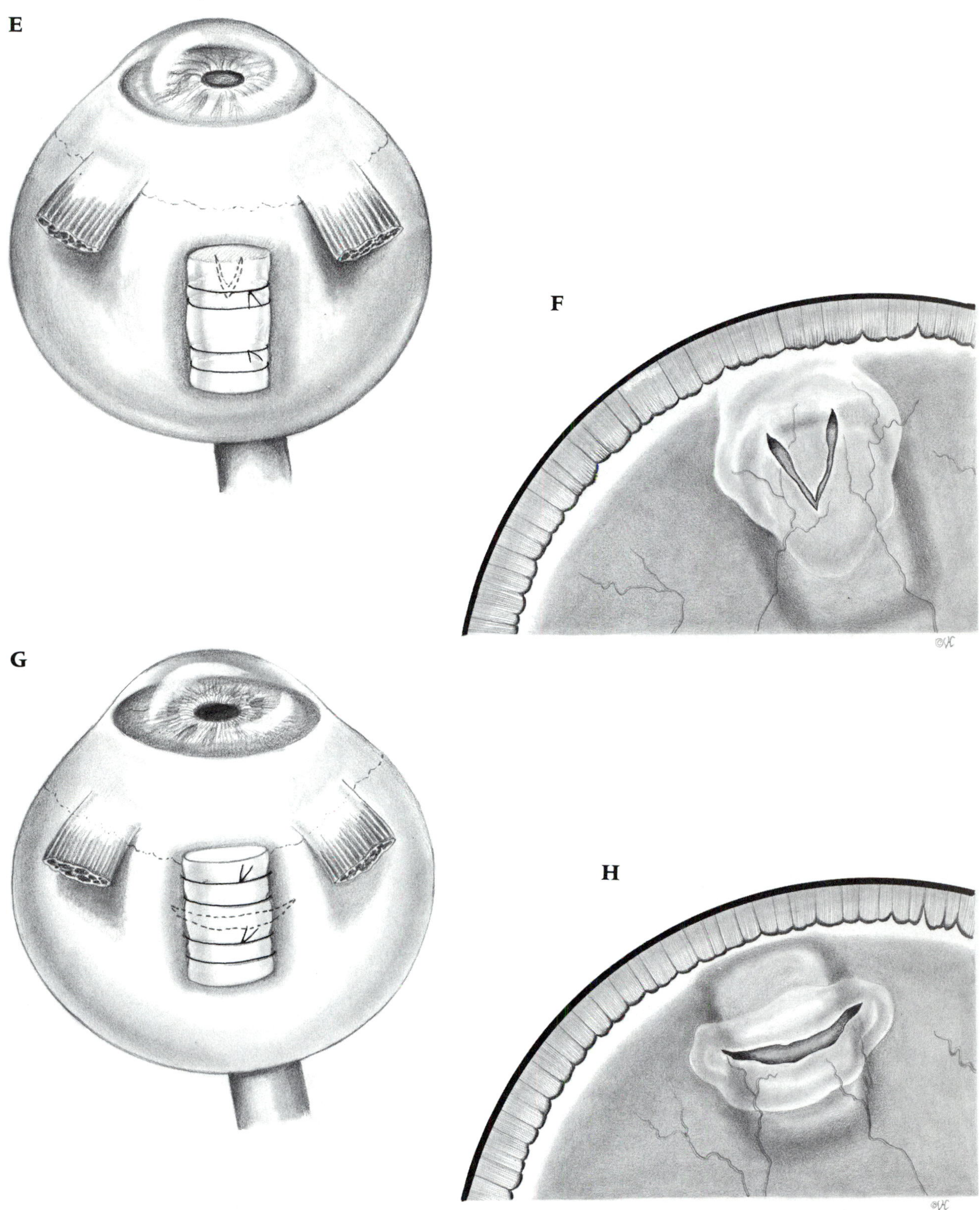

FIGURE 39-4, cont'd

Continued.

The better solution to this problem is the placement of a circumferentially oriented sponge buckle whose apex lies immediately posterior to the posterior lip of the break and whose ends extend beyond the margins of the break (Fig. 39-4, *I*). The sutures are placed at a wider distance than the width of the buckle so that when they are tightly tied (Fig. 39-4, *J*) the buckle is wedged into the wall of the eye and the retinal tear is sealed (Fig. 39-4, *K*). Residual subretinal fluid will be absorbed in the postoperative period ranging in time from hours to a few days. Cryosurgery can be done before the placement of the buckle, or laser photocoagulation can be performed once the tear is tightly sealed on the indented buckle with complete resorption of the subretinal fluid (Fig. 39-4, *L*).

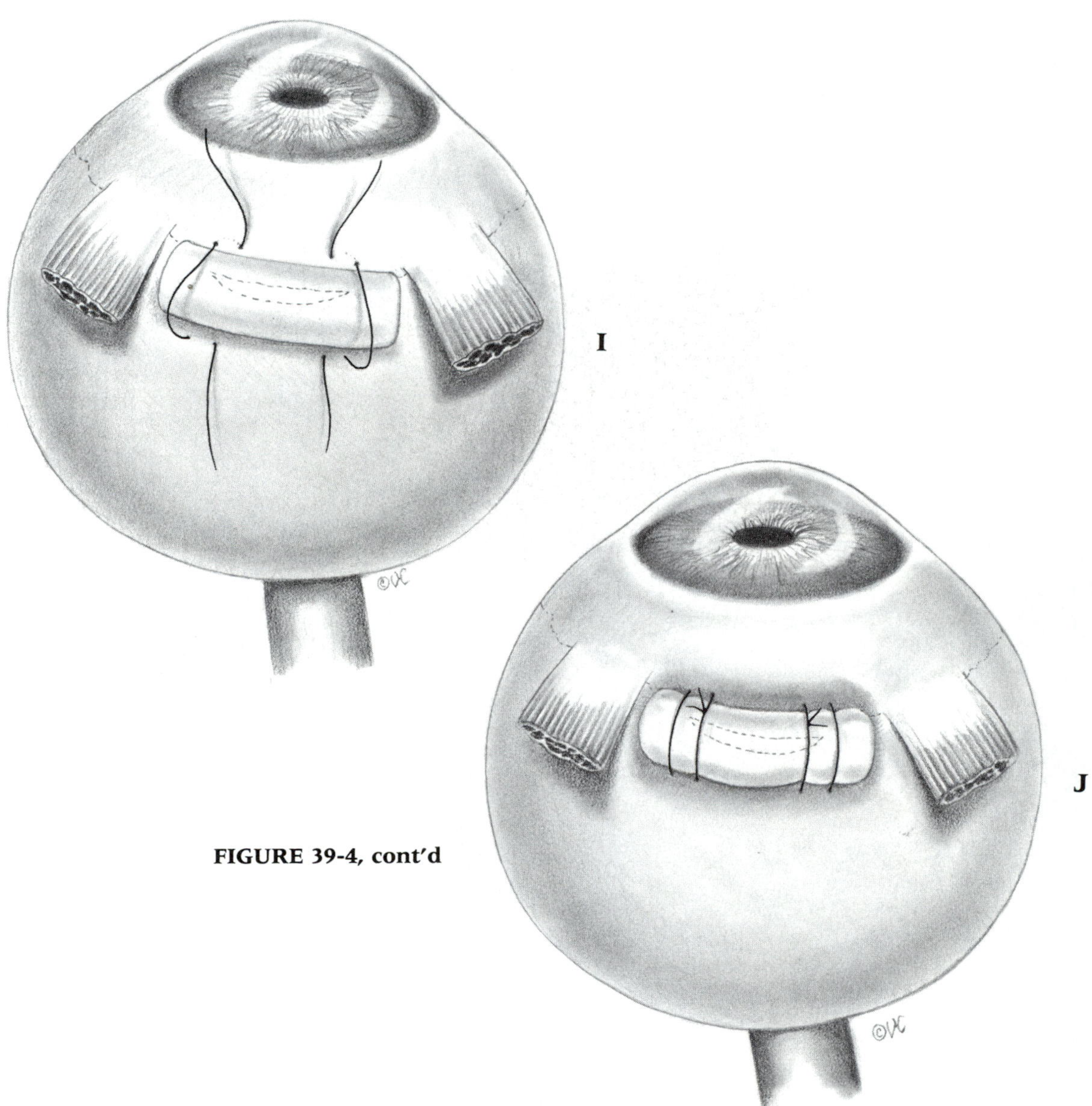

FIGURE 39-4, cont'd

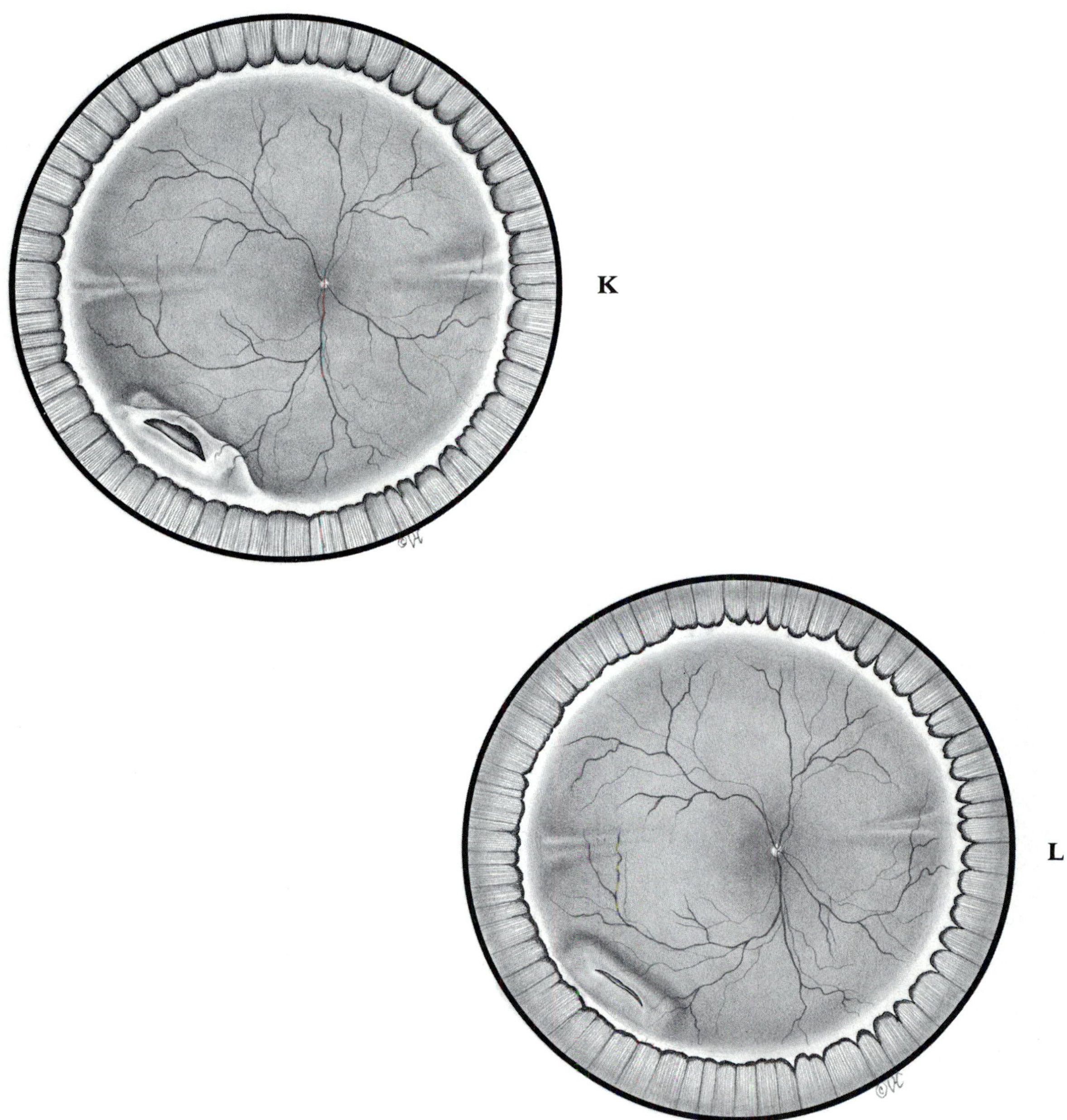
K
L

Complications of circumferential buckle

The leading complication of circumferential buckling is placement of the buckle so that the posterior margin of the tear lies on the posterior slope of the buckle (Fig. 39-5, *A*). The buckle will take the position symmetrically placed between the two sutures. The buckle will not move any closer to the posterior suture than it will to the anterior suture when the sutures are tied (Fig. 39-5, *B*). This placement will leave the posterior margin of the tear open and will permit the passage of fluid into the subretinal space (Fig. 39-5, *C*).

Placement of a circumferential buckle too far posteriorly (Fig. 39-5, *D*) leaves the front margin of the tear unsealed and permits subretinal fluid to accumulate (Fig. 39-5, *E*).

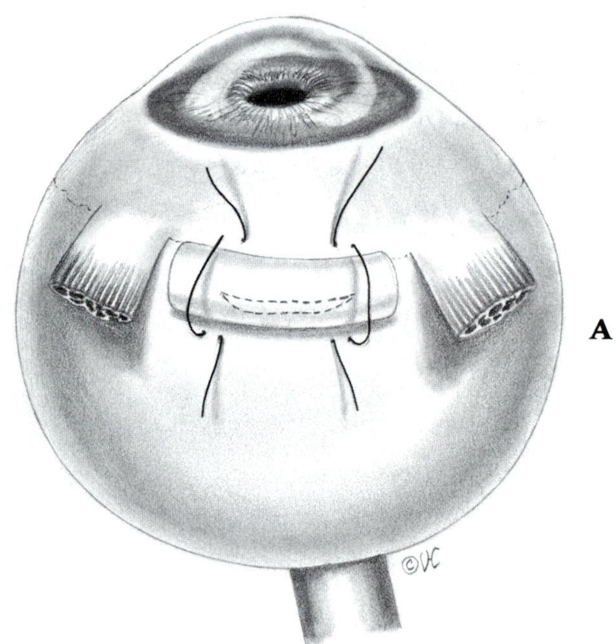

FIGURE 39-5. Complications of circumferential buckle.

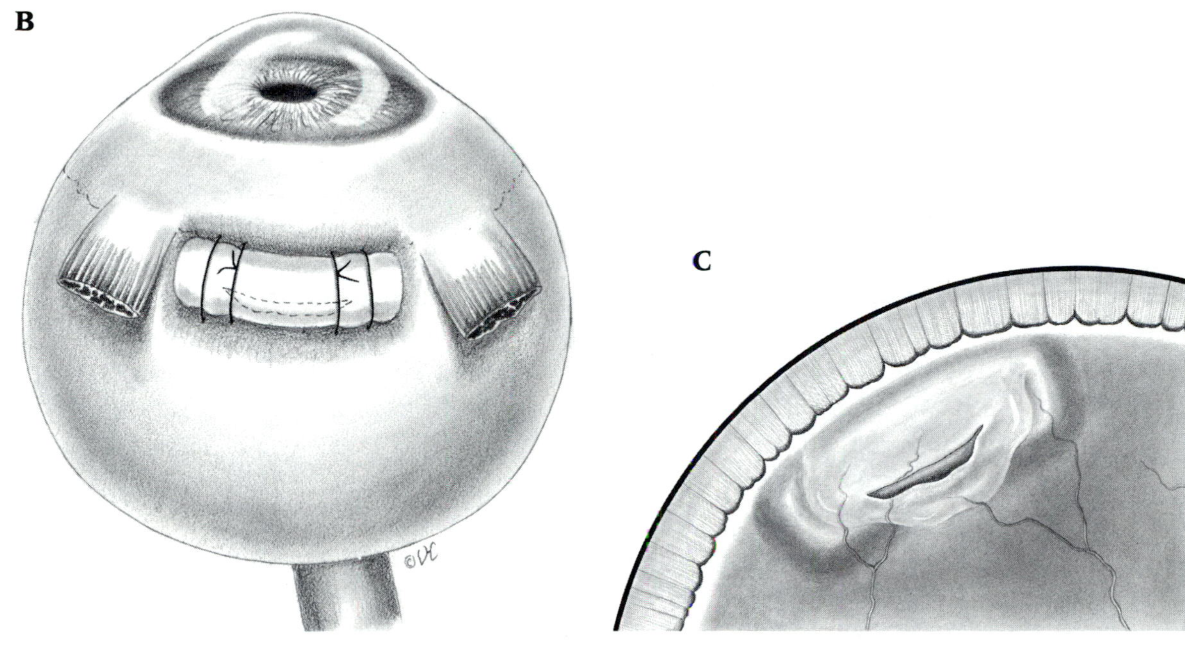
B
C

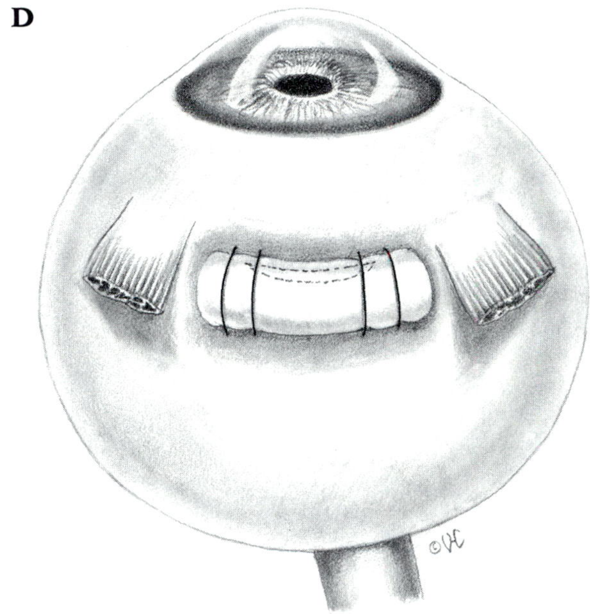
D

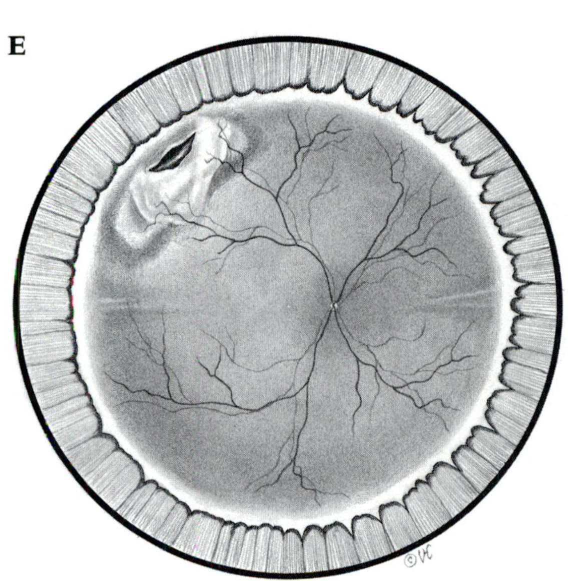
E

Explant Combined with Encircling Band

The placement of an explant beneath an encircling band is a good method of management of a retinal break. The band helps to maintain the permanence of the scleral indentation by the explant. The explant alone tends to lose its indentational height after the passage of several months because of erosion of scleral sutures.

Imbricating sutures must be placed over the explant in order to wedge it into the sclera (Fig. 39-6, *A*). Notice that the sutures are wider than the explant so that when they are tied the explant is wedged into the sclera (Fig. 39-6, *B*). Permanent sutures of 5-0 Mersilene are excellent for this purpose with a spatula needle. The encircling band is pulled tight against itself only after the explant is wedged into the eye wall. Tie the band to itself also with a permanent suture. The band must be mounted into the wall of the eye in each quadrant with another permanent suture, which can also be of 5-0 Mersilene. If the buckle is placed squarely beneath the tear so that it extends beyond both the anterior and posterior and the lateral margins and is indented to cause relative closure with the band lying in a circle holding the explant in place (Fig. 39-6, *C*), it is unnecessary to drain subretinal fluid. In the postoperative days, the subretinal fluid will be absorbed and the tear will adhere to the buckle (Fig. 39-6, *D*). Scarring of the tear onto the buckle can be done at the time of surgery using cryocoagulation to produce a white reaction in the retina surrounding the tear or it can be done at approximately 4 to 6 weeks postoperatively by laser. After initial resolution of the fluid, the retina gradually settles completely flat and is prepared for laser attachment to the site of the tear (Fig. 39-6, *E*). In phakic eyes, neither cryosurgery nor laser is necessary if the tear is well sealed at the buckle. The permanence of the combination of an explant mounted beneath an encircling band relieves the traction on the tear and prevents the reopening of the tear despite the absence of a chorioretinal effusion.

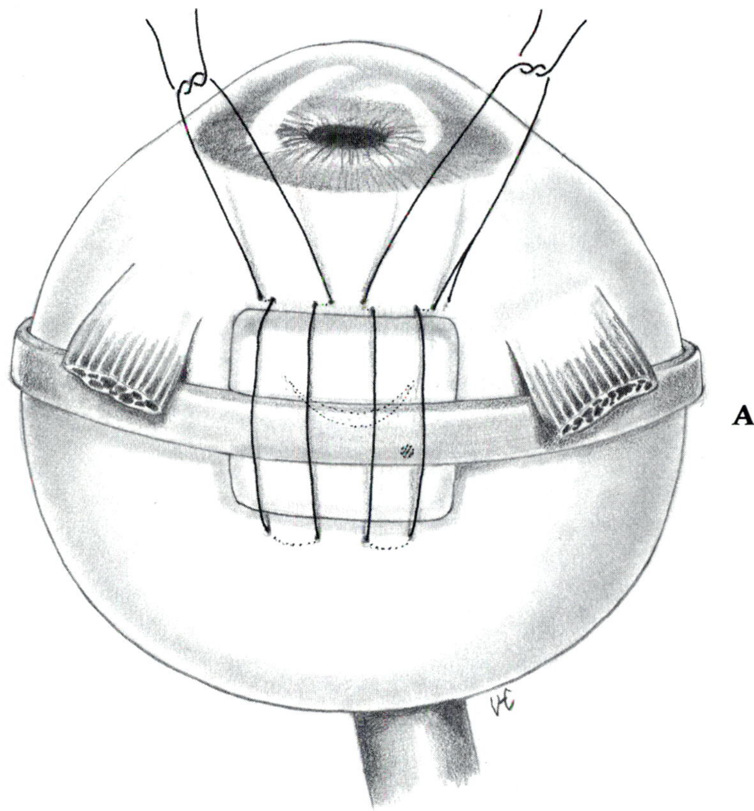

FIGURE 39-6. Explant combined with encircling band.

Continued.

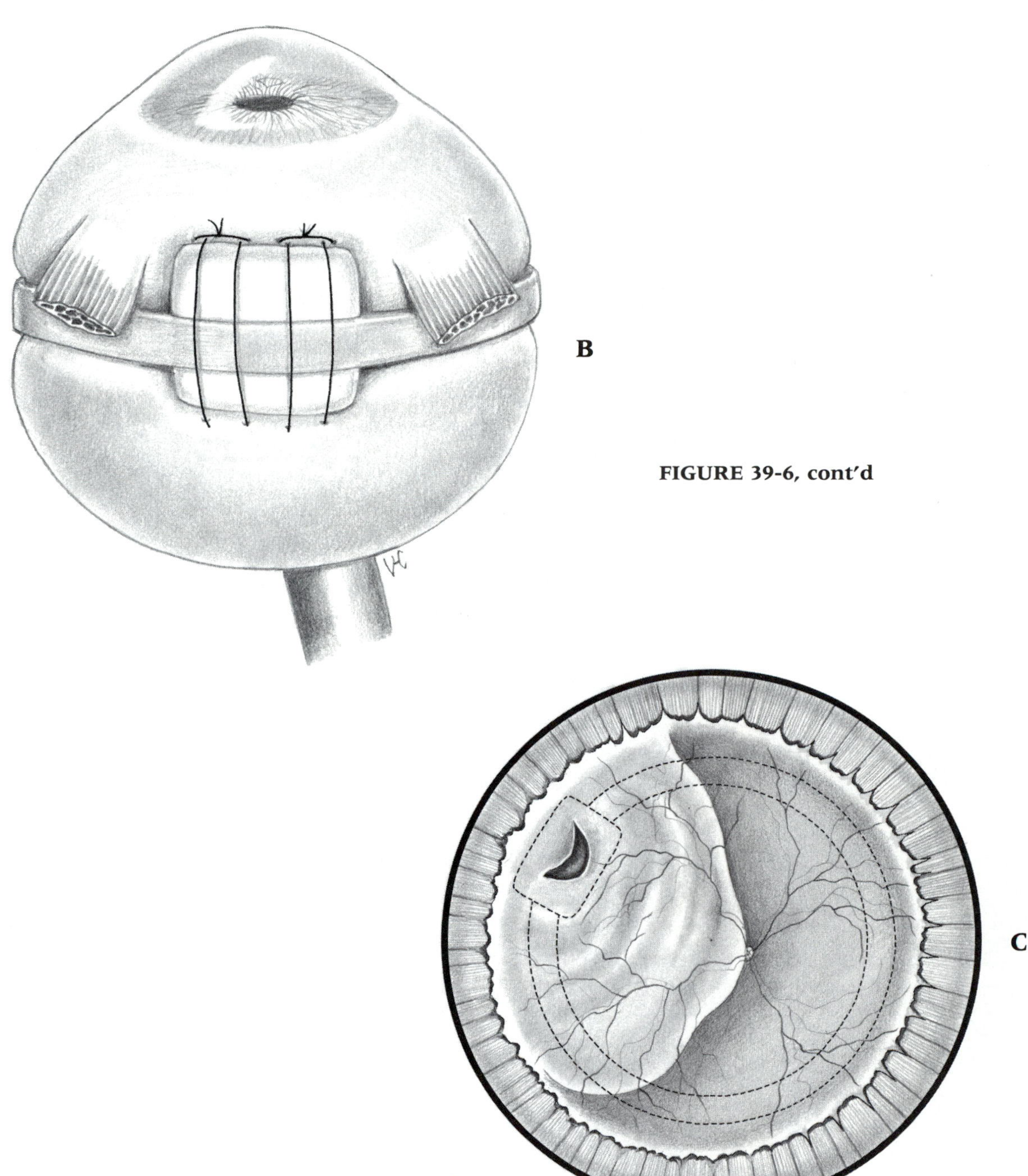

FIGURE 39-6, cont'd

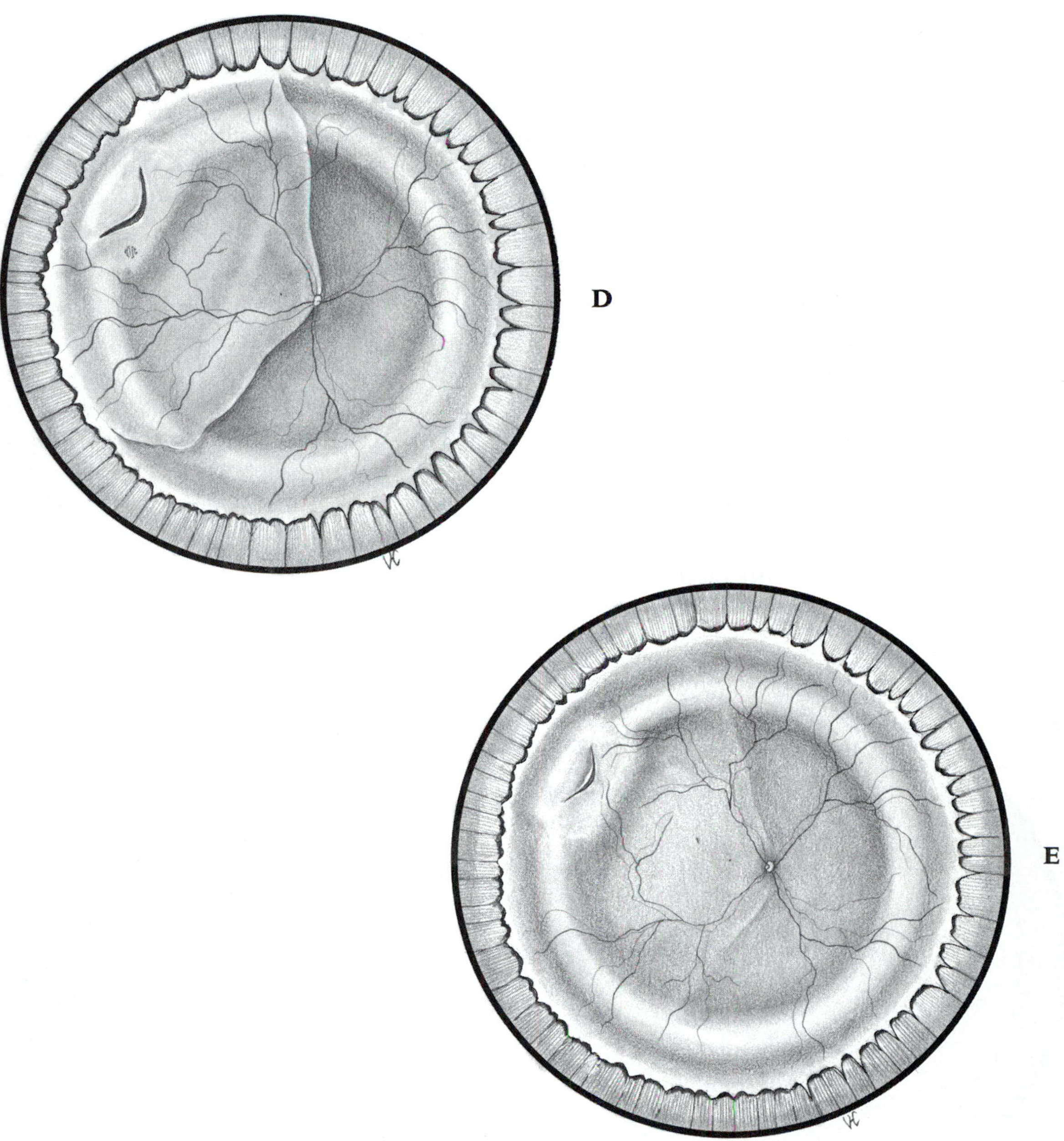
D
E

Balloon Buckling

Balloon buckling requires placement of the balloon directly beneath the break regardless of the configuration of the detachment (Fig. 39-7, *A*). Place the balloon into the sub-Tenon's space through a small incision. Using the binocular indirect ophthalmoscope, localize it so that the apex of the balloon lies directly beneath the tear (Fig. 39-7, *B*). Inflate the balloon at surgery as much as possible without excessively raising the intraocular pressure to risk damage to the ocular circulation. At surgery, it may be possible only to inflate the balloon adequately to see a small indentation whose apex extends toward the retinal tear (Fig. 39-7, *C*). On the day after surgery, inflate the balloon further. On subsequent postoperative days, continue to inflate the balloon as much as intraocular pressure allows until the balloon seals the retinal break (Fig. 39-7, *D*). Once the subretinal fluid is resorbed, usually 1 to 3 days after sealing of the tear, apply laser photocoagulation to the margins of the tear (Fig. 39-7, *E*). Approximately 2 days later, deflate the balloon and remove it. Over the ensuing 2 to 3 weeks, the laser zone will form pigmented scars and the tear is sealed (Fig. 39-7, *F*). Should the tear reopen during the healing process, permanent buckling should be undertaken immediately.

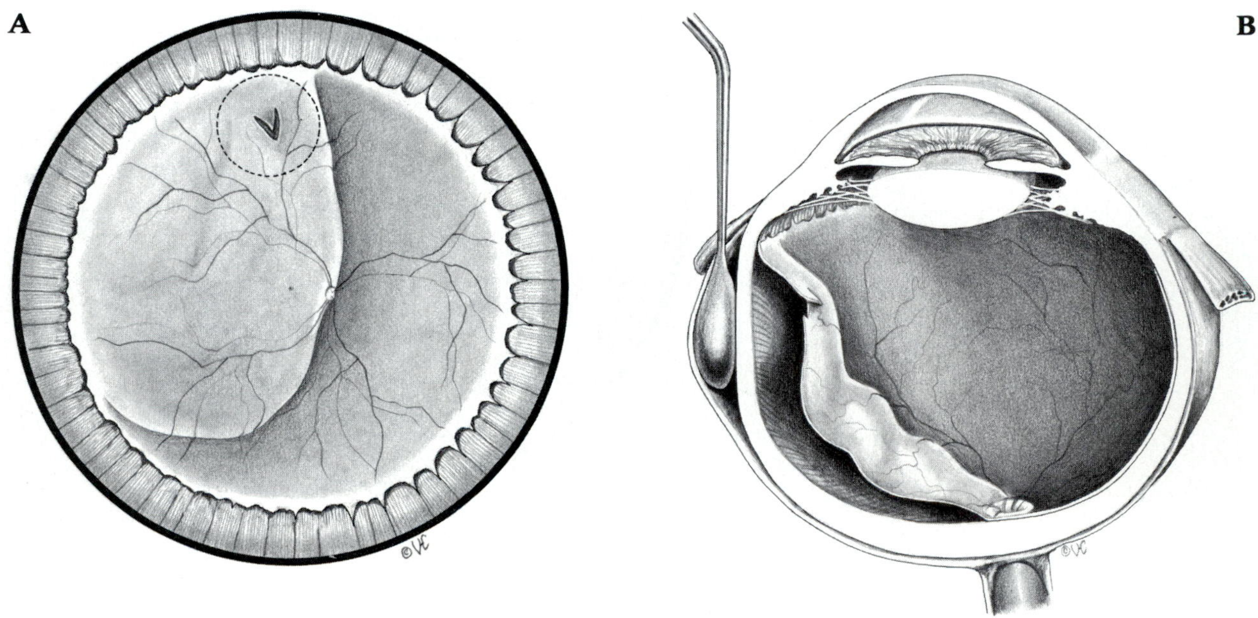

FIGURE 39-7. Balloon buckling.

C

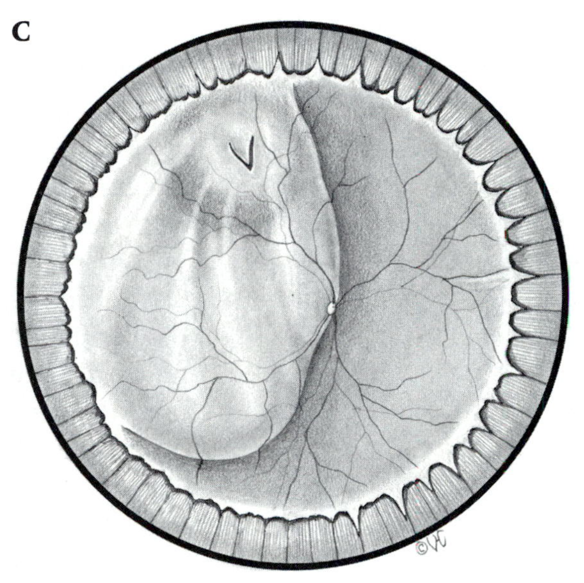

D

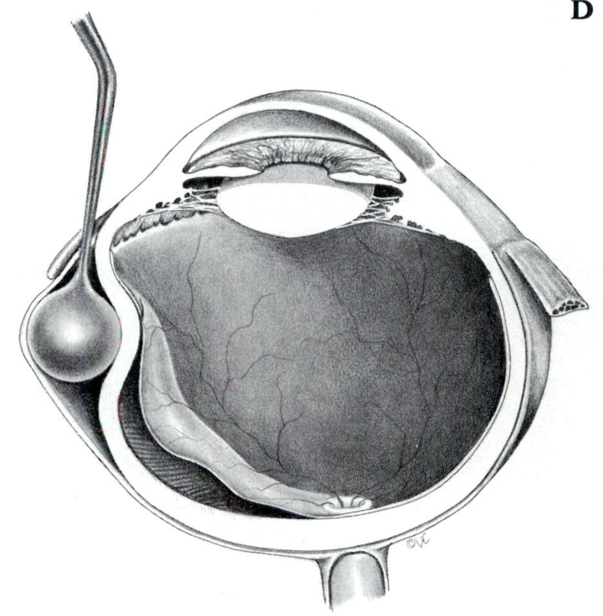

E

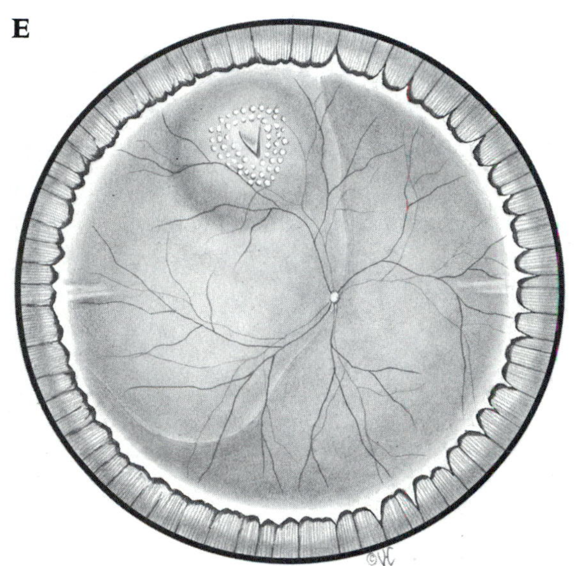

F

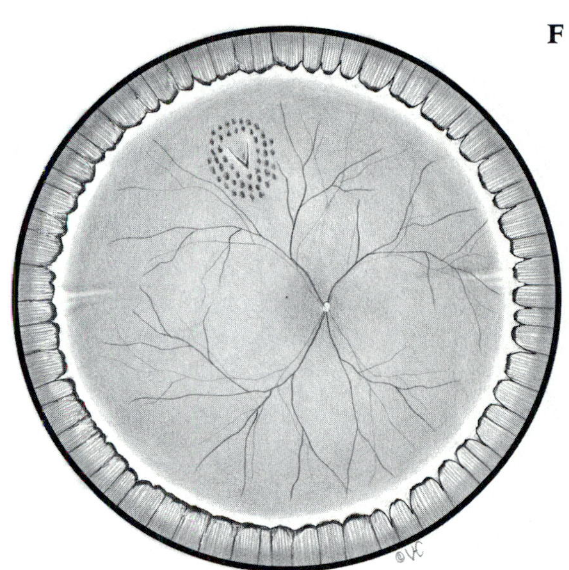

Management of a Large Single Break with Elevated Posterior Lip and Partial Retinal Detachment

A large retinal tear with a partial retinal detachment presents the problem of how best to seal the tear without necessitating the drainage of subretinal fluid. The large width and anteroposterior length of the tear pose a problem for buckling (Fig. 39-8, *A*). Circumferential buckling poses a risk of producing the "fish-mouth" phenomenon wherein the apex of the posterior lip of the tear becomes elevated as the retina is indented. One approach is to place two meridional sponge buckles next to each other under a single set of overlying imbricating sutures (Fig. 39-8, *B*). The advantage of this arrangement is to avoid the fish-mouthing phenomenon that would have occurred at the posterior margin of the tear with a circumferential buckle. To make up for the narrow width of a single meridional buckle, the two buckles are placed next to each other. To ensure a smooth contour of the internal shape of the buckle, the sponges are placed next to each other beneath the single set of sutures. When the sutures are tightened, the buckle is wedged into the wall of the eye to create an indentation (Fig. 39-8, *C*). The indentation produced by the double buckling need not bring about complete sealing of the tear at the time of surgery (Fig. 39-8, *D*). Relative sealing of the break will produce flattening of the detachment in the postoperative days (Fig. 39-8, *E*). Either cryocoagulation performed at the time of surgery or laser photocoagulation in the postoperative period can produce a final scar.

Permanent buckling at the site of the tear can be achieved when an encircling band overlying the meridional sponge buckles is added. The band is tied to itself to create an indentation that keeps the sponge buckles permanently indented. The encircling band should be sutured to the sclera once in each quadrant with a permanent suture (Fig. 39-8, *F*). The encircling band preferentially should lie over the meridional buckles near the posterior margin of the break (Fig. 39-8, *G*). Even without drainage of subretinal fluid, the retina will seal flat as the subretinal fluid is absorbed in the postoperative days. With a permanent buckle, a chorioretinal adhesion is unnecessary in a phakic eye. In an aphakic eye, the adhesion should be achieved either with cryocoagulation at the time of surgery or laser photocoagulation postoperatively.

A

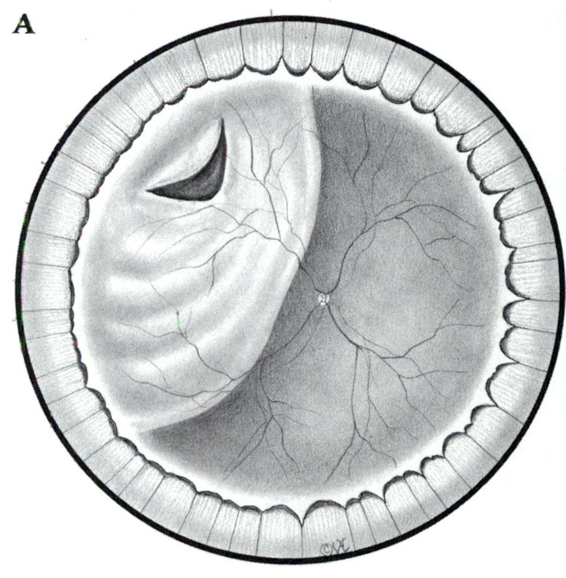

B

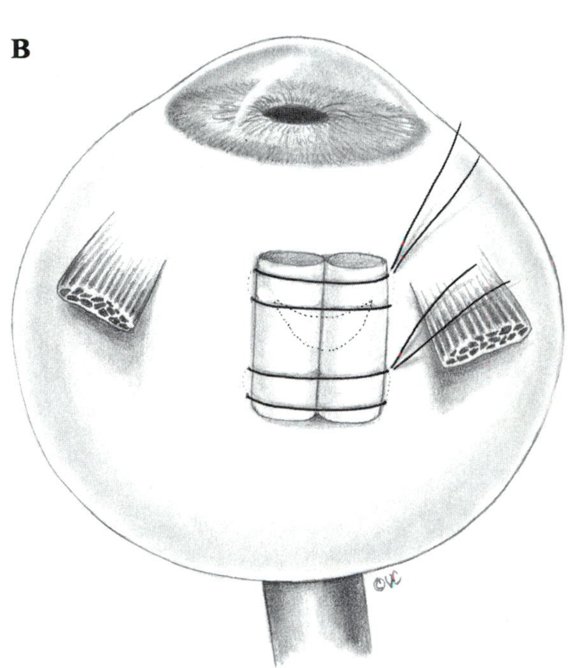

C

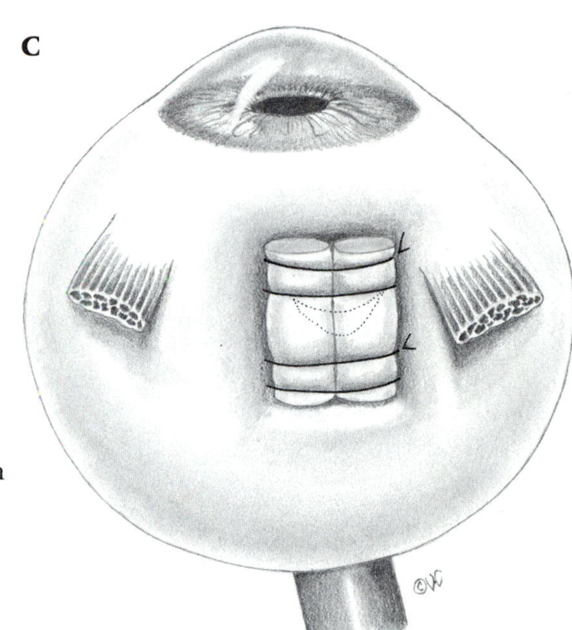

FIGURE 39-8. Management of a large single break with elevated posterior lip and partial retinal detachment.

Continued.

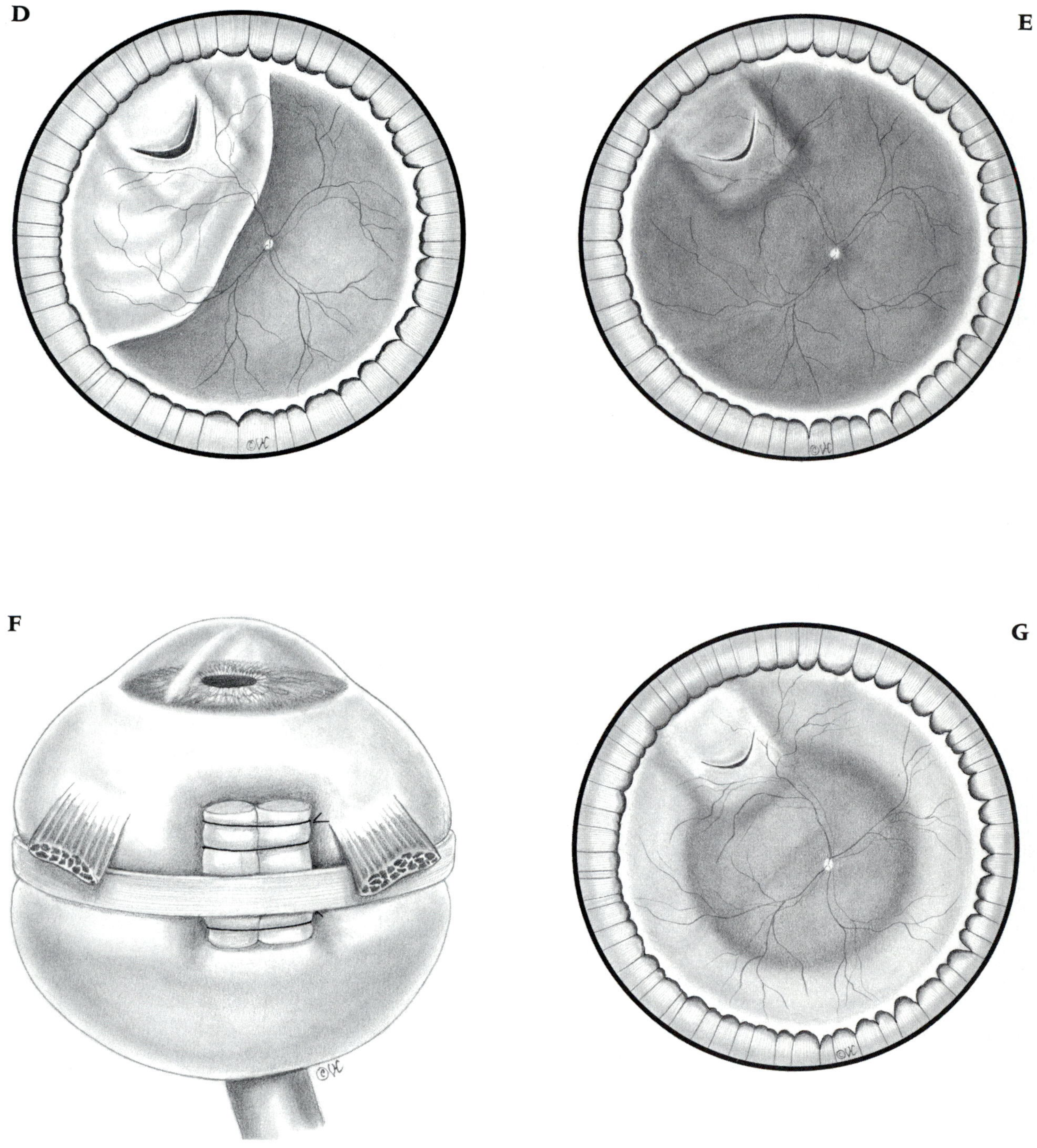

FIGURE 39-8, cont'd

CHAPTER 40

Giant Retinal Tear

Giant retinal tears are grouped together because they extend more than 90 degrees. Most giant tears show elevation of the posterior margin with 50% of the tear above the horizontal meridian (Fig. 40-1). The tear lies near the ora serrata. The anterior margin shows slight elevation, whereas the posterior margin is relatively immobile because of its attachment to the vitreous and because of the retinal contraction from an epiretinal membrane. Severe inversion of the posterior edge of a giant tear can make the underside of the retina visible to ophthalmoscopy. The immobility of the posterior lip of the inverted type of giant tear gives it a poor prognosis for retinal reattachment.

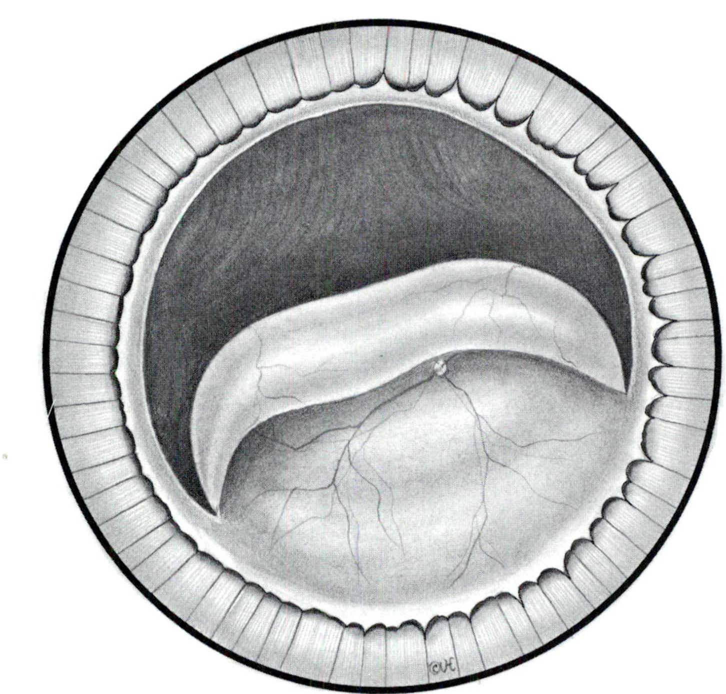

FIGURE 40-1. Giant retinal tear with 50% of tear above the horizontal meridian.

The second type of large retinal tear, the *dialysis,* shares with the giant tear a length extending more than 90 degress and a location near the ora serrata. The posterior edge shows only slight elevation with neither the organized vitreous attachment nor epiretinal membrane formation characteristic of the true giant tear. The mobility of the posterior lip of a dialysis tear differs greatly from the immobility of the posterior lip of a giant tear; for this reason the success rate of surgical treatment of dialyses exceeds that of giant tear. The importance of distinguishing between giant tear and dialyses, both of which can be spontaneous or the result of trauma, is that the treatment of the giant retinal tear is a major surgical undertaking, usually warranting vitrectomy surgery; a dialysis responds well to scleral buckling.

ETIOLOGY

Of giant retinal tears, 80% are spontaneous and 20% are secondary to trauma. The age of diagnosis ranges from 1 year to 63 years with the average at 32 years of age. A family history of retinal detachment is present in approximately 20% of cases. About 80% of patients with giant tears are myopic, with a third of the myopic group having a correction greater than 6 diopters. Fully half of patients with a giant retinal tear have a retinal detachment, a large single retinal tear, or multiple retinal tears in the opposite eye. The time span between detachment in the first eye and detachment in the fellow eye ranges from 1 to 10 years with an average of 4.5 years. The presence of lattice degeneration in the affected and the opposite eye shows a strong relationship to giant retinal tears.

The fundamental cause of spontaneous giant retinal tears probably is similar to that of horseshoe tears. Vitreous contraction along a section of the posterior margin of the vitreous base produces an initial ripping of the retina usually at the time of posterior vitreous detachment. The large size of the tear may result from the combination of abnormally tight vitreoretinal adhesion combined with vulnerability of a thinned and rigid retina at sites of lattice degeneration. The immobility of the posterior flap results from contraction of the remnant adherent posterior hyaloid and the formation of epiretinal membranes secondary to the proliferation of retinal pigment epithelial cells or glial cells along the inner or the outer surface of the posterior aspect of the retinal tear. Traumatic giant retinal tears appear to result from the same vitreous contraction that causes the spontaneous variety except that traumatic tears often are associated with complete vitreous base avulsion rather than posterior vitreous detachment. In neither the spontaneous nor the traumatic cases does the posterior lip of the tear have any direct adhesion to the vitreous body. This lack of adhesion differs from the adhesion of the vitreous base to the anterior margin of the posterior lip of the retinal tear in a dialysis.

Vitrectomy with Intraocular Gas

The posterior flap of a giant retinal tear is almost always inverted by epiretinal membrane formation and hyaloid contraction. Although gravity can evert the posterior flap in many cases, the flap will remain everted only in rare cases that permit treatment with laser or cryoprobe without scleral buckling or vitrectomy. In the vast majority of cases where the flap is rigidly inverted, pars plana vitrectomy (see Chapter 23) should be used to free surface membranes from the retina and remove hyaloid adhesions (Fig. 40-2, *A*). Once the flap is unfolded, the retina will fall back toward the wall of the eye (Fig. 40-2, *B*). Cryocoagulation should be placed in a wide band for the length of the giant break so that an adhesion will form in the entire zone of the break in the postoperative 2 weeks. An alternative method that avoids the risk of pigment scatter and recurrent membrane formation from cryocoagulation is to place laser photocoagulation to the margins of the break either during surgery by endophotocoagulation or, more commonly, postoperatively when the retina is tightly settled against the eye wall.

Once the retina is loosened by vitrectomy, an expansile intraocular gas bubble can be introduced (Fig. 40-2, *C*). As the gas bubble expands, it will force the retina against the eye wall and permit laser photocoagulation to the margins of the break. The bubble should be chosen to provide a duration of at least 21 days in order to allow a permanent scar to form between the retina and pigment epithelium before the spontaneous retraction of the bubble. Placement of the bubble requires a complete gas-fluid exchange of the intraocular contents, a subject discussed on pp. 453 to 459. As the bubble resorbs, much of the giant tear may remain sealed against the wall of the eye, but a small section may show a tendency for partial retraction away from the eye wall (Fig. 40-2, *D*). Failure to seal this area of retraction will permit complete reopening of the giant tear. Placement of a sponge meridional buckle in an area where the retina cannot remain attached to the eye wall after resorption of the gas bubble can produce a seal in that region and maintain a seal in the other regions of the tear until a final pigmented scar forms (Fig. 40-2, *E*).

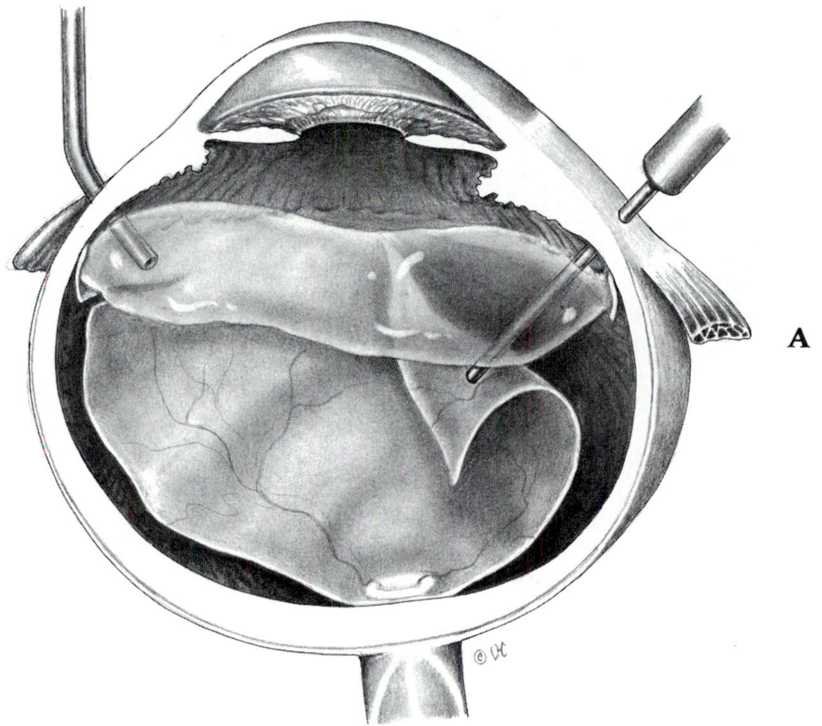

FIGURE 40-2. Vitrectomy with intraocular gas.
Continued.

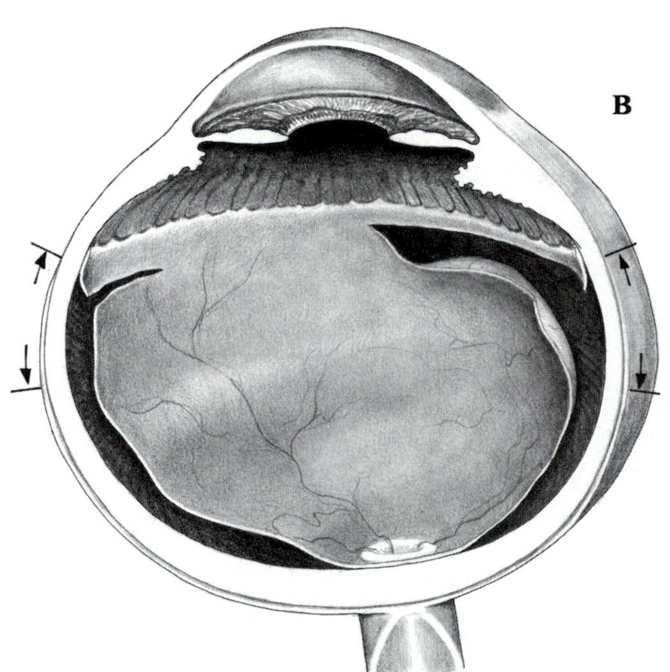

FIGURE 40-2, cont'd

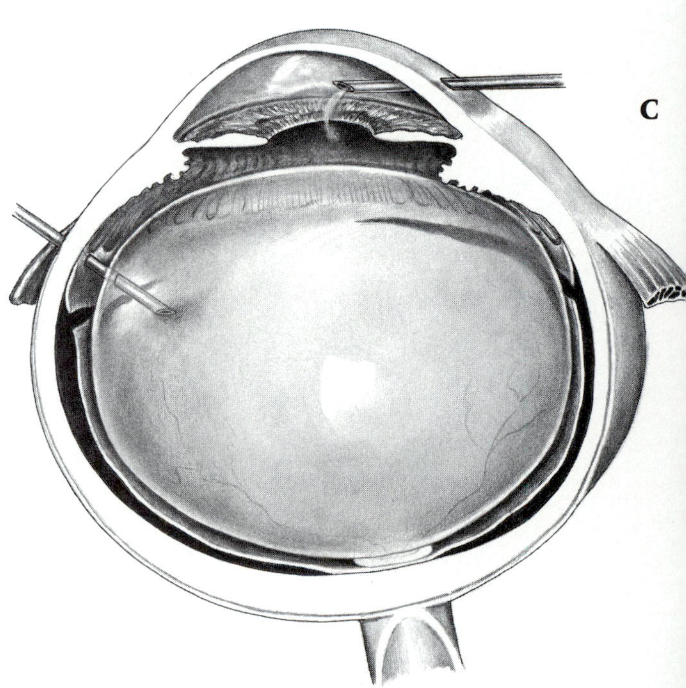

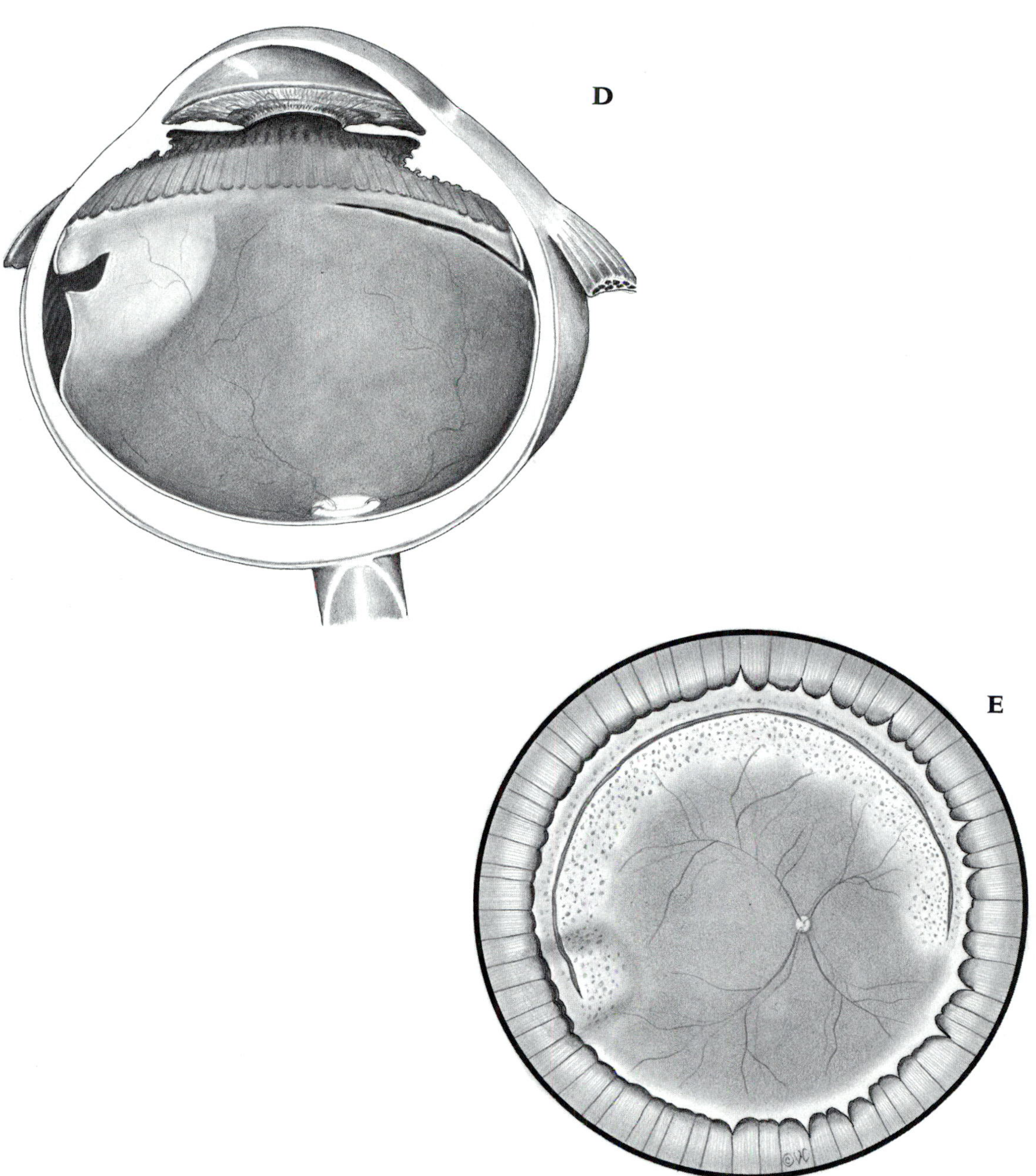
D
E

Simultaneous Vitrectomy, Gas Injection, and Scleral Buckling

This operation is necessary for cases where preoperative gravitational positioning shows a strong predilection for the flap to become reinverted after initial unfolding. This phenomenon is most common in retinal tears that are greater than 180 degrees in length.

With the patient in the supine position, place a broad silicone explant whose width will extend from the ora serrata to a point approximately 4 to 6 mm posterior to the posterior margin of the break after the break settles against the eye wall (Fig. 40-3, *A*). Cryocoagulation can be done before placement of the buckle or laser can be performed postoperatively. Laser is preferable because of its lesser tendency to stimulate epiretinal membrane formation.

Next, perform lensectomy (see p. 420) and pars plana vitrectomy. The lensectomy is necessary because of the need for a complete gas-fluid exchange. The long duration of the postoperative gas bubble would produce a cataract. The anterior vitreous and the vitreous base should be left intact (Fig. 40-3, *B*). With the retina now mobile, after the vitrectomy, the patient should be placed in the prone position and a gas-filled exchange performed in order to unroll the retina against the wall of the eye. After expansion of the gas bubble with the patient in the prone position postoperatively, the retina should seal against the wall of the eye (Fig. 40-3, *C*). At this time, laser photocoagulation should be performed as soon as orbital swelling permits.

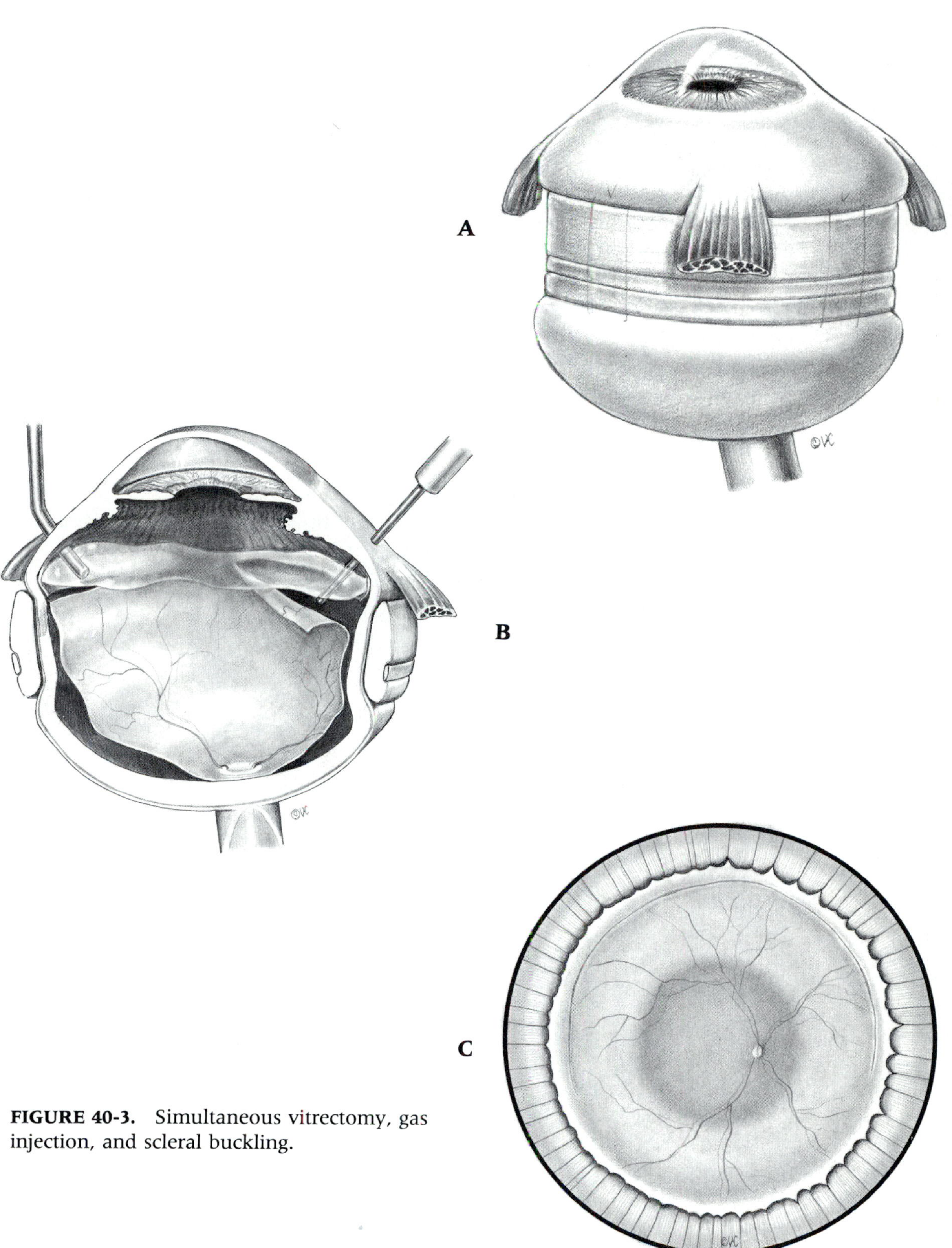

FIGURE 40-3. Simultaneous vitrectomy, gas injection, and scleral buckling.

Complications

The most frequent problem in combining buckling with vitrectomy in giant retinal breaks is to create excessive indentation by the buckle. The indentation reduces the intraocular diameter so greatly that folds form in the retina (Fig. 40-4, *A*). The folds can lead to reaccumulation of subretinal fluid. To prevent this problem, the buckle should be broad but not highly indented.

The management of the fold (Fig. 40-4, *B*) consists in placement of a meridional buckle beneath the encircling buckle. Place a meridional buckle at the original surgery under any area of retina that shows significant residual folds after placement of the gas bubble. Suture the meridional buckle to the sclera to form a deep indentation in order to tampon the retinal meridional fold and to prevent distortion of the encircling indentation of the broad overlying buckle (Fig. 40-4, *C*). The indentation of the meridional sponge smooths the retinal contour (Fig. 40-4, *D*) and prevents the reaccumulation of subretinal fluid. Reopening of any sector of the tear toward a meridional fold as the bubble is being resorbed warrants meridional buckle placement.

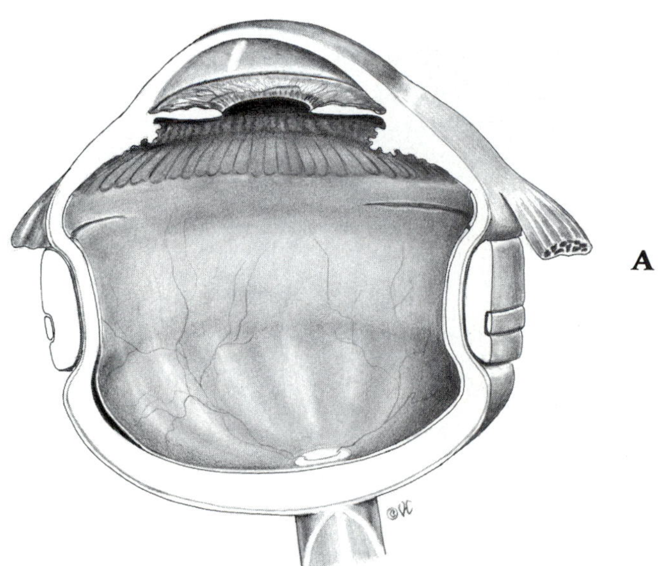

FIGURE 40-4. Postoperative complications.

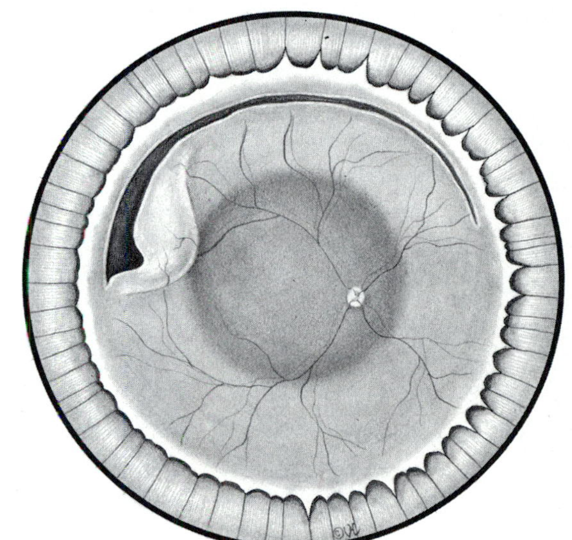

B

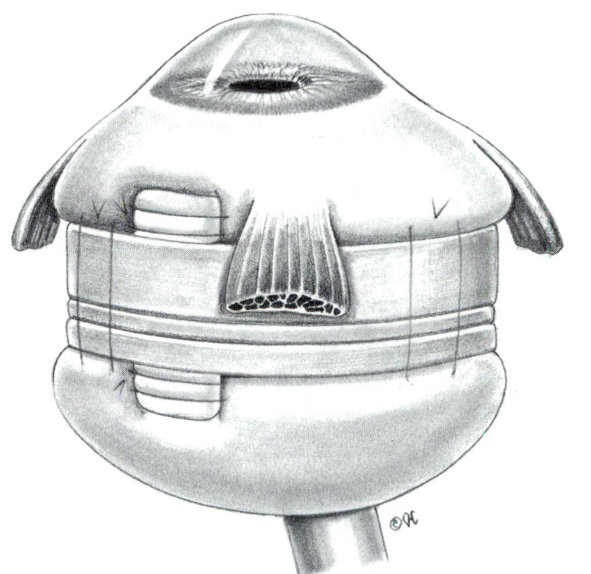

C

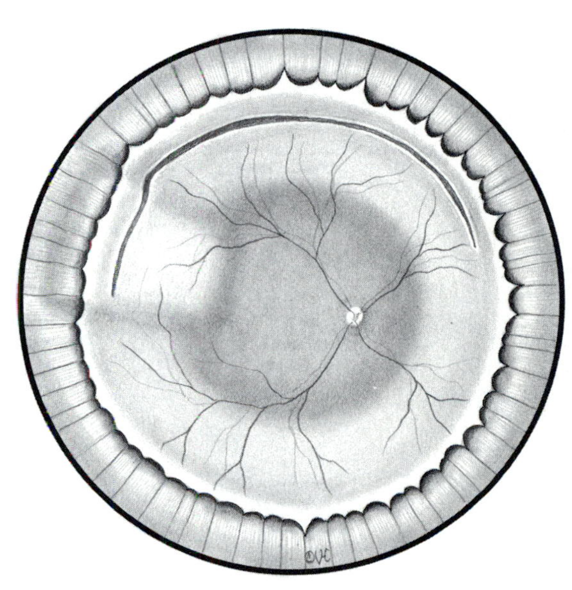

D

Scleral Buckling with Diathermy

For cases where the retinal flap does not show a strong tendency to revert to its folded position after gravitation, scleral dissection implant with diathermy can be successful and can eliminate the need for vitrectomy and lensectomy with gas bubble. The scleral dissection should extend at least 6 mm posterior to the anterior margin of the posterior flap of the retinal tear (Fig. 40-5). The diathermy bed should extend to cover both the posterior and anterior margins of the tear. The diathermy bed should extend the entire length of the tear. Drain subretinal fluid posterior to the tear. Incarceration of the retina as part of the drainage procedure has the advantage of stabilizing the retinal position. The buckle should be tightened only enough to produce tamponade of the tear. Do not tighten it to the point of producing radial retinal folds.

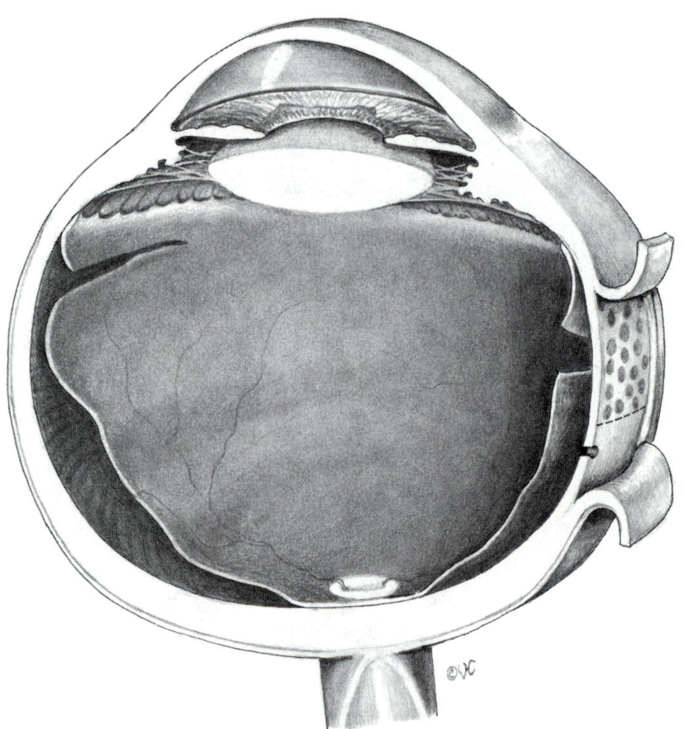

FIGURE 40-5. Scleral buckling with diathermy.

CHAPTER 41

Angiomatosis Retinae

Angiomatosis retinae and von Hippel's disease are alternative names for the phacomatosis of retinal angioma. The occurrence of this condition together with hemangioblastoma of the cerebellum, medulla, or spinal cord constitutes the syndrome of von Hippel-Lindau disease. The angioma of the retina is a benign tumor rather than part of a generalized retinal vascular disease and is transmitted in an autosomal dominant genetic pattern with incomplete penetrance.

NATURAL HISTORY

Although present at birth as hamartomatous collections of small nests of angioblastic and astroglial rest cells, retinal angiomas do not grow sufficiently large for clinical detection until the second or third decade of life. Some angiomas can remain latent throughout life with discovery only on autopsy. At first, the angioma is not associated with abnormalities in the capillary bed of the adjacent retina and fails to show specific feeding or draining channels. The angioma originates in the inner retina and eventually grows to occupy the full retinal thickness. With its enlargement the angioma shows arteriovenous communications that cause the hypertrophy of specific capillary feeders and draining venules. The vascular system forms a high-flow fistula with hypertrophy of a single arteriole and a single venous channel to serve the tumor. In full size, the feeder arterty and vein are enlarged during the entire course from the optic disc to the angioma. The shunting mechanism of the tumor is responsible for the alteration of the circulatory state producing dilatation, tortuosity, and sclerosis of the large feeder vessels. With severe shunting, circulatory stasis occurs in the capillary bed of the adjoining retina and microaneurysms form in response to the ischemia. Capillary-bed ischemia leads to intraretinal edema, cystoid degeneration, hemorrhage, and even serous retinal detachment if the circulatory shunting is severe enough.

A peripheral angioma can produce maculopathy consisting of lipid exudates but not of edema. Theoretically the exudates result from shunting of blood circulation from the macular capillary bed to the angioma. Frequently there is no observable link between the exudate at the fovea and the angioma.

Macular edema can develop with both small and large angiomas in concomitance with lipid exudation. Eradication of the angioma leads to rapid resolution of the edema and slow resorption of the lipid at the macula with a degree of improvement in macular function dependent on the extent of destruction of the cellular elements in the macula during the long period of edema accumulation.

Without treatment, the angioma can lose its vascular competence and show breakdown of the blood-retinal barrier with both intraretinal and subretinal exudation, exudative retinal detachment, vitreous hemorrhage, vitreous contraction, and retinal detachment. Uveitis, cataract, and glaucoma are the results of this exudative process. Spontaneous resolution of an angioma is very rare.

HISTOPATHOLOGY

Digestion studies with trypsin show that the angiomas begin as small proliferations of endothelial cells between an arterial and a venule in the retinal capillary bed. Astrocytes that are vacuolated with lipid are interspersed between the capillaries, an indication that the lesions are not pure hemangioblastomas but rather they consist of both vascular and glial cells.

CLINICAL APPEARANCE

Angiomatosis retinae can appear at any age from premature infancy up to the sixth decade of life. Most commonly, it presents at 25 years of age, when the patient develops decreased visual acuity because of subretinal exudation, preretinal hemorrhage in the macula, or vitreous hemorrhage. The classic findings are the triad of angioma, enlarged feeder vessels, and subretinal exudate. The stage of progression determines the relative significance of each component of the triad.

An angioma can show no mass in its earliest clinically recognizable stage. The angioma may resemble a cluster of capillary vessels and microaneurysms or only a small intraretinal hemorrhage. Rarely the early lesion is identifiable as a small arteriovenous malformation. The angioma is present most commonly in the temporal periphery but can grow anywhere, even at the macula or the disc. Angiomas are multiple in 33% of affected eyes and bilateral in up to 50% of cases.

In the early stage, the feeder vessels are subtle in appearance. The normal appearance of the microvasculature surrounding the angioma in the early stage differentiates the angiomatosis from the telangiectasis of Coats's disease. Fluorescein angiography is best for this distinction. Usually, the flat angioma grows slowly until it presents a small, slightly elevated, red nodule with only the feeding vein in prominence. Exudate may accumulate in a small amount on the angioma's red surface. Further growth of the angioma produces the classic appearance of a red nodule with its base on the retina and elevation by as much as 5 mm above the retinal surface. The angioma's surface shows small, irregular dilated vessels with enormously widened feeder vessels, both arteries and veins, leading to the angioma. Fluorescein angiography demonstrates profuse leakage at the angioma. Red preretinal hemorrhage later occurs at the surface of the angioma and can extend to the macula or burst into the vitreous. The hemorrhage results from proliferative retinopathy on the surface of the angioma. Eventually, lipid and serous exudation from the angioma accumulate to such a great extent that the retina is totally detached with subsequent onset of uveitis, absolute glaucoma, and finally phthisis bulbi.

CATEGORIZATION AND INDICATIONS FOR SURGERY

The natural history of angiomatosis retinae is the basis for its clinical categorization (Table 41-1). Surgery is indicated for all stages of angioma formation.

TABLE 41-1
Classification of angiomatous retinae

Type	Characteristics
Embryonic	Hamartoma Barely observable pink red spot No patent vessels No fluorescein leakage No feeder vessels
Young angioma	Slight elevation of pink red nodule Patent vessels Fluorescein leakage Feeder vessels minimally enlarged
Mature angioma	Elevated spherical nodule Exudate at angioma and macula Hemorrhage from surface vessels Profuse fluorescein leakage Prominent feeder vessels Microaneurysms and dropout in circumangioma capillary bed
Degenerative angioma	Exudative detachment of part of the retina
Terminal angioma	Total exudative retinal detachment Cataract Phthisis

From Sigelman J: Angiomatosis retinae. In Sigelman J: Retinal diseases, Boston, 1984, Little, Brown & Co.

Photocoagulation

The earliest stage of angiomatosis (Fig. 41-1, *A*) is an indication for laser photocoagulation. Argon green is the best wavelength because of its absorption by pigment and hemoglobin. Using a 200 or 500 μm spot size with a duration of 0.5 seconds, start treatment with a 100-milliwatt power coagulation aimed directly at the angioma (Fig. 41-1, *A*). Increase the power of the treatment gradually by 25-milliwatt increments until a gray-white reaction results. Then place overlapping coagulations over the surface of the angioma (Fig. 41-1, *B*). Once the entire lesion has been covered with the gray-white reaction, it is safe to increase the power of the laser by approximately 20% of the power level of the initial treatment. The initial surface coagulation of the angioma deceases the risk of explosive hemorrhage from the high-energy burns necessary for coagulation of the outer portion of the angioma (Fig. 41-1, *B*). In a stage 1 angiomatosis, the initial treatment will be able to destroy the entire thickness of the angioma; in stage 2, successive laser treatments separated by a period of approximately 3 weeks are necessary to produce full-thickness destruction.

The success of treatment can be determined approximately 2 months after treatment. A satisfactory outcome, showing pigmentation and diminished elevation of the angioma, absence of fluorescein leakage, and resolution of macular edema indicate that no further treatment is necessary (Fig. 41-1, *C*). Continued fluorescein leakage (not staining) indicates the presence of persistent angiomatous tissue, which requires additional photocoagulation. Although the macular edema should be resorbed, decreased visual acuity can persist because of irreversible degeneration that occurred during the period of edema.

A

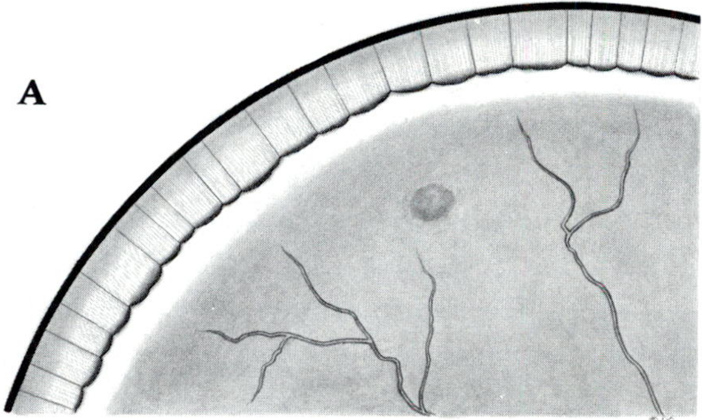

B

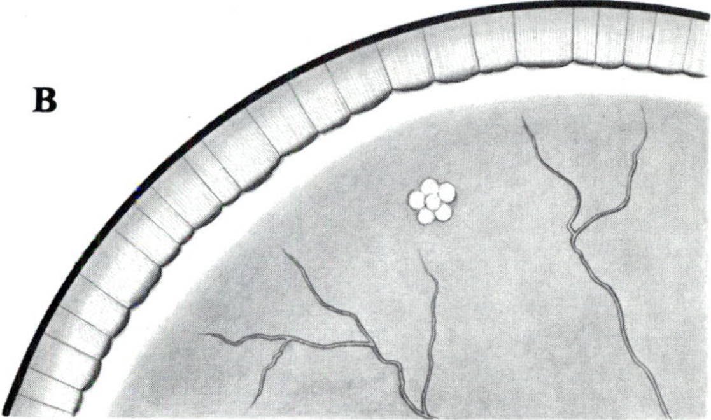

C

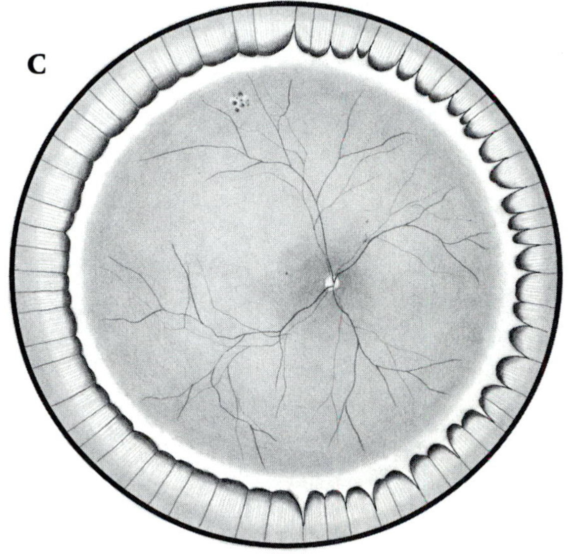

FIGURE 41-1. Laser treatment.

Continued.

For stage 3 angiomatosis, photocoagulation should be directed only to the angioma and its surrounding telangiectatic vessels (Fig. 41-1, *D* and *E*). Only when there is no hemorrhage on the surface does argon green become the wavelength of choice because the green light is absorbed by the blood in the angioma. If hemorrhage covers the surface of the tumor, krypton red is the preferable wavelength because it passes through the surface hemorrhage to be absorbed by the pigment within the angioma. With either wavelength, use photocoagulation to coagulate the angioma and the rim of telangiectatic retina surrounding it (Fig. 41-1, *F*). Do not photocoagulate either the feeder vessels or the edematous macula (Fig. 41-1, *G* and *H*). Pretreatment with low-energy laser decreases the risk of hemorrhage when the higher energy is subsequently used. With krypton red laser, do not attempt to whiten the surface of the hemorrhagic angioma because the energy necessary to produce such total coagulation risks further hemorrhage. Avoid intense coagulation around the rim of the angioma because of the risk of choroidal rupture and hemorrhage.

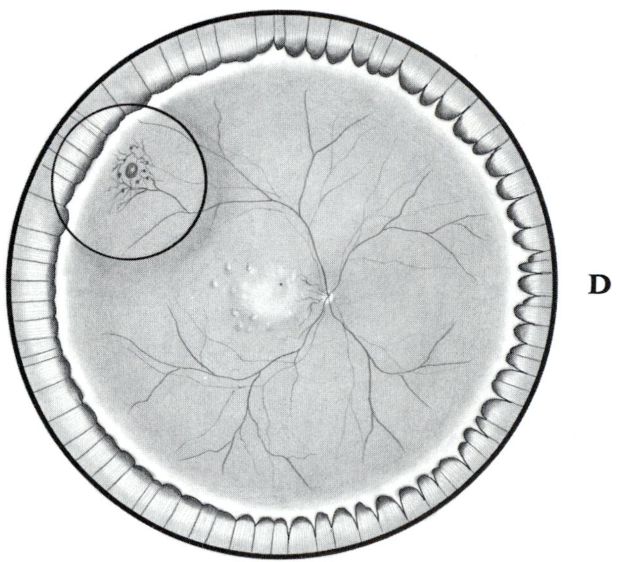

FIGURE 41-1, cont'd

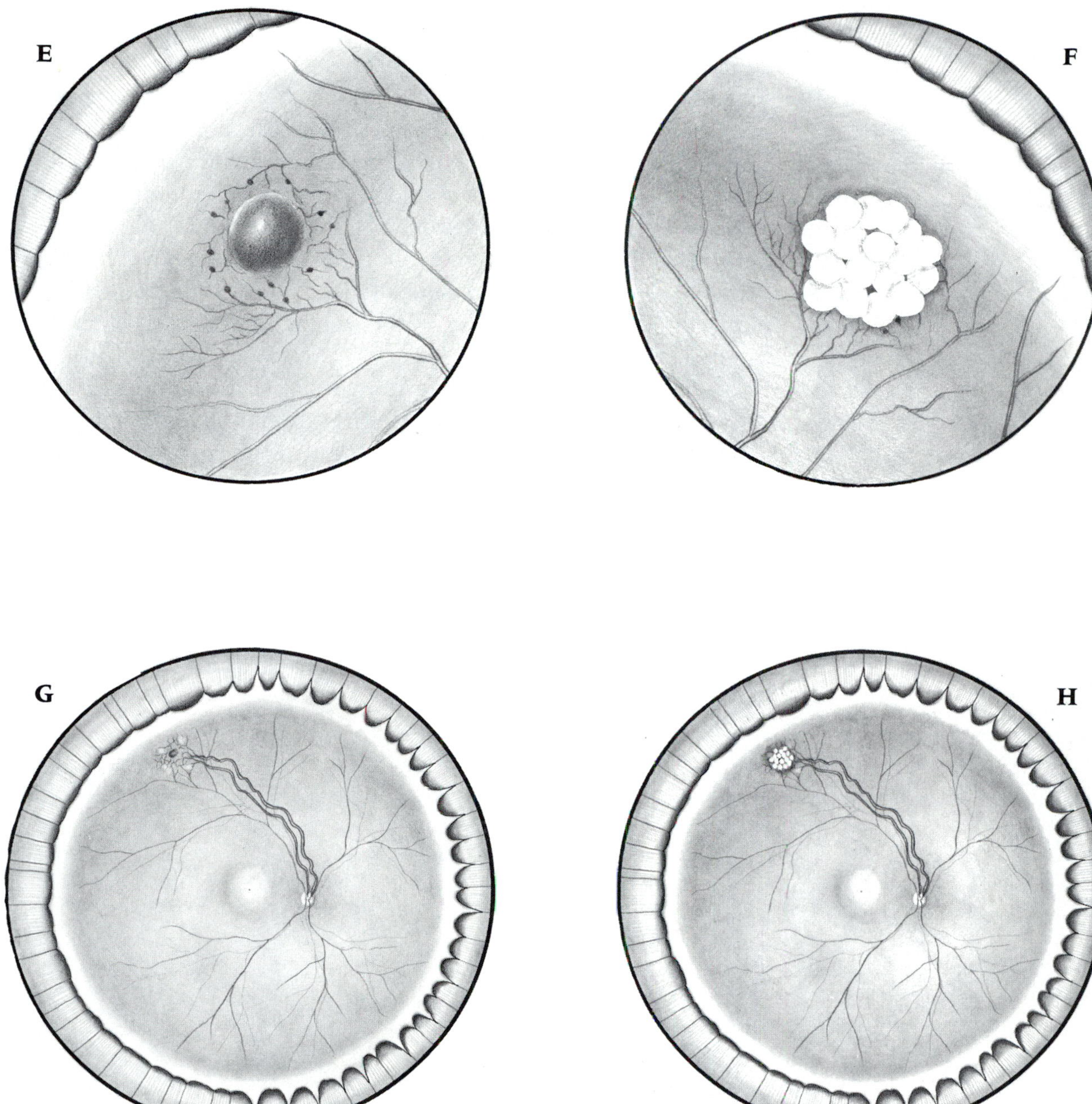
E
F
G
H

Follow-up study

Immediately after treatment, angiomas that were white originally without hemorrhage tend to appear pink because of the dilatation of the coagulated blood vessels. Angiomas that were red originally, because of overlying hemorrhage or dense packing of vessels near the surface, appear whiter because of the coagulation of the hemorrhage and the vessels. One month after treatment, determine whether or not treatment has produced a permanent scar at the angioma. Although pigmentation and shrinking of the angioma are favorable signs, attenuation of the feeder vessels and absence of fluorescein leakage from the angioma are the only reliable indices that the angioma is totally scarred. Angiography of the telangiectatic perimeter shows pigmentation and vessel closure. If the angioma remains pink 1 month after photocoagulation, repeat the treatment. The power level of the laser must be reduced for retreatment because of the increased energy absorption by the pigment.

Six months after closure of the angioma, the lesion should appear as a pigmented scar, the exudate surrounding the angioma should have diminished or disappeared, the feeder vessels should be atrophic, and the macula should be dry (Fig. 41-2).

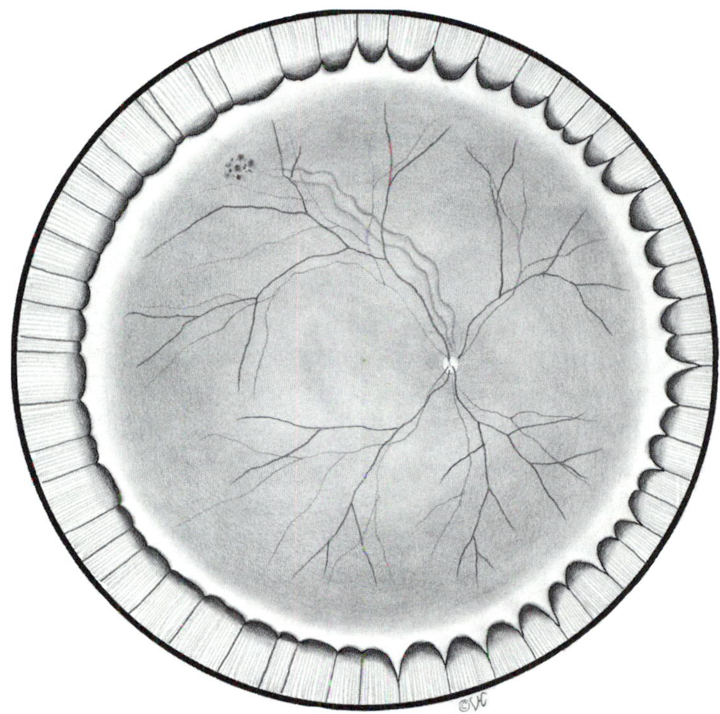

FIGURE 41-2. Follow-up observation.

Surgery for Stage 4 Angiomatosis

Angiomas in stage 4 accompanied by partial exudative detachment of the retina should receive primary treatment with laser photocoagulation to the surface of the angioma in an attempt to coagulate both the angioma and its surface neovascularization (Fig. 41-3, *A*). In cases with little exudate, laser photocoagulation can be successful if the treatment is repeated at 3-month intervals until the residual external portion of the tumor is obliterated.

Cases with pronounced exudative detachment necessitate treatment by scleral buckling and coagulation of the angioma. After exposure of the sclera in the standard pattern for scleral buckling surgery, localize the point on the sclera corresponding to the angioma. Attempt cryocoagulation using the binocular indirect ophthalmoscope. If the freeze from the cryoprobe is able to permeate the angioma, whitening will appear on the angioma's inner surface. If the subretinal exudative fluid presents too great a thermal barrier, penetrating diathermy should be risked. Puncture through the sclera directly into the tumor for large lesions (Fig. 41-3, *B*). Execute the puncture with a diathermy needle 1.5 mm in length. This length, approximately 0.5 mm longer than the thickness of the sclera, allows the needle to penetrate through the subretinal exudate into the angioma without perforating the retina. Once the needle penetrates the sclera, apply the diathermy current at a low-power setting for 1 second. After withdrawing the needle, use ophthalmoscopy to determine if the angioma has begun to whiten. If no whitening appears, repeat the puncture with an increase in power and time duration of treatment until the angioma shows the first sign of whitening, indicating that the coagulation has penetrated to the surface of the angioma and the surface neovascularization. When the first whitening is produced, terminate the current application immediately, for excessive diathermy application increases the hazard of hemorrhaging by the angioma. The sclera overlying the area for diathermy treatment must be resected so that focal full-thickness scleral necrosis is prevented. Occasionally, transscleral diathermy through a scleral dissection bed can cause whitening of the angioma without the necessity for penetration. If whitening is produced, do not penetrate the sclera. Perform diathermy treatment of the dissected scleral bed before puncture to diminish the risk of choroidal hemorrhage.

After puncture, perform scleral buckling to support the area of puncture and angioma (Fig. 41-3, *C*). This is done with a solid silicone explant mounted on an encircling silicone band.

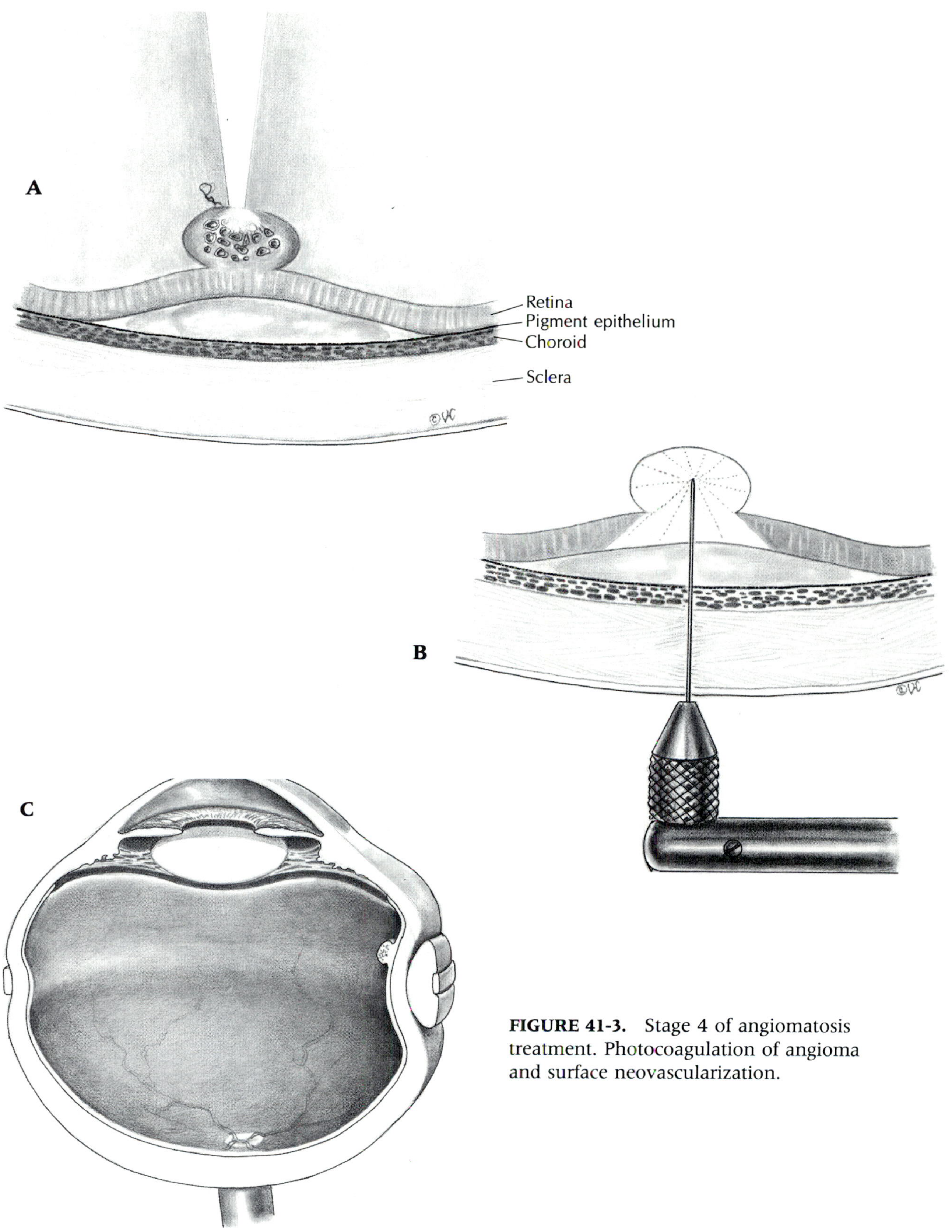

FIGURE 41-3. Stage 4 of angiomatosis treatment. Photocoagulation of angioma and surface neovascularization.

Cryosurgery

Cryosurgery using a temperature higher than −80° C can cause atrophy of the angioma if the cryocoagulation is repeated with multiple-freeze-thaw episodes. Temperature less than −80° C risks the production of excessive uveitis and exudation. Because freezing depends on heat transfer from the angioma to the site of the cryoprobe on the external scleral wall, indentation of the scleral wall toward the retina must be performed with the cryoprobe (Fig. 41-4, *A*). If whitening is achieved, three freeze-thaw cycles should be done. If the cryoprobe cannot reach close enough to the angioma to overcome thermal barrier (Fig. 41-4, *B*), drain subretinal fluid, along with an intravitreal injection to prevent hypotony (Fig. 41-4, *C*). Then perform the cryocoagulation when the sclera can be brought closer to the retina (Fig. 41-4, *D*). Scleral buckling should be done after the cryoprocedure.

Cryosurgery is preferable to transscleral diathermy because of the severe risk of hemorrhage from the diathermy.

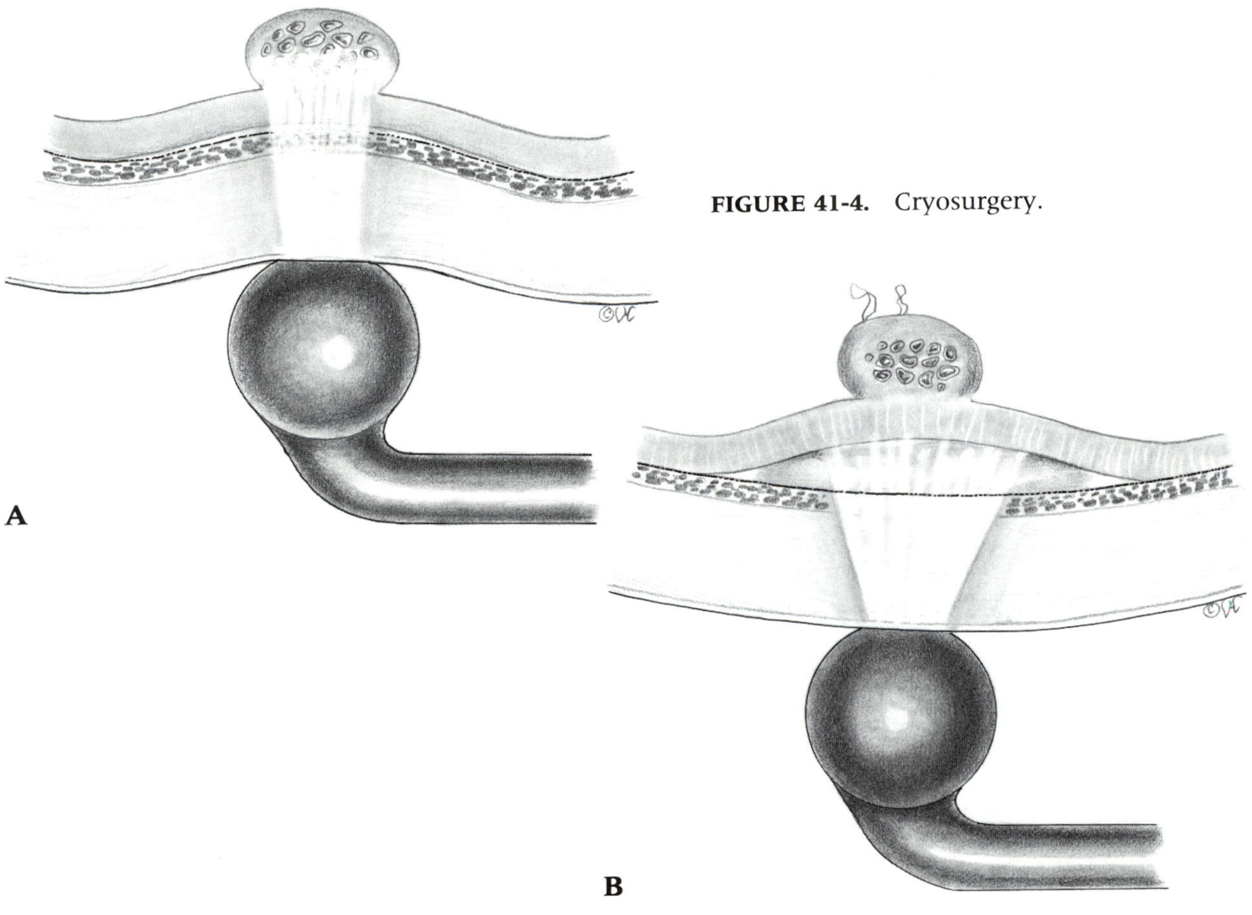

FIGURE 41-4. Cryosurgery.

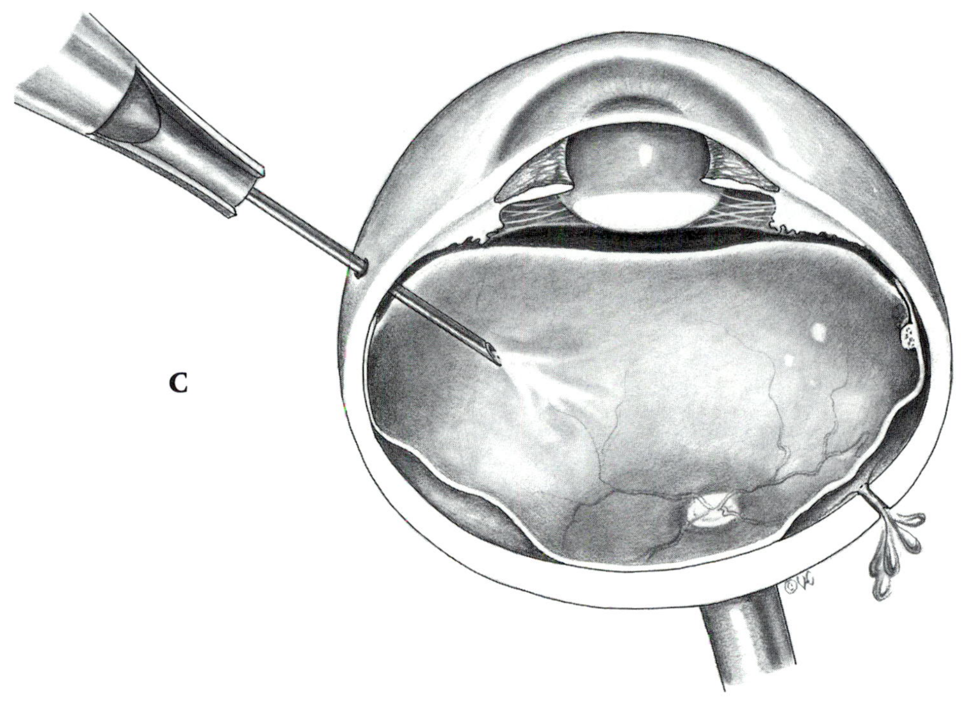

C

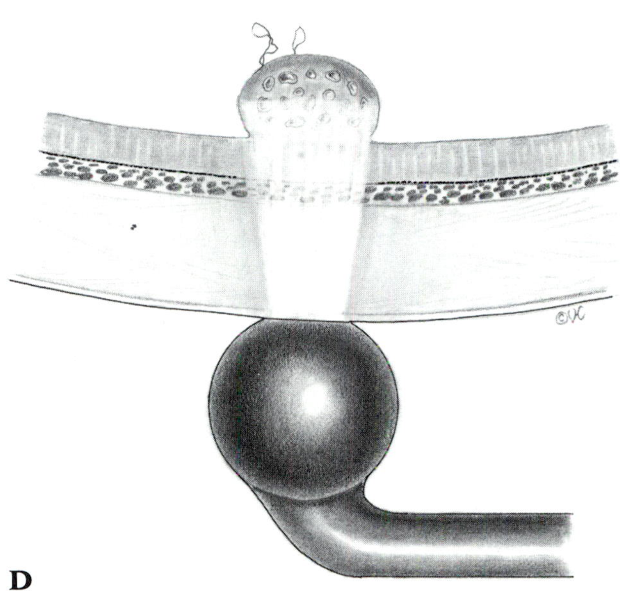

D

FOLLOW-UP STUDY

After 3 months the feeder vessels to the angioma should show some attenuation from their preoperative state. In addition, the exudation should be somewhat less. As long as the retinal condition looks improved, there is no need to repeat surgery. If exudation begins to reaccumulate or the feeder vessels continue to look highly developed, surgery should be repeated.

COMPLICATIONS

The leading complication from both transscleral cryosurgery and transscleral diathermy or penetrating diathermy is failure of the procedure to produce atrophy of the angioma. If atrophy does not occur within 3 months after the surgery, the procedure should be repeated in some form to produce coagulation of the angioma.

Cryocoagulation carries the risk of worsening the exudation. This risk is usually temporary.

The major complication of transscleral diathermy is hemorrhage from the angioma. This complication can be minimized by careful placement of the diathermy needle and use of minimum diathermy energy.

CHAPTER 42

Sickle Cell Retinopathy

Sickle cell retinopathy is the combination of primary closure of normal retinal circulation and the resultant growth of abnormal blood vessels in patients with specific hemoglobin defects. The neovascularization associated with sickle cell retinopathy is distinct from that associated with diabetes mellitus and the other ischemic retinopathies (Takayasu's disease and carotid occlusive disease). Sickle cell retinopathy produces neovascularization predominantly in the preequatorial retina in comparison to the other ischemic retinopathies, which cause neovascularization principally in the postequatorial retina. The pattern of sickle cell retinopathy is geographically discrete, with infarction of the discrete regions of the retinal capillary bed adjacent to other infarcted regions that show no abnormalities. This geographic pattern contrasts with the diffuse retinal vascular disease caused by diabetes and the ischemic retinopathies. Of the eight known groups of hemoglobinopathies—AA, SS, AS, SC, CC, AC, S-thal, and SF—it is Sc disease (sickle hemoglobin C disease) and S-thal (sickle cell thalassemia) that are the two major causes for significant clinical disorders.

ETIOLOGY

Sickle cell retinopathy results from the abnormal rheology of the erythrocytes in the affected patient groups. The erythrocytes containing an abnormal hemoglobin can adopt a crescentic, elongated sickle-shaped configuration in the presence of abnormally low oxygen tension. With sickling, the erythrocytes lose their suppleness and become abnormally rigid, and so they cannot pass through small-caliber blood vessels. The resultant blockage stops erythrocyte flow and causes ischemia, hypoxia, and eventually necrosis of the affected tissues. The secondary hypoxia exacerbates the sickling. The role of oxygen tension explains the predilection of sickling in capillary occlusion in the peripheral area of the retina and, secondarily, at the macula, where retinal capillary oxygen tensions are lowest.

The site of primary blockade appears to be the arteriole-capillary junction. This causes the proliferative and nonproliferative manifestations of sickle retinopathy: (1) salmon-patch hemorrhages resulting from intraretinal bleeding at the site of obstruction, (2) a black sunburst spot resulting from the residual pigment from hemorrhage, (3) iridescent spots resulting from the residue of intraretinal or preretinal hemorrhage, and (4) loss of macular function from acute infarction. Vitreous hemorrhage can occur secondary to preretinal hemorrhage at the site of acute infarction.

The most devastating consequence of capillary closure is proliferative retinopathy. The neovascularization is a response to retinal ischemia anterior to the point of arterial closure. The zone of peripheral retinal ischemia produces a sharp border at the junction of the normal and ischemic retina. Arteriovenous shunt vessels form across the border of necrotic capillaries and microaneurysms that develop at the posterior margin of the zone of capillary closure. Buds of neovascularization from the zone of patent vessels immediately posterior to the blocked capillaries appear first within the retina and gradually grow to the surface of the retina and eventually progress into the vitreous where they appear as a fan of vessels derived from a single stem and give rise to the "sea-fan" appearance. Eventually, vitreous fibrosis and vitreous contraction pull on the bands, leading to tractional retinal detachment, schisis, retinal holes, and vitreous hemorrhage.

NATURAL HISTORY AND CLASSIFICATION

Proliferative sickle retinopathy (PSR) progresses in a relatively orderly sequence in five stages. These phenomena occur primarily during the third and fourth decades of life, though PSR has been noted as early as the second decade. Stages 1 and 2 occur late in the second decade, with the subsequent stages occurring in the third and fourth decades, as shown in Table 42-1.

Proliferative sickle retinopathy is progressive. Lack of apparent change in a single patient can be deceptive because of the slow rate of progression: the disease may idle at one stage for as long as a decade, but progression to the next stage can then occur rapidly with SC hemoglobinopathy. Patients in the third decade usually have not progressed beyond stage 3 retinopathy, whereas patients in the fourth decade usually have reached stage 4 or 5. Pregnancy can accelerate progression.

TABLE 42-1
Stages of Proliferative Sickle Retinopathy

Stage 1	Occlusion of arterioles in the peripheral retina
Stage 2	Anastomoses between the arterioles and venules bypass occlusions
Stage 3A	Neovascularization within and on the surface of the retina
Stage 3B	Elevation of neovascularization to form "sea fans"
Stage 4	Vitreous hemorrhage
Stage 5A	Rhegmatogenous retinal detachment
Stage 5B	Traction retinal detachment

From Sigelman J: Sickle cell retinopathy. In Sigelman J: Retinal diseases, Boston, 1984, Little, Brown & Co.

INDICATIONS FOR PHOTOCOAGULATION

All cases of stages 3, 4, and 5 sickle retinopathy should be treated. Treatment of stages 1 and 2 could retard progression to stage 3, but the treatment of early stages remains experimental; the slow progression of untreated retinopathy from stages 1 and 2 to stage 3 makes it difficult to evaluate the efficacy of treatment.

Laser Treatment of Stage 2

Photocoagulation at this stage aims to destroy the entirety of the ischemic peripheral retina anterior to the line of demarcation that separates the perfused from the nonperfused retina. Argon laser photocoagulation can be used with a 200 μm spot size and duration of 0.5 second with a gradual increase of a power level from an initial setting of 100 milliwatts until each burn produces whitening of the retina. Extend the burns contiguously around the ischemic periphery. Scleral indentation is unnecessary because the treatment can terminate peripherally at approximately 1.5 mm from the ora serrata. Krypton red laser could also be used but would necessitate anesthesia injection.

Photocoagulation of Stage 3

Laser treatment of the neovascular stage aims to coagulate the neovascularization in order to prevent its further growth. At stage 3A, with neovascularization within or on the surface of the retina, the laser treatment should be aimed directly at the flat neovascularization. Argon green laser photocoagulation should be used with a 200 or 500 μm spot size for a 0.5-second duration with a gradual increase in power from an initial setting of 100 millimeters until each burn produces an almost dense white reaction. During the photocoagulation, the neovascularization becomes more pronounced as its red color is highlighted by the laser burns. The photocoagulation should be aimed directly at the neovascularization and the immediately surrounding retina (Fig. 42-1, *A*).

Edema will obscure the laser reaction until, gradually, approximately 3 to 4 weeks after treatment, pigment will begin to accumulate at the site of the laser coagulation (Fig. 42-1, *B*). Fluorescein angioscopy at this time will demonstrate whether neovascularization has been sealed. If fluorescein leakage persists, the laser treatment should be repeated to the same zone.

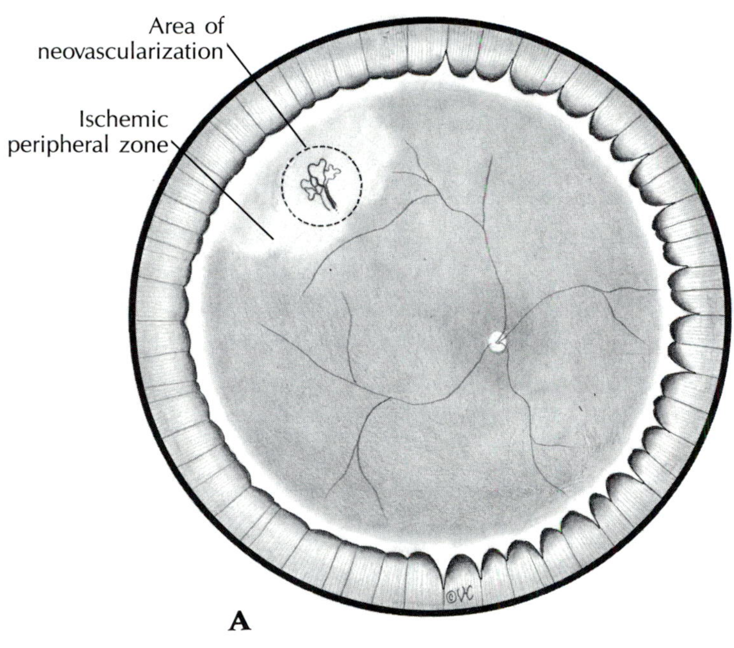

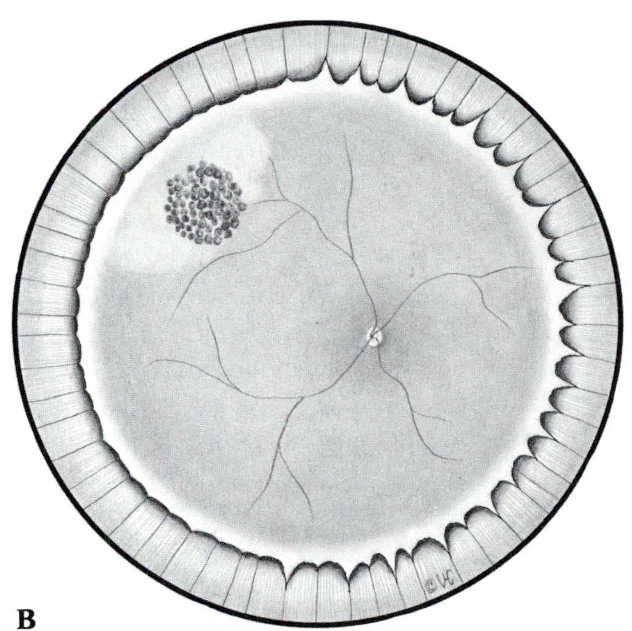

FIGURE 42-1. Photocoagulation of stage 3.

Laser Photocoagulation of Elevated Neovascularization or "Sea Fans"

Photocoagulation of stage 3B presents the difficulty of the elevation of the sea fans away from the retina by their attachment to the posterior hyaloid (Fig. 42-2, *A*). The separation of the sea fan from the pigment epithelium prevents transfer of the photocoagulation energy from the pigment epithelium to the fans. Direct laser photocoagulation to the sea fan is not likely to cauterize the sea fan because of poor energy absorption by the blood vessels. Additionally, photocoagulation directly to an elevated sea fan can create vitreous hemorrhage by producing contraction of the vitreous with secondarily increased traction on the sea fans.

Instead of direct photocoagulation to the sea fan, photocoagulation to the feeding vessels is a safer and more effective means of producing permanent closure of the sea fan.

Begin by photocoagulating the feeder artery using argon green laser with a spot size of 100 or 200 μm and duration of 0.5 second with a power setting gradually elevated from 100 milliwatts until a white reaction results. Place photocoagulations along the feeder artery where it is flat against the pigment epithelium rather than where the artery is elevated toward the sea fan (Fig. 42-2, *B*). Arterial closure should be attempted before venous closure to eliminate blood flow and diminish the risk of hemorrhage. Each photocoagulation of the feeding artery must be done gradually to produce permanent closure without hemorrhage. Initially, aim the laser photocoagulation so that it straddles the artery in order to maximize the energy absorption at the site of the artery (Fig. 42-4, *C*). Continue the photocoagulation under direct observation until the artery goes into spasm as seen against the white background of the initial laser reaction (Fig. 42-2, *D*). Stop the photocoagulation and continue to observe the artery at the laser. Initially, the artery will appear sealed or severely narrowed (Fig. 42-4, *E*). After 1 to 3 minutes, the artery most likely will begin to reopen at the site of photocoagulation (Fig. 42-2, *F*). Repeat the photocoagulation immediately to that site (Fig. 42-2, *G*). Continue the photocoagulation until no strand of artery remains within the whitened area (Fig. 42-2, *H*). Continue with this procedure throughout approximately 800 to 1000 μm length of the artery.

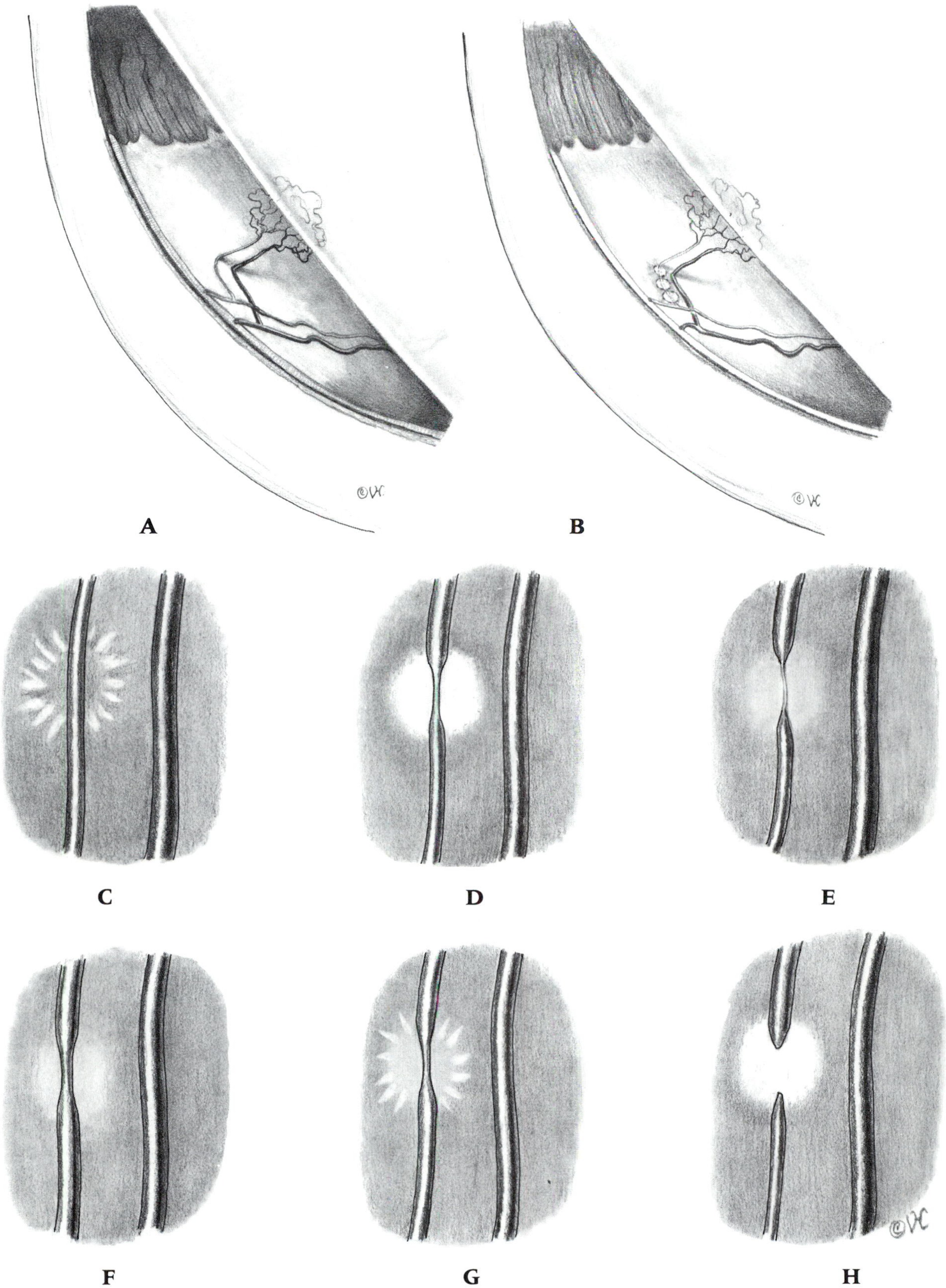

FIGURE 42-2. Laser photocoagulation of elevated neovascularization or sea fans.

Continued.

If much of the artery is elevated toward the sea fan (Fig. 42-2, *I*), laser photocoagulation should not be aimed at the elevated artery or at the sea fan. An alternative means of treatment is photocoagulation of the sea fan and the artery immediately adjacent to the sea fan during indentation of the sclera (Fig. 42-2, *J*). Using the Eisner indentation funnel or any similar funnel, move the indenter until the sea fan and the immediately adjacent artery are in touch with the pigment epithelium. Then begin photocoagulation of the feeding artery adjacent to the sea fan to produce arterial closure. If the sea fan can be brought against the pigment epithelium, continue the photocoagulation to include the sea fan (Fig. 42-2, *K*). Then continue with photocoagulation along the draining vein in the area of indentation using the same technique as that used for closure of the artery (Fig. 42-2, *L*). Closure of the sea fan will be simpler than closure of either the artery or vein during the treatment session. Fewer repeat photocoagulations will be necessary to produce whitening of the sea fan if it can be juxtaposed to the pigment epithelium.

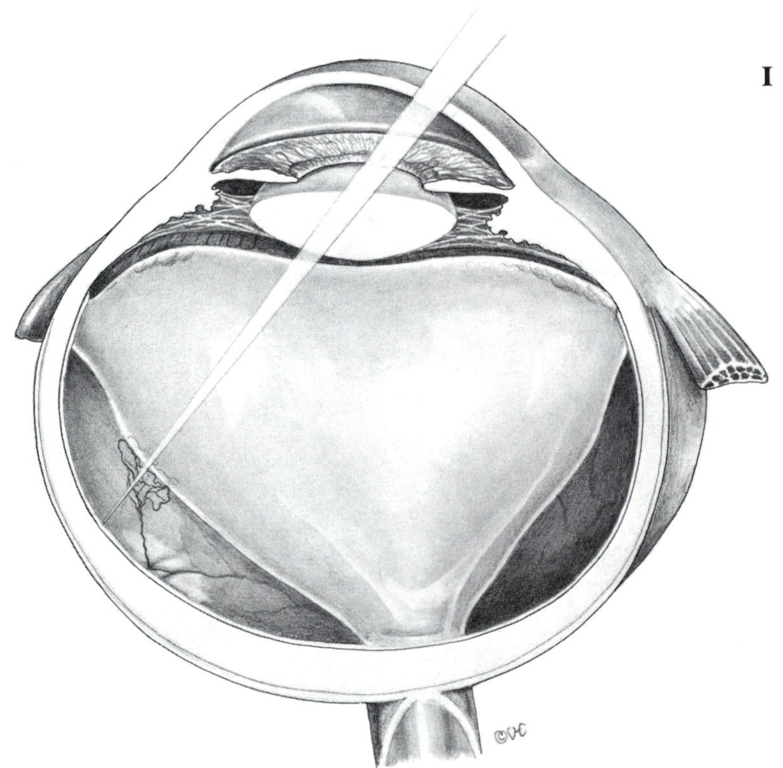

FIGURE 42-2, cont'd

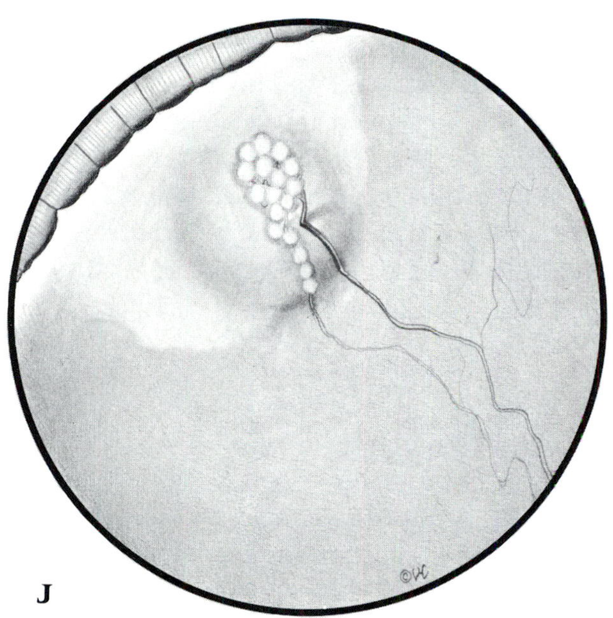

J

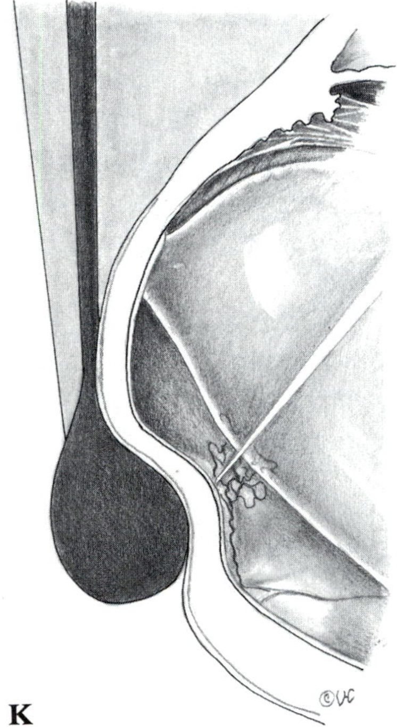

K

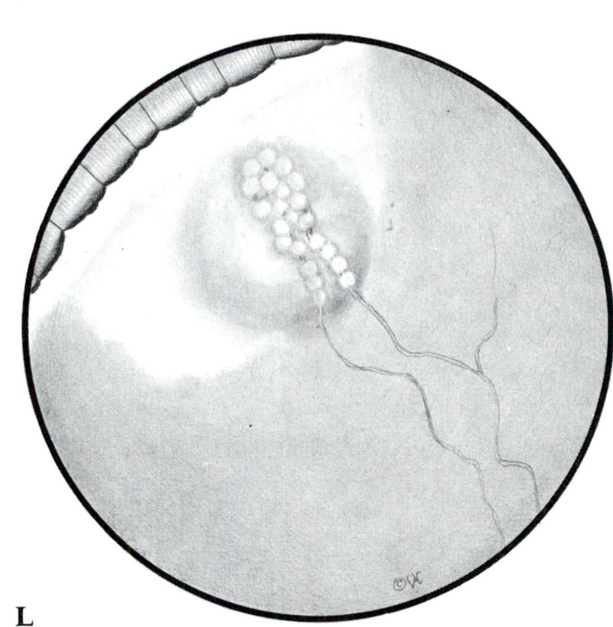

L

Photocoagulation of elevated complexes of sea fans

The elevated complex of sea fans presents the difficulty of multiple feeding and draining systems (Fig. 42-3, *A*). Failure to close any of the family of feeding vessels results in persistence of the sea fan.

Begin photocoagulation along the feeder arteries in the same manner as the treatment of a single elevated sea fan (Fig. 42-3, *B*). After photocoagulating the feeding arterioles, perform the similar photocoagulation on all the sets of draining venules with care that the photocoagulation is on the venules in the area of retina attached to the pigment epithelium rather than in the elevated retina (Fig. 42-3, *C*), unless the indentation method is used to permit photocoagulation of the elevated vessels and sea fan.

FOLLOW-UP STUDY

Inspection of the photocoagulation zone 4 to 6 weeks after the laser treatment should show pigmentation and closure of the feeder vessels. Pigment can obscure the treated vascular segments even if they remain patent. Change of the color of the sea fan from pink to an avascular white is a significant sign of closure. Fluorescein angioscopy is the most accurate means of determining whether sea-fan perfusion persists. If there is continued circulation, treatment should be repeated to the patent feeding vessels with additional consideration given to indentation technique for direct treatment of the sea fans.

COMPLICATIONS

Vitreous hemorrhage occurs in approximately 14% of cases and is the most significant complication. If hemorrhage occurs during treatment, increase both the size and the power of the laser spot, aim it at the site of hemorrhage and apply continuous photocoagulation until a white scar appears in the hemorrhagic material and the hemorrhage can be observed to have ceased. Most postoperative hemorrhages do not require repeat photocoagulation.

Dense vitreous hemorrhage, traction retinal detachment or retinoschisis, or rhegmatogenous retinal detachment either before or after laser photocoagulation indicates the need for scleral buckling surgery almost always combined with vitrectomy to retrieve the traction caused by the adhesions of the posterior hyaloid to the elevated sea fans.

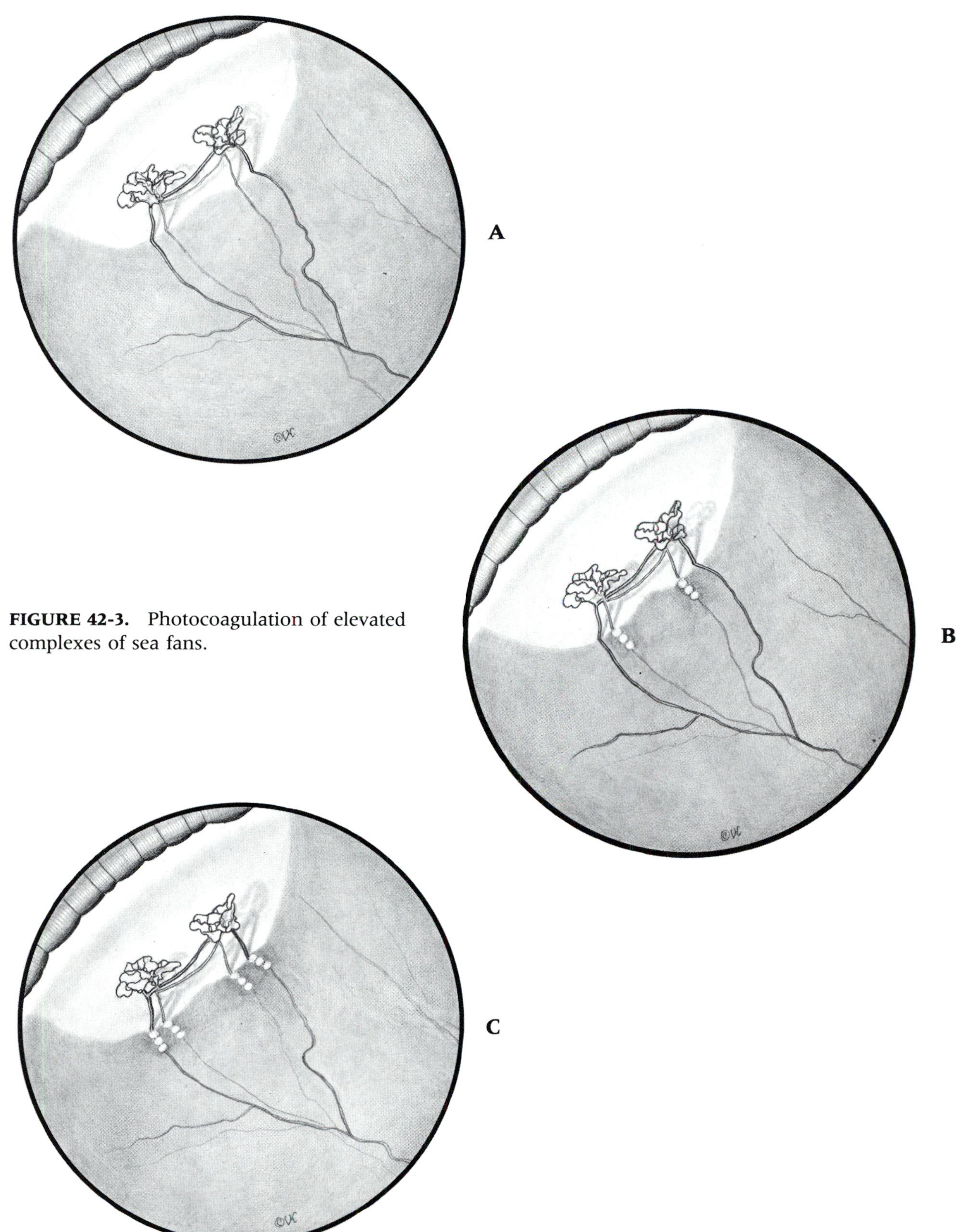

FIGURE 42-3. Photocoagulation of elevated complexes of sea fans.

Peripheral Scatter Photocoagulation

Scatter treatment to the ischemic retinal periphery has been shown to be effective in almost all cases of stage 3B retinopathy; almost none of 40 treated eyes have progressed to a more advanced stage after treatment. The scatter treatment must include the entire zone of ischemic peripheral retina. The treatment surrounds but does not directly treat the sea fan.

Before treatment, identify the ischemic retinal zone, using either fluorescein angiography, angioscopy, or biomicroscopy to observe the change from normal color retina to a yellowish atrophic zone (Fig. 42-4, *A*). The sea fans are located usually at the margin between the perfused and nonperfused retina.

Treat with argon green laser using 200 to 500 μm burns with a spot duration of 0.1 to 0.5 second and power ranging from 100 to 400 milliwatts until a gray but not dense white reaction results. Space the burns approximately one burn width apart. In each of three treatment sessions, place approximately 300 to 400 burns so that there is a total of approximately 1000 burns at the completion of all the treatment sessions. Extend the photocoagulations to surround neovascular areas that lie posterior to the usually geometric line of demarcation (Fig. 42-4, *B*).

Krypton red laser can also be used for peripheral scatter technique. It has the advantage of producing less vitreous heating than argon green does. The krypton treatment resembles that of argon except that krypton requires a sub-Tenon's anesthesia injection because of the pain from the choroidal involvement from the krypton coagulation. Use krypton treatments of 200 or 500 μm for a duration of 0.2 to 0.5 second with power ranging from 150 to 500 milliwatts to produce a yellow-white but not dense white burn.

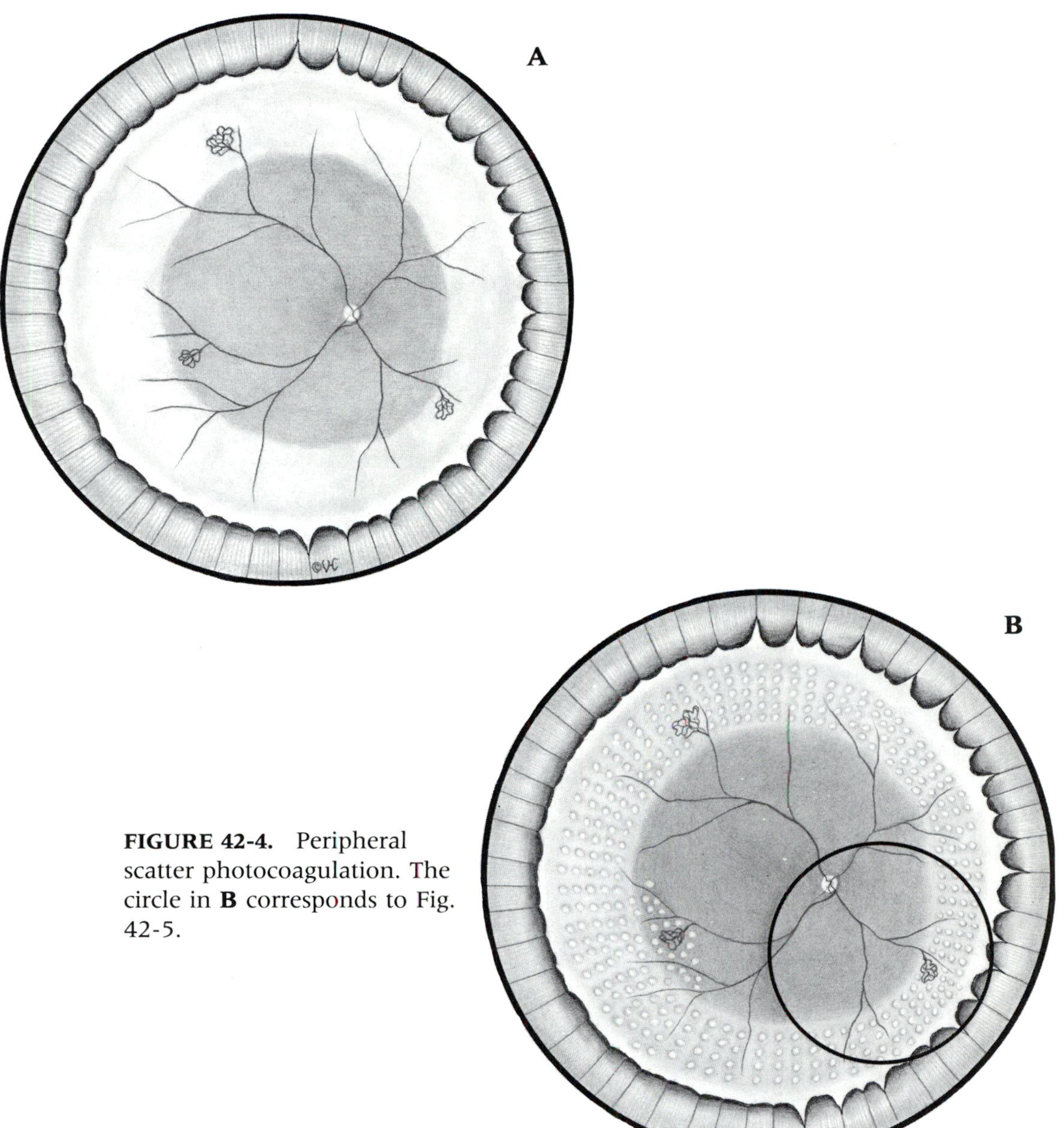

FIGURE 42-4. Peripheral scatter photocoagulation. The circle in **B** corresponds to Fig. 42-5.

FOLLOW-UP STUDY

By approximately 6 weeks after photocoagulation the burns will show pigment and the sea fans should show shrinkage. The sea fans will not disappear because of residual glial and vascular tissue, which will form a scar. Fluorescein angioscopy or angiography will show whether the sea fan is nonperfused (Fig. 42-5). Continued perfusion of the sea fan warrants either a repeat of the peripheral photocoagulation or direct photocoagulation of the feeder vessels and perhaps of the sea fan itself.

Treatment of Stage 5 (Retinal Detachment)

Retinal detachments occurring in sickle cell retinopathy are predominantly rhegmatogenous and result from small tears at the base of the fibrovascular growth to the sea fans. These detachments show a significant tractional component. Scleral buckling surgery carries hazards in these patients because of the risk of anterior-segment necrosis, which occurs in approximately 71% of patients with SC disease but only 3% of patients with other hemoglobinopathies showing this complication. Transfusion therapy and hyperbaric environment for surgery diminish this risk along with other precautions against constriction of the ocular circulation. Vitrectomy now provides the backbone for retinal detachment surgery in the sickling group because of its ability to eliminate the tractional component.

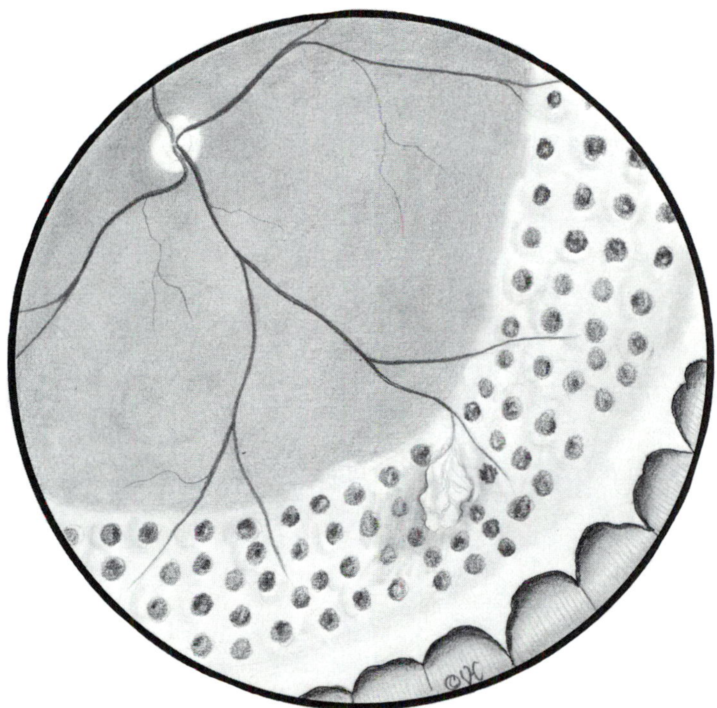

FIGURE 42-5. Follow-up observation.

CHAPTER 43

Proliferative Diabetic Retinopathy

Proliferative diabetic retinopathy refers to the growth of neovascularization from the retina or optic disc in response to diminished perfusion and increased ischemia in the diabetic retina. Proliferative retinopathy is not unique to diabetes and can complicate all other forms of retinopathy that involve ischemia: branch retinal vein occlusion, central retinal vein occlusion, pulseless disease, carotid artery insufficiency, and the hemoglobinopathies. The neovascular proliferation in diabetic retinopathy, however, is the most prevalent and devastating form of neovascularization and is potentially amenable to treatment. The photocoagulation treatment of proliferative diabetic retinopathy is one of the most dramatic recent advances in retinal therapy. Panretinal photocoagulation has converted a disease prognosis of almost certain severe visual loss or even blindness to one of preservation of useful vision.

The reason for separating proliferative changes from the other retinal complications of diabetes and the other ischemic retinopathies is that proliferative retinopathy has a behavior pattern that is common to all the diseases in which it occurs and is distinct from the exudative circinate retinopathy and macular edema that can also occur in retinal disease and can involve breakdown of the blood-retinal barrier.

PATHOGENESIS

The earliest observable change in diabetic retinopathy is the loss of intramural pericytes in the retinal capillaries. As the pericytes disappear, the normal one-to-one ratio of pericytes to endothelial cells diminishes and the capillary wall loses its structural integrity. Thin outpouchings are the first visible sign of diabetic retinopathy, which is microaneurysms that are distributed randomly throughout the arteriolar and venular sides of the capillary network. Eventually the walls of the microaneurysms degenerate by thickening and ultimately disappearance of the endothelial cells. The progressive closure of the capillary bed secondary to the endothelial cell degeneration leads to retinal ischemia and hypoxia in the areas of nonperfusion. *Ischemic foci* are areas of capillary nonperfusion surrounded by shunt vessels and microaneurysms. The clinical hallmarks of the development of ischemic foci are cotton-wool spots and intraretinal hemorrhages. The rapid development of cotton-wool spots and hemorrhages indicates the onset of extensive capillary closure and indicates that the development of neovascularization will soon follow.

Exudative retinopathy differs from proliferative retinopathy because it develops from the leakage of the microaneurysms and capillaries at the margins of the ischemic foci and is not a direct response to ischemia. Exudative retinopathy is related to proliferative retinopathy only to a variable degree. In type I diabetics, neovascularization is the predominant response to capillary disease and nonperfusion, whereas exudation is the predominant response in type II diabetics.

NATURAL HISTORY

Neovascularization develops after a minimum of approximately 15 years of diabetes. At its earliest stages, the neovascularization is intraretinal. Eventually the neovascularization perforates through the internal limiting membrane to proliferate along the retina's anterior surface with adherence of the proliferative vessels to the posterior hyaloid where they first undergo a rapid cycle of growth. The vessels may regress spontaneously, or they may continue to proliferate. Once the vessels appear on the posterior hyaloid, the potential tractional relationship between the hyaloid and the retina persists regardless of whether there is further neovascularization. When the vitreous undergoes a partial or complete detachment, the vessels are dragged forward to produce the two dreaded complications of proliferative retinopathy: retinal detachment and vitreous hemorrhage. Initially, the tractional force can produce retinoschisis. The retina may become covered on its surface by glial and fibrous proliferation in response to the neovascularization. The slower than normal progression of the separation of the vitreous in diabetics can gradually produce tractional separations at the macula or elsewhere. Spontaneous regression of the neovascularization with clearing of vitreous hemorrhage after completion of the posterior vitreous detachment occurs in only approximately 15% of cases. Photocoagulation treatment should not be given to those few cases that undergo spontaneous resolution.

Neovascularization can present as either rapidly growing or slowly growing. The florid type of retinopathy can develop so rapidly that change occurs within weeks. This usually occurs in eyes with extensive capillary closure.

In contrast to the rapid type, slow proliferative retinopathy is associated with less conspicuous retinal lesions and a smaller percentage of retinal area showing ischemia. Disc neovascularization occurs predominantly in eyes with extensive capillary closure, whereas disc neovascularization is rare in eyes with minimal capillary closure.

PROLIFERATION

Proliferation evolves through three distinct stages with a span of approximately 5 years between the early and the advanced stage. If the optic disc is involved, fine vessels appear from the capillary network on its surface. These vessels soon establish connections with larger veins. Retinal neovascularization grows more slowly, requiring 1 to 4 years before it progresses to the next stage.

The second stage of proliferation is characterized by rapid growth of the neovascularization of the connective tissue surrounding it. During the second stage, hemorrhagic activity increases dramatically, and hemorrhage is likely to occur during the first 2 years of this period. Rubeosis iridis and neovascular glaucoma are frequent concomitants to this rapid progression stage.

Proliferative retinopathy enters its third stage on an average of 1.6 years after the onset of the rapid growth stage. In the third stage the neovascularization shows regression and atrophy with contraction of the connective tissue elements surrounding it. Visual deterioration occurs from tractional retinal detachment or mechanical obstruction of the fundus by condensation of connective tissue rather than from hemorrhage.

The urgency of treatment of proliferative retinopathy results from the finding that 60% of patients experience progression of the retinopathy with considerable visual impairment over 5 years, whereas only 30% remain stable and 10% regress. The visual consequences of retinopathy are severe. Fifty percent of patients develop vision reduction to the level of 20/200 or less within 5 years of onset; 100% of patients with disc neovascularization are blind in at least one eye within 10 years; 75% of patients with peripheral neovascularization are blind in at least one eye within 10 years. Both juvenile and adult onset diabetes have a 50% risk, approximately, of blindness in an eye with proliferative retinopathy within 5 years of the onset of neovascularization. Although diabetic maculopathy causes a gradual loss of acuity over a period of months to years, proliferative retinopathy can cause a patient's visual acuity to change from 20/20 to 20/400 in minutes.

INDICATIONS FOR PHOTOCOAGULATION

The visual loss from vitreous hemorrhage secondary to neovascularization is so severe and relatively irreversible that prophylactic photocoagulation is the best treatment. Effective photocoagulation makes it possible for the diabetic patient to retain some vision for the 6-year average life expectancy after the onset of neovascularization.

The most significant prospective study of photocoagulation shows that the risk of severe vision loss (visual acuity less than 20/200) without photocoagulation far exceeds the risk of visual loss from argon laser panretinal photocoagulation in eyes with specific high-risk characteristics, including the following:

1. Presence of neovascularization equaling or exceeding one-fourth to one-third disc area in extent at the disc regardless of the presence or absence of vitreous hemorrhage or preretinal hemorrhage
2. Presence of vitreous hemorrhage or preretinal hemorrhage with less extensive new vessels and neovascularization at the disc less than one-fourth disc area
3. Neovascularization elsewhere on the retina (NVE) larger than one-half disc diameter.

Severe visual loss in eyes that meet these criteria is 26% during a 24-month observation period. The risk is reduced to 11% by panretinal photoablation. These data indicate that panretinal photoablation should be performed in eyes with these risks as soon as the diagnosis is made.

In eyes with proliferative retinopathy without the high-risk characteristics, photoablation produces more than a 50% reduction (from 7% to 3%) in the rate of severe visual acuity loss. Photocoagulation treatment of eyes in this low-risk group is attractive because it can prevent eyes from progressing to the high-risk group, which is not uniformly controllable in 12% of cases wherein the panretinal photoablation fails. Treatment of low-risk cases must be undertaken with care because the treatment can reduce visual acuity by as much as two lines and produce constriction of visual field along with nyctalopia.

Photocoagulation for rapid capillary closure is an option that should be considered for patients who are unreliable for follow-up study. The possible progression from rapid capillary closure to high-risk neovascularization can be so fast that hemorrhage can intervene and preclude photocoagulation if the patient is not seen at intervals of 3 months or less.

Laser Technique

The laser technique for proliferative retinopathy of the disc and retina is *panretinal photoablation*. The aim of the photoablation is to destroy enough of the ischemic retina to bring about regression of neovascularization.

Photocoagulation should be used in a way to maximize the chance of neovascular regression and minimize the risks of hemorrhage and macular dysfunction. Although argon green, dye yellow, and krypton red wavelengths are efficacious, krypton red has the theoretical advantage of producing less vitreous heating than what would result from argon green. Yellow is absorbed by blood and is contraindicated in the presence of vitreous hemorrhage. Vitreous heating could result in hemorrhage because contraction of the vitreous can exert tractional force on the attached neovascular fronds causing them to rupture and bleed (Fig. 43-1, *A*). The risk of hemorrhage is also diminished when the photocoagulation is aimed at the retina and not at the neovascularization, which is elevated from the retina and can absorb only little of the photocoagulation energy.

Sub-Tenon's anesthesia should be considered for use with the argon green wavelength and should always be used with the krypton red wavelength to prevent pain. Freedom from pain will permit the placement of a large number of sufficiently intense burns to bring the neovascularization under control within three or four treatment sessions.

With krypton red, use a 200 or 500 μm spot size for 0.5 second to produce a medium yellow-white reaction rather than an intense white reaction. The intensity of the center of the coagulation spot determines the degree of retinal destruction. Inadequate intensity will fail to produce whitening, whereas excess intensity will spread the whitening to the margins of the burn. The ideal treatment spot leaves a rim of moderately treated tissue surrounding a central core of intense treatment (Fig. 43-1, *B*).

A

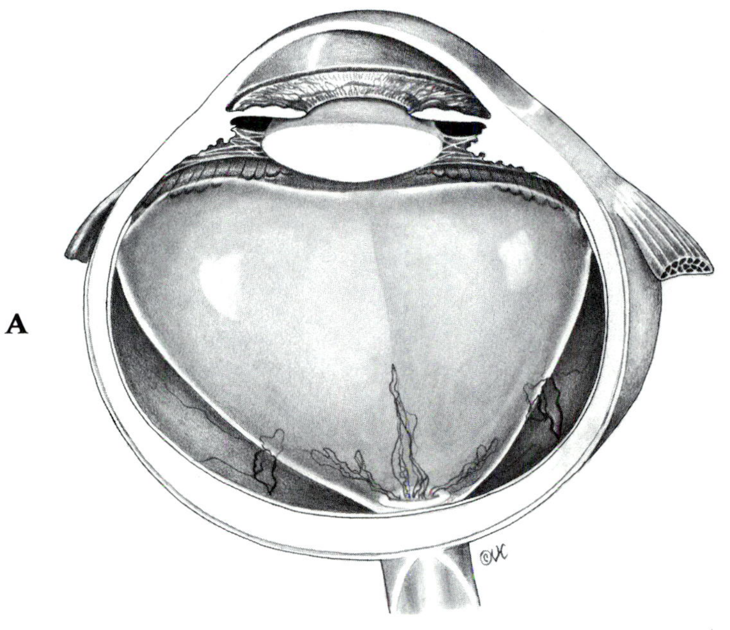

B

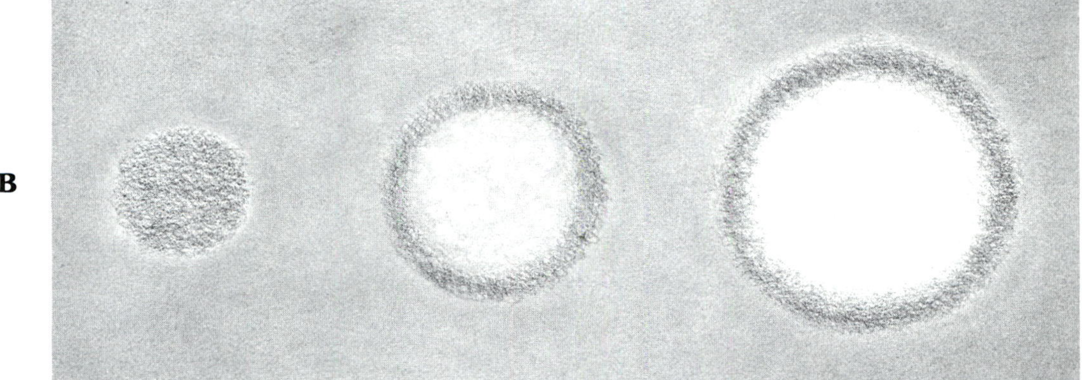

FIGURE 43-1. Panretinal photoablation.

Continued.

Argon green (the 200 or 500 μm spot) coagulation should be used for 0.5 second at a power setting to produce an almost white reaction.

With both types of coagulation, not only avoid treatment directly to elevated fronds of neovascularization, but also avoid areas of tractional retinoschisis, which can surround the elevated neovascular fronds.

The laser coagulations can be placed either through a Rodenstock lens, which provides an excellent view of most of the fundus except for the far periphery, or the Goldmann three-mirror lens. It is especially good for the far retinal periphery but is difficult to use for the midperiphery.

The photocoagulation sessions should be divided by approximately 2 to 5 weeks to permit resolution of inflammation after the coagulation. A systematic approach to treatment can include the placement of laser coagulation to the inferior retina during the primary treatment. This has the advantage of having already protected the inferior retina should vitreous hemorrhage occur and subsequently settle inferiorly, blocking laser access of the inferior retina. In the second and third sessions the superior retina can be completed (Fig. 43-1, *C*). An alternative plan divides the fundus into four sectors, with the primary sector in the nasal retina where it is safest for the operator to experiment with the retinal reactions to the laser burns (Fig. 43-1, *D*). The advantage of the third plan (Fig. 43-1, *E*) is that the primary treatment surrounds the posterior pole. This plan diminishes the risk for the beginning operator to accidentally photocoagulate into the macula while using the three-mirror lens. The subsequent three coagulation sessions complete the treatment to the periphery.

Regardless of the method chosen, the goal is to completely coagulate the fundus with burns that are slightly separated from each other. The separation maintains some degree of peripheral retinal vision and diminishes nyctalopia. The burns toward the posterior pole should be made smaller than the burns in the periphery (Fig. 43-1, *F*).

For focal photocoagulation of the neovascularization, the photocoagulation technique is the same as that for panretinal photocoagulation but should be aimed only at the specific area of the ischemic retina that stimulates the neovascular growth. The retinal area requiring treatment usually lies immediately peripherally to the neovascularization. Photocoagulation should treat the entire region of ischemic retina but should avoid coagulation of the adjacent elevated neovascularization where treatment is unnecessary and can cause vitreous hemorrhage.

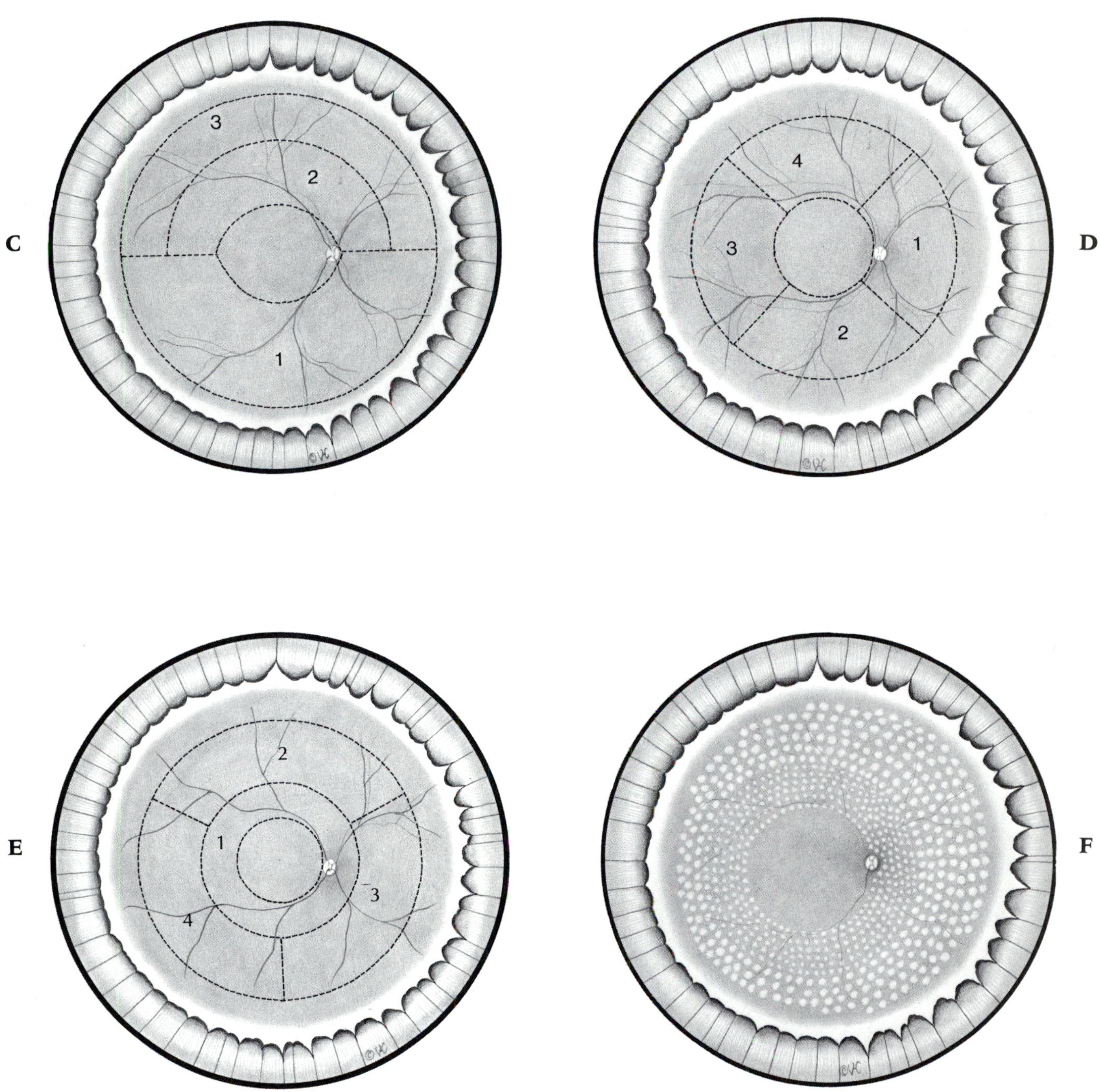

FIGURE 43-1, cont'd

FOLLOW-UP STUDY

Successful panretinal or focal treatment should produce a regression of neovascularization within 1 month after photocoagulation. The fronds of neovascularization should appear attenuated, and the previously dilated retinal vein should appear more normal in caliber. Pigmented scars will appear at each photocoagulation spot. If neovascularization does not involute, at least partially, by at least 4 weeks after completion of treatment, photocoagulation should be repeated with an energy input high enough to produce retinal whitening at each photocoagulation spot. The aim of the repeated treatment is destruction of the full retinal thickness at each treatment site rather than the partial retinal thickness destruction that was used in the initial treatment to spare nerve fiber layer function. Regression of neovascularization can be subtle; that is, the neovascularization may persist because of ghost vessels and glial tissue contraction. With successful treatment, the neovascularization should become pale and finer in caliber than it was before treatment (Fig. 43-2).

COMPLICATIONS

Failure to involute the neovascularization is the leading complication. Vitreous hemorrhage can result from rupture of the vessels and necessitates rephotocoagulation when the hemorrhage clears. Krypton red wavelength is necessary in the presence of residual hemorrhage. Should the hemorrhage not clear after 6 months, vitrectomy is warranted.

Choroidal neovascularization is a rare complication of photocoagulation. The avoidance of strong photocoagulation burns diminishes the risk of this complication.

Constriction of visual field, nyctalopia, macular edema, and macular striae are the other complications of panretinal photocoagulation.

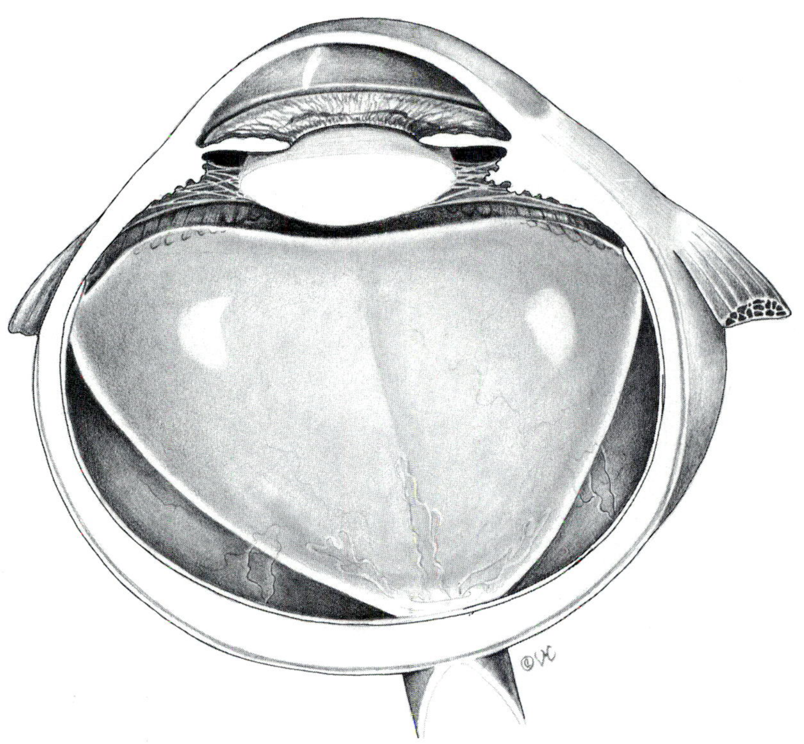

FIGURE 43-2. Successful treatment. Compare with Fig. 43-1, **A**.

PART SEVEN

OPHTHALMIC PLASTIC SURGERY

Richard R. Tenzel

CHAPTER 44

General Comments

The following chapters on oculoplastic surgery outline my preferred technique for each deformity, under the realization that there are other operations that may correct these abnormalities.

The preferred anesthetic is a 50-50 mixture of 2% lidocaine (Xylocaine) and 0.75% bupivacaine (Marcaine) both with epinephrine. One part of this mixture is combined with nine parts of a balanced saline solution and given as a preliminary injection. After 2 minutes, a full-strength anesthetic mixture is injected. A total volume of anesthetic should be kept at a minimum so as not to distort the anatomy of the lids.

Hemostasis is accomplished with wet-field cautery with use of a tip that does not completely close.

Specifics of patient evaluation and preparation, as well as pertinent surgical anatomy, are discussed as appropriate to each procedure.

Many techniques of anatomic dissection for lid repair are used in multiple procedures. You will be referred back to these descriptions and drawings in the context of lid surgical procedures. Two of these are medial and lateral canthal tendon fixation. They may be used in cosmetic blepharoplasty with lower lid laxity, ectropion, or entropion. Primary closure of the lid margin is used with lacerations, small lid defects, and semicircle flaps.

SURGICAL ANATOMY

The anatomy can be conveniently broken down into the upper lid and the lower lid. Study the structures in Figs. 44-1 and 44-2.

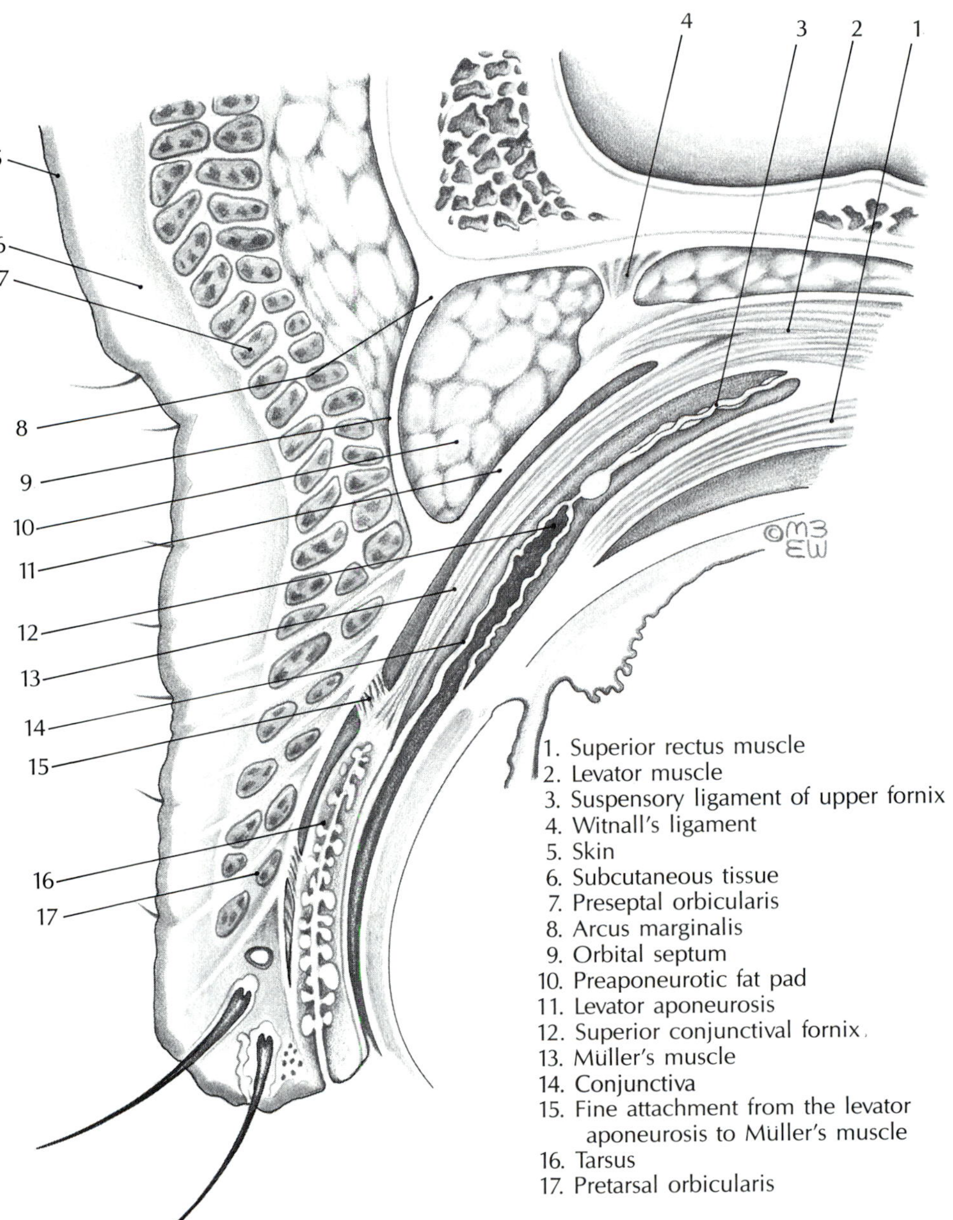

FIGURE 44-1. Anatomy of upper lid.

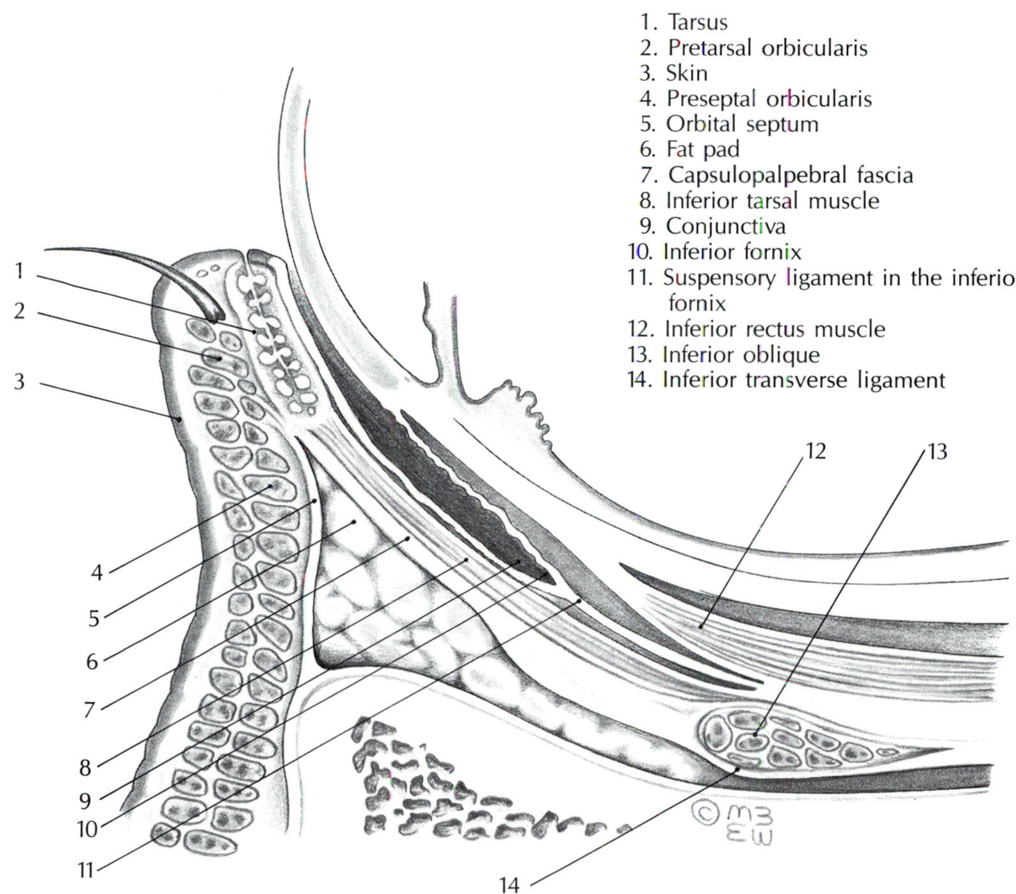

FIGURE 44-2. Anatomy of lower lid.

STANDARD TECHNIQUES FOR OPHTHALMIC PLASTIC PROCEDURES

Lateral canthal tendon fixation

A 2 mm lateral canthotomy is performed (Fig. 44-3, *A*). A full-thickness cut of the lower lid is made in the canthotomy (Fig. 44-3, *B*). The lid is overlapped (Fig. 44-3, *C*) and the redundant lid is excised (Fig. 44-3, *D*). Three 7-0 Vicryl sutures are placed from the lateral cut edge of the tarsus to the medial cut edge of the lateral tendon. This tendon is immediately anterior to the conjunctiva (Fig. 44-3, *E*). The muscle layer is closed with buried sutures of 7-0 Vicryl (Fig. 44-3, *F*). If this is just a lateral shortening, the skin is closed with interrupted or continuous sutures (Fig. 44-3, *G*). When a skin or skin muscle flap has been created before the lateral shortening, the lid margin can be left without sutures.

Fig. 44-3, *H,* shows the preoperative appearance of a patient who had had a lower lid blepharoplasty where the surgeon had not recognized the lateral canthal laxity. Fig. 44-3, *I,* shows the postoperative appearance on repair of the right eye in an attempt to match the left eye.

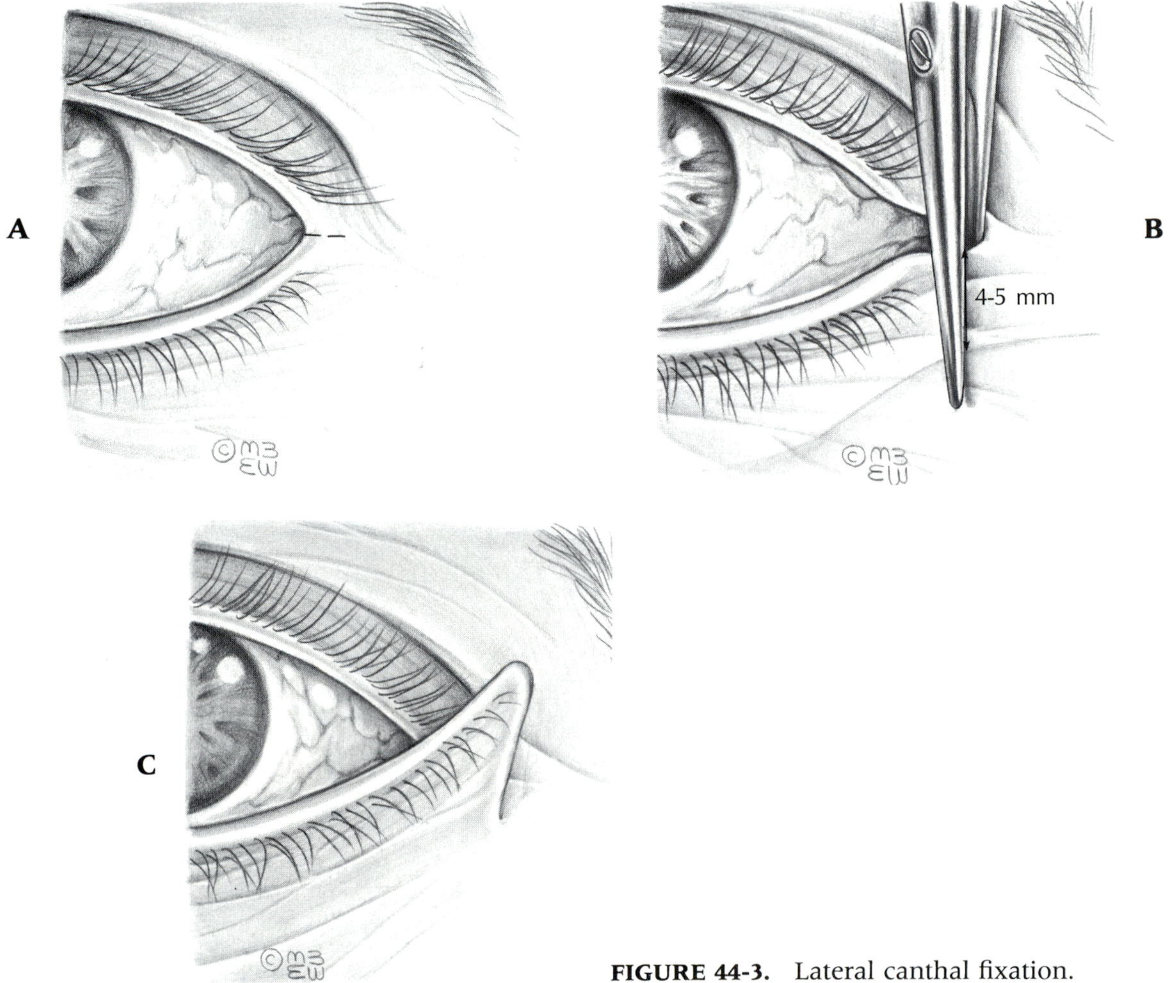

FIGURE 44-3. Lateral canthal fixation.

D

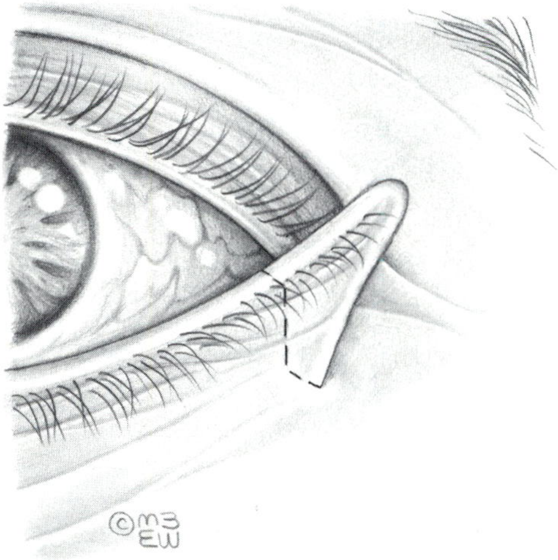

E

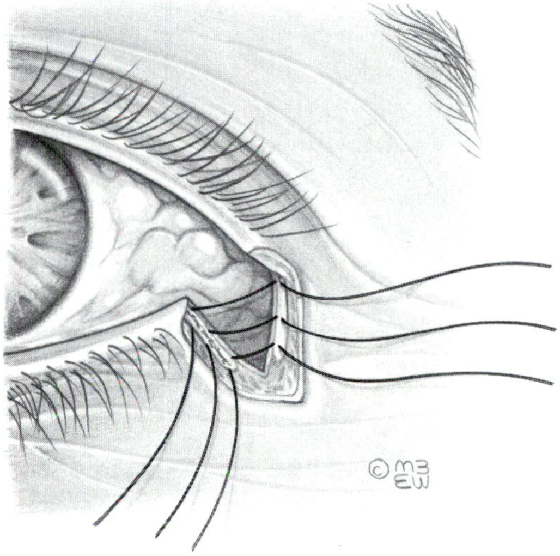

F

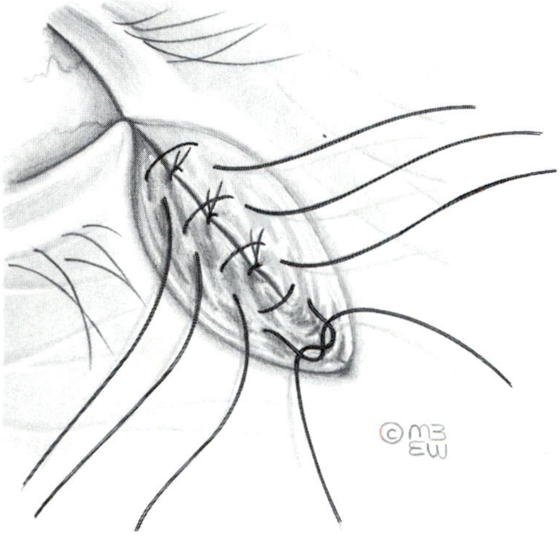

G

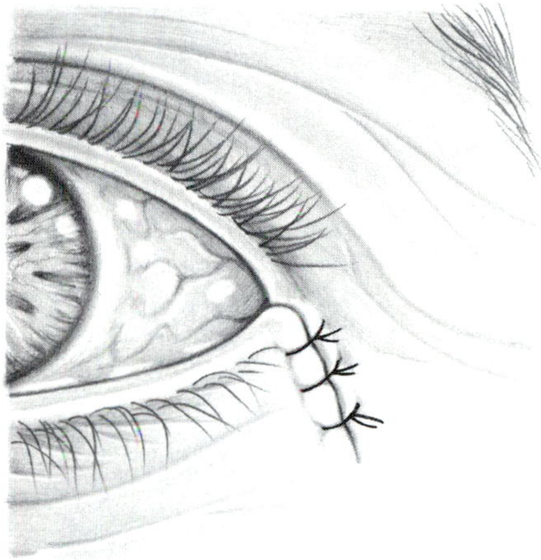

H

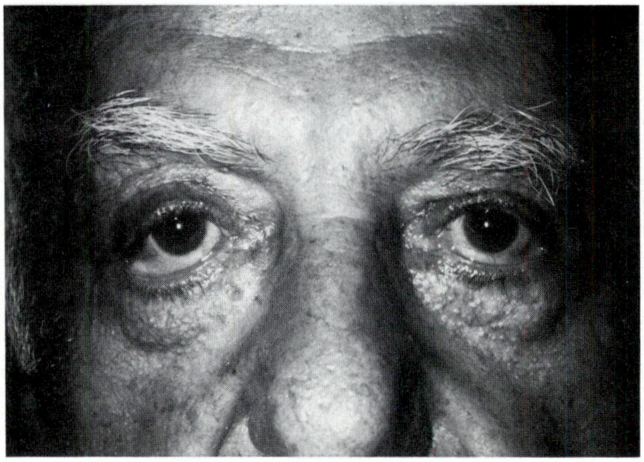

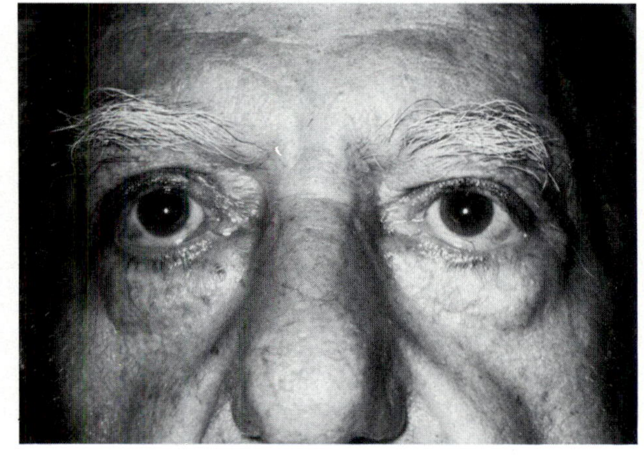

I

Medial canthal tendon fixation

An incision is made at the mucocutaneous junction from just inside the medial canthus to 4 mm lateral to the punctum (Fig. 44-4, *A*). A very superficial skin flap dissection reveals the medial tendon at the most medial aspect of the incision (Fig. 44-4, *B*). A 6-0 Mersilene suture goes into the muscle 3 mm laterally to the punctum and takes a partial-thickness bite of the tarsus. The needle goes back beneath the muscle and takes a second partial-thickness tarsal bite creating a whip stitch. Both needles of the double-armed suture then go beneath the muscle and through the medial tendon (Fig. 44-4, *C*). They are tied beneath the tendon. The skin is closed with "wipe-off" sutures (Fig. 44-4, *D*). A "wipe-off" suture takes a very small bite of the skin at each edge of the wound and is tied very tightly. These sutures will fall out in 5 to 7 days but should not be used on patients with darkly pigmented skin because they may cause cross-hatching.

Fig. 44-4, *E,* shows the preoperative appearance of a patient with a slight punctate ectropion with the medial portion of the lid away from the globe. Fig. 44-4, *F,* shows the appearance after medial canthal tendon repair for laxity.

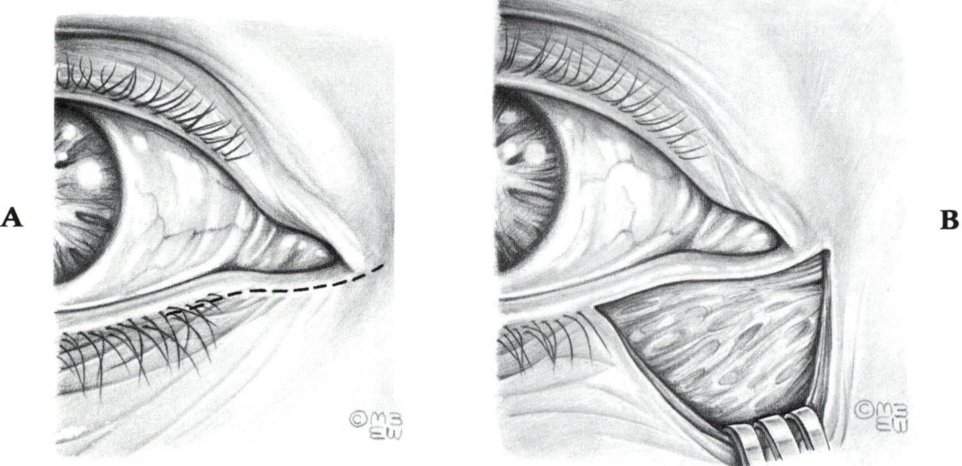

FIGURE 44-4. Medial canthal fixation.

C

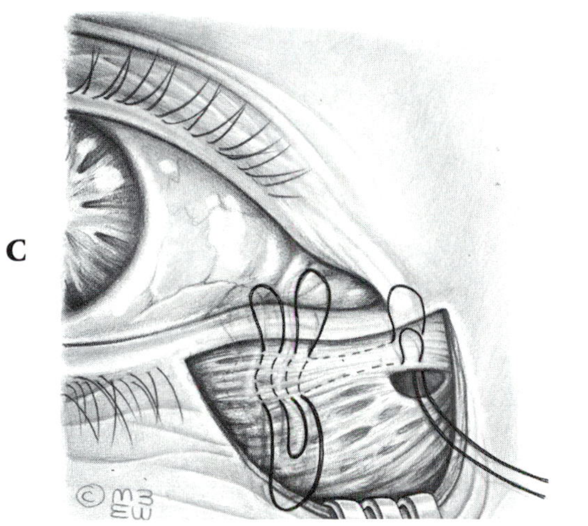

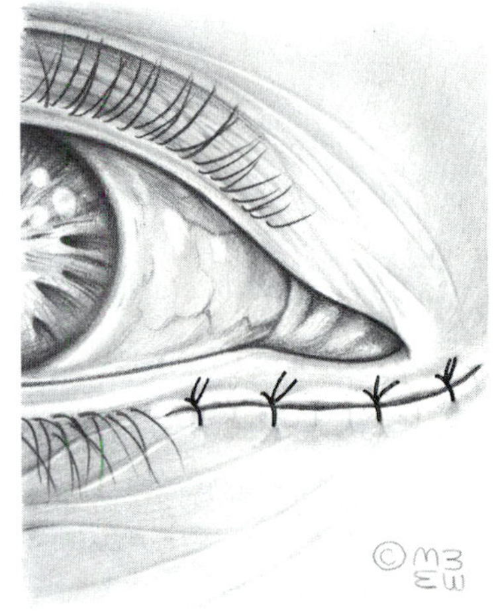

D

E

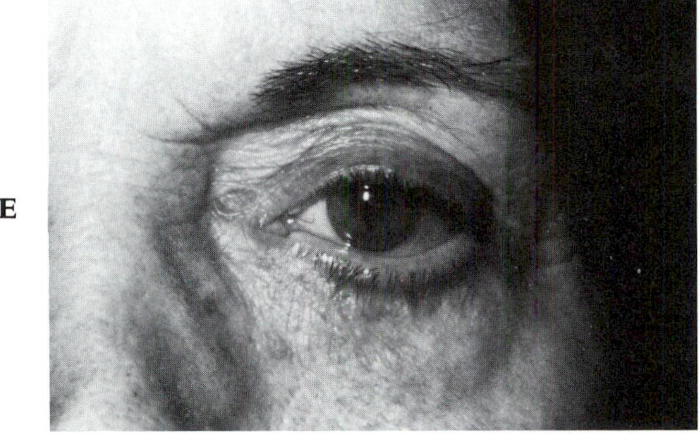

F

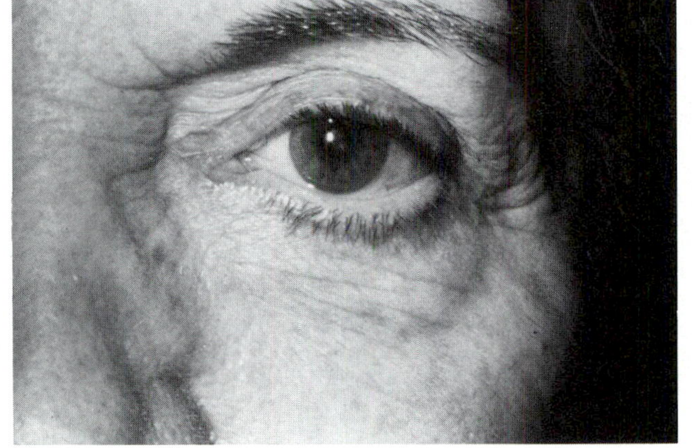

Primary repair of lid margin

This is the basic closure technique for a laceration or defect of the lid margin that can be closed primarily. Fig. 44-5, *A,* shows the lid margin defect. The first suture (*1*) (Fig. 44-5, *B*) enters immediately anterior to the posterior lid margin 3 mm from the cut edge and exits in the anterior tarsal fascia 3 mm from the lid margin and then enters the opposite side of the wound 3 mm from the lid margin in the anterior tarsal fascia and exits just anterior to the posterior lid margin 3 mm from the cut edge. A 7-0 Vicryl suture (*2*) is placed in a partial-thickness manner in the tarsus adjacent to but not through this suture. By crossing suture 2, suture 1 on the lid margin is easily closed.

Once the suture on the posterior lid margin has been tied, it is clamped onto a hemostat (Fig. 44-5, *C*). The suture is put on a stretch pulling the lid margin into an overcorrected position. This brings all opposing parts of the lid together so that interrupted partial-thickness tarsal sutures of 6-0 or 7-0 Vicryl can be used to close the tarsus (Fig. 44-5, *D*). The same suture material is used to close the orbicularis oculi muscle (Fig. 44-5, *E*). All knots are directed anteriorly in the upper lid. In the lower lid the muscle sutures have the knots buried. The second lid margin suture, just posterior to the lashes, as well as the suture beneath the lashes are now placed into position. The two lid margin sutures are tied beneath the suture beneath the lashes to prevent corneal abrasion, and the skin is closed with a continuous suture of 6-0 polypropylene (Fig. 44-5, *F* and *G*).

The skin sutures are removed in 4 to 5 days, and the lid margin sutures are removed in 8 to 10 days.

Fig. 44-5, *H,* shows the preoperative appearance of a patient with a small basal cell in the medial third of the left lower lid. Fig. 44-5, *I,* shows the appearance after excision of tumor with primary closure.

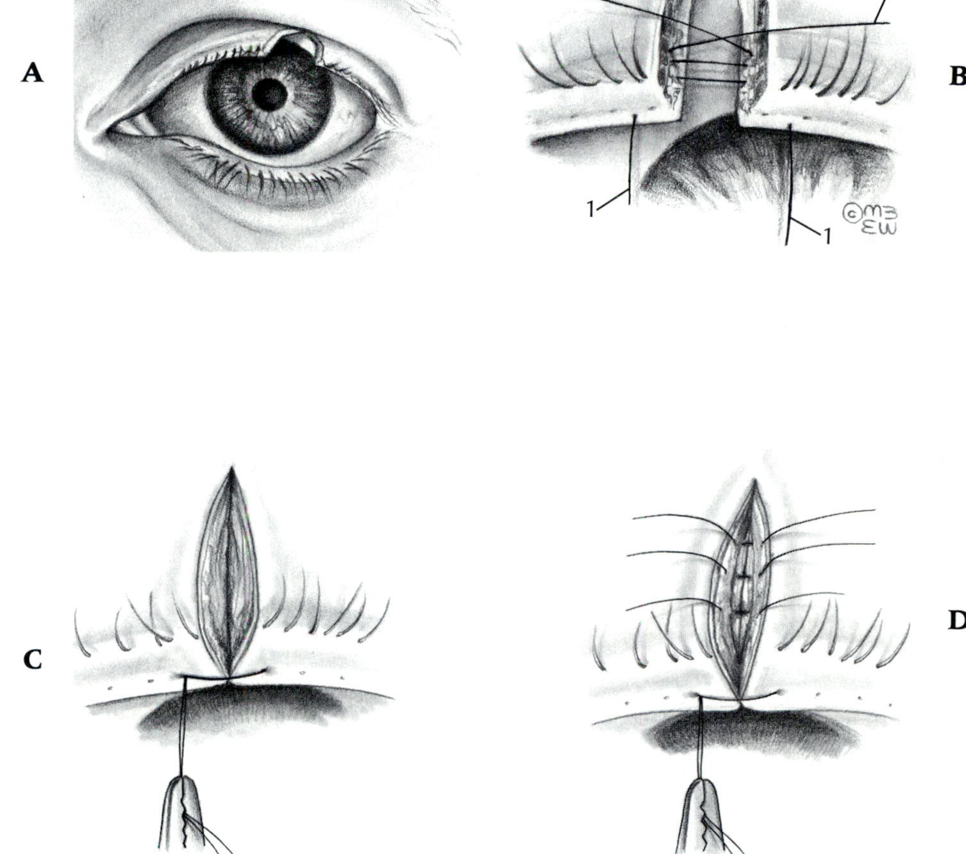

FIGURE 44-5. Transmarginal excision and repair.

Continued.

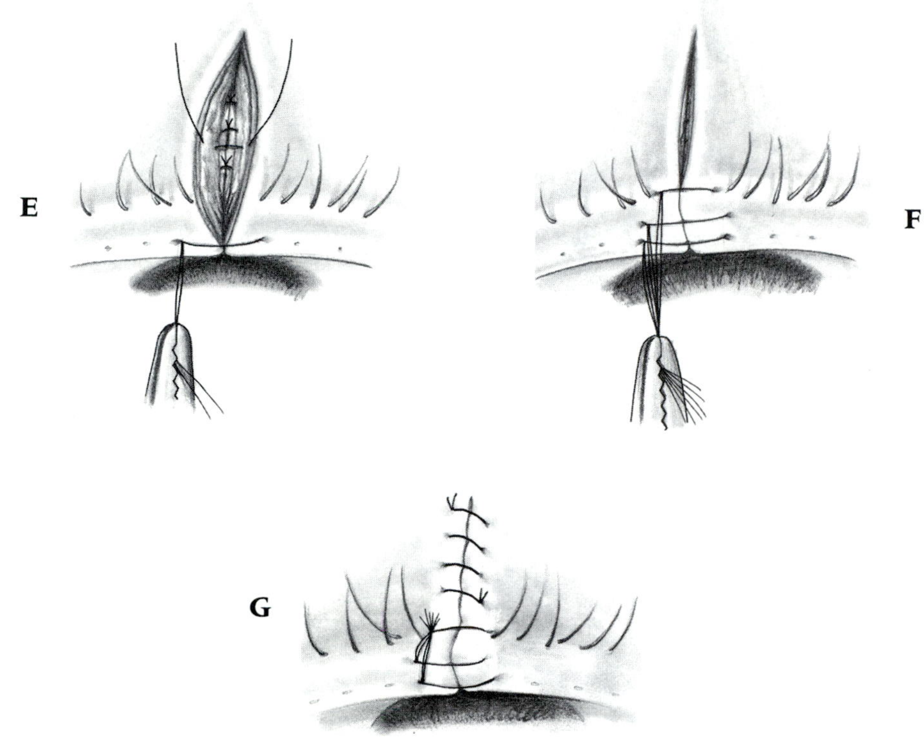

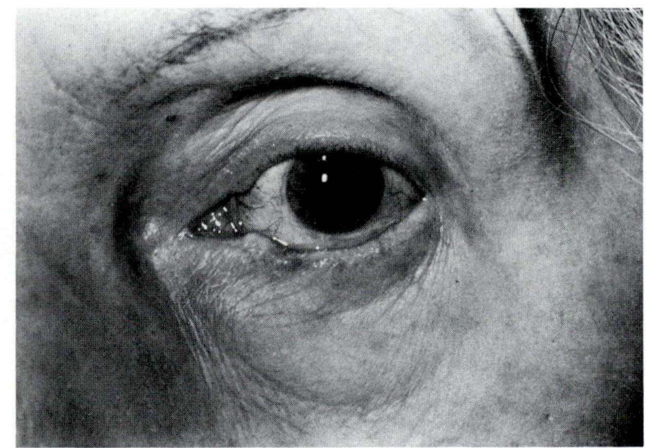

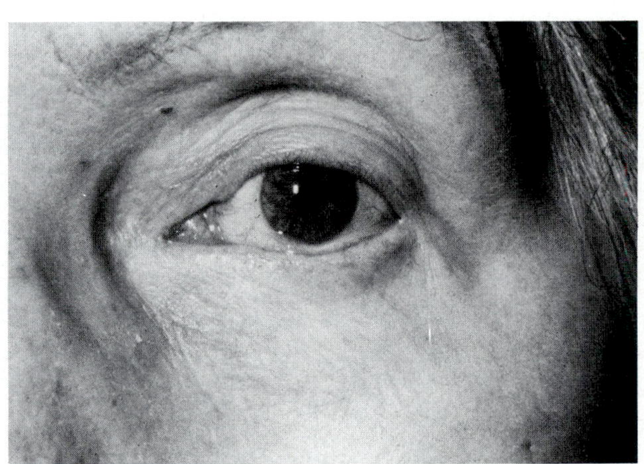

FIGURE 44-5, cont'd

CHAPTER 45

Cosmetic Blepharoplasty and Entropion

BROWS AND UPPER LIDS

Patient evaluation starts with an explanation to the patient as to what can or cannot be accomplished with surgery. Realistic expectations on the part of the patient and surgeon are necessary prerequisites to a happy, satisfied patient. Complications must be explained, and these should include such things as loss of vision, lower lid ectropion, ptosis, and scar deformity.

Basic secretory function testing should be performed on all patients undergoing upper lid surgery. Below 10 mm of wetting means anything from undercorrection, the use of a technique that limits skin excision, to even advising against surgery depending upon surgical judgment.

Preoperative photographs and field testing help with insurance claims and patients' impressions that a deformity resulted from the surgery whereas it was really a preexisting condition.

The examination of a patient for cosmetic blepharoplasty starts at the brows. In the female the cilia should be above the orbital rim, whereas in the male they should be at the rim. If the cilia are below the desired height, the brow must be elevated to accomplish a proper result in upper lid blepharoplasty.

Brow Elevation

There are several techniques for brow elevation. The coronal flap (Fig. 45-1, *A*) is a gull-shaped incision 3 cm from the hairline going through the galea aponeurotica. One makes the dissection between the galea and the periosteum, going down to and cutting the corrigator and procerus muscles. Blocks of frontalis muscle are removed between the supraorbital vessels and nerves to maintain better fixation to the periosteum and prevent brow droop. Tightening is accomplished by excision of the anterior hair flap until symmetry of the brow is achieved. The deep wound is closed with interrupted sutures of 3-0 Vicryl, and the hair is closed with staples. If only the tail of the brow is ptotic, the incision can be made at the third frown line into the temporal hair so that this corner is elevated (Fig. 45-1, *B*). Again, the deep wound is closed with interrupted sutures, but 6-0 Vicryl is sufficient in this area. The skin is closed with a continuous suture of 6-0 Prolene (polypropylene).

The easiest technique for elevation of the brow is the superciliary approach, where the inferior line is placed in the upper hairline of the brow (Fig. 45-1, *C*). The brow is elevated to the desired level. This is marked out with a marking pen, and just the skin and subcutaneous tissues are excised. An M-plasty can be done at the medial aspect so that the two brow incisions do not meet. The deep wound must be closed with a double row of buried 6-0 Vicryl sutures and the skin with 6-0 Prolene.

Any crease in the forehead can be used to conceal the scar for elevation of the brow. This is particularly true in men who might have pronounced frown lines. The incision goes slightly above the frown line, and the frown line is excised with the inferior skin, and a new frown line is formed with wound closure.

Fig. 45-1, *D,* is the appearance before coronal flap operation; *E,* postoperative elevation of brow; *F,* preoperative appearance on patient with seventh nerve palsy on the right; *G,* after elevation of the right brow with a superciliary incision.

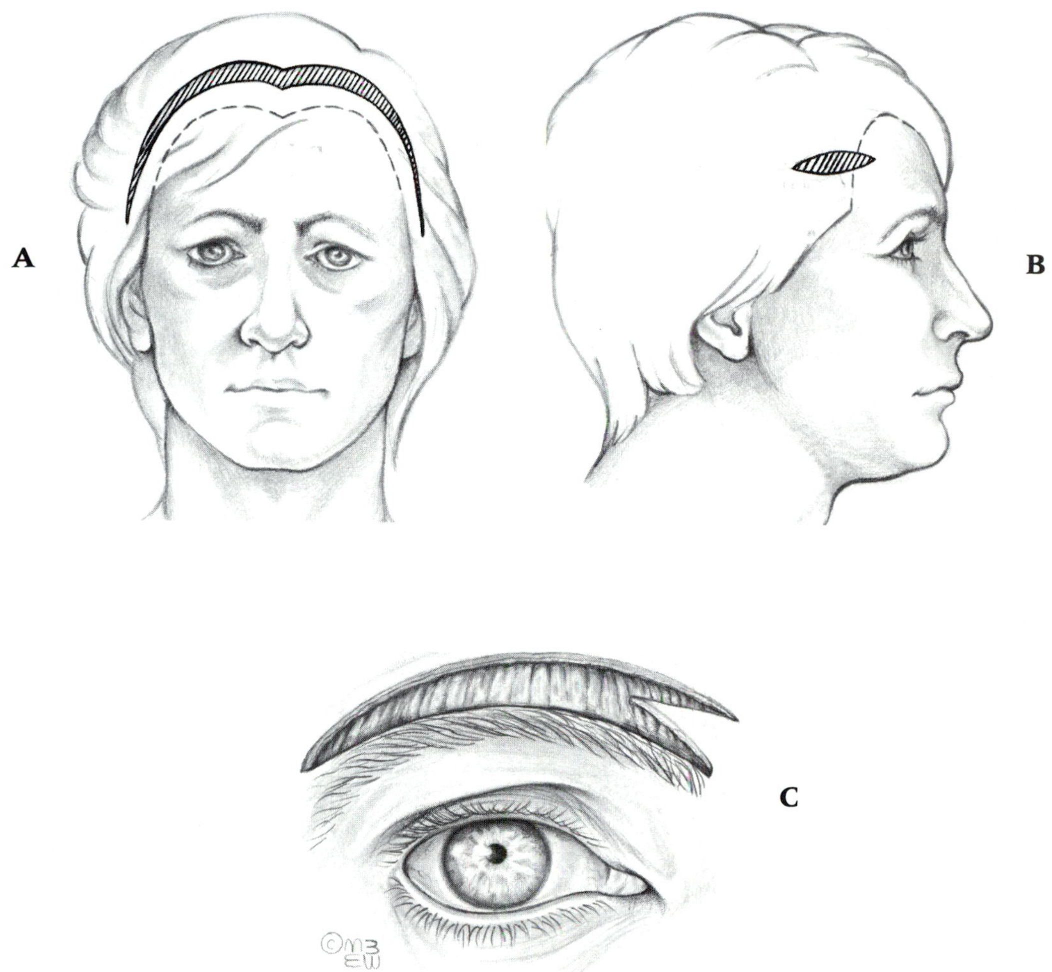

FIGURE 45-1. Brow elevation.

Continued.

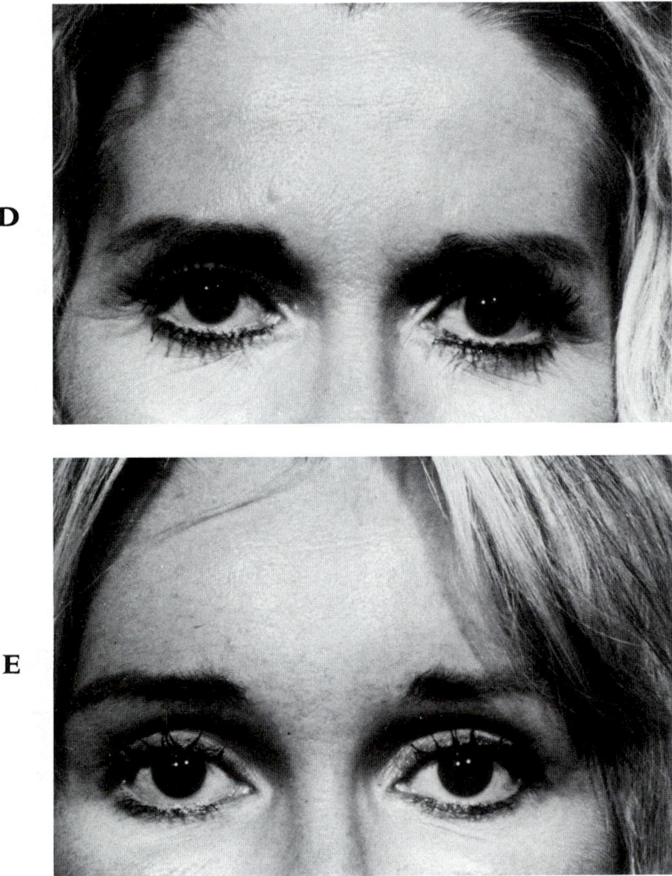

FIGURE 45-1, cont'd

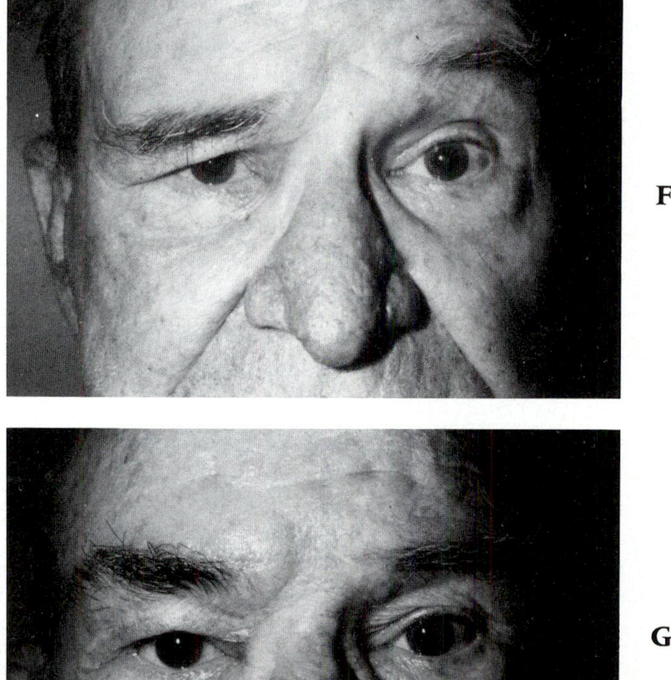

FIGURE 45-1, cont'd

Upper Lid Blepharoplasty

If there is noticeable upper lid skin redundancy, it should be gently lifted from the lashes and the level of the lid margin checked to rule out a true ptosis. The most common technique that I use in the upper lid is one where the lid crease is reformed. The lids are marked out 10, 9, and 8 mm from the central, temporal, and nasal lash base in a woman and 1 mm less on each measurement in a man. A pair of Green's fixation forceps grasps the skin, and only the redundant skin that can be grasped in the forceps without causing lash eversion is marked out with a marking pen (Fig. 45-2, *A*). The medial inferior mark goes to the punctum and then continues superonasally, where it is joined by the superior mark. Temporally it goes beyond the orbital rim to elevate the lateral portion of the lateral canthus. An incision is made in the premarked lines either with a Bard-Parker blade (Fig. 45-2, *B*) or with a razor knife starting from the most dependent portion and continuing to the highest level of the lid to prevent the blood from erasing the premarked lines. I prefer to remove the skin (Fig. 45-2, *C*) and muscle in separate layers with scissors (Fig. 45-2, *D*). Care must be taken in removal of the muscle layer to prevent damage to the levator aponeurosis. Open the orbital septum across the lid by putting pressure on the lids, buttonholing the orbital septum, and cutting between the orbital rim and levator aponeurosis (Fig. 45-2, *E* and *F*). There are two fat pockets in the upper lid—medial and central. The medial fat pocket has a finer, whiter type of fat than the central pocket does. The amount of fat that can be made to prolapse with pressure on the lids is clamped with a hemostat, cut, cauterized, and grasped with a forceps while the hemostat is removed to make sure there is no bleeding before the fat is allowed to drop back into the orbit (see Fig. 45-3, *E* to *H*).

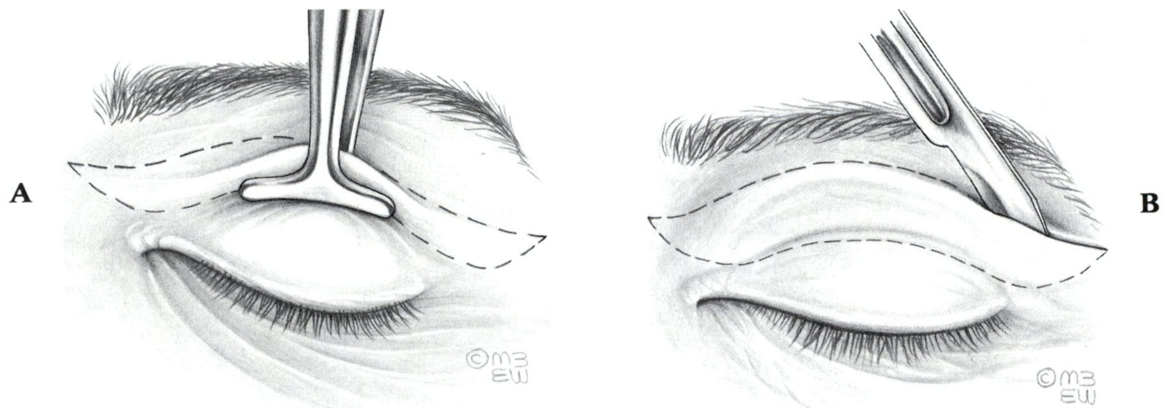

FIGURE 45-2. Upper lids.

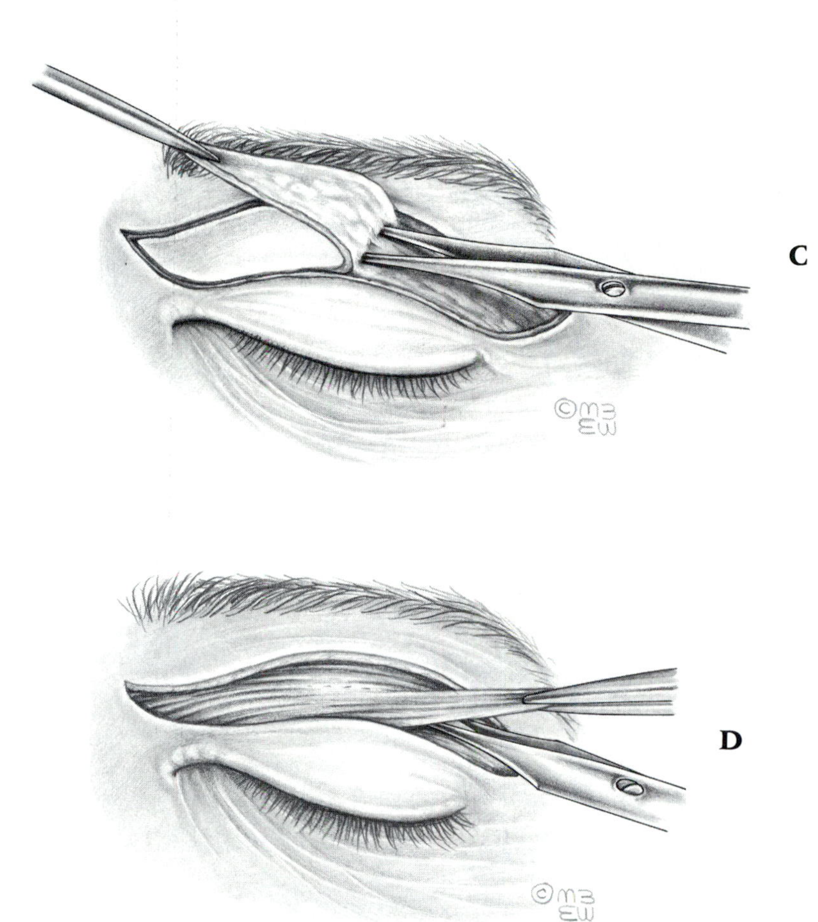

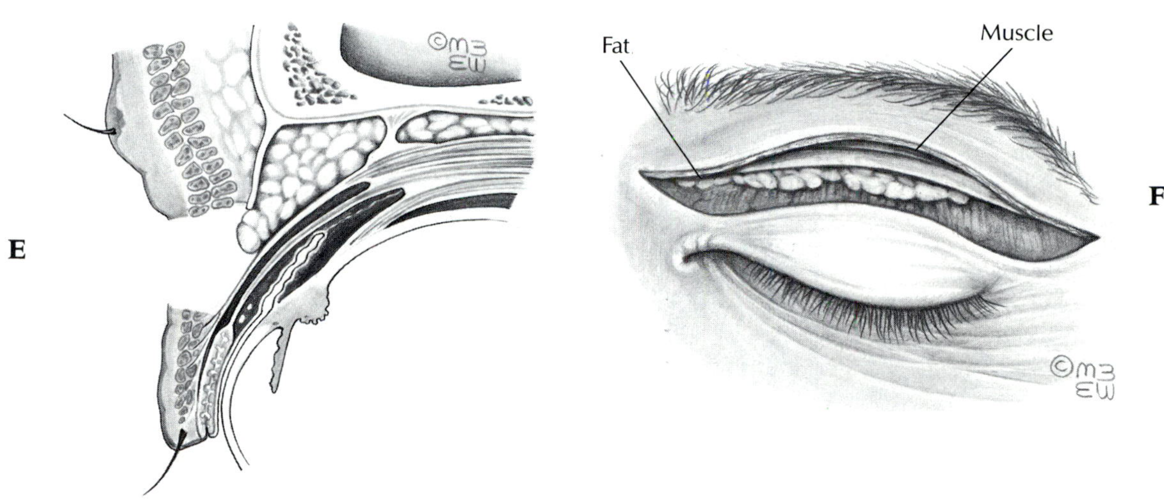

FIGURE 45-2, cont'd

Continued.

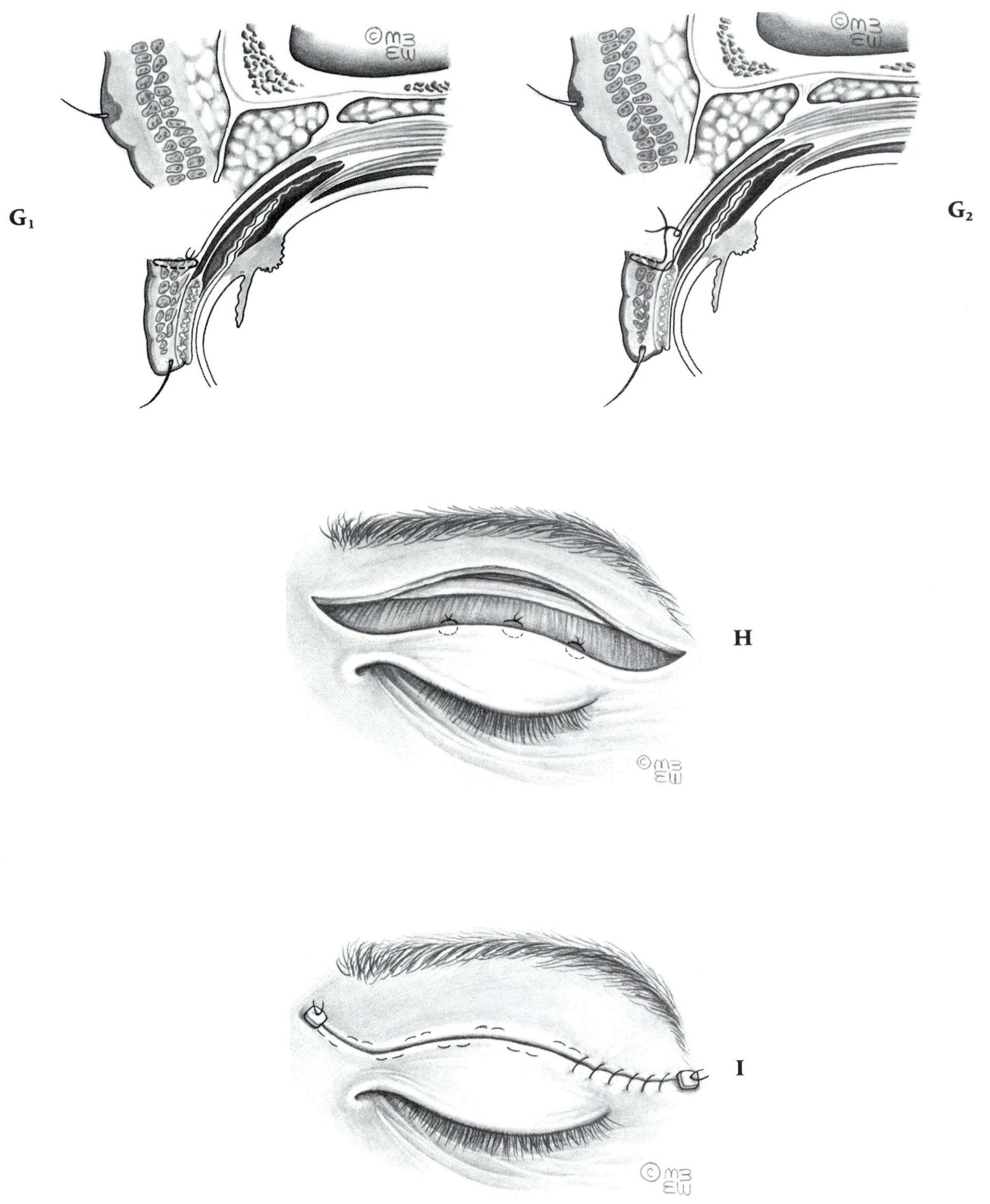

FIGURE 45-2, cont'd

J

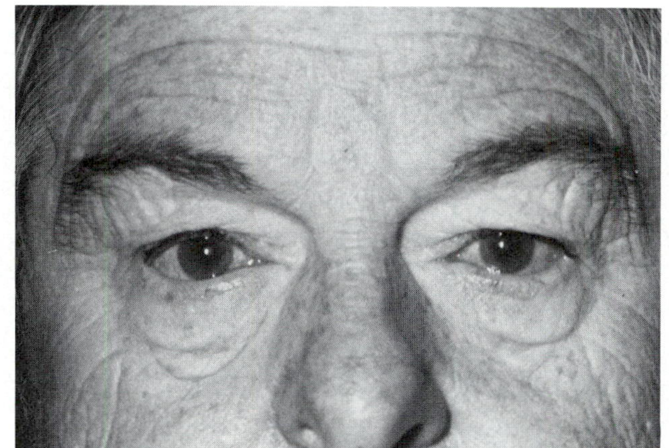

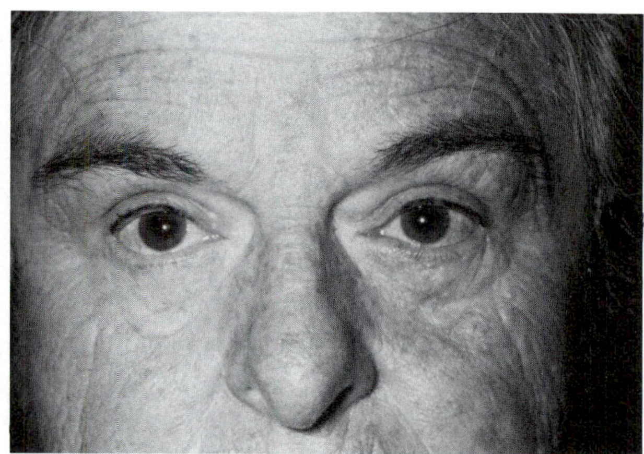

K

Fixation of the superior portion of the inferior skin flap is made to either the levator aponeurosis (high lid crease technique) (Fig. 45-2, G_1) or to the tarsus (anchor blepharoplasty) (Fig. 45-2, G_2). In the anchor blepharoplasty technique, the levator aponeurosis is divided and incorporated with the suture going to the upper edge of the inferior skin flap. Care must be taken that the lid fixation suture goes to the subcutaneous tissue immediately beneath the skin, not to just the muscle, to prevent loss of the lid crease. Three sutures are used to obtain a symmetric lid crease (Fig. 45-2, *H*). More can be used if desired. The medial skin is closed with a subcuticular suture of 6-0 polypropylene. When the closure approaches within six lashes of the lateral canthus, the needle is brought out of the skin and continues as an over-and-over suture (Fig. 45-2, *I*). The end is tied to a rubber band.

Fig. 45-2, *J,* is a preoperative view of upper lid blepharoplasty; *K,* postoperative appearance.

LOWER LID BLEPHAROPLASTY AND ENTROPION REPAIR

Since my "standard" technique for entropion repair is almost identical to that of lower lid cosmetic blepharoplasty with lateral tendon laxity, they will be described together with the addition of lower lid retractor repair used only in patients with entropion, and other techniques.

In the treatment of spastic or involutional lower lid entropion, the advantages of the "standard" procedure are a very low recurrence rate after 5 years, an excellent-looking lid with the removal of excess fat and skin, and, especially, usefulness in the treatment of recurrent entropion. There are less effective but good procedures that can also be used.

Lower Lid Blepharoplasty

In evaluating a patient for lower lid blepharoplasty, grasp the lower lid with the fingers and pull anteriorly (Fig. 45-3, *A*). If there is more than 1 cm separation between the globe and the lid, a horizontal lid-tightening procedure should be done. If the punctum moves laterally to the limbus, a medial fixation must be performed with or without the lateral fixation, depending on the laxity of the lateral tendon as well. My preferred technique of lower lid blepharoplasty is the skin-muscle flap. An incision is made temporally at about a 30-degree angle at the lateral canthus (Fig. 45-3, *B*) and carried through the skin and muscle. The flap is formed with blunt dissection beneath the muscle plane with scissors (Fig. 45-3, *C*). One blade of the scissors is then placed in the pocket, another is placed beneath the lashes, and open the flap by cutting the tissue immediately beneath the lashes (Fig. 45-3, *D*). There are three fat pockets in the lower lid, compared to two pockets in the upper lid (Fig. 45-3, *E*). Open the fat pockets by putting pressure on the lids and buttonholing a pocket (Fig. 45-3, *F*). The orbital septum is opened across the lower lid. The fat is made to prolapse with pressure on the lids. The fat is clamped with a hemostat, cut (Fig. 45-3, *G*), and cauterized. The pedicle is grasped with forceps before the hemostat is released to make certain there is no bleeding before the fat is allowed to drop back into the orbit (Fig. 45-3, *H*). If there is lid laxity involving the medial tendon, a medial tendon repair is performed (see Fig. 44-4). First the medial superficial skin flap is formed (see Fig. 44-4, *A* and *B*), then the lateral skin muscle flap (see Fig. 45-3, *B* to *D*), and then the two flaps are joined. The fat is excised, and then the medial tendon is repaired (see Fig. 44-4, *C*).

If there is lateral tendon laxity, the lateral tendon resection is performed (see Fig. 44-3, *A* to *F*) at this stage of the operation. The procedure is continued with redundant skin excision.

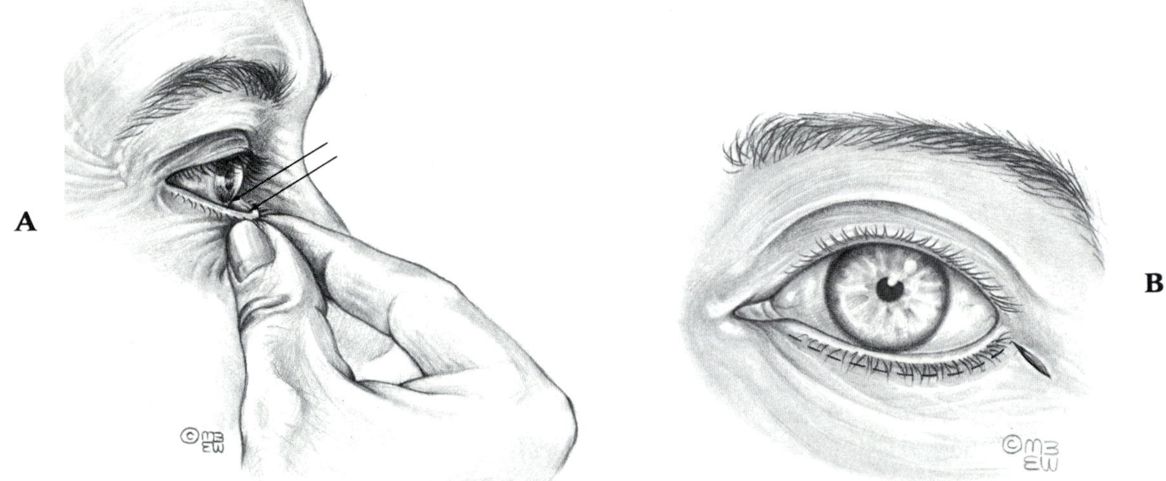

FIGURE 45-3. Lower lid cosmetic blepharoplasty.

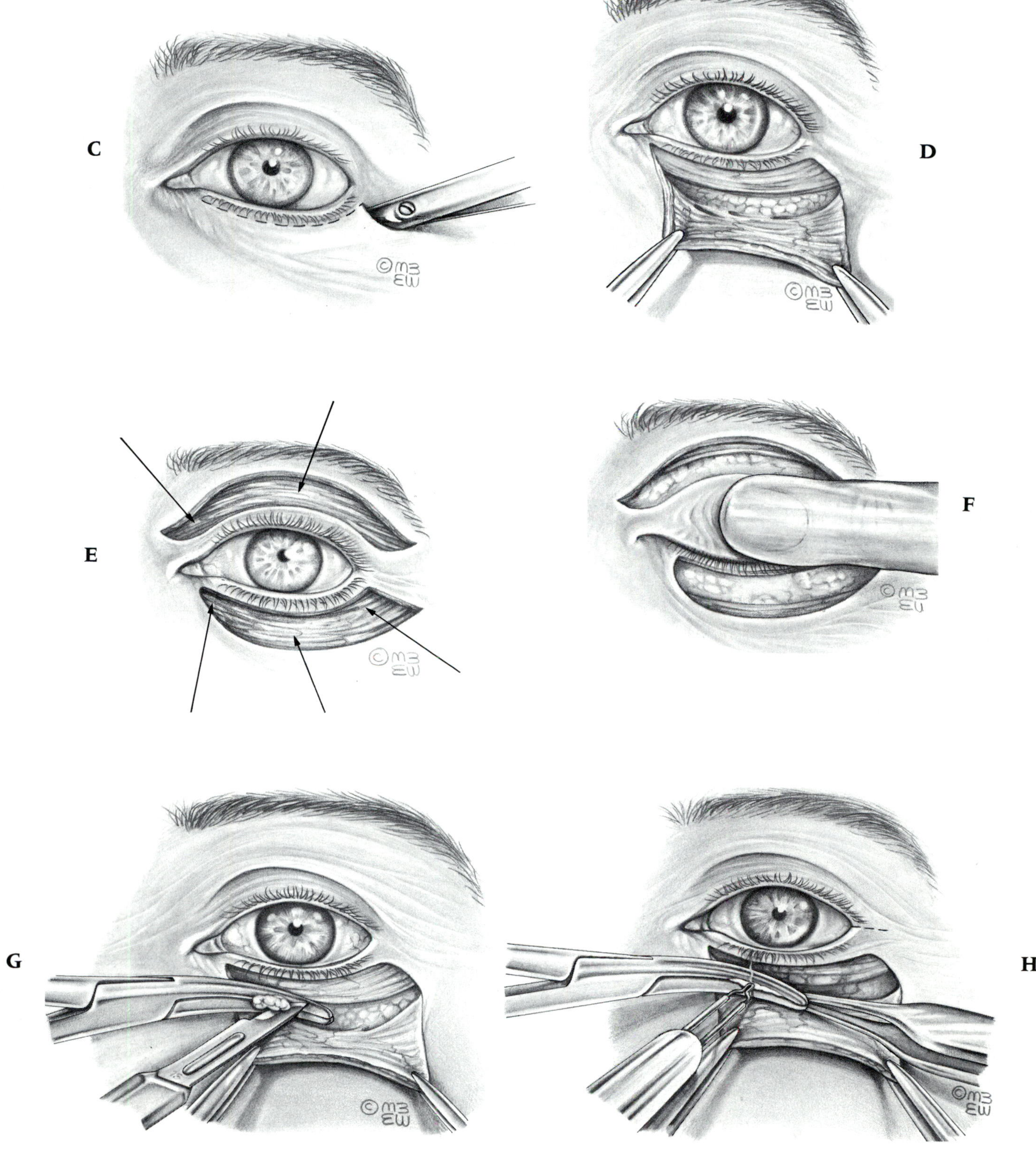
C
D
E
F
G
H

Standard Entropion Repair

My classic repair of an entropion is a lower lid blepharoplasty with a lateral tarsal tendon resection and the addition of sutures from the lower lid retractors to the pretarsal orbicularis. At least three interrupted 7-0 Vicryl sutures are placed from the lower lid retractors to the inferior edge of the orbicularis muscle (Fig. 45-4, *A*). One suture is in the center of the lid, one lateral to the punctum, and one medial to the lateral canthus. After the sutures are tied, the lid margin should not be able to be forcefully rotated into an entropion position. The procedure is then continued as in a standard lower lid blepharoplasty with the skin excision. Fig. 45-4, *B,* shows involutional entropion of the left lower lid; *C,* close-up of the patient preoperatively; *D,* postoperative appearance; *E,* close-up of the left lower lid postoperatively.

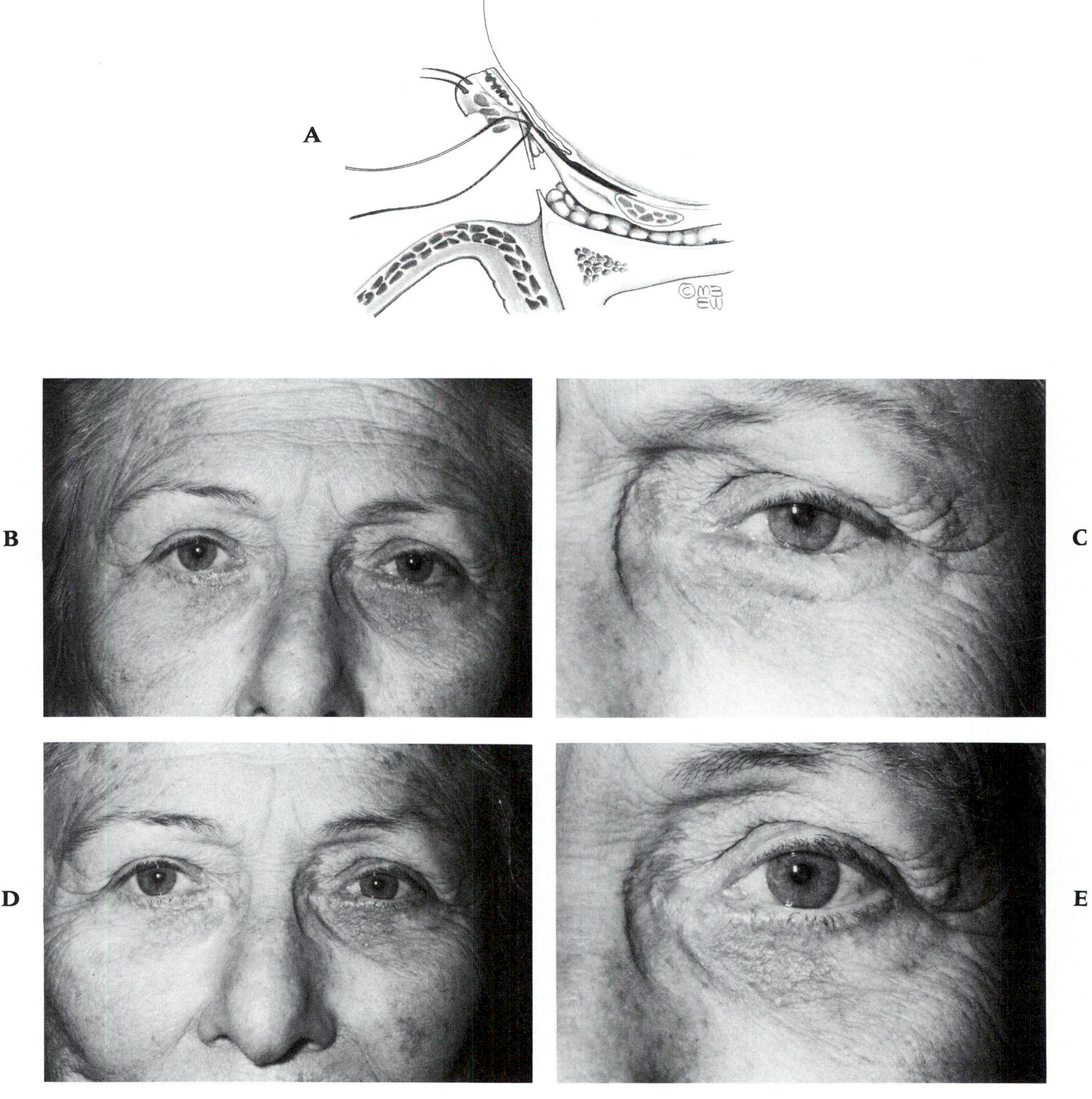

FIGURE 45-4. Standard entropion repair for lower lid entropion.

Redundant Skin Excision

Ascertain the amount of redundant skin by using posteroinferior pressure on the globe through the upper lid or having the patient look up at the time of the procedure. These techniques flatten out the depression of the lower lid to prevent excess skin excision (Fig. 45-5, *A* and *B*). The skin is draped over the wound. A second cut is made temporally, and the flap is rotated into position (Fig. 45-5, *C*). The excess skin is removed. All bleeding is stopped before closure, and the wound is closed with a continuous suture of 6-0 polypropylene with very small bites widely scattered across the lower lid and then with a vertical mattress closure on the temporal portion of the wound (Fig. 45-5, *D*). The deep bites are looped with pullout sutures of 6-0 polypropylene so that the mattress sutures might be easily removed. The dotted circles show the positions of the lid retractor sutures in entropion repair. Fig. 45-5, *E*, shows the preoperative appearance on the patient before lower lid blepharoplasty; *F*, postoperative appearance.

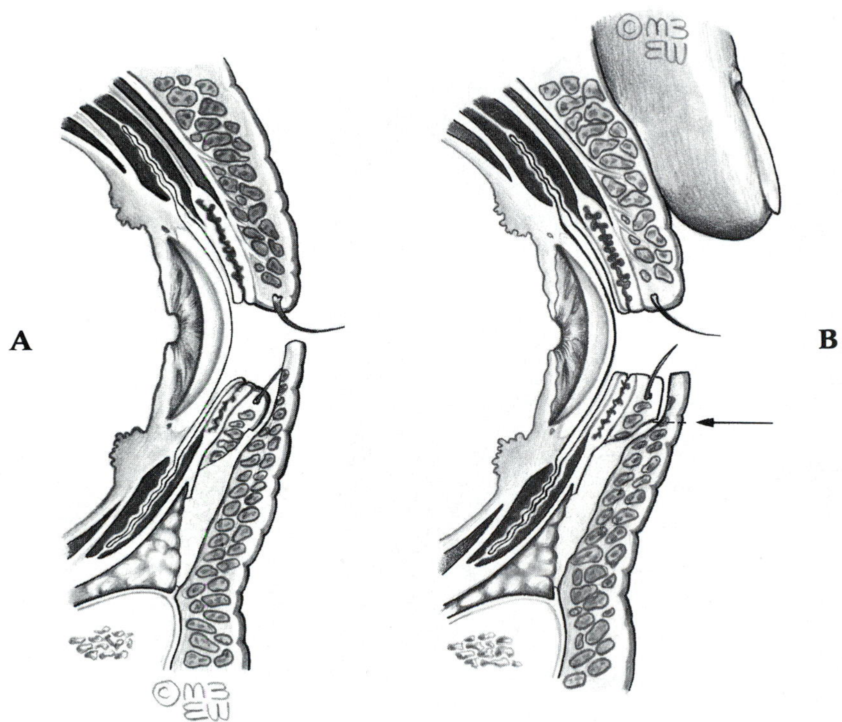

FIGURE 45-5. Redundant skin excision.

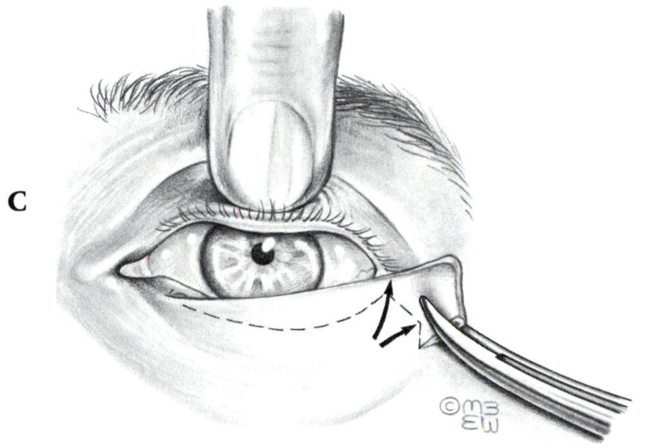

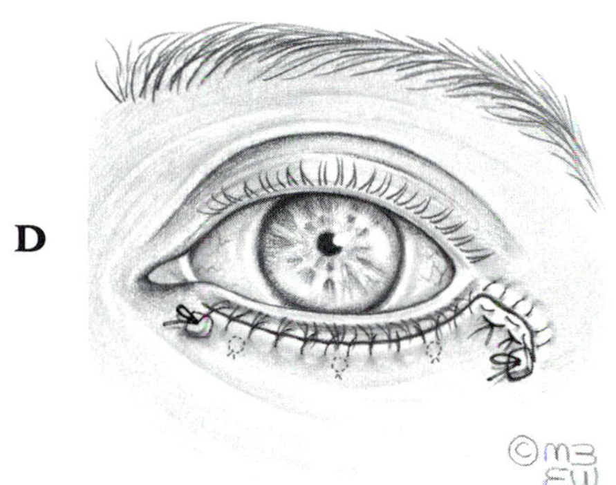

E

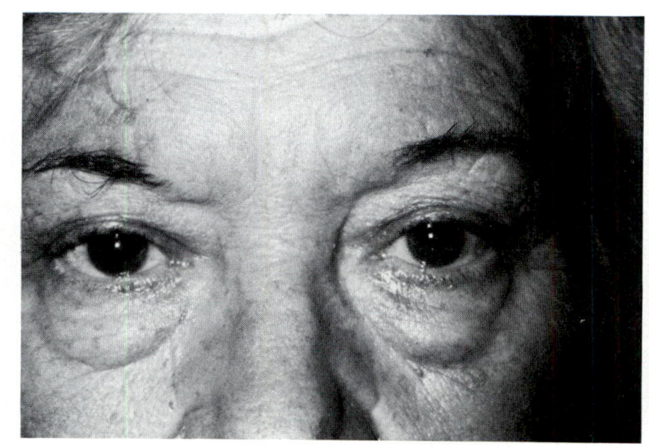

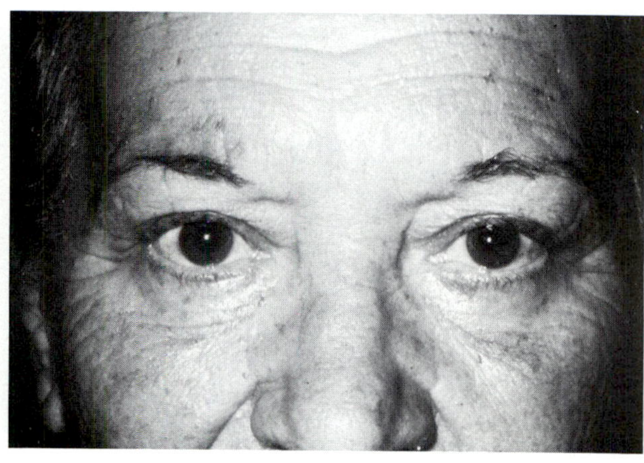

F

Other Techniques for Involutional Entropion

Simplified entropion procedure

A simplified entropion procedure is performed by placement of a chalazion clamp on the lid at the junction of the central and lateral thirds of the lid. A 10 mm base-down triangle is removed from the tarsus. A second smaller triangle is removed inferiorly for closure (Fig. 45-6, *A*). Two to three interrupted 6-0 Vicryl sutures are placed so that the knots are anterior to the tarsus (Fig. 45-6, *B*). There will be a slight bulge on the lid margin that goes away within 2 to 3 weeks (Fig. 45-6, *C*).

This technique is especially useful on debilitated patients, those on anticoagulant therapy, or patients who cannot have the appearance of having had recent eyelid surgery.

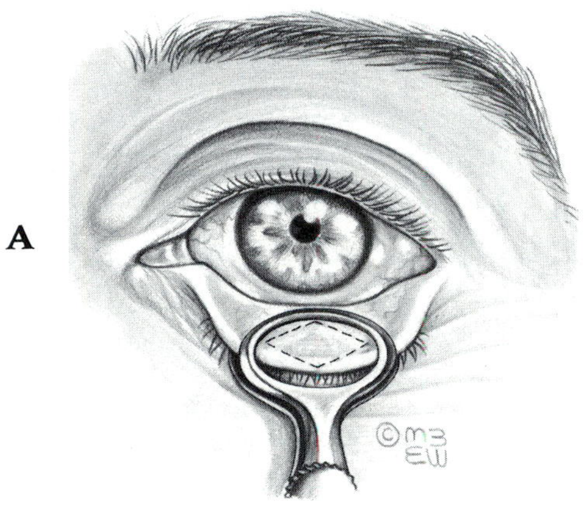

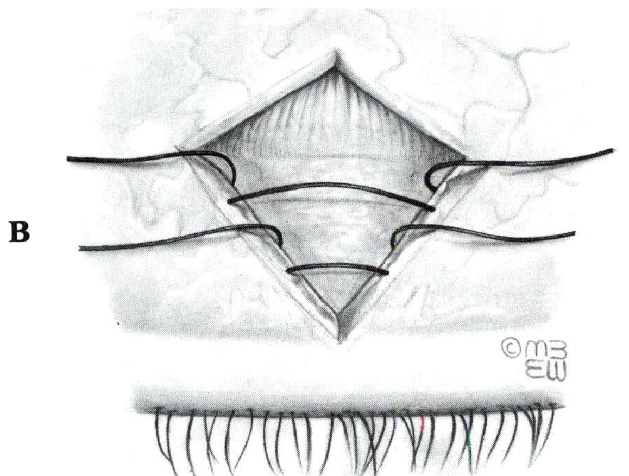

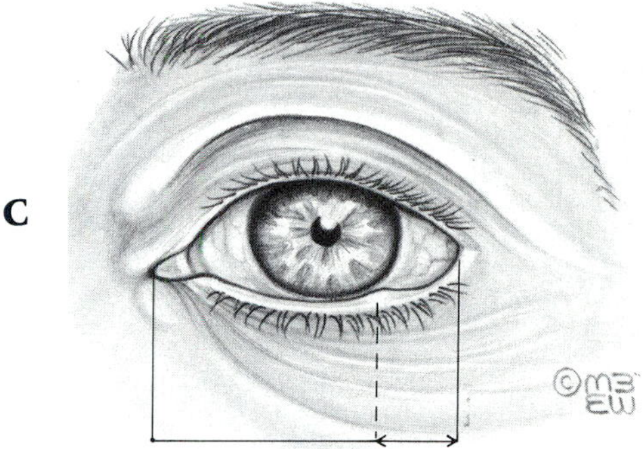

FIGURE 45-6. Base-down triangle.

Repair of entropion after intraocular surgery

An incision is made at the junction of the central and lateral thirds of the lid, 3 mm from the lid margin, exposing the orbicularis muscle (Fig. 45-7, *A*). A double-arm 5-0 polypropylene suture is used as a whip stitch around the muscle, giving a good firm attachment to the muscle (Fig. 45-7, *B*). A second incision is made over the anterior orbital rim inferotemporally to the first incision (Fig. 45-7, *C*). Again, the deeper orbicularis muscle that is attached to the underlying tissues is isolated. Each arm of the suture near the lid margin is carried subcutaneously to exit through the second wound, then takes a whip stitch around the orbicularis, and is tightened until the lid is in the slightly overcorrected position (Fig. 45-7, *D*). The wound is closed with small interrupted sutures of 7-0 silk (Fig. 45-7, *E*).

As the title indicates, this procedure is especially useful in spastic entropion occurring after intraocular surgery. During the procedure there is no pressure placed on the globe. All of the surgery is from the skin side, and the procedure is very easy and quick. Unfortunately there is frequently inflammation around the sutures, and they have to be removed, but, by then, the irritative phenomenon of the ocular surgery has usually passed and the lid stays corrected.

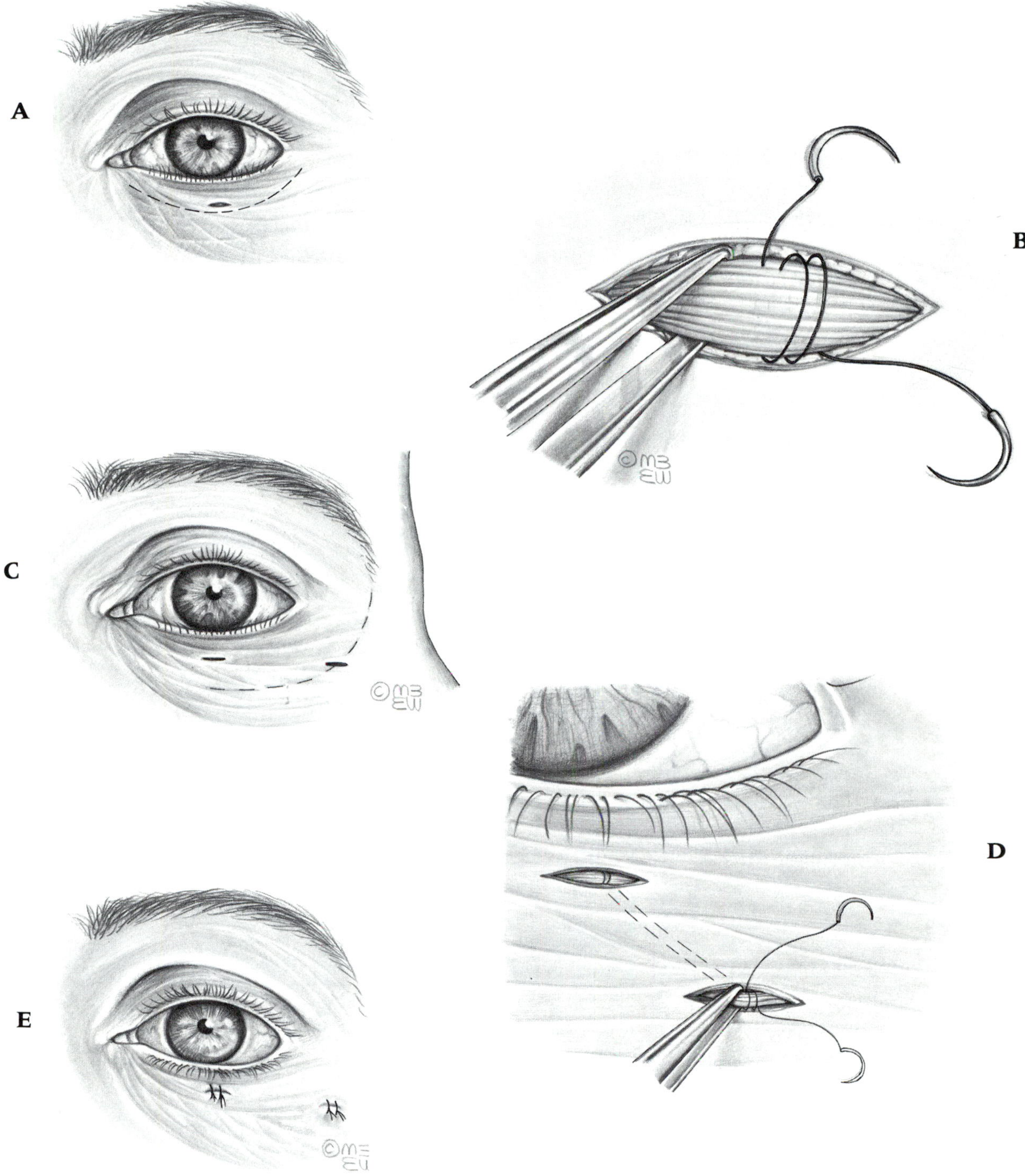

FIGURE 45-7. Modified Wheeler technique by suture.

Cicatricial Entropion of the Lower Lid

The earliest sign of cicatricial lower lid entropion is a section of trichiasis in the center of the lid. The way to differentiate this type of entropion from true trichiasis is to follow the path of meibomian glands starting at the medial or lateral part of the lid. In cicatricial entropion the meibomian gland orifices move from the center of the lid margin toward the conjunctival surface and may actually be on the posterior lid surface.

A lid plate behind the lid protects the globe. Silk sutures, 4-0, are placed through the lid 4 mm from the lid margin, 3 mm medial and 3 mm lateral to the area of entropion (Fig. 45-8, *A*). An incision is made through the skin and muscle of the lid between these sutures staying parallel to the lid margin (Fig. 45-8, *B*).

The lid is everted over the lid plate. An incision is made through the conjunctiva and tarsus between the sutures, again staying parallel to the lid margin (Fig. 45-8, *C*).

The two incisions are joined, giving a through-and-through transverse blepharotomy (Fig. 45-8, *D*). The 4-0 silk sutures are removed and used as horizontal mattress sutures (Fig. 45-8, *E*). They enter the skin just inferior to the lashes. Staying anterior to the tarsus, they exit through the wound, go into the small remaining portion of the tarsus in the lower lid or, if tarsus is not present, into the lower lid retractors, exit on the conjunctiva, and go back into the conjunctiva. Again picking up either the tarsus or lower lid retractors, they exit through the lower wound, enter the upper wound, staying anterior to the tarsus, and exit through the skin beneath the lashes. When these sutures are tied, the lid should be in a mild ectropion position. The skin can be left open or closed with small interrupted sutures of either 4-0 silk or 7-0 silk (Fig. 45-8, *F*). Fig. 45-8, *G*, shows the preoperative appearance of a cicatricial entropion of the right lower lid; *H*, postoperative appearance.

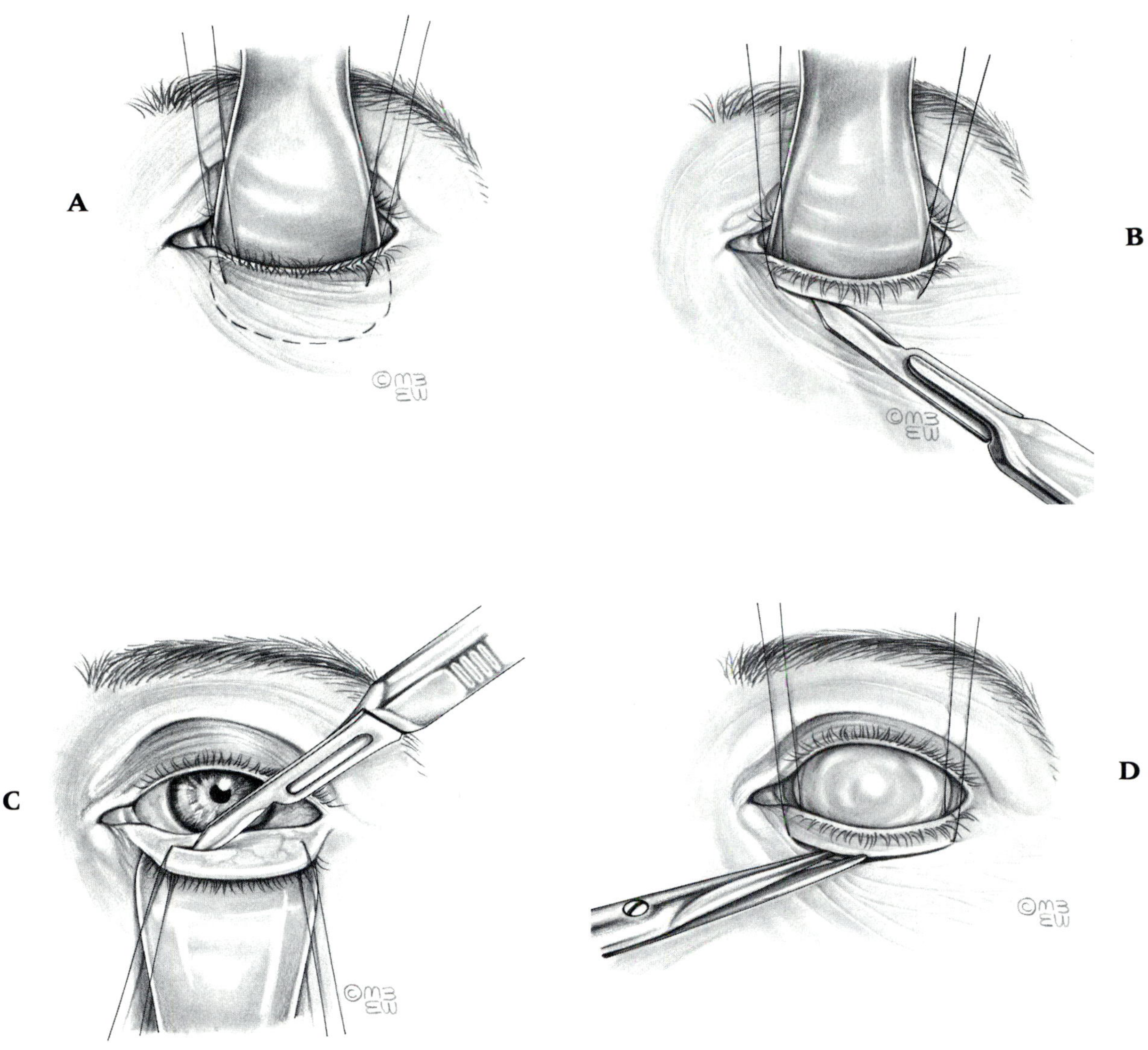

FIGURE 45-8. Modified Wies technique.

Continued.

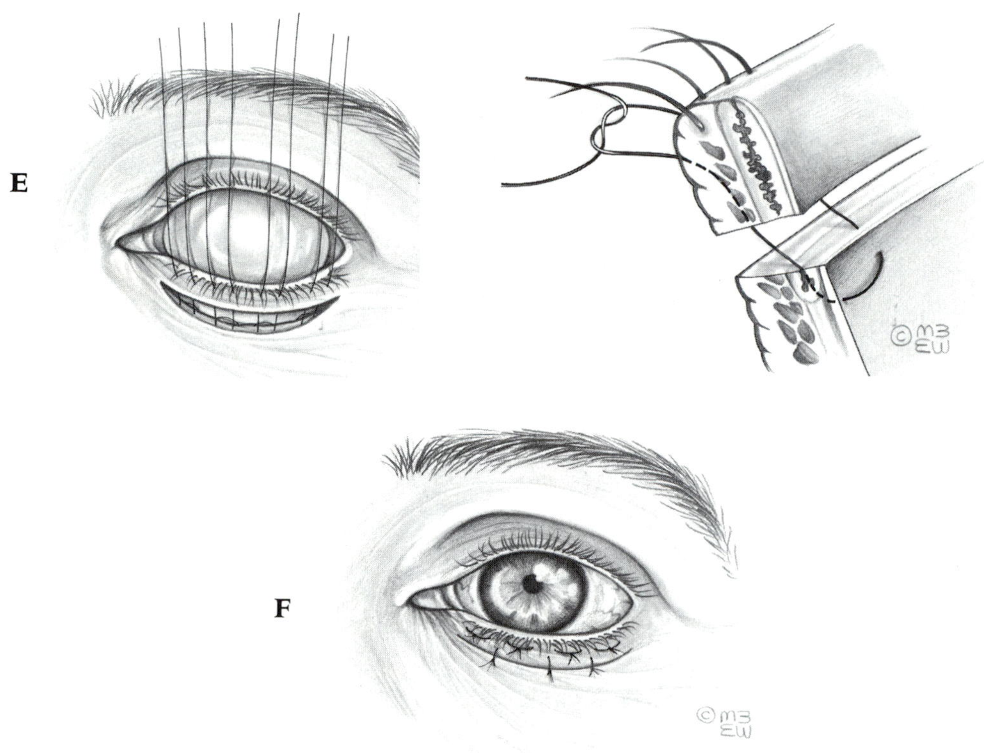

FIGURE 45-8, cont'd

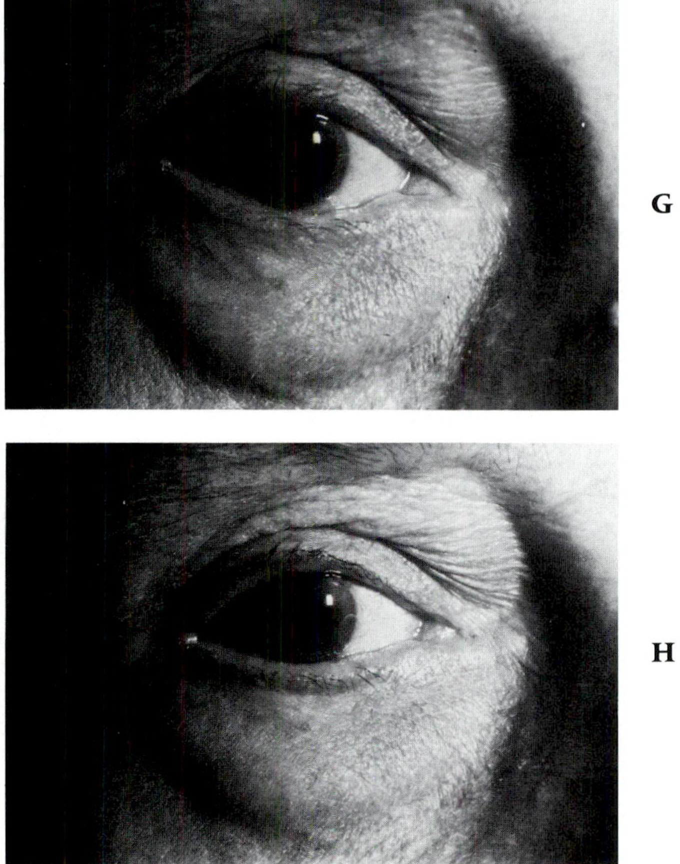

FIGURE 45-8, cont'd

Upper Lid Entropion with Graft

The upper lid is everted, and an incision is made across the lid 6 mm from the lid margin through the conjunctiva, tarsus, and levator aponeurosis (Fig. 45-9, *A*). A 6 to 8 mm block of tissue, either sclera, tarsus, or upper palate, is placed into the defect. A horizontal mattress suture enters the skin just above the lashes, comes out of the wound with a partial-thickness tarsal bite, enters the graft in a horizontal fashion, takes another partial-thickness tarsal bite, and exits through the skin. These horizontal mattress sutures are placed completely across the lid, causing eversion of the lashes. A second row of sutures enters the skin approximately 6 mm higher than the first row and takes a partial-thickness bite in the tarsus, takes a horizontal partial-thickness bite in the graft, comes through the tarsus, and exits through the skin (Fig. 45-9, *B*). These sutures are removed in 10 days. It is easier to do this type of suturing with a spatula needle and a 6-0 silk or a 6-0 Mersilene suture.

Fig. 45-9, *C,* shows the preoperative appearance of an entropion of the right upper lid; *D,* preoperative close-up of the right eye; *E,* postoperative view; *F,* close-up appearance of the right upper lid.

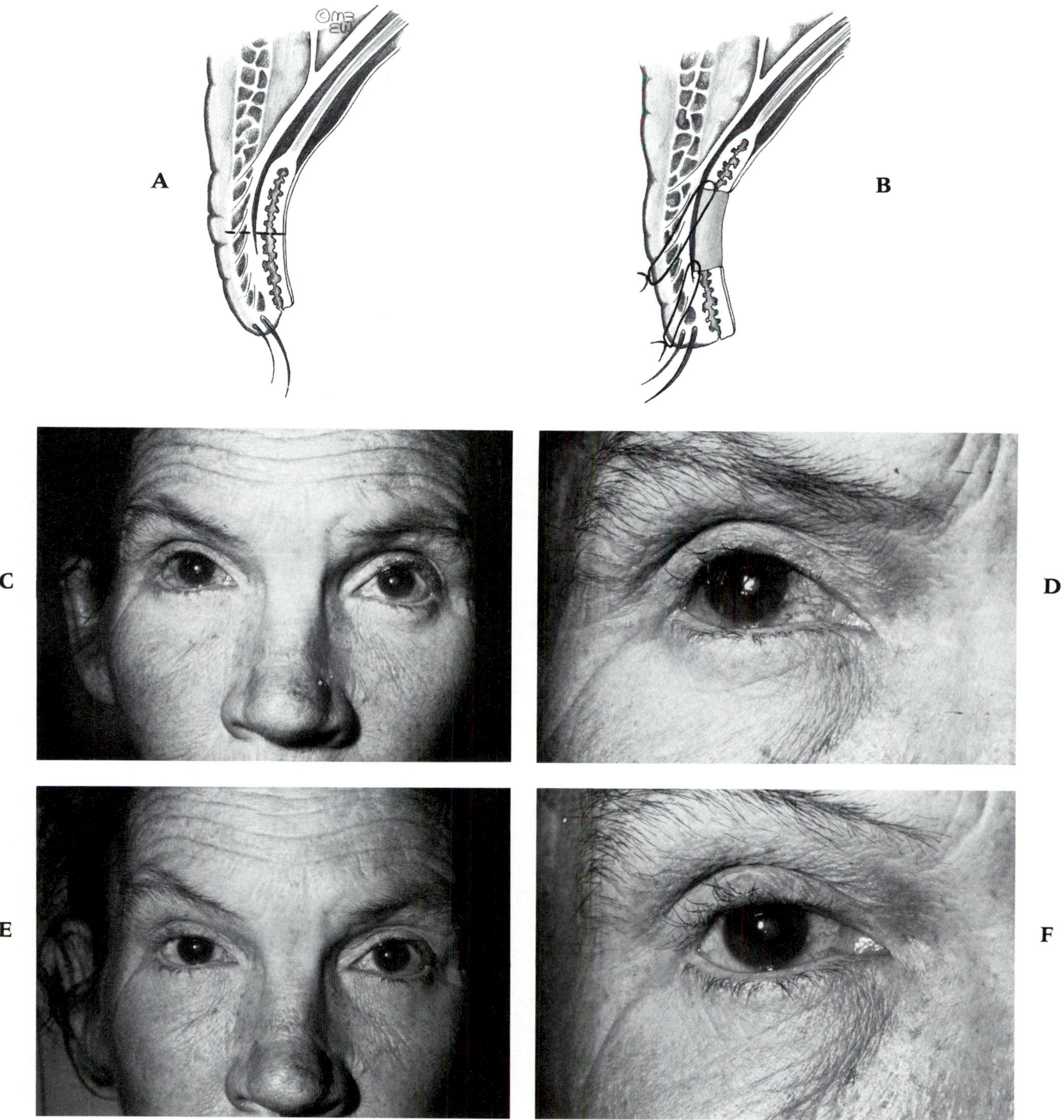

FIGURE 45-9. Upper lid entropion repair with grafts.

Treatment of Severe Cicatricial Upper and Lower Lid Entropion

The upper and lower lids are split at the gray line for a distance of 7 mm. Care must be taken to be posterior to all cilia and not to cut any lash roots. The tarsal margin of both the upper and the lower lids is excised, and the lower lid lashes are excised (Fig. 45-10, *A*). The two edges of the tarsus are sewed together with a continuous suture of 9-0 nylon (Fig. 45-10, *B*). The upper and lower lids are sutured to the tarsus, with an approximately 8 mm distance being left between the two margins. A full-thickness mucous membrane graft is taken from the mouth and sutured between the lid margins totally across the tarsus (Fig. 45-10, *C*). After 1 month the lids are opened in the center line (Fig. 45-10, *D*). This procedure is reserved for those severe cases of entropion occurring after Stevens-Johnson syndrome, ocular pemphigus, and so on. If the patient has acquired distichiasis with metaplasia of the meibomian glands, these fine hairs are excised after the lid is split.

Fig. 45-10, *E*, is a close-up appearance on the patient after Stevens-Johnson syndrome with metaplastic meibomian glands and severe entropion; *F*, post-operative view after the lids are opened.

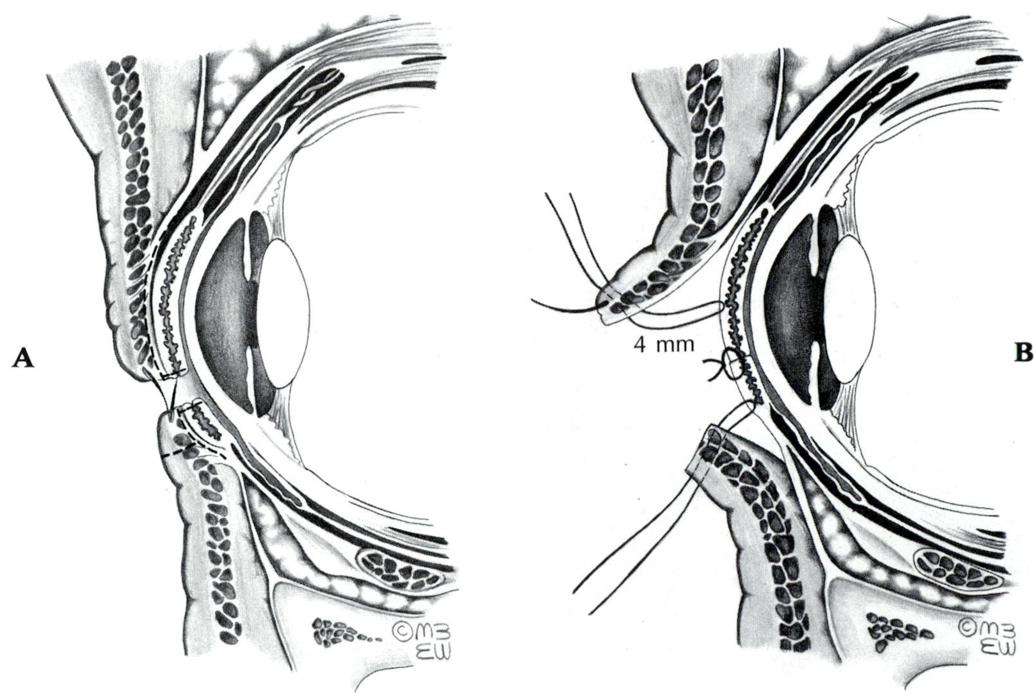

FIGURE 45-10. Severe upper and lower lid entropion repair.

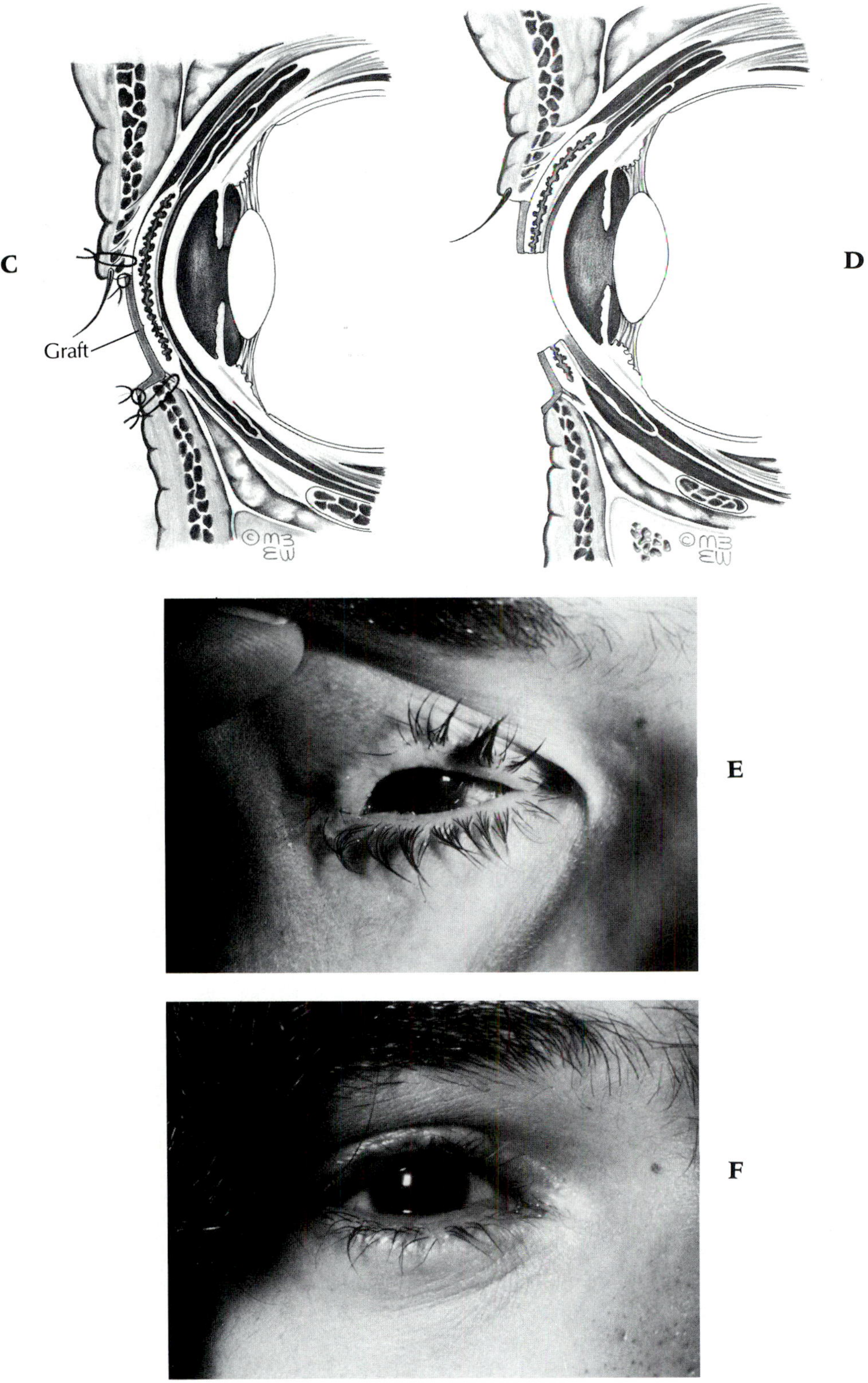
C
Graft
D
E
F

CHAPTER 46

Ectropion

Ectropion is divided into two parts: involutional and cicatricial. In my experience, involutional ectropion starts with a medial and superior shift of the lower lid as evidenced by the punctum moving in that direction. The upper lid can then slide behind the lower lid, and the resulting increasing ectropion is caused by the mechanical action of the upper lid pushing the lower lid margin away from the globe. At the completion of any corrective procedure for involutional ectropion, the upper lid should not be able to slide behind the lower lid. Failure to remedy this finding will usually result in a surgical failure.

Ectropion Repair

Mild lid laxity can be repaired as in Fig. 44-3. If there is punctal ectropion as well, the lower lid retractor shortening as described in Fig. 46-2 can be used. Because the lateral canthal sling procedure fixes the tarsus to the temporal periosteum, as the ectropion gets worse, the operation becomes easier. The fixation to the outside of the rim gives an excellent hold to the tarsus. Bringing the tarsus through the buttonhole of the upper lid places the lateral margin firmly against the globe.

Lateral Canthal Sling Procedure

A canthotomy is made to the orbital rim (Fig. 46-1, *A*). The inferior arm of the canthal tendon is then cut at the rim (Fig. 46-1, *B*). The lid is draped across the upper lid, and a point is marked on the lower lid where it crosses the beginning of the canthotomy of the upper lid (Fig. 46-1, *C*). Up to this point, the lid margin is removed (A in Fig. 46-1, *D*), the lashes are excised, the skin is separated from the muscle, and the conjunctiva is removed from the posterior surface of the tarsus (Fig. 46-1, *E*). A suture can be placed in the end of the tendon for easier handling of tissue (Fig. 46-1, *F*).

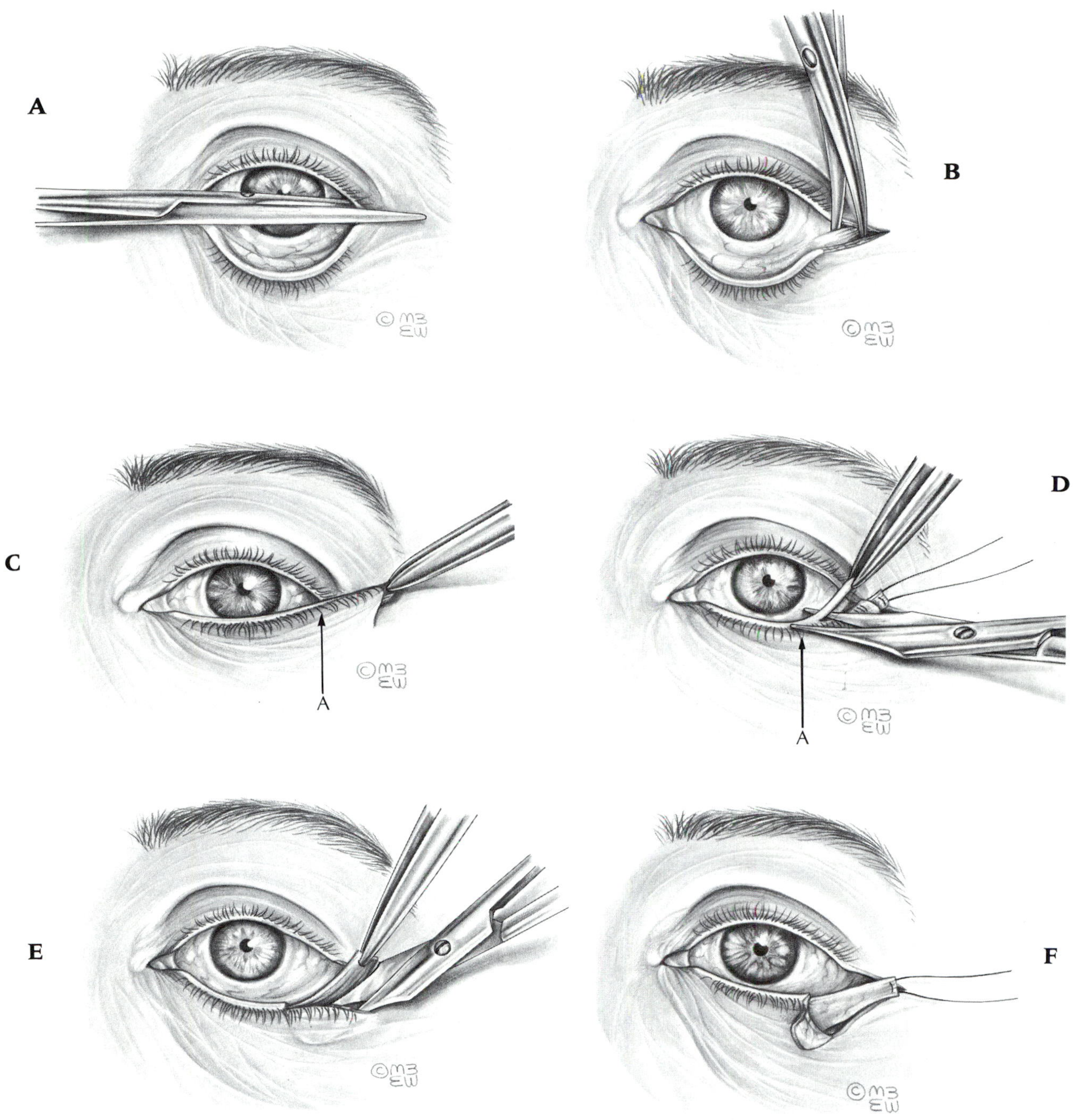

FIGURE 46-1. Lateral canthal sling.

Block shortening of the conjunctiva and lower lid retractors

If there is a severe marginal ectropion, an addition is made to the procedure with a 6 to 7 mm excision of conjunctiva and lower lid retractors. The conjunctiva is picked up 3.5 mm below the tarsus with two forceps. Two hemostats are placed across these tissues at the base of the tarsus, giving a 7 mm excision (Fig. 46-2, *A*). A 6-0 polypropylene (Prolene) suture enters the skin medially and comes out beneath the hemostat, goes beneath the hemostat at a 45-degree angle to exit through the other side, goes back in almost the same hole, again making a 45-degree path beneath the hemostat, and continues across the lid. This pattern leaves very little suture material on the conjunctival surface (Fig. 46-2, *B*). When the lateral end of the wound is reached, the suture is brought out on the skin and tied over a rubber band. The hemostats are removed, and the excess conjunctiva and lower lid retractors are excised (Fig. 46-2, *C*).

Fig. 46-2, *D,* is a full-face view showing severe marginal ectropion; *E* and *F,* preoperative close-up appearance; *G,* postoperative appearance of the patient; *H* and *I,* close-up appearance of the lids postoperatively.

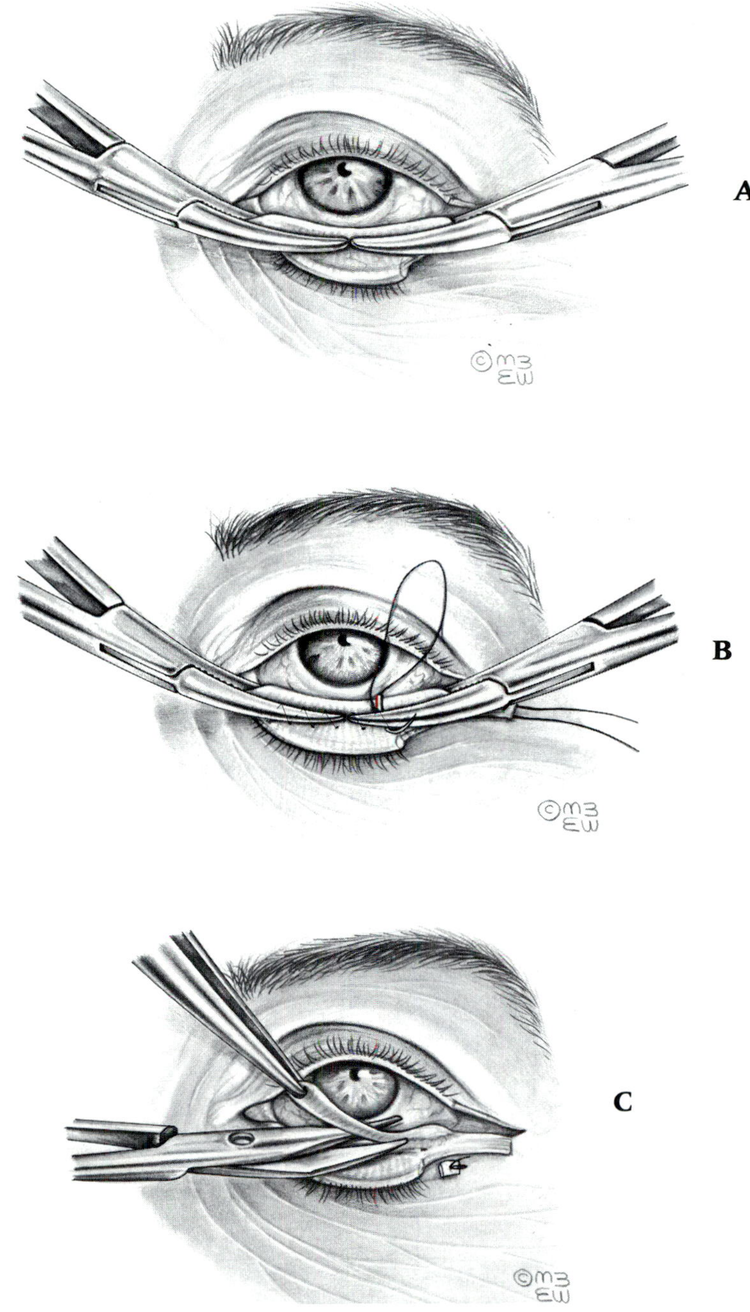

FIGURE 46-2. Lower lid posterior retractor repair.

Continued

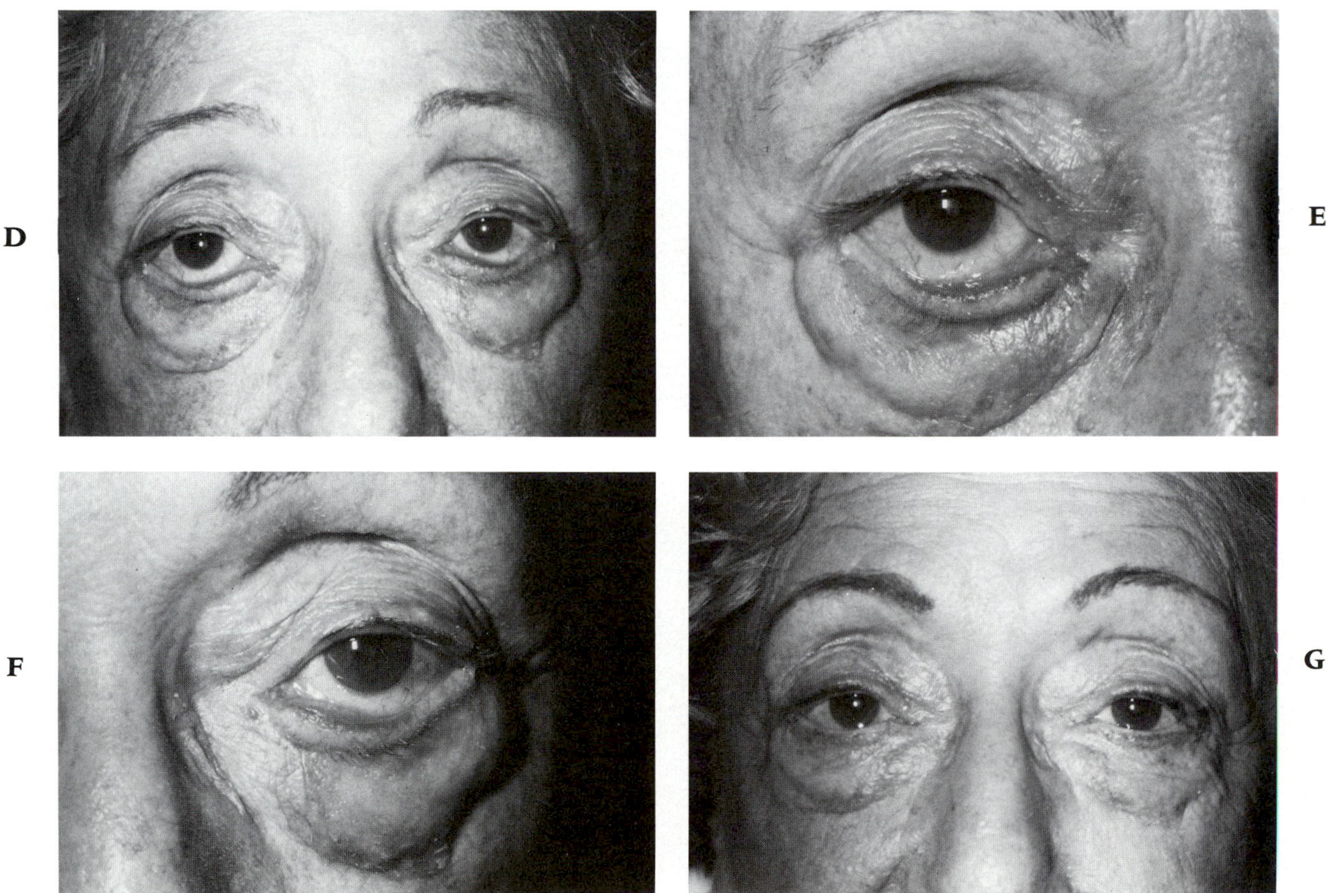

FIGURE 46-2, cont'd

H

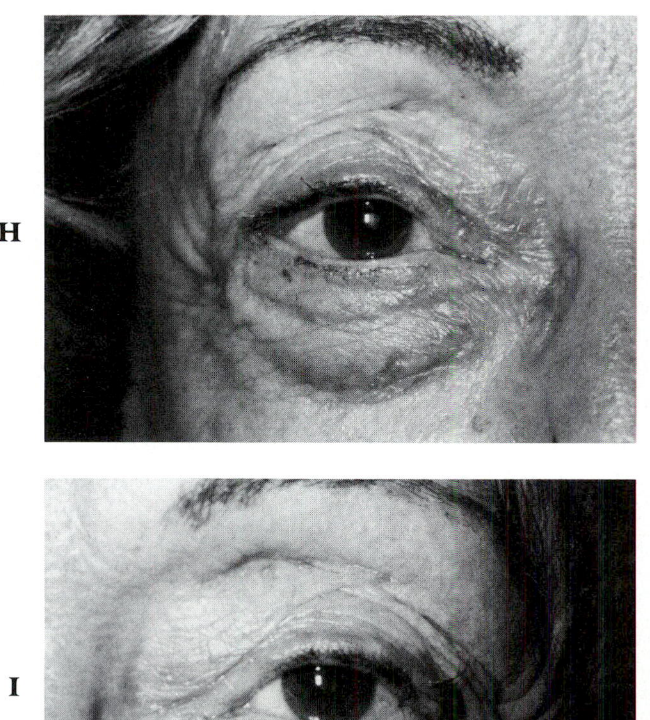

I

FIGURE 46-2, cont'd

Continuation of sling procedure

The periosteum is exposed at the lateral orbital rim (Fig. 46-3, *A*) by blunt dissection, and a buttonhole is made in the remaining arm of the canthal tendon (Fig. 46-3, *B*). The lower arm is brought through this buttonhole (Fig. 46-3, *C*) and sutured to the periosteum with a whip stitch of 5-0 nylon on a small half-circle spatula needle (Fig. 46-3, *D*). The level should correspond to the level of the lateral canthus on the fellow eye. A second suture is placed superiorly and temporally to the first suture just for better support (Fig. 46-3, *E*), and the lateral canthus is closed with a full-thickness vertical mattress suture tied over a cotton pledget (Fig. 46-3, *F*). This suture stays in place for 8 to 10 days. The remaining wound is closed with either deep sutures or 6-0 Vicryl and a continuous suture of 6-0 polypropylene on the skin or else near-far-far-near sutures of 6-0 polypropylene. These sutures and the continuous suture to the lower lid retractors are removed in 5 days.

Fig. 46-3, *G,* is the preoperative appearance of the patient before repair of the right lower lid; *H,* postoperative repair of the right lower lid.

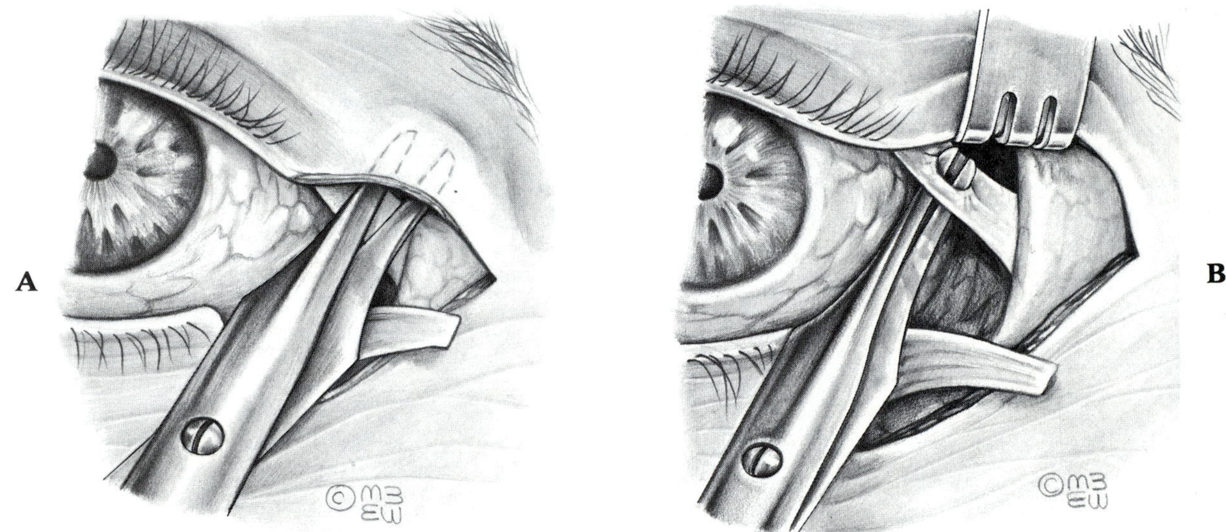

FIGURE 46-3. Continuation of sling procedure.

C

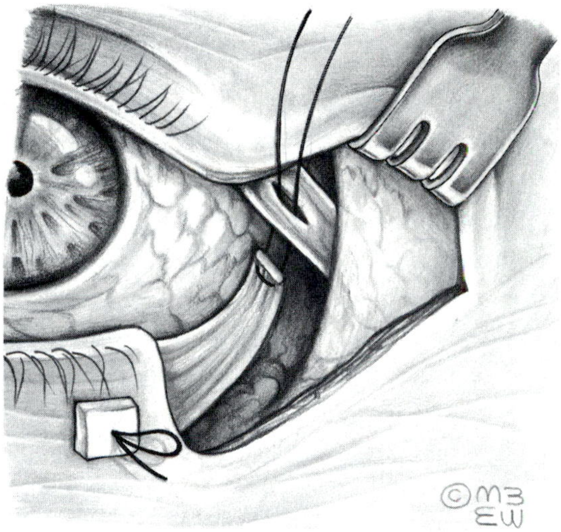

D

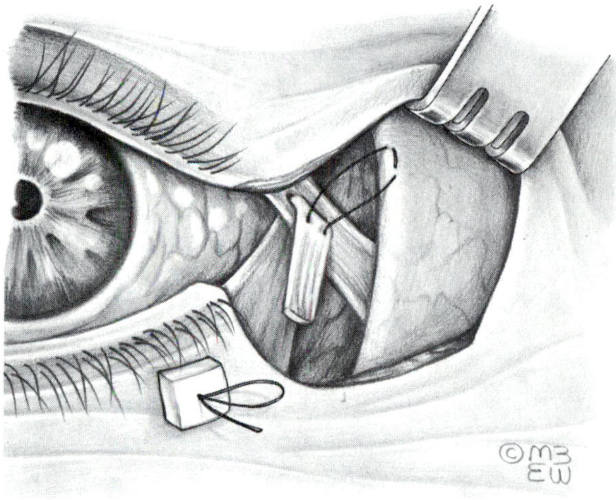

E

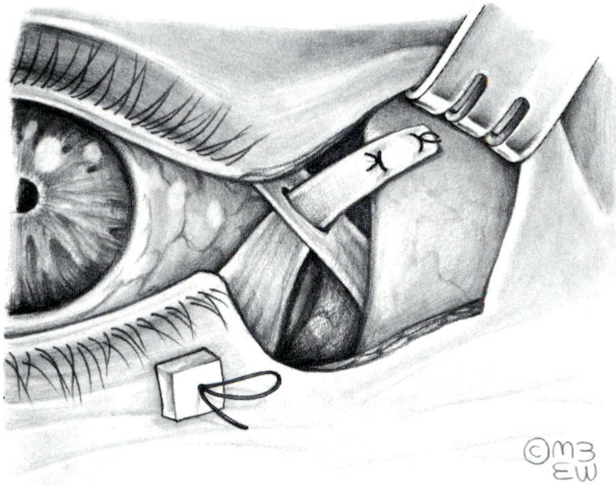

F

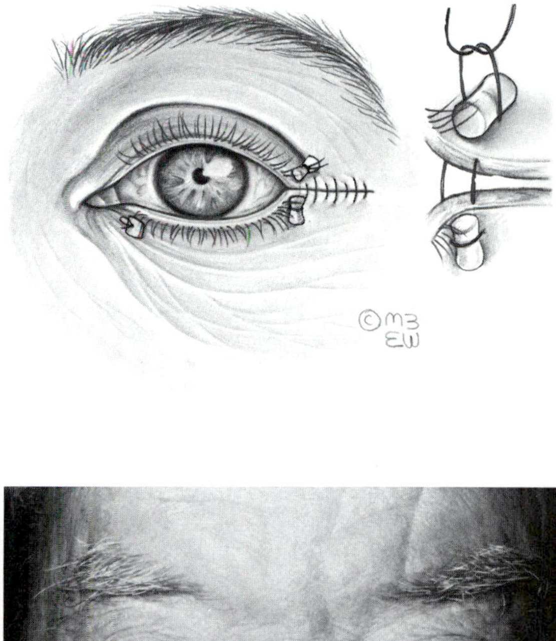

G

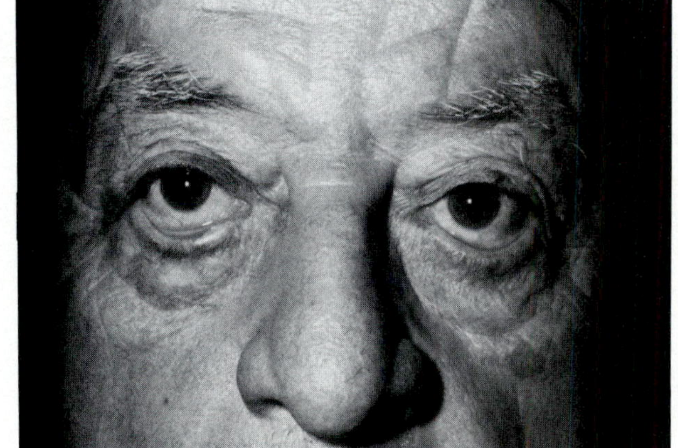

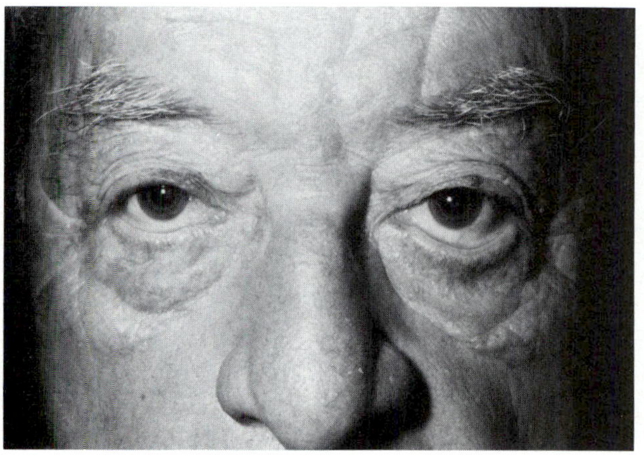

H

Cicatricial Ectropion

Lower lid ectropion

In a mild ectropion secondary to lid laxity, an incision is made beneath the lashes (Fig. 46-4, *A*) and the skin is undermined (Fig. 46-4, *B*). A tarsal tendon resection is done at the lateral canthus as described in Fig. 44-3. The skin is closed with a continuous 6-0 polypropylene suture (Fig. 46-4, *C*).

If there is a shortage of skin (Fig. 46-4, *D*), two 4-0 silk traction sutures are placed just beneath the lashes. Skin dissection is carried out until the lid can be brought up into the overcorrected position (Fig. 46-4, *E*). The tarsal tendon resection is performed as in Fig. 44-3, and the two traction sutures are used to bring the lid back into the overcorrected position. A large skin graft is placed into the defect and sutured with two continuous 6-0 polypropylene sutures. One arm of each of the 4-0 silk sutures is placed below the graft (Fig. 46-4, *F*). A Telfa bolus is inserted beneath these sutures, and the sutures are tied over the bolus (Fig. 46-4, *G*). The bolus is removed after 48 hours, and the graft sutures are removed in 5 to 7 days.

A basic rule of repair of cicatricial lower lid ectropion is to do a horizontal lid shortening. I now prefer to do this as described in Fig. 44-3, but the trans-marginal shortening can be performed as described in Fig. 44-5.

If the ectropion is after previous lower lid surgery and there was unrecognized laxity of the medial canthal tendon, this may have to be repaired also. This repair is described in Fig. 44-4.

Fig. 46-4, *H,* is a preoperative cicatricial ectropion of the right lower lid after blepharoplasty; *I,* close-up of the right eye; *J,* postoperative appearance of the patient; *K,* close-up of the right eye postoperatively.

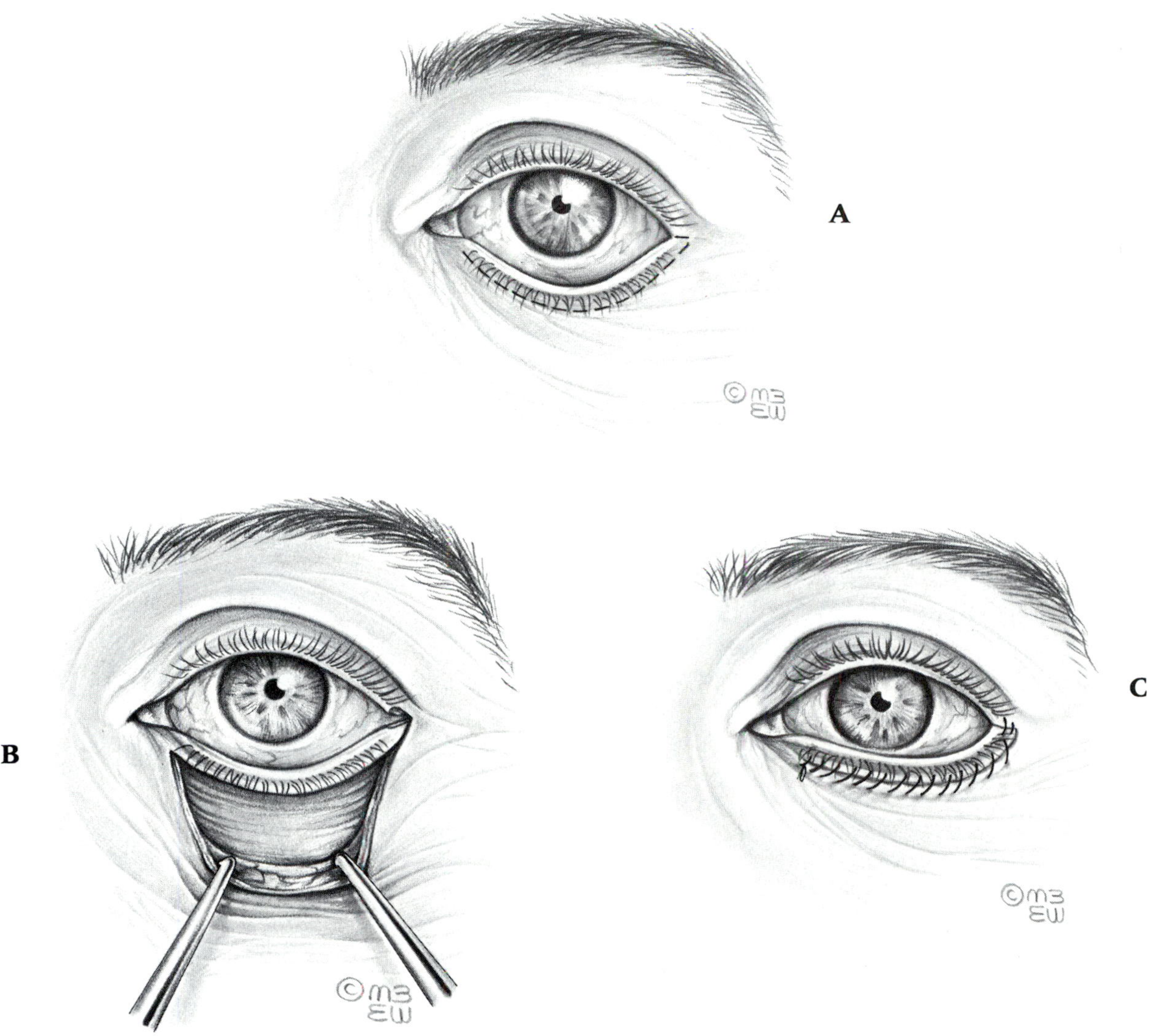

FIGURE 46-4. Cicatricial ectropion of the lower lid.

Continued.

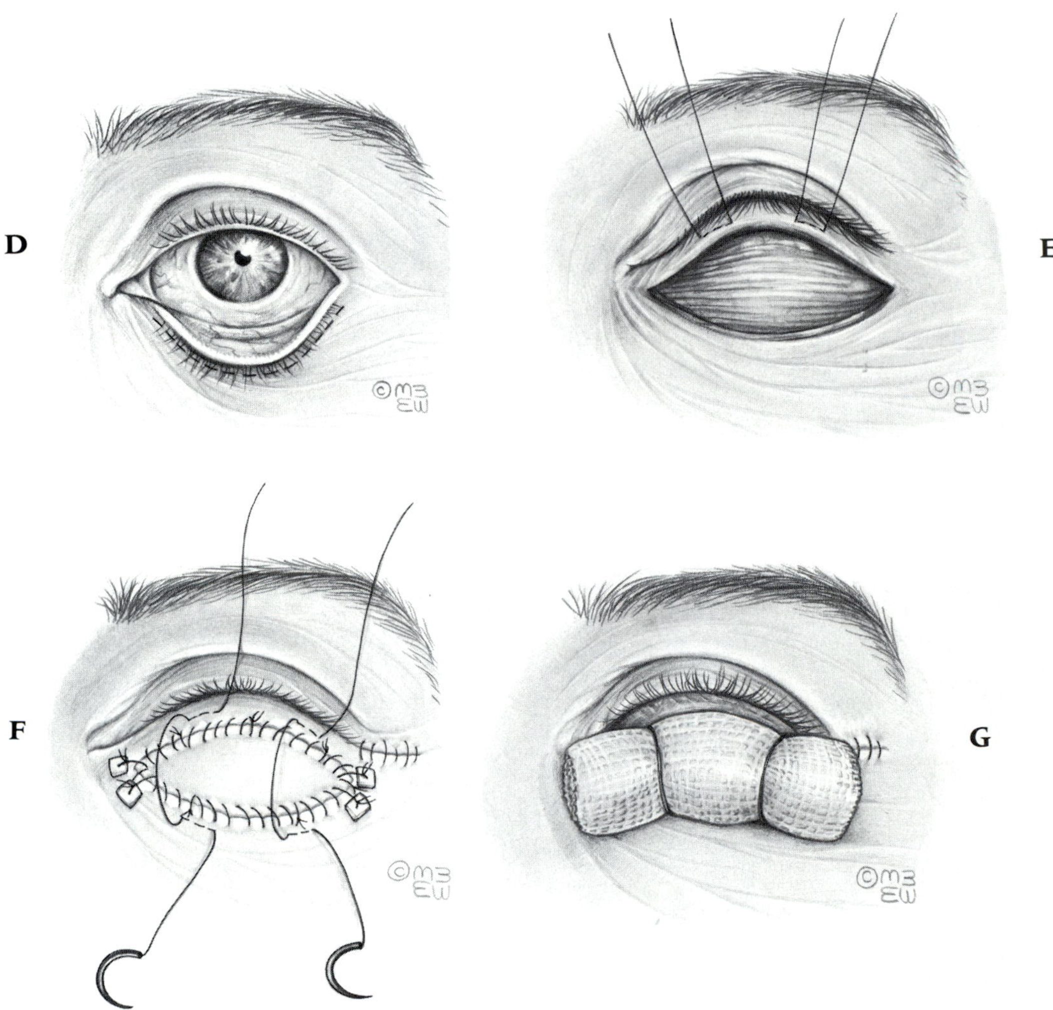

FIGURE 46-4, cont'd

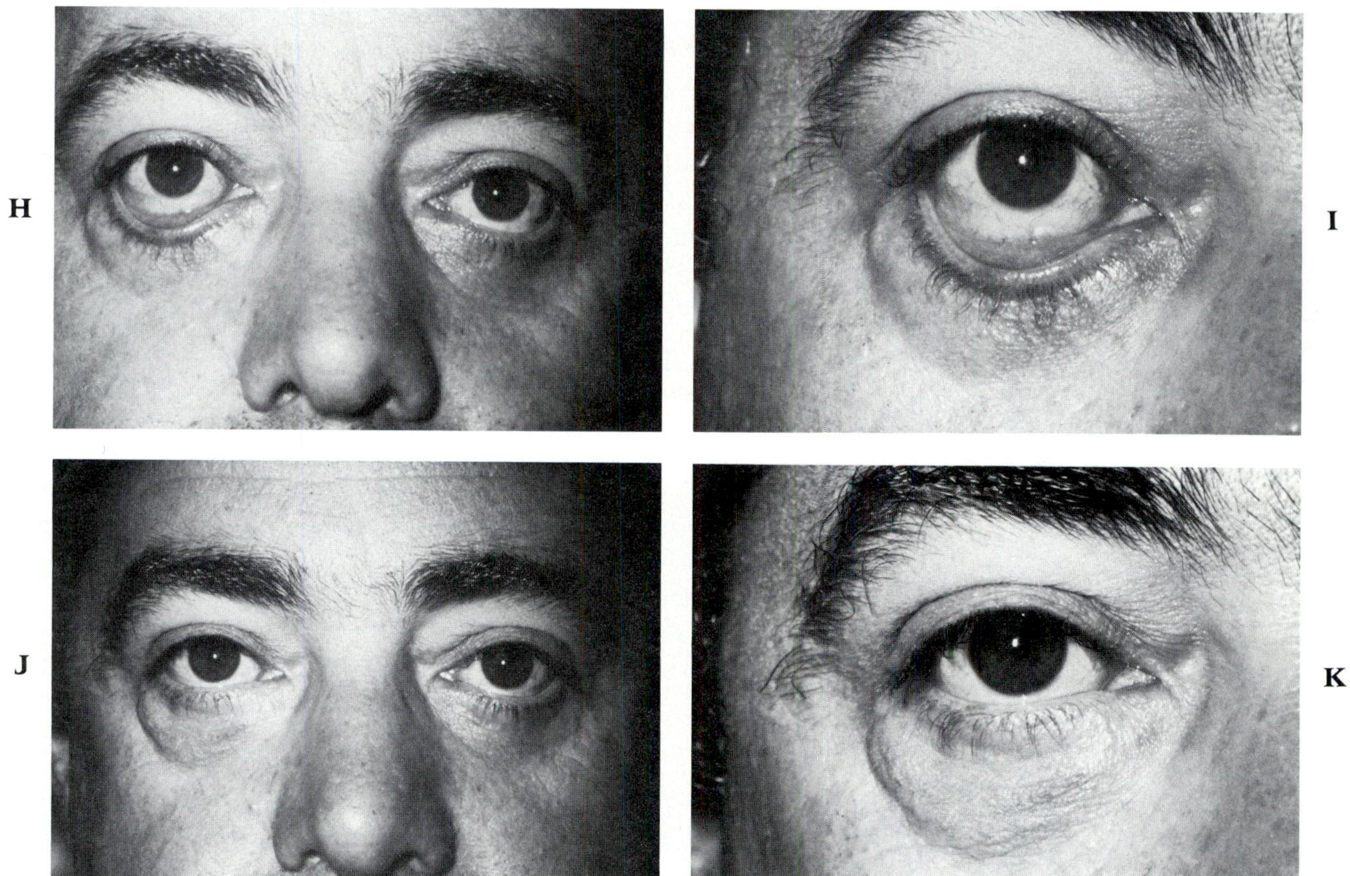

FIGURE 46-4, cont'd

Upper lid ectropion

Upper lid ectropion is usually secondary to a cicatrix. The lid may not be in the true ectropion position but just be unable to close. The basic rule in repair of ectropion of the upper lid is to open the orbital septum totally across the lid because the orbital septum is frequently shortened with the scar formation.

The scar (Fig. 46-5, *A*) is excised, and the orbital septum is opened (Fig. 46-5, *B*). The lid is brought down over the lower lid into an overcorrected position, and a graft is sutured into the defect with continuous sutures of 6-0 polypropylene. Two 4-0 silk sutures straddle the graft (Fig. 46-5, *C*). A Telfa bolus is placed beneath these sutures, and the sutures are tied over the bolus, which is removed after 48 to 72 hours (Fig. 46-5, *D*).

Fig. 46-5, *E*, shows a patient after having had a skin graft on the right upper lid for trauma, *F*, close-up on the right eye with attempted closure; *G*, after repair with a large skin graft; *H*, close-up demonstrating full closure postoperatively.

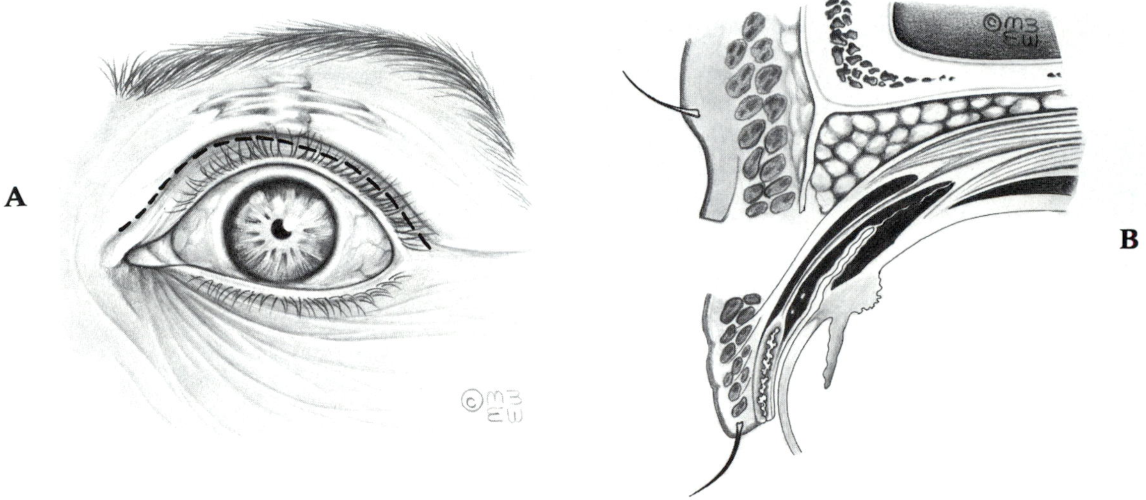

FIGURE 46-5. Cicatricial ectropion of the upper lid.

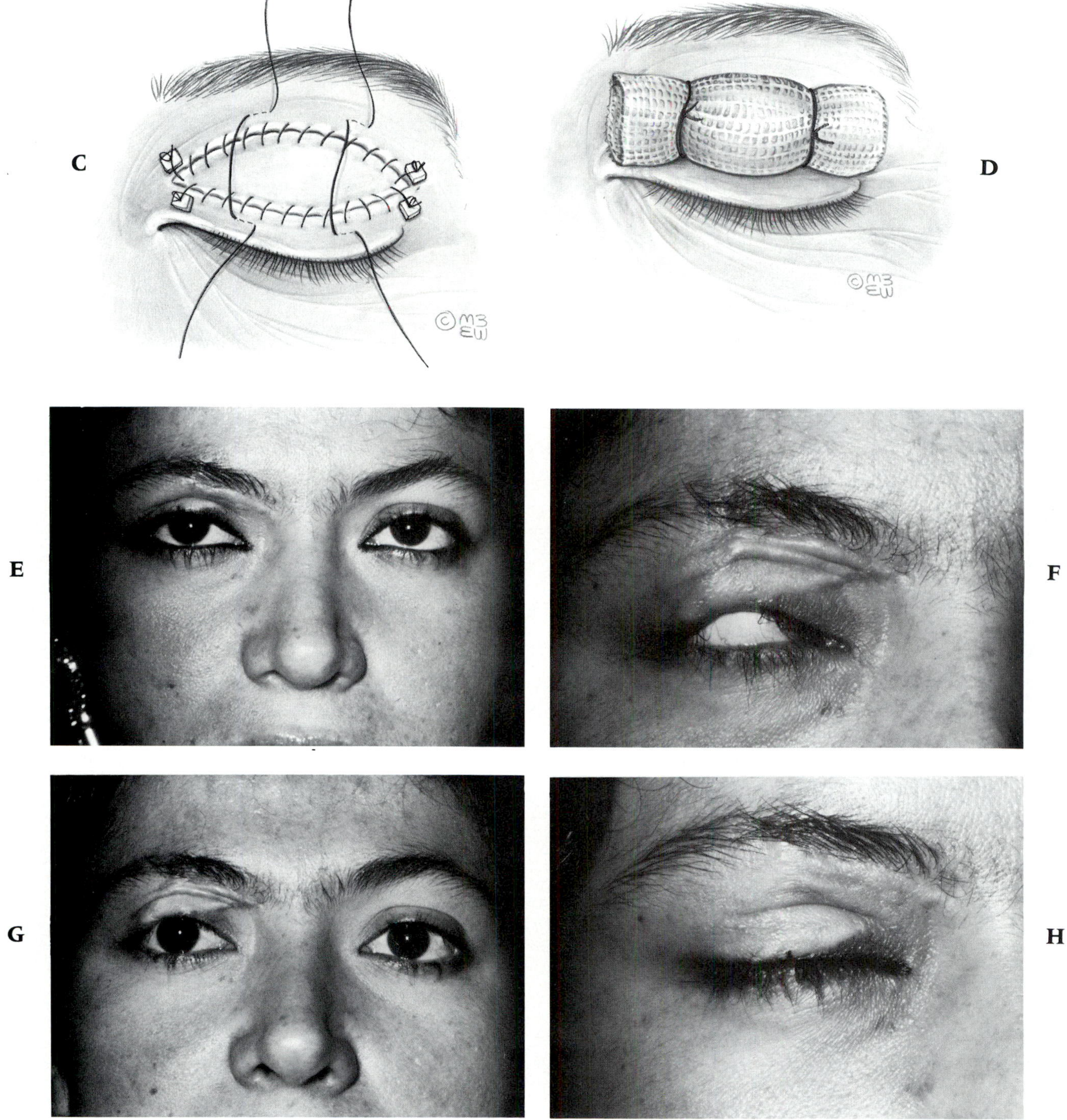
C
D
E
F
G
H

CHAPTER 47

Lid Reconstruction

Loss of a fourth of either the upper or lower lid can usually be repaired by primary closure described in Fig. 44-5.

Larger defects, up to half of the lid, that cannot be closed primarily can be repaired with a semicircular flap (Figs. 47-1 and 47-2) *if* they have at least 2 mm of normal lateral lid margin remaining. Frequently, up to two thirds of a lower lid defect can be repaired with this flap.

If the defect extends into the lateral canthus, the temporal hinged tarsal conjunctival flap (Fig. 47-3) is my procedure of choice. I prefer this technique on those patients who have enough skin to repair the anterior lamella as an advancement skin flap.

In extensive defects of the lower lid, or where there is not enough skin to repair the anterior lamella as an advancement flap, the use of the superiorly hinged tarsal conjunctival flap is preferred (Fig. 47-4). This same type of flap is also used for reconstruction of a lid defect extending into the medial (Fig. 47-5) and lateral (Fig. 47-6) canthi.

Semicircular Flap for Lower Lid Defects

Fig. 47-1, *A,* illustrates a defect in the lower lid of a half to two thirds of the horizontal lid margin. Outline a skin-muscle flap starting at the lateral canthus. The flap does not extend beyond the line that would be the continuation of the eyebrow inferiorly. The skin muscle flap is retracted inferiorly, and a canthotomy to the orbital rim is performed at the lateral canthus (Fig. 47-1, *B*). The canthal tendon to the lower lid is cut at the orbital rim. A triangulation is taken out of the bottom of the lid margin defect (Fig. 47-1, *C*), and the defect is closed as one would a primary laceration (Fig. 44-5). It is most important that the new lower lid margin be extremely tight. The lid is pulled firmly temporally, and where it crosses the beginning of the canthotomy of the upper lid, the lateral canthus is reformed with a full-thickness vertical mattress suture (Fig. 47-1, *D*). The suture goes full thickness through the normal upper lid, coming out on the conjunctiva, takes a deep bite of the new lid, and comes back with a partial-thickness bite in the tendon at the angle. Either the skin muscle flap is brought back into position and closed with vertical mattress sutures of 6-0 silk, or the muscle layer is closed with buried sutures of 6-0 Vicryl and the skin is closed with a continuous suture of 6-0 Prolene.

Fig. 47-1, *E,* is the preoperative appearance of the patient with a basal cell carcinoma of the right lower lid; *F,* close-up of the right eye preoperatively; *G,* postoperative appearance; *H,* close-up of the right eye after semicircular flap.

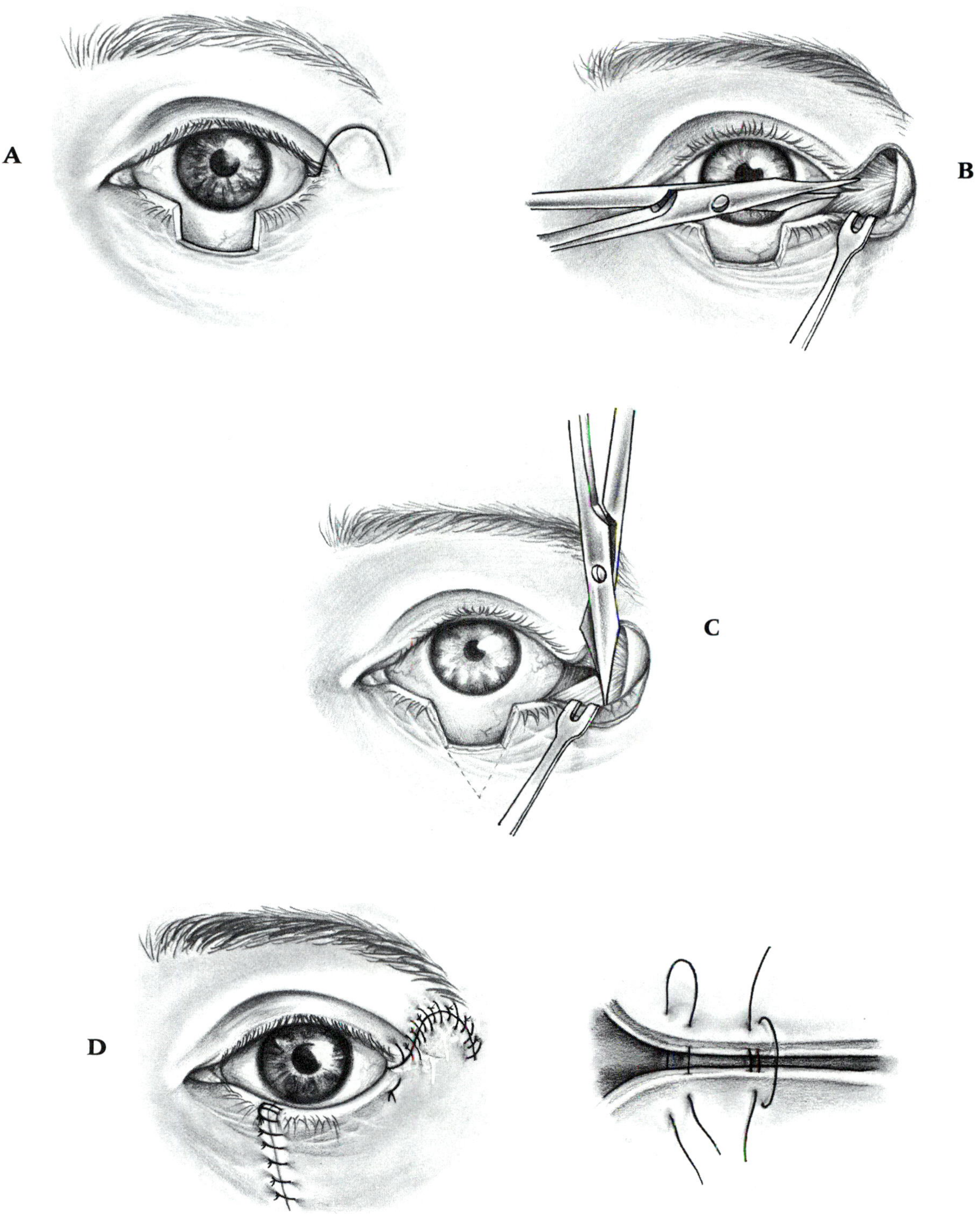

FIGURE 47-1. Semicircular flap for lower lid.

Continued.

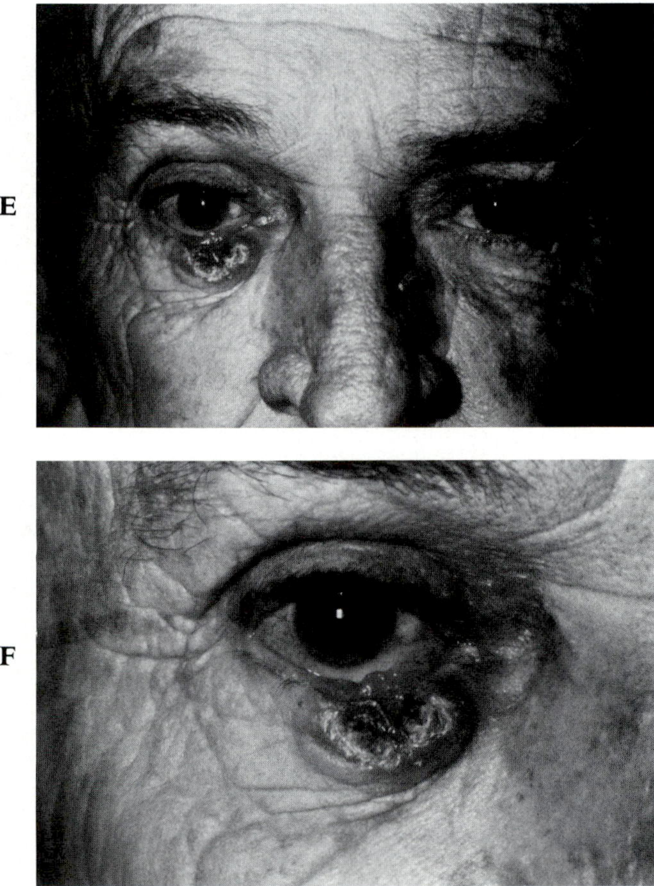

FIGURE 47-1, cont'd

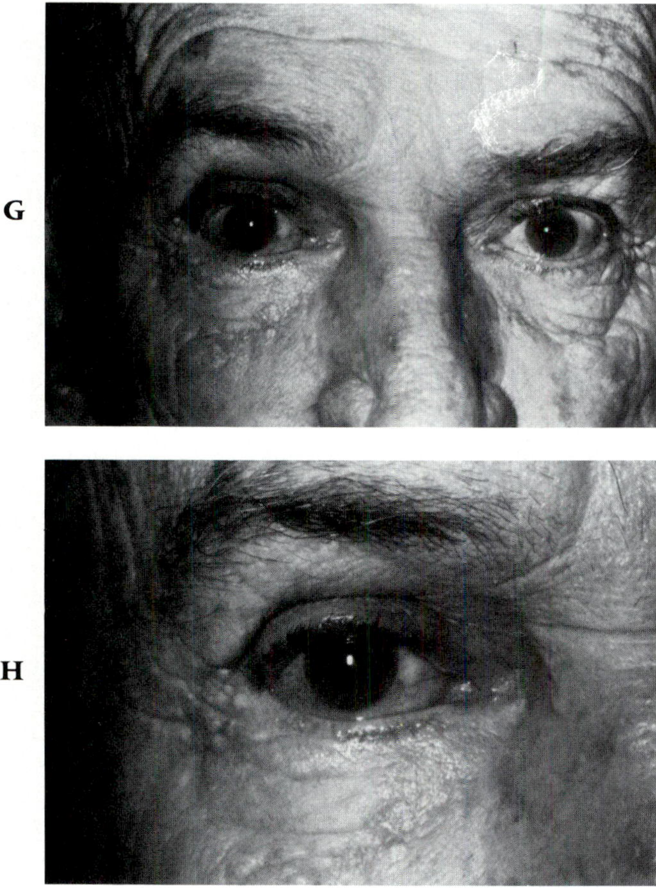

FIGURE 47-1, cont'd

Semicircular Flap for Upper Lid Defects

This repair is almost exactly like that described for the lower lid defects (Fig. 47-1) except in the upside-down position. Fig. 47-2, *A,* illustrates a defect in the upper lid from a fourth to a half of the lid. A skin-muscle flap is outlined at the lateral canthus. This flap does not extend beyond the line that would be the continuation of the eyebrow inferiorly. The skin-muscle flap is retracted superiorly, and a canthotomy to the orbital rim is performed at the lateral canthus (Fig. 47-2, *B*). The canthal tendon to the upper lid is cut at the orbital rim. A triangulation is taken out of the top of the lid margin defect (Fig. 47-2, *C*), and the defect is closed as one would a normal laceration (Fig. 44-5). The new lid margin is elevated to the limbus, and where the new lid crosses the beginning of the canthotomy in the lower lid, the lateral canthus is reformed with a full-thickness vertical mattress suture (Fig. 47-2, *D*). The suture goes full thickness through the normal lid, coming out on the conjunctiva, takes a deep bite of the new lid, and comes back with a partial-thickness bite in the lower tendon at the angle. The skin-muscle flap is brought back into position and closed with either vertical mattress sutures, or the muscle layer is closed with buried sutures of 6-0 Vicryl and the skin is closed with a continuous suture of 6-0 polypropylene.

The skin sutures are removed in 4 to 5 days, and the lateral canthal angle suture and lid margin sutures are removed in 8 to 10 days.

Fig. 47-2, *E,* is the preoperative appearance with a basal cell carcinoma occupying the lateral half of the left upper lid; *F,* close-up of the eye preoperatively; *G,* postoperative appearance; *H,* close-up of the eye postoperatively.

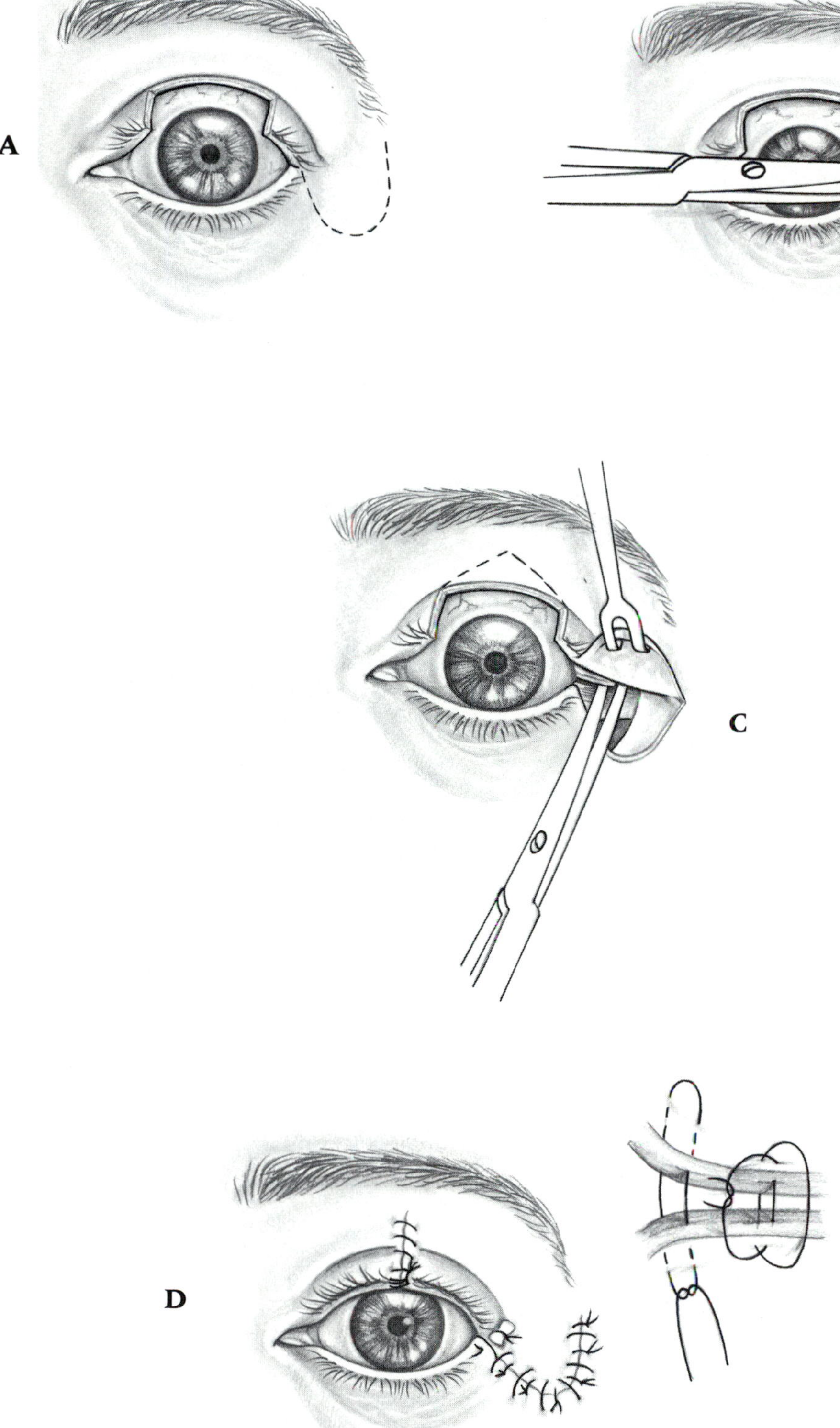

FIGURE 47-2. Semicircle flap for upper lid.

Continued.

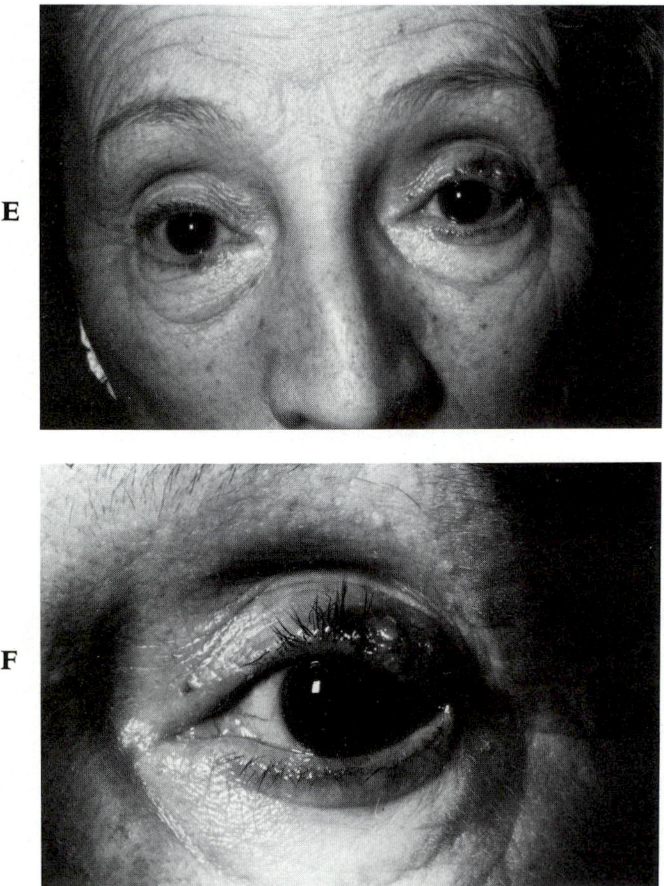

FIGURE 47-2, cont'd

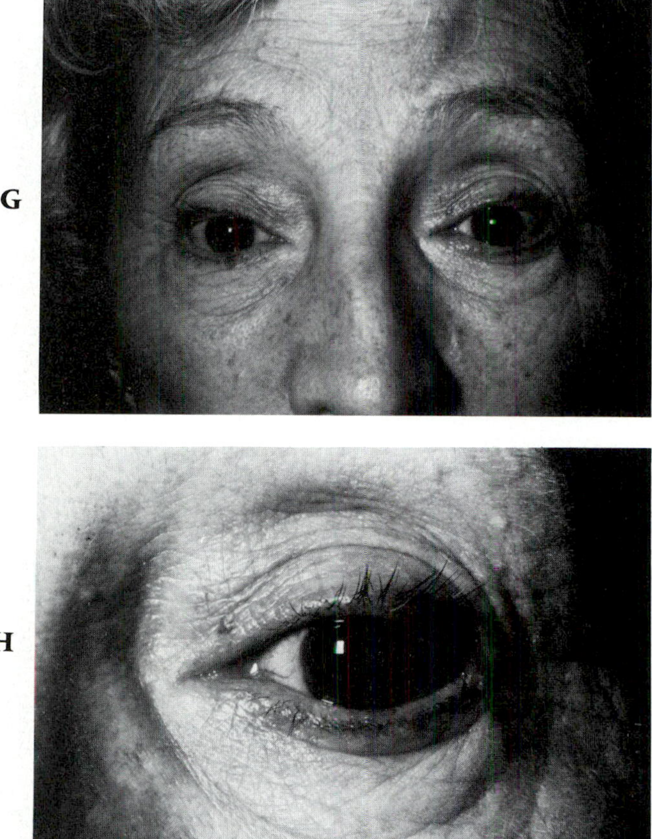

FIGURE 47-2, cont'd

Temporal Hinged Tarsal Conjunctival Flap

A 3 to 4 mm wide tarsal conjunctival flap is taken from the midportion of the tarsus of the upper lid (Fig. 47-3, *A*) and is left with its blood supply coming from the lateral portion of the wound rather than superiorly. The flap is rotated into position in the defect of the lower lid (Fig. 47-3, *B*) and is anchored as described in Fig. 47-4, *E* to *G*. The upper wound is closed with partial-thickness tarsal interrupted sutures of 6-0 polypropylene that are tied on the skin. The partial-thickness tarsal bites prevent corneal abrasion. The anterior lamella is repaired with an advancement skin flap inferiorly (Fig. 47-3, *C*). The wound is closed (Fig. 47-3, *D*) with interrupted sutures of 7-0 silk.

Fig. 47-3, *E*, is the preoperative appearance of a basal cell occupying the lateral two thirds of the right lower lid; *F*, close-up of the eye preoperatively; *G*, postoperative appearance after a Beard-Hewes tarsoconjunctival flap; *H*, post-operative close-up of the eye.

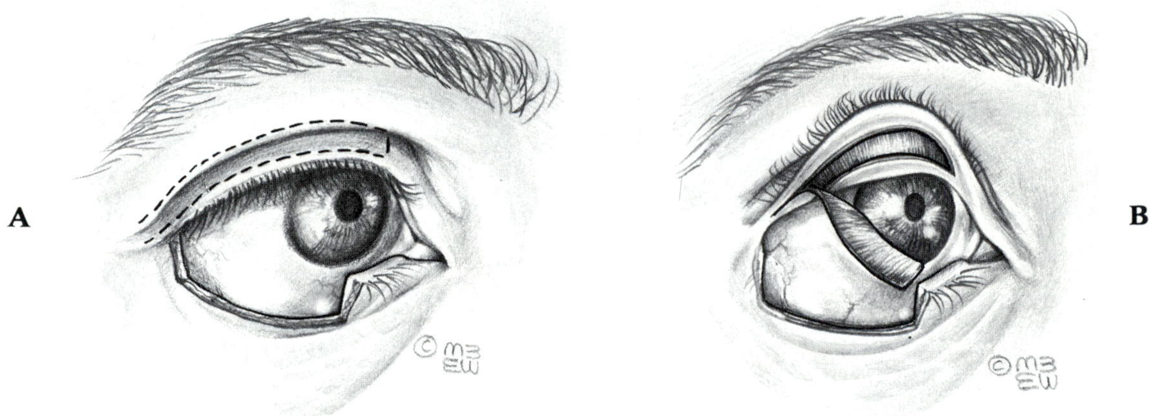

FIGURE 47-3. Beard-Hewes tarsoconjunctival flap for lower lids. (From Smith BC, Della Rocca RC, Nesi FA, Lisman RD: Ophthalmic plastic and reconstructive surgery, St Louis, 1987, The CV Mosby Co.)

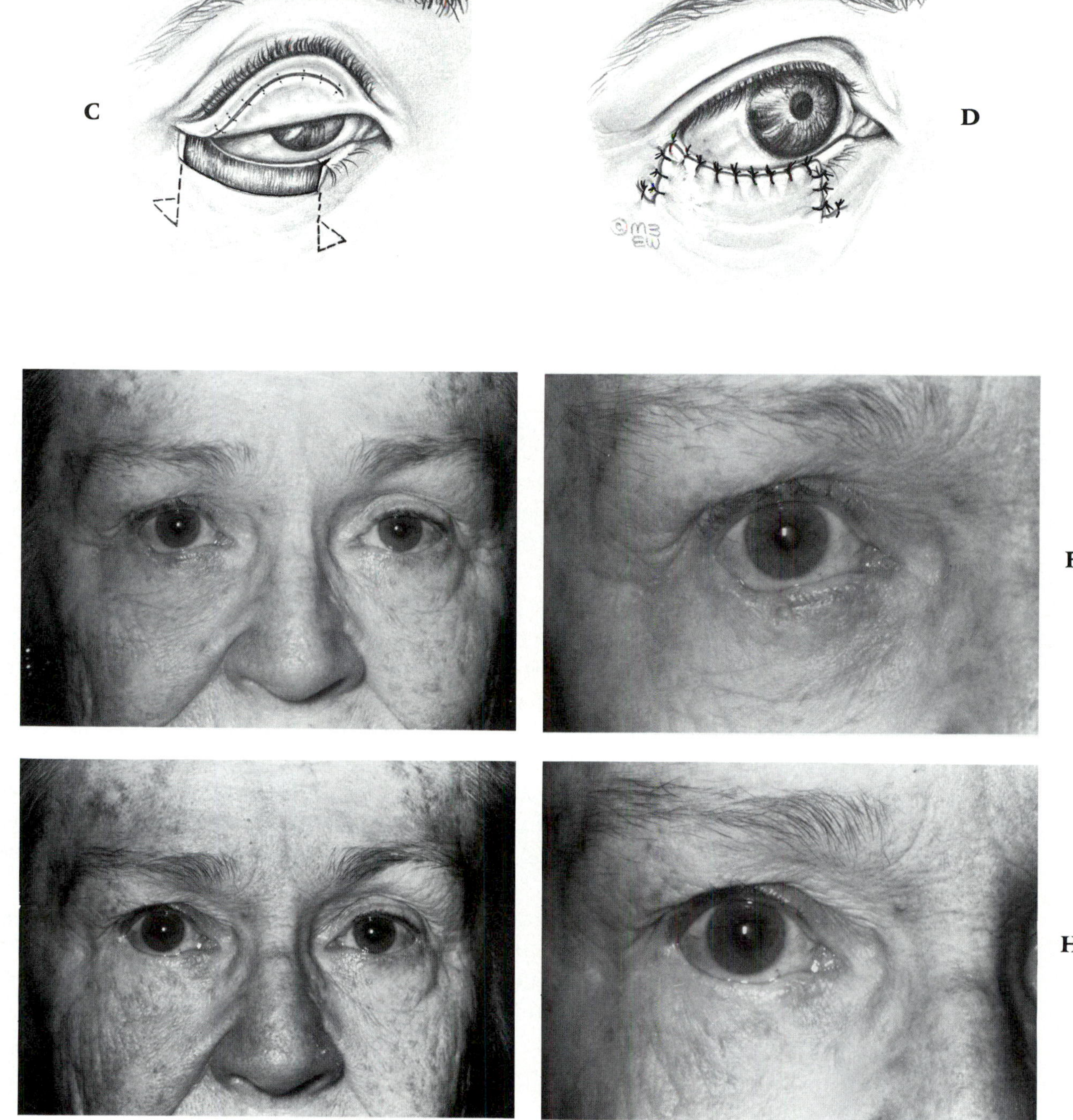
C
D
E
F
G
H

Tarsal Conjunctival Flap for Lower Lid Defects

Fig. 47-4, *A*, illustrates a tumor to be excised. The tumor is excised and the lids are pulled together to allow one to see the minimal amount of tarsal conjunctival flap necessary for a lid reconstruction (Fig. 47-4, *B*). The tarsal conjunctival flap is outlined in the lid (Fig. 47-4, *C*), staying 3 mm from the lid margin. Fig. 47-4, *D*, shows a profile of the incision. The dotted lines indicate the plane of dissection. If Müller's muscle is to be included in the tarsal conjunctival flap, dissection is carried between Müller's muscle and the conjunctiva. If Müller's muscle is to be left in place, dissection is between Müller's muscle and the levator aponeurosis. The tarsal conjunctival flap is brought into the lower lid (Fig. 47-4, *E*). The inferior margin of the flap is sutured to the conjunctiva and the lower lid retractors with a continuous suture of 8-0 chromic. A side view of the tarsal conjunctival flap extending down to the lower lid is illustrated in Fig. 47-4, *F*. The tarsal conjunctival flap is anchored to the remaining lower lid (Fig. 47-4, *G*). The lid is split at the gray line for a distance of 2 to 3 mm. Each arm of a double-arm 6-0 silk suture enters the skin of the lid, exits the apex to the groove, takes a full-thickness bite in the tarsal conjunctival flap, reenters the apex of the wound, and exits on the skin where the suture is tied over a cotton bolus. The anterior lamella is repaired with an advancement flap of the lower lid (Fig. 47-4, *H*) or free skin graft (Fig. 47-4, *I*).

In 4 to 6 weeks the tarsal conjunctival flap is opened where it exits at the tarsus (Fig. 47-4, *J*). The lower lid is left slightly on the high side, approximately 1 mm, to allow for slight contracture. The rest of the flap is trimmed for the contour of the lower lid. The patient is asked to open the eyes, and the contour of the upper lid is checked to the fellow eye (Fig. 47-4, *K*). If there is elevation or notching of the upper lid, the lid is everted over a Desmarres retractor (Fig. 47-4, *L*), and all scar bands to the lid are separated. This is especially true of the medial and lateral corners from where the flap was taken. This dissection is continued until the contour and elevation of the operated eye matches the fellow eye (Fig. 47-4, *M*).

Fig. 47-4, *N*, is the preoperative appearance of a patient with a tumor occupying two thirds of the right lower lid; *O*, close-up of the eye preoperatively; *P*, postoperative appearance after resection of two thirds of the lower lid and repair with a tarsoconjunctival flap and a free skin graft; *Q*, close-up of the eye postoperatively.

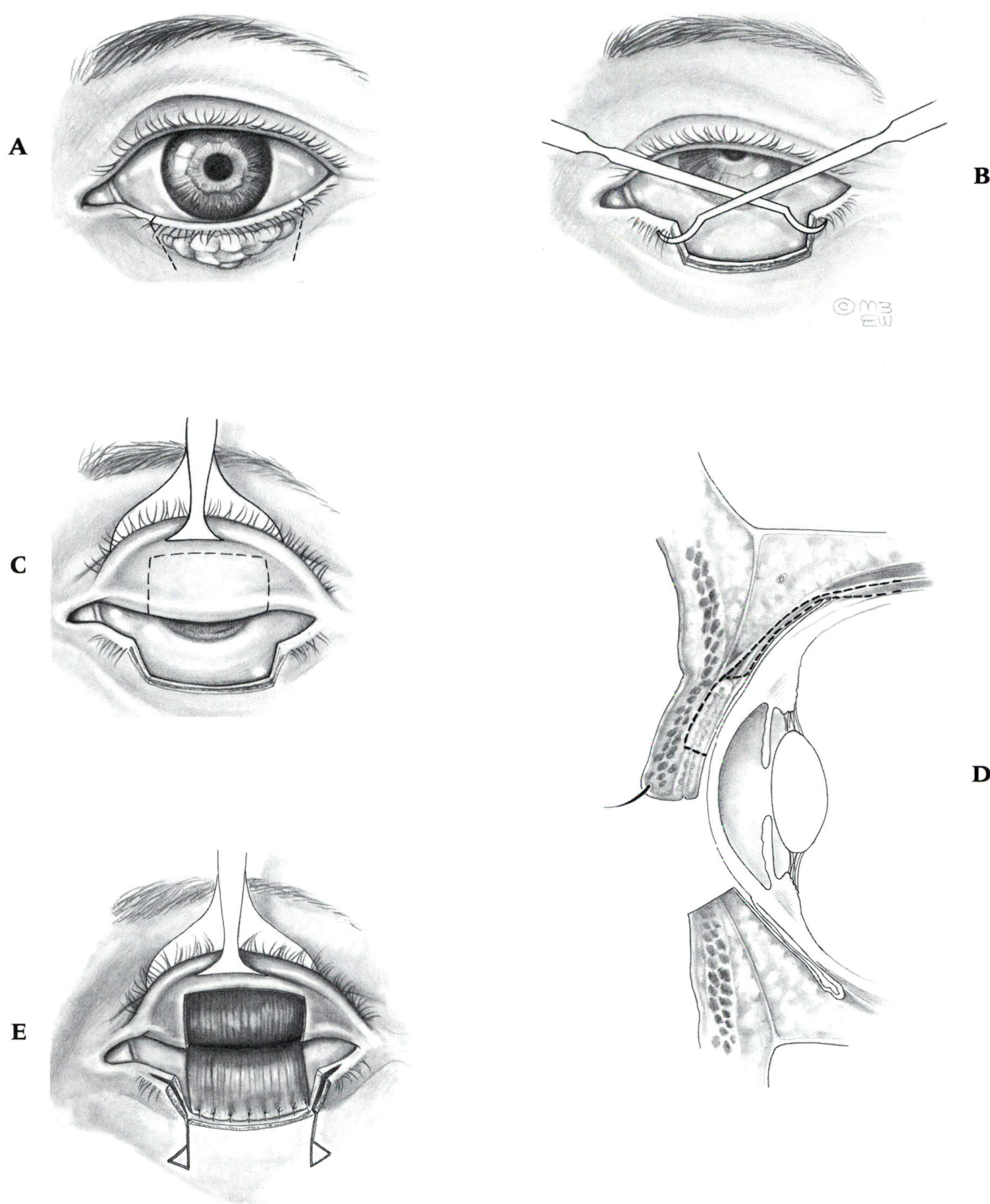

FIGURE 47-4. Tarsoconjunctival flap for lower lids after Köllner-Hughes technique. (From Smith BC, Della Rocca RC, Nesi FA, and Lisman RD: Ophthalmic plastic and reconstructive surgery, St Louis, 1987, The CV Mosby Co.)

Continued.

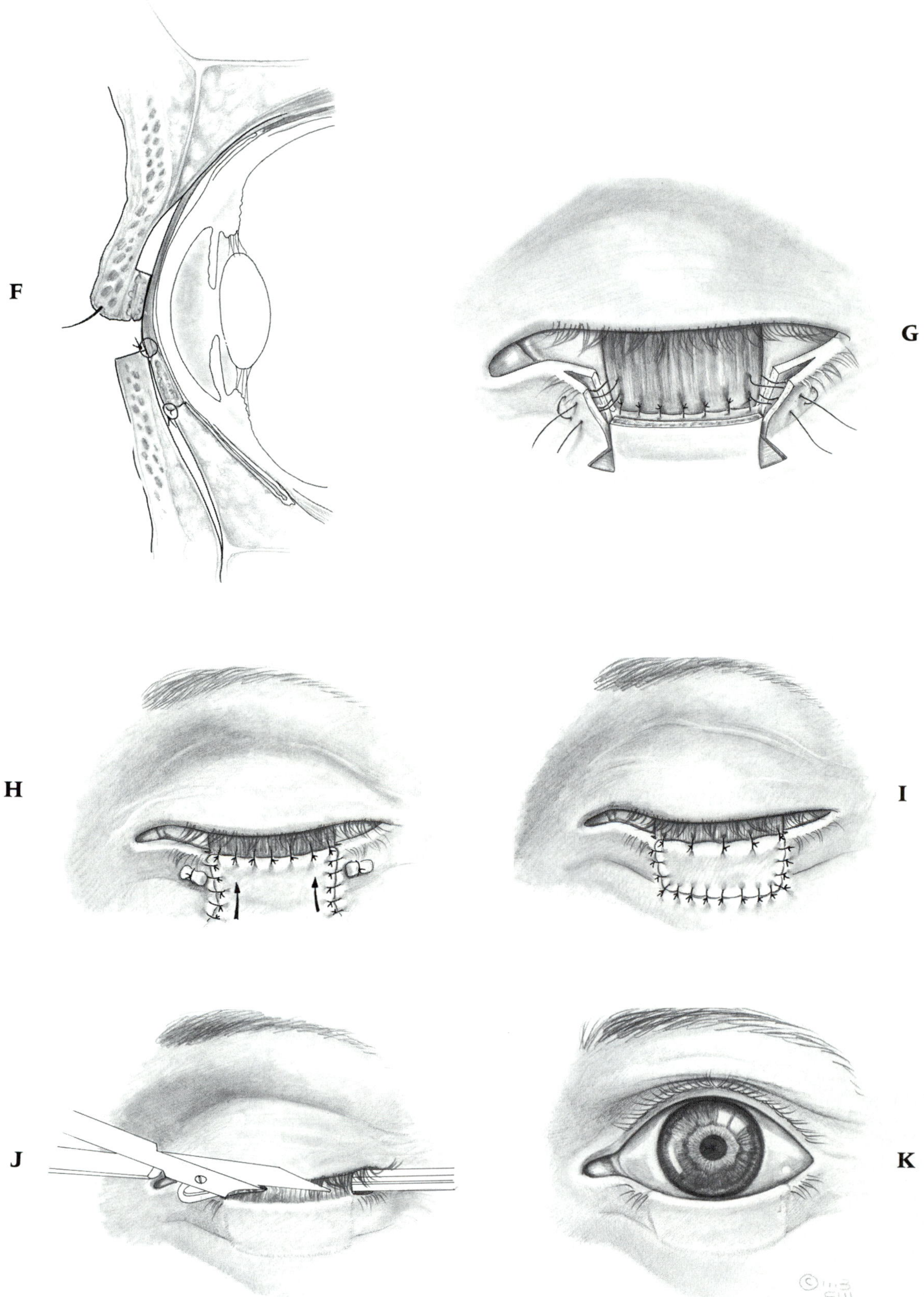

FIGURE 47-4, cont'd

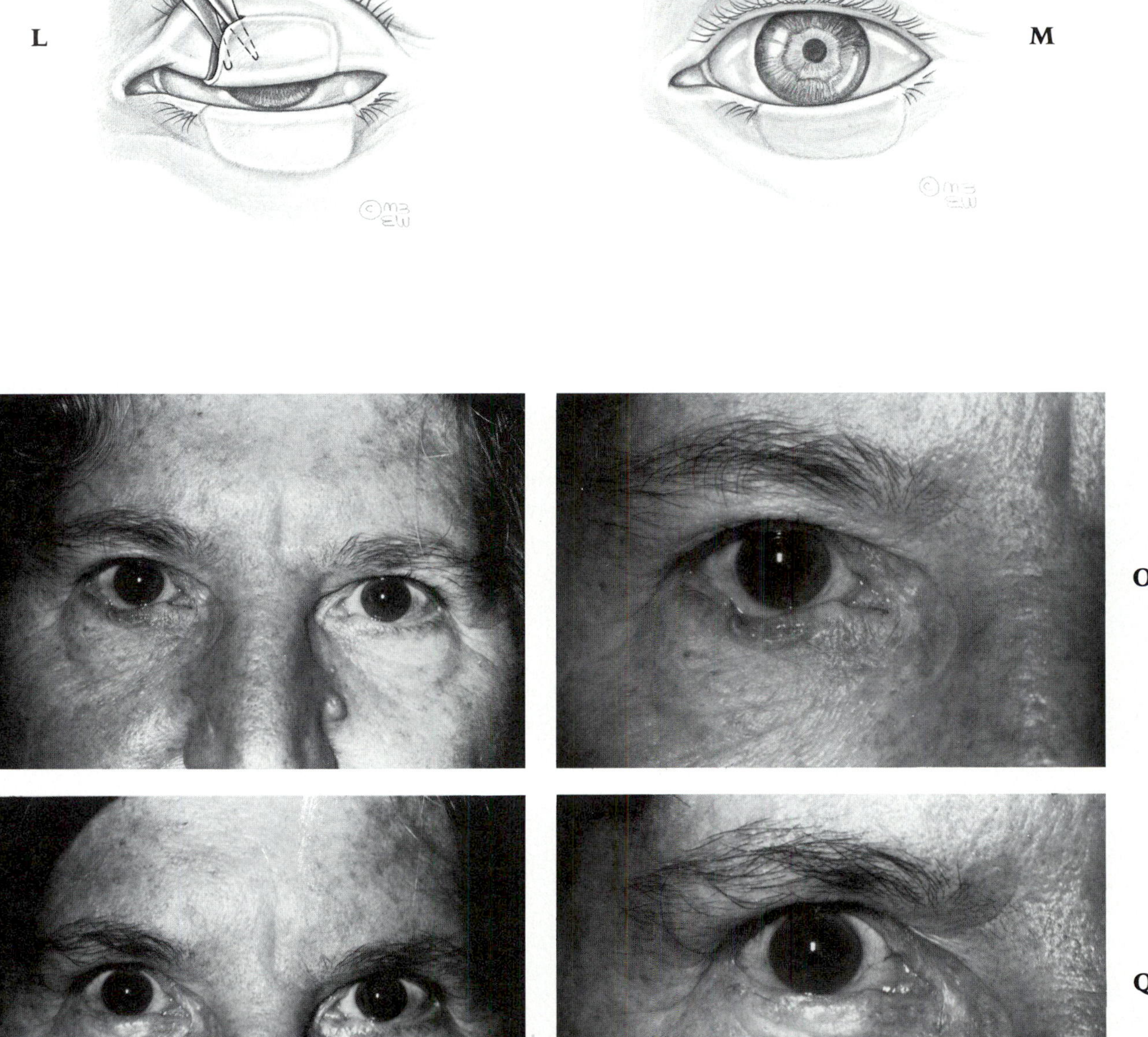

FIGURE 47-4 cont'd

Tarsal Conjunctival Flap for Lower Lid and Medial Canthal Defects

The tumor is outlined (Fig. 47-5, *A*) and excised (Fig. 47-5, *B*). The tarsal conjunctival flap is taken from the remaining lid (Fig. 47-5, *C*), staying 3 mm from the lid margin. The flap is rotated into position (Fig. 47-5, *D*) and anchored to the medial periosteum or bone. The periosteum can be brought over as a flap to form a new medial canthal tendon (Fig. 47-5, *E*). The lateral portion of the tarsal conjunctival flap is anchored into the remaining lid as described in Fig. 47-4, *E* to *G*. The anterior lamella is repaired with a free skin graft. The graft is sutured into place with a few interrupted sutures of 7-0 silk and then continuous sutures of 6-0 polypropylene. Silk sutures, 4-0, are placed in the skin straddling the graft (Fig. 47-5, *F*), a Telfa bolus is placed under the sutures, and the sutures are tied over the bolus (Fig. 47-5, *G*). This bolus is left in place for 48 to 72 hours. The opening of the tarsal conjunctival flap is accomplished as in Fig. 47-4, *J* to *M*.

Fig. 47-5, *H,* is the preoperative appearance of a patient with a recurrent basal cell carcinoma occupying the medial third of the upper lid, the medial canthus, and two thirds of the lower lid; *I,* close-up of the eye preoperatively; *J,* postoperative appearance after tarsoconjunctival flap and free skin graft from beneath the arm; *K,* close-up of the eye postoperatively.

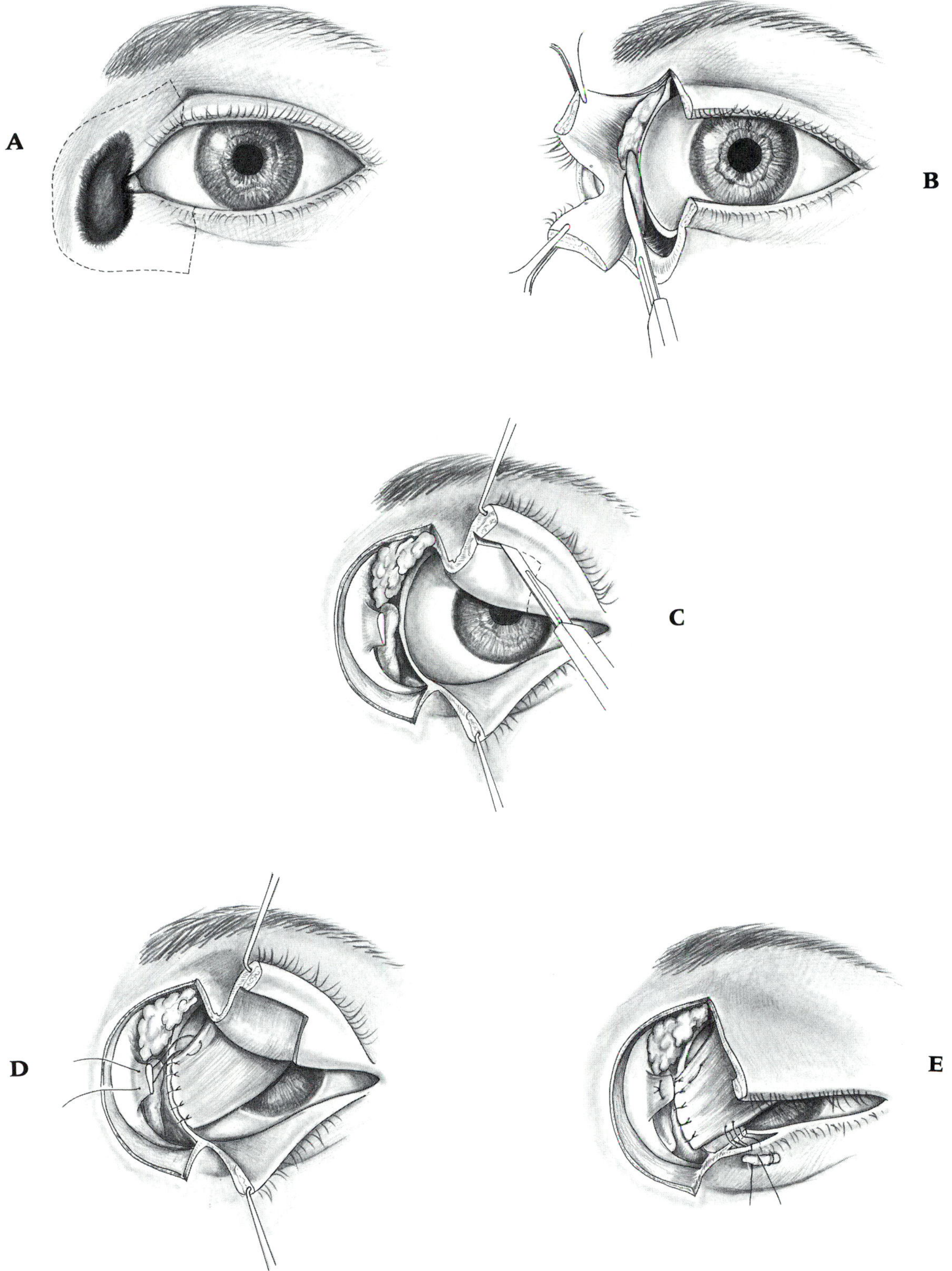

FIGURE 47-5. Smith modification, tarsoconjunctival flap for medial canthus and lower lid. (From Smith BC, Della Rocca RC, Nesi FA, and Lisman RD: Ophthalmic plastic and reconstructive surgery, St Louis, 1987, The CV Mosby Co.)

Continued.

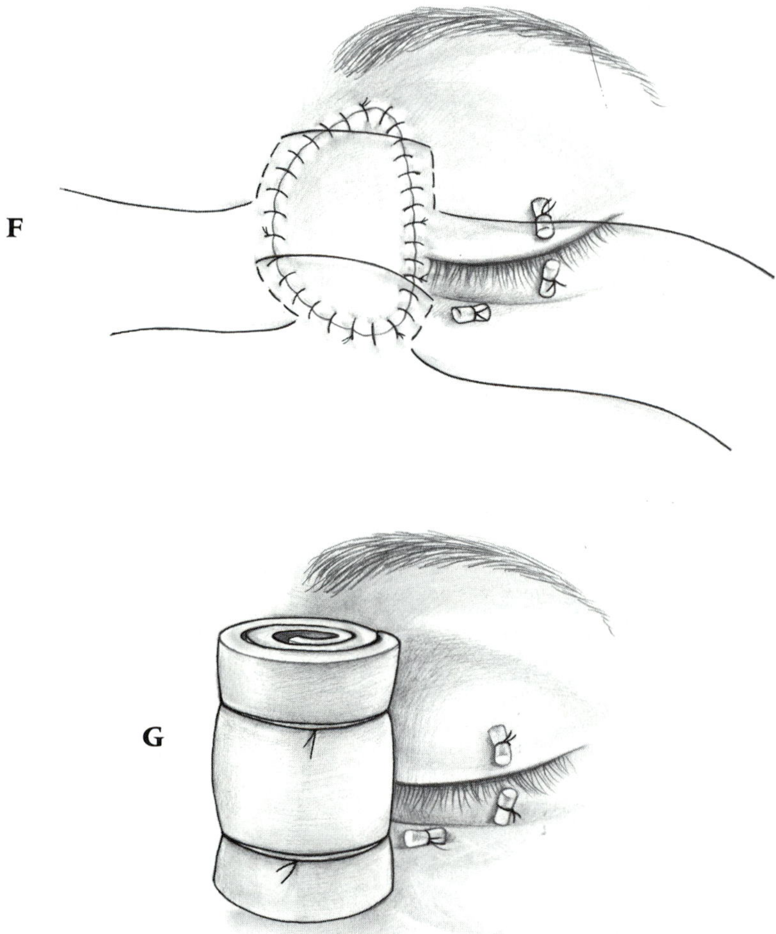

FIGURE 47-5, cont'd

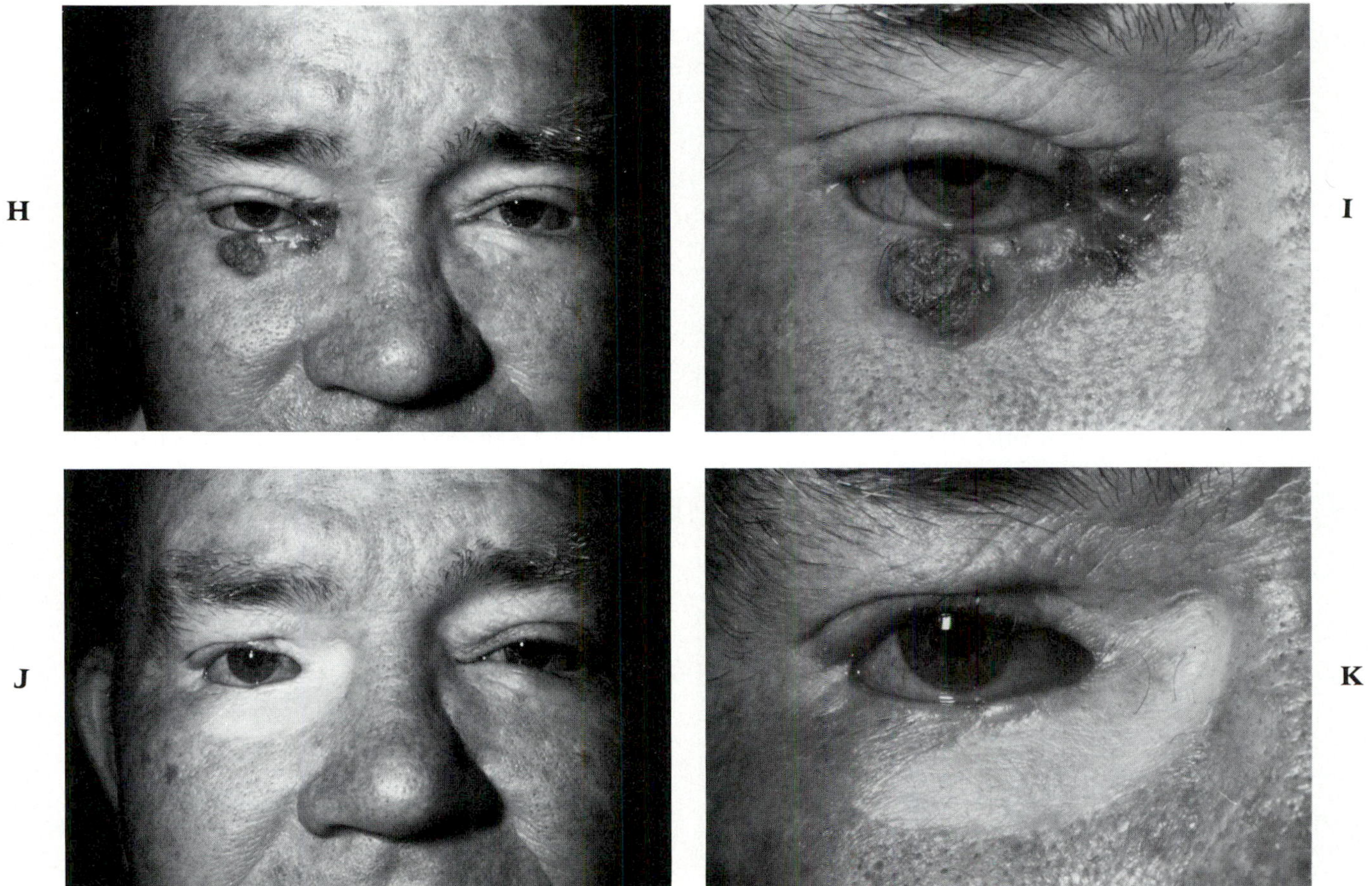

FIGURE 47-5, cont'd

Tarsal Conjunctival Flap for Lower Lid and Lateral Canthal Defects

The lesion to be excised is illustrated in Fig. 47-6, *A,* and excised in Fig. 47-6, *B.* The tarsal conjunctival flap is formed (Fig. 47-6, *C*), brought into the defect, and anchored to the remaining portion of the lid as described in Fig. 46-5, *E* to *G.* A periosteal flap is formed laterally to reconstruct a new lateral canthal tendon (Fig. 47-6, *D*) and sutured to the tarsal conjunctival flap. The anterior lamella can be repaired by dissection of a lateral skin flap (Fig. 47-6, *E*) and rotation of it into position. Continuous sutures of 6-0 Prolene are used to close the defect (Fig. 47-6, *F*). Alternative repair for the anterior lamella is a free skin graft (Fig. 47-6, *G*) as shown in Fig. 47-5, *F* and *G.* The flap is opened in 4 to 6 weeks as shown in Fig. 47-4, *J* to *M.*

Fig. 47-6, *H,* is the preoperative appearance of the patient with recurrent basal cell carcinoma of the upper lid, lateral canthus, and most of the lower lid; *I,* close-up of the eye postoperatively; *J,* postoperative appearance after tarsoconjunctival flap from the upper lid and reconstruction with a free skin graft from beneath the arm; *K,* close-up of the eye postoperatively.

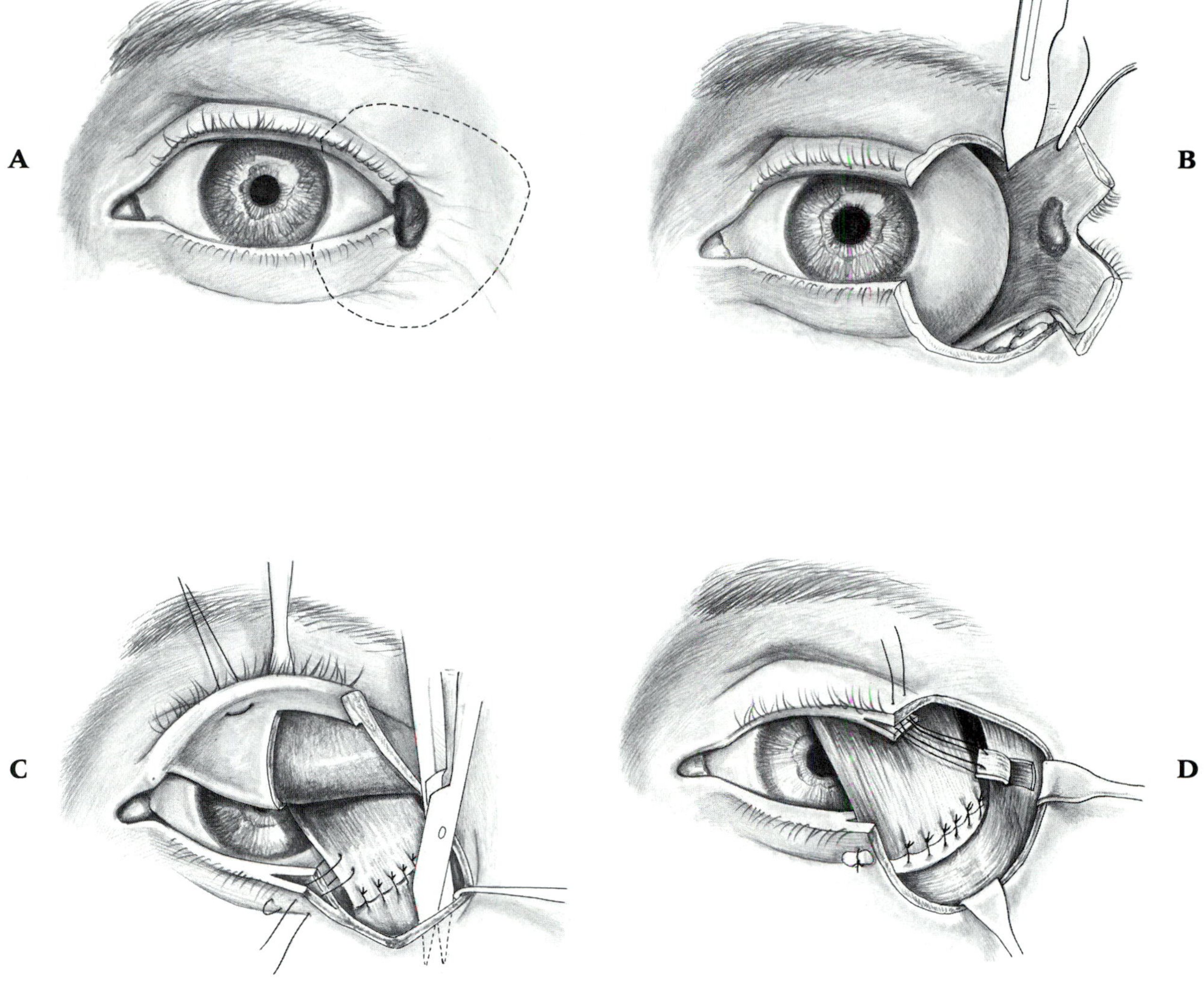

FIGURE 47-6. Smith modification, tarsoconjunctival flap for lateral canthus and lower lid. (From Smith BC, Della Rocca RC, Nesi FA, and Lisman RD: Ophthalmic plastic and reconstructive surgery, St Louis, 1987, The CV Mosby Co.)

Continued.

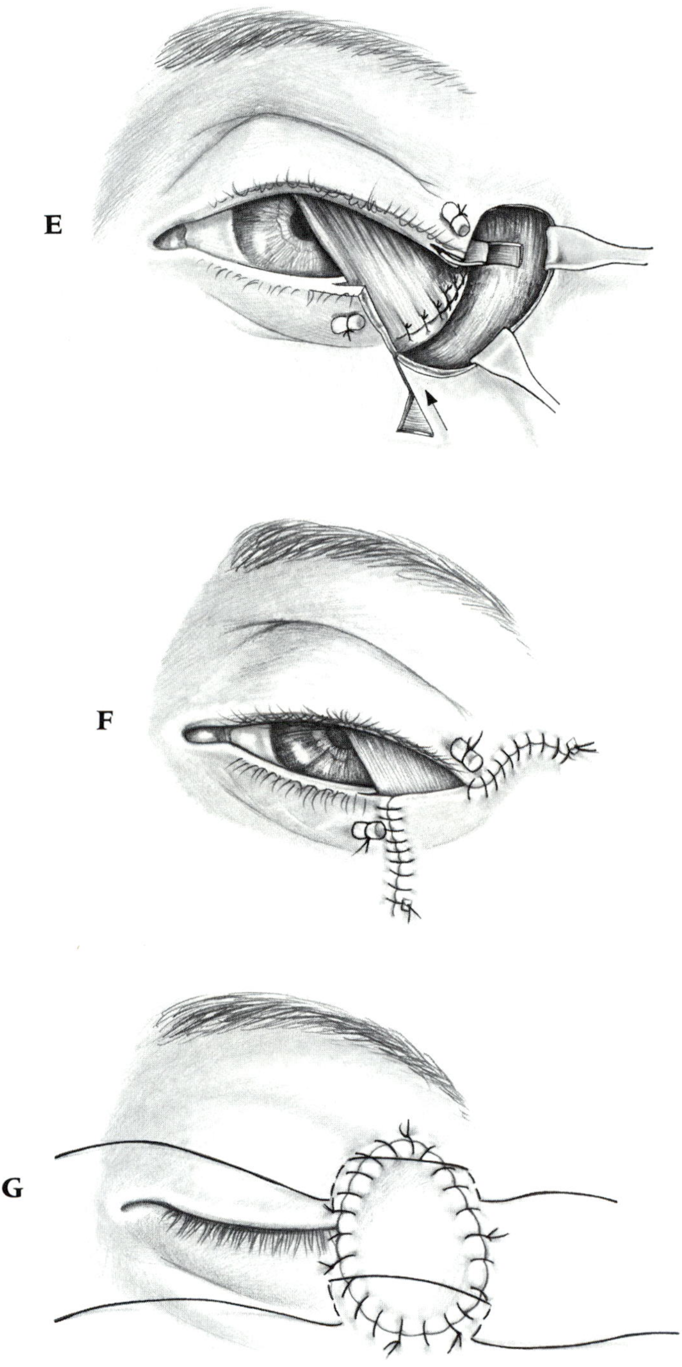

FIGURE 47-6, cont'd

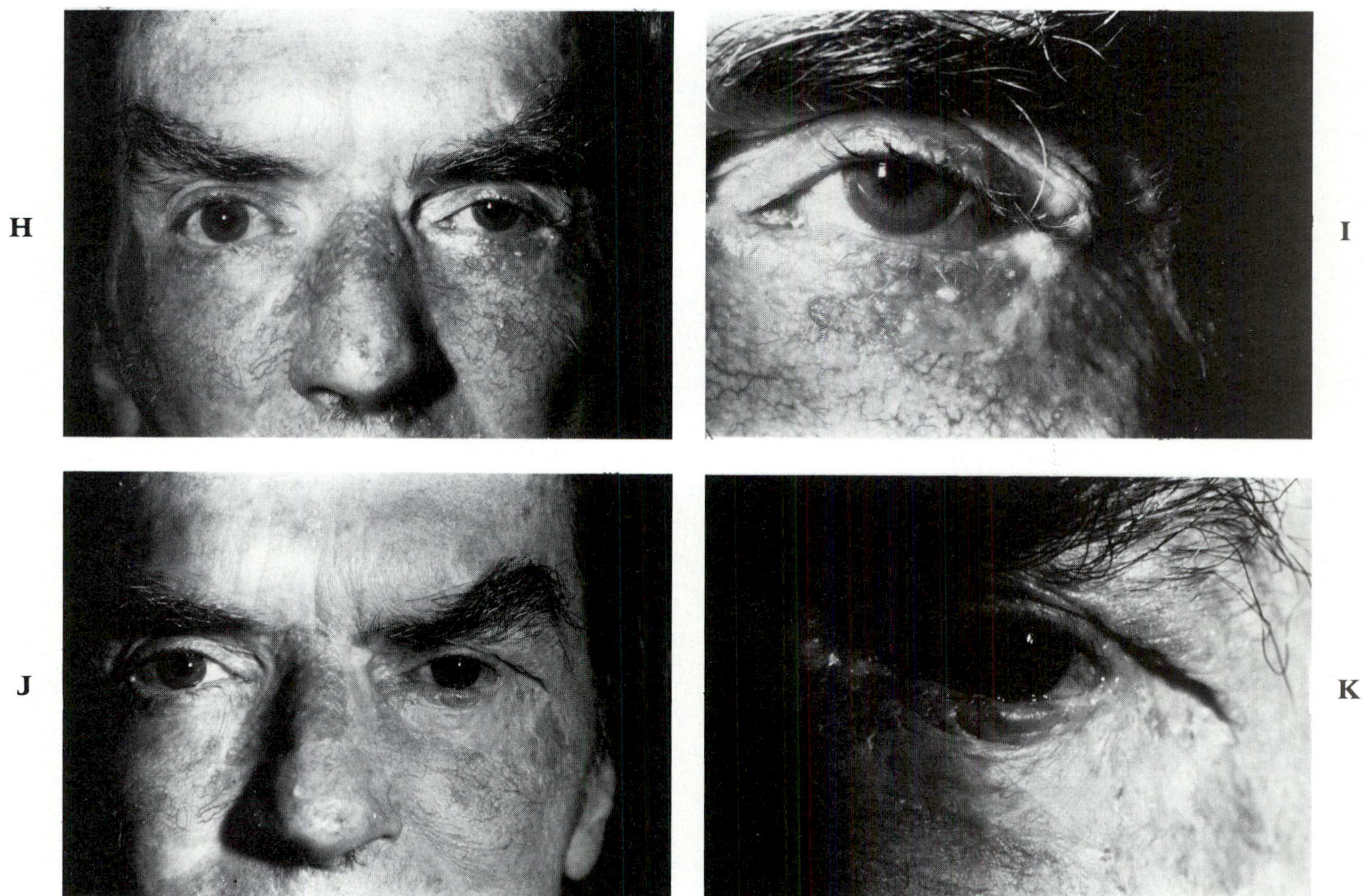

H I J K

FIGURE 47-6, cont'd

Cutler-Beard Technique for Upper Lid Defects

The Cutler-Beard technique is an excellent technique for repair of full-thickness upper lid defects of over one half of the lid. Below the defect in the upper lid (Fig. 47-7, *A*) parallel lines are drawn for the desired amount of flap to be brought into the upper lid. The cutting of the superior edge of the full-thickness flap is performed as was the transverse blepharotomy incision in cicatricial entropion of the lower lid (Fig. 45-8, *A* to *D*). A full-thickness vertical incision is made inferiorly on each side of the horizontal lid incision (Fig. 47-7, *B*), mobilizing a full-thickness lid flap to be brought into the defect of the upper lid. Fig. 47-7, *C*, is a side view illustrating the intact lower lid margin and the full-thickness flap from the lower lid placed in the upper lid defect. The tarsus from the upper lid is sutured to the conjunctiva and the lower lid retractors with interrupted sutures of 7-0 Vicryl (Fig. 47-7, *D*); be certain that none of the sutures go full-thickness through the lid to cause corneal abrasion. The muscle layer is closed with interrupted sutures of the same material and the skin with interrupted or continuous sutures of silk or synthetic material. In 6 to 8 weeks the new lids are opened (Fig. 47-7, *E*), and the upper lid is contoured to match the fellow eye. The lower lid margin will have become tubed. This is opened with scissors until a normal appearance of the lower lid is obtained. The lower lid is repaired (Fig. 47-7, *F*) with interrupted sutures of 7-0 Vicryl in the posterior portion of the lid and the skin with a continuous suture of 6-0 polypropylene.

The upper lid is left open to heal. Frequently corneal abrasions can result from the very fine skin hairs of the new upper lid, and these can be treated with cryosurgery to the lid margin. A thermocouple is placed immediately beneath the skin, and the skin is frozen to −20° C, allowed to thaw, and refrozen to −20°.

Fig. 47-7, *G*, is the preoperative appearance of a patient with a large basal cell carcinoma of the left upper lid; *H*, close-up of patient preoperatively; *I*, postoperative appearance after the Cutler-Beard flap is opened; *J*, close-up of the eye postoperatively.

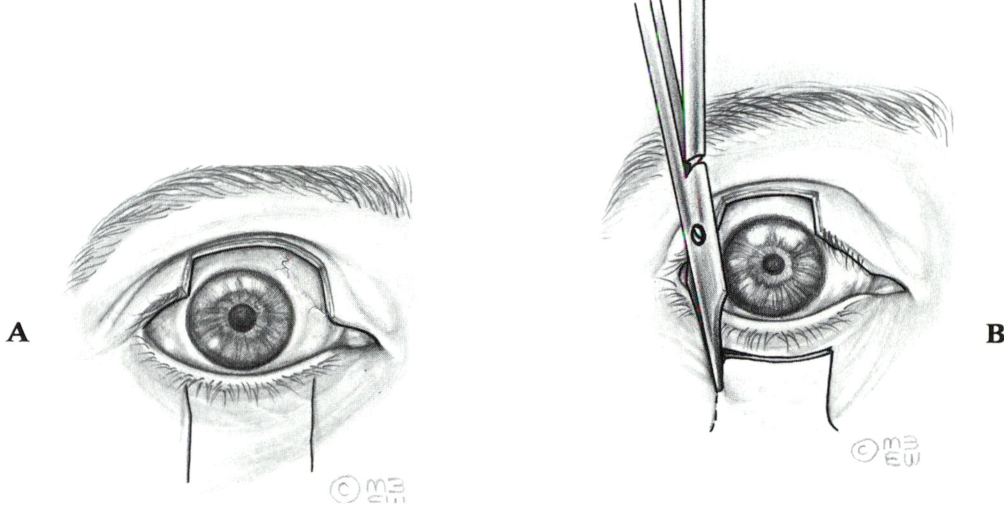

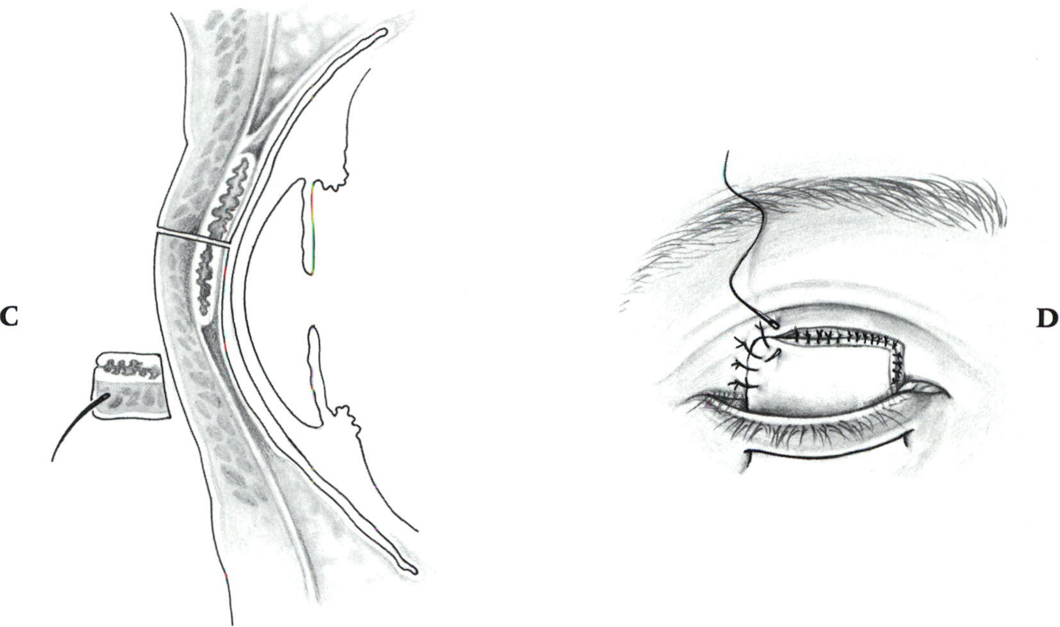

FIGURE 47-7. Cutler-Beard flap for upper lid reconstruction. (From Smith BC, Della Rocca RC, Nesi FA, and Lisman RD: Ophthalmic plastic and reconstructive surgery, St Louis, 1987, The CV Mosby Co.)

Continued.

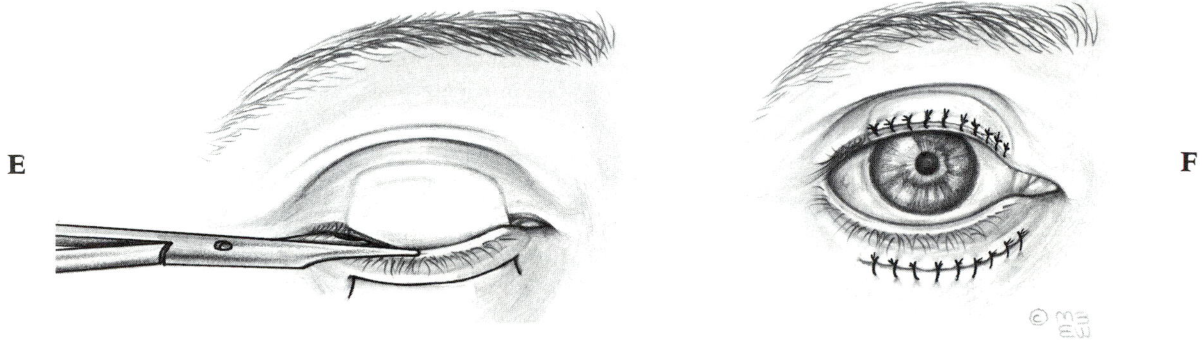

G H

I J

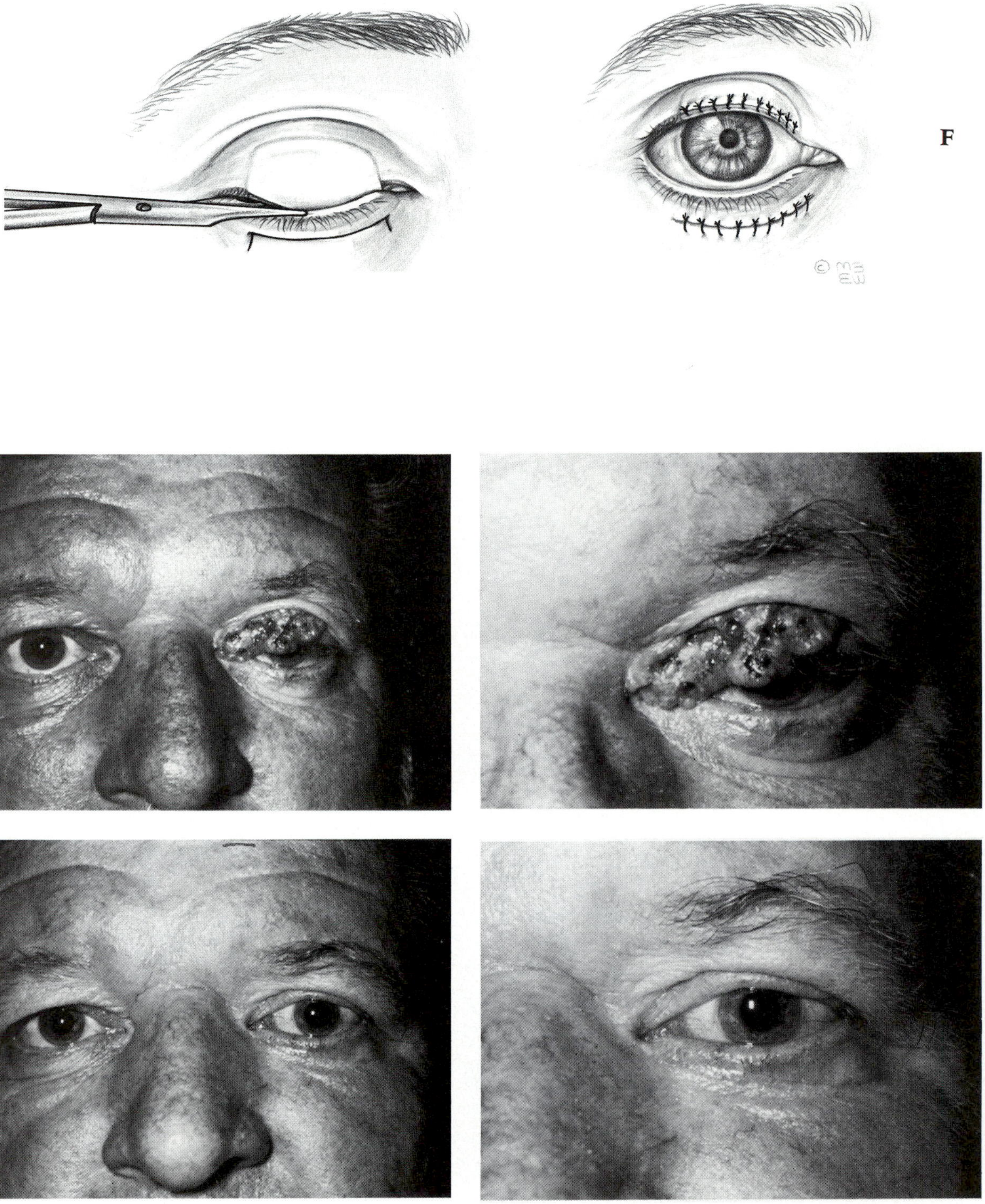

FIGURE 47-7, cont'd

CHAPTER 48

Ptosis and Levator Aponeurosis Surgery

PTOSIS

The most common complications of ptosis repair are undercorrection or overcorrection. The use of selected techniques for different types of ptosis helps minimize these complications. A simplified classification is to divide ptosis into congenital and acquired ptosis. *Congenital ptosis* can be further subdivided into mild, moderate, or severe.

Mild ptosis is defined as 1 to 2 mm of ptosis with excellent levator function of over 15 mm. If a drop of 10% phenylephrine (Neo-Synephrine) HCl instilled into the eye raises the lid to the same level as that in the fellow eye, a conjunctival Müller's muscle excision (see Fig. 48-3) can be performed. If there is no response to the drop, a posterior-approach levator resection (see Fig. 48-4) limited to a 10 to 11 mm excision of conjunctiva, Müller's muscle, and levator aponeurosis is indicated.

A moderate ptosis is defined as 2 to 3 mm of ptosis with a levator function of over 7 mm. In those patients a posterior approach to the levator resection (see Fig. 48-4) is performed with a 13 mm excision.

A severe ptosis is defined as more than 3 mm of ptosis with or without a levator function of 6 mm or less. In these patients an external levator–Müller's muscle resection with advancement (see Fig. 48-7) can be done or a frontalis fixation (see Fig. 48-2) can be done. If the patient has a syndrome of blepharophimosis, ptosis, and epicanthus inversus, a frontalis fixation is the procedure of choice.

In those patients with the Marcus-Gunn phenomenon the treatment depends on the amount of lid elevation with movements of mouth, jaw, or tongue. With mild synkinesis the patient is treated as one with a congenital ptosis. With moderate to severe excursions, the levator muscle is cut from the lid and the lid is elevated with frontalis muscle fixation.

Acquired ptosis is divided into those patients without or with muscular dystrophy, that is, chronic progressive external ophthalmoplegia, myasthenia gravis, and so on.

The procedure of choice in acquired ptosis without muscular dystrophy is resection or plication of the levator aponeurosis from the anterior approach (see Fig. 48-6). The use of sharp dissection exposing the levator aponeurosis will usually demonstrate a very diaphanous aponeurosis, which probably accounts for the ptosis.

In patients with muscular dystrophy the use of the Silastic-sling frontalis fixation (see Fig. 48-1) is a fairly effective procedure. In this type of patient the end point in tightening the sling is to just have the lids closed. This position allows the patient to close the eye in sleep.

Frontalis Fixation with Silastic Sling

Two 2 mm incisions are made 2 mm above the lash line, one at the medial limbus and the other 2 mm lateral to the lateral limbus. The brow is elevated with a finger, and where a small crease is formed in the forehead a third incision, approximately 4 mm wide, is made (Fig. 48-1, *A*) down to the periosteum. A straight Keith needle threaded with the silicone elastic sling is placed into the nasal lid incision and made to go superoposteriorly until it meets the orbital bone. The needle comes over the rim of the orbit and exits through the brow incision (Fig. 48-1, *B*). This technique secures a posterior placement of the sling. The other end of the silicone material is threaded on the needle and goes in the medial and out the lateral incision and then reenters the lateral incision to come out of the brow, repeating the medial maneuver. A Watzke cuff is placed over the ends of the suture, and they are tightened until the desired height is obtained. A 6-0 polypropylene (Prolene) suture is tied over the cuff to further secure the slings (Fig. 48-1, *C*).

This operation is particularly good on patients with chronic progressive external ophthalmoplegia or myasthenia gravis where there is poor ocular movement. The end point on these patients is to tighten the sling until the lid is just closed. There should be no opening with sleep.

Fig. 48-1, *D*, shows the primary position of a patient with chronic progressive external ophthalmoplegia; *E*, upgaze; *F*, downgaze; *G*, primary postoperative position of patient with Silastic sling of the upper lids; *H*, upgaze; *I*, downgaze; *J*, patient with excellent closure of the eyes.

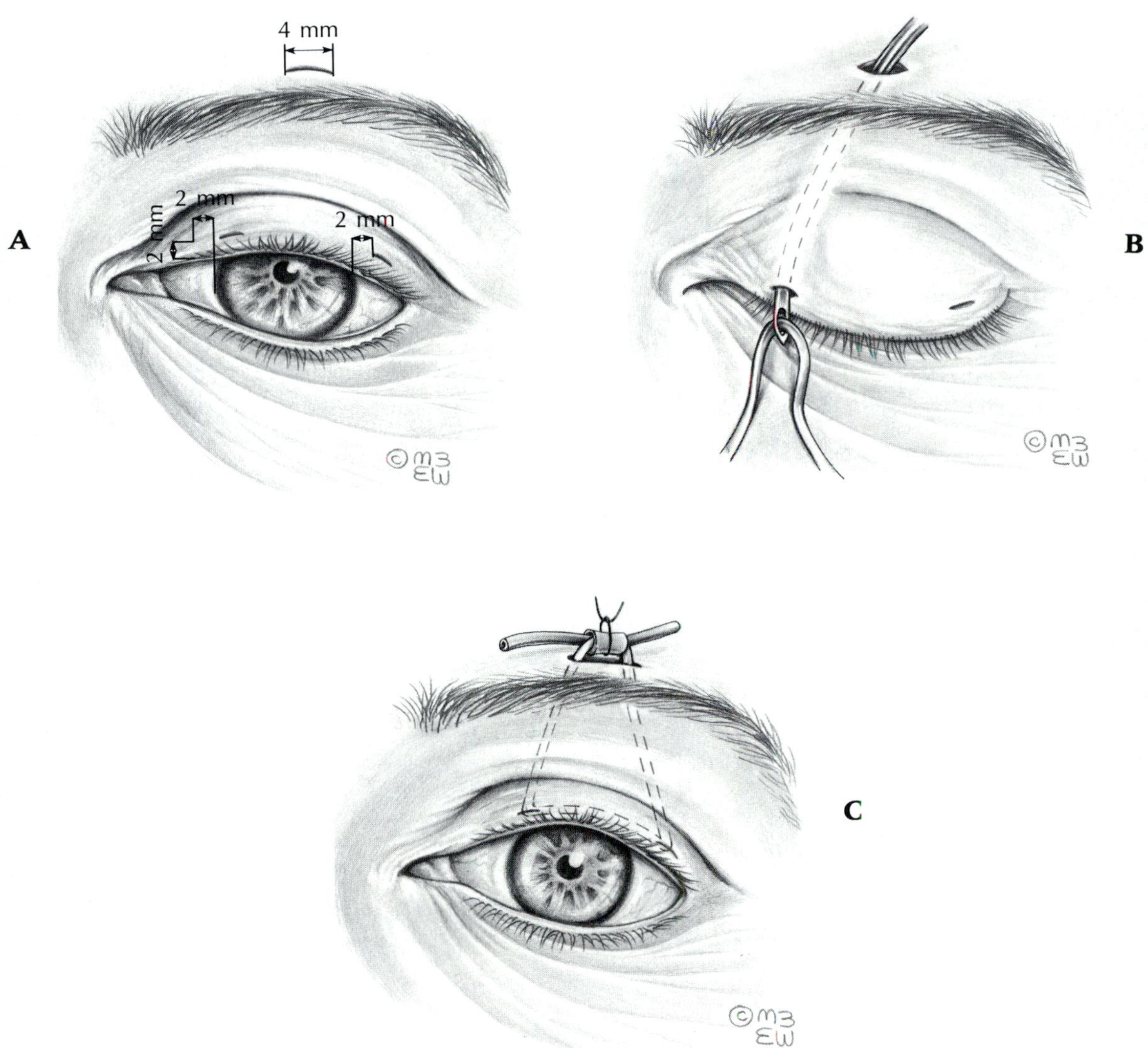

FIGURE 48-1. Silastic sling. (From Smith BC, Della Rocca RC, Nesi FA, and Lisman RD: Ophthalmic plastic and reconstructive surgery, St Louis, 1987, The CV Mosby Co.)

Continued.

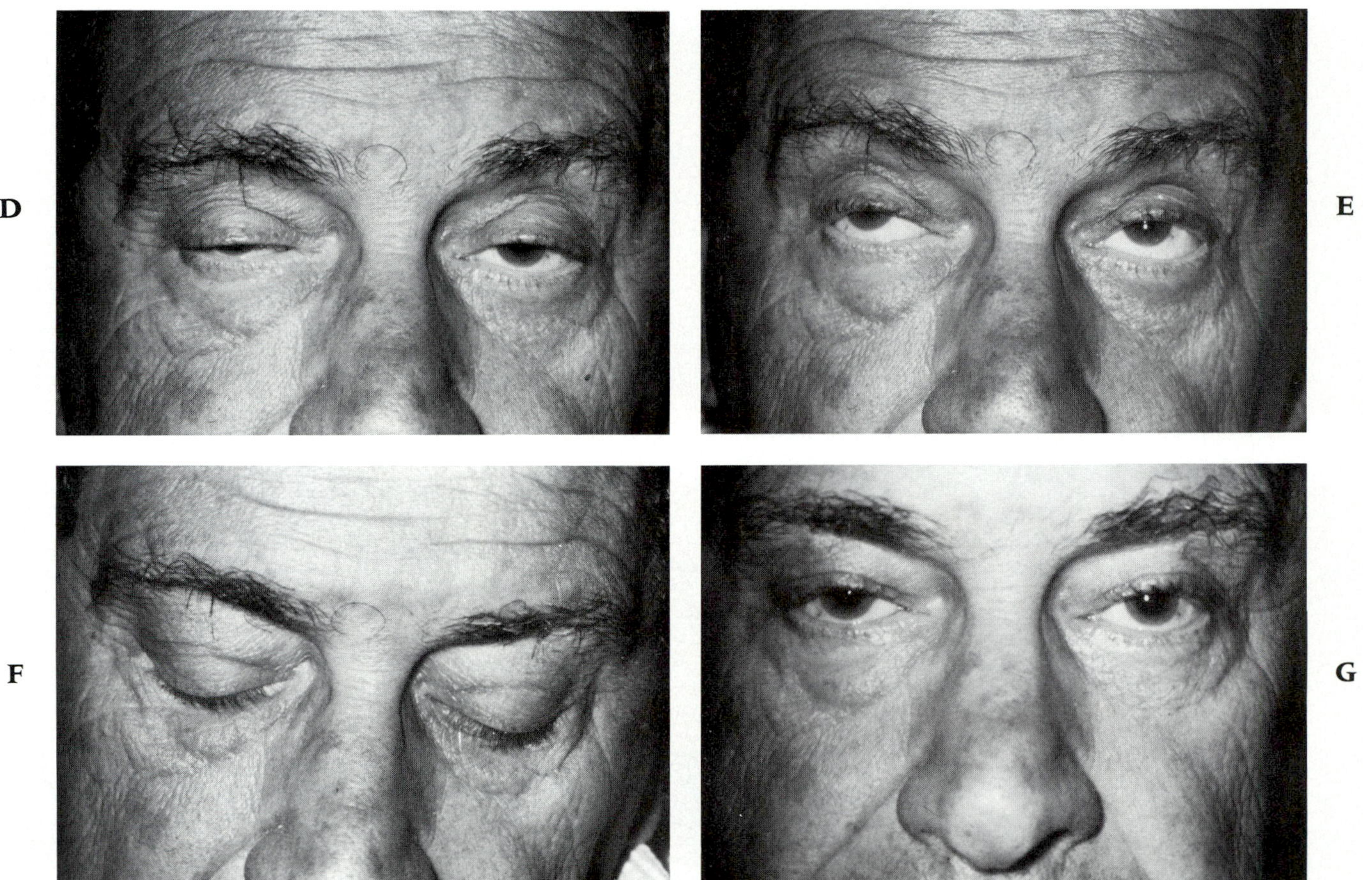

FIGURE 48-1, cont'd

H 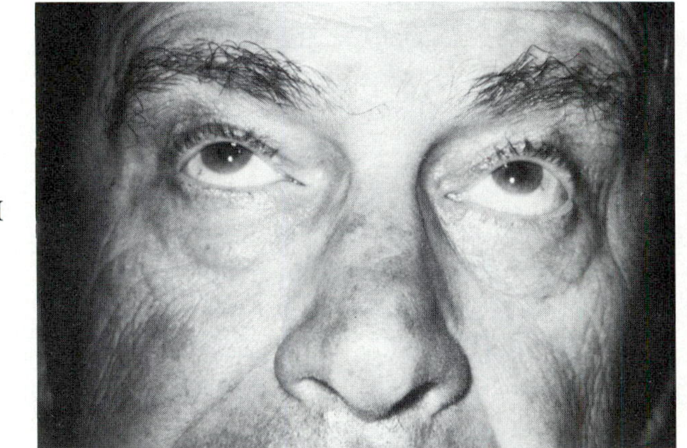

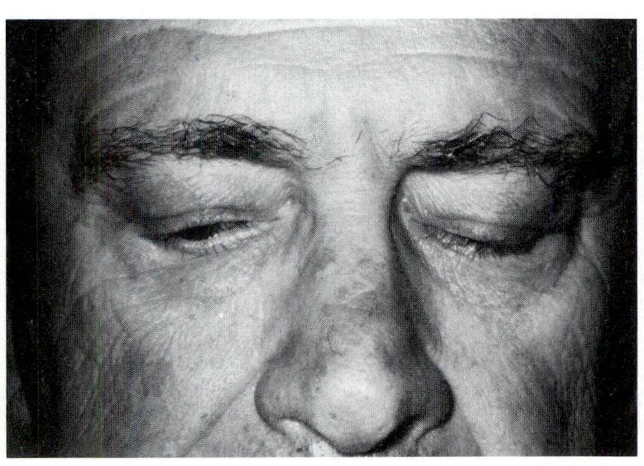 I

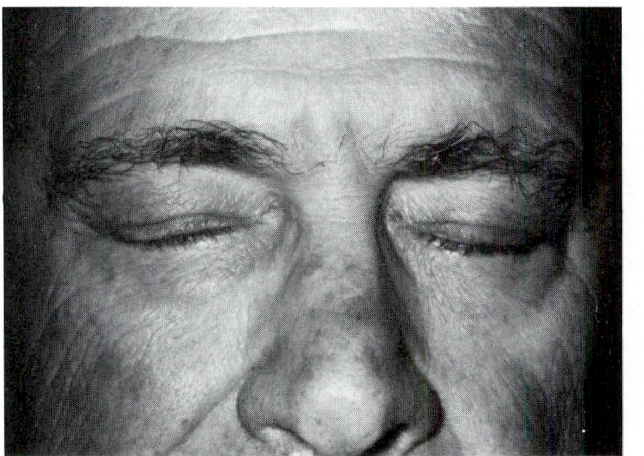 J

FIGURE 48-1, cont'd

Frontalis Fixation with Fascia Lata

Frontalis fixation is indicated in some patients with ptosis and very poor levator function. This technique is particularly useful in patients with blepharophimosis, ptosis, and epicanthus inversus and in those with Turner's syndrome.

The upper lids are marked into thirds. Three incisions are made in each lid 2 mm from the lid margin. The first two incisions are 4 mm in length. The first incision is made 1.5 mm medially to the medial mark. The second incision is made 1.5 mm laterally to the lateral mark. The third incision extends from 1.5 mm laterally to the medial mark to 1.5 mm medially to the lateral mark. There are also three incisions of the forehead. The medial and lateral incisions are placed in the crease that is formed when the brow is passively elevated. The central incision is 6 mm higher than the medial and lateral incisions. Autogenous fascia lata is taken from the leg, or donor fascia is used. The fascia is placed on a straight Keith 2134-8 needle. The needle goes into the nasal lid incision, heading posteriorly toward the anterior roof of the orbit. Once the roof of the orbit is met the needle then comes anteriorly over the orbital rim and exits through the medial brow incision (Fig. 48-2, *A*). The other arm of the fascia is threaded on the needle, goes into the medial wound, comes out of the central wound (Fig. 48-2, *B*), reenters the central wound, and, with the same technique as previously described, exits through the medial brow incision. A second piece of fascia is placed in the lateral wound and repeats the type of placement as with the first fascia to form two triangles with the base just above the lid margin (Fig. 48-2, *C*). Each of these triangles is tightened and tied to give the lid good height and curvature. One arm of each of the pieces of fascia is then brought out through the central forehead incision (Fig. 48-2, *D*), and these arms are adjusted and tied to give better curve and contour (Fig. 48-2, *E*). When tying the fascia, place a suture of 6-0 Prolene (polypropylene) beneath the fascia. A single loop is tied in the fascia. The suture is tied over this loop. A second loop is placed in the fascia, and the suture is tied again. This step will prevent the fascia from slipping. The end point of the procedure is to have the lid in the desired position, Fig. 48-2, *F,* shows the preoperative appearance of the patient in the primary position; *G,* upgaze; *H,* downgaze; *I,* primary position of patient after fascia lata repair for ptosis; *J,* upgaze; *K,* downgaze.

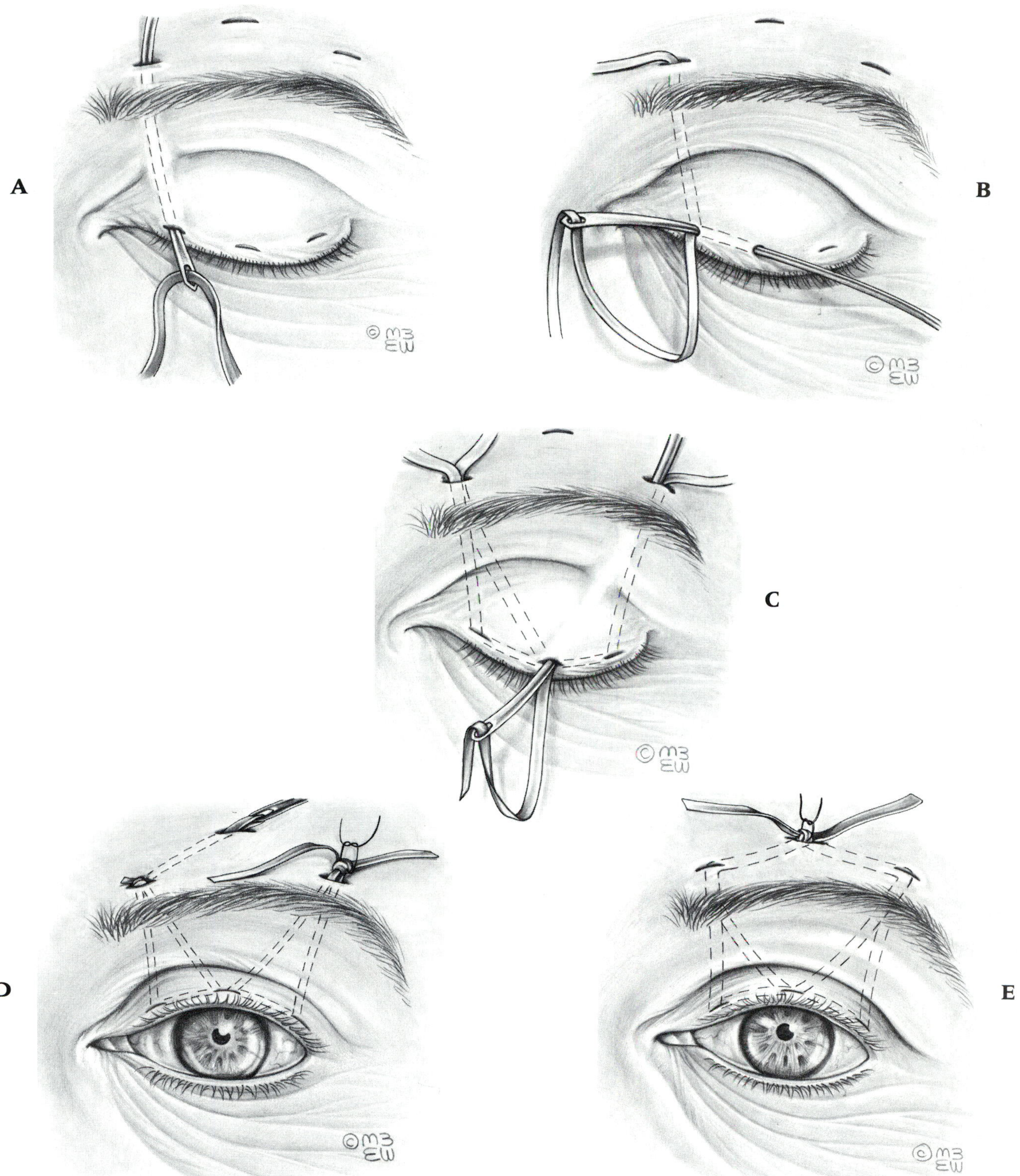

FIGURE 48-2. Crawford technique for fascia lata frontalis fixation. (From Smith BC, Della Rocca RC, Nesi FA, and Lisman RD: Ophthalmic plastic and reconstructive surgery, St Louis, 1987, The CV Mosby Co.)

Continued.

F

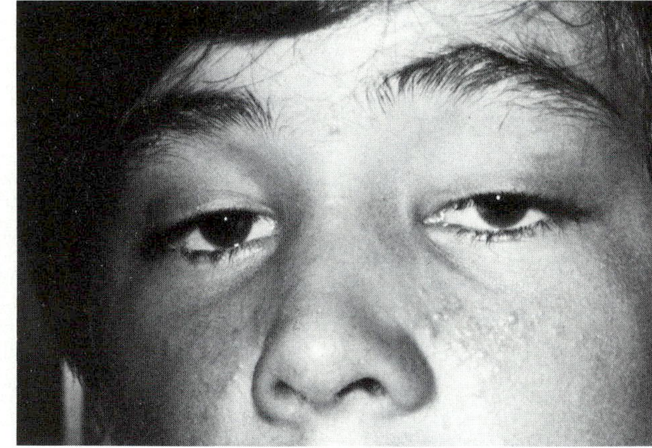

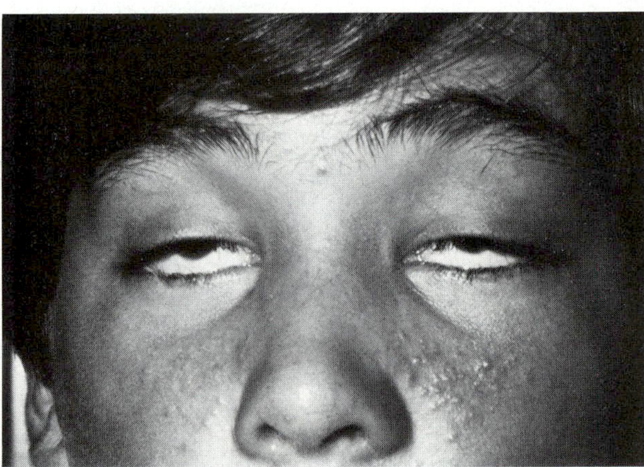

G

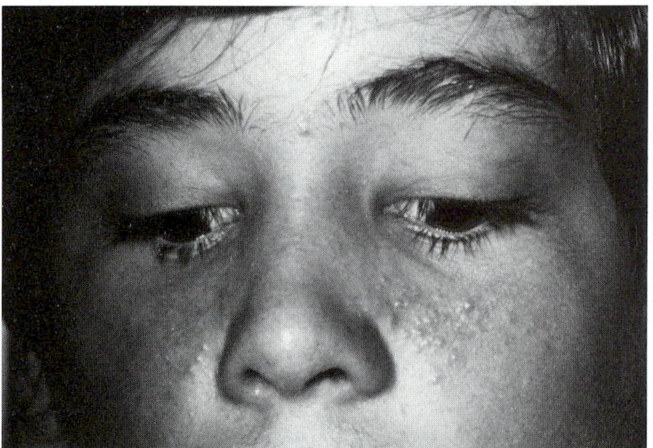

H

FIGURE 48-2, cont'd

I

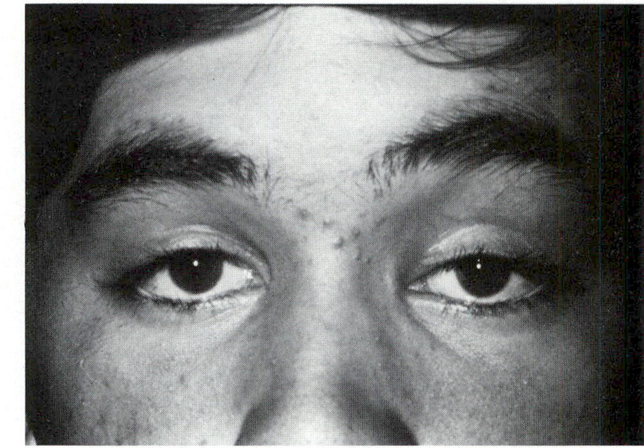

J

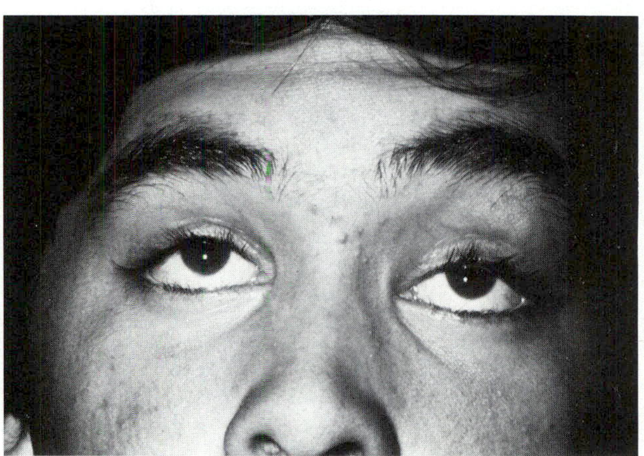

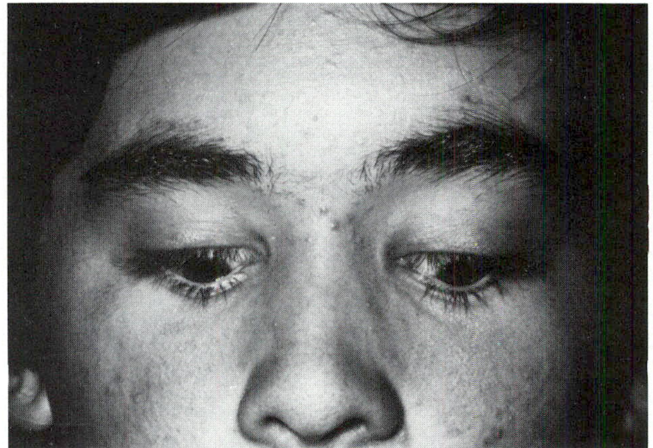

K

FIGURE 48-2, cont'd

Müller's Muscle and Conjunctival Excision

The conjunctiva is picked up with two forceps 4 mm above the upper edge of the tarsus. Two clamps are placed across the base of this tissue, one medial and one lateral (Fig. 48-3, *A* and *B*). A 6-0 Prolene (polypropylene) suture enters the skin of the lid and exits behind the clamp. It traverses the wound by going at a 45-degree angle through the tissues. Each entrance into the conjunctiva is at the exit of the previous wound so that essentially no suture material is exposed on the conjunctival surface. Once the suture reaches the other end of the wound, it is brought out on the skin (Fig. 48-3, *C* and *D*). The clamps are removed and the redundant conjunctiva and Müller's muscle are excised (Fig. 48-3, *E*). The suture goes back into the wound, having been draped over a cotton pledget, and continues to the opposite side in a subconjunctival serpentine fashion (Fig. 48-3, *F*). The suture exits through the skin near the original point of entrance and is tied to the other end over a cotton pledget (Fig. 48-3, *G*). The suture should be removed in 4 or 5 days.

Fig. 48-3, *H,* shows a patient in primary position with a mild ptosis of the right upper lid; *I,* upgaze; *J,* downgaze; *K,* postoperative appearance after conjunctival müllerectomy; *L,* upgaze; *M,* downgaze.

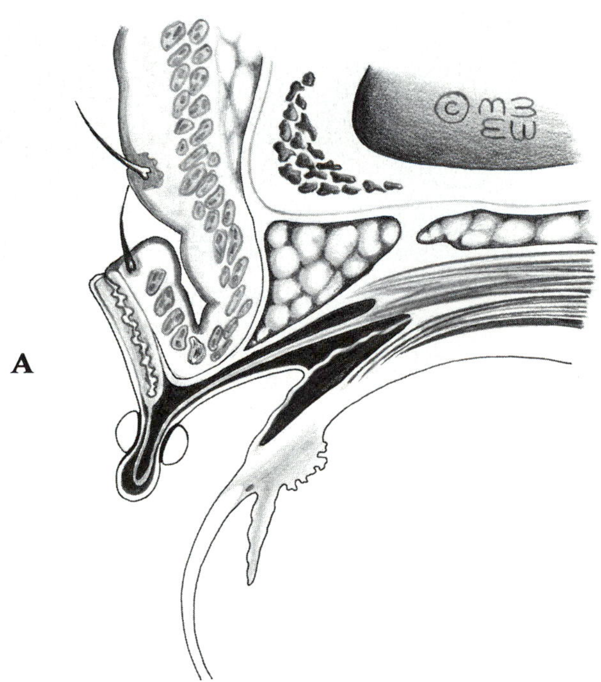

FIGURE 48-3. Conjunctival müllerectomy.

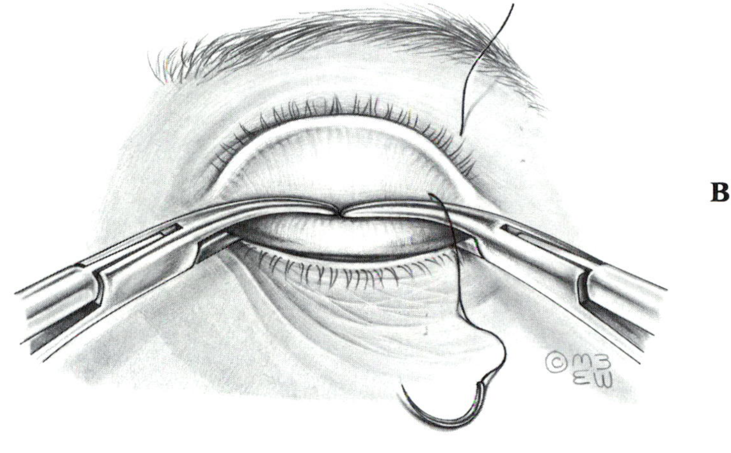
B

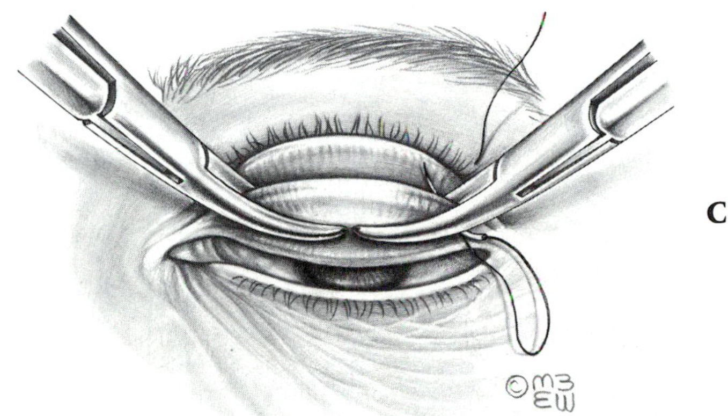
C

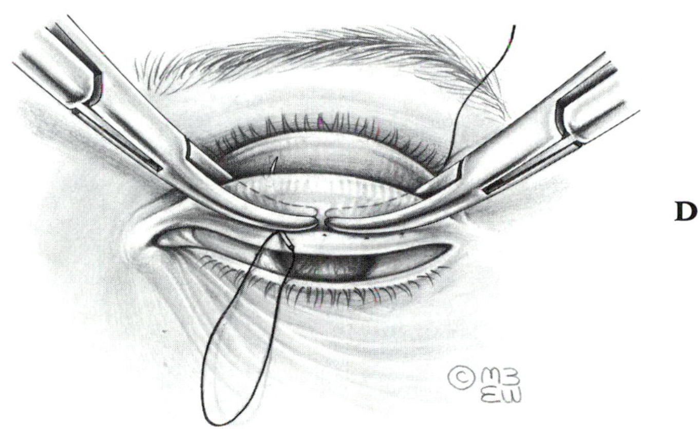
D

FIGURE 48-3, cont'd

Continued.

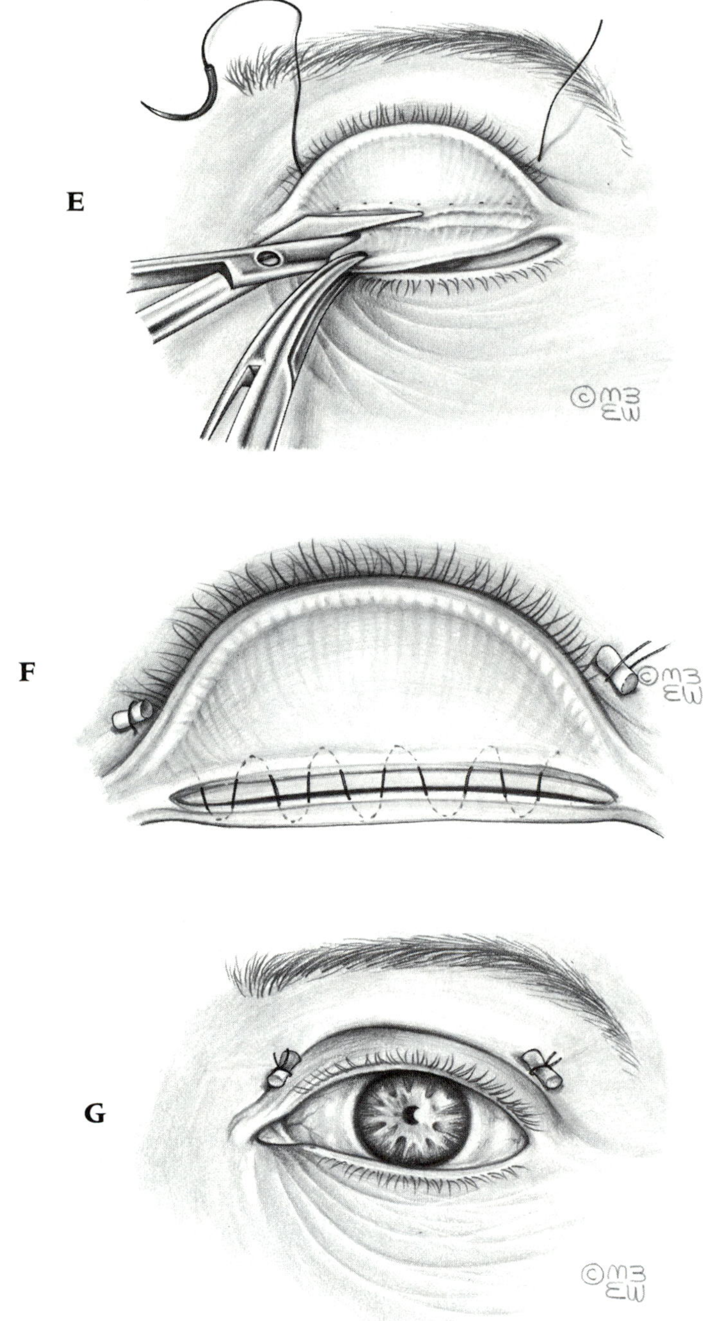

FIGURE 48-3, cont'd

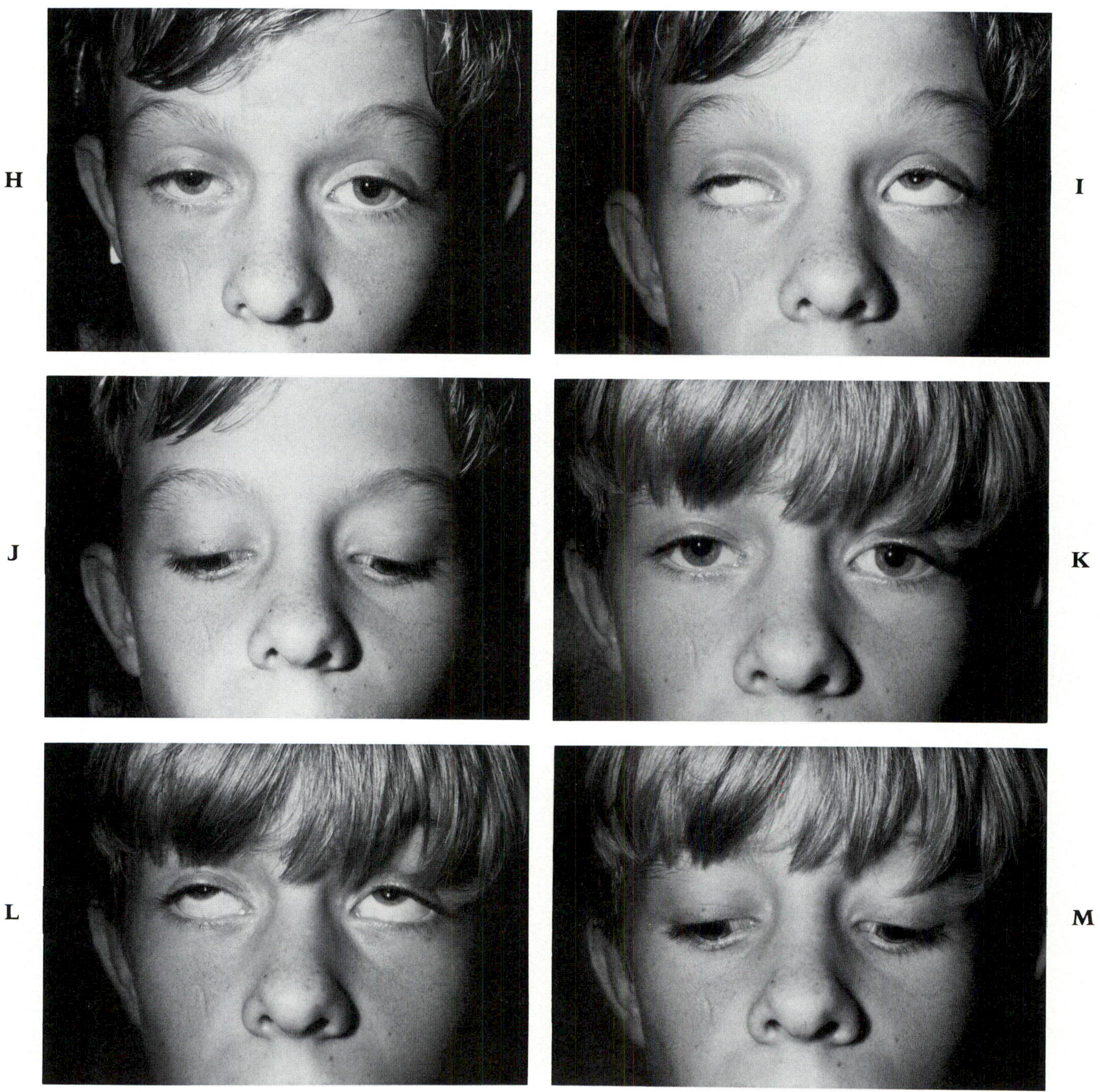

FIGURE 48-3, cont'd

Internal Approach to Levator Resection with Müller's Muscle and Conjunctiva

The upper lid is everted over a Desmarres retractor, and a buttonhole is made at the upper edge of the medial tarsus through the conjunctiva, Müller's muscle, and the levator aponeurosis. Blunt scissors are then passed across the lid in this plane (Fig. 48-4, *A*) until they reach the other side, where a second buttonhole is made. The scissors are withdrawn while a Cryle clamp is advanced across the lid. The clamp is placed just at the upper border of the tarsus (Fig. 48-4, *B*). The clamp will encompass the conjunctiva, Müller's muscle, and the levator aponeurosis (Fig. 48-4, *C*). The tissues distal to the clamp are cut, and the orbital septum is opened across the lid. Sutures are placed, usually so that a 13 mm resection is produced. However, if the patient has a levator function of 13 to 14 mm, the resection is only 11 mm. Four double-arm horizontal mattress sutures of 4-0 silk are placed across the wound. Each needle goes through the conjunctiva, Müller's muscle, and the levator aponeurosis. One arm of each suture takes a partial-thickness bite at the upper edge of the tarsus, and then both sutures exit just behind the lashes (Fig. 48-4, *D* and *E*). The sutures should be placed symmetrically across the lid so that the tension is distributed equally. The redundant aponeurosis is excised with scissors (Fig. 48-4, *F*), and the sutures are tied over cotton pledgets (Fig. 48-4, *G*). The sutures are removed at 5 days. The result of the ptosis surgery will not be seen until 6 weeks after surgery. There will be some splinting of the lid and undercorrection present for at least 2 weeks.

Fig. 48-4, *H,* shows the primary position on the patient with bilateral mild congenital ptosis; *I,* upgaze; *J,* downgaze; *K,* postoperative appearance after bilateral internal approach for a levator resection; *L,* upgaze; *M,* downgaze.

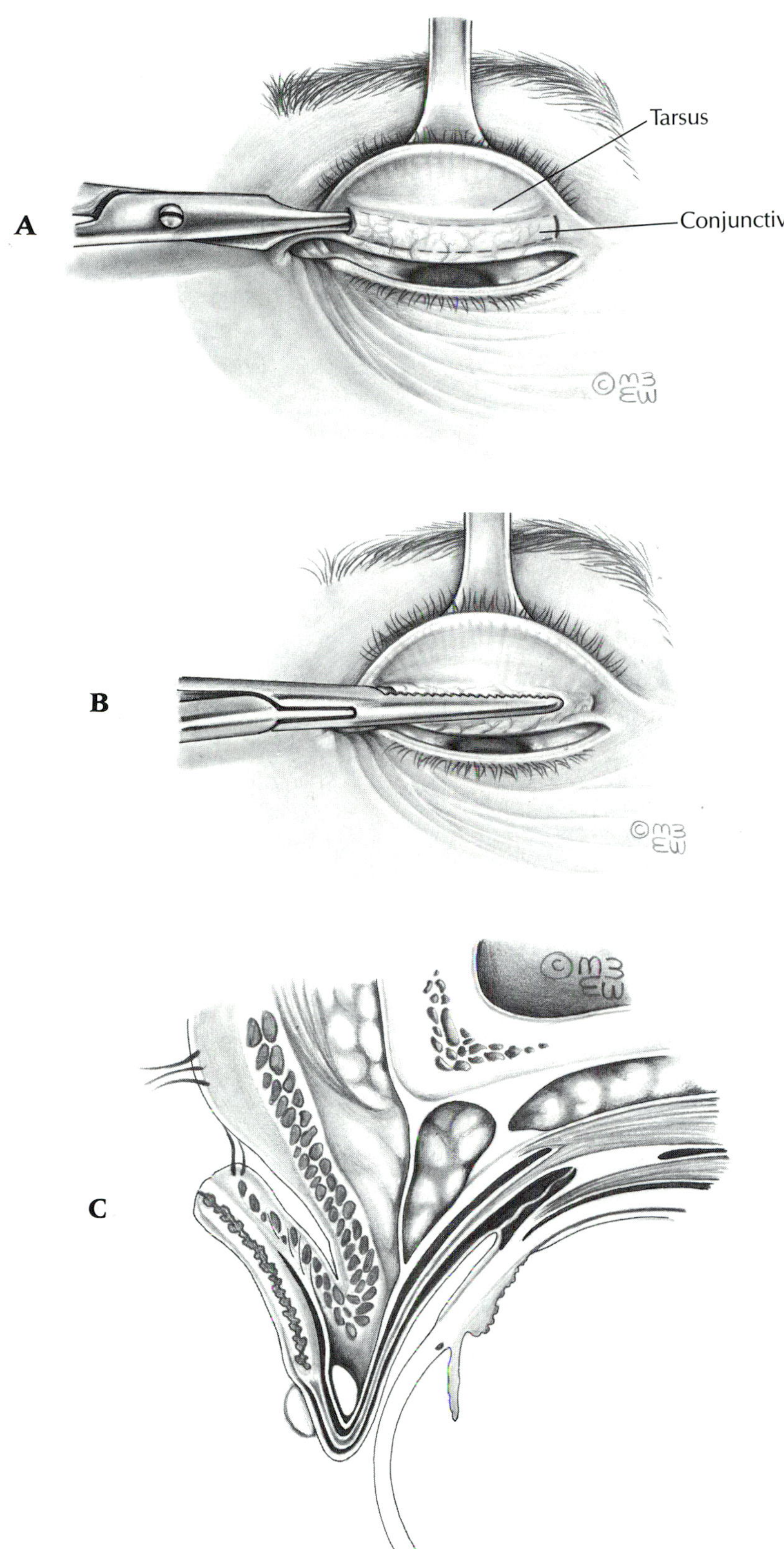

FIGURE 48-4. Internal approach to levator resection—modified Iliff technique.

Continued.

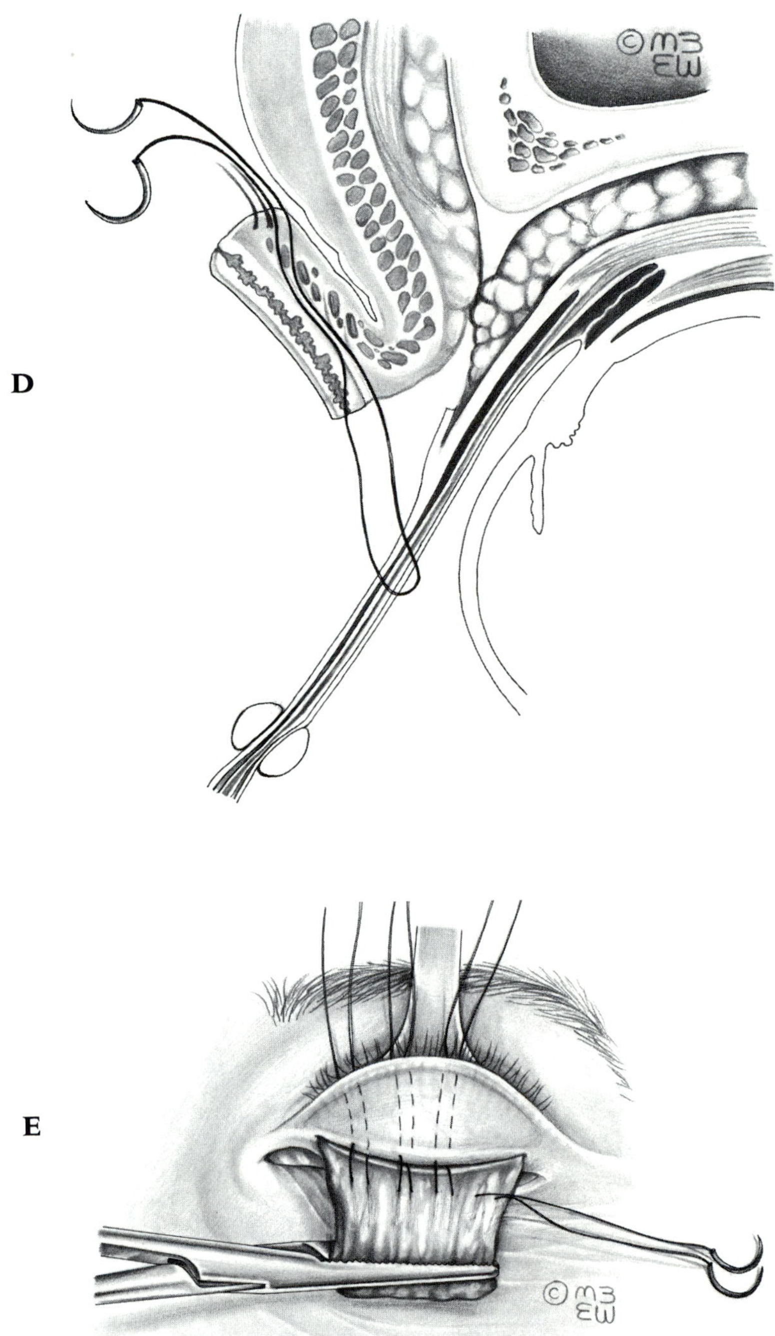

FIGURE 48-4, cont'd

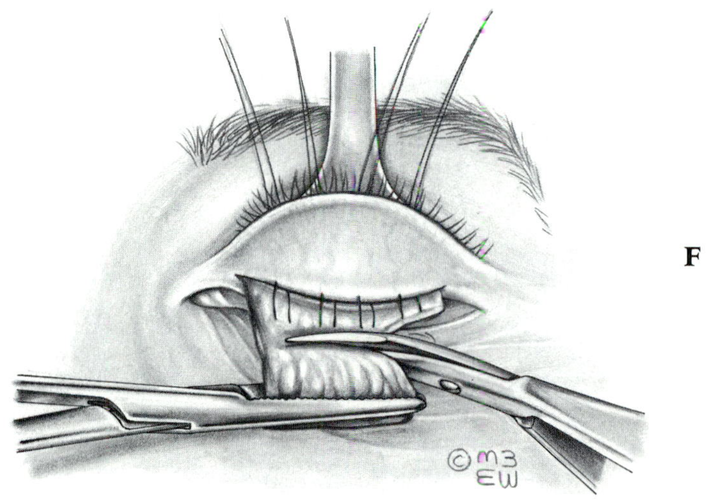

F

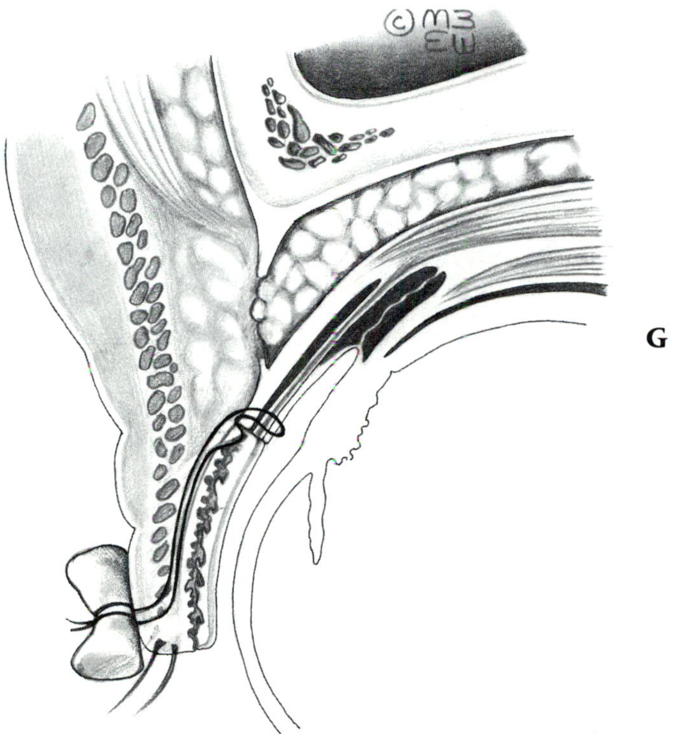

G

FIGURE 48-4, cont'd

Continued.

H

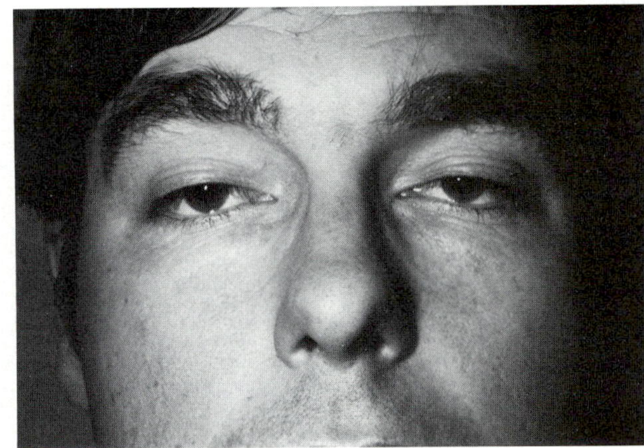

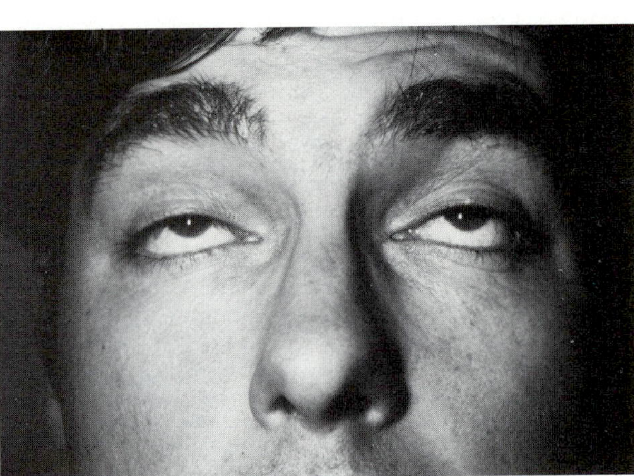

I

J

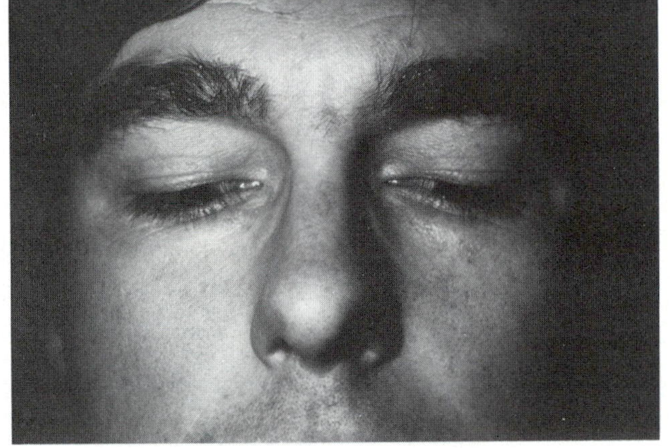

FIGURE 48-4, cont'd

K

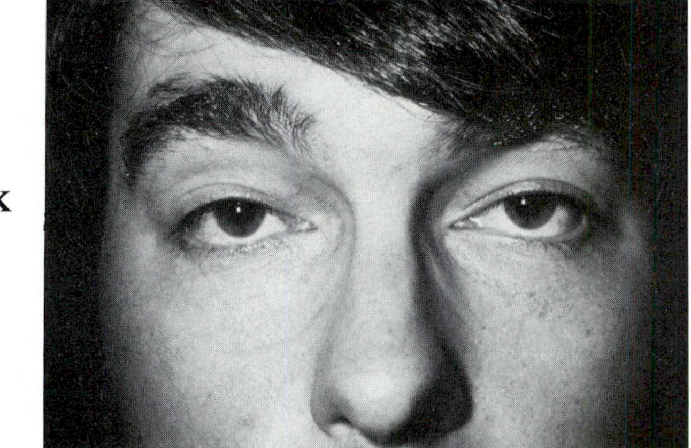

L

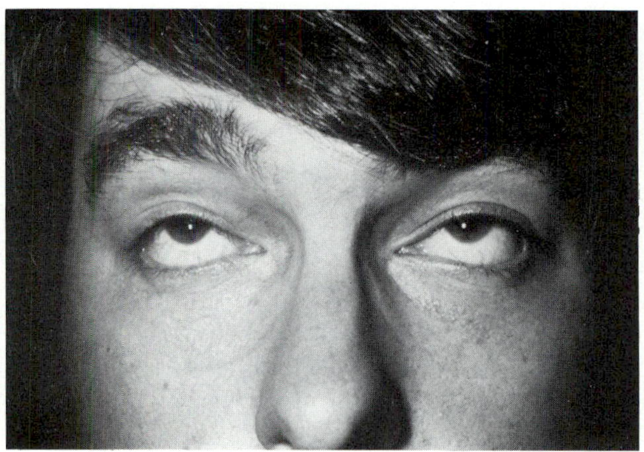

M

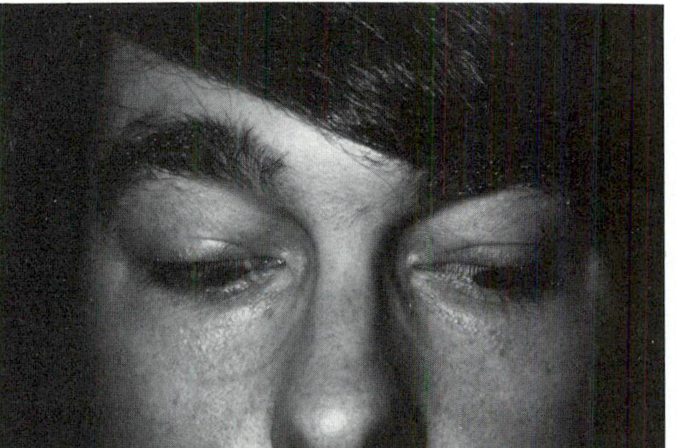

FIGURE 48-4, cont'd

LEVATOR APONEUROSIS SURGERY

Surgery on the levator aponeurosis is performed under local anesthesia for titration surgery. In the upright position the patient is asked to open the eyes and look at applicator sticks. The height of the lid margins are noted. The lid margin height is then checked with the patient in the supine position to see if there is a change. If there is no change, all lid levels are checked in the supine position.

Exposure of the Levator Aponeurosis

The lid crease is marked on the lid (Fig. 48-5, *A*). In a unilateral case the crease is matched to the fellow eye. In bilateral surgery the lid is divided into thirds. The central measurement in women is 10 mm from the base of the lashes, the lateral is 9 mm, and the nasal is 8 mm. In men or women with small eyes the heights are 1 mm less. An incision is made with a razor knife through the skin (Fig. 48-5, *B*). Both sides of the wound are picked up with forceps to cut the subcutaneous tissue under tension (Fig. 48-5, *C*) and cut with scissors, revealing the orbicularis muscle (Fig. 48-5, *D*). A strip of orbicularis muscle is either removed or incised (Fig. 48-5, *E*). The dissection is carried superiorly beneath the orbicularis muscle until the orbital septum is exposed (Fig. 48-5, *F*). With pressure on the lids the fat bulging beneath the septum is buttonholed and opened across the lid (Fig. 48-5, *G* and *H*) revealing the levator aponeurosis beneath the septum.

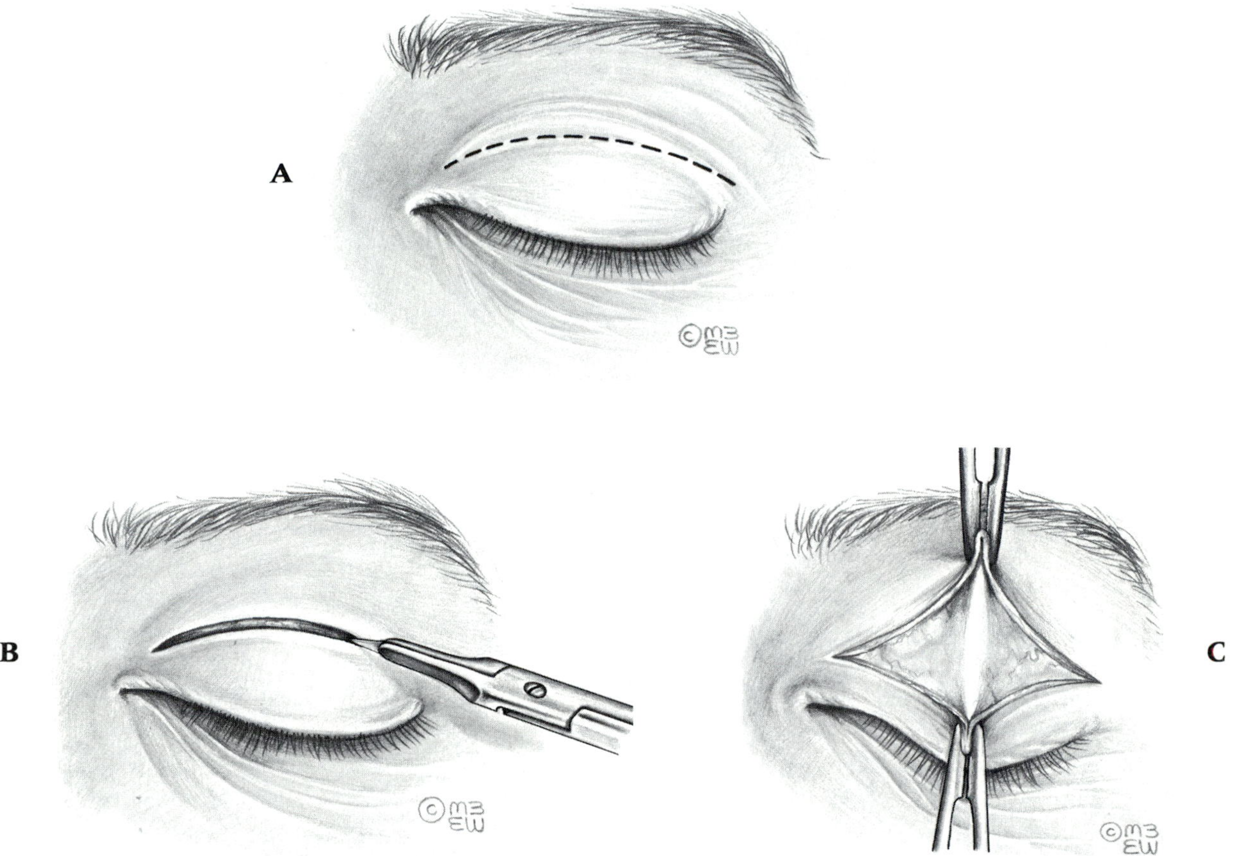

FIGURE 48-5. External approach to levator aponeurosis.

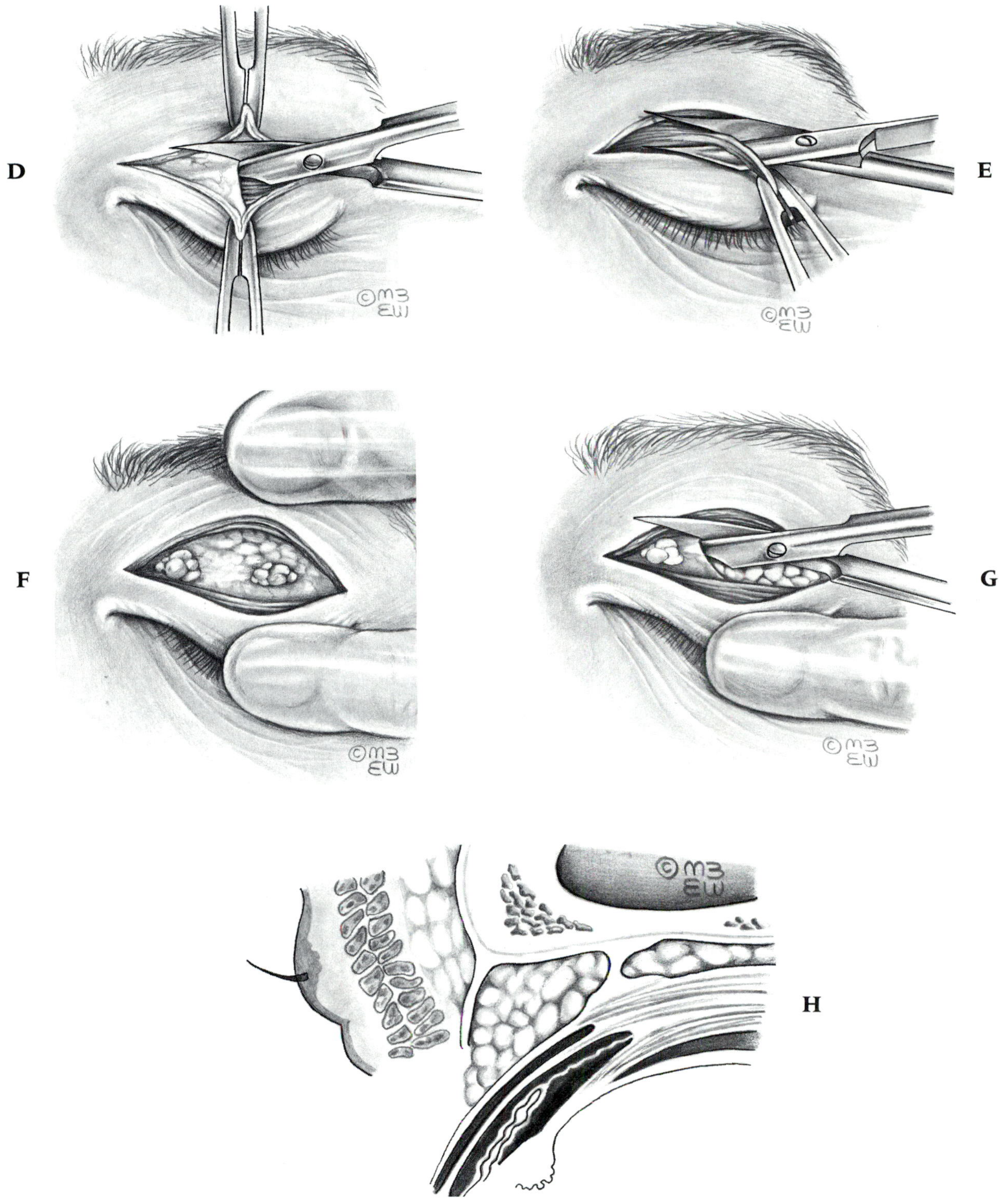
D
E
F
G
H

Aponeurosis Resection for Acquired Ptosis

Titration surgery is used. The levator is exposed, and the orbital septum is opened as in Fig. 48-5. After the orbital septum has been opened, the patient is again asked to look at applicator sticks (Fig. 48-6, *A*), and the difference from the preoperative lid height is noted. If there is a lowering of the lid margin (rarely), the lid is undercorrected by the amount of lowering. If the lid is higher (very frequently), the lid is overcorrected by the amount of rise. The levator aponeurosis is then opened across the midface of the tarsus and dissected from the tarsus (Fig. 48-6, *B*). When the dissection reaches the upper edge of the tarsus, one sees very fine attachments to Müller's muscle (Fig. 48-6, *C*), which are then separated with blunt and sharp dissection (Fig. 48-6, *D*), freeing the levator from the underlying Müller's muscle. The three original measurements for formation of the lid crease are marked on the tarsus for the placement of three 6-0 double-armed Mersilene sutures. After placement of each suture in the tarsus, the lid is everted to make certain the suture was only partial thickness in the tarsus. The central suture is placed first (Fig. 48-6, *E* and *F*), brought through the levator aponeurosis (Fig. 48-6, *G*), and temporarily tied. Check the lid height by having the patient look at the applicator sticks (Fig. 48-6, *H*), and make adjustments until the lid height is as desired. The medial and lateral sutures are placed in the tarsus and then continue on through the aponeurosis. The lid curvature is adjusted with these sutures. The sutures are tied, the redundant aponeurosis is excised, and a running 6-0 Mersilene suture is used to suture the cut edge of the aponeurosis to the aponeurosis continuing to the lid margin (Fig. 48-6, *I*). One arm of each of the sutures into the tarsus goes through the upper edge of the inferior skin flap and is tied beneath the orbicularis muscle, so that the lid crease is re-created. Fig. 48-6, *J*, shows all sutures in place. The skin is closed with a subcuticular suture of 6-0 polypropylene tied over rubber bands (Fig. 48-6, *K*).

Fig. 48-6, *L*, shows the preoperative appearance with ptosis of the right upper lid after cataract extraction; *M*, upgaze; *N*, downgaze; *O*, postoperative appearance after aponeurosis repair of the right upper lid; *P*, upgaze; *Q*, downgaze.

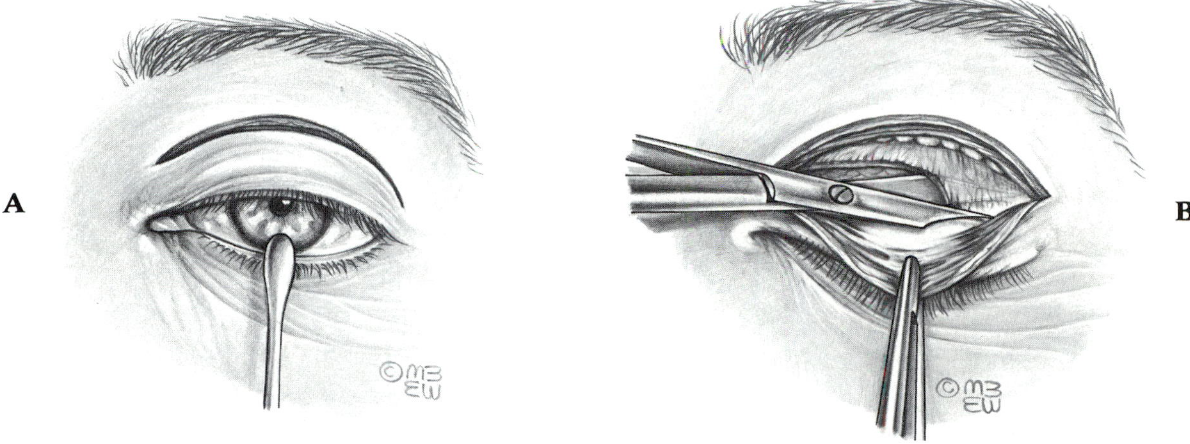

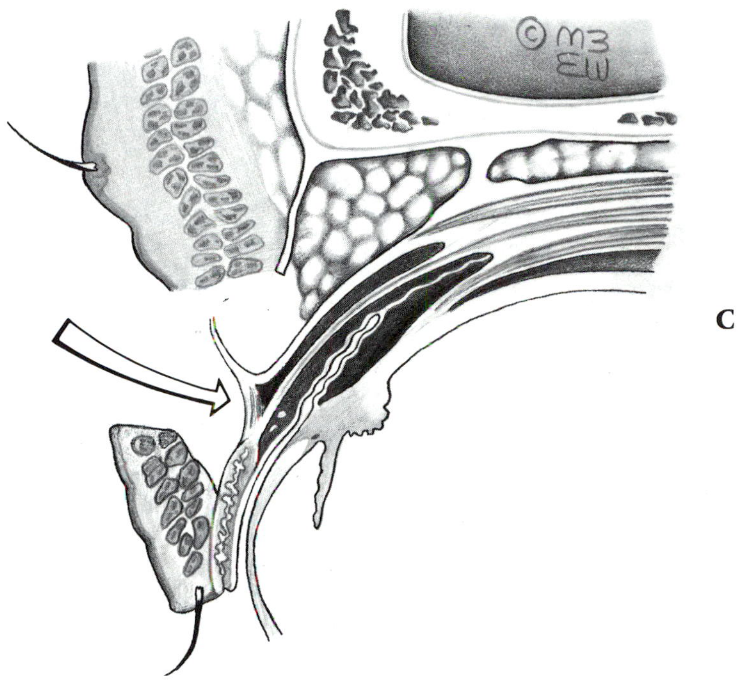

FIGURE 48-6. Isolated aponeurosis resection.

Continued.

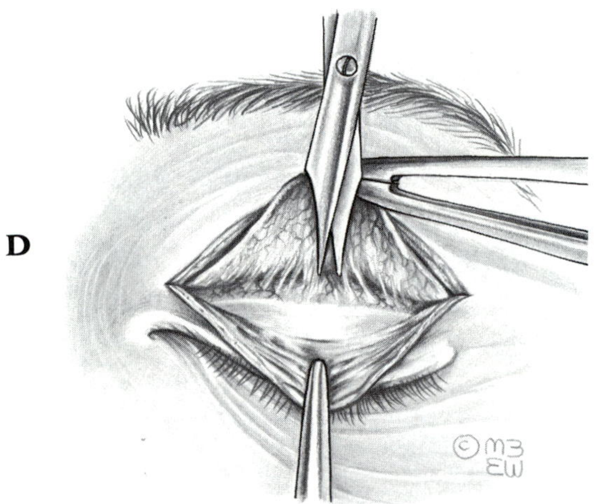

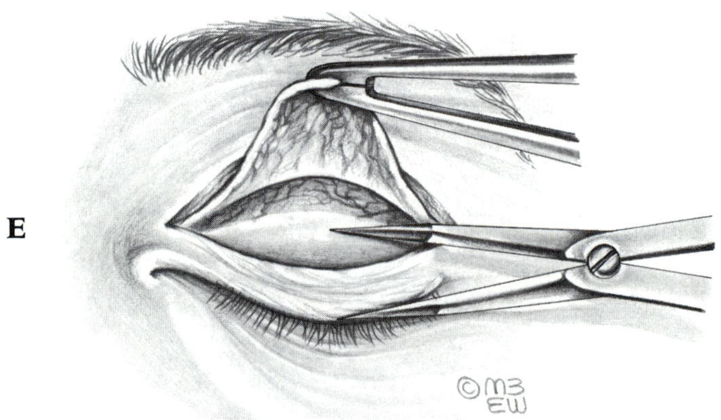

FIGURE 48-6, cont'd

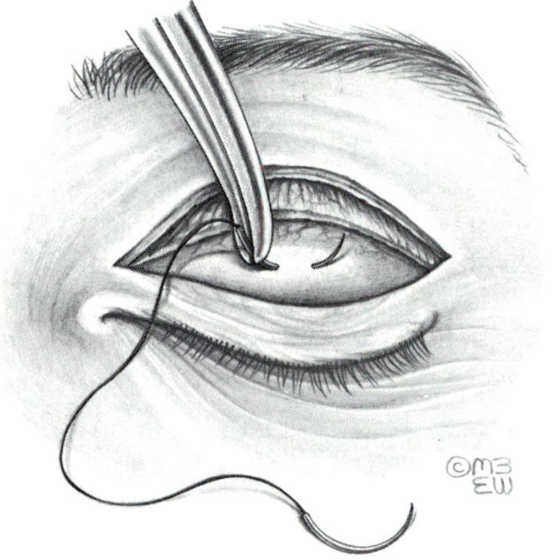

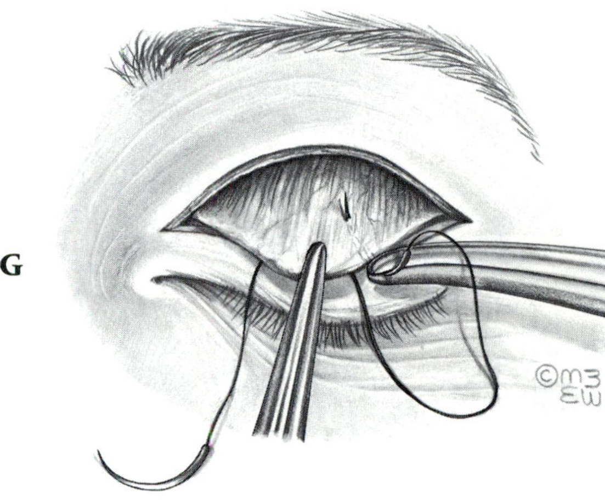

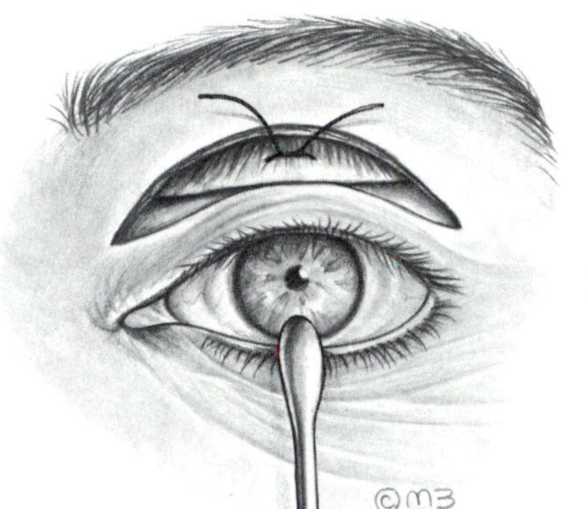

FIGURE 48-6, cont'd

Continued.

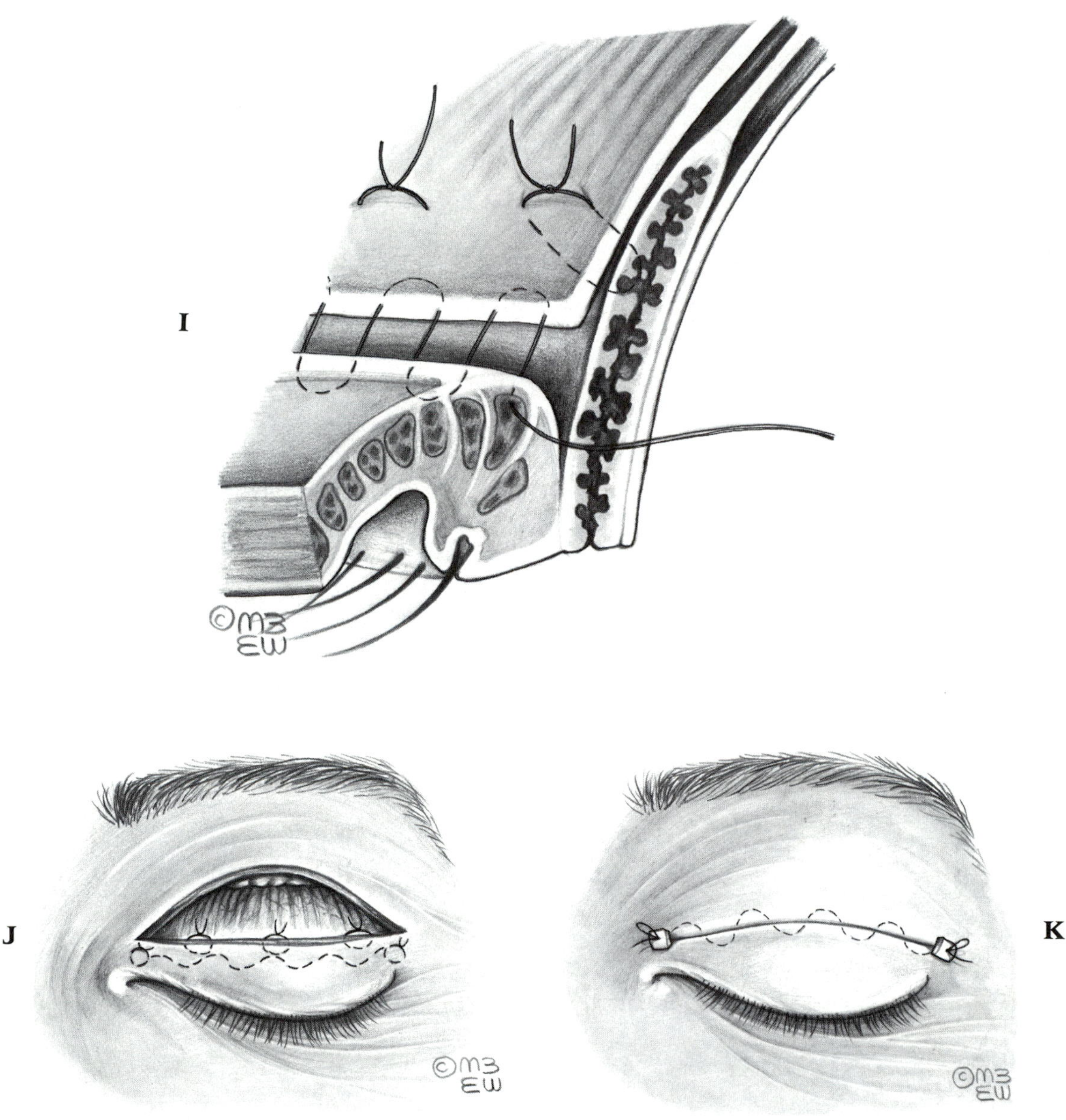

FIGURE 48-6, cont'd

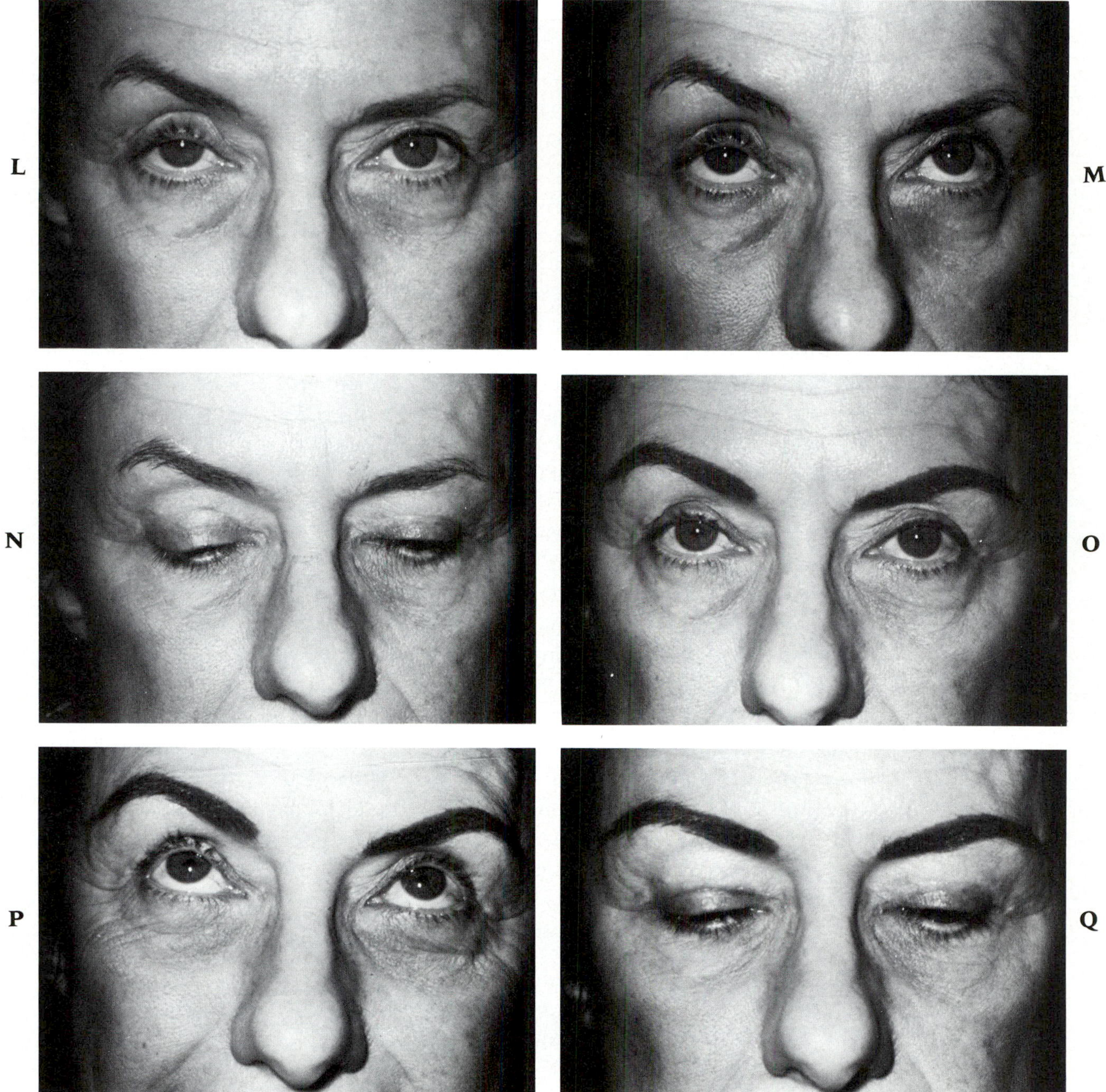
L
M
N
O
P
Q

Levator Aponeurosis–Müller's Muscle Resection and Advancement

The levator is exposed and the orbital septum is opened as in Fig. 48-5. The orbicularis muscle, below the skin incision, is excised to the base of the lashes (Fig. 48-7, *A*). The levator aponeurosis is cut and separated from the anterior surface of the tarsus. When the dissection reaches the upper edge of the tarsus and Müller's muscle, a Desmarres retractor is placed beneath the lid and the conjunctiva is made taut (Fig. 48-7, *B*). Dissection is carried upward between the conjunctiva and Müller's muscle, so that both the levator aponeurosis and Müller's muscle are freed. Three double-armed 6-0 Mersilene sutures are placed partial thickness in the tarsus (Fig. 48-7, *C*) just above the lashes. The sutures are brought through Müller's muscle and the levator aponeurosis (Fig. 48-7, *D*). The height of the resection is determined by the contour and level of the lid. If there is from 3 to 6 mm of levator function, the lid margin is placed at the final desired position. If there is 0 to 3 mm of levator function, the lid is overcorrected 1 mm. Three or four interrupted 4-0 chromic sutures then go through the upper edge of the tarsus, exiting on the levator aponeurosis at the desired lid crease height, and then one arm of each suture goes through a skin edge (Fig. 48-7, *E*). This step gives a second line of fixation of the levator aponeurosis, closes the skin, reforms the lid crease as well as everts the lashes. Two 4-0 silk sutures are then placed in a horizontal mattress fashion 4 mm beneath the lashes of the lower lid coming out of the gray line. These are placed over cotton pledgets and taped to the brow (Fig. 48-7, *F*), so that the lower lid is brought up to protect the cornea. A light dressing is placed on the eye for 48 hours, and then the sutures holding the lower lid to the brow are removed. Artificial tear drops and protection at night are used until the cornea can tolerate the additional exposure.

Fig. 48-7, *G*, shows congenital ptosis of the left upper lid with poor levator function; *H*, upgaze; *I*, downgaze; *J*, postoperative appearance after maximum levator resection without cutting of horns of the levator aponeurosis; *K*, upgaze; *L*, downgaze.

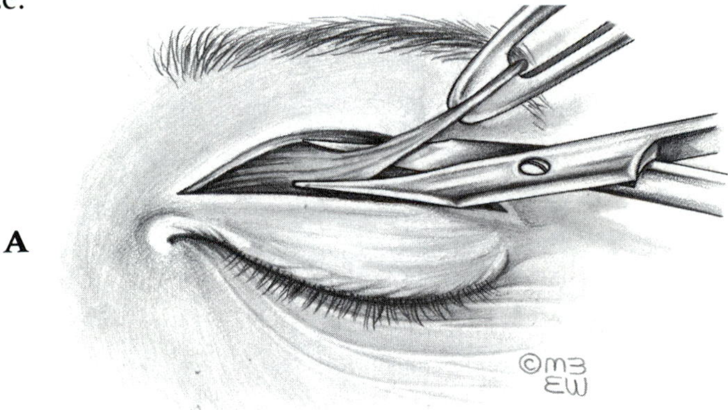

FIGURE 48-7. Aponeurosis with Müller's muscle resection.

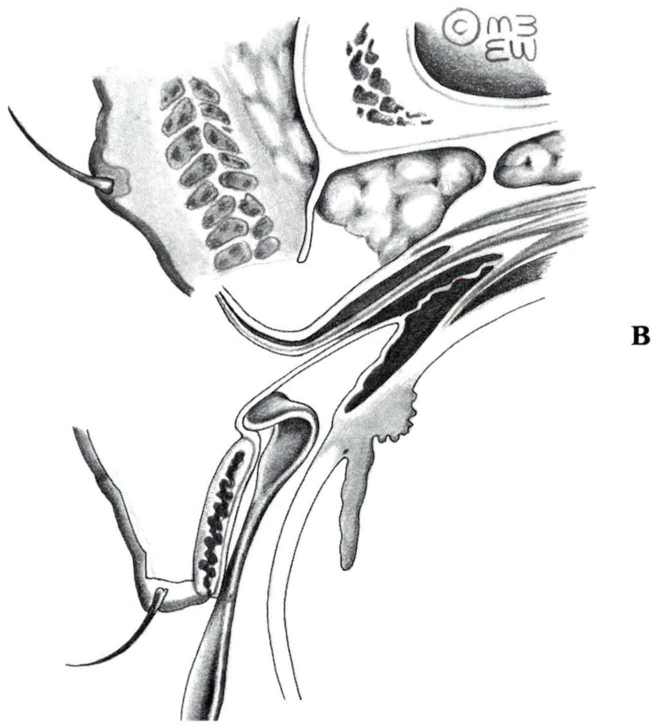

B

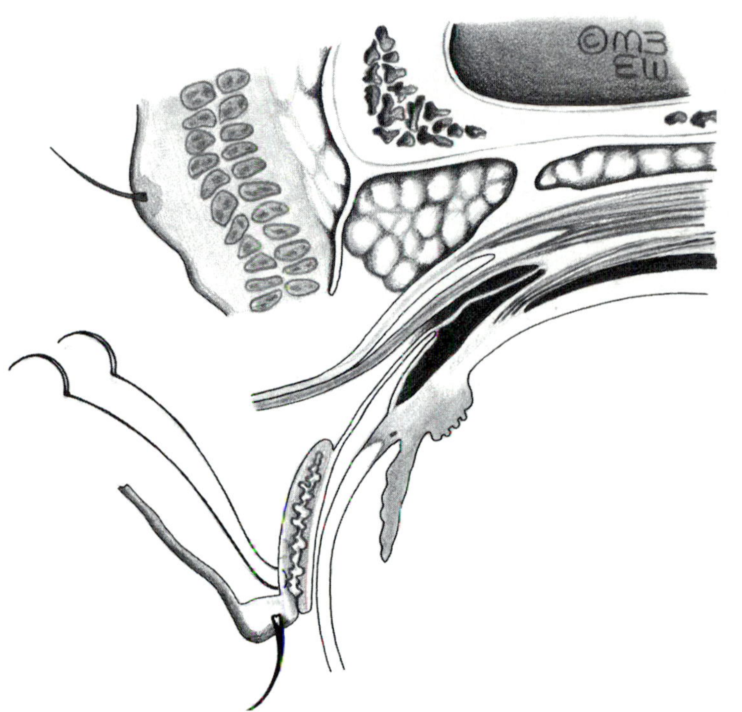

C

Continued.

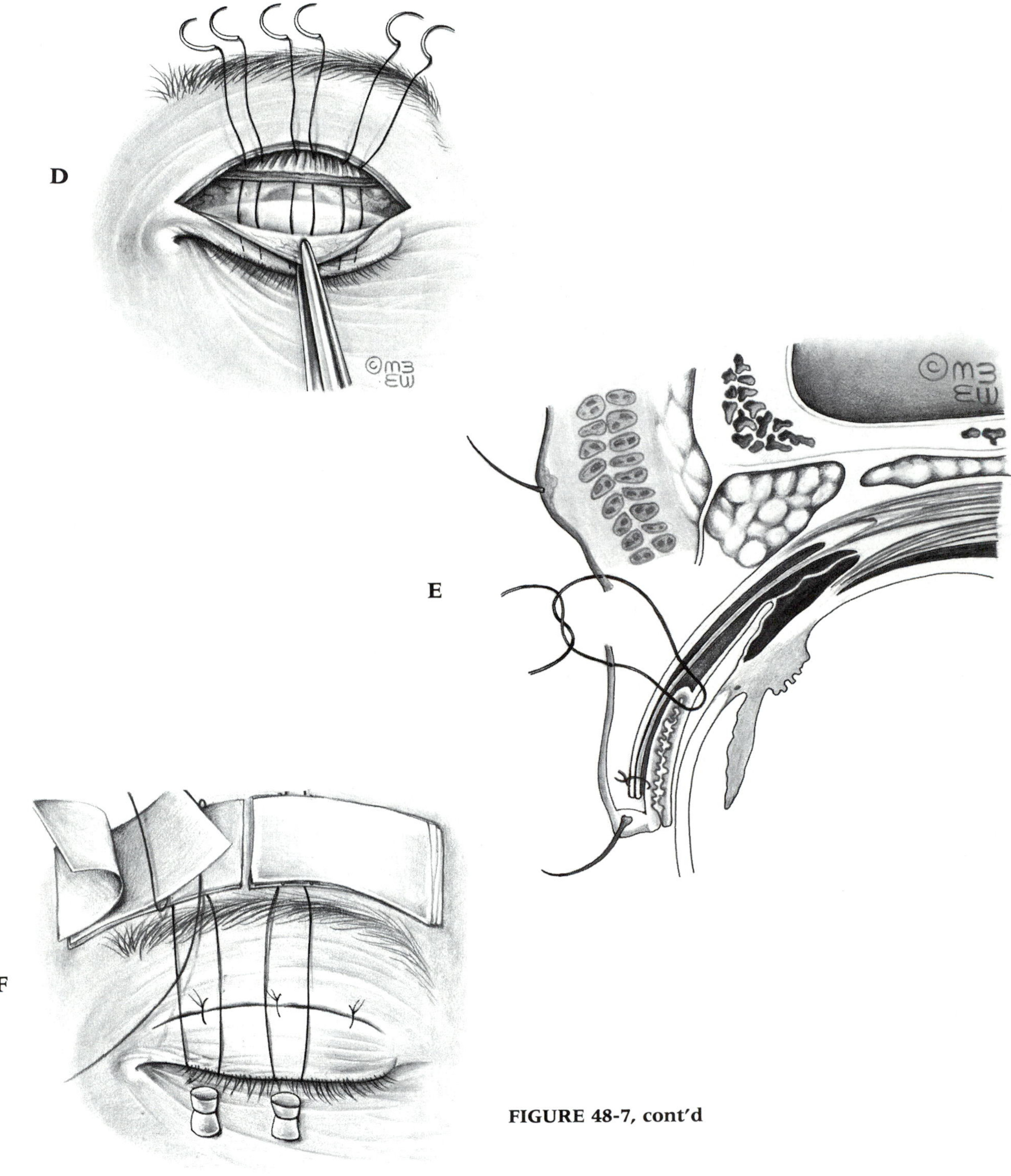

FIGURE 48-7, cont'd

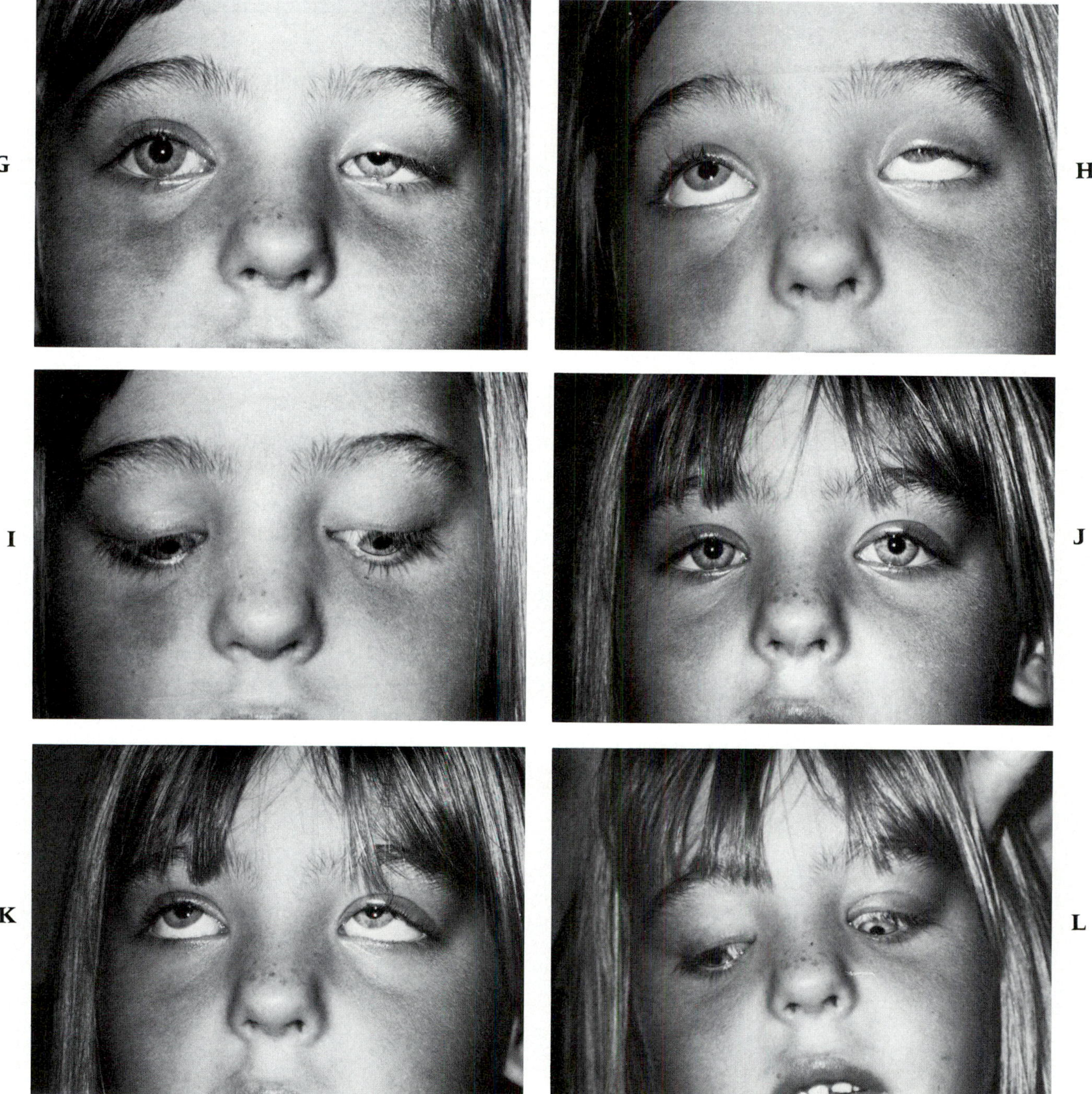
G
H
I
J
K
L

Levator Aponeurosis–Müller's Muscle Recession

This is a titration technique, and is the procedure of choice for correction of lid retraction secondary to thyroid eye disease. As described in Fig. 48-5, the orbital septum is opened across the lid and the levator aponeurosis is exposed. The levator aponeurosis is cut and dissected from the tarsus. When Müller's muscle is reached, a Desmarres retractor is placed behind the upper edge of the tarsus, making the conjunctiva taut so that Müller's muscle and the levator aponeurosis can be recessed en bloc (Fig. 48-8, *A*). The recession is initially confined to the lateral two thirds of the lid. During the surgery the patient is asked to open the eyes repeatedly so that the level of the lids can be seen by the surgeon (Fig. 48-8, *B*). If it is found that more nasal dissection is necessary, it is done a small segment at a time to prevent nasal overcorrection. When the desired end point is reached, 1 mm higher than the final desired position, place a double-arm 6-0 Mersilene suture at the upper edge of the tarsus, making certain that the needle takes only a partial-thickness bite and is brought through the lid retractors so that the retractors will not recede farther into the orbit postoperatively (Fig. 48-8, *C*). The lid crease is reformed with three interrupted horizontal mattress sutures of 6-0 Mersilene. Each suture takes a partial-thickness tarsal bite, goes through the muscle at the upper edge of the inferior skin flap, comes out just beneath the skin, goes back through, and is tied under the muscle (Fig. 48-8, *D* and *E*). These sutures will keep the lid crease at its proper position. The skin is closed with a continuous suture of 6-0 polypropylene.

Fig. 48-8, *F,* shows the preoperative appearance patient with thyroid eye disease; *G,* postoperative appearance after recession of the upper lid retractors bilaterally.

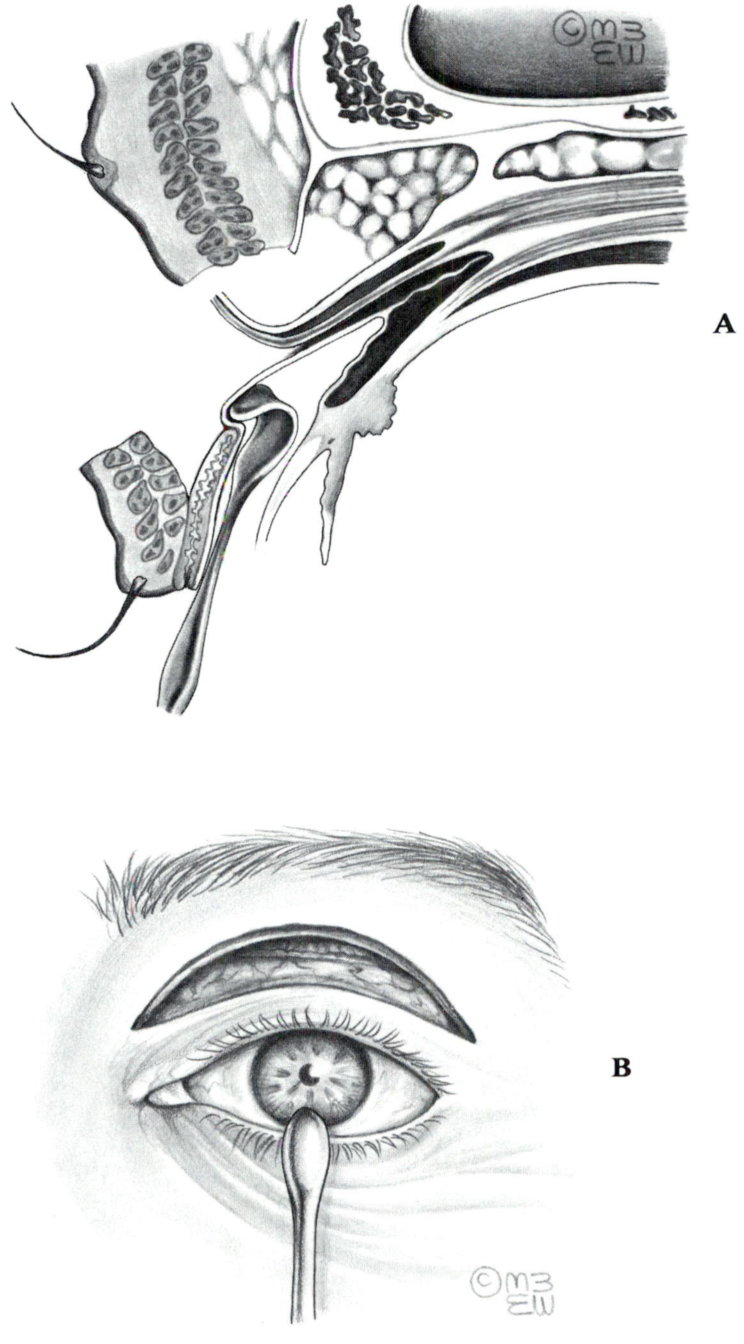

FIGURE 48-8. Recession of the upper lid retractors.

Continued.

C

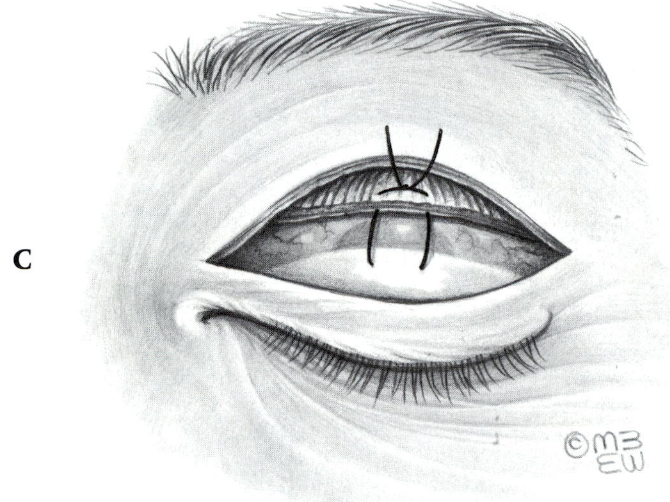

D

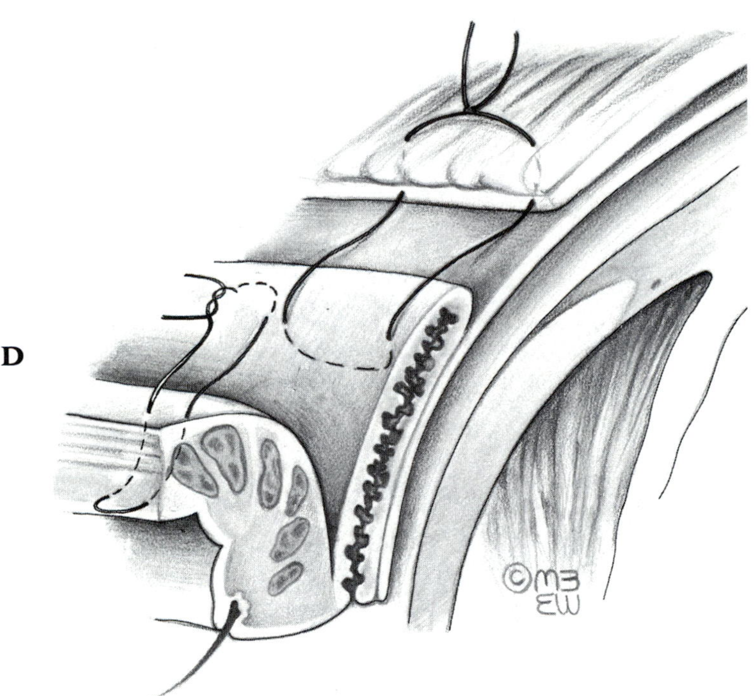

FIGURE 48-8, cont'd

E

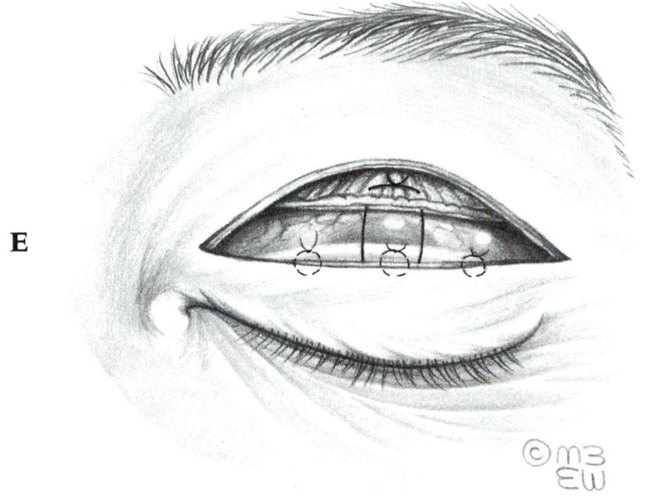

F

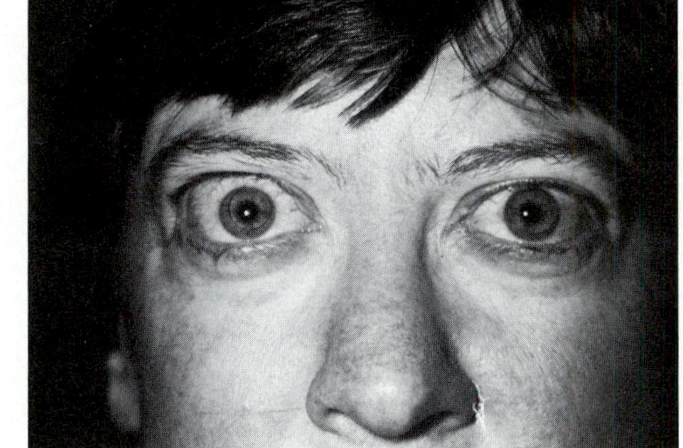

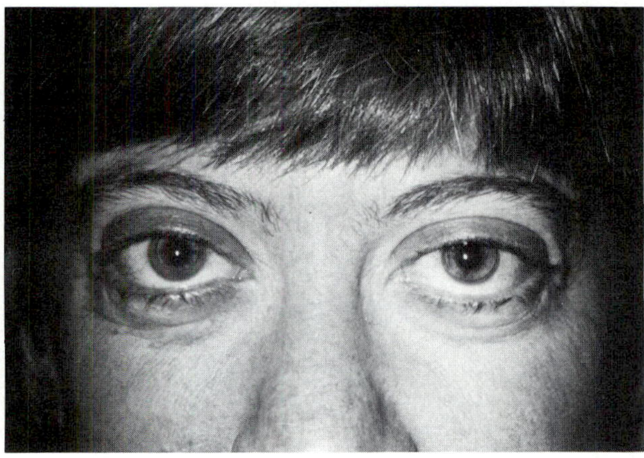

G

Formation of a Lid Crease

The lid-crease technique can be used for loss of a lid crease or Caucasianizing of the Oriental eye. The lid crease location is marked on the skin. An incision is made through the skin. Dissection is carried superiorly and inferiorly beneath the skin for 2 mm (Fig. 48-9, *A*). This is shown in the diagram with the slotted lines. A triangular block of tissue is excised with its apex at the tarsus (Fig. 48-9, *B*). The superior edge of the inferior skin flap is sutured to the tarsus (Fig. 48-9, *C*). These sutures can also include the inferior edge of the upper skin flap, but the step is not necessary. Any fat or orbital septum is removed from this area so that the skin can be attached to the tarsus.

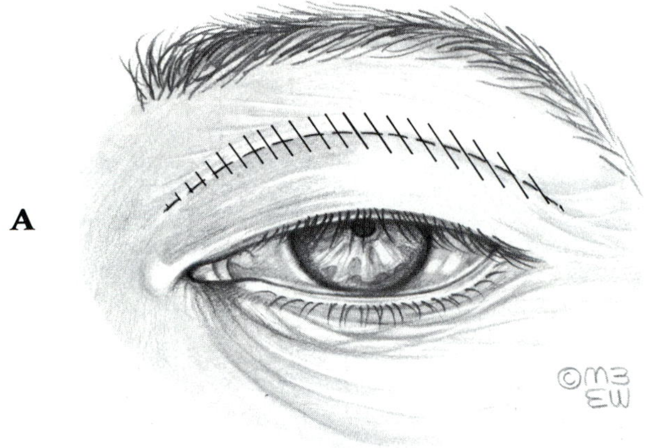

FIGURE 48-9. Lid crease formation.

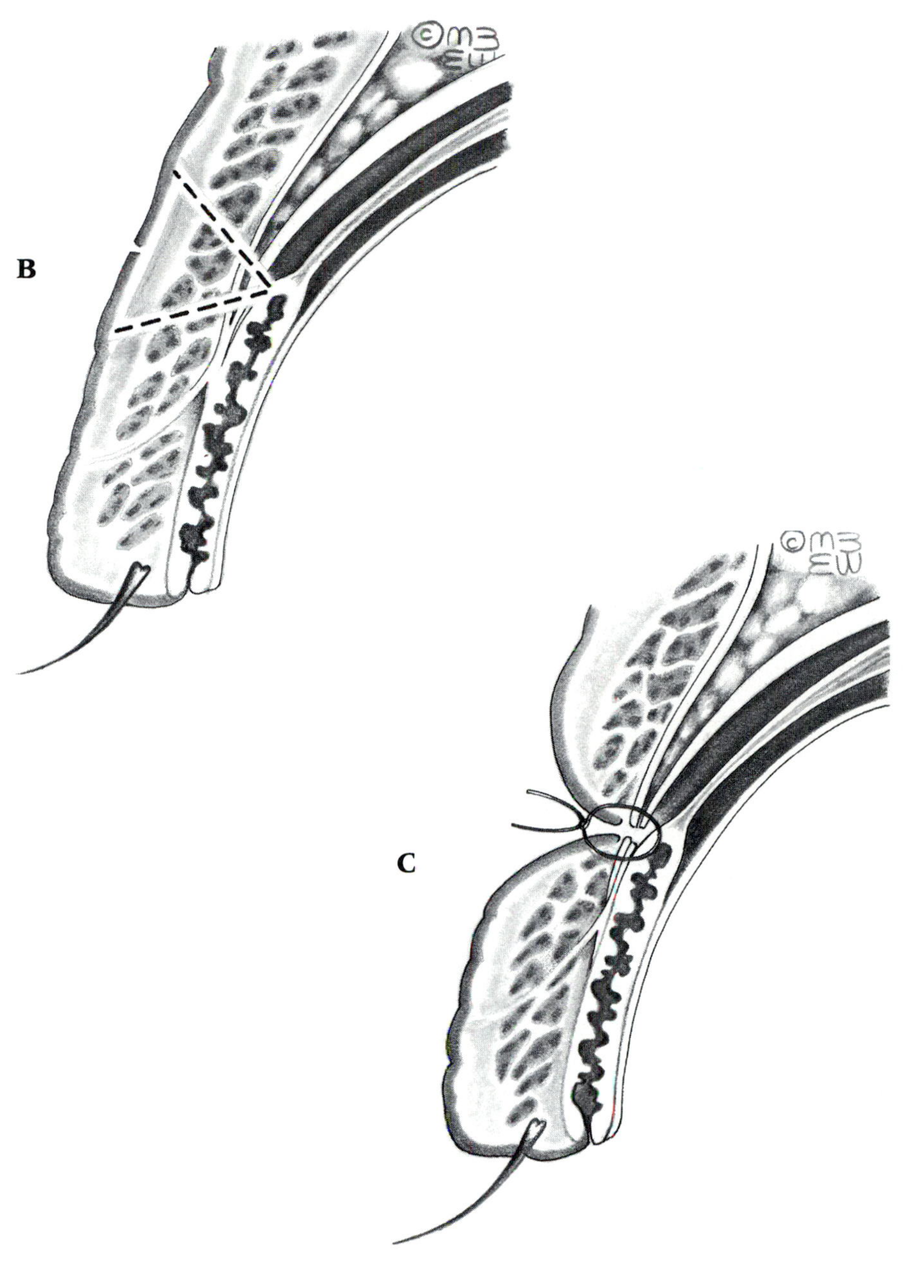
B
C

CHAPTER 49

Miscellaneous Procedures

The greater the exophthalmos, the harder it is to maintain a good result from recession of the lower lid retractors. In a patient with thyroid eye disease and considerable exophthalmos, I use a scleral graft larger than 2½ times the desired elevation.

My techniques for dacryocystorhinostomy and conjunctivodacryocystorhinostomy are only slightly modified in comparison to those published by other authors. The major change is in the construction of two very large flaps, as described in this section. Remember it is usually necessary to trim these flaps. They must be taut after suturing.

Recession of Lower Lid Retractors

An incision is made through the conjunctiva at the lower edge of the tarsus, and the conjunctiva is dissected from the lower lid retractors beyond the reflection of the inferior fornix, by cutting of the fascial connections to the inferior fornix. Dissection then goes through the lower lid retractors at the lower edge of the tarsus and continues down the anterior face of the orbital septum (Fig. 49-1, *A*). This path allows the lower lid retractors to recede into the orbit en bloc. If necessary, the orbital septum is cut. A strip of sclera 2½ times the amount of desired recession is placed into the defect and sutured to the upper edge of the lower lid retractors with a continuous suture of 6-0 Vicryl (Fig. 49-1, *B*). A 6-0 polypropylene (Prolene) suture enters the skin 4 mm from the lid margin, takes a partial-thickness bite of the tarsus, takes a bite at the upper edge of the scleral graft, takes a subconjunctival bite of the conjunctiva, goes back through the sclera, takes a horizontal partial-thickness bite in the tarsus, goes back through sclera, takes another subconjunctival bite in the conjunctiva, and continues across the lid, thereby connecting the upper edge of the sclera to the tarsus and bringing the conjunctiva over the scleral graft (Fig. 49-1, *C*). When the end of the lid is reached, the suture is brought out on the skin and tied. This suture is left in place for 5 days.

Fig. 49-1, D, shows the preoperative appearance of patient with retraction of the left lower lid after maximum inferior rectus recession for fibrosis of the inferior rectus muscle; *E*, postoperative appearance after lower lid recession and scleral graft insertion.

A

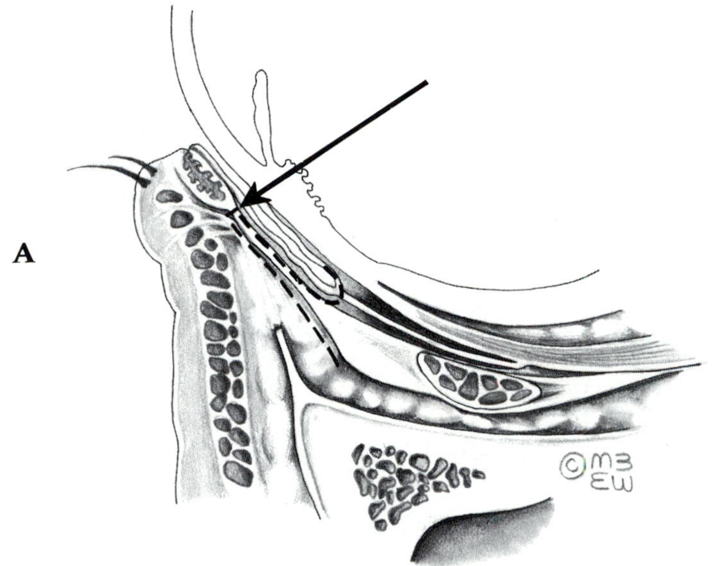

FIGURE 49-1. Recession of lower lid retractors.

B

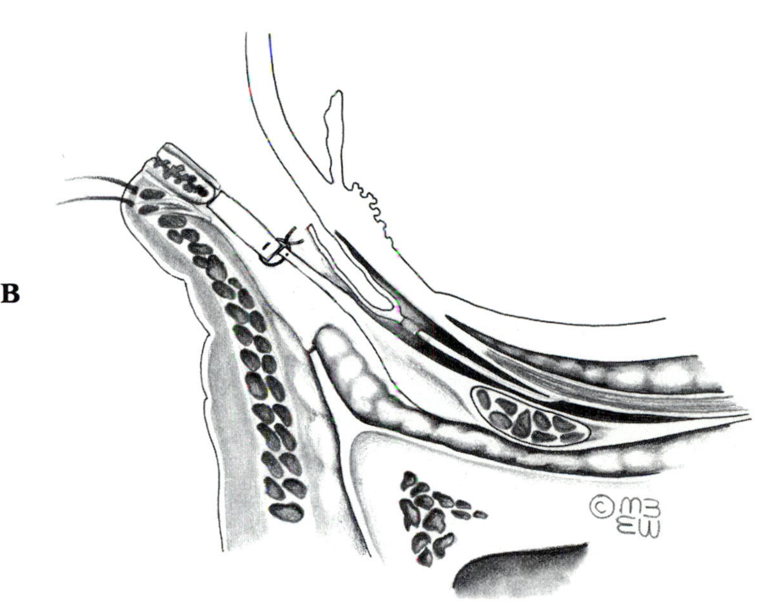

Continued.

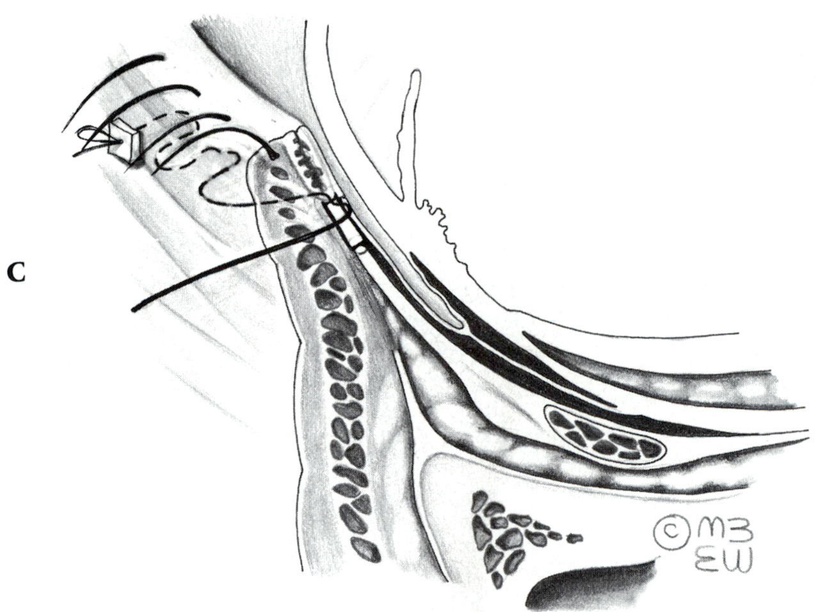

FIGURE 49-1, cont'd

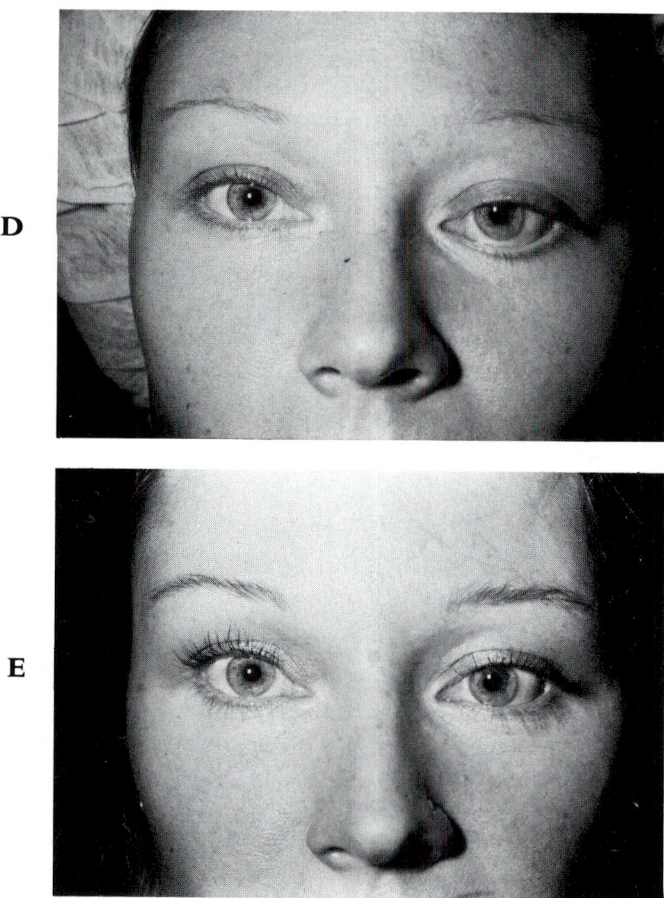

FIGURE 49-1, cont'd

Dacryocystorhinostomy

An incision is made at the inferior orbital rim, including the lower third of the medial canthal tendon (Fig. 49-2, *A*). The incision goes through the periosteum, which is reflected anteriorly and posteriorly off the crest (Fig. 49-2, *B*). A large osteotomy is made in the bone of the nose straddling the anterior crest, and the medial wall of the nasolacrimal duct is then removed (Fig. 49-2, *C*). Once the osteotomy has been made, the circumference of the opening is injected with 2% Xylocaine (lidocaine) with epinephrine, and the anesthetic is placed between the remaining bone and the periosteum for hemostasis. Fig. 49-2, *D*, illustrates the opening of the osteotomy from the nasal side. If the middle turbinate is in the way of the osteotomy, it is removed. The lacrimal sac is incised very anteriorly and reflected posteriorly. The nasal mucosa is incised very posteriorly and reflected anteriorly (Fig. 49-2, *E*). This step creates two very large flaps of mucosa (Fig. 49-2, E_1). In closure, the flaps must be tight and usually need to be trimmed. The excess sac mucosa can be sent for pathologic examination. After closure of the posterior flaps with interrupted sutures of 6-0 Vicryl, the patency of the canaliculi is checked, so that one can make certain that they open into the osteotomy. Sutures are placed into the anterior flaps (Fig. 49-2, *F*) and tied (Fig. 49-2, *G*). The periosteum is closed with interrupted sutures of 6-0 Vicryl, and the superior orbicularis muscle is closed with buried sutures going from the depth of the wound to just beneath the skin (Fig. 49-2, *H*). Such closure helps to prevent postoperative bowstringing. The muscle layer of the inferior third of the wound is closed in two layers rather than one. The skin is closed with a continuous suture of 6-0 polypropylene (Fig. 49-2, *I*). Packing is placed in the nose if there is considerable bleeding.

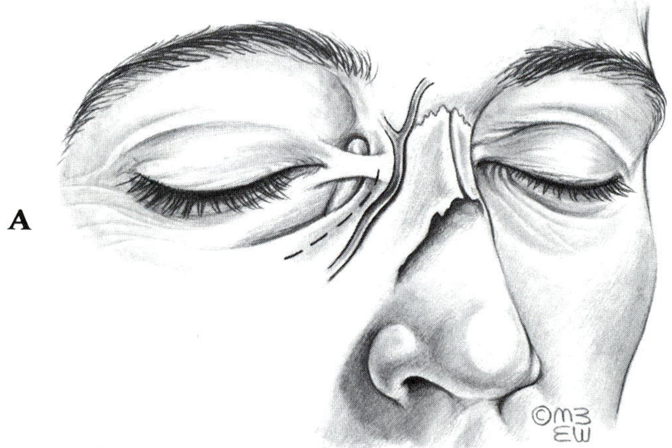

FIGURE 49-2. Dacryocystorhinostomy.

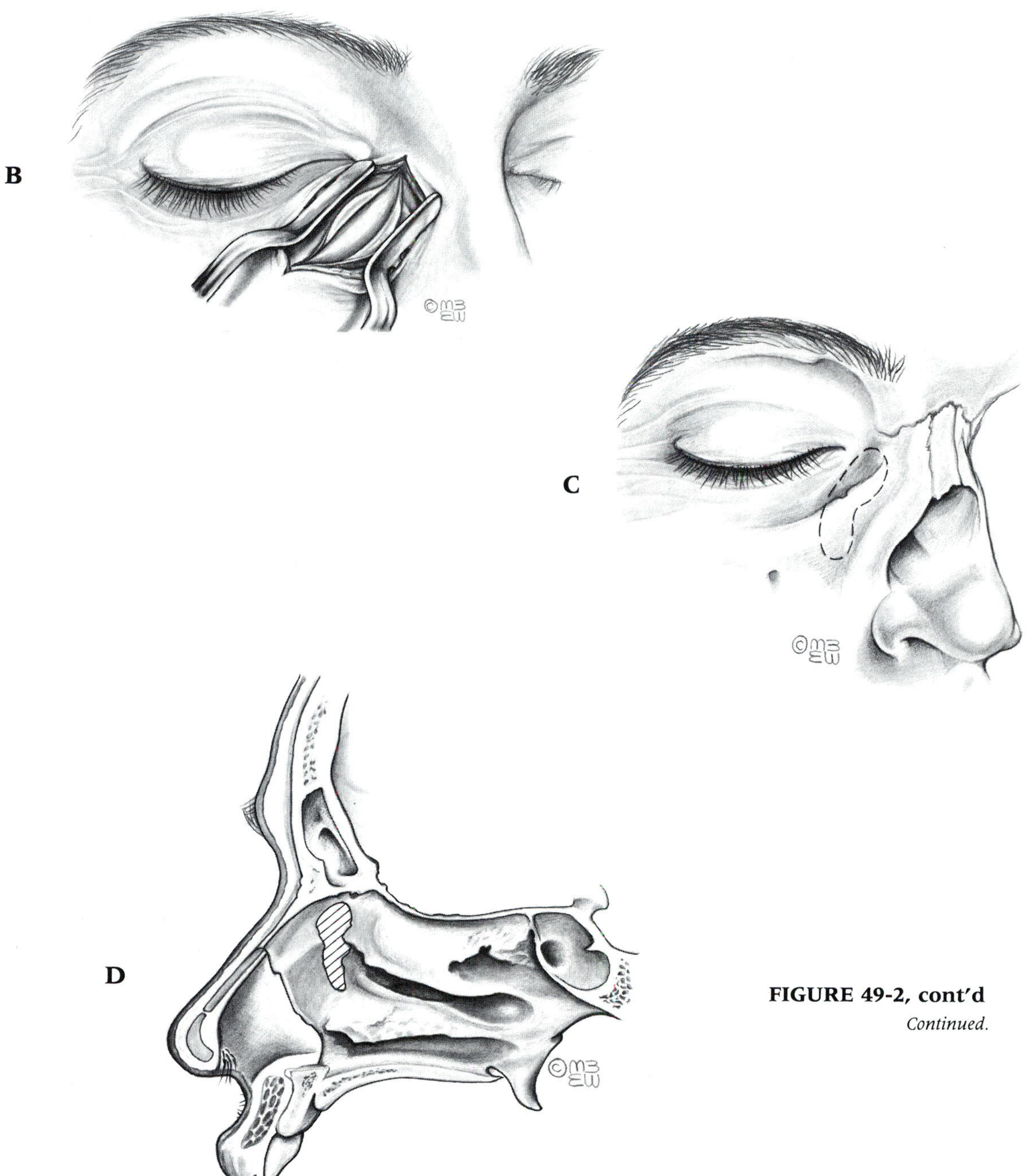

FIGURE 49-2, cont'd
Continued.

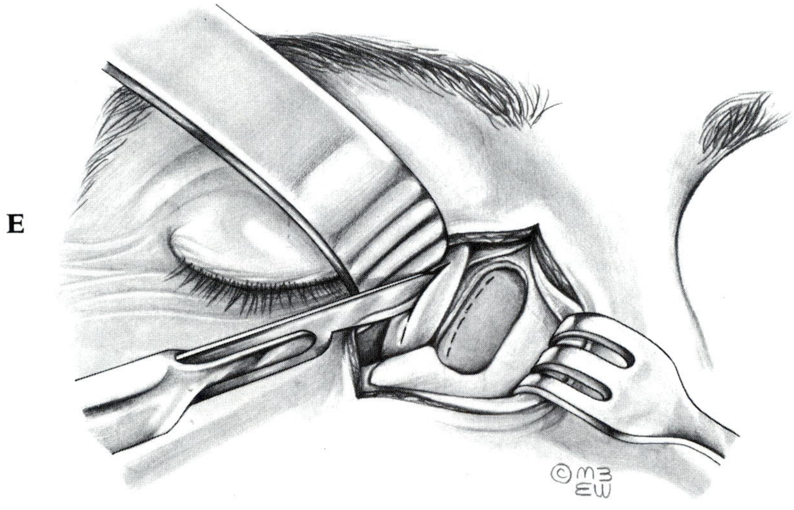

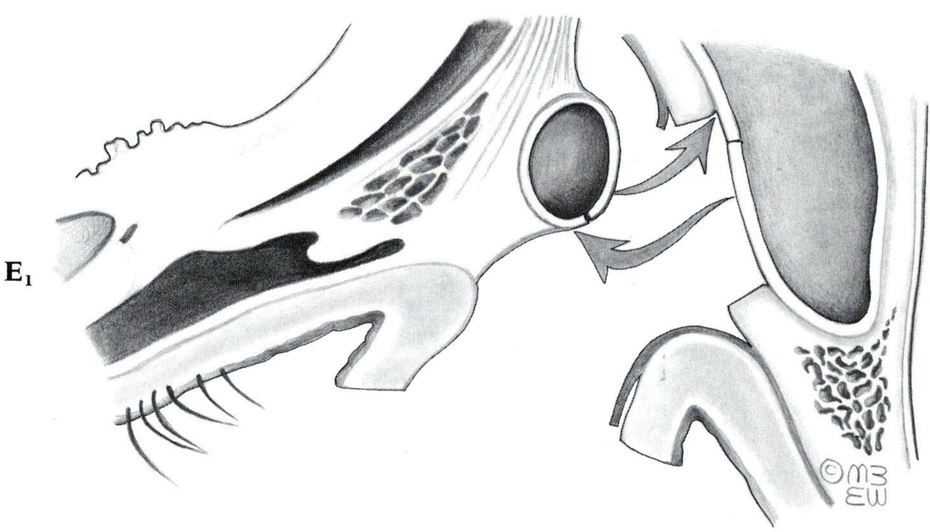

FIGURE 49-2, cont'd

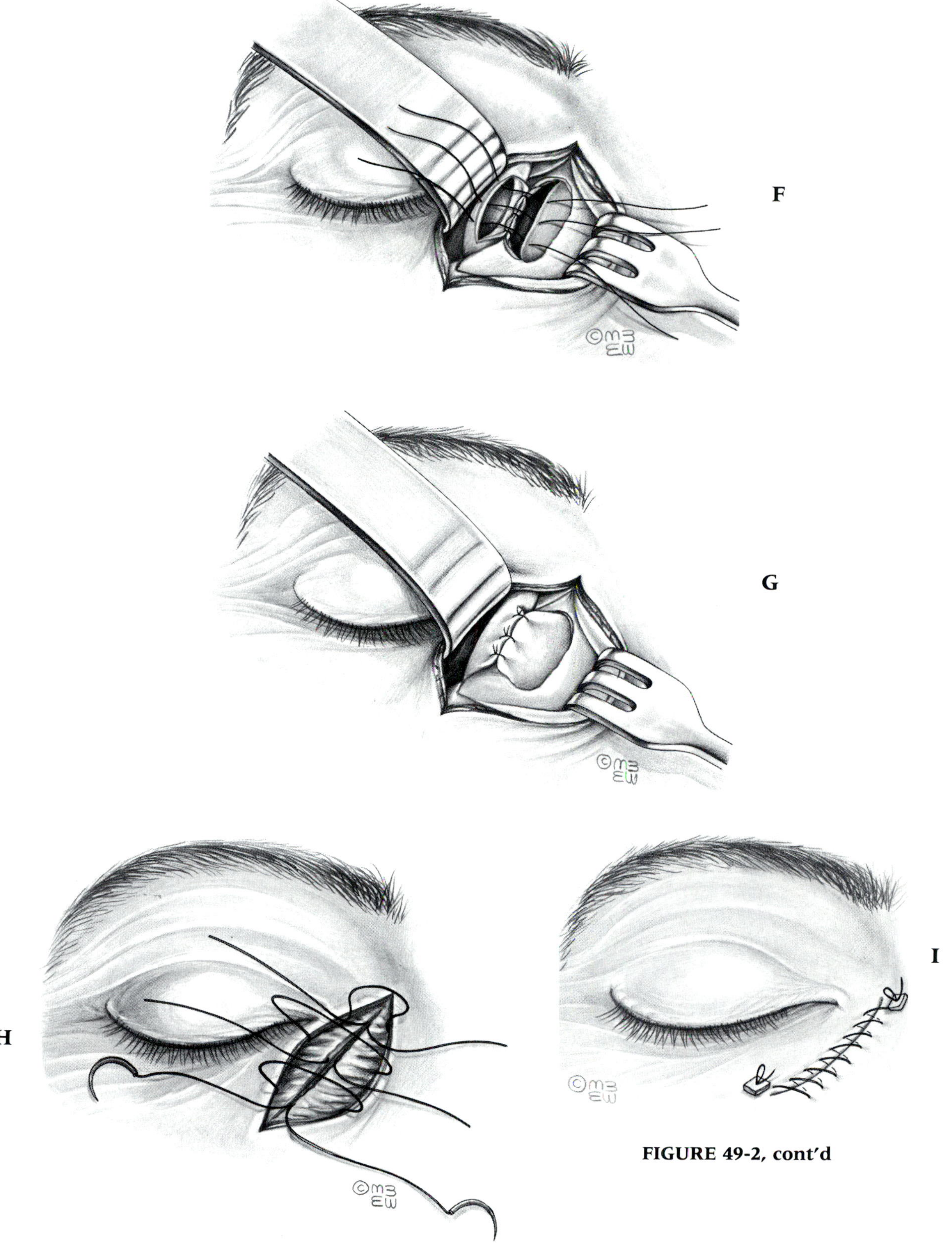

FIGURE 49-2, cont'd

Conjunctivodacryocystorhinostomy

If a Jones tube is necessary, it is inserted after the posterior flaps are in place (Fig. 49-2, *A* to *F*). A portion of the caruncle is excised *(dotted lines)*, and an 18-gauge needle is placed in the medial canthus going into the osteotomy. When the needle is in the proper position, it is followed with a Graefe knife (Fig. 49-3, *A*), and either a polyethylene 200 tubing or a glass Jones tube is placed into the opening (Fig. 49-3, *B*). I prefer a long PE 200 tubing that rests parallel to the septum and keeps the conjunctival opening in the correct position. The remainder of the closure is the same as that in a standard dacryocystorhinostomy (Fig. 49-2, *F* to *H*).

A

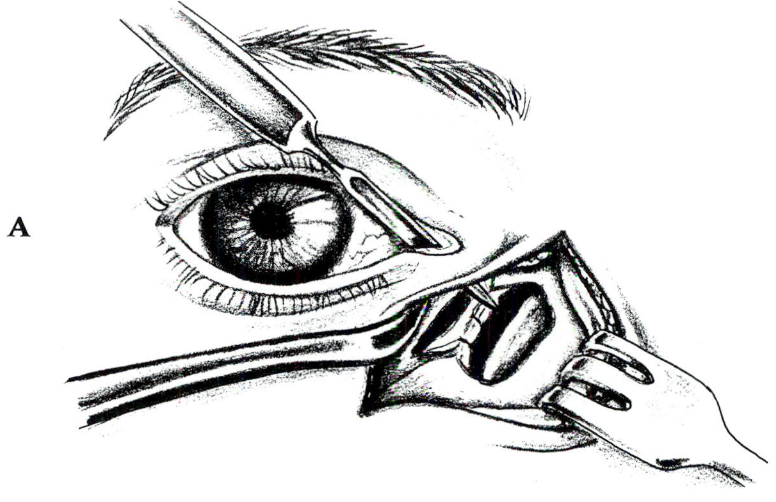

B

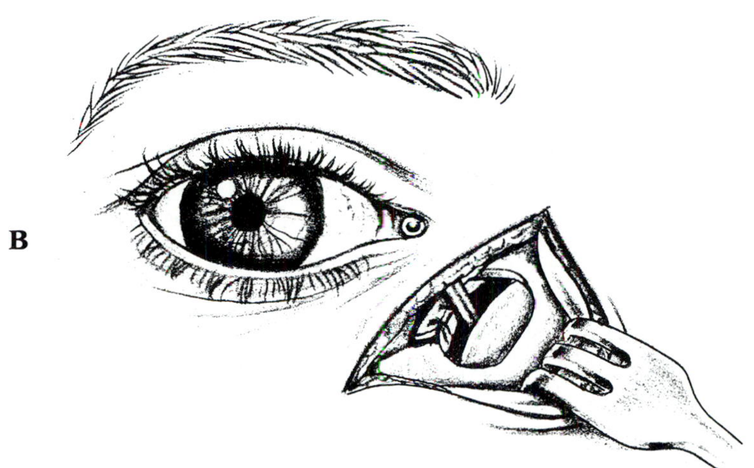

FIGURE 49-3. Conjunctivodacryocystorhinostomy.

Skin Grafts

The donor site of choice to replace facial skin is skin from the upper lids. The maximum size of the graft can be determined when the skin is grasped with Green's fixation forceps until just before lash eversion occurs. A marking pen is used to outline the graft on the lid. The lines are incised with a razor knife, and the skin graft is removed with scissors (Fig. 45-2, *A* to *C*). The donor site is closed with a subcuticular suture of 6-0 polypropylene (Fig. 45-2, *I*).

The second best site for a facial color match is the postauricular skin. The graft straddles the crease of the ear. After the graft has been marked out, it is incised with a Bard-Parker knife and excised with scissors. The closure is formed with a continuous deep to subcutaneous suture of 6-0 Vicryl. The first suture is taken with the knot buried. The suture continues from the depth of the wound to just beneath the skin, goes across the wound, enters just beneath the skin, and exits through the depth of the wound. The suture is pulled tight and held under tension by the assistant. The next suture is placed in the same fashion, the wound edges are pushed together, and the assistant releases the previous suture. The suture is pulled tight, and the assistant once again keeps tension on the suture. When the end of the wound is reached, the suture goes back into the depth of the wound on the same side where the last suture exited. The suture comes out beneath the skin edge, goes across the wound beneath the skin edge, exits deeply, and then is tied to the previous suture, so that the knot is again placed in the depth of the wound. No further sutures are needed in the postauricular area.

The third site for a skin graft to the face is a full-thickness graft from beneath the arm. Even though it is not a good color match, the skin will have had very little sun exposure but may be necessary in those patients who have severely sun-damaged skin. The skin beneath the arm is marked out, incised with a Bard-Parker blade and excised with scissors. The subcutaneous tissues are closed with interrupted sutures of 6-0 Vicryl, and the skin wound itself is closed with staples. These are removed in 8 to 9 days.

The grafts are fixed into the defect with several interrupted sutures of 7-0 silk and sutured with continuous sutures of 6-0 polypropylene. Silk sutures, 4-0, are placed into the normal tissue on each side straddling the graft. A bolus is placed beneath these sutures, and the sutures are tied over the bolus, so that the entire graft is firmly pressed against its vascular bed. (See Fig. 46-4, *F* and *G*.)

Mucous Membrane Grafts

If mucous membrane lining is needed on the palpebral surface, a full-thickness lid mucosal graft is used. The lower lip is anesthetized and clamped with a towel clip on each edge of the lip. The lip is blown up with either saline or very dilute anesthetic until the mucosa is very tight, and a full-thickness graft is outlined with a marking pen. The lines are incised with a razor knife, and the graft is taken full-thickness with scissors.

If the mucosa is needed on the bulbar surface, a partial-thickness 0.4 mm graft is taken with a Castroviejo keratotome. The lips are clamped and injected as one would with a full-thickness graft, and the keratotome is brought firmly across the lip. While the partial-thickness graft is being cut, additional cuts may have to be made on each side of the blade. Before the graft is cut free from the lip, two sutures are placed into the graft to identify the epithelial surface for correct placement on the globe.

Neither the full-thickness nor the partial-thickness donor site need be closed. Chloraseptic (total phenol 1.4% solution) mouth wash is used for any pain to the lip.

PART EIGHT

ORBITAL SURGERY

Robert C. Della Rocca

CHAPTER 50

Surgical Anatomy

The orbital cavities are paired bony structures that are centered just above the horizontal midline of the face. The entrance to the orbit is approximately 40 mm in width and 35 mm in height. The volume of the orbit is 30 cc, whereas that of the globe is only 6.5 cc. The seven bones that contribute to the orbital vault are the frontal, zygoma, maxilla, lacrimal, ethmoid, sphenoid, and palatine. They are covered by a periosteal lining referred to as the "periorbita."

The orbital rim is a solid structure made up of the frontal bone superiorly, the prominent zygomatic bone temporally, and the maxilla inferiorly and nasally. The medial rim is formed by the frontal bone. The lacrimal fossa is the space between the anterior and posterior lacrimal crests, which contains the lacrimal sac. It extends inferiorly to the entrance of the nasolacrimal duct.

The orbital rim is very thick compared to the orbital walls and offers protection to the orbital contents (Fig. 50-1). Essentially the rim is made up by the frontal, zygomatic, and maxillary bones. The sturdy and prominent zygomatic bone makes up the greater part of the lateral orbital rim.

The infraorbital nerve exits from the infraorbital canal approximately 6 to 8 mm below the orbital rim in adults and 3 mm below the rim in young children. Lying between the greater and lesser wings of the sphenoid bone is the superior orbital fissure. The inferior orbital fissure lies between the orbital floor and lateral wall posteriorly (Fig. 50-2, *A*). In the depression between the anterior lacrimal crest and the posterior lacrimal crest lies the lacrimal sac (Fig. 50-2, *B*).

The roof of the orbit is composed primarily of the orbital plate of the frontal bone and a small posterior contribution by the lesser wing of the sphenoid bone. It is concave when compared to the other orbital walls. The lacrimal gland is housed in a depression on the anterolateral aspect of the roof. Medially the trochlea exists near the junction of the superior and medial walls approximately 5 mm behind the orbital rim. The frontal sinuses are located above the orbital plate of the frontal bone. Mucoceles can form in the frontal sinus when the nasofrontal duct is obstructed.

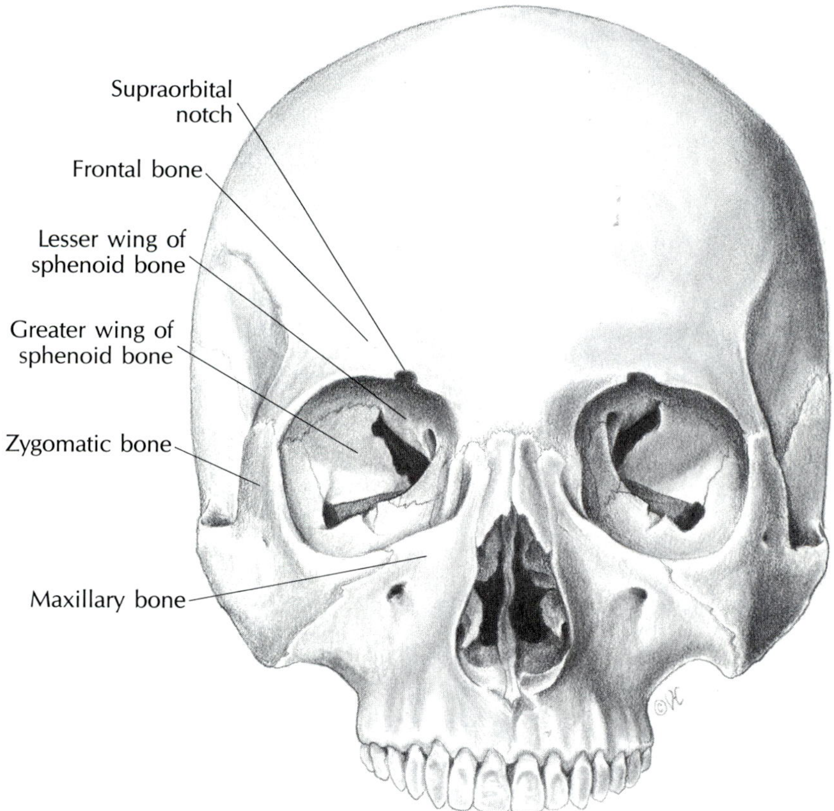

FIGURE 50-1. Anatomy of orbital rim.

A

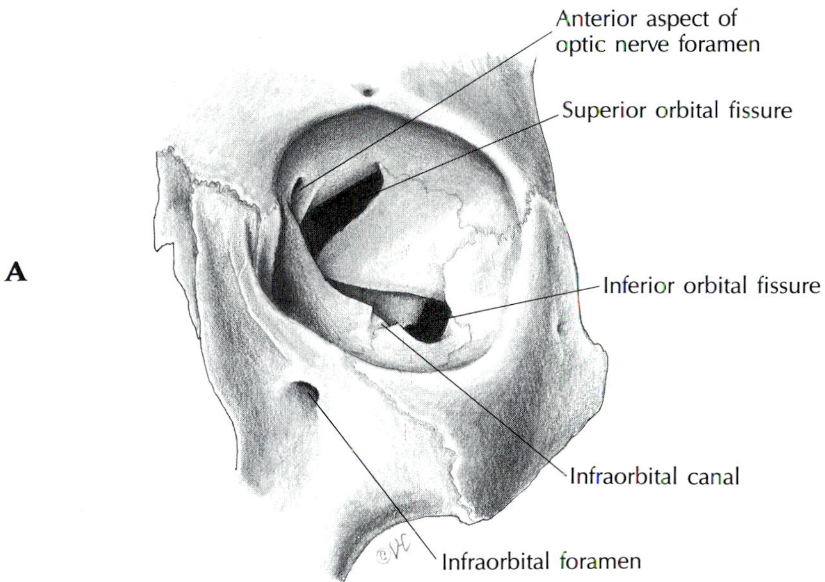

B

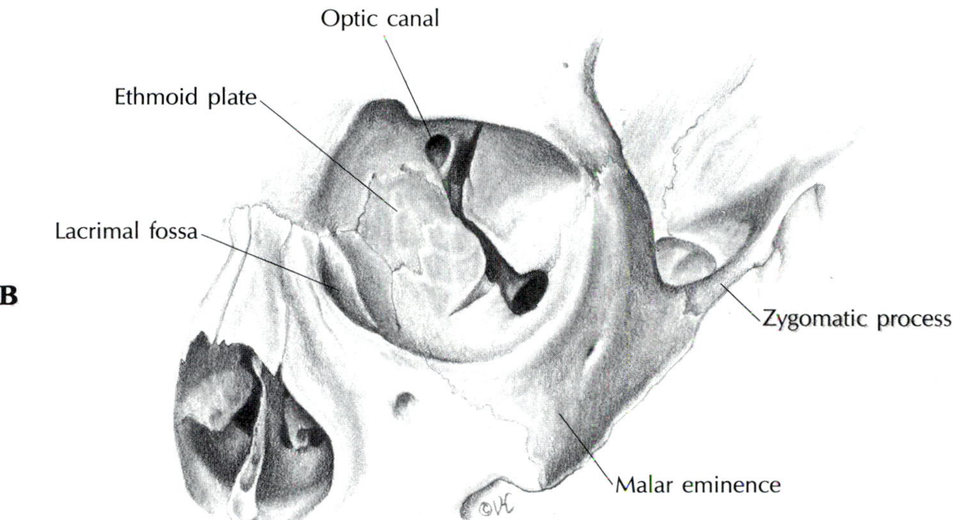

FIGURE 50-2. Medial view of lateral wall.

A coronal cut of the orbits also demonstrates the intimate relationship between the orbits and sinuses (Fig. 50-3). Immediately beneath the orbital floor is the maxillary sinus. The thin medial wall separates the orbits from the ethmoid sinuses. The wall between the frontal sinus and orbit will erode secondary to large mucocele formation.

Of the four walls of the orbit, the medial wall is the only one that has an oblong rather than a triangular shape. From anterior to posterior, it is composed of the frontal process of the maxillary bone, the lacrimal bone, the orbital plate of the ethmoid bone, and the body of the sphenoid.

The orbital plate of the ethmoid bone has the distinction of being the thinnest bone in the orbit, measuring only 0.2 to 0.4 mm in thickness. It is referred to as the lamina papyracea. The anterior and posterior ethmoidal foramina are found in or just above the suture line between the ethmoid and frontal bones approximately 18 and 35 mm behind the orbital rim respectively.

Congenital as well as acquired dehiscences may occur in the thin orbital plate of the ethmoid bone and along with the ethmoidal foramina may act as a communicating tracts between the ethmoid sinuses and the orbit. These may predispose the orbit to developing orbital cellulitis or abscess when there is infection in the adjacent sinuses. Orbital abscesses are usually found in the subperiorbital space.

The sagittal view in Fig. 50-4, *A*, shows the orbital plate of the frontal bone, the ethmoid bone, and the lacrimal fossa (Fig. 50-4, *B*). The anterior and posterior ethmoidal arteries leave the orbit through the anterior and posterior foramina.

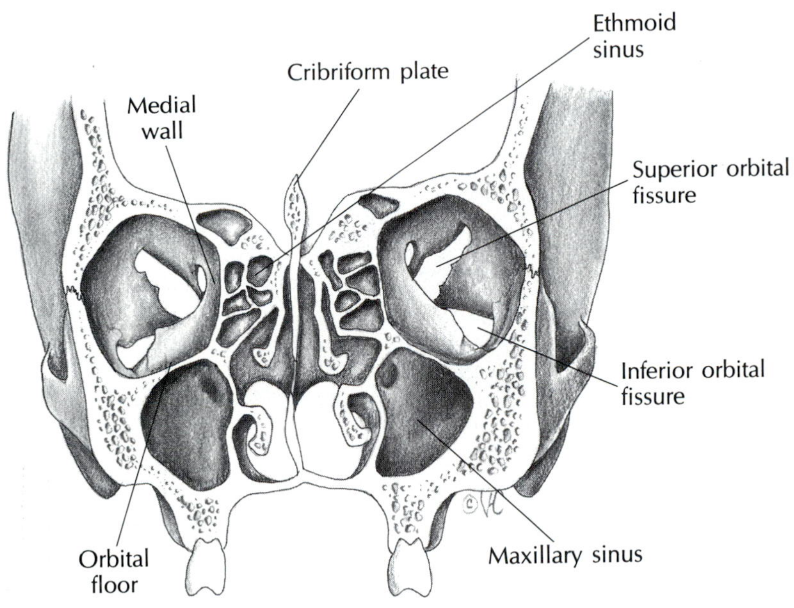

FIGURE 50-3. Coronal cut of orbits.

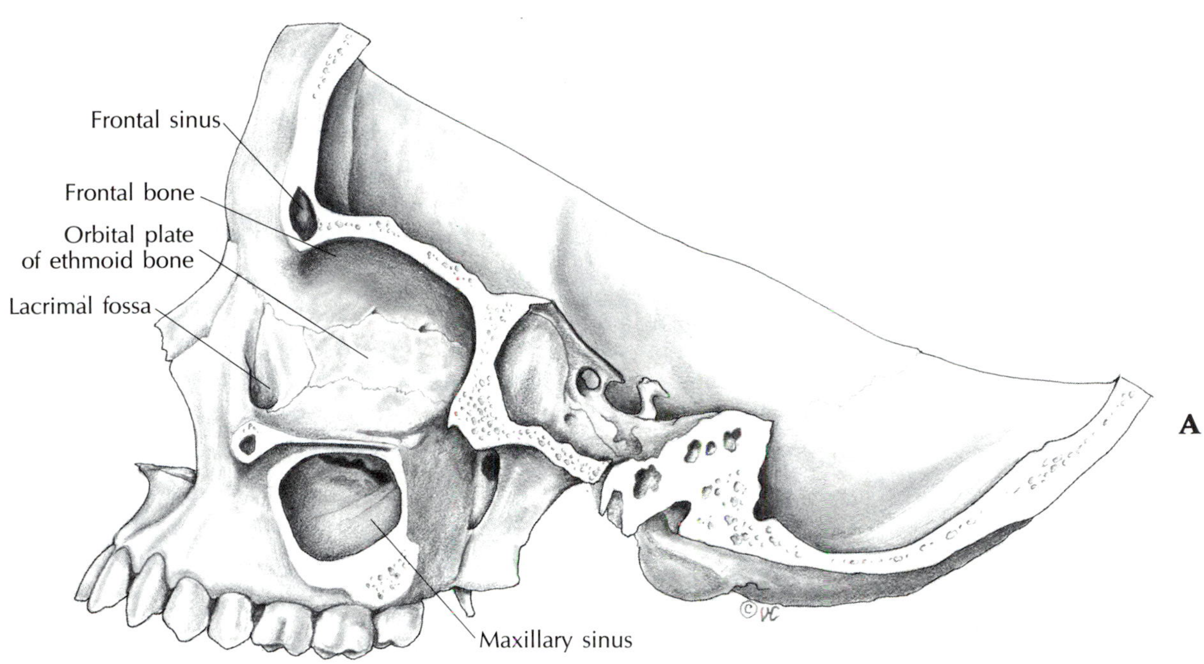

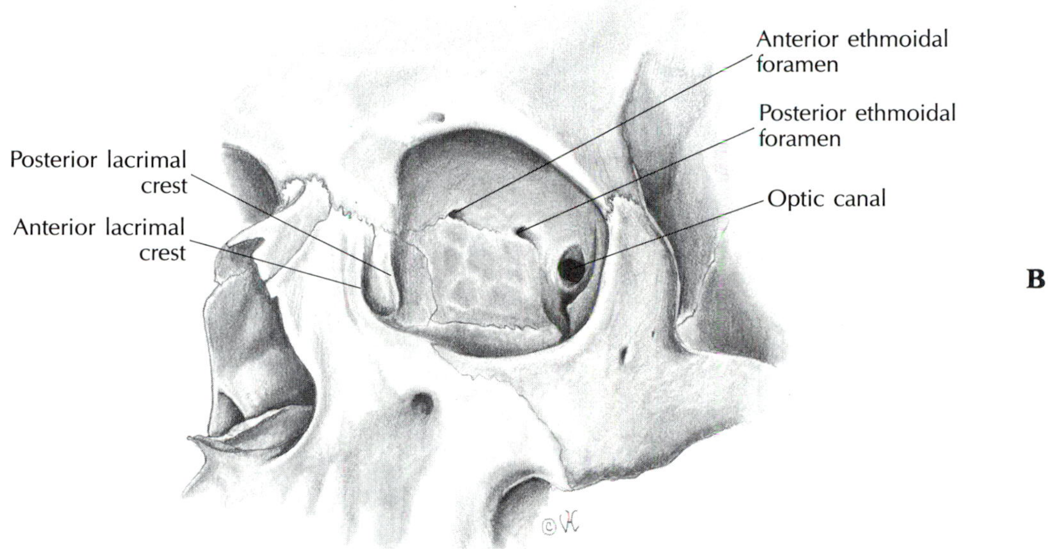

FIGURE 50-4. **A,** Sagittal view of medial orbital wall, sphenoid sinus, and sella turcica. **B,** Medial wall of the orbit.

The intranasal view in Fig. 50-5 demonstrates the relationship of the turbinates. The nasolacrimal duct exits below the inferior turbinate in the anterior third of the inferior meatus. Above the inferior turbinate are the middle and superior turbinates.

The orbital floor is triangular in shape and made up of three bones—the maxilla, zygomatic, and palatine. The inferior orbital fissure is a space bordered by the maxilla and palatine bones nasally and the greater wing of the sphenoid temporally. It begins at the apex and extends anteriorly and laterally to a point approximately 20 mm from the orbital rim. During surgery to repair an orbital floor fracture, the fissure is a landmark representing a limit to posterior subperiorbital dissection. The infraorbital sulcus is a depression in the maxilla beginning at the inferior orbital fissure and extends anteriorly to the center of the orbital floor. Here it becomes the infraorbital canal. The floor of the orbit is thinnest medial to the infraorbital canal where blow-out fractures more frequently occur.

With the transverse view of the orbital floor shown in Fig. 50-6, the inferior orbital fissure can be seen to lie parallel to the lateral orbital wall. The infraorbital groove begins at the inferior orbital fissure and courses anteriorly, becoming the infraorbital canal. The nasolacrimal duct enters the orbital floor anteromedially. The floor is thinnest medial to the canal. The canal courses obliquely and inferiorly to exit at the infraorbital foramen below the orbital rim.

The lateral wall of the orbit is the strongest of the four walls. It is made up of the prominent zygomatic bone anteriorly and the greater wing of the sphenoid posteriorly. Like the orbital roof and the floor, it is roughly triangular in shape. The lateral orbital tubercle, a small elevation of bone found just inside the lateral orbital rim, is notable because of its attachments to several important structures. These include the lateral canthal tendon, the lateral horn of the levator aponeurosis, Lockwood's suspensory ligament of the globe, and the check ligament of the lateral rectus muscle.

The greater wing of the sphenoid bone, which lies behind the zygoma, is thinner than the zygoma. As one follows the greater wing posteriorly, however, it becomes separated from the orbital roof by the superior orbital fissure.

Lying temporal to the lateral orbital wall is the temporal fossa through which the temporalis muscle passes. The attachments of this muscle to the lateral orbital rim are severed when the rim is removed during a lateral orbitotomy. The anterior aspect of the greater wing of the sphenoid borders the temporal fossa. As one moves posteriorly, the sphenoid wing becomes part of the anterior wall of the middle cranial fossa.

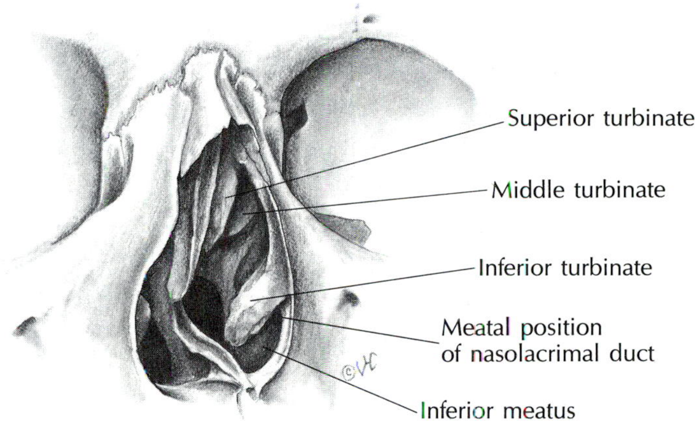

FIGURE 50-5. Intranasal view of orbital of turbinates.

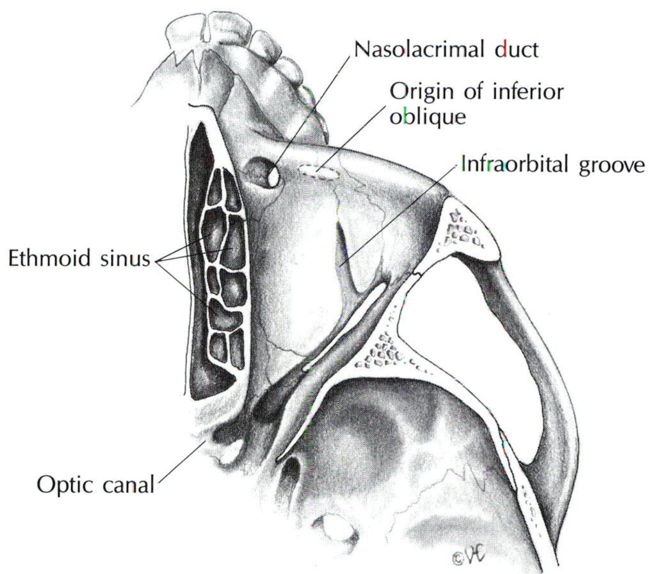

FIGURE 50-6. Transverse view of orbital floor.

Fig. 50-7, *A*, shows a lateral view of the skull. Tripod fracture involves the zygomatic and maxillary bones as well as the zygomatic process.

Fig. 50-7, *B*, shows the temporalis muscle, which courses inferiorly in the temporal fossa just lateral to the orbit. It attaches to the coronoid process.

Fig. 50-7, *C*, shows the masseter as it extends from the mandible to the zygomatic process. If the fractured zygoma impinges on the coronoid process, movement of the mandible will be limited, perhaps leading to trismus.

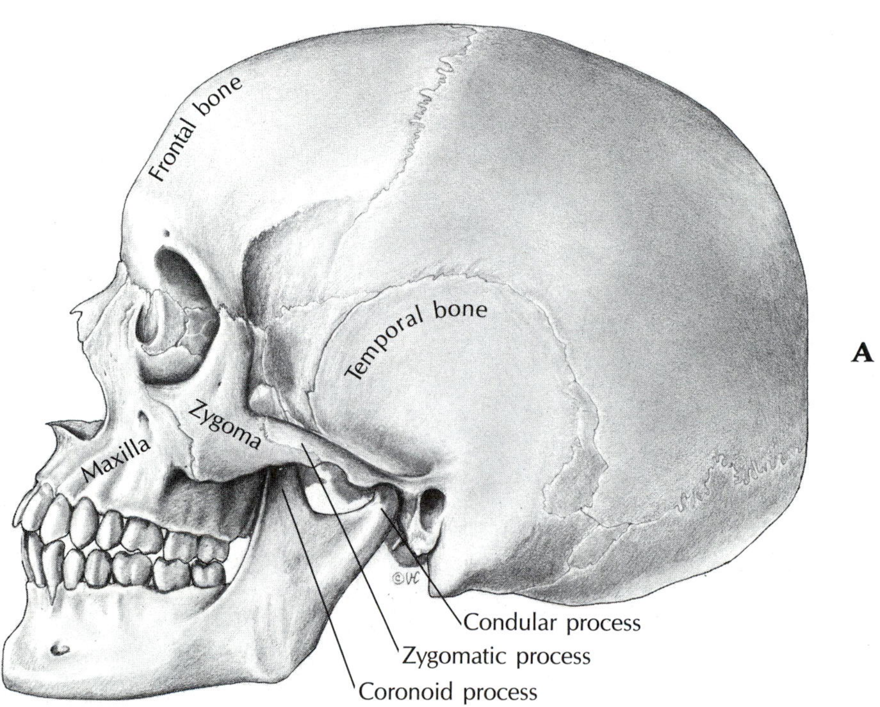

FIGURE 50-7. **A,** Lateral view of the skull. **B,** View with temporalis muscle. **C,** View with masseter and temporalis muscles.

B

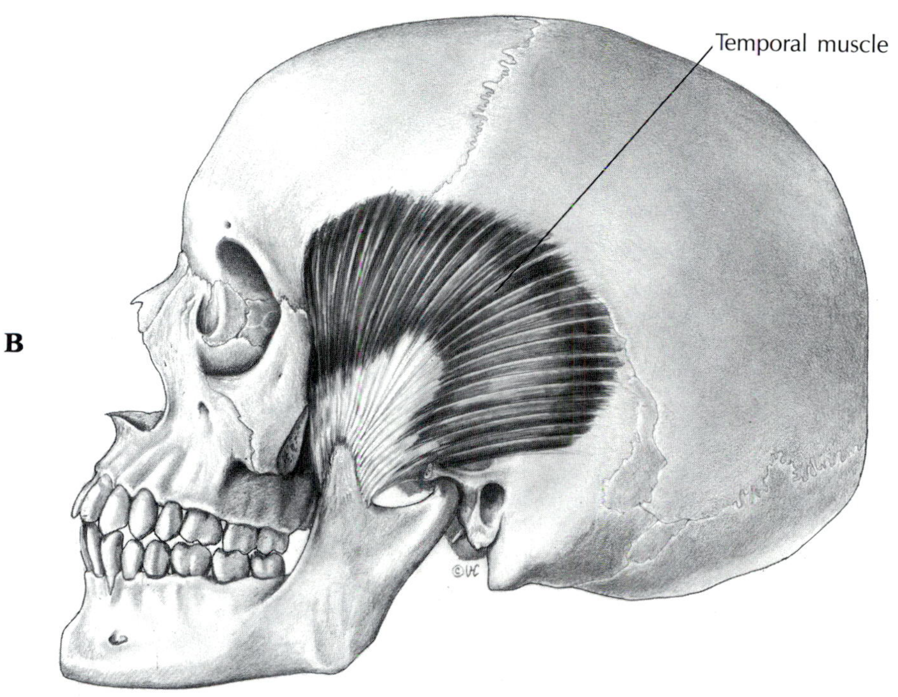
Temporal muscle
©VC

C

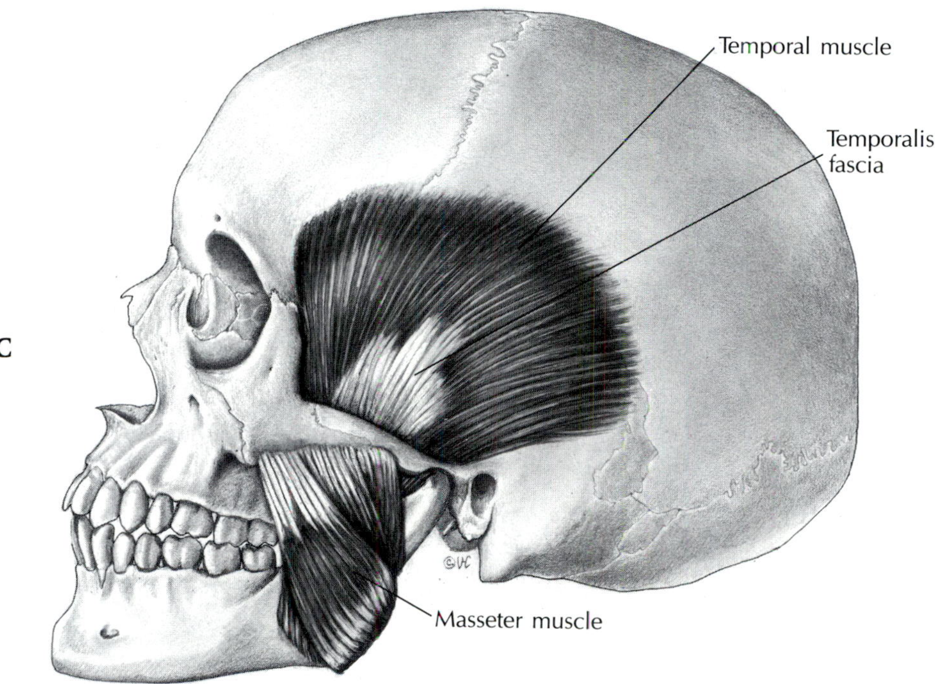
Temporal muscle
Temporalis fascia
Masseter muscle
©VC

Fig. 50-8 shows the anterior wall of the maxilla and orbital rim cut away to show the maxillary sinus and relation between medial wall and orbital floor. The Caldwell-Luc maxillary approach allows for good exposure of the posterior medial wall and orbital floor.

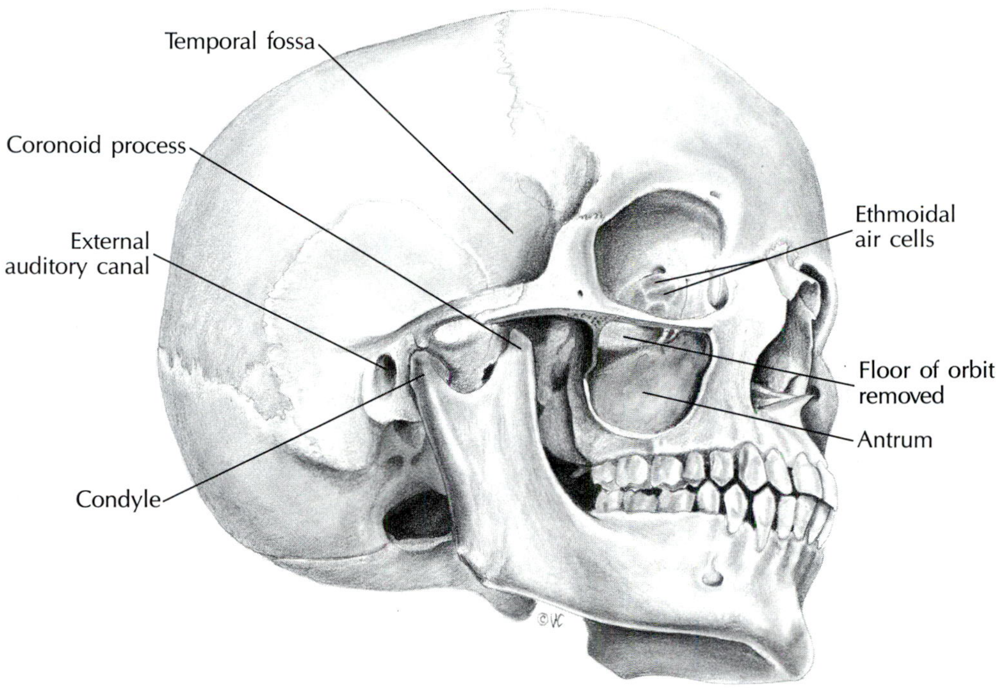

FIGURE 50-8. Oblique view of skull with anterior wall of maxilla and orbital rim cut away.

The superior transverse ligament supports the eyelids and the globe. It extends through the lacrimal gland and inserts laterally on the superior portion of the lateral orbital wall. Medially it inserts at the trochlear region.

As shown in Fig. 50-9, the inferior oblique muscle arises from the anterior floor of the orbit just lateral to the ostium for the nasolacrimal duct and courses beneath the inferior rectus muscle. Whitnall's ligament supports the levator complex and upper eyelid. The inferior oblique muscle is unique among the extraocular muscles because of its anterior origin. It extends beneath the inferior rectus muscle to insert on the posterotemporal aspect of the globe. Lockwood's ligament supports the globe inferiorly. It is formed by sheath condensation of the inferior rectus and inferior oblique muscles. Fig. 50-10 illustrates how the inferior oblique inserts on the globe posterolaterally near the inferior edge of the lateral rectus muscle.

The check ligaments are fascial structures that extend from the sheaths of the rectus muscles to the corresponding orbital wall. They are found anterior to the equator and tend to be better developed for the medial and lateral rectus muscles. They do not in fact limit the action of the muscles but act as one of the structures responsible for supporting the globe. Between adjacent rectus muscles is a thin connective tissue structure referred to as the "intermuscular membrane." This membrane joins the rectus muscles in helping to form the muscle cone of the orbit.

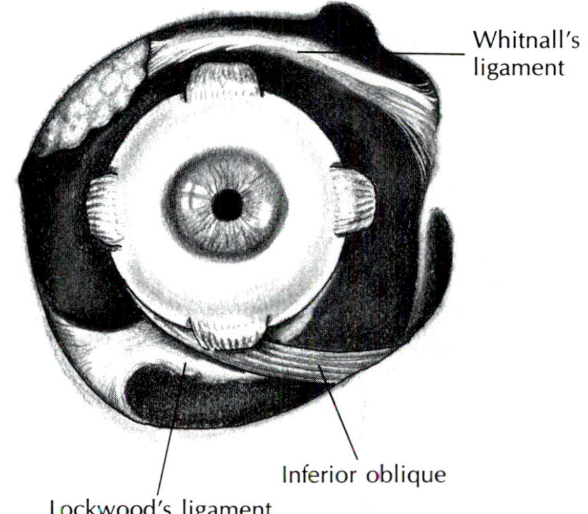

FIGURE 50-9. Anterior view of inferior oblique muscle, Lockwood's ligament, and Whitnall's ligament.

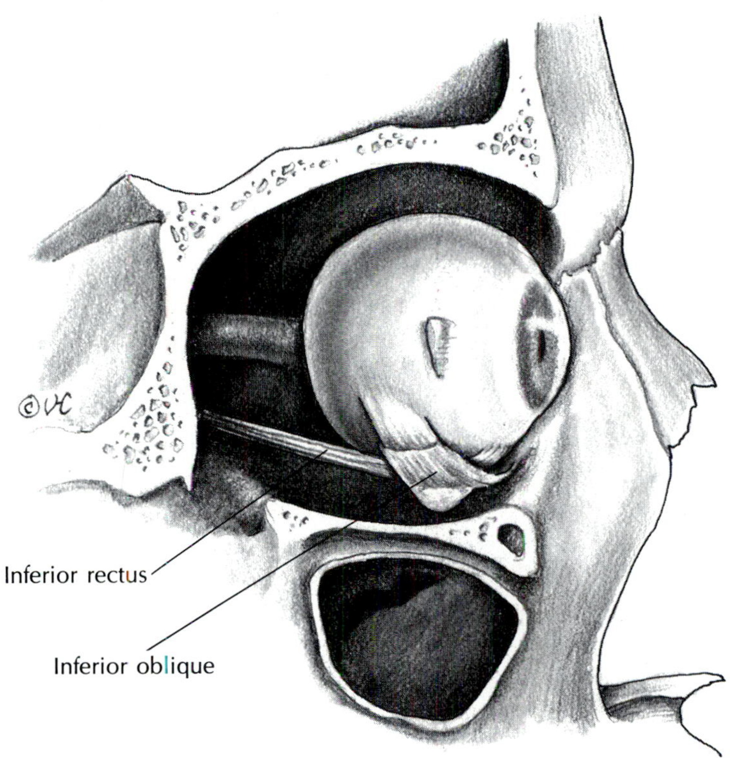

FIGURE 50-10. Lateral view of globe and inferior oblique.

Fig. 50-11 shows the lacrimal sac as it lies within the lacrimal fossa. The numerous connections between the orbital structures and the orbital walls can be seen. Tenon's capsule, lying posterior to the point where it is pierced by the rectus muscles, is referred to as "posterior Tenon's capsule" whereas that lying anterior is "anterior Tenon's capsule."

Tenon's capsule is a connective tissue structure covering the globe from the limbus to the optic nerve. It is firmly fixed to the globe anteriorly, where it fuses with the overlying conjunctiva near the limbus. It is penetrated by the rectus muscles posterior to the equator. It reflects onto the rectus muscles to envelope them and allows free movement of the muscle within this covering.

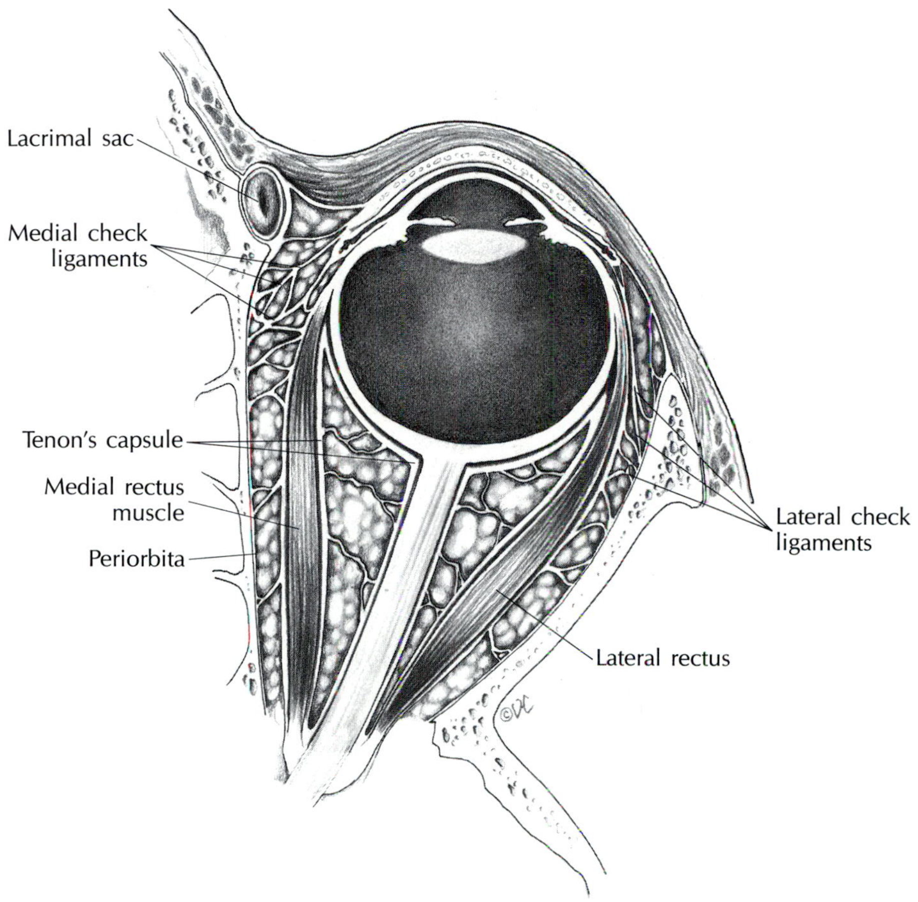

FIGURE 50-11. Transverse view of globe and intraorbital tissue.

Fig. 50-12 is a sagittal view of orbital soft tissue and demonstrates that Tenon's capsule is a connective tissue layer covering most of the globe. It extends from the optic nerve to the limbus and is penetrated by the rectus muscles posterior to the equator. There are several diffuse connective tissue septa between the orbital structures and the orbital wall as described by Koorneef. These septa help support the position of the globe within the orbit and may transmit nerves and blood vessels. Notice the position of the levator muscle and its aponeurosis at the level of Whitnall's ligament. There is an abrupt change in direction of the levator from horizontal to vertical at this point.

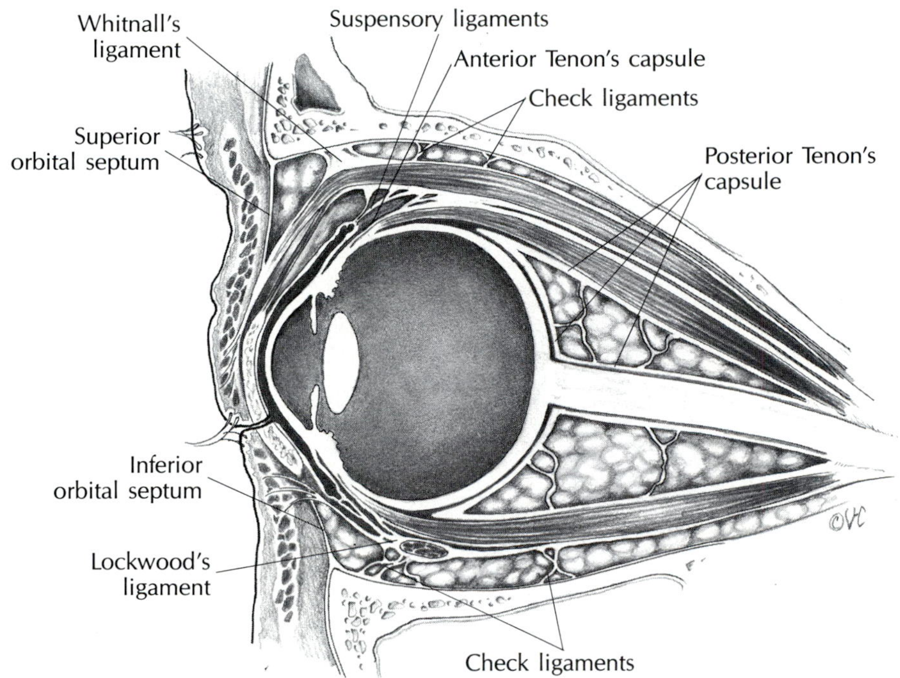

Fig. 50-13 illustrates where the lacrimal gland is housed behind the orbital rim superotemporally. It is separated into orbital and palpebral lobes by the lateral extension of the levator aponeurosis. The anterior portion of Tenon's capsule fuses with the overlying conjunctiva near the limbus.

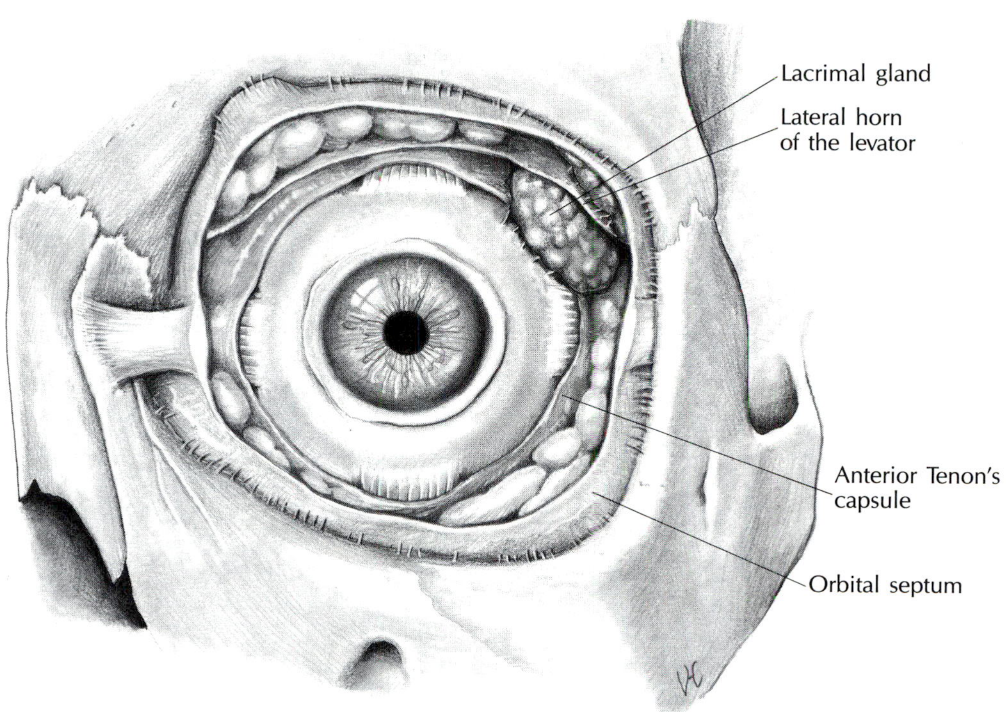

FIGURE 50-13. Anterior view of orbit, adnexa, and intraorbital tissue.

Fig. 50-14 shows the area within the muscle cone that is referred to as the central surgical space (III). The peripheral surgical space lies between the muscle cone and the periorbita (II). The potential space lying between the periorbita and the bone is the subperiorbital space (I). It becomes apparent when the periorbita is separated from the orbital walls. We refer to these spaces when we describe the surgical technique in this part.

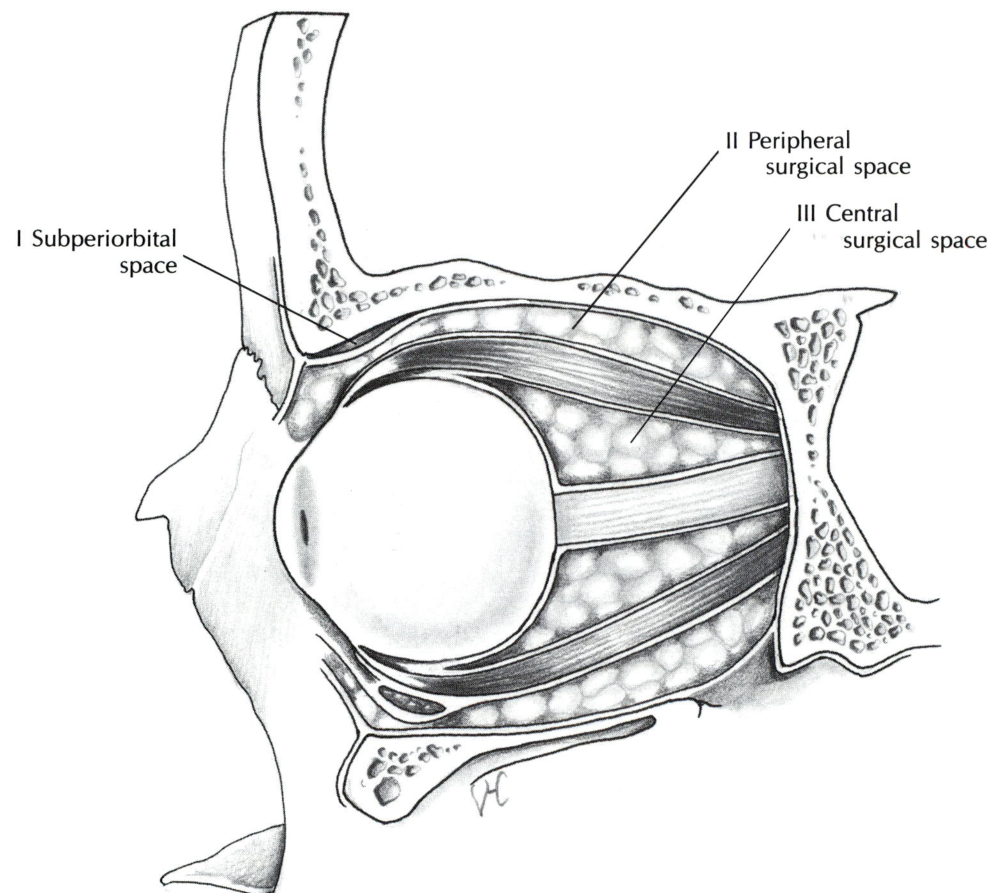

FIGURE 50-14. Surgical spaces of the orbit.

CHAPTER 51

Orbital Floor Fractures

Orbital floor fractures are classified into two categories—direct fractures and indirect fractures. Direct fractures of the orbital floor are posterior extensions of inferior orbital rim fractures, frequently associated with tripod fractures. Indirect fractures of the orbital floor are not associated with an inferior orbital rim fracture and are commonly referred to as "blow-out fractures." They are the most common type of orbital fractures treated by the ophthalmologist.

The evaluation of a patient with an orbital floor fracture involves a detailed history, complete ocular and orbital examination, and appropriate radiographic studies. Orbital floor fractures are managed only after systemic trauma and intraocular trauma have been addressed. A complete ophthalmic evaluation is performed. This includes visual acuity determination, pupil, adnexal and motility evaluation, biomicroscopy, and ophthalmoscopy. Neurosensory facial evaluation and nasal examination are also completed. Hyperesthesia or hypesthesia of the face and gums is noted. Rhinorrhea is ruled out after the injury. Serial exophthalmometry measurements are done to help determine if enophthalmos exists and is changing.

BLOW-OUT FRACTURES

The mechanism associated with the cause of blow-out fractures was established by Smith and Regan. Although the bony orbital rim protects the globe from a force created by a nonpenetrating object greater in diameter than the orbital entrance, the orbital contents are compressed posteriorly toward the orbital apex. This sudden increase in intraorbital pressure, if great enough, will break the fragile intraorbital bones at their weakest point. The weakest point of the orbital floor is medial to the infraorbital canal. Another mechanism causing an orbital-floor fracture occurs because a striking object causes a compressive force at the inferior rim. This directly buckles the orbital floor, causing it to break. In either case, the degree of increased orbital pressure determines whether intraorbital contents will prolapse through the orbital floor fracture into the maxillary sinus.

The diagnosis of a blow-out fracture of the orbital floor is suggested by the clinical findings of globe malposition, limitation of ocular movement, or perhaps also infraorbital nerve hypesthesia or paresthesia. Subcutaneous emphysema and orbital emphysema indicate communication between the orbit, sinuses, and nose. It usually results from a fracture of the medial orbital wall. With large orbital floor fractures, globe ptosis results from herniation of orbital soft tissues into the maxillary sinus (Fig. 51-1).

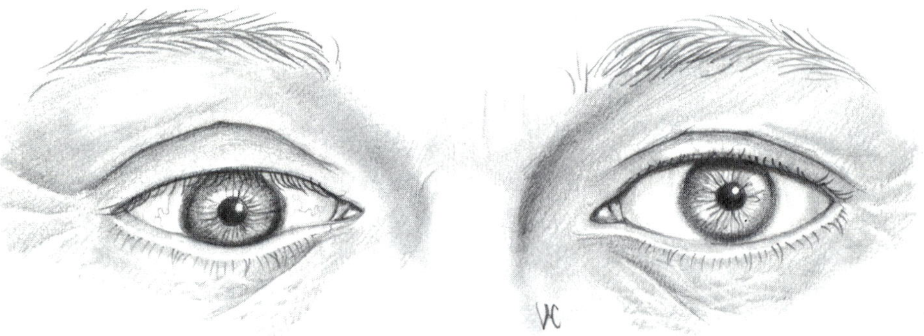

FIGURE 51-1. Globe ptosis resulting from herniation of orbital soft tissues into the maxillary sinus.

X-ray films and computerized tomographic (CT) scans are indispensable in the diagnosis and management of orbital floor fractures. They allow one to (1) localize the fracture site and demonstrate the degree of displacement, (2) evaluate the paranasal sinuses, and (3) identify orbital emphysema. The Waters and intermediate views are particularly useful in evaluation of the orbital floor, orbital rim, and maxillary sinus. Coronal and axial CT scans provide more detailed information on fracture localization and the relationship of soft tissue, including the extraocular muscles to the fracture. Transverse and true coronal views are important and useful when one is determining the need and approach for surgery.

Vertical muscle imbalance is suggestive of entrapment of the inferior rectus or inferior oblique muscles. Limitation of both horizontal and vertical eye movements can be associated with diffuse orbital edema, orbital hemorrhage, or paresis.

The administration of systemic corticosteroids is helpful in clarifying the clinical course of the fracture patient. If there is no muscle entrapment, motility limitation will usually improve with this treatment. Forced duction tests (Fig. 51-2) can be performed when there is restriction of motility. Pain, spasm, orbital edema, and orbital hemorrhage can, however, give false-positive findings.

In the forced duction test, after local or topical anesthesia is applied, the insertion of the inferior rectus muscle is grasped. As the eye is pulled superiorly, the patient is asked to look in a superior direction. Forced duction tests are repeated at the start of surgery with the patient under general anesthesia. They should again be repeated during fracture exploration and repair so that the effect of surgery can be evaluated.

With definite muscle entrapment early exploration is appropriate. When symptoms and signs of the fracture are improving, the patient is observed closely.

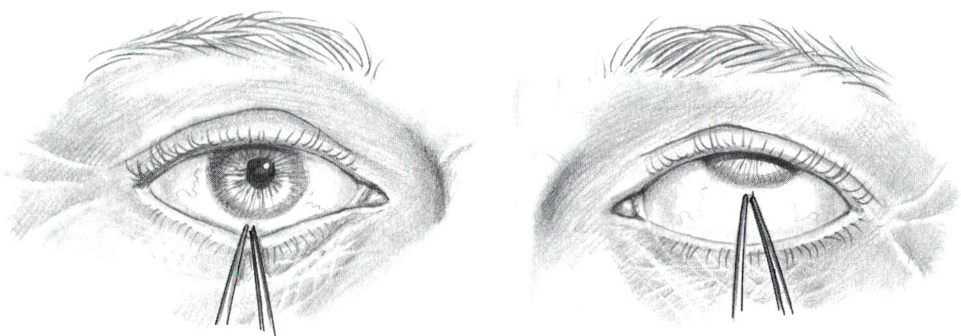

FIGURE 51-2. Forced duction test.

Surgical Procedure

Surgical repair of radiographically documented blow-out fractures is indicated in patients with (1) persistent diplopia and restriction of ocular motility or (2) significant enophthalmos, or both.

Surgical repair of blow-out fractures is usually delayed 10 to 14 days, a period that permits subsidence of orbital edema and reevaluation of the clinical findings. Various surgical approaches to the orbital floor exist. Here is offered a description of the subciliary approach. The transconjunctival approach to the orbit is discussed in the chapter on orbital decompression and is an effective approach to repair of orbital floor fractures. The Caldwell-Luc approach to the maxillary sinus can be a useful adjunctive procedure for repair of orbital floor fractures.

Complications of surgery include persistent diplopia, infraorbital nerve damage, and lower eyelid retraction. Less commonly, the patient may experience implant migration, and infrequently there is visual loss.

Fig. 51-3, *A*, shows how the flap is undermined to the inferior orbital margin after the subciliary incision is made with the eyelid held in stretch superiorly. The pretarsal orbicularis is left intact and dissection is continued beneath the orbicularis muscle with Stevens scissors (Fig. 51-3, *B*). Care is taken to leave the orbital septum essentially intact down to the orbital rim.

The orbital rim is then exposed (Fig. 51-3, *C*). The periosteum is incised 2 to 3 mm below the orbital rim with a no. 15 blade. In the child the incision is made closer to the rim to avoid damaging the infraorbital nerve, which exits closer to the rim than in an adult. The periosteum is then elevated until the fracture is identified.

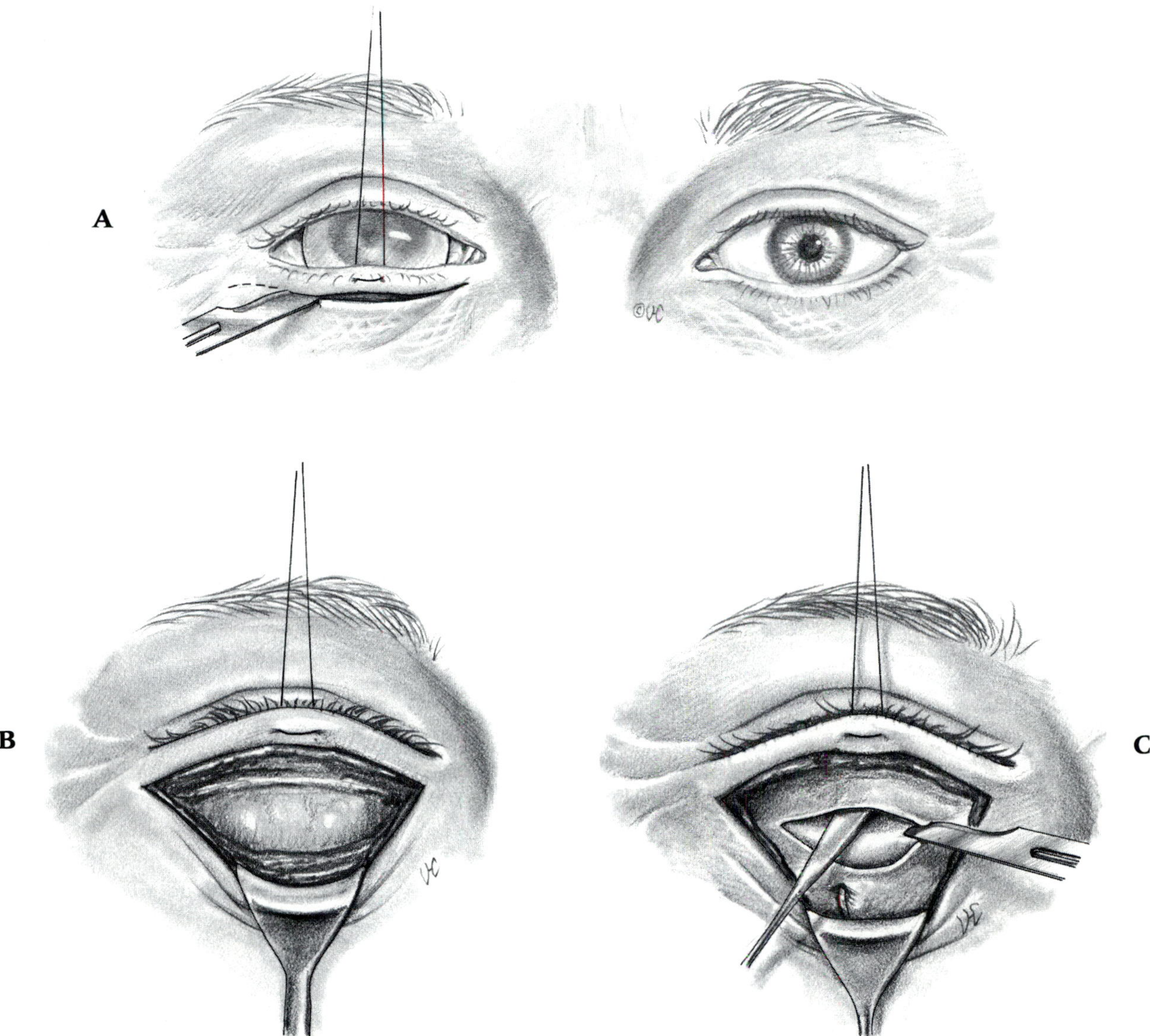

FIGURE 51-3. Surgical sequence for repair of blowout fracture.

Continued.

The entrapment is shown in Fig. 51-3, *D*. Exposure of the blow-out fracture with entrapped inferior rectus is obtained with a ribbon retractor and a Desmarres retractor. Excessive and steady pressure on the globe with the retractor should be avoided.

Incarcerated soft tissue is released from the fracture site by a "hand-over-hand" technique using periosteal elevators (Fig. 51-3, *E*). It may be necessary to extend the fracture by removing small pieces of bone around entrapped tissue to facilitate its removal. Repeat forced duction testing is done at this time to evaluate the status of globe restriction.

After the dimensions of the fracture are identified and measured, a sulfameter (sulfametin, Supramid) implant (0.4 mm) is cut to size and placed over the fracture (Fig. 51-3, *F*). The periorbita is sufficiently freed from the bone so that the implant can be placed under it, supported by bone around the edges of the fracture.

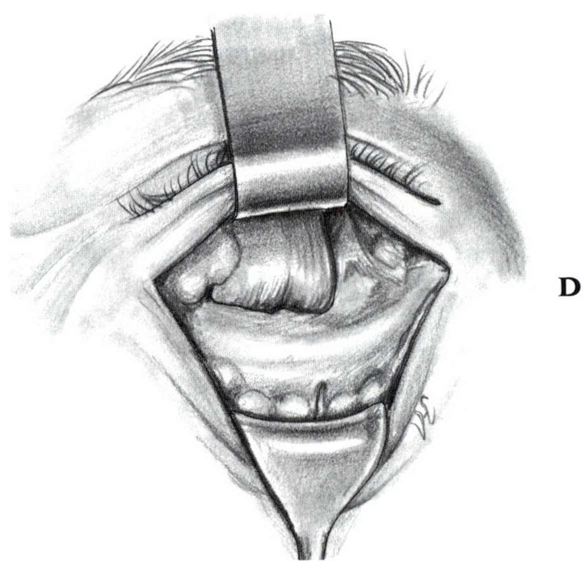

FIGURE 51-3, cont'd

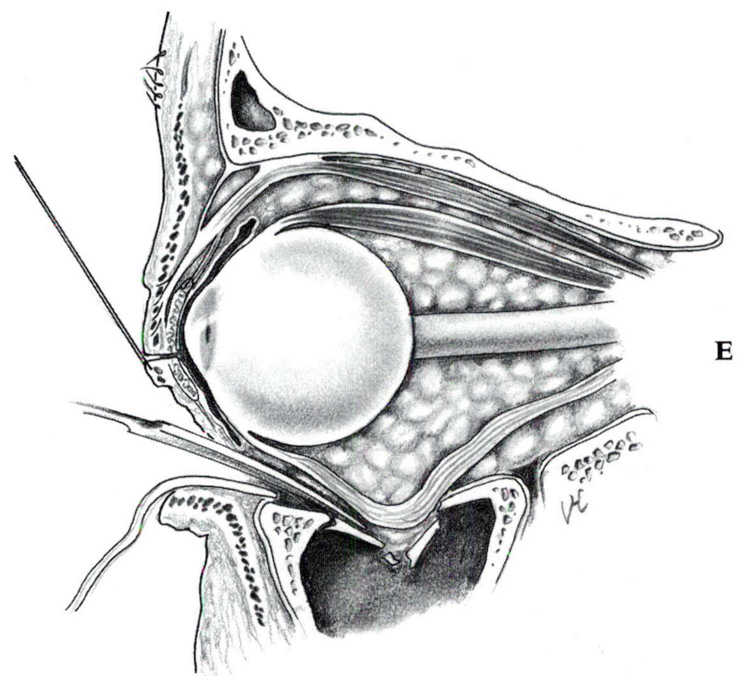

E

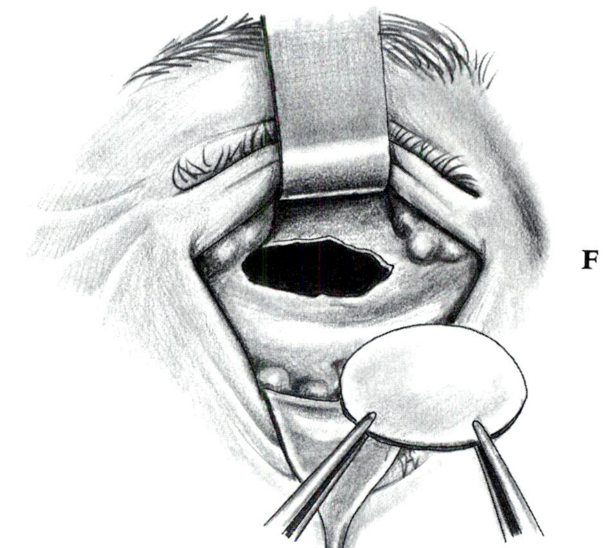

F

Continued.

Proper positioning of the implant is then checked (Fig. 51-3, *G*). The anterior edge of the implant rests inside the infraorbital rim. The implant should be stable. Forced ductions are again repeated to rule out the possibility that the implant is restricting movement of the globe. At times it is necessary to wire or suture the implant in position.

The periosteum is closed with interrupted 5-0 chromic catgut sutures (Fig. 51-3, *H*). Before this is done, complete hemostasis is the orbit is obtained. If blood or debris in the maxillary sinus has accumulated, a nasal antrostomy is done.

The subciliary incision is closed with an interrupted or running 6-0 nylon suture (Fig. 51-3, *I*).

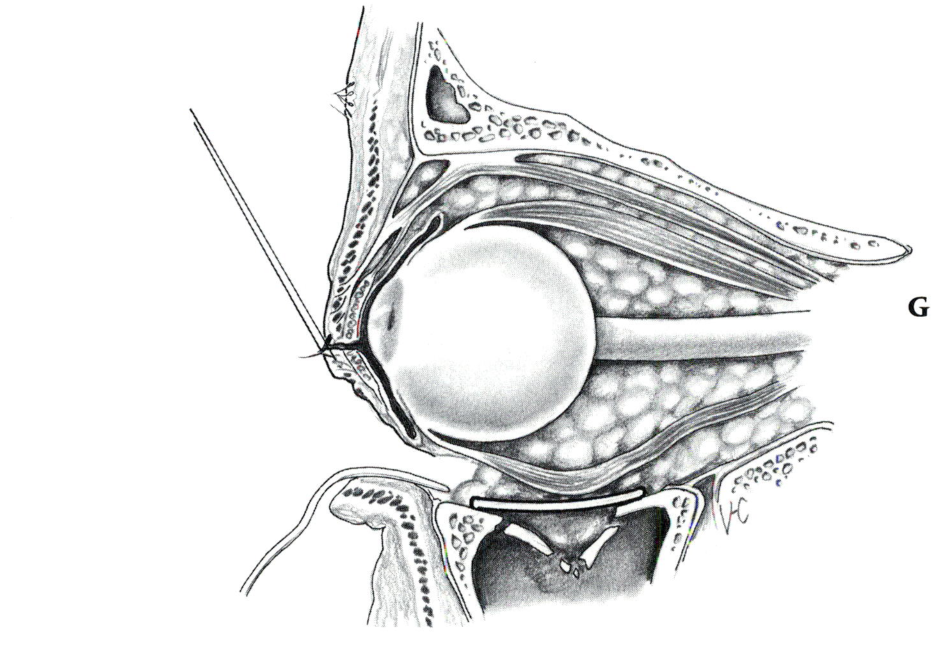

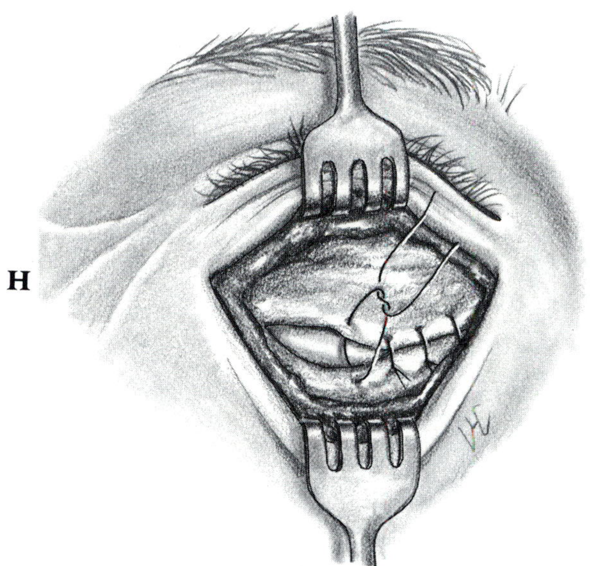

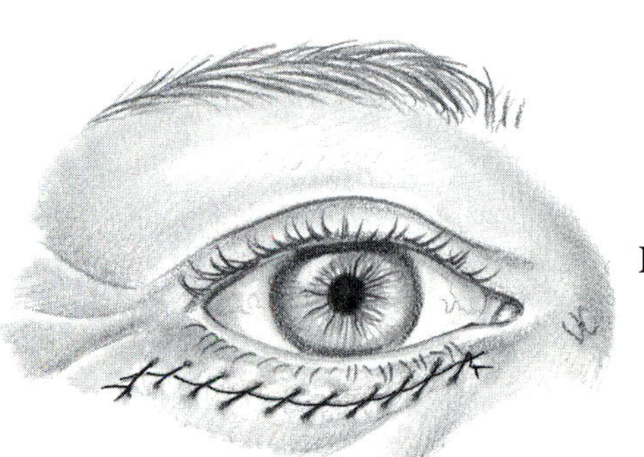

FIGURE 51-3, cont'd

CHAPTER 52

Zygomaticomaxillary Fractures

The zygomatic, or malar, bone is responsible for the prominence of the cheek, which is an important feature in the facial skeleton. It helps to protect orbital contents from traumatic forces. Both the lateral and Lockwood's suspensory ligaments are attached to the zygomatic bone at the lateral orbital tubercle. Patients with fractures and displacement of the zygomatic bone may present with cosmetic deformities including malar flattening, displacement of the lateral canthal angle, and globe ptosis. The anatomic relationships of the zygomatic bone, the zygomatic arch, the mandible, and the temporalis and masseter muscles govern normal movement of the mandible. Fractures and dislocations of the zygomatic bone or zygomatic arch can disturb these relationships and interfere with normal mastication.

A tripod fracture is a fracture involving the zygomatic bone. As the name implies, it involves fractures at three sites: (1) the zygomaticofrontal suture, (2) the zygomaticomaxillary suture, and (3) the zygomatic arch. With displaced zygomatic fractures there is usually a fourth and fifth fracture site, the orbital floor and the anterior wall of the maxillary sinus.

Fig. 52-1 shows a tripod fracture. With completely displaced tripod fractures there is a fracture at (1) the zygomaticofrontal suture, (2) the zygomaticomaxillary suture, (3) the zygomatic arch, (4) the inferior orbital floor, and (5) the anterior wall of the maxilla.

Zygomatic fractures are classified according to the type of displacement, the direction of displacement, and the site of fragment attachment. They can be nondisplaced, incompletely displaced, or completely displaced. If incompletely displaced, the zygoma will be hinged at either the zygomaticofrontal suture or at the zygomaticomaxillary suture. Completely displaced fractures have no sites of attachment. The direction of displacement of the detached site is dependent on the direction of the traumatic force. Forces from above can cause downward displacement of the zygoma, creating a gap deformity at the lateral orbital rim, inferior displacement of the lateral canthal angle, retraction of the lower lid, and a step deformity of the inferior orbital rim. Forces from below can cause superior displacement, creating "telescoping" of bone fragments at the lateral orbital rim. If there is a displaced fracture of the zygomatic arch, pain on mastication may be significant. Since there is a close relationship between the zygoma and coronoid process, the displaced zygoma may impinge on the coronoid process thereby limiting movement of the mandible.

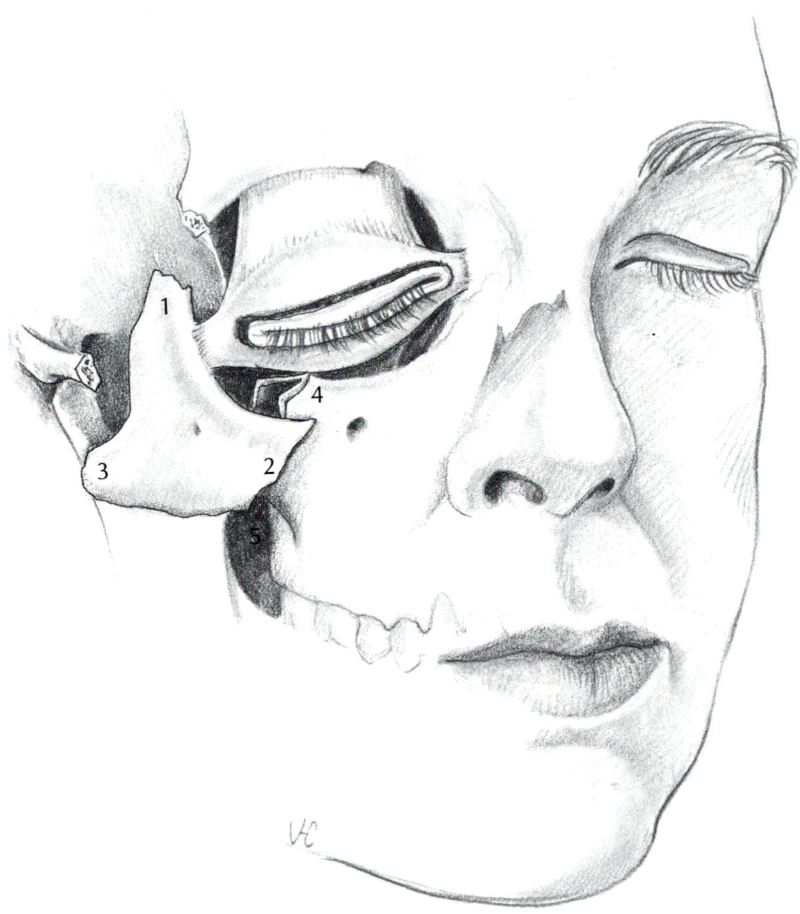

FIGURE 52-1. Tripod fracture.

Fig. 52-2 illustrates inferior displacement of the lateral canthal angle associated with displacement of the zygomatic bone. The lateral canthal tendon is attached to the lateral orbital tubercle, which lies 4 mm inside the lateral orbital rim. If the lateral orbital rim is fractured, these structures may be displaced inferiorly.

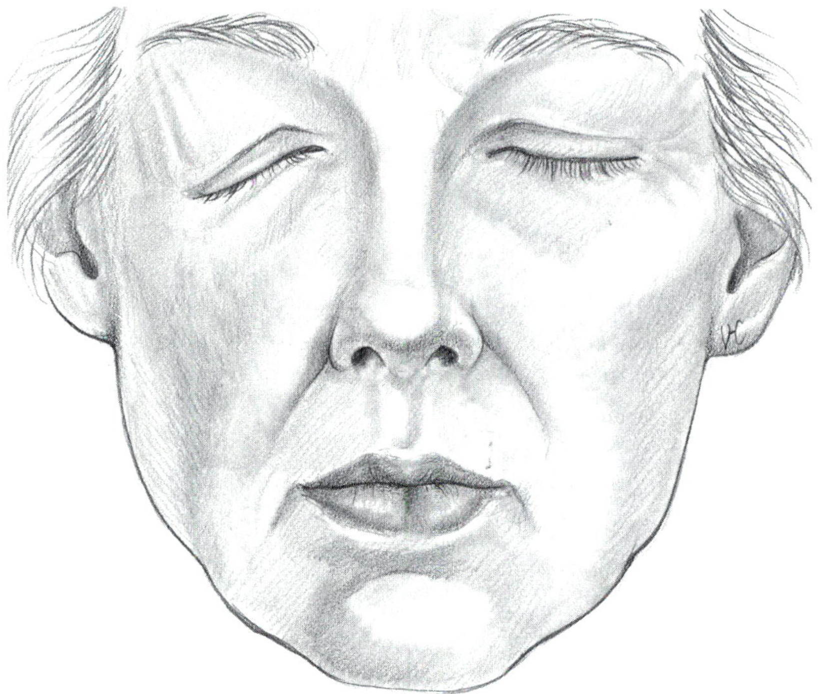

FIGURE 52-2. Inferior displacement of the lateral canthal angle.

A finger is used to palpate the inferior orbital rim. Step-down rim displacement is detected with palpation (Fig. 52-3, *A*). Intraoral palpation will help to define the degree of zygomatic bone and coronoid process displacement (Fig. 52-3, *B*).

PRINCIPLES OF TREATMENT

Surgery is indicated for restoration of normal zygomatic arch anatomy (1) to relieve persistent pain on mastication, (2) to ensure stable positioning of the lateral canthus and Lockwood's ligament, (3) to prevent irreparable complications of enophthalmos or diplopia in muscle entrapment, and (4) to restore normal cosmetic facial contours particularly when there is persistent malar flattening.

If pronounced deformities exist, surgical repair can be done within 24 to 48 hours after the injury. In less dramatic cases, surgical repair of tripod fractures can be delayed 7 to 10 days after the injury to allow for decrease of orbital edema while motility function is observed. Inspection, direct rim, and intraoral palpation precede detailed radiographic evaluation. CT scanning, including transverse and coronal views, best define the fractures and relationship to orbit tissue and extraocular muscles.

Many techniques for surgical repair of tripod fractures exist. Both fracture reduction and fixation must be performed for adequate healing and stabilization of the fractures. The method selected depends on the type of fracture, the amount of fragment displacement, and surgeon preference. The ophthalmologist, oculoplastic surgeon, and general plastic surgeon usually prefer a periorbital approach. The otolaryngologist and oral surgeon prefer the oral approach. To repair a complex tripod fracture, a combined transorbital and oral approach may be indicated. The use of bone-fixation miniplates is effective in repairing complex and severe tripod fractures. The plates enhance fracture stabilization.

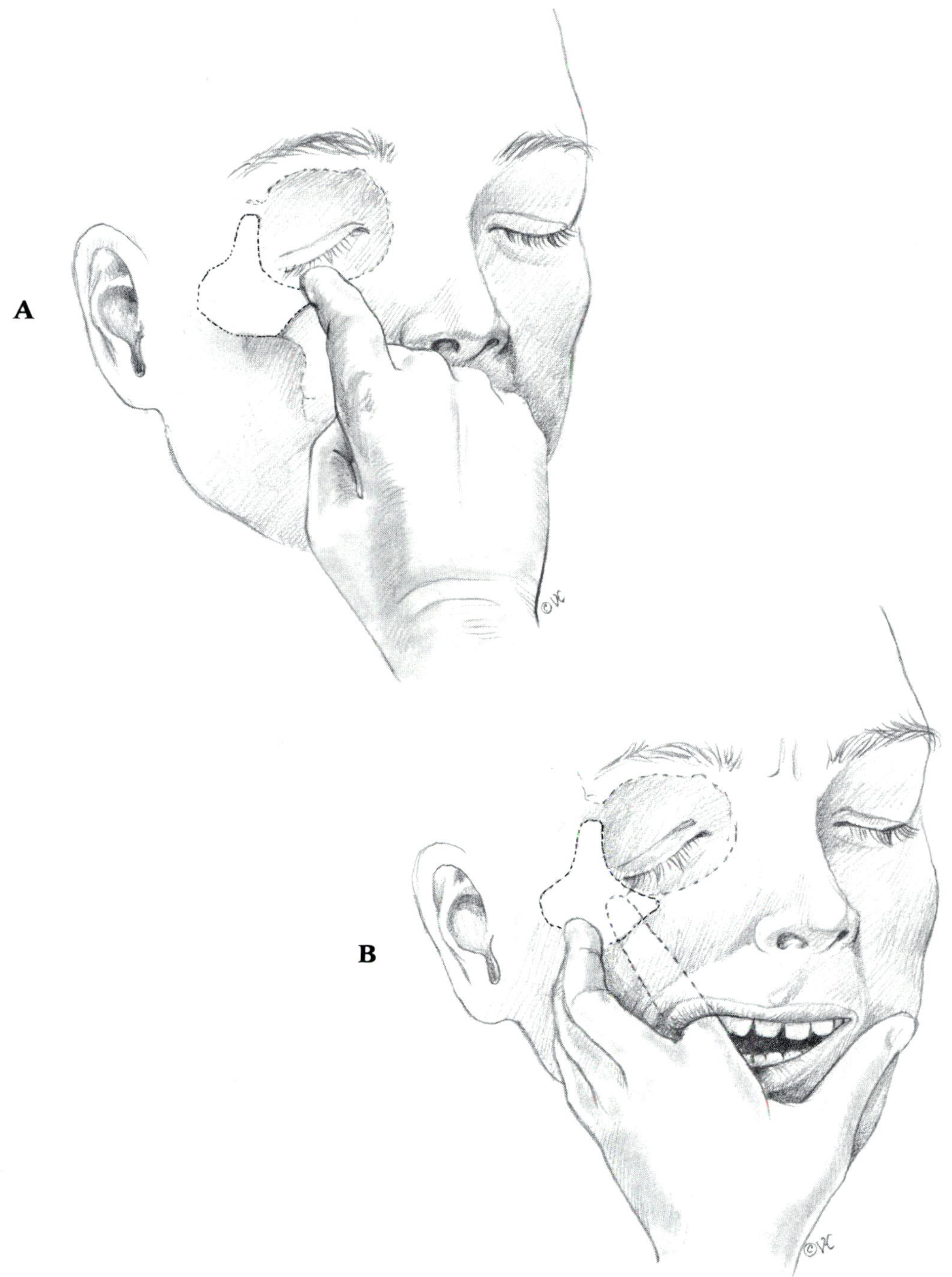

FIGURE 52-3. Orbital rim and zygoma palpation.

Periorbital Approach

Surgical management utilizing a periorbital approach for reduction with internal fixation with interosseous wiring is discussed here. A technique using two incisions, one over the zygoma and a subciliary approach to the orbital floor, is described. The transconjunctival approach to the orbit (described for orbital decompression) is effective for repair of zygomaticomaxillary fractures. It allows for good exposure of the zygomatic and orbital rim and floor fracture sites. The fractures can be repaired with this single incision. For exposure of the lateral orbital rim the canthal incision extends over the zygoma continuing the completed transconjunctival fornix incision.

The Gillies temporal approach is shown in Fig. 52-4, *A*. The elevator is passed beneath the temporalis fascia extending below the zygomatic bone after penetrating the attachment of the temporalis muscle to the zygoma. The elevator will help mobilize displaced fractures. The zygoma is palpated during its reduction to help direct the displaced bone into better position.

Combined subciliary floor and supralateral incisions allow for direct exposure of the zygomaticofrontal and zygomaticomaxillary fractures. The periosteum covering the zygomaticofrontal displacement is freed up while the orbital floor is approached as described with orbital floor fractures. It may be necessary to osteotomize malunited fracture sites in long-standing unoperated cases.

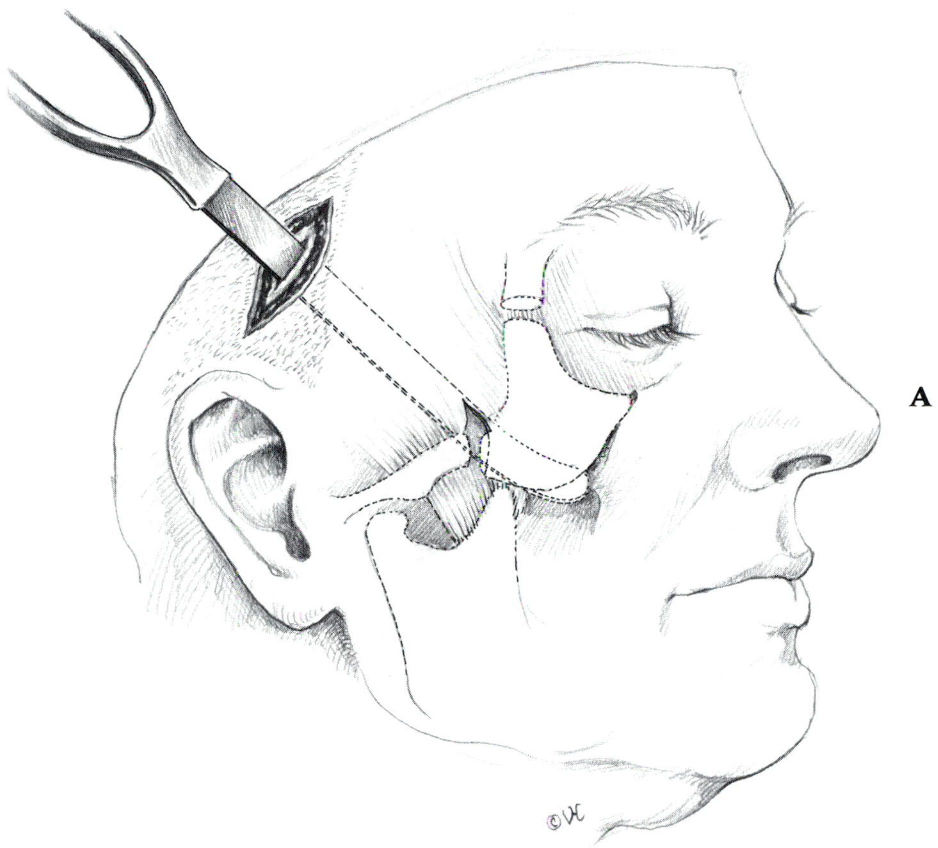

FIGURE 52-4. Surgical techniques for repair of tripod fractures.

Continued.

The elevator is passed through a supralateral incision beneath the zygomatic bone (Fig. 52-4, *B*). It is used to reduce and elevate the depressed bone. Elevators are also used to mobilize and help rotate the displaced zygoma through the supralateral, anterior orbit (Fig. 52-4, *C*), and transoral approach (Fig. 52-4, *D*).

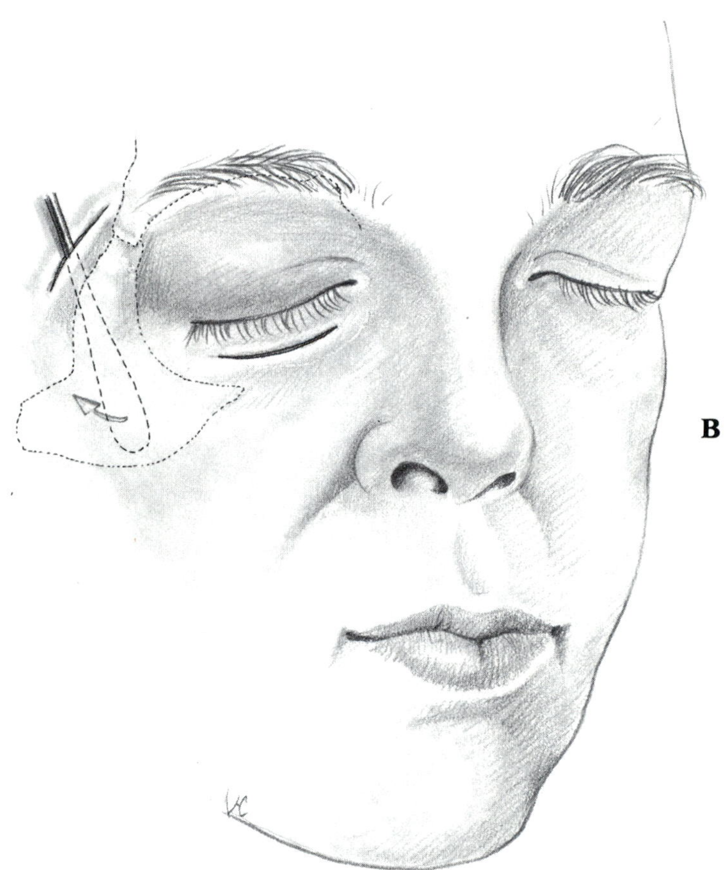

FIGURE 52-4, cont'd

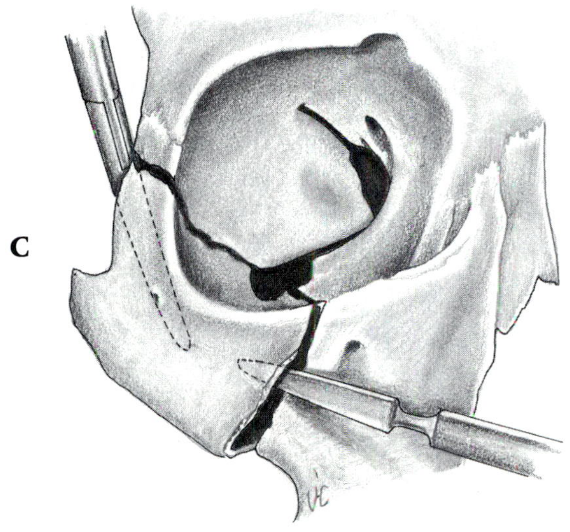
C

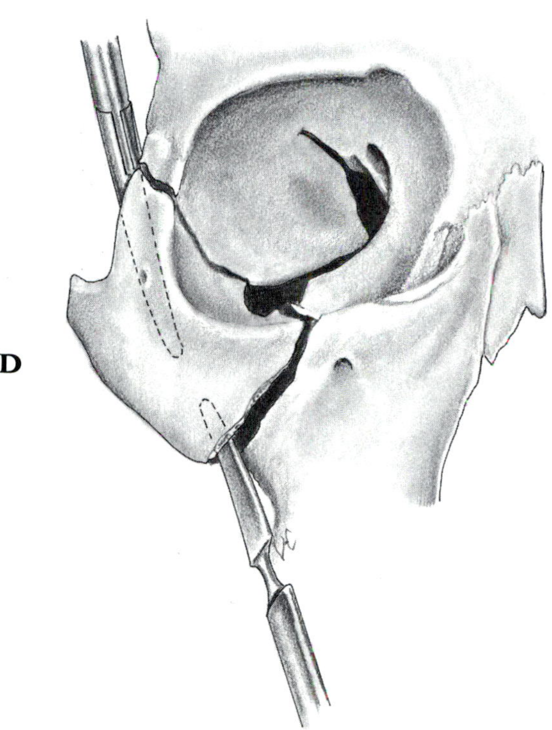
D

Continued.

Displaced fractures are then reduced (Fig. 52-4, *E*). Orbital floor fracture is apparent and enlarged after the maneuver shown in Fig. 52-4, *C* and *D*, has been done. It is important to expose the orbital floor when the zygomatic maxillary fractures are reduced to avoid potential damage to orbital tissue when the fractures are reduced.

Wire holes are made into bone before passage of wire on either side of reduced zygomaticofrontal and zygomaticomaxillary fractures is necessary (Fig. 52-4, *F*). Wire at zygomatic frontal fracture site is twisted to stabilize the reduced fracture.

An alloplastic implant or autogenous bone graft is designed to cover the floor fracture after the tripod fracture sites are reduced and wire is fixed (Fig. 52-4, *G*).

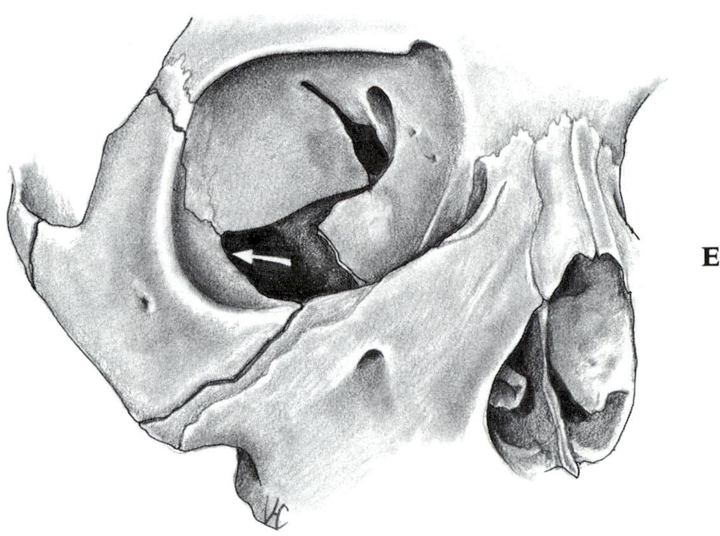

FIGURE 52-4, cont'd

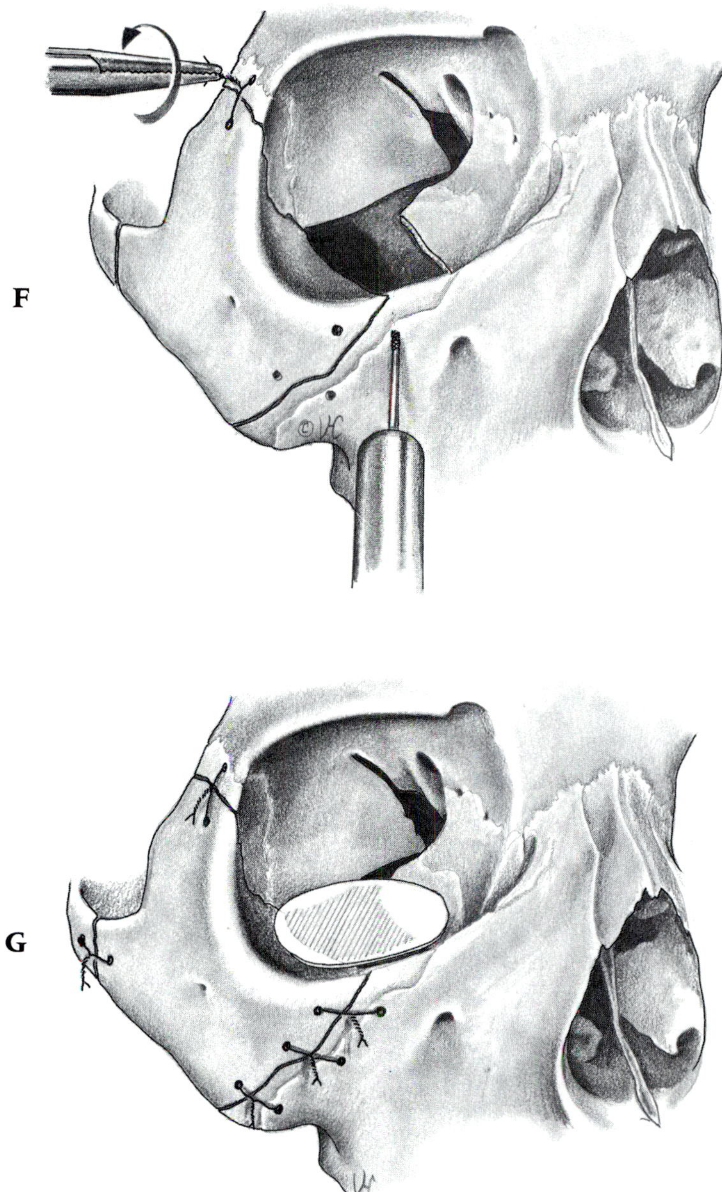
F
G

CHAPTER 53

Surgery for Orbital Tumors

The surgical approach into the orbit is dictated by a variety of factors including the location, size, and type of the lesion in question. In addition the surgical objective (excision, biopsy, or drainage) will also influence the type of entry into the orbit.

PATIENT EVALUATION AND PREPARATION

A careful history and physical examination of the orbit will help to classify and localize the lesion (inflammatory, vascular, or neoplastic). Among the important factors considered are the age of the patient, onset of symptoms, degree of proptosis, and globe displacement. The orbit is palpated between the globe and the orbital rims. Anterior tumors can be palpated and defined with the fingertips. Diagnostic techniques including computerized tomographic scanning, ultrasonography, and magnetic resonance imaging allow for more precise tumor localization. The lesion can then be classified into the neoplastic, inflammatory, or vascular category, and the appropriate surgical approach can then be planned.

PRINCIPLES OF TREATMENT

The first priority of orbital exploration is to determine whether an incisional biopsy or complete excision of the tumor is indicated. Well-encapsulated lesions are usually completely excised, whereas infiltrative or diffuse lesions are biopsied. For biopsy sufficiently large pieces of tissue are taken to ensure satisfactory histopathologic evaluation.

Aspirin or aspirin-containing products are stopped 10 to 14 days before surgery. Patients with bleeding abnormalities or tendencies are carefully evaluated preoperatively.

In this section three basic surgical approaches to the orbit are described: (1) anterior orbitotomy, (2) transcutaneous medial orbitotomy, and (3) lateral orbitotomy. These approaches either alone or in combination are sufficient to approach most orbital lesions with maximal exposure and minimal trauma. Consider that the subperiorbital space lies between the orbital walls and periorbita, the peripheral surgical space between the periorbita and the intermuscular septum and muscles, and the central surgical space within the intermuscular septum behind the globe.

Anterior Orbitotomy

The anterior orbitotomy approach allows access to lesions in either the subperiorbital or anterior peripheral surgical space. The majority of these lesions can be palpated near the orbital rim. Inflammatory tumors, lymphomas, and cystic masses are among the more common lesions encountered in the anterior orbit. Lacrimal gland masses can be biopsied with this approach. For complete resection of large encapsulated masses this approach may have to be combined with either a medial or lateral orbitotomy. Although frontal sinus mucoceles usually involve the anterior orbit, they are best treated with a combined orbit and sinus approach usually with an osteoplastic flap.

A skin incision for superior anterior orbitotomy is made just inferior to the brow (Fig. 53-1, *A*). Although the limits of the incision are modified according to the location of the lesion, the incision should follow the natural brow contour and remain inferior to the brow cilia. Superiorly, the supraorbital nerves and vessels and trochlear bundle should be avoided. The length of the incision will depend on the extent of the lesion and whether the mass is to be biopsied or completely excised.

With the edges of the skin and subcutaneous tissues retracted by use of 4-0 silk sutures and rakes, the periosteum is incised above the orbital margin (Fig. 53-1, *B*). It is reflected off the bone with a Freer elevator. Medially the supraorbital and supratrochlear nerves can be identified and protected if necessary.

With the orbital contents retracted anteriorly and inferiorly, the lesion is localized by palpation.

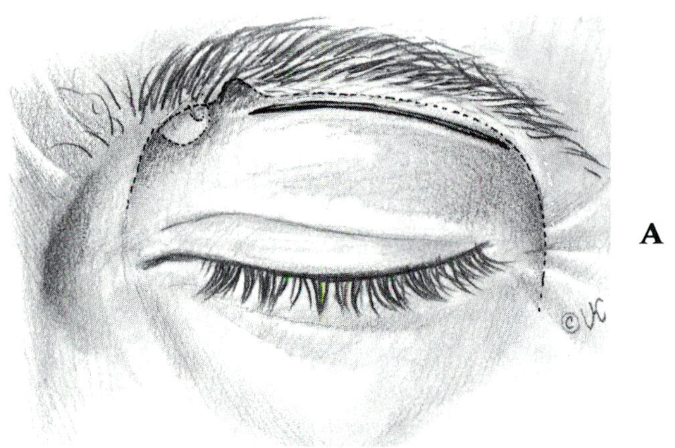

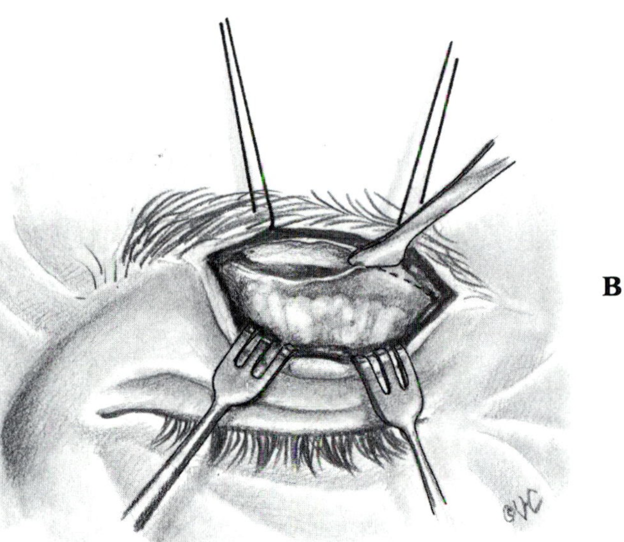

FIGURE 53-1. Anterior orbitotomy.
Continued.

After the periorbita has been reflected from the orbital rim, the periorbita directly over the lesion is incised in an anteroposterior direction and the mass is exposed. A forceps grasps the mass, and a blade is used to excise part of the infiltrative lesion (Fig. 53-1, *C*). It is important to excise a sufficiently large piece of tissue for histologic evaluation.

Fig. 53-1, *D*, shows the sagittal view of anterior orbitotomy. This approach allows one to enter the peripheral surgical space while avoiding major orbital structures. Since the lesion is close to the levator and superior rectus muscles, careful dissection directly above and toward the lesion will allow for biopsy or excision while limiting the chance of injury to these adjacent structures.

After biopsy or removal of the lesion, the periorbita is closed with interrupted absorbable sutures (Fig. 53-1, *E*). Complete hemostasis is established before the periorbita is closed with 4-0 chromic sutures. With lacrimal gland biopsy, special attention is given to establishing hemostasis because of the vascularity of the gland.

The skin edges are reapproximated with interrupted nonabsorbable 6-0 or 5-0 nylon sutures (Fig. 53-1, *F*). Deeper subcutaneous layers and skin are closed in separate layers.

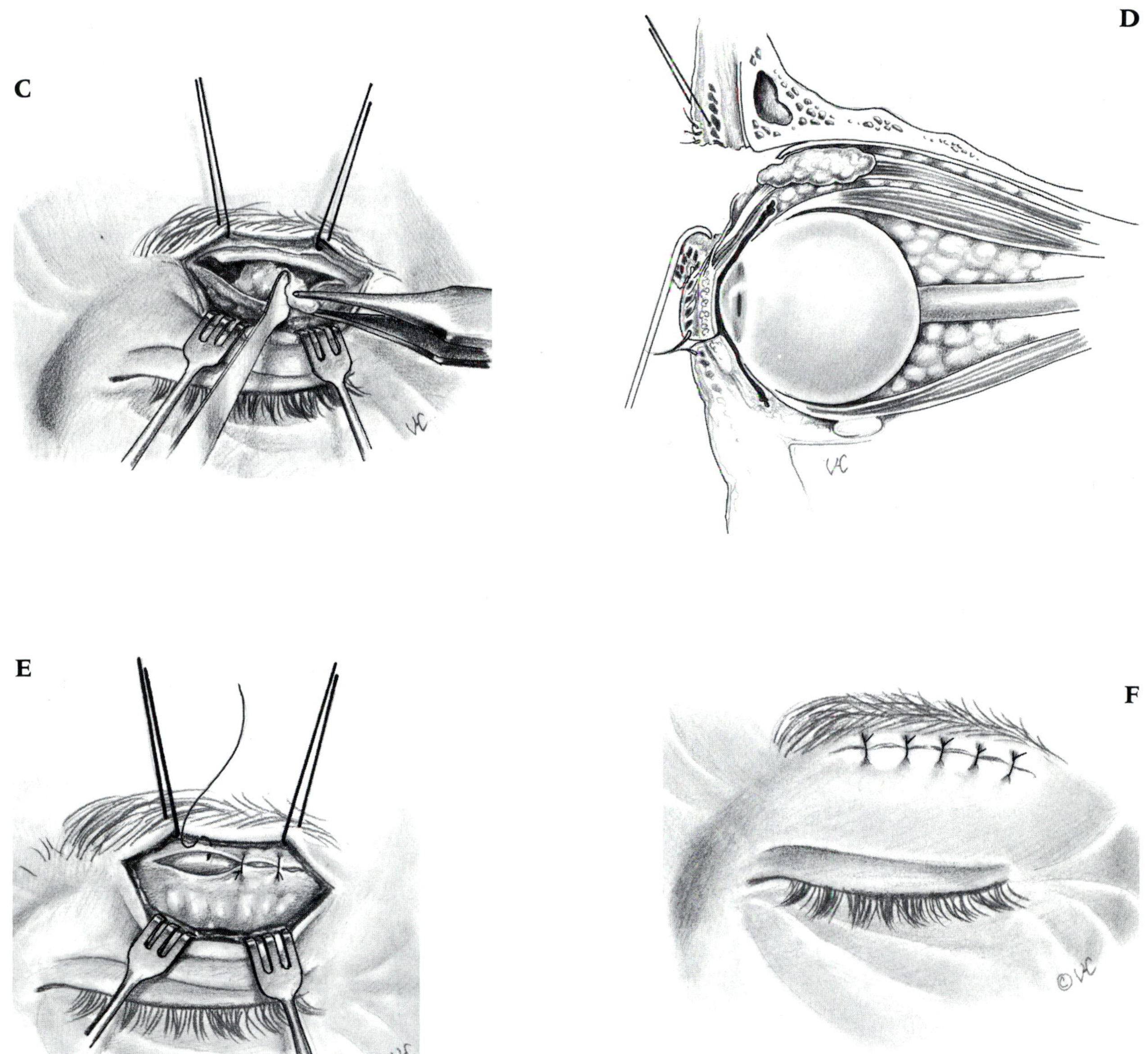

FIGURE 53-1, cont'd

Medial Orbitotomy

The transcutaneous medial orbitotomy approach allows access to the medial subperiorbital region and peripheral surgical space. It is useful in allowing drainage of subperiosteal abscesses and excision or biopsy of tumors along the medial wall that may extend from the ethmoid sinuses. For larger posterior lesions this procedure can be combined with a lateral orbitotomy with zygoma removal to allow for more surgical space medially. Repair of isolated medial wall fractures is best achieved with this technique. To avoid a "bowstring" scar along the medial canthus, one can use a lazy-Z-plasty skin incision.

Fig. 53-2, *A*, shows a lazy-Z-plasty incision for the medial orbitotomy. This incision in the medial canthus limits the chance of a bowstring scar that may occur with a standard curvilinear incision (Lynch incision). The trochlea and medial canthal tendon represent the superior and inferior limits of the skin incision. The points of the incision are joined wth a no. 11 Bard-Parker blade.

After subcutaneous dissection is done, the medial tissues are retracted with 4-0 silk sutures while fine rake retractors are used laterally. The periorbita overlying the medial wall is exposed.

After subcutaneous dissection, the edges of the incision are retracted with 4-0 silk sutures and a rake to expose the underlying periosteum (Fig. 53-2, *B*).

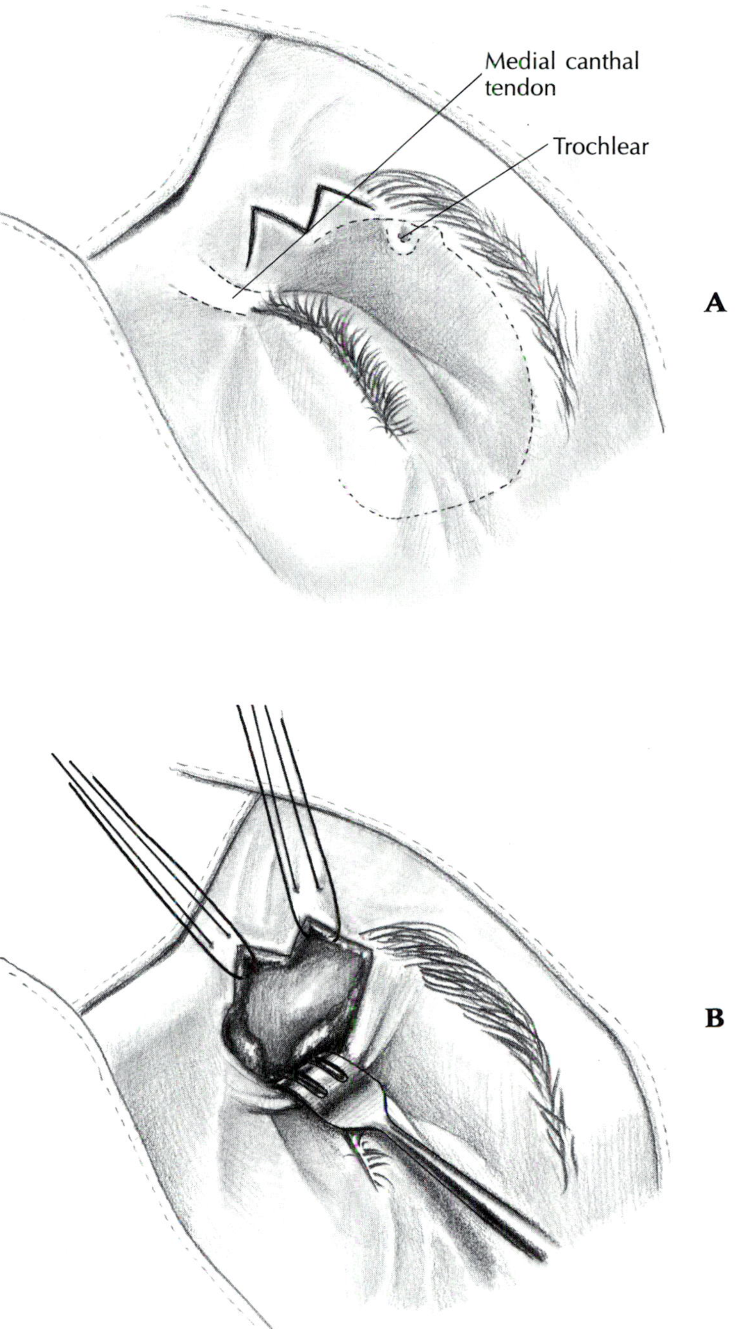

FIGURE 53-2. Medial orbitotomy.

Continued.

The medial periorbita is incised vertically and reflected off the bone (Fig. 53-2, *C*). Malleable retractors are used to expose the lesion. If the mass lies within the peripheral surgical space, the periorbita is opened adjacent to it. The anterior ethmoidal artery and nerve are transmitted through their respective foramina at the junction of the frontal and ethmoid bones.

The lesion is carefully dissected from surrounding structures (Fig. 53-2, *D*). When dissection is carried posteriorly, the ethmoidal vessels are identified and may be cauterized, or tantulum clips are applied to them for hemostasis. For additional exposure the medial canthal tendon may be tagged and cut away from its origin.

The edges of the periorbita are sutured with interrupted absorbable material (Fig. 53-2, *E*). If the medial canthal tendon was previously removed, it is re-attached to its origin with 4-0 or 5-0 Prolene sutures.

Fig. 53-2, *F,* shows skin closure. Meticulous skin and subcutaneous closure is necessary to achieve a good cosmetic result and thereby limit the possibility of "webbing" in the canthus.

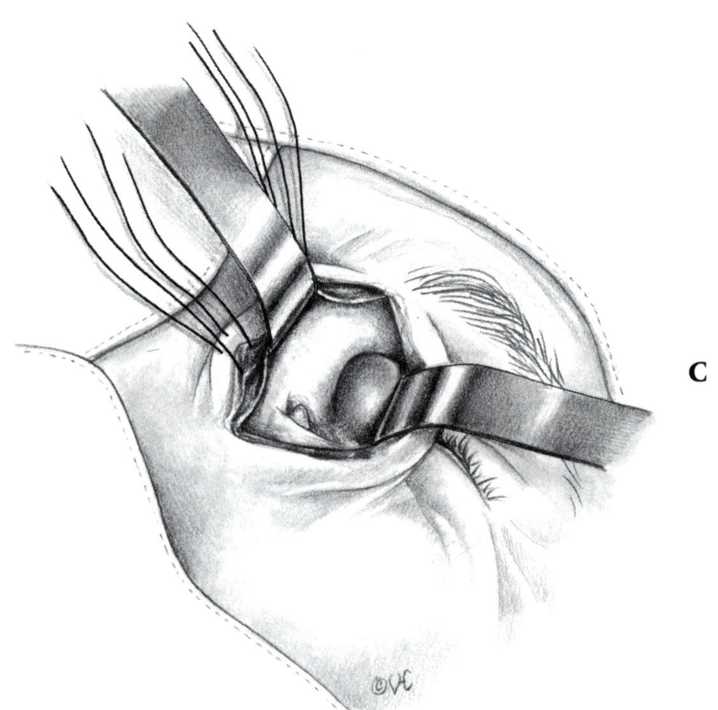

FIGURE 53-2, cont'd

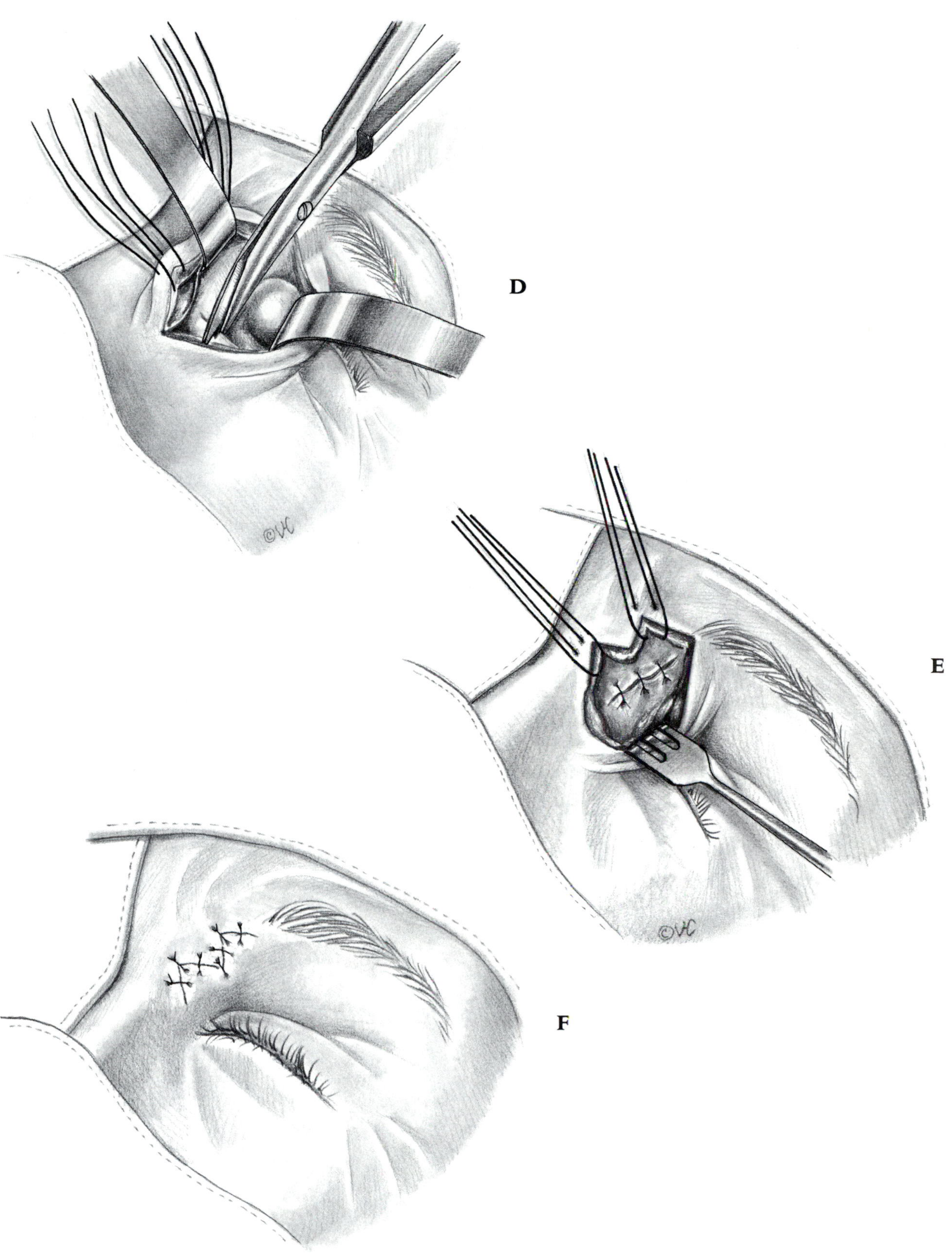
D
E
F
©VC
©VC

Lateral Orbitotomy

The lateral subperiorbital, peripheral, and central surgical spaces are explored with the lateral orbitotomy. Among the lesions most commonly encountered laterally are well-defined lesions such as cavernous hemangioma, dermoid cyst, a lacrimal fossa mass, or infiltrative lesions including lymphomas and pseudotumors. Optic nerve lesions including optic sheath meningioma can also be approached with a lateral orbitotomy or with the transconjunctival medial approach. The lateral orbital rim is removed when resection of large or deeply situated orbital lesions is required. With removal of the rim and part of the sphenoid bone, the lateral orbital apex can be reached. The lateral orbitotomy can be combined with a transconjunctival orbitotomy to reach deeper medial lesions that extend toward the apex in the central surgical space.

A "lazy-S" (Wright-Stallard) skin incision for lateral orbitotomy is shown in Fig. 53-3, *A*. The superior aspect of the incision begins in the lateral area of the brow. The incision is carried inferiorly along the orbital rim and terminates at the level of the zygomatic arch. The length of the incision can vary depending on the location and size of the lesion. Before the skin is incised, a suture is passed beneath the lateral rectus muscle to help identify the muscle during intraorbital dissection. A suture is also passed around the superior or inferior rectus muscle depending on the site of the orbital lesion.

Sharp and blunt dissection through the subcutaneous and orbital orbicularis muscle layers is completed (Fig. 53-3, *B*). The skin-muscle flaps are undermined to expose the periosteum along the lateral orbital rim and temporalis fascia.

A

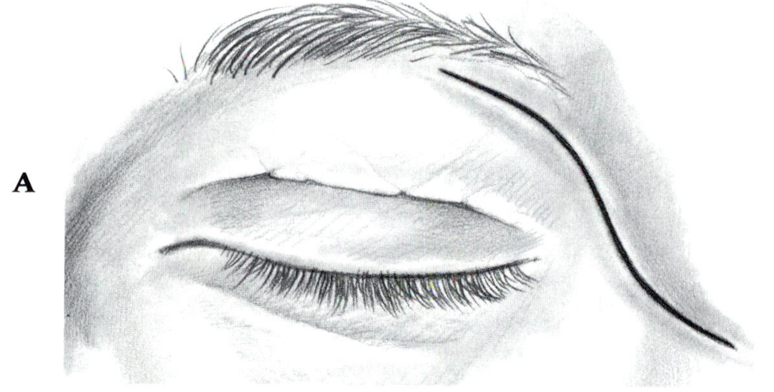

B

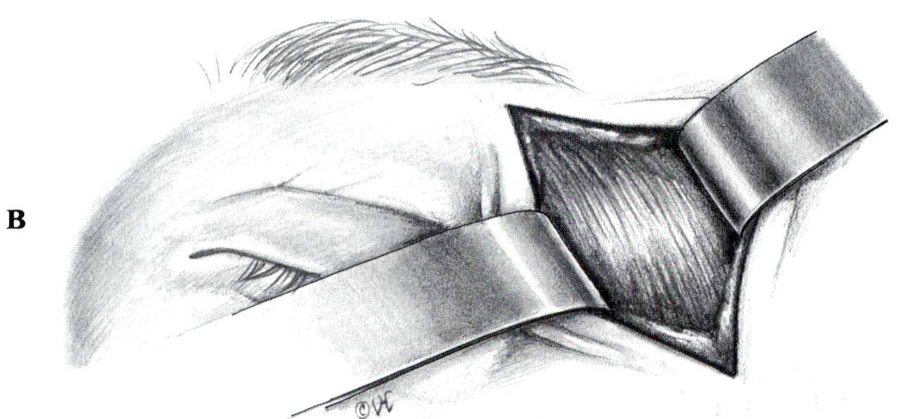

FIGURE 53-3. Lateral orbitotomy.

Continued.

The temporalis fascia and lateral rim periosteum are exposed (Fig. 53-3, *C*). Continuous or single 4-0 silk traction sutures are placed beneath the skin-muscle flaps for retraction and exposure. Malleable or rake retractors are also used for this purpose. Bleeders are now cauterized.

The periosteum is incised vertically approximately 5 mm from the medial edge of the lateral rim (Fig. 53-3, *D*). Oblique relaxing incisions are made at the superior and inferior edges of the vertical incision. A periosteal elevator is used to reflect the periosteum laterally and medially to expose the bone. The insertion of the lateral canthal tendon is identified, tagged with a suture, and removed from the bone.

The superior and inferior extent of bone removal is marked (Fig. 53-3, *E*). The superior border is usually slightly above the frontozygomatic suture, and the lower border just above or at the zygomatic arch. The distance between the two cuts is modified according to the nature and size of the orbital lesion.

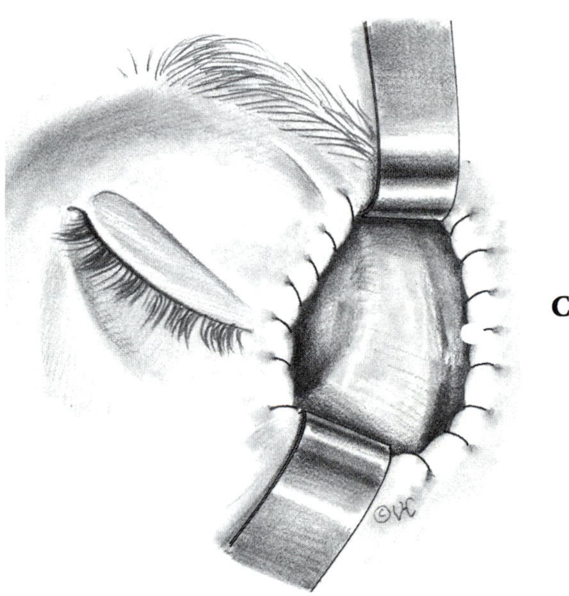

FIGURE 53-3, cont'd

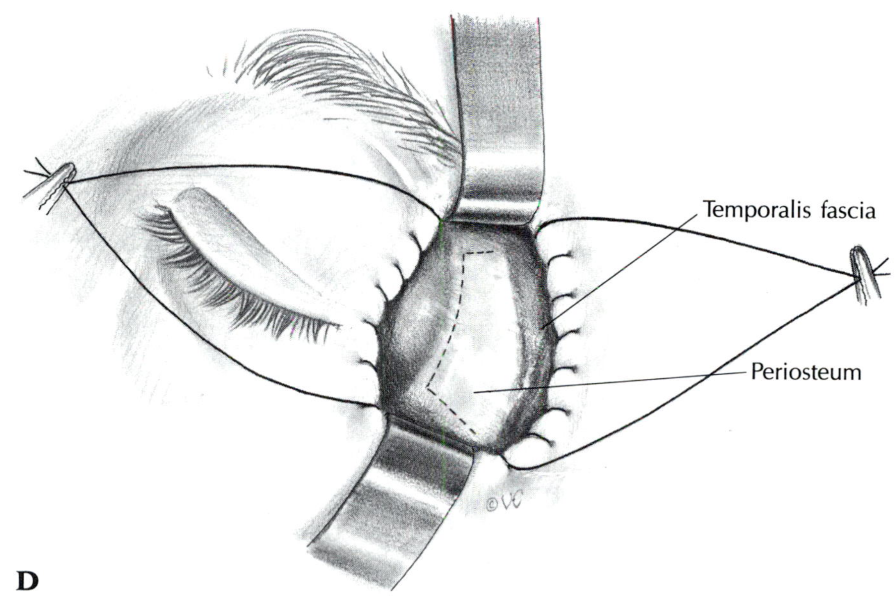

D

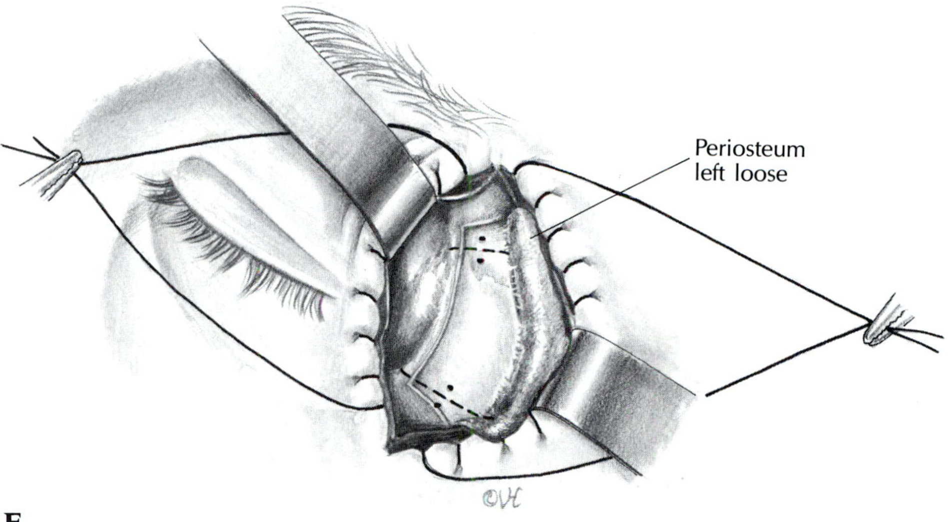

E

Continued.

In preparation for lateral orbital rim removal, the temporalis fascia and periorbita along the lateral wall is separated from the bone (Fig. 53-3, *F*). A cutting cautery can be used to separate the temporalis muscle from the bone. Before the bone is cut with a Stryker saw, drill holes are placed on either side of the proposed bone cuts. These allow for later placement of suture or fixation wires when the bone is replaced.

With malleable retractors in place to protect the orbital contents and globe, a Stryker saw is used to cut the lateral area of the rim between the drill holes (Fig. 53-3, *G*). The rim is loosened vertically and horizontally with an osteotome. After the cuts are made in the lateral orbital rim, an Allis clamp or large hemostat is used to remove the bone (Fig. 53-3, *H*). The rim is then grasped with an Allis clamp or hemostat, removed, and placed into an antibiotic solution. As necessary a portion of the anterior sphenoid bone is removed with a straight rongeur. Bone wax may be applied to bleeding points on the bone.

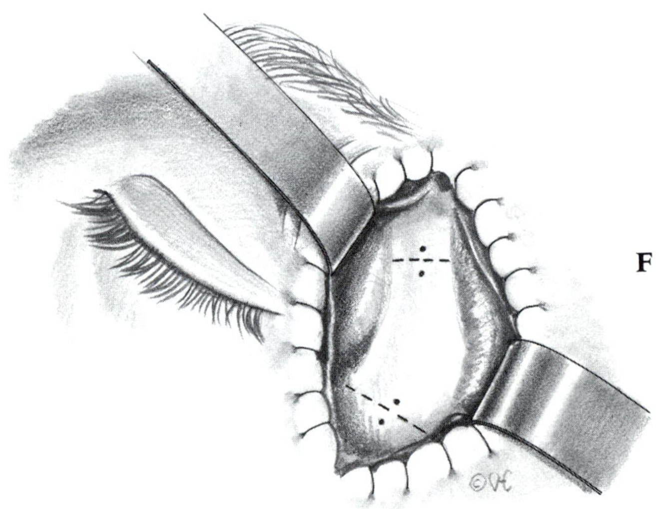

FIGURE 53-3, cont'd

G

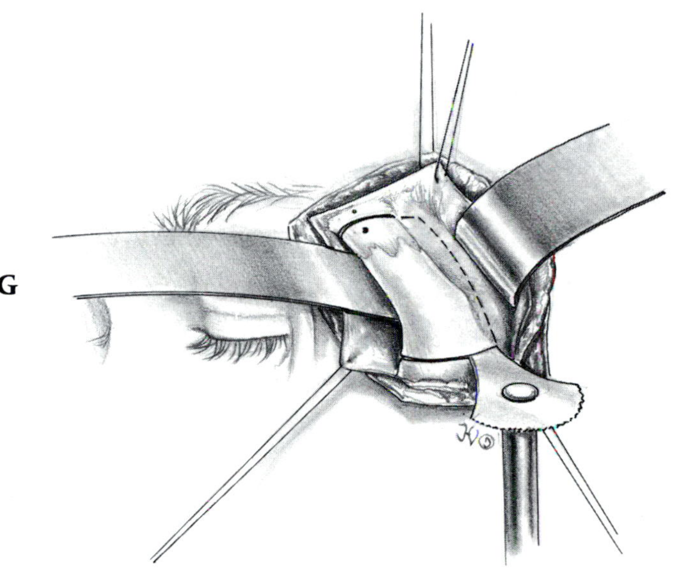

H

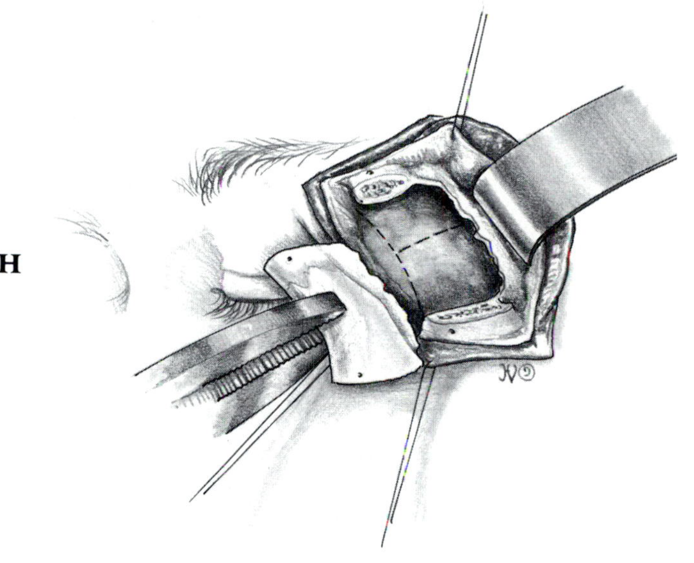

Continued.

Tent the periorbita with two forceps before cutting into it (Fig. 53-3, *I*). Make an anteroposterior incision in the underlying periorbita while avoiding the lacrimal gland and lateral rectus.

With gentle traction on the lateral rectus tendon suture, the belly of the muscle is identified and retracted out of the field. As the periorbital incision is completed, establish complete hemostasis to avoid bleeding into the orbit when the tumor is being exposed.

Gentle finger palpation is helpful in localizing the lesion (Fig. 53-3, *J*). If the mass of the lesion lies within the central surgical space, overlying orbital fat is retracted or shrunken with light bipolar cautery. The cautery is used on fat directly over the lesion. It should not be used in the deep orbit away from the mass.

With gentle retraction of the lateral rectus muscle, the lesion is exposed (Fig. 53-3, *K*). The belly of the lateral rectus muscle is retracted with a 5-0 silk suture or Silastic band. A well-defined mass is exposed.

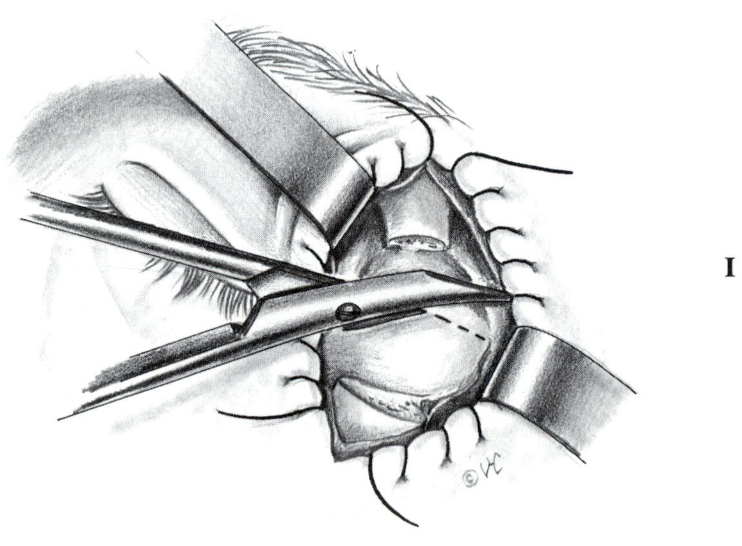

FIGURE 53-3, cont'd

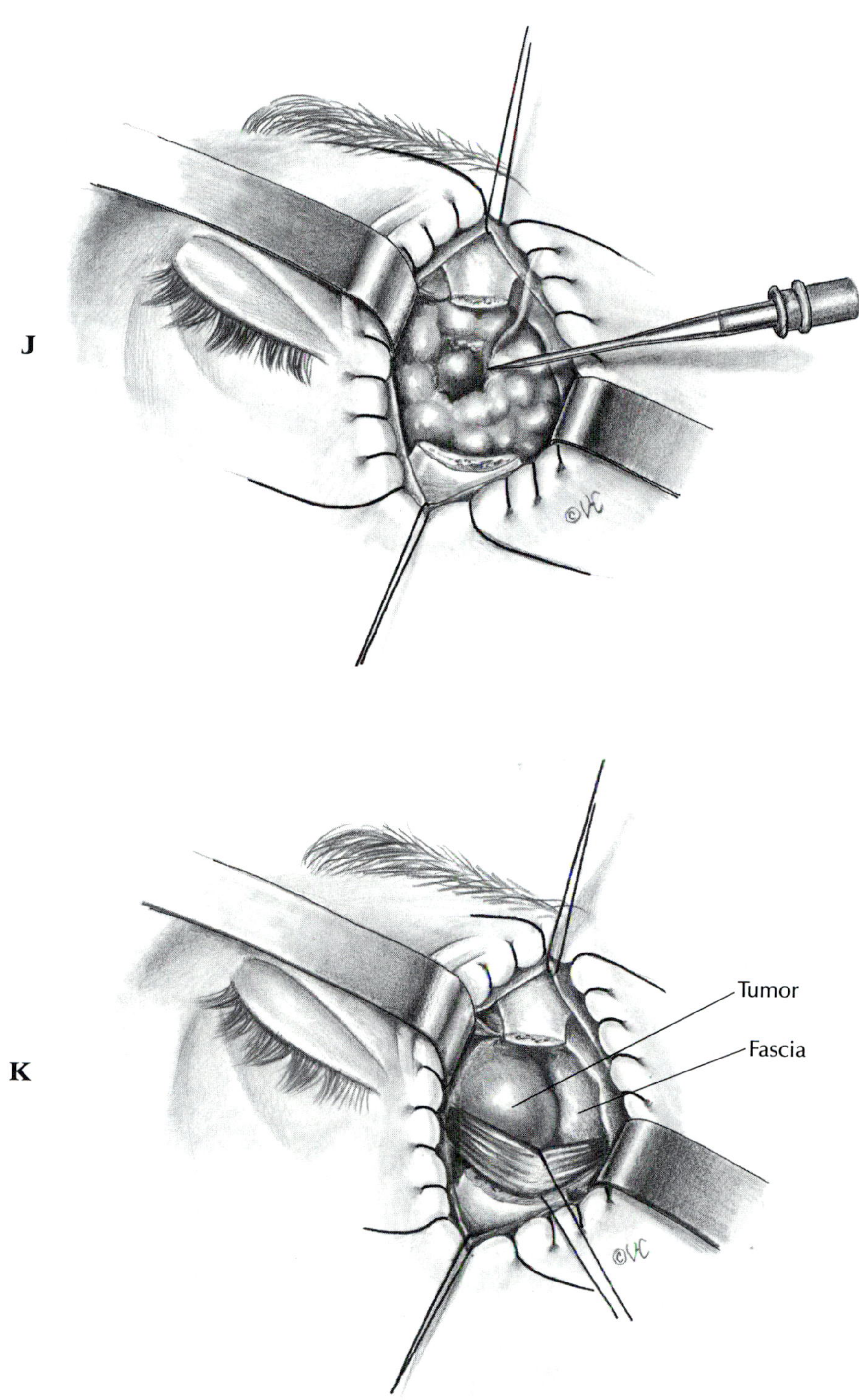

Continued.

Sharp dissection with microscissors and blunt dissection are used to free the tumor from surrounding orbital structures (Fig. 53-3, *L*). Cottonoid sponges are placed around the lesion to separate it from the surrounding structures during its excision and to prevent the accumulation of blood in the orbital apex.

If the lesion is well encapsulated, a cryoprobe may be used for gentle traction on the mass while it is being excised. The removal of diffuse vascular lesions with larger vessel supply is often aided by the use of a CO_2 laser. The determination to biopsy or completely excise the lesion is usually made preoperatively. After biopsy or removal of the lesion, the surgical site is irrigated with an antibiotic-steroid solution.

After the lesion is biopsied or excised and complete hemostasis has been established, the lateral orbital rim is put into position and stainless steel wires or 4-0 Prolene sutures are placed into the preplaced holes (Fig. 53-3, *M*). The periorbita is closed anteriorly with 4-0 chromic sutures.

L

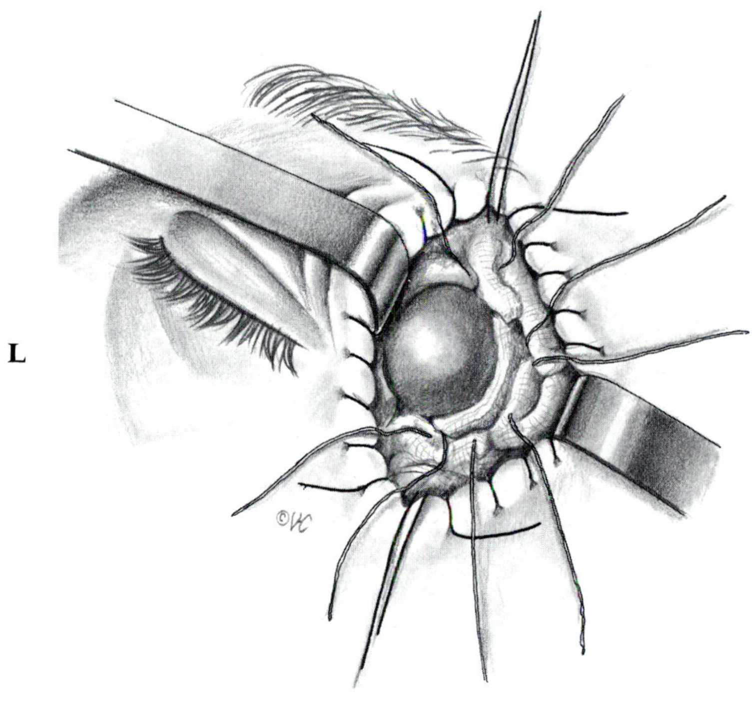

M

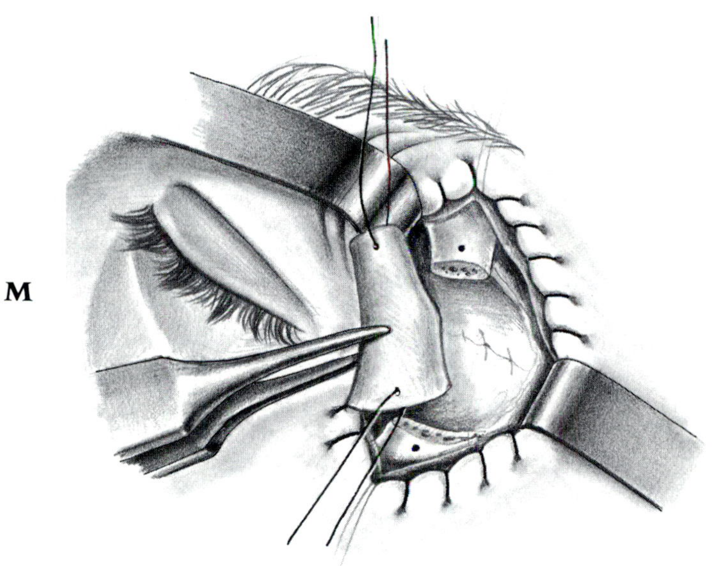

FIGURE 53-3, cont'd

Continued.

Wire fixation of the lateral rim is completed (Fig. 53-3, *N*). The ends of the wire are cut and buried into the drill holes. Pull up on the ends of the wire as it is being twisted and tightened. 4-0 Prolene sutures may also be used to fix the bone segment. If the lesion is malignant and there is evidence of periosteal or bony involvement, the bone is not replaced; additional removal of bone and periorbita may be necessary, and this is achieved with a high-speed burr. The lack of lateral orbital bone replacement typically creates minimal depression over the zygoma.

A butterfly drain is placed postoperatively (Fig. 53-3, *O*). It is positioned in the peripheral surgical space, and the outer layer of periosteum is sutured over it. The end of the drain is tunneled through subcutaneous tissues and brought out through a stab incision in the lateral malar region and sutured to the skin.

The subcutaneous and skin layers are sutured separately, and the butterfly drain is attached to a Vacutube (Fig. 53-3, *P*). The drain is removed in 24 hours or when sanguinous drainage has subsided. A moderately firm dressing is placed over the incision site.

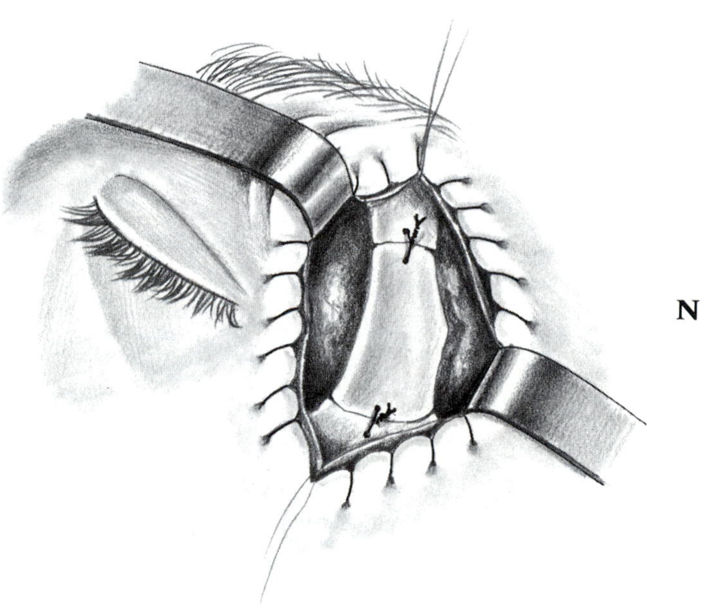

FIGURE 53-3, cont'd

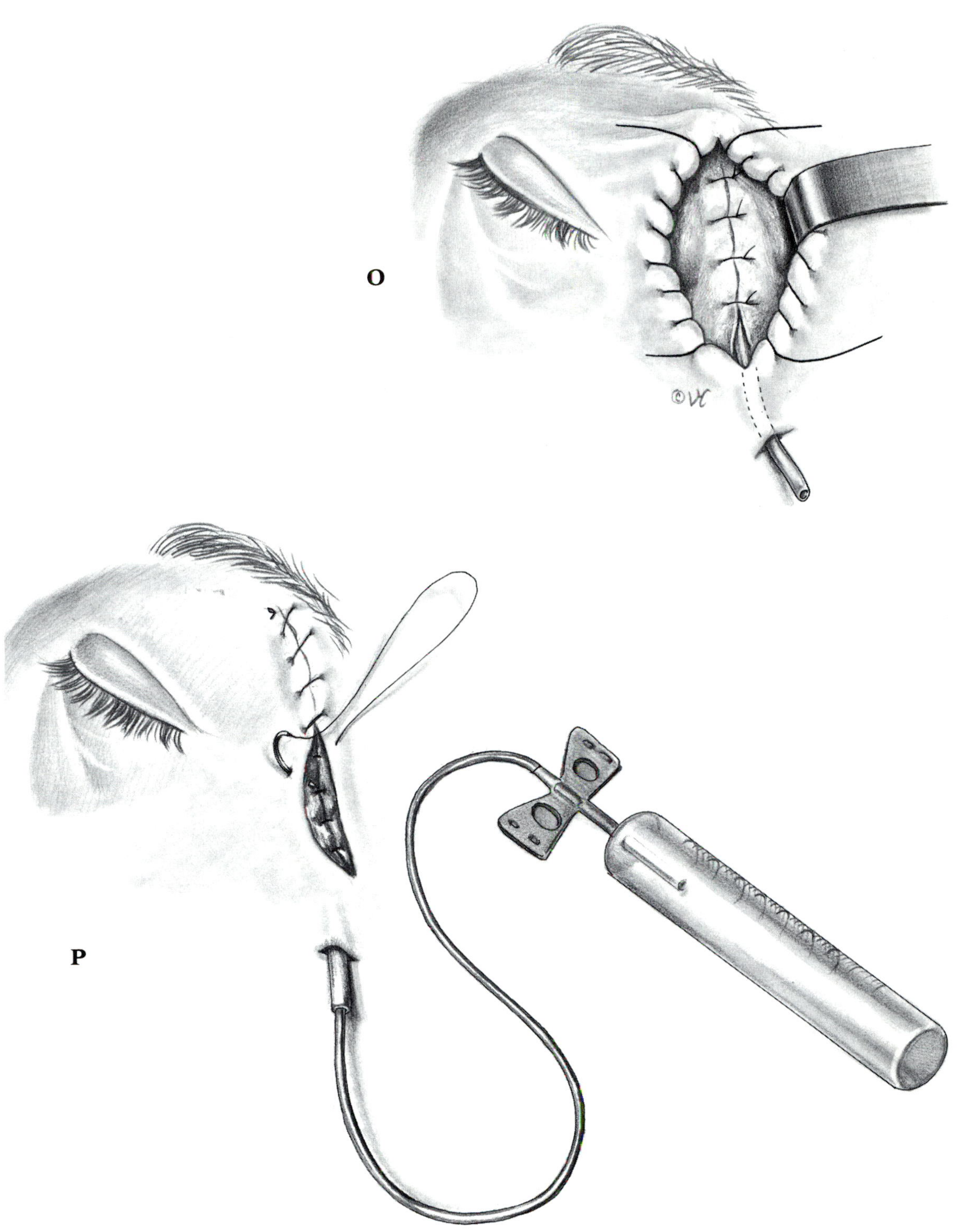
O
©VK
P

CHAPTER 54

Orbital Decompression

Dysthyroid orbitopathy, the most frequent cause of exophthalmos, can cause a myriad of ocular and orbital problems. The most common findings include eyelid retraction and lagophthalmos, exposure keratopathy, restrictive strabismus, exophthalmos, and optic neuropathy. After using medical intervention to its optimal effect, surgery is frequently necessary to improve the patient's deformity and function. The eyelids, extraocular muscles, and bony orbit are the three main surgical targets of the dysthyroid orbit. If orbital decompression is planned, it usually represents the first step in the treatment and rehabilitation of the dysthyroid orbit, with extraocular muscle or eyelid surgery (or both) following later.

INDICATIONS

The indications for surgical intervention fall into two categories, functional and cosmetic. Optic nerve dysfunction is a paramount indication for prompt treatment. Anatomically, this usually occurs because of apical crowding of the optic nerve by the hypertrophic extraocular muscles. It is believed that inflammatory and toxic factors may contribute to optic neuropathy, particularly with acute active dysthyroid orbital inflammation. The use of systemic corticosteroids in high doses (prednisone 100 to 200 mg) is suggested as a first step in treatment. Response to this treatment is expected within 5 to 7 days. Orbital decompression is necessary when there is orbital apex crowding around the nerve or the response to corticosteroid therapy is inadequate or transient.

PREOPERATIVE EVALUATION

Prospective patients for decompression should undergo vigorous preoperative optic nerve function evaluation. This includes visual fields, color vision testing, and if possible visual evoked potentials. When optic nerve dysfunction exists, bone removal in these cases is completed far posteriorly with posterior ethmoidectomy and removal of the orbital floor and if necessary the lateral wall. The infraorbital nerve is left intact. This allows for enlargement of the bony orbit, prolapse of the orbital soft tissue, and decompression of the orbital apex. Multiple incisions into the periorbita and "teasing" of orbital fat into the sinuses are critical to volumetric expansion of the orbit. In functional cases this again should be maximal in an attempt to create the largest expanse of soft-tissue volume. Essentially the same surgical technique is used for cosmetic decompression, except here reasonably symmetric position of globes is a priority. Expansion of the orbital apex is not required in this latter instance. Intraoperative and postoperative antibiotics should be maintained with broad-spectrum coverage for prophylaxis against sinusitis and cellulitis for 2 weeks.

Important points in the evaluation of the dysthyroid orbit that pertain to surgical planning are axial proptosis, vertical disparity of the globes, and motility restriction. Patients with exophthalmos are studied with computerized tomography and possibly ultrasound imaging. Those with asymmetric exophthalmic orbits are candidates for decompression, possibly including two-wall decompression on the lesser side and three-wall decompression on the more severely involved side. For each eye, removal of bone and release of periorbita and orbital fat into the sinuses depends on the degree of exophthalmos.

PRINCIPLES OF TREATMENT

The decision to utilize a transorbital approach versus combined orbital-transantral approach is a matter of preference. Good results can certainly be obtained by both methods. Advocates of the combined orbital transantral approach indicate that more effective posterior bone resection and apical decompression is accomplished because of better exposure of the medial wall. The orbital approach allows for better visualization and control of the orbital tissue and protection of the infraorbital nerve. The combined approach is particularly effective in patients with significant optic neuropathy.

At the close of the procedure drains are inserted into the maxillary sinus and at times directly into the orbit. A medium to firm dressing can be applied for 1 hour postoperatively to displace the orbital fat into the sinus. The dressing is removed, and a preliminary visual check is done. Dressing application may provide additional control of symmetry postoperatively. Should some asymmetry and proptosis persist in the first postoperative day, a dressing applied to the orbits can enhance further prolapse of the orbital fat into the sinus during the first 24 hours. Orbits usually become stabilized in 3 to 4 months, and should second- and third-stage reconstruction for the extraocular muscle and eyelid abnormalities be required, they can be treated at that time.

Three-Wall Decompression; Fornix-Orbit Approach

Lateral canthotomy is done after traction sutures have been placed in the upper and lower eyelids (Fig. 54-1, *A*).

Completion of an inferior crus cantholysis gives "free-swinging" lower eyelid flap in preparation for the transfornix conjunctival incision (Fig. 54-1, *B*). Dissection into the subconjunctival and precapsulopalpebral space is done in preparation for the fornix incision (Fig. 54-1, *C*).

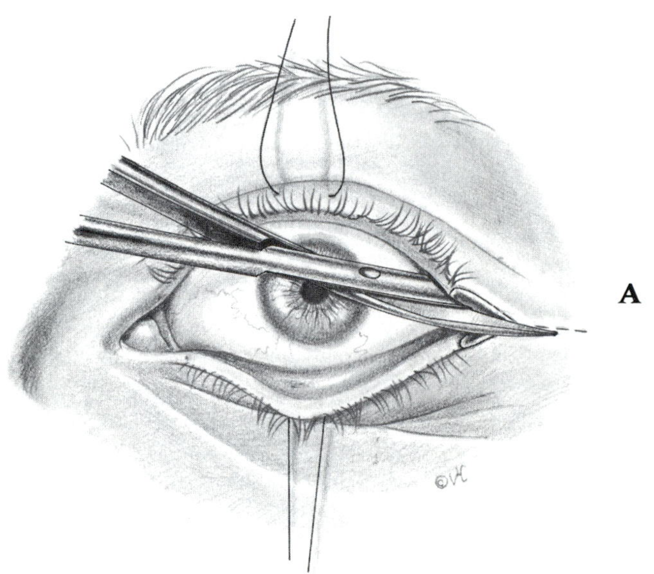

FIGURE 54-1. Three-wall decompression, fornix-orbit approach.

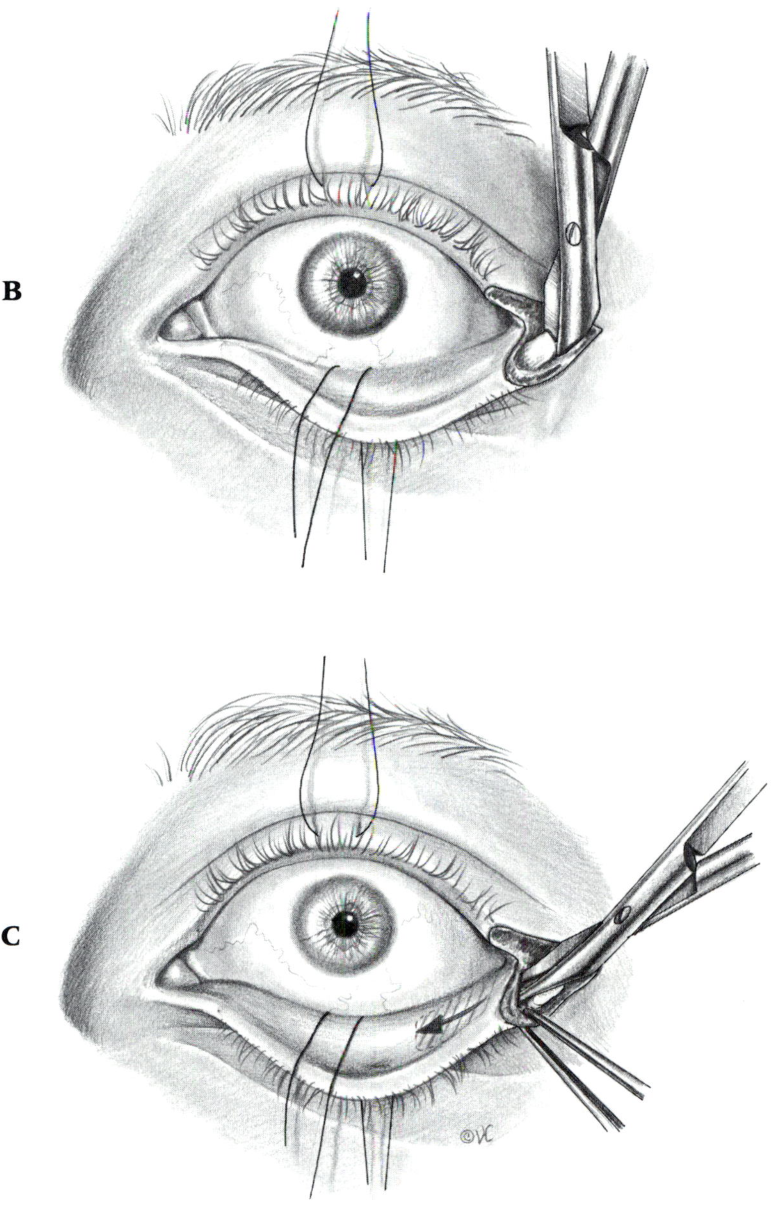

Continued.

Fig. 54-1, *D,* shows extension of the palpebral conjunctival incision 3 mm superior to the fornix across the eyelid. The eyelid retractors are severed. Incision extends to a point just medial to the punctum level. Bleeding points are cauterized with a fine unipolar cautery.

Conjunctival and lower lid retractor flap is attached to upper eyelid with 5-0 silk suture to facilitate exposure of inferior orbital rim (Fig. 54-1, *E*). During surgery this suture will be loosened to allow for the pupil to be checked. The incision line into the periorbita is marked by the serrated line.

Incision of periorbita is made with a no. 15 blade above the foramina of the infraorbital nerve (Fig. 54-1, *F*).

Reflection of periorbita "unzips" the floor of the orbit (Fig. 54-1, *G*). A Freer elevator is used to separate the periorbita from the orbital floor.

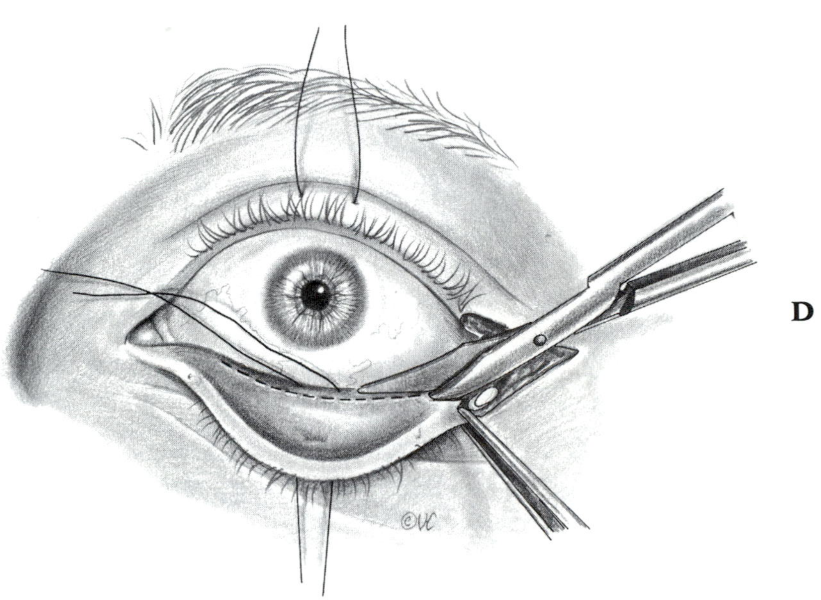

FIGURE 54-1, cont'd

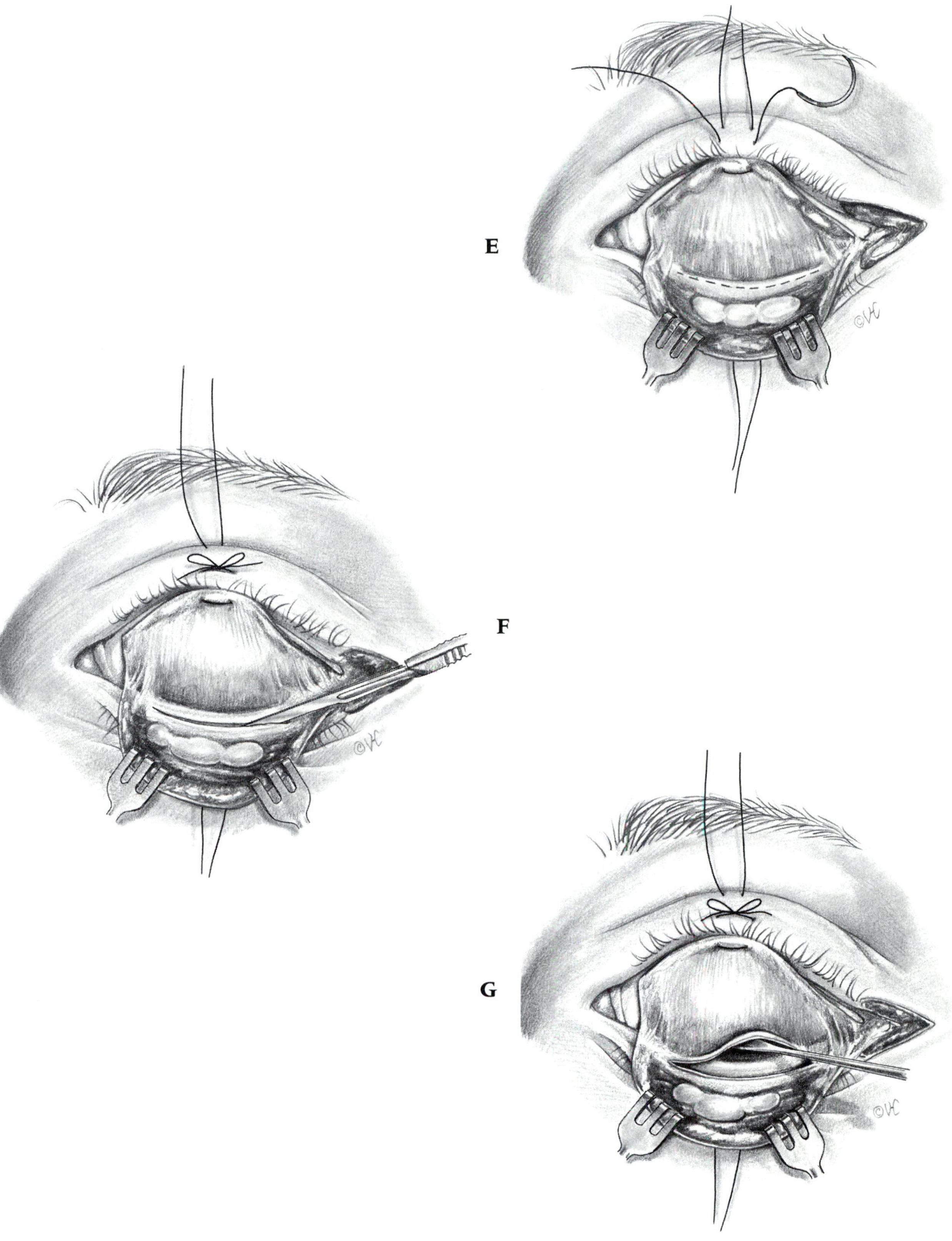

Continued.

For three-wall orbital decompression, retraction of soft tissue from the zygoma allows for periorbital incision to extend over the zygoma contiguous with inferior rim incision (Fig. 54-1, *H* and *I*).

An oscillating saw is used to complete osteotomies of the zygoma (Fig. 54-1, *J*). Globe and soft tissue are protected with malleable retractors.

The rongeur helps to break off the lateral wall after an osteotomy parallel to the orbital rim osteotomies shown in Fig. 54-1, *J,* was made (Fig. 54-1, *K*).

The rongeur is then used to clip off part of the lateral wall (Fig. 54-1, *L*).

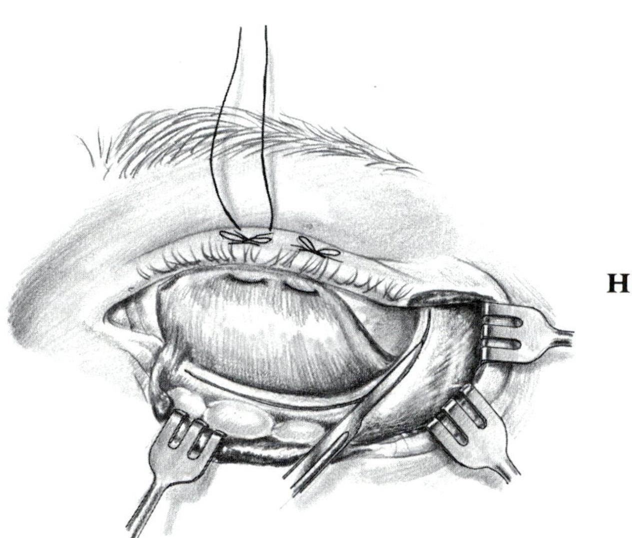

FIGURE 54-1, cont'd

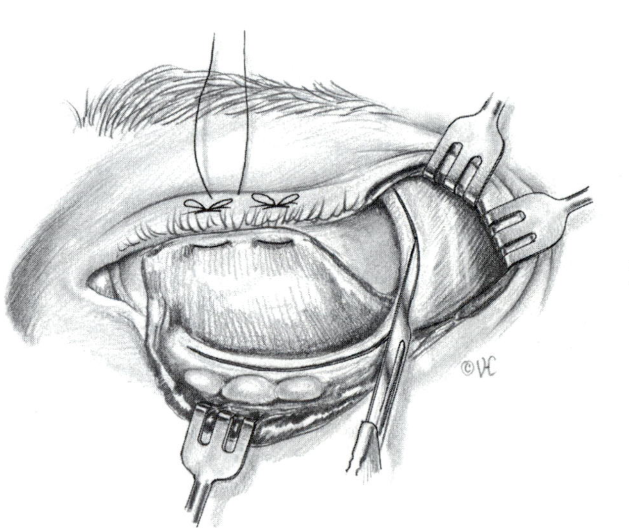

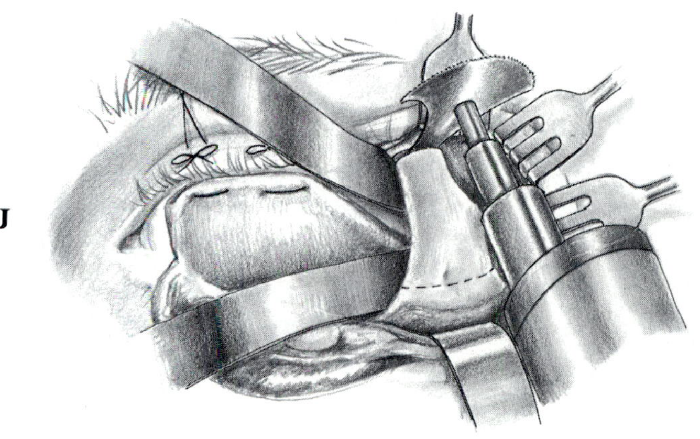

J

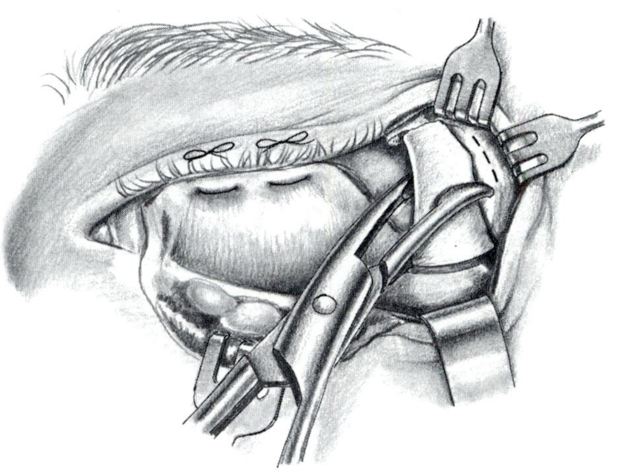

K

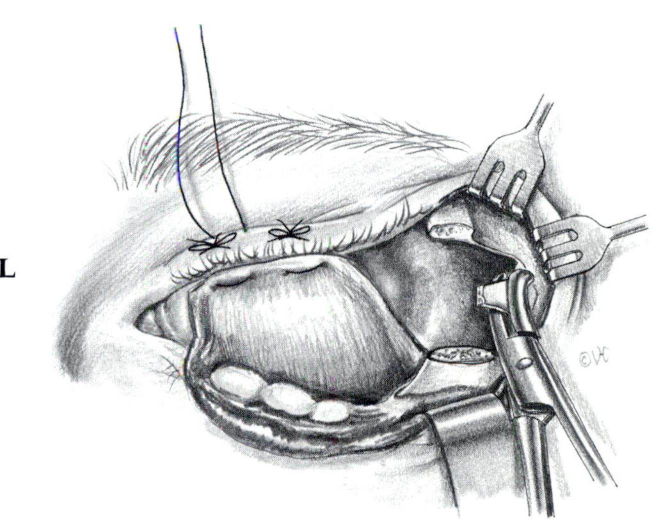

L

Continued.

Fig. 54-1, *M,* shows an outline of orbital floor to be removed. The bulk of it involves the floor medial to the infraorbital nerve. The infraorbital nerve is kept intact.

Fig. 54-1, *N,* shows a schematic coronal view of the orbit after removal of a substantial part of the orbital floor, medial wall, and lateral wall. Periorbital incisions allows for prolapse of fat into ethmoid and maxillary sinuses. The periorbital incisions can be made with a myringotomy knife and extended with Wescott scissors. Periorbita incisions are made from a posterior to anterior direction. The fat can be gently teased into the sinuses with a forceps.

A large curved hemostat or trochar is used to make entry transnasally to the antrum of the maxillary sinus (Fig. 54-1, *O*). It is passed along the floor of the nose posterior to the membranous portion of the nasolacrimal duct.

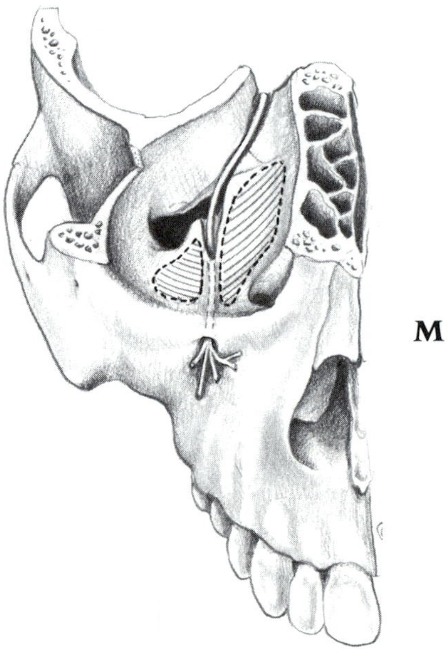

FIGURE 54-1, cont'd

N

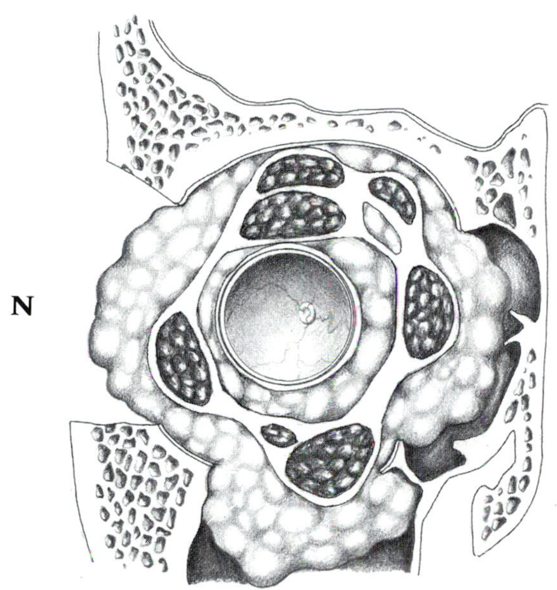

O

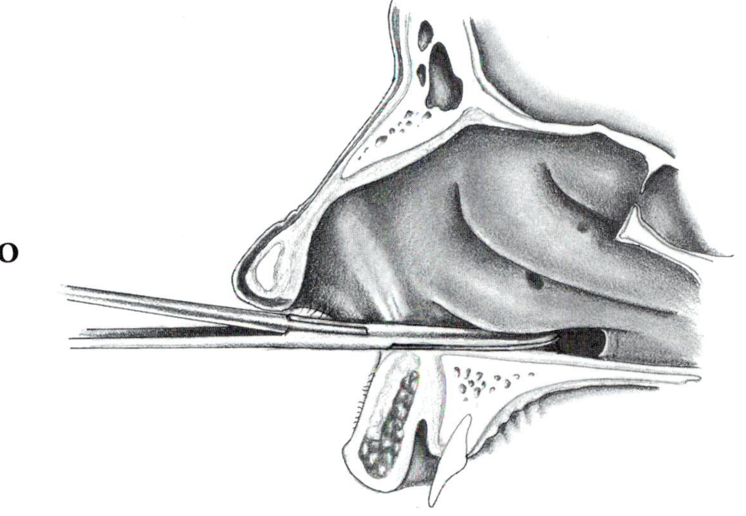

Continued.

Fig. 54-1, *P,* shows a Foley catheter drain inserted transnasally into the maxillary sinus.

A schematic coronal view of a completed three-wall decompression with nasoantral drain and fluid-inflated catheter balloon in the maxillary sinus is shown in Fig. 54-1, *Q*.

The conjunctival fornix incision is closed with running 6-0 chromic sutures (Fig. 54-1, *R*). 5-0 Prolene suture is used to attach the lateral aspect of the eyelid to the periosteum. This suture will help define the lateral canthus.

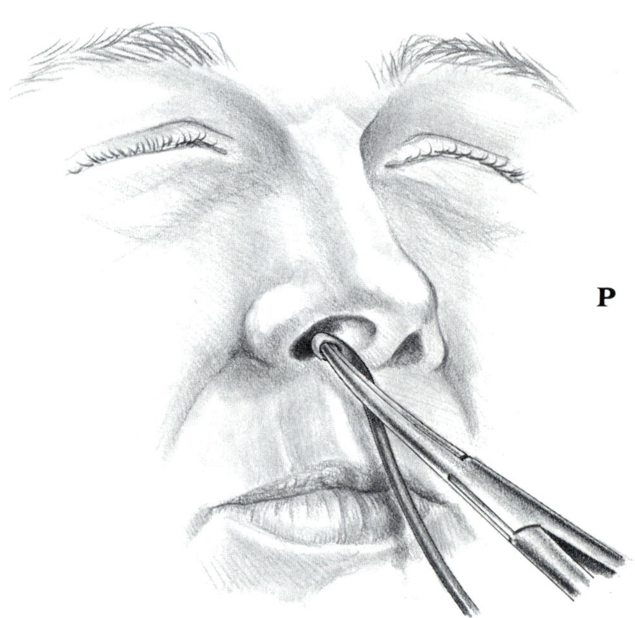

FIGURE 54-1, cont'd

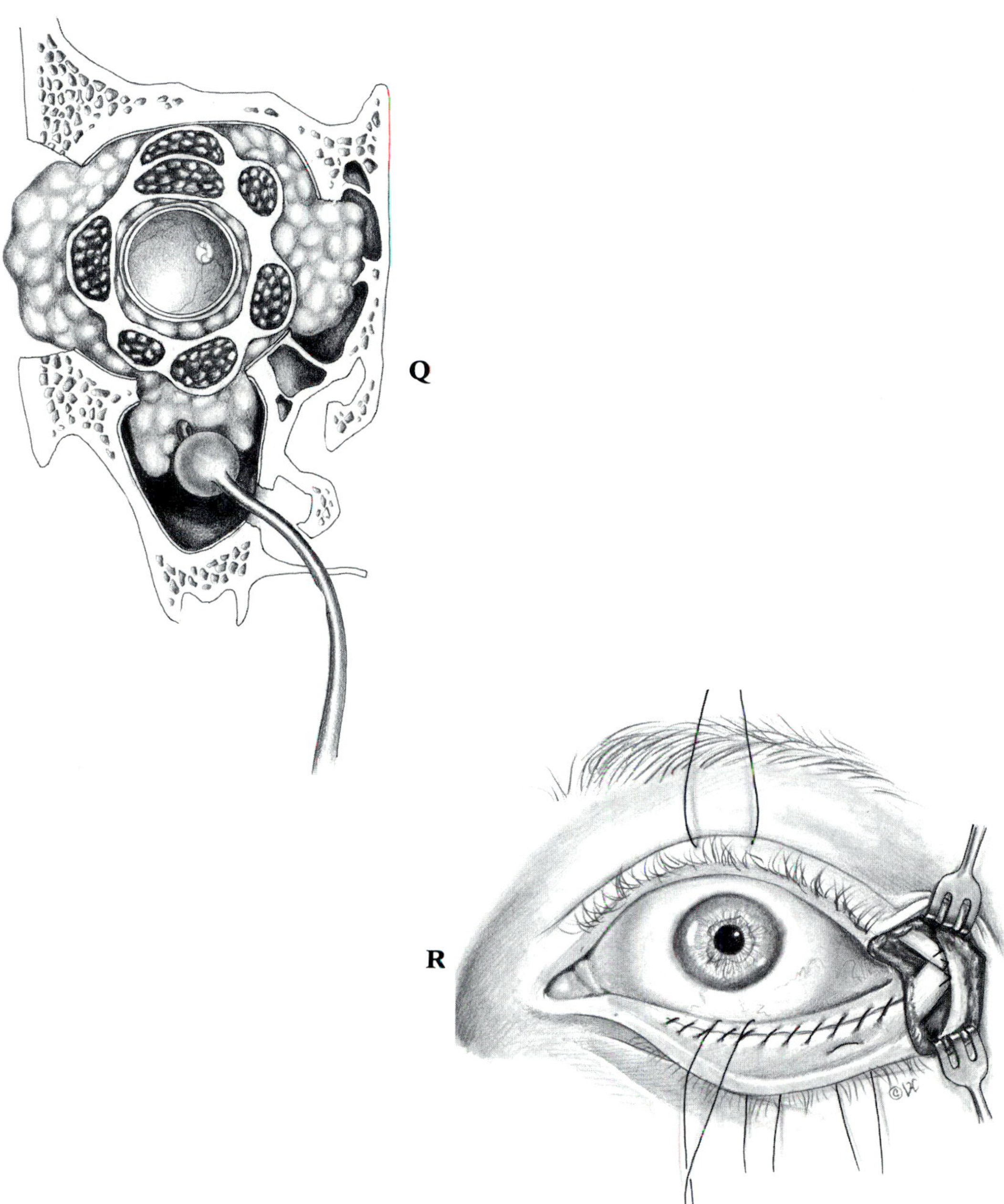
Q
R

Combined Orbit-Transantral Approach

As an alternative to the transconjunctival approach, the lower eyelid crease incision is suitable to expose the orbital rim and orbital floor as described in the orbital fracture section (Fig. 54-2, *A*). The anterior approach precedes the transantral approach.

At the site of gingival mucosal incision for Caldwell-Luc approach, the incision begins near the fourth incisor (Fig. 54-2, *B*). Mucosa is reflected superiorly so that the anterior wall of the maxilla is exposed (Fig. 54-2, *C*). Mucosa is retracted and the infraorbital nerve is identified in preparation for entry into the maxillary sinus (Fig. 54-2, *D*). The infraorbital nerve and canal are left intact when anterior maxillary bone is removed.

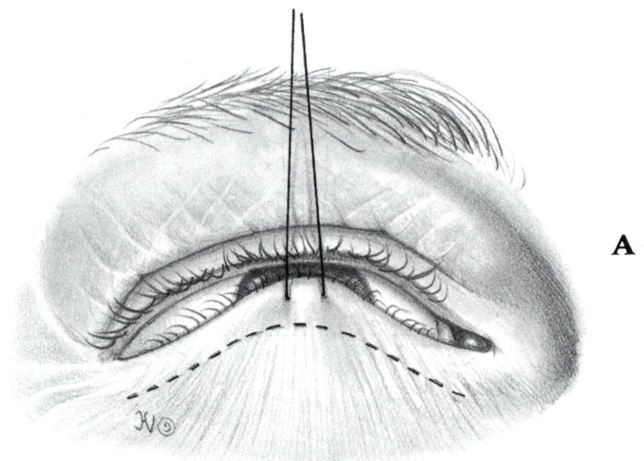

FIGURE 54-2. Combined orbital-transantral approach.

B

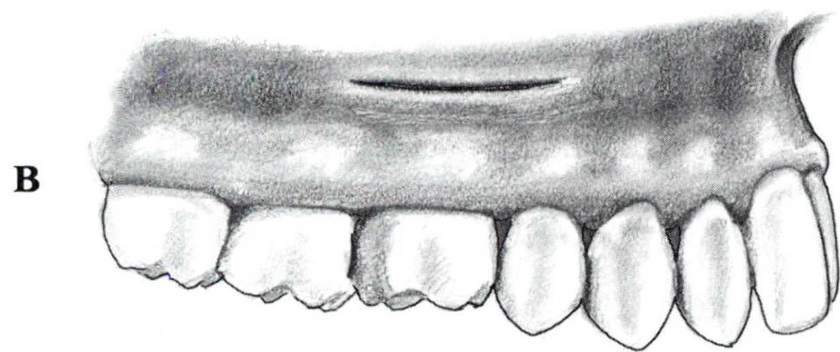

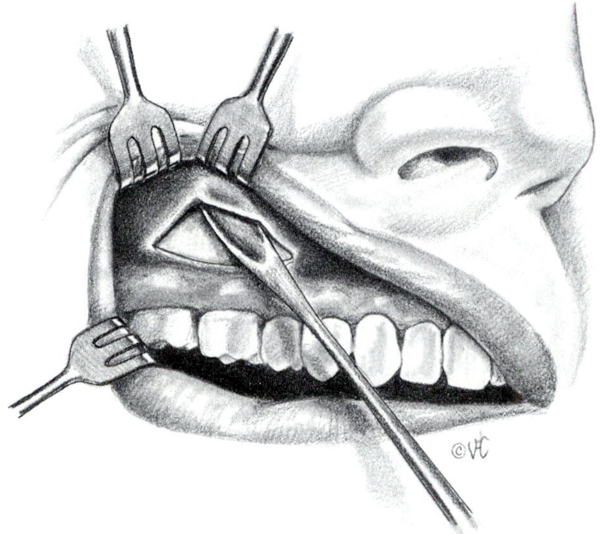

C

D

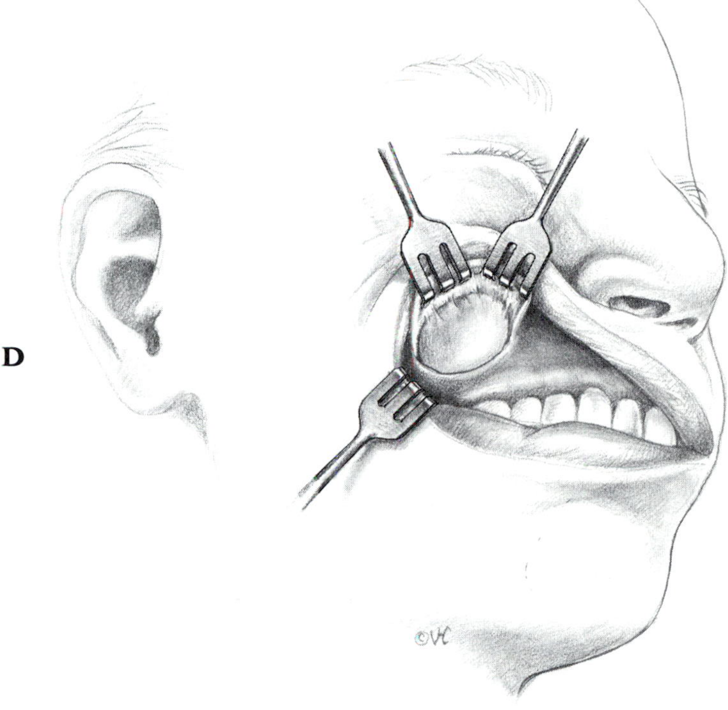

Continued.

Fig. 54-2, *E,* shows the removal of part of the anterior maxillary wall with osteotome and rongeurs to expose the antrum. The removal of the medial orbital wall and ethmoidectomy are done through the antral approach (Fig. 54-2, *F*). With this approach bone can be removed posteriorly with good exposure. Intact periorbita and orbital tissue contents are reflected away and protected by malleable retractors when bone is removed.

Combined orbit-transantral approach allows for good exposure when the posterior floor and medial wall are removed. The orbital floor is removed with the orbital approach, and the medial wall is removed with the transantral approach to within 10 mm of the optic canal. Citelli and straight rongeurs are used to remove small segments of bone, with the retracted periorbita being left intact (Fig. 54-2, *G*).

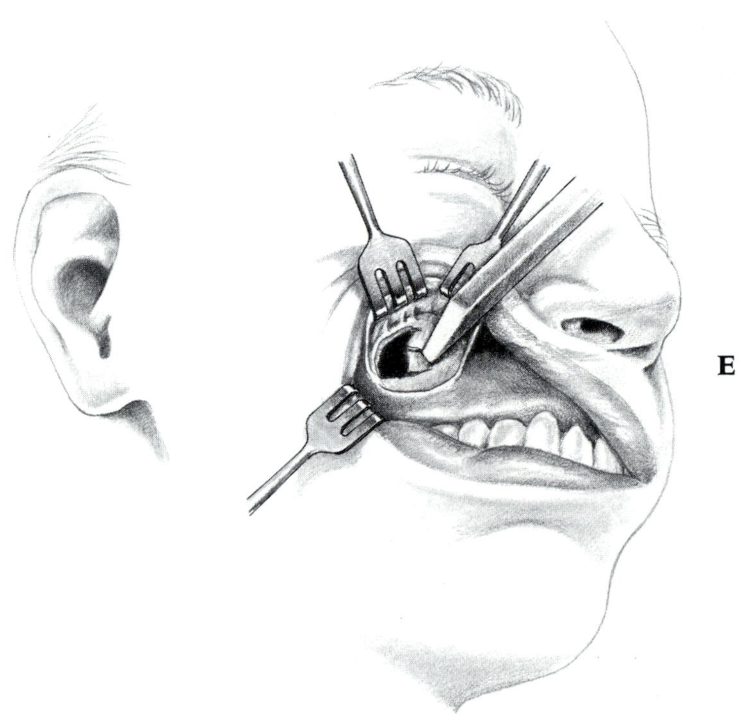

FIGURE 54-2, cont'd

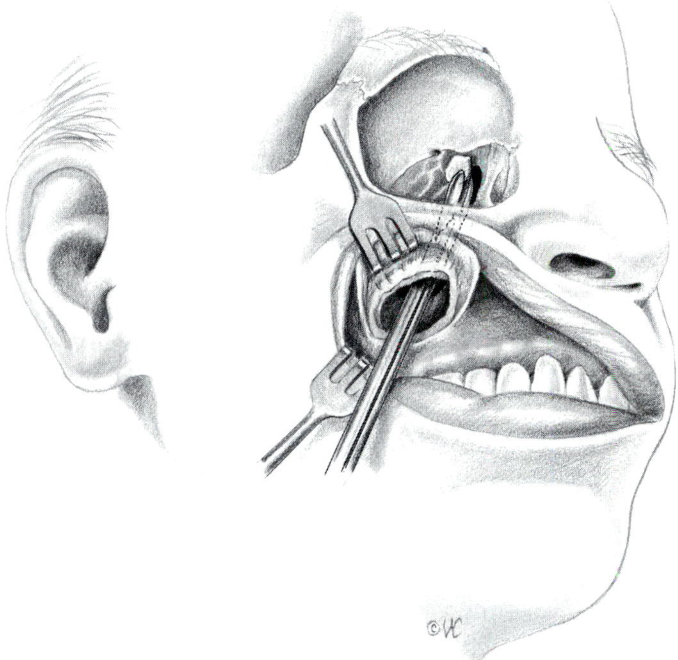

F

G

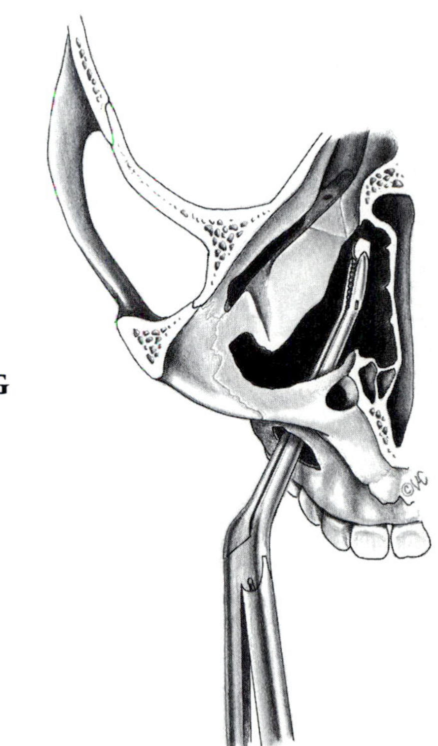

Continued.

Fig. 54-2, *H*, shows the orbit after removal of bone for three-wall decompression. Periorbital incisions are made, and fat is prolapsed into the sinuses.

The gingival incision is closed with 3-0 chromic sutures (Fig. 54-2, *I*).

H

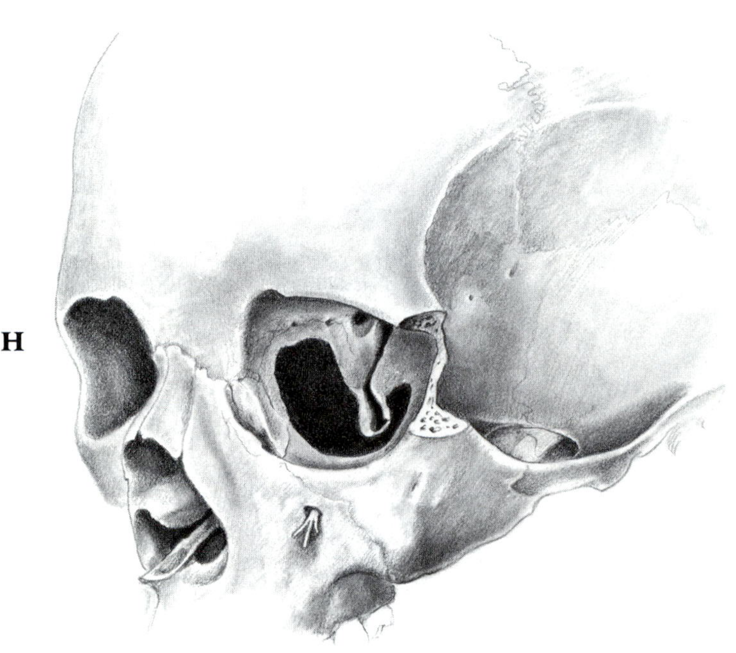

I

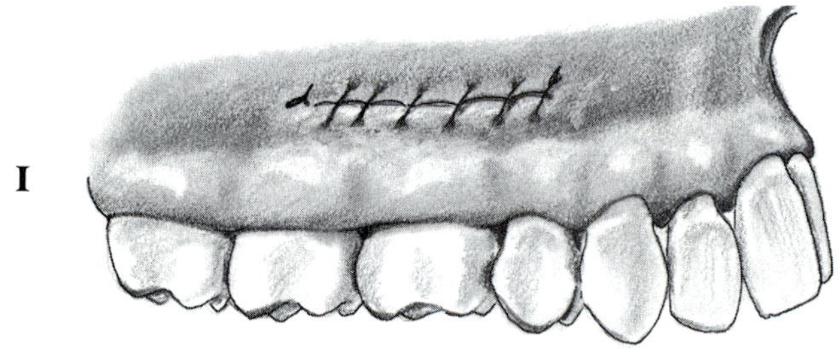

FIGURE 54-2, cont'd

CHAPTER 55

Orbital Exenteration

Orbital exenteration involves removing the globe, orbital contents, and additional periocular tissue as indicated by the nature and location of the underlying disease. Among the most common diseases for which an exenteration is performed are the following: (1) malignant tumors of the eye and adnexa, (2) malignant tumors extending into the orbit from the cranium or paranasal sinuses, and (3) widespread *Mucor* or other fungal infections.

Less commonly, modified exenteration is indicated for recurrent deforming congenital or benign orbital tumors and possibly severe orbital and socket contracture.

More commonly, orbital exenteration is performed to remove a life-threatening neoplasm or infection. Examples of primary orbital tumors that may require this include basal cell carcinoma, squamous cell carcinoma, melanoma, lacrimal gland adenocarcinoma, and meibomian gland carcinoma. Rhabdomyosarcoma once treated by exenteration is now effectively treated by radiation, chemotherapy, or both. A multidisciplined approach to exenteration may be necessary if the disease extends beyond the orbit. A combined approach with neurosurgical colleagues is used when there is intracranial involvement. Intraorbital extension of a maxillary sinus squamous cell carcinoma requires a combined approach with the head and neck surgeon. Immunocompromised patients with mucormycosis involving the orbit, paranasal sinuses, and cranium often require exenteration. Indeed it may be lifesaving in these patients.

Exenteration is occasionally performed in the treatment of benign orbital tumors such as a diffusely infiltrating neurofibroma or a rapidly growing and extensive meningioma.

Exenteration is an option in the management of severely contracted anophthalmic sockets when standard surgery has failed or is impractical.

For malignancy, margin-controlled removal of all diseased tissue while sparing uninvolved tissue is the primary goal of orbital exenteration. However, effort is made to maximize potential for the later use of an ocular or orbital prosthesis. Modified exenteration of the orbital contents with preservation of the eyelids and conjunctiva may allow the patient to wear a conventional prosthesis. Radical exenteration will require a customized exenteration prosthesis for rehabilitation of the patient.

Exenteration Procedure

The location of the skin (or conjunctival) incision is determined by the nature and location of the underlying disease (Fig. 55-1, *A*). If the eyelids are free of disease, the tarsus and eyelid margins may be spared to allow an ocular prosthesis to be fitted.

Sometimes uninvolved eyelid skin can be used to line the socket. Important structures such as the supraorbital neurovascular bundle and medial canthal tendon are shown. Fig. 55-1, *B,* shows the skin incised at the predetermined site with a scalpel beginning laterally. The incision is extended to the orbital rim with the skin margins retracted (Fig. 55-1, *C*). A cutting blade of the electrocautery unit is effective in cutting down to the periosteum on the orbital rim while minimizing bleeding. The dissection to the orbital rim is completed (Fig. 55-1, *D*). Medially the angular vessels need to be identified and ligated.

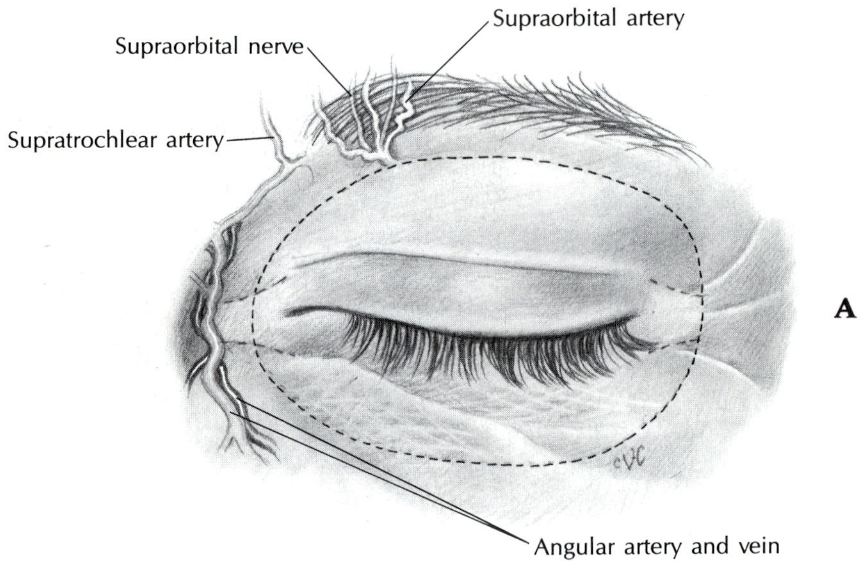

FIGURE 55-1. Exenteration procedure.

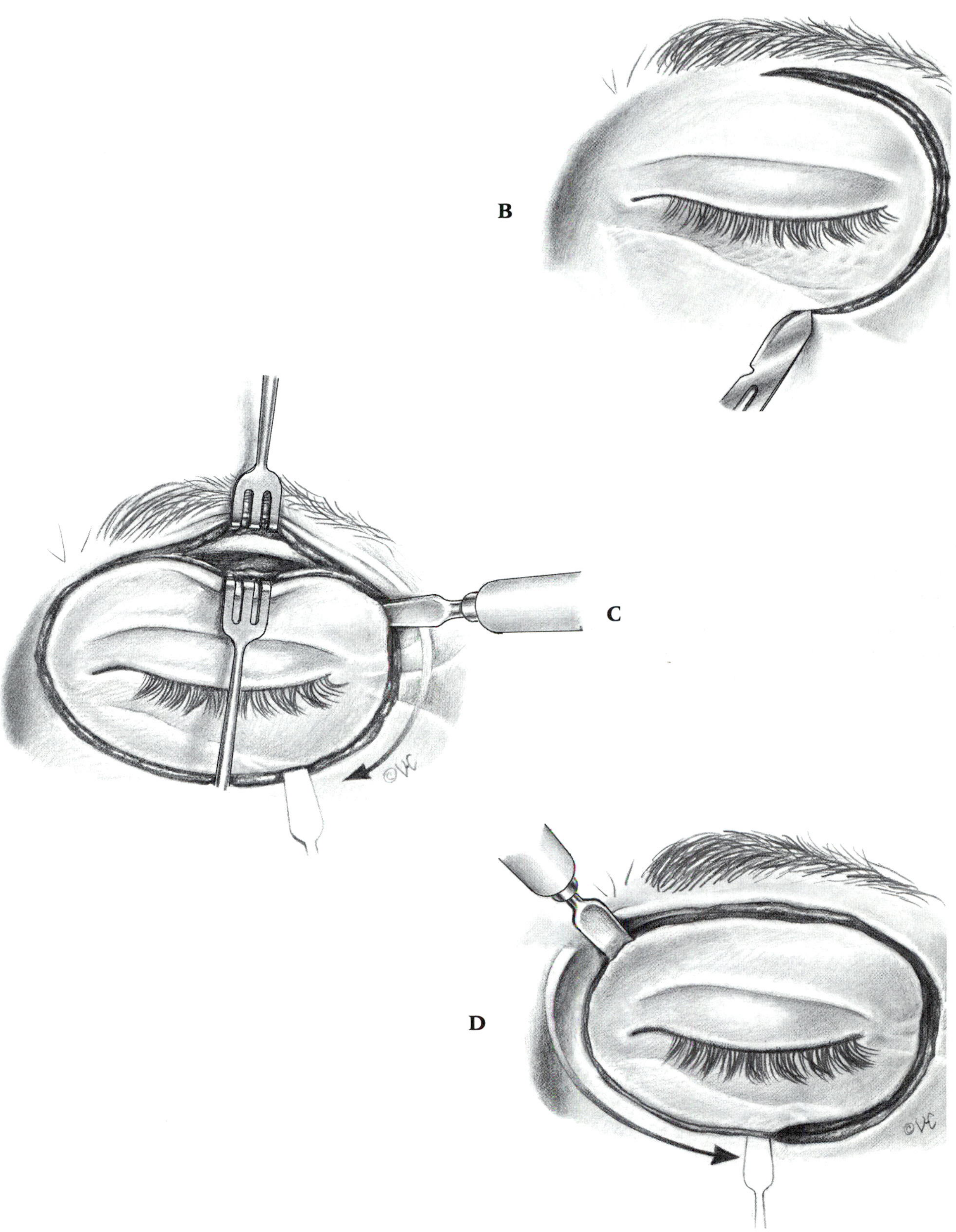

Continued.

After the periosteum is incised and retracted, traction sutures are used to facilitate exposure as the periorbita is elevated (Fig. 55-1, *E*) and dissection proceeds to the orbital apex. The tip of a suction handpiece, surrounded by a gauze pad, is used to bluntly separate the periorbita from the orbital bones. Care is taken to avoid fracturing the walls and entering into the adjacent sinuses.

The optic nerve and ophthalmic artery are positioned between the tips of an opened curved hemostat (Fig. 55-1, *F*). The clamp is closed, crushing the structures close to the optic foramen. Enucleation or Metzenbaum scissors are used to cut the optic nerve anterior to the positioned clamp (Fig. 55-1, *G*). Metal clips, suture ties, or electrical coagulation will help secure hemostasis in the apex (Fig. 55-1, *H*).

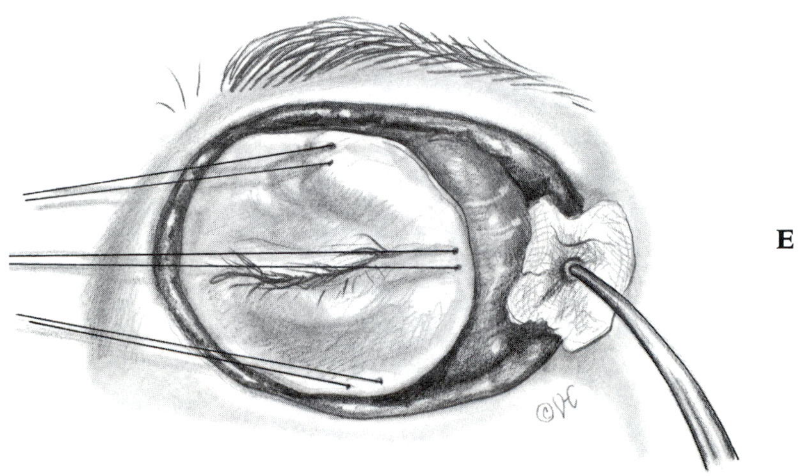

FIGURE 55-1, cont'd

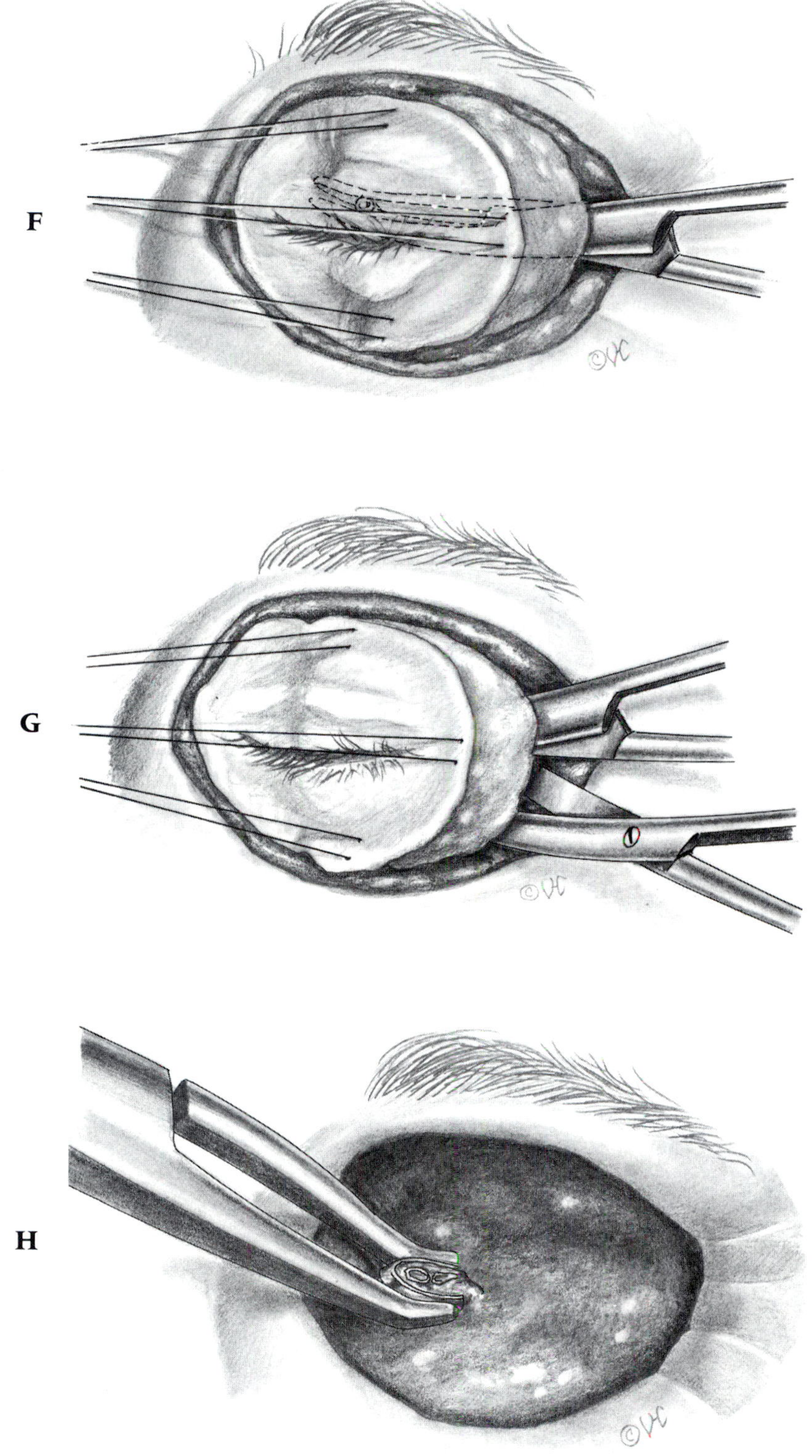

Continued.

A split-thickness skin graft, taken from the inner thigh, is positioned over the exenterated orbit (Fig. 55-1, *I*). The graft can be incised to allow for drainage. The graft is sutured at the orbital margins. Then the skin-grafted socket is lined with nonadherent gauze or Telfa (Fig. 55-1, *J*). Petrolatum gauze is then used to be firmly packed and conformed to the exenterated orbit. A pressure adhesive dressing is applied to the socket (Fig. 55-1, *K*).

The dressing is removed on postoperative day 4 unless severe pain or fever exists, at which time it is removed sooner. Wound hygiene with diluted hydrogen peroxide solution can be applied to the socket until healing is complete. Customized prothesis evaluation can begin approximately 8 weeks postoperatively. The use of silicone rubber in the fabrication of an orbital prosthesis has allowed for the development of more realistic prostheses. With these improved products available, prosthesis fitting and use should be actively encouraged.

Several options exist in the management of the orbit after exenteration. The socket can be allowed to granulate without skin grafts. The healing is prolonged and sometimes incomplete though the socket is more easily observed for recurrent tumor growth with socket granulation. Full-thickness skin grafting directly onto bone is of less value because of graft necrosis secondary to inadequate nutrition. Temporalis muscle can be transferred into the orbit to fill the orbital volume. It can be used when a portion of the orbital rims have been resected. With all exenteration procedures, continued observation to detect tumor recurrence is important.

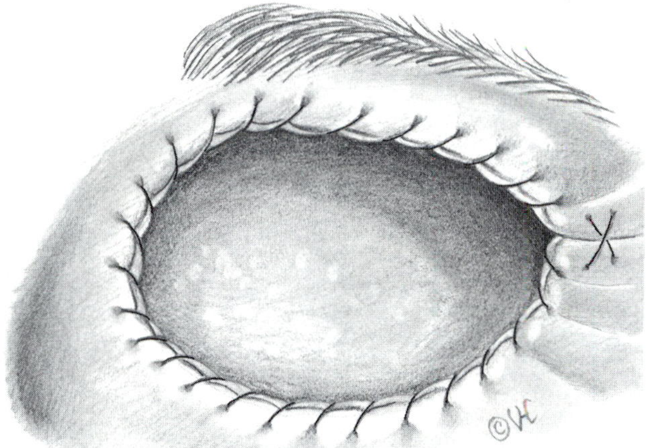

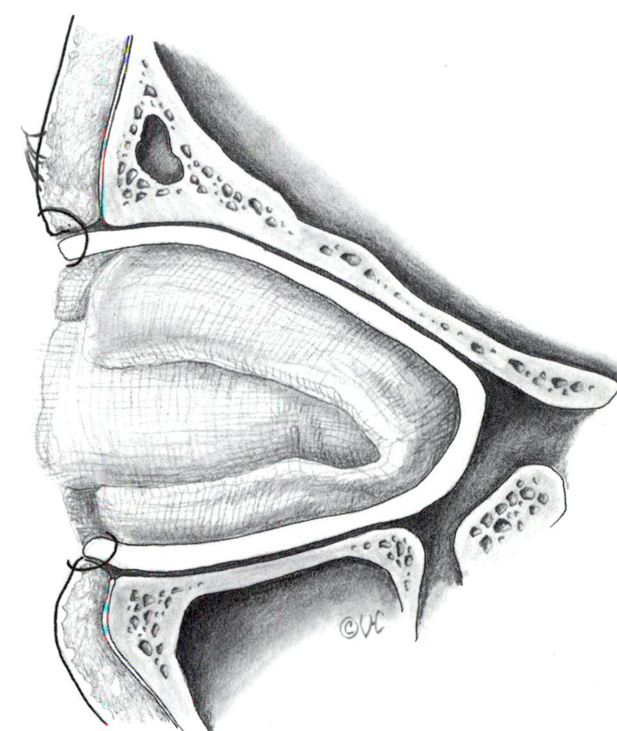

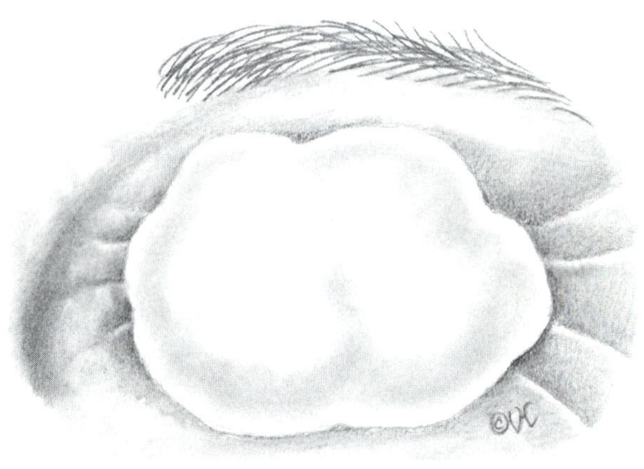

FIGURE 55-1, cont'd

CHAPTER 56

Enucleation

Postenucleation goals include a natural and symmetric prosthetic appearance, perhaps some prosthesis motility, and little if any socket discharge. No one procedure answers all these requirements, as evidenced by the numerous surgical techniques advocated over the years. After surgery, close collaboration between the ophthalmologist and the ocularist is important so that one can obtain the best cosmetic results with the ocular prosthesis while decreasing the possibility of secondary socket repair.

INDICATIONS FOR ENUCLEATION

Enucleation is indicated in extensively traumatized globes, particularly when there is a large posterior globe rupture or extensive lacerations involving the cornea, ciliary body, and sclera when both light projection and perception are lost. An enucleation is also indicated in blind, severely painful, deformed or disfigured globes, which develop secondary to absolute glaucoma, detached retina, or chronic inflammation. Ultrasonography is done preoperatively to help rule out an intraocular tumor.

Two strong indications for enucleation are nontreatable intraocular tumors and unrepairable injured globes where there is concern for developing sympathetic ophthalmia. Alternative therapy for lesions such as malignant melanomas and retinoblastomas including the use of radiation plaques has altered the need for enucleation in some cases of intraocular tumors.

Severely traumatized and disorganized globes, with associated deformities of the socket, present a challenge to the surgeon in restoring the socket to allow for the successful wearing of a prosthetic eye. With severe trauma every effort is made to attempt repair of the globe. Enucleation is done if globe lacerations are extensive and vision is not salvageable and is done within 10 days after injury because of the threat of sympathetic ophthalmia.

PATIENT PREPARATION

Preoperatively, the patient is advised concerning the advantages and disadvantages of an enucleation procedure and the fitting and wearing of a prosthesis. An appointment is scheduled with the ocularist, 3 to 4 weeks after the procedure. Aspirin and aspirin-related products are stopped at least 10 to 14 days before surgery.

ANESTHESIA AND PREPARATION

General anesthesia is preferred. If general anesthesia is medically contraindicated, a local anesthesia supplemented by neuroleptic analgesia may be used. For local anesthesia, a 3 to 6 ml retrobulbar injection extending into the apex of the orbit with a 1 : 1 mixture of 2% lidocaine with epinephrine (1 : 100,000 or 1 : 200,000) and 0.75% bupivacaine (Marcaine) is given with a long, blunted needle. Infiltration with lidocaine and epinephrine may be useful with general anesthesia to facilitate vasoconstriction to improve hemostasis and provide a longer postoperative period of analgesia.

Before prepping and draping the patient, the surgeon should again verify the correct eye to be enucleated. If the involved globe has an intraocular tumor, in an otherwise normal-appearing globe indirect ophthalmoscopy is performed before the procedure is begun.

Enucleation Technique

A double-armed 4-0 silk superior fornix traction suture is placed through the superior fornix and through the eyelid and is secured by a hemostat (Fig. 56-1, *A*). This suture will pass through the aponeurosis, and Müller's muscle and helps identify the superior extent of dissection into the fornix.

A 360-degree limbal peritomy of conjunctiva and Tenon's capsule is performed (Fig. 56-1, *B*). Care is taken to preserve as much conjunctiva and Tenon's capsule as possible.

Conjunctiva and Tenon's capsule are dissected posteriorly to the rectus muscles by use of a blunt-tipped Westcott scissors (Fig. 56-1, *C*). The conjunctiva and Tenon's capsule, which are joined approximately 2 to 3 mm from the limbus, are dissected as one layer. Steven's scissors or blunt-tipped Westcott scissors are then inserted into each quadrant, between the muscles, to free the attachments of Tenon's capsule to the globe.

The muscle hook is passed around the four individual rectus muscles (Fig. 56-1, *D*). A double-armed 5-0 suture (Vicryl or Dexon) is then weaved through the muscle 2 mm posterior to its insertion, with both arms of the suture being locked. The muscle is then amputated anterior to the suture.

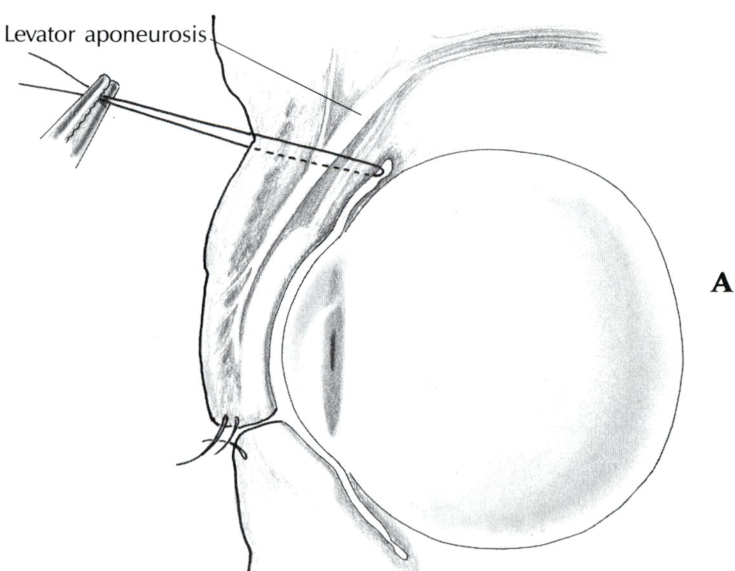

FIGURE 56-1. Enucleation technique.

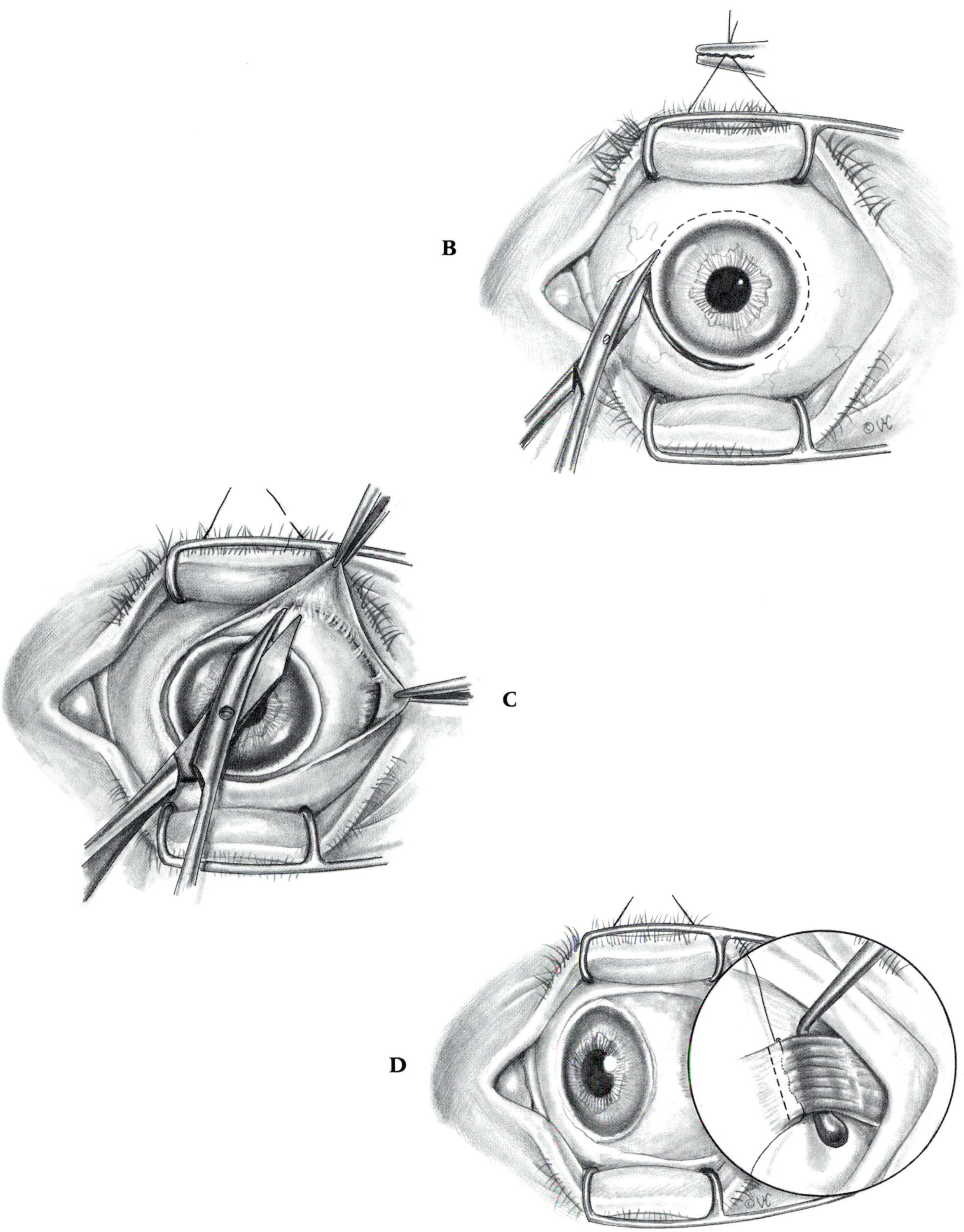

Continued.

A traction suture is placed through the remaining stump of the lateral and medial rectus muscles. These traction sutures promote fixation and rotation of the globe. During the isolation of the superior and inferior rectus muscles, avoid excessive superior and inferior dissection to limit the chance of postoperative ptosis, or damage to Lockwood's suspensory ligament.

After all the rectus muscles have been cut from their insertions, the superior oblique muscle is visualized when the stump of the superior rectus muscle is grasped and the globe is rotated inferiorly and temporally. The whitish tendon of the superior oblique muscle courses medially to laterally, just posterior to the superior rectus stump. The tendon may be hooked with a small tenotomy hook. The superior oblique muscle is then amputated near its insertion to the globe and allowed to retract (Fig. 56-1, *E*).

To expose the inferior oblique muscle, the stump of the lateral rectus muscle is rotated medially and superiorly while Tenon's capsule is retracted inferiorly (Fig. 56-1, *F*). The muscle is then isolated and divided within 5 mm of its insertion. It can be sutured to the inferior border of the lateral rectus to provide additional support for the implant and inferior fornix.

A firm adhesion exists between Tenon's capsule and the dural sheath of the optic nerve. The globe is gently retracted with forceps or perhaps traction sutures. An incision is then made through Tenon's capsule, adjacent to the optic nerve, just large enough to pass the scissors blades into the muscle cone (Fig. 56-1, *G*).

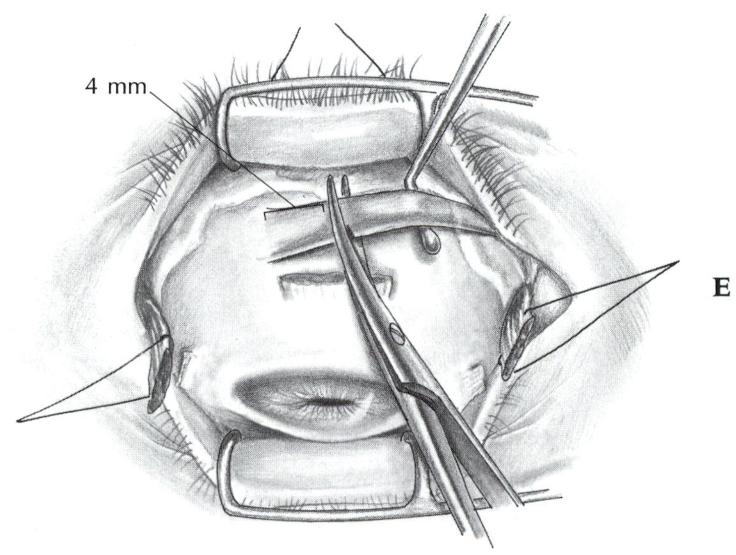

FIGURE 56-1, cont'd

F

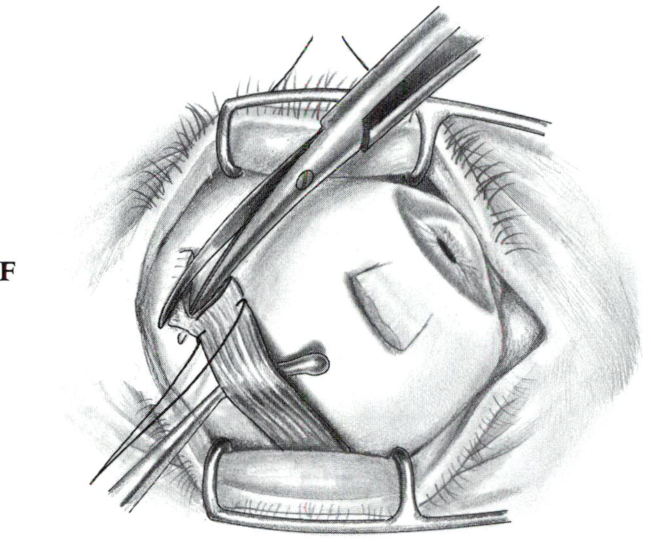

G

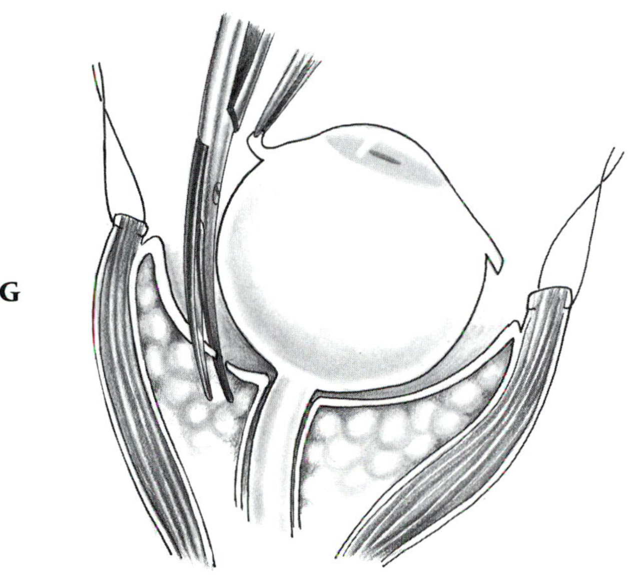

Continued.

A curved Kocher type of hemostat is then maneuvered through the opening in posterior Tenon's capsule to clamp the optic nerve at the desired level (Fig. 56-1, *H*). The enucleation scissors blades are inserted just in front of the hemostat straddling the optic nerve. While one maintains forward traction with sutures or a locking forceps on the horizontal muscle stumps, the neurectomy is performed (Fig. 56-1, *I*). The globe is inspected to ensure that it is intact and that there is no gross tumor extension. It is then wrapped in a moist sponge and sent to the laboratory immediately to begin histopathology evaluation.

A tonsil snare can also be used for the neurectomy (Fig. 56-1, *J*). It has the advantage of crushing the optic nerve and its vessels, decreasing the chance of hemorrhage. The wire of the snare passes over the globe within Tenon's capsule, with care being taken to avoid including orbital tissue other than the optic nerve in the snare. The ratchet screw is tightened, and the snare loop is closed, severing the optic nerve and vessels. The snare is not used when an intraocular tumor exists, since it may create a rapid increase in the intraocular pressure possibly causing spread of the tumor into the circulation.

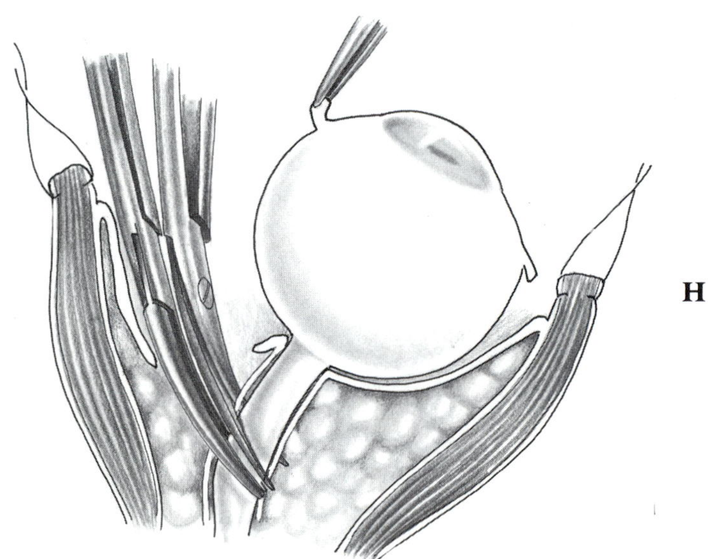

FIGURE 56-1, cont'd

I

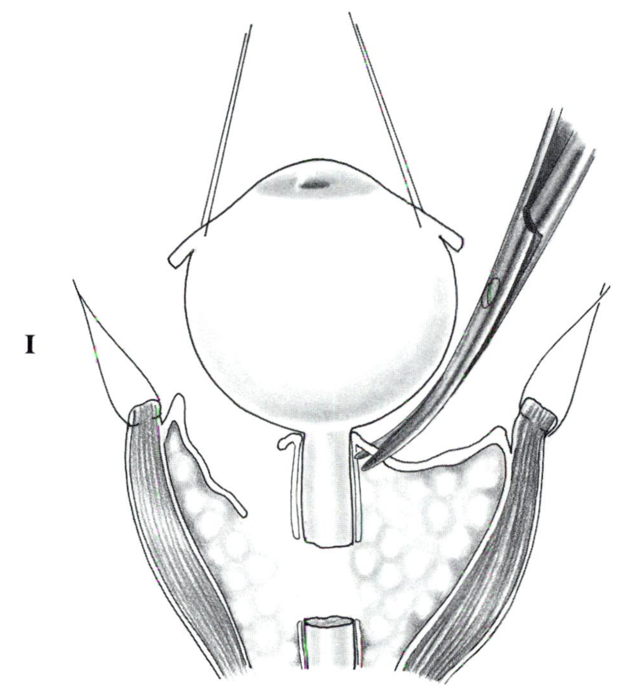

J

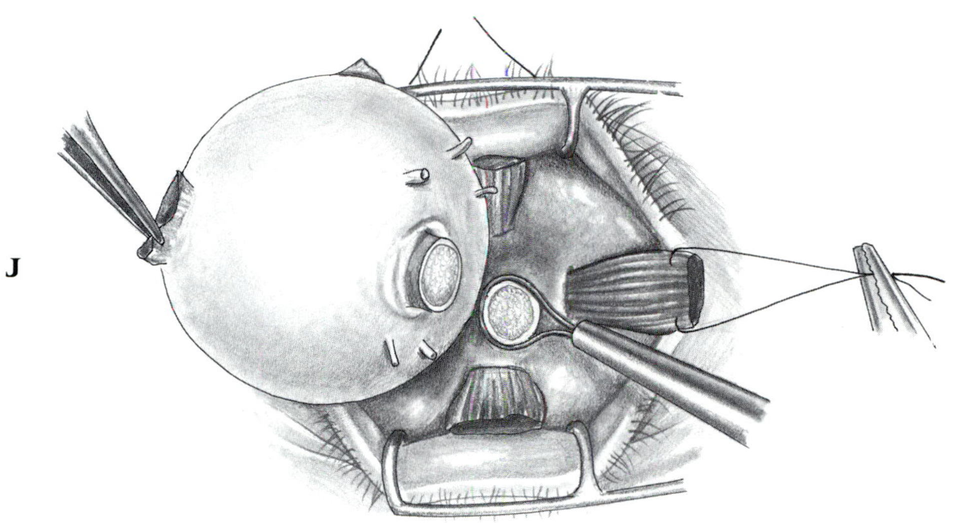

Continued.

If attempts to perform the neurectomy fail, this failure is usually secondary to faulty positioning of the enucleation scissors. No cutting is done until it is certain that the scissors blades surround the optic nerve. Hemostasis is obtained by firm packing of the orbit with a moist 4×4 inch gauze sponge and the application of digital pressure for 5 minutes. The pack is then gently removed. If bleeding persists, an absorbable gelatin sponge (Gelfoam), oxidized cellulose (Oxycel), microfibrillar collagen (Avitene), or thrombin can be applied to the deep socket. Cautery is used if bleeding vessels are identified. Complete hemostasis is necessary to prevent postoperative hemorrhage, which may lead to increased incidence of pain, infections, and implant migration.

The appearance of the socket after enucleation has been performed is shown in Fig. 56-1, *K*. With the lid speculum in place 5-0 Vicryl or Dexon sutures have been placed through medial and lateral rectus muscles. The inferior oblique muscle may now be sutured to the inferior border of the lateral rectus muscle, 8 to 10 mm posterior to its anterior end. The anterior layer of Tenon's capsule is divided from the posterior layer at the level where the rectus muscles exit. The opening in posterior Tenon's can be extended if necessary for insertion of the implant.

Enucleation with insertion of the implant deep to the posterior layer of Tenon's capsule has some advantages. With placement behind posterior Tenon's layer the implant is placed within the intraconal space. This creates two strong barrier layers anterior to the implant, decreasing the chance of extrusion and implant migration. A larger implant can be placed behind the posterior Tenon's layer. The implant can be as large as 20 to 22 mm in diameter. If the rent in the posterior capsule is not large enough, it is enlarged to permit the passage of the implant. The proper size of the implant is determined by the ease with which Tenon's capsule may be reapproximated. Too large an implant bows forward and may make the socket fornices shallow and thus make it difficult to maintain the prosthesis.

The spherical implant is placed into position behind posterior Tenon's layer (Fig. 56-1, *L*). A 20 to 22 mm implant usually fits easily into the apex. The posterior layer of Tenon's capsule is now closed with "vest-over-pants closure" in a horizontal plane with 5-0 Vicryl or Dexon interrupted sutures (*C* in Fig. 56-1, *L*). Then the horizontal rectus muscles are sutured up to the anterior surface of posterior Tenon's layer (*A* and *B* in Fig. 56-1, *L*). The vertical recti are not sutured to this surface and are allowed to retract.

K

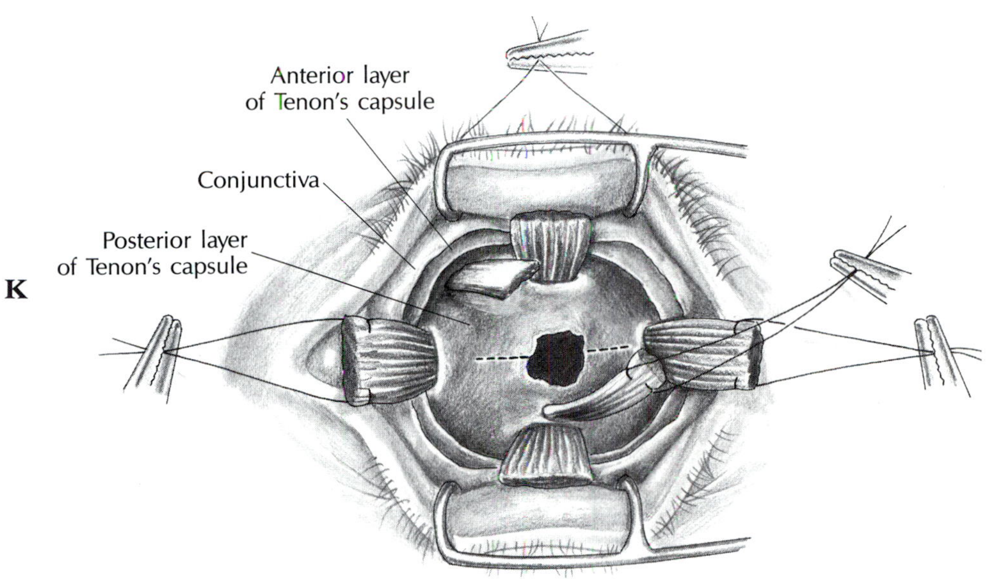

L

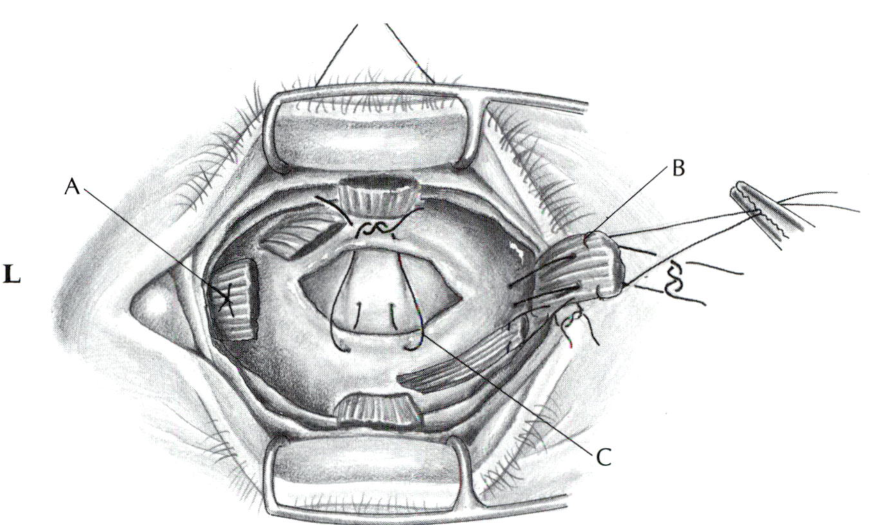

FIGURE 56-1, cont'd

Continued.

Anterior Tenon's layer is closed after the conjunctiva is separated from it (Fig. 56-1, *M*). This allows for sufficient mobilization of conjunctiva decreasing the chance of shortening the fornices.

The conjunctiva is then sutured with a running or interrupted 6-0 plain or chromic sutures (Fig. 56-1, *N*).

A transparent conformer with several drainage perforations is then placed in the cul-de-sac. The size of the conformer should be large enough to fill the fornices but should not place any tension on the conjunctival wound. The conformer will help maintain the fornices and avoid prolapse of the conjunctiva. The placement of temporary tarsorrhaphy sutures at the medial third and lateral third of the eyelids will also help decrease the possibility of conjunctival prolapse. A pressure dressing is applied and allowed to remain in place for 2 to 3 days unless there is significant postoperative pain or fever.

M

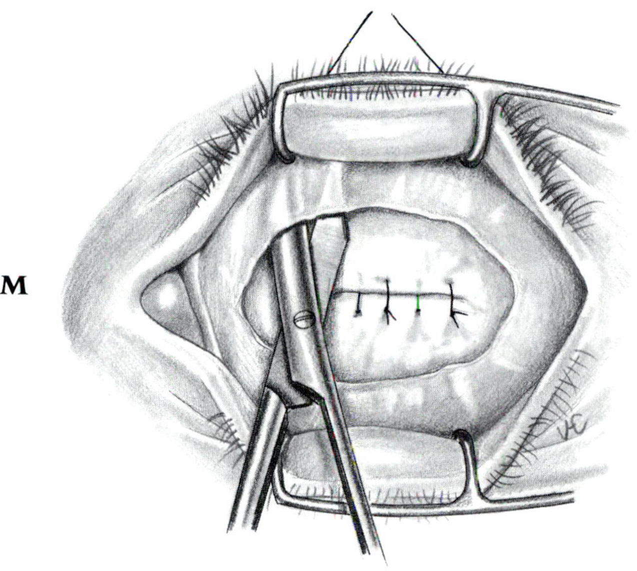

N

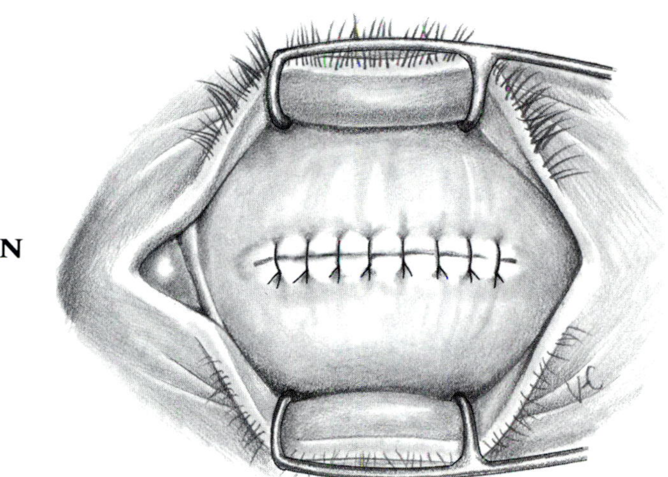

FIGURE 56-1, cont'd

Postoperative Care

After the first dressing, have cool compresses applied. The conformer remains in the socket until the socket is ready for prosthesis fitting, which is begun in the fourth or fifth postoperative week. The patient is instructed to replace the conformer if it becomes displaced. Without it, the fornices may become shallow secondary to the postoperative edema, inflammation, and adhesions.

Proper hygiene of the socket is important. Patients are instructed to thoroughly clean their hands before touching the prosthesis or socket. Ideally the prosthesis is removed only several times a year for inspection. To produce maximum comfort, minimal discharge, and socket irritation, the prosthesis should be highly polished and contain no rough edges.

CHAPTER 57

Evisceration

Evisceration, the removal of the intrascleral contents, does not invade the orbit. In the preantibiotic era evisceration was performed for panophthalmitis associated with intraocular infection and irreparable vision loss, rather than enucleation. It was done to avoid the spread of infection along the severed optic nerve and nerve sheath (potential subarachnoid space).

Evisceration generally provides greater motility of the prosthesis. There is also less chance for development of an enophthalmic appearance, deepening of the supratarsal sulcus, and atrophy of the orbit soft tissue. Typically there is a less adverse effect on the eyelids and socket because of the undisturbed suspensory ligaments and Tenon's capsule, which may be disturbed with enucleation.

INDICATIONS

Indications for evisceration include eyes blinded by absolute glaucoma or uveitis. Intraocular tumor is ruled out by direct visualization, ultrasonography, CAT scan, or magnetic resonance imaging. Evisceration is advised when a virulent endophthalmitis resistant to antibiotic therapy destroys vision. In such cases, evisceration without the insertion of an implant is the procedure of choice.

CONTRAINDICATIONS

Contraindications to evisceration include the possibility of sympathetic ophthalmia, the possibility of intraocular tumor, phthisis bulbi with noticeable shrinking of the globe, and advanced degeneration of the globe. An evisceration should not be performed if the globe has been severely lacerated. Enucleation rather than evisceration is recommended when histologic examination of the globe is particularly important. Certainly there are ophthalmologists who strongly advise against evisceration for this latter reason.

Evisceration with retention of the cornea permits the use of a larger implant to replace the orbital volume. This will necessitate the use of a scleral shell or thin prosthesis to prevent corneal necrosis and permit a good cosmesis. If the cornea is thin or ulcerated, it should be excised. The spherical implant to be placed within the sclera is usually not larger than 16 mm in diameter. The implant should not fit tightly, since scleral shrinkage occurs in the postoperative healing period, and erosion of the implant through the cornea or sclera is a concern.

ANESTHESIA

The procedure is generally performed under general anesthesia for patient comfort and psychologic reasons but may be performed under local anesthesia if necessary. Retrobulbar injection of 3 ml of a 1:1 mixture of lidocaine hydrochloride with epinephrine (1:100,000) and bupivacaine hydrochloride (Marcaine HCl) in conjunction with general anesthesia may help reduce bleeding and provide an extended period of postoperative analgesia for several hours.

Evisceration with Retention of the Cornea

An incision is made through the conjunctiva and Tenon's capsule, approximately 6 mm from the superior limbus, so that a 120-degree limbus-based flap is created (Fig. 57-1, *A*). A 5-0 Vicryl suture is woven through the superior rectus tendon a few millimeters from its insertion. The superior rectus is detached from its insertion. With the muscle retracted, a transverse scratch-down incision is made approximately 2 mm posterior to the superior rectus insertion through the sclera, but not the choroid. The incision is extended 150 degrees around the superior part of the globe with a scissors.

A long cyclodialysis spatula is then passed anteriorly, between the sclera and choroid, so that the firm uveal attachments located at the scleral spur can be lysed. The tip of the spatula is seen in the anterior chamber (Fig. 57-1, *B*). The spatula is then swept around to lyse all the scleral spur attachments and rotated 360 degrees to separate the choroid from the sclera posteriorly.

An evisceration spoon is inserted between the sclera and choroid, and the remaining attachments are scraped off while the assistant fixates the globe (Fig. 57-1, *C*). The intraocular contents are then delivered by scooping of the specimen with a large evisceration spoon. Bleeding from the central retina artery may be encountered and can generally be controlled by direct pressure with gauze packing. The remaining uveal tissue is meticulously removed with forceps, curette, or a gauze wrapped about one's finger. Extreme care must be taken to remove all uveal tissue and obtain complete hemostasis. The cornea is then everted, and the endothelium is scarified with a curette or a scalpel blade.

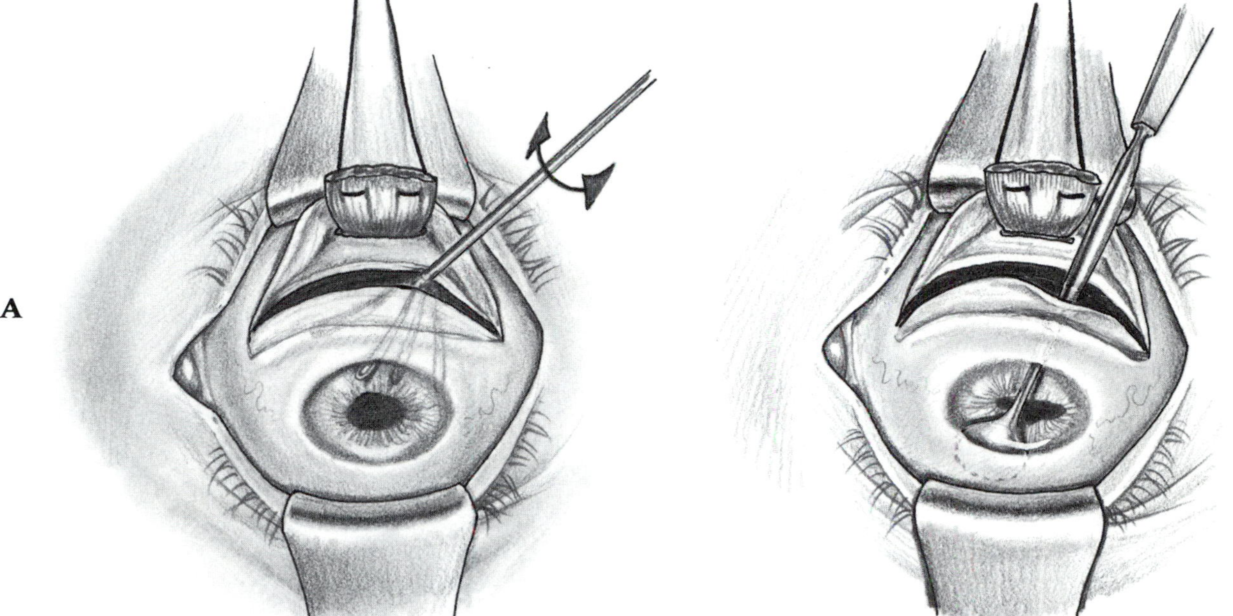

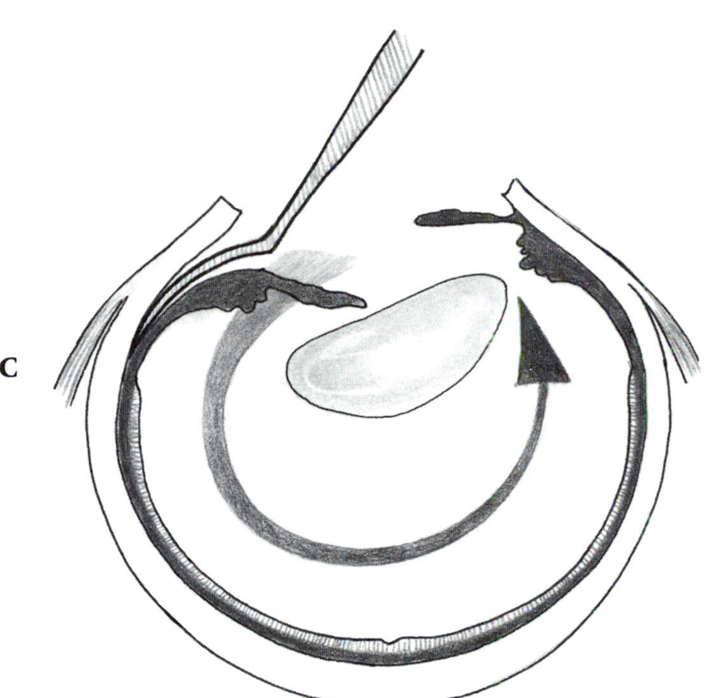

FIGURE 57-1. Evisceration with retention of the cornea.

Continued.

A plastic or silicone intraocular implant may be inserted into the scleral shell (Fig. 57-1, *D*). The implant should not be larger than 14 to 16 mm. This size allows the wound edges to be reapproximated without tension on the wound but snug enough to fit into the scleral shell without leaving significant dead space in which fluid may accumulate or infection develop. The scleral cavity is irrigated with antibiotic solution.

The scleral wound edges are reapproximated with multiple horizontal mattress sutures of 4-0 Mersilene or Prolene sutures (Fig. 57-1, *E*). The superior rectus muscle is reinserted with a 5-0 Vicryl suture.

Tenon's capsule and the conjunctiva is closed with a running 6-0 chromic or plain catgut suture (Fig. 57-1, *F*).

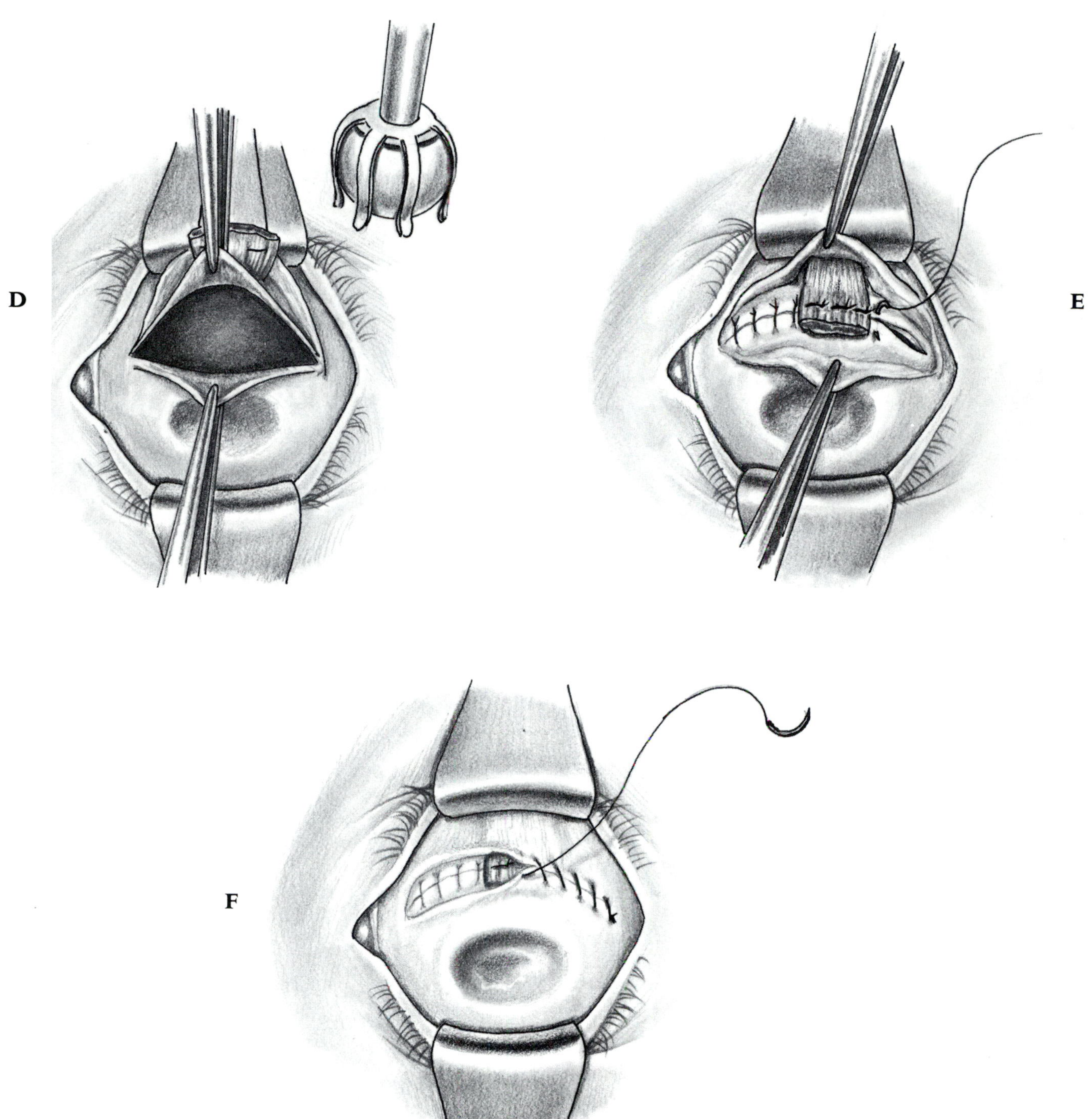

FIGURE 57-1, cont'd

Evisceration with Keratectomy

A 360-degree peritomy is performed and the Tenon's capsule and conjunctiva are undermined and dissected away from the limbus (Fig. 57-2, *A*). The anterior chamber is entered at the 12 o'clock position at the limbus, and the cornea is completely excised with scissors.

The contents of the globe are then eviscerated and the interior of the scleral shell is treated as previously described to meticulously remove all uveal tissue (Fig. 57-2, *B*). Small triangles of sclera are excised at the 3 and 9 o'clock positions, so that the round wound is converted into an ellipse for closure without dog ears. The intraocular contents are then removed as described in Fig. 57-1, *C*.

A 14 to 16 mm intraocular implant (plastic or silicone) is inserted, and the scleral wound is reapproximated horizontally with multiple mattress sutures of 4-0 Mersilene or Prolone sutures (Fig. 57-2, *C*).

Tenon's capsule and the conjunctiva is reapproximated horizontally with 6-0 chromic suture (Fig. 57-2, *D*).

DRESSING AND POSTOPERATIVE CARE

A solid conformer is used when the cornea has been removed. When the cornea is retained, a doughnut conformer is placed in the socket to avoid corneal irritation and possibly necrosis, which may occur with the solid prosthesis. With evisceration there is a decreased incidence of conjunctival prolapse, mucosal shrinkage, or fornix contracture.

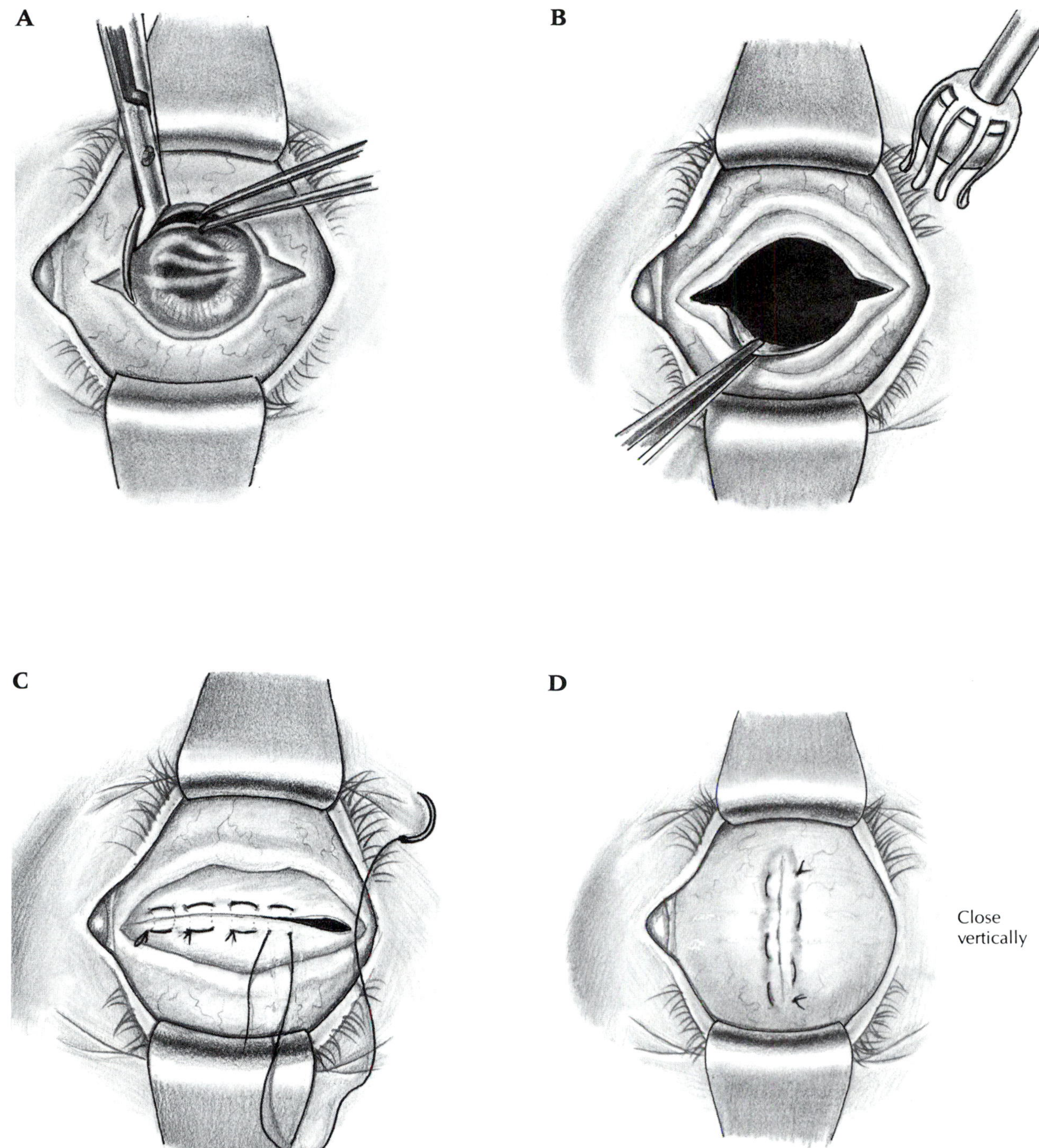

FIGURE 57-2. Evisceration with keratectomy.

CHAPTER 58

Socket Reconstruction

The normal globe occupies a volume of 6 to 7 cc and sits 2 mm behind a line drawn from the superior to the inferior orbital rims. It is suspended within the orbit by muscles, fascia, and fat, which give it motility to help maintain the fornices and support the eyelids in their proper position.

Enucleation upsets the balance between these structures. After enucleation the globe is usually replaced by spherical implants, which occupy a volume of 2 to 3 cc and a prosthesis of about 2 cc. Clearly this does not fully replace the volume removed during enucleation. Because the implant does not have the dynamic attachments and movements as a globe, motility is decreased and there is a tendency for implant migration. The prosthesis can exert a downward gravitational force, thereby not adequately supporting the upper eyelid and exerting pressure on the lower eyelid. This can lead to sulcus and fornix abnormality.

The optimum implant should be lightweight and inert, such as polymethylmethacrylate, measure 16 to 20 mm in diameter, and sit centrally within the orbit. It should support the upper eyelid but not impinge upon the fornices. Integrated mesh implants and implants larger than 20 mm have a tendency to become extruded and are generally avoided. The prosthesis should be thin, sitting in the plane of the opposite cornea and supporting the upper eyelid. Before proceeding with the surgical correction of a socket problem, an ocularist can attempt to correct some of these problems by refitting the prosthesis. Except for cases involving an extruding implant, ocularist evaluation is suggested.

EVALUATION OF THE ANOPHTHALMIC SOCKET

The anophthalmic socket should be compared to the normal orbit. Exophthalmometry reading may be helpful in comparing the plane of the prosthesis with the contralateral globe. The depth of the superior sulcus should be measured. The eyelids are examined for ptosis and laxity. Look for eyelid closure and its extent over the prosthesis. The eyelid margin is examined for entropion and trichiasis. The fit, size, contour, and edges of the prosthesis are evaluated.

After removal of the prosthesis the covering of the implant and the depth of the fornices are checked. A culture is taken of any socket discharge. While a glove is worn, the position of the implant is palpated within the orbit. Motility of the implant is evaluated both with and without the prosthesis in place.

Preoperative photographs, including a full-face photograph and close-up photographs of the orbit, both with and without the prosthesis are taken before socket surgery is performed.

SOCKET PROBLEMS

Extruding implant

Extrusion of the implant can occur in the early or late postoperative period. Early extrusion is attributable to wound separation. Late extrusion is characterized by gradual thinning of the tissue overlying the implant with ultimate exposure of the implant. More frequently, this problem can be associated with excessively large implants, usually over 20 mm in diameter, with integrated or mesh implants, and with migration of the implant causing pressure necrosis of the overlying tissue.

In the early stages, when there is a small defect, the edges of conjunctiva and Tenon's capsule can be sutured together or a scleral patch graft can be placed over the implant. When a large portion of the implant is exposed because some degree of socket contracture exists, additional tissue must be added to the socket, along with replacement of the implant. An excellent way of managing this problem is with a dermis-fat graft. This replaces the extruding implant and adds orbital volume by contributing tissue to the center of the socket. The fornices are well maintained, and motility may be preserved by suturing of the extraocular muscles to the dermis.

Contracted socket

A contracted socket can occur because of scar tissue formation within the socket, associated with infection or chemical injury such as a lye burn.

Mild socket contraction is characterized by shortening of the tarsus and conjunctiva with secondary entropion and with the lashes turning inward against the prosthesis. This frequently can be corrected with eyelid and marginal rotation. To lengthen the posterior surface of the eyelid, one can use a mucous membrane graft or autogenous cartilage graft.

Severe degrees of contraction involve loss of the fornices. A prosthesis with a small lip must be fit, and this problem is usually characterized by embarrassing extrusion of the prosthesis. In extreme cases a prosthesis cannot be worn at all. Additional tissue, preferably buccal mucous membrane, must be added to the contracted fornix. When loss of a fornix occurs because of implant migration, the implant is removed and a dermis-fat graft or sclera-covered implant replaces it in a preferred position.

In the most severe instances of socket contraction, total socket reconstruction must be performed by use of a "C-shaped conformer" with extensive replacement of tissue.

Loss of the inferior fornix is not an uncommon problem in the anophthalmic socket. This can occur secondary to conjunctival contraction and scarring or migration of the implant.

Enophthalmic anophthalmos

The enophthalmic anophthalmos syndrome is characterized by the following:

1. Enophthalmos
2. Deep superior eyelid sulcus
3. Lower eyelid ptosis
4. Upper eyelid ptosis

It is caused by the loss of orbital volume, atrophy of orbital fat, and abnormal distribution of the orbital contents inferiorly and posteriorly because of gravity. Ptosis is caused by lack of support of the upper eyelid. Constant downward pressure of the unsuspended prosthesis eventually causes laxity and ptosis of the lower eyelid.

Scleral Patch Graft for Extruding Implant

An extruding orbital implant that is exposed by only a 3 or 4 mm dehiscence can be covered with a scleral patch to reinforce Tenon's capsule and conjunctiva.

As Fig. 58-1, *A*, shows, the dehiscence is enlarged in a horizontal direction by use of Westcott scissors. The edges of the exposed area are excised to create a viable surgical margin. Thinned conjunctiva overlying the implant is excised.

Conjunctiva is separated from Tenon's capsule and dissected into the fornices (Fig. 58-1, *B*), so that flaps of conjunctiva and Tenon's capsule are created. Silk sutures, 6-0, are placed through the edge of conjunctiva for traction and exposure. An oval piece of sclera, slightly larger than the defect, is fashioned from the donor eye. Uveal tissue should be carefully cleaned from its inner surface.

Tenon's capsule is sutured over the implant, and the scleral patch graft is sutured to the surface of Tenon's capsule with 5-0 chromic sutures (Fig. 58-1, *C*). If Tenon's capsule cannot be completely closed, the scleral graft is placed over the implant and is sutured to the underlying Tenon's capsule at least 4 mm from its edge. The scleral graft will overlap Tenon's capsule.

The conjunctiva is closed over the scleral implant with a running 6-0 plain catgut suture in a horizontal direction (Fig. 58-1, *D*). It is important for conjunctiva to cover the graft to facilitate the blood supply to the free scleral graft.

At the conclusion of surgery a doughnut-shaped conformer is inserted into the socket to maintain the fornices. Antibiotic drops are administered four times daily for 5 days. A new prosthesis is fitted in 3 or 4 weeks.

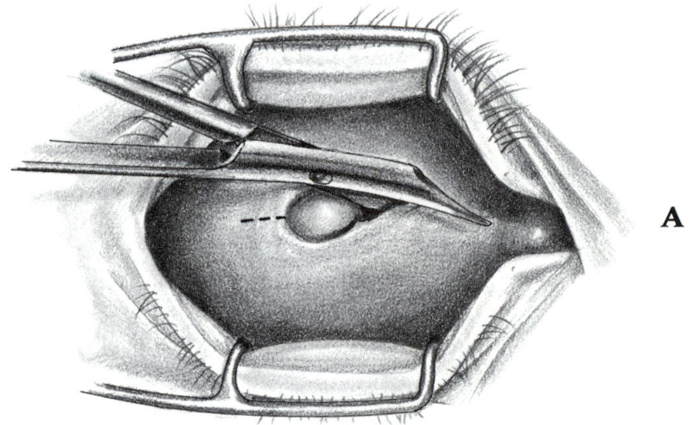

FIGURE 58-1. Scleral patch graft.

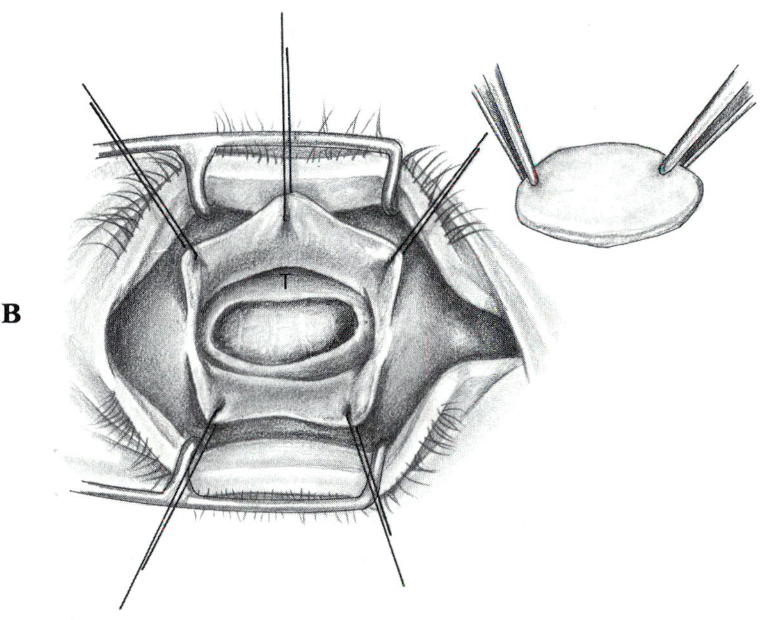
B
T

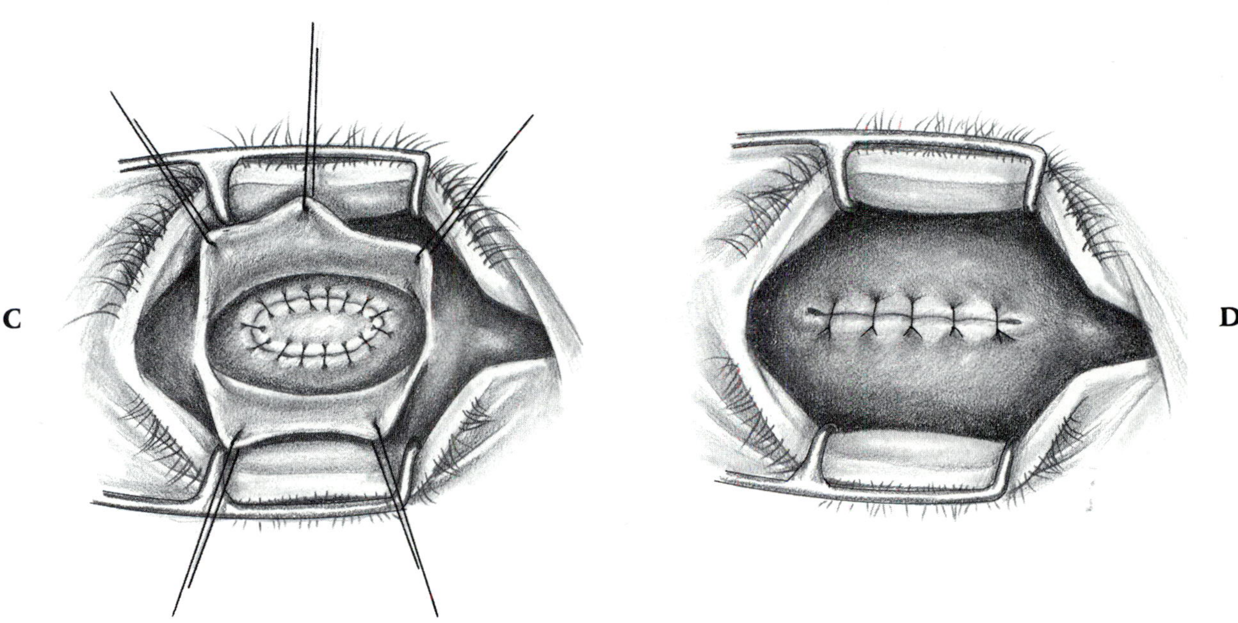
C
D

Dermis-Fat Graft for Extruding Implant

A good primary enucleation can be performed by insertion of a plain plastic or silicone sphere. However, exposed, extruding, and migrated implants of significant degree will require removal and replacement. Dermis-fat grafts have been used for secondary implantation with good results. They supply tissue to the deep socket as well as adding tissue to replace lost conjunctiva. Dermis-fat grafts do not migrate and can provide increased motility. A variable amount of postoperative atrophy does occur.

An implant that is exposed more than 4 or 5 mm with thinned conjunctiva or where a patching procedure has failed will require removal and replacement with a dermis-fat graft (Fig. 58-2, *A*). Integrated and mesh implants may have a higher incidence of extrusion than inert spherical implants have.

The operation is usually performed under general anesthesia. A wire speculum is inserted between the eyelids. Using a Westcott scissors, enlarge the opening in a horizontal direction, removing abnormally thinned tissue while freshening the edges of the remaining conjunctiva and Tenon's capsule (Fig. 58-2, *B*). The anterior surface of the implant is sufficiently exposed. A Freer elevator is used to shell out the original implant. Adhesions to the mesh will have to be cut. Care should be exercised superiorly to avoid damaging the levator complex. An identifying 4-0 silk suture can be passed above the edge of the tarsus through the levator complex to help identify it and prevent injury to it. The implant is completely removed with adherent capsule surrounding the implant.

An attempt is made to expose the four rectus muscles (Fig. 58-2, *C*). If the muscles themselves cannot be completely isolated, they may be identified within surrounding orbital tissue. Most of the pseudocapsule remaining in the socket after the implant has been removed should be excised so that there is good healthy tissue from which the graft can receive its blood supply. Incisions are made into the remaining capsule to allow blood vessels to enter the recipient site. A 5-0 absorbable double-arm suture is placed through each muscle or muscle bundle that has been isolated. Saline-soaked gauze is inserted into the orbit.

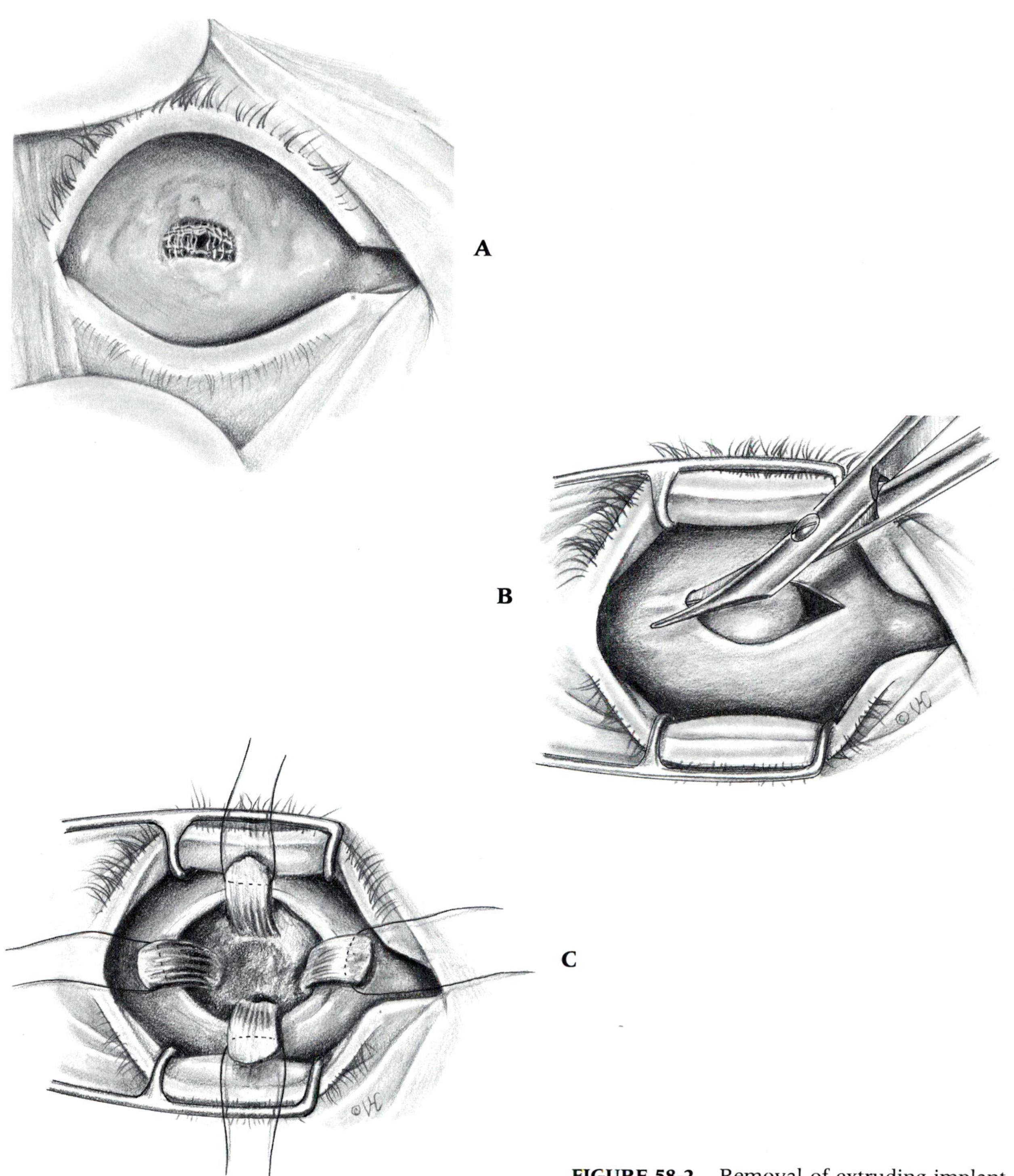

FIGURE 58-2. Removal of extruding implant.

At the outset of the operation the buttocks and thigh are prepped with Betadine (povidone-iodine complex) soap, Betadine solution, and draped (Fig. 58-3, *A*). The optimal donor site to obtain the dermis-fat graft contains abundant subcutaneous fat and will be hidden by a woman's bikini. A good area to take the graft is from the lateral aspect of the buttock.

The graft is outlined as a circular area 20 mm in diameter. It is deepithelialized with use of a razor blade knife (Fig. 58-3, *B* and *C*) or a fine diamond burr attached to a Hall air drill (Fig. 58-3, *B*) to expose the underlying dermis.

The edge of the dermabrided area is incised through the dermis by use of a no. 10 scalpel (Fig. 58-3, *D*). The scalpel is then extended deeper into the fat to a depth of 30 or 40 mm. An alternative and perhaps preferred procedure is to raise the dermis slightly from the donor site and cut deeper under direct visualization by use of Stevens scissors, thereby delivering a graft of appropriate size from the wound. With either technique, the base of the graft is cut with a scissors. The graft is placed directly into the socket bed and secured in position. Active bleeding vessels within the donor site are then cauterized, and saline packing is inserted.

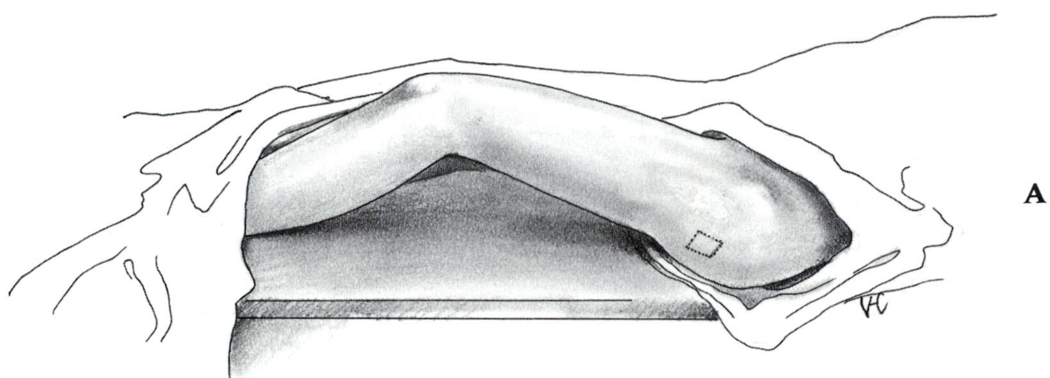

FIGURE 58-3. Harvesting dermis fat graft.

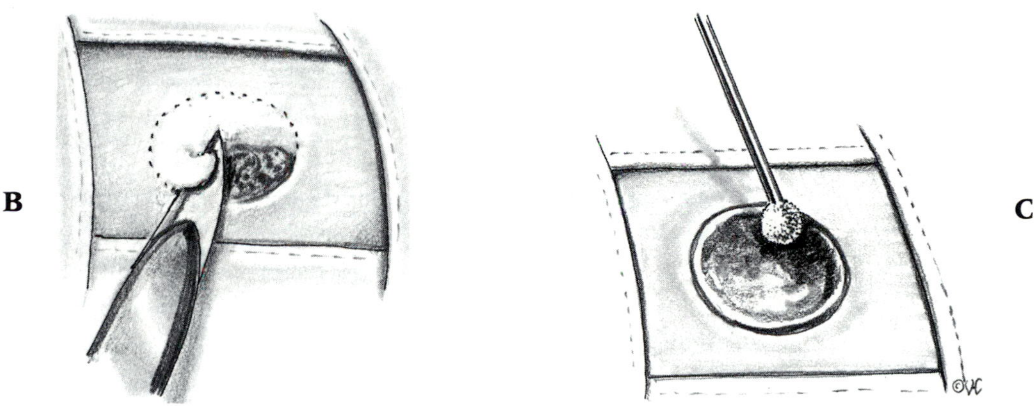

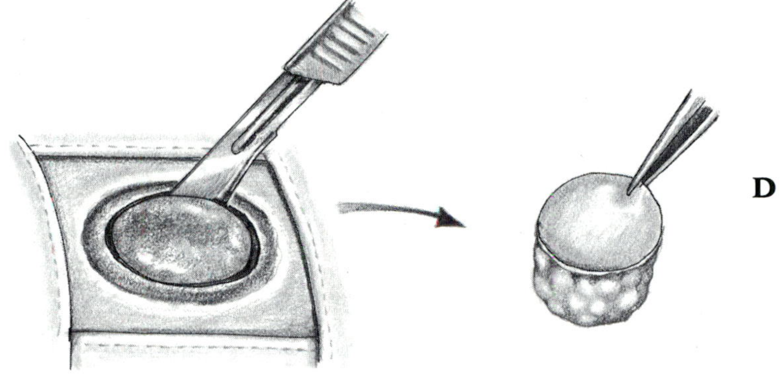

Continued.

Excess fat is excised to allow for proper graft fit. The previously placed double-arm sutures from each muscle bundle are placed firmly through the posterior edge of the dermis and tied (Fig. 58-3, *E*). Additional 5-0 chromic or Vicryl sutures are inserted to suture the dermis to Tenon's capsule and conjunctiva so that the fat is buried in the orbit. Some 6-0 plain catgut sutures may also be used to suture the dermis to the conjunctiva. A doughnut-shaped conformer is placed into the socket to maintain the fornices in the early postoperative period.

Bleeding vessels within the donor site are cauterized, and 3-0 chromic sutures are used to close the fat and deeper tissue (Fig. 58-3, *F*). The skin and subcutaneous tissue are closed with 3-0 nylon vertical mattress sutures. Four-0 nylon sutures or staples can be used to approximate the skin edges. Telfa is placed on the wound, followed by fluff gauze and an Elastoplast dressing.

In the sagittal plane the dermis-fat graft, which measures approximately 20 mm in diameter and 35 to 40 mm in depth, is seen within the muscle cone (Fig. 58-4). A doughnut-shaped conformer helps maintain the fornices.

An adhesive pressure dressing is applied to the orbit for a few days. Oral and topical antibiotics are given for 1 to 2 weeks. Epithelium usually grows over the dermis within 1 to 2 months, at which time a new prosthesis can be fit.

The pressure dressing on the donor site is removed in 48 hours, and a light dressing is applied. Nylon sutures or staples are removed in 10 to 14 days.

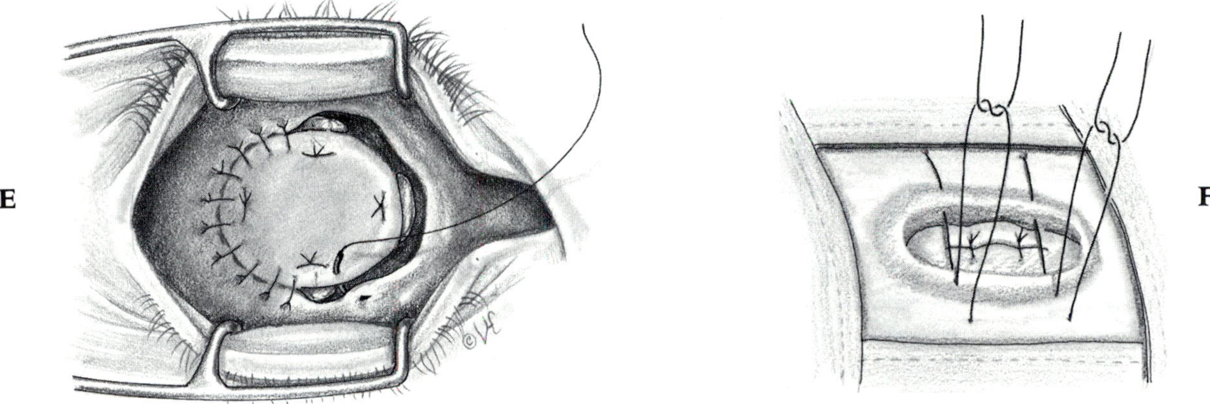

FIGURE 58-3, cont'd

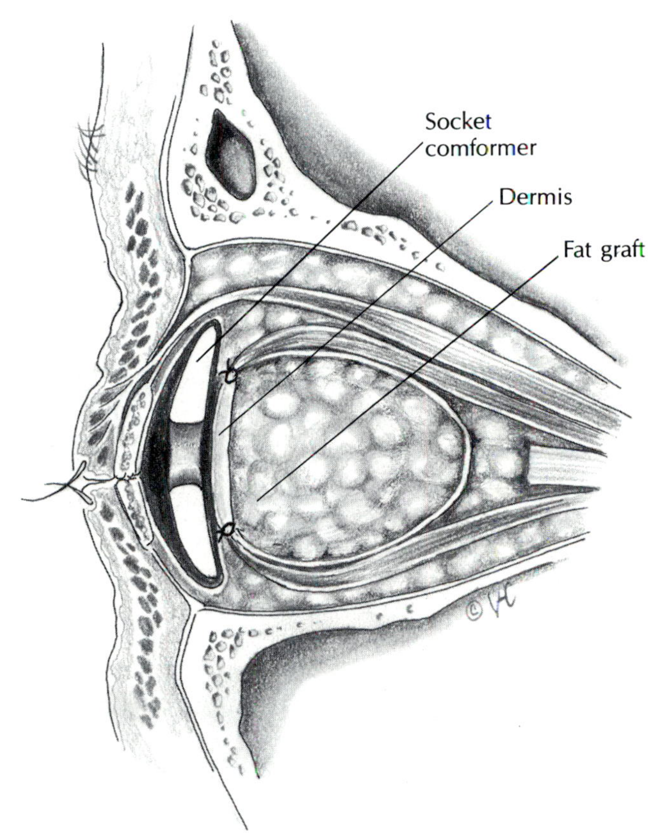

FIGURE 58-4. Dermis fat graft within the socket.

Procedure for Contracted Fornix

In the patient with a shortened inferior fornix, clinically the prosthesis is seen to rest virtually on the lower eyelid margin (Fig. 58-5, *A*). The lower eyelid is retracted with the lashes turned inward toward the prosthesis. Removing the prosthesis reveals a very shallow inferior fornix. The patient will complain that the implant keeps "popping out."

An injection of 2% lidocaine (Xylocaine), 0.75% bupivacaine (Marcaine) with 1:200,000 epinephrine and hyaluronidase (Wydase) is applied into the fornix to decrease intraoperative bleeding and postoperative pain. The new fornix is formed inferior to the tarsus (Fig. 58-5, *B*). An incision, as shown, is made through the conjunctiva and eyelid retractors with use of a no. 15 scalpel toward the orbital rim extending from the caruncle to the lateral canthus (Fig. 58-5, *C*). Subconjunctival scar tissue in the area should be excised. With the lower eyelid on stretch the size of the defect is measured by insertion of an elliptic piece of Telfa as a template into the fornix and by estimation of the mucosal graft size. Depending on the degree of contraction the Telfa template can measure up to 25 or 30 mm long and 15 mm wide.

A mucosal graft is taken from the lower lip (Fig. 58-5, *D*), and cheek mucosa may also be used. The Telfa mold is placed on the inner aspect of the lip and outlined with a marking pencil or scalpel. Care is taken to remain at least 5 mm from the buccal sulcus, frenulum, and vermilion border of the lip. If cheek mucosa is taken, one should identify the parotid duct opening, in front of the upper second molars, to preserve its integrity. The same anesthetic mixture used in the socket is injected into the donor site. Gauze sponges are placed in the pharynx and lateral aspect of the mouth to prevent swallowing or aspirating blood. The lip is retracted with towel clips, placed at the corner of the mouth and center of the lower lip. If a mucotome is available, a 0.5 mm thick graft is used.

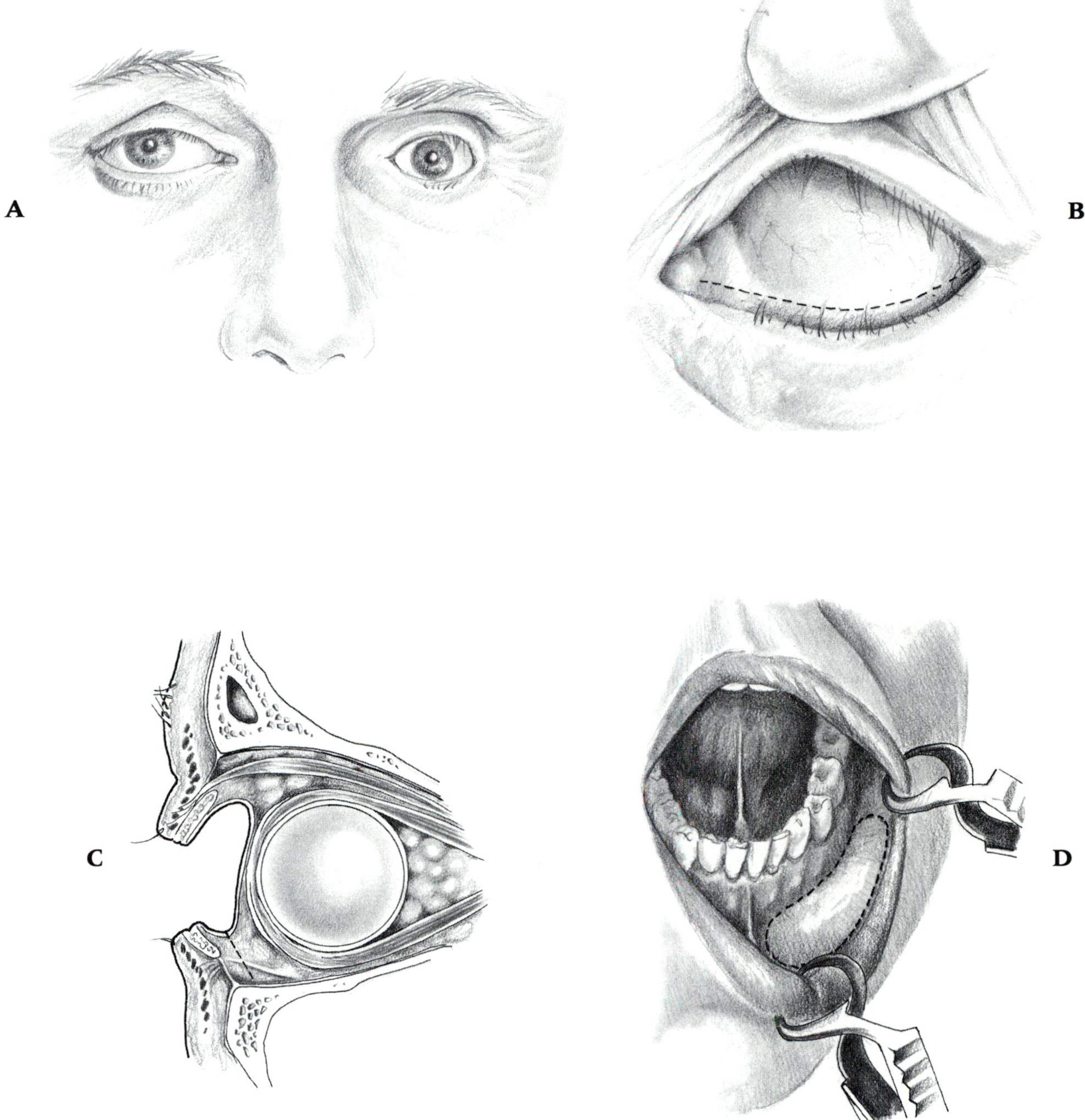

FIGURE 58-5. Surgery for contracted fornix.

Continued.

As Fig. 58-5, *E* and *F*, show, in frontal and sagittal views, 5-0 chromic, Vicryl, or Dexon sutures are used to suture the graft at each end. A running suture is used to suture the anterior edge to the eyelid and conjunctiva and the posterior edge to the bulbar conjunctiva.

A 3 mm retinal sponge is cut to fit into the newly created fornix. Two double-armed 4-0 nylon sutures on a long thin needle such as the FS-1 (Ethicon) is placed through the retinal sponge, laterally, centrally, and medially, with 4 mm between each arm (Fig. 58-5, *G*). Both arms of the suture are placed through the sponge and then through the center of the graft down toward the orbital rim, taking a bite into periosteum and coming out through the skin overlying the orbital rim. Each suture is tied tightly over a cotton bolster (Fig. 58-5, *H*). This stent serves to keep the graft firmly against its recipient bed and deepens the fornix.

The patient's prosthesis or a conformer, which has been soaking in sterilizing solution, is reinserted into the socket. A double-armed 4-0 silk suture placed through the lower eyelid margin is taped to the forehead for the first 48 hours to keep the lower eyelid in upward traction. Topical antibiotics and a light dressing are applied.

A soft, bland diet is eaten until the donor site heals. Lidocaine (Xylocaine) viscous mouthwash can be given before meals. A regular diet is usually started in 3 to 5 days. Oral antibiotics are given for 1 week.

The stent is left in the lower cul-de-sac for 6 to 8 weeks, after which a new prosthesis is fitted.

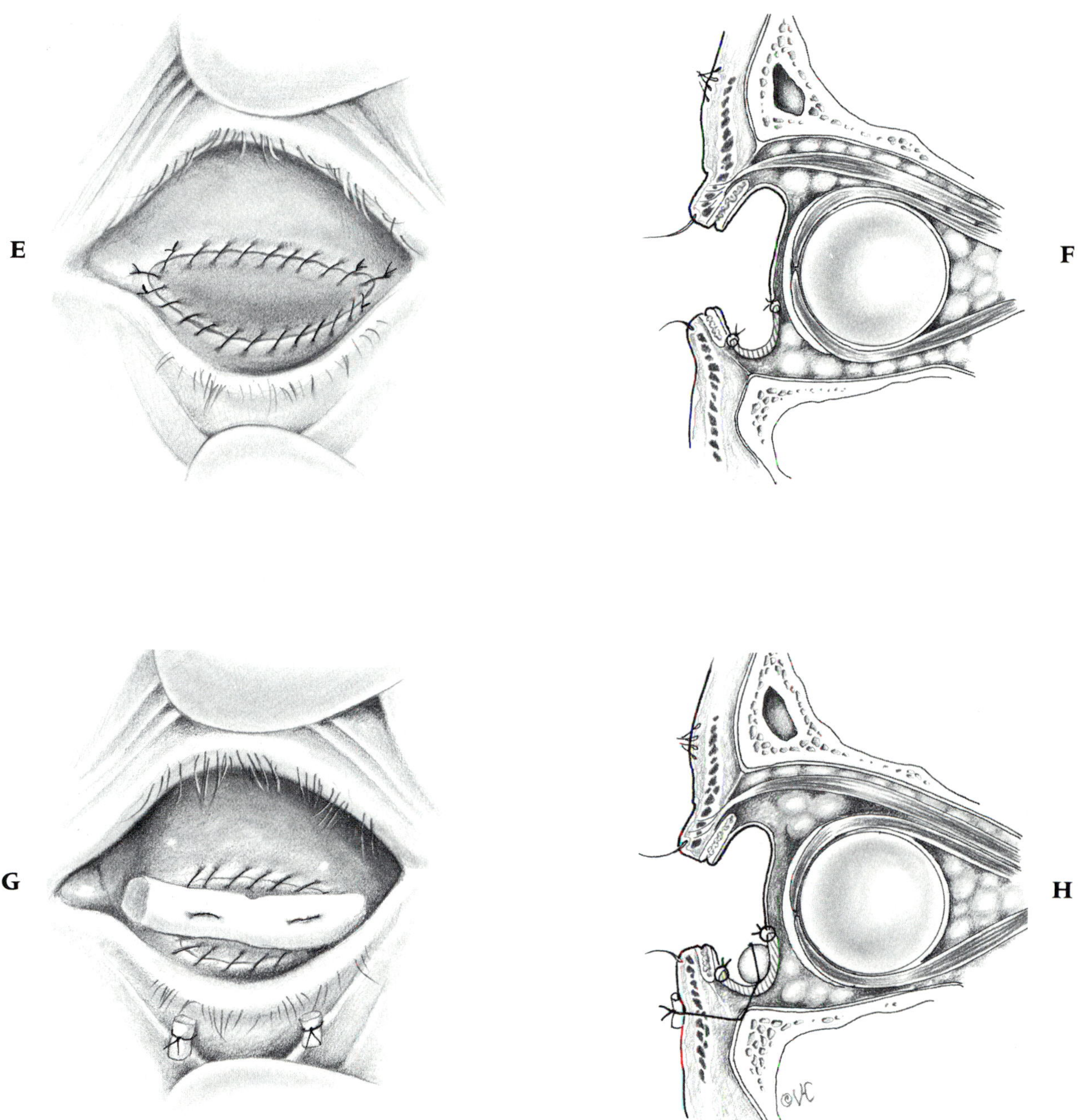

FIGURE 58-5, cont'd

Procedure for Enophthalmic Anophthalmos

Correction of the volume loss with resultant enophthalmos and deep superior sulcus is accomplished when volume is added to the orbit. Many materials have been described to accomplish this, such as bone, glass beads, injectable silicone, Teflon sleds, inflatable silicone expanding implants, and methyl methacrylate molded at the time of surgery. They are placed within the orbit to displace the orbital contents anteriorly and superiorly.

Lower eyelid ptosis (eyelid retraction and ectropion) can be repaired with a medial canthal tendon plication combined with a lateral tarsal strip procedure, or a fascia sling between the canthal tendons. If, after volume is added and the lower eyelid is tightened, the upper eyelid is still ptotic, a ptosis procedure is indicated.

We favor the use of the Teflon sled* to add volume and solve the problems of enophthalmic anophthalmos. The sled is shaped like a dogsled, with most of the volume placed posteriorly, behind the orbital implant, to push the orbital contents forward and upward. Sleds come in three sizes, all of which should be available at the time of surgery.

Clinically these patients have a sunken appearance to the prothesis with a deep superior sulcus, apparent retracted lower eyelid, and upper eyelid ptosis (Fig. 58-6, *A*).

---

*Available from John J. Kelley, Ocularist, 1930 Chestnut Street, Philadelphia, PA 19103.

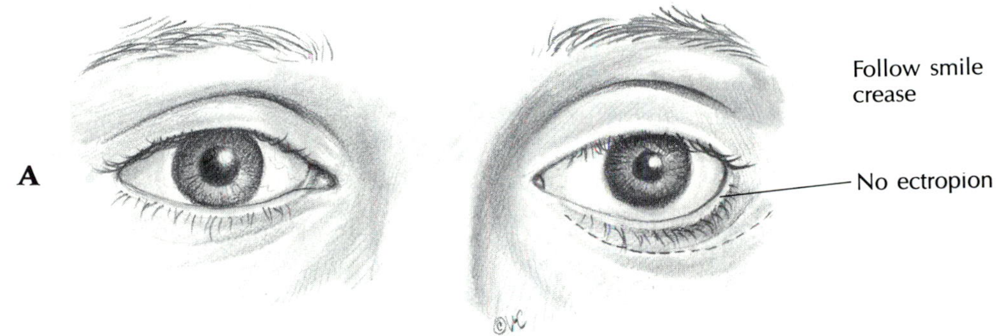

FIGURE 58-6. Repairs of enophthalmic anophthalmos.
Continued.

The eyelid crease incision, as shown by the dotted line, can be used to approach the orbital floor and subperiorbital space. The approach is the same as for an orbital floor fracture wherein a blepharoplasty or lid-crease incision is made in the lower eyelid in a stepwise fashion (Fig. 58-6, *B*). A skin muscle flap is reflected from the septum. The orbital rim is exposed, and an incision is made on its anterior surface. The periorbita is elevated posteriorly, with as much of the orbital floor being exposed as possible. The Teflon implant with fenestrations, which has been gas sterilized and soaked in antibiotic solution, is placed along the orbital floor with the prominent segment posterior to the orbital implant.

When the implant is determined to be in good position under the periosteum, it is removed and two 1 mm drill holes are made in the orbital rim about 5 to 8 mm apart corresponding to the fenestration (Fig. 58-6, *C*). The implant is replaced after a 28-gauge stainless steel wire is placed through the holes in the anterior surface of the implant after it passes the rim holes. The wire edges are twisted by use of a clamp and cut, and the ends are turned downward into one of the fenestration holes. If the implant has a tendency to override the edge of the orbit, a few millimeters of its anterior edge can be excised. The implant should sit just behind the orbital rim without signs of posterior pressure pushing it forward.

The periosteum is closed over the implant with 4-0 or 5-0 absorbable sutures. The skin is closed with a running 6-0 silk or nylon suture. The patient's prosthesis is reinserted into the socket. A mild pressure dressing is applied. Oral antibiotics are administered for 1 week postoperatively.

After correction of the volume deficiency, the lower eyelid retraction if present can be corrected. Subsequent upper eyelid ptosis repair can be considered if residual ptosis remains.

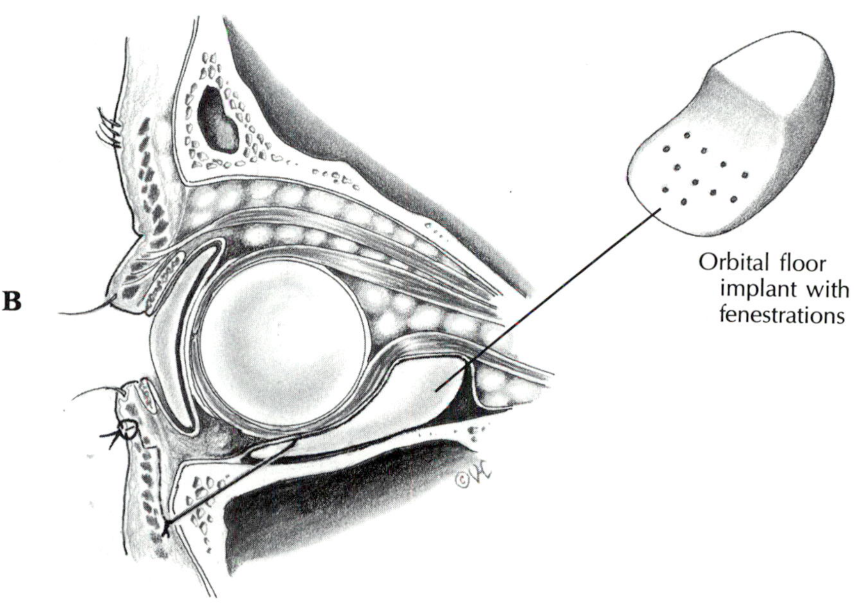

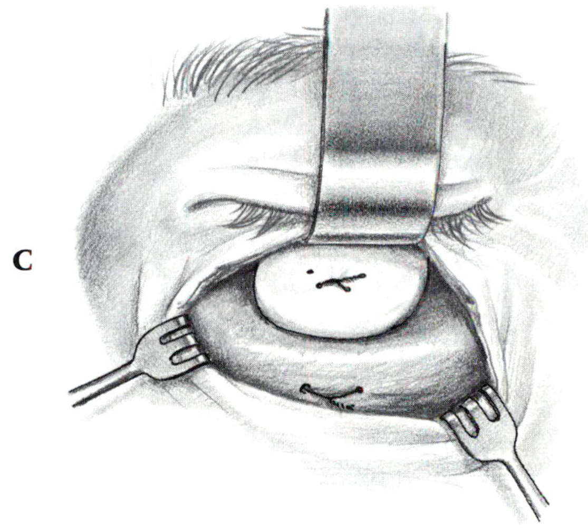

FIGURE 58-6, cont'd

Total Socket Reconstruction

Patients with severe socket contracture such as those with lye burns exhibit considerable contracture of the fornices and are unable to wear a prosthesis. The socket may be totally obliterated so that the eyelids are fused together and to the posterior orbital tissue. A very aggressive approach must be taken in these patients to supply an adequate amount of tissue to rebuild the socket and establish the fornices so that the prosthesis may be worn. A useful procedure has been described by Putterman and Scott. Mucosal tissue is taken from the cheek and lip to line the socket. Split-thickness skin grafts may also be used if adequate mucosa is not available.

In reconstruction of a socket the fornices must extend posteriorly into the orbit along the superior and inferior orbital rims to properly hold a prosthesis. Specially designed conformers must be obtained preoperatively to create this type of socket.* The conformers are available in numerous sizes. A complete set should be obtained and gas sterilized preoperatively. The conformer has superior and inferior extensions to help create the necessary fornix depths and posterior extensions into the orbit. There is a central hole for drainage of fluid and numerous holes superiorly and inferiorly to suture the conformer in place. If there is evidence of socket infection, it should be cultured and treated with the appropriate antibiotic before surgery. General anesthesia is preferred for this procedure.

The clinical picture reveals very shallow or even totally obliterated fornices in the left eye (Fig. 58-7, *A*). Frequently a prosthesis cannot be fitted into the socket. The eyelids may be fused together or to the posterior socket tissue.

The sagittal view shows noticeable contraction of the fornices and the area into which the fornices are to be expanded superiorly, inferiorly, and posteriorly (Fig. 58-7, *B*). It is not enough to create fornices in both the upward and downward direction. Expansion must extend posteriorly into the orbit to create a pocket wherein the prosthesis can be maintained. With use of a combination of sharp dissection with scissors and blunt dissection with cotton applicators, a plane is created within the orbital tissue. Dissection close to the levator aponeurosis is avoided, to limit the possibility of damaging it.

Incisions 2 cm long are made over the inferior orbital rim and over the superior orbital rim down to the bone (Fig. 58-7, *C*). After the rims are exposed, two drill holes are made with a dental drill in the central aspect of each incision 1 cm apart. The broken lines show the extent of dissection within the socket. It may be necessary to remove submucosal scar tissue to prepare for the conformer to be fixed to the orbital rims.

---

*Available from Robert Scott, Ocularist, 111 N. Wabash Avenue, Chicago, IL 60602.

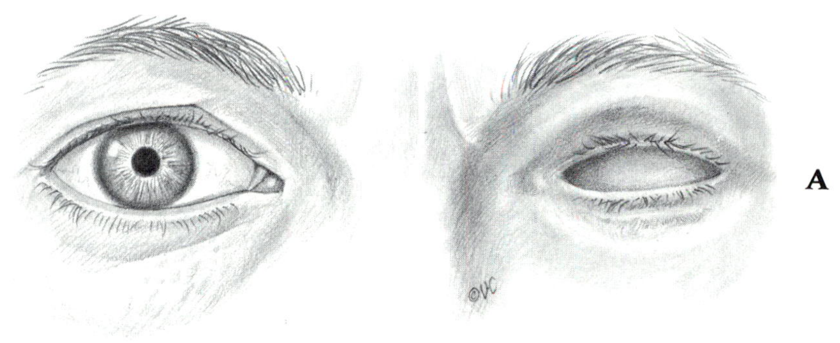

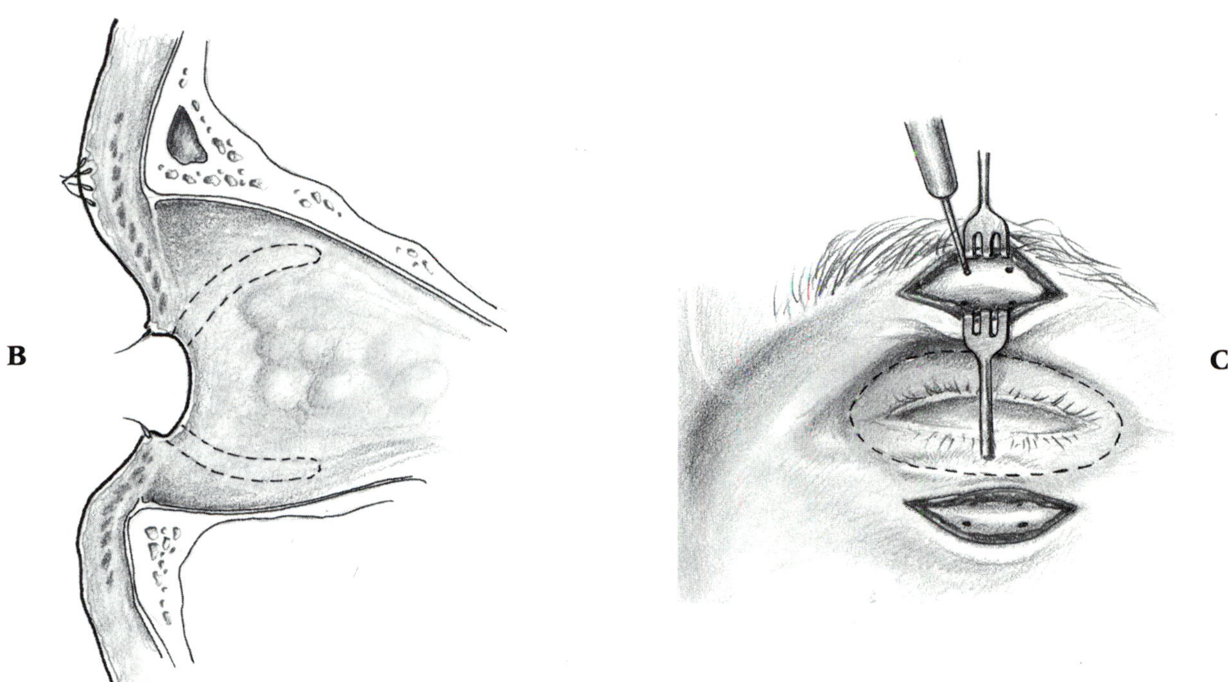

FIGURE 58-7. Total socket reconstruction.

Continued.

The appropriate conformer is placed into the newly created socket. A 2-0 Mersilene, Prolene, or Supramid suture is passed through the holes in the inferior orbital margin from its anterior surface inward (Fig. 58-7, *D*). Free surgical needles are placed on the suture ends to bring the sutures through fornices to enter the inferior peripheral holes of the conformer externally to internally and through the central holes from internally to externally. A similar suture is placed through the superior orbital rim and the superior holes in the conformer.

A large mucous membrane graft is taken from the inner aspect of the cheek and adjacent upper and lower lips (Fig. 58-7, *E*). Here cheek is retracted with two towel clips, and a submucosal injection of 2% Xylocaine, 0.75% Marcaine, and if necessary 1:200,000 epinephrine is used. This will expand the mucosal surface and allow for graft harvesting. A full-thickness graft, large enough to completely cover the conformer, is outlined with a scalpel and undermined to keep the graft as thin as possible with a sharp iris scissors. Care is taken to avoid the parotid duct opening and the edge of the vermilion. Bleeding vessels in the donor site are cauterized. Fat is removed from the posterior surface of the graft to make the graft as thin as possible. The graft is placed into antibiotic solution. If there is not adequate mucosa a 0.012-inch split-thickness skin graft may be used, preferably from the inner aspect of the thigh.

The graft is placed around the conformer with the mucosal surface against the conformer (Fig. 58-7, *F*). The raw surface is outward. Small holes are made in the graft to accompany the fixation sutures. The graft is sutured together using 5-0 chromic or Vicryl sutures so that the entire conformer is covered.

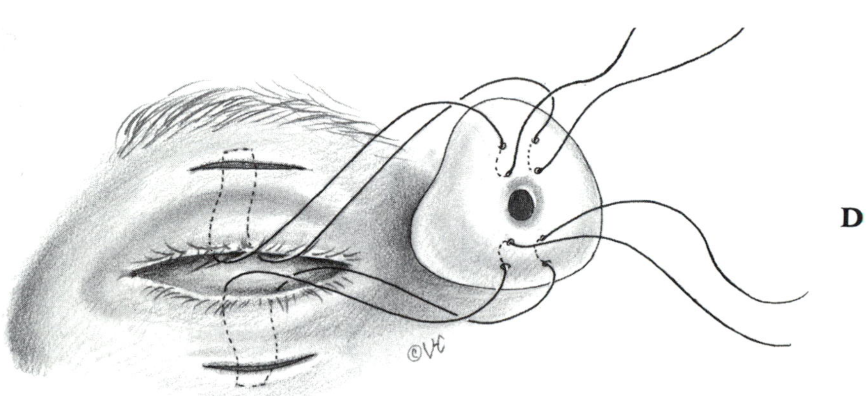

FIGURE 58-7, cont'd

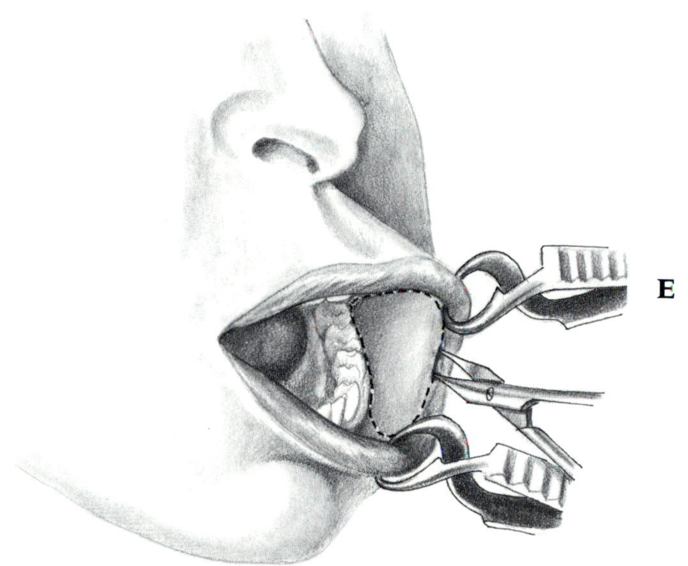

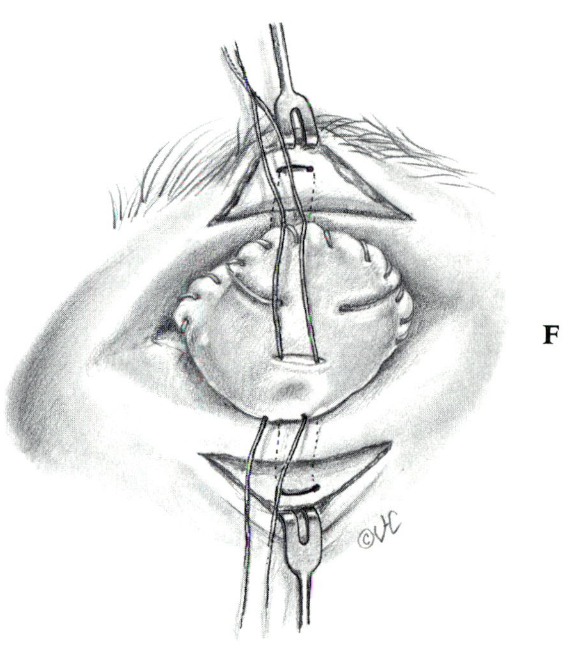

Continued.

The conformer, with its mucosal covering, is placed into the socket as the 2-0 nonabsorbable sutures are pulled tight and tied (Fig. 58-7, *G*). The periosteum over the orbital rims are closed with 4-0 chromic sutures. The subcutaneous tissue is closed with 5-0 absorbable sutures and the skin with 6-0 nylon sutures. The broken line shows the conformer and extension into the fornices encased by the graft within the newly created socket.

A two-pillar suture tarsorrhaphy is performed by use of 4-0 silk double-armed sutures (Fig. 58-7, *H*). Both arms are placed through the skin, muscle, and anterior tarsus 4 mm above the eyelid margin, 5 mm apart, and are brought out through the gray line. They enter the opposite eyelid at the gray line, come out through the skin 4 mm below the eyelid margin, and are tied over cotton or silicone bolsters to close the eyelid. One suture is placed between the medial and central third of the eyelids, the other between the lateral and central third. The sutures are left in for 3 to 4 weeks.

In the presence of severe socket contracture the tarsorrhaphy is performed by removal of the epithelial surface of the eyelid margins before the intermarginal sutures are placed. Such removal will allow for a longer-standing tarsorrhaphy.

The sagittal section in Fig. 58-7, *I*, shows the C-shaped conformer in place forming deep superior and inferior fornices. The 2-0 Mersilene suture is seen anchoring the conformer to the orbital rim.

Postoperatively the patient is given oral and topical antibiotics for 3 weeks. The cheek donor site usually heals within 2 weeks. A soft bland diet should be eaten in the early postoperative course. Viscous xylocaine can be used to decrease pain. If there is evidence of contracture of the cheek, the patient can stretch it by opening the mouth widely and massaging it with the tongue.

The sutures anchoring the customized conformer are cut, and the conformer is removed in 6 months. A standard clear-plastic conformer is inserted, and an ocular prosthesis is fit 3 weeks later.

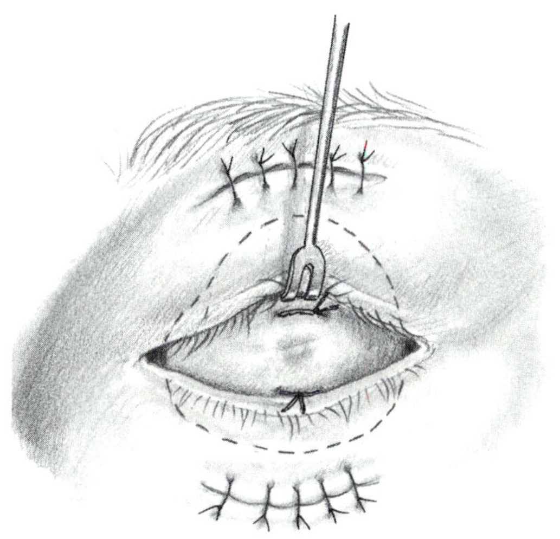

G

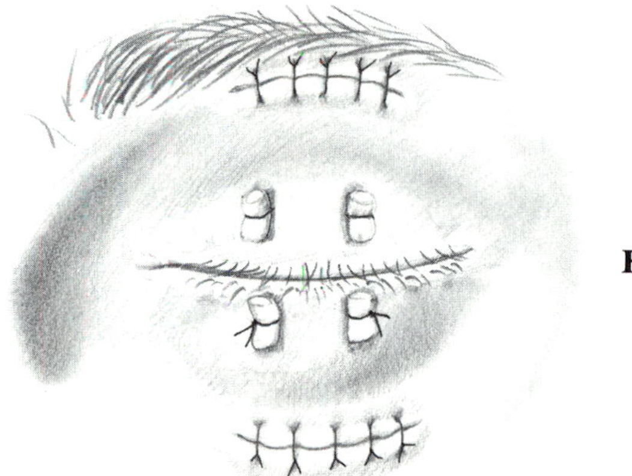

H

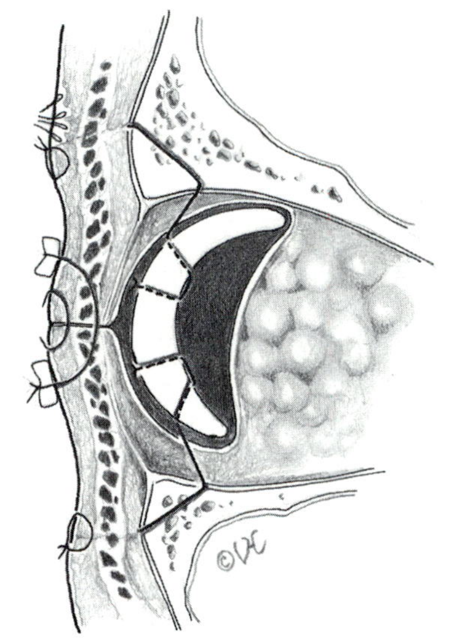

I

FIGURE 58-7, cont'd

Bibliography

PART ONE

Chapter 1

Apple DJ, Mamalis N, Loftfield K, Googe JM, Novak LC, Kavka-Van Norman D, Brady SE, and Olson RJ: Complications of intraocular lenses: a historical and histopathological review, Surv Ophthalmol 29:1, 1984.

Apple DJ and Olson RJ: Closed-loop anterior chamber lenses, Arch Ophthalmol 105:19, 1987.

Arentsen JJ, Donoso R, Laibson PR, and Cohen EJ: Penetrating keratoplasty for the treatment of pseudophakic corneal edema associated with posterior chamber lens implantation, Ophthalmic Surg 18:514, 1987.

Arffa RC, Barron BA, and McDonald MB: Optics of lamellar refractive keratoplasty. In Duane TD and Jaeger EA, editors: Duane's clinical ophthalmology, New York, 1988, JB Lippincott Co., vol. 1.

Arffa RC, Busin M, Barron BA, McDonald MB, and Kaufman HE: Epikeratophakia with commercially prepared tissue for the correction of aphakia in adults, Arch Ophthalmol 104:1467, 1986.

Barraquer JI: Modificación de la refracción por medio de inclusiones intracorneales, Arch Soc Am Oftal Optom 4:229, 1963.

Barraquer JI: Queratomileusis para la corrección de la miopía, Ann Inst Barraquer 5:209, 1964.

Barraquer JI: Keratomileusis for myopia and aphakia, Ophthalmology 88:701, 1981.

Barron BA: Prosthokeratoplasty. In Kaufman HE, Barron BA, McDonald MB, and Waltman SR, editors: The cornea, New York, 1988, Churchill Livingstone.

Barron BA, Busin M, Page C, Bergsma DR, and Kaufman HE: Comparison of the effects of Viscoat and Healon on postoperative intraocular pressure, Am J Ophthalmol 100:377, 1985.

Belmont SC and Troutman RC: Compensating compression sutures in wedge resection, J Refractive Surg 1:104, 1985.

Binder PS: Intraocular lens powers used in the triple procedure: effect on visual acuity and refractive error, Ophthalmology 92:1561, 1985.

Binder PS: Selective suture removal can reduce postkeratoplasty astigmatism, Ophthalmology 92:1412, 1985.

Binder PS: The triple procedure: refractive results: 1985 update, Ophthalmology 93:1482, 1986.

Bores LD: Historical review and clinical results of radial keratotomy, Int Ophthalmol Clin 23:93, 1983.

Bourne WM, Davison JA, and O'Fallon WM: The effects of oversize donor buttons on postoperative intraocular pressure and corneal curvature in aphakic penetrating keratoplasty, Ophthalmology 89:242, 1982.

Brightbill FS, Kaufman HE, and Levenson JE: A vitreous suction cutter for aphakic keratoplasty, Am J Ophthalmol 76:331, 1973.

Brightbill FS, Polack FM, and Slappey T: A comparison of two methods for cutting donor corneal buttons, Am J Ophthalmol 75:500, 1973.

Busin M, Arffa RC, McDonald MB, and Kaufman HE: Intraocular lens removal during penetrating keratoplasty for pseudophakic bullous keratopathy, Ophthalmology 94:505, 1987.

Busin M, Halliday BL, Arffa RC, McDonald MB, and Kaufman HE: Precarved lyophilized tissue for lamellar keratoplasty in recurrent pterygium, Am J Ophthalmol 102:222, 1986.

Buxton JN and Norden RA: Adult penetrating keratoplasty: indications and contraindications. In Brightbill FS, editor: Corneal surgery: theory, technique, and tissue, St Louis, 1986, The CV Mosby Co.

Buzard KA, Haight D, and Troutman R: Ruiz procedure for post-keratoplasty astigmatism, J Refract Surg 3:40, 1987.

Cohen KL, Holman RE, Tripoli NK, and Kupper LL: Effect of trephine tilt on corneal button dimensions, Am J Ophthalmol 101:722, 1986.

Crawford GJ, Stulting RD, Waring GO, VanMeter WS, and Wilson LA: The triple procedure: analysis of outcome, refraction, and intraocular lens power calculation, Ophthalmology 93:817, 1986.

Dietze TR and Durrie DS: Indications and treatment of keratoconus using epikeratophakia, Ophthalmology 95:236, 1988.

Feldman ST and Brown SI: Reduction of astigmatism after keratoplasty, Am J Ophthalmol 103:477, 1987.

Fine M: Therapeutic keratoplasty, Trans Am Acad Ophthalmol Otolaryngol 64:786, 1960.

Fine M: Penetrating keratoplasty in aphakia, Arch Ophthalmol 72:50, 1964.

Foulks GN, Perry HD, and Dohlman CH: Oversize corneal donor grafts in penetrating keratoplasty, Ophthalmology 86:490, 1979.

Gasset AR: Lamellar keratoplasty in the treatment of keratoconus: conectomy, Ophthalmic Surg 10:26, 1979.

Gelender H: Corneal endothelial cell loss, cystoid macular edema, and iris-supported intraocular lenses, Ophthalmology 91:841, 1984.

Gundersen T: Conjunctival flaps in the treatment of corneal disease with reference to a new technique of application, Arch Ophthalmol 60:880, 1958.

Hagan JC: A comparative study of the 91Z and other anterior chamber intraocular lenses, Am Intraocul Implant Soc J 10:324, 1984.

Hagan JC: Complications while removing the IOLAB 91Z lens for the UGH-UGH+ syndrome, J Am Intraocul Implant Soc 10:209, 1984.

Hall JR and Muenzler WS: Intraocular lens replacement in pseudophakic bullous keratopathy, Trans Ophthalmol Soc UK 104:541, 1985.

Heidemann DG, Sugar A, Meyer RF, and Musch DC: Oversized donor grafts in penetrating keratoplasty: a randomized trial, Arch Ophthalmol 103:1807, 1985.

Hessburg PC and Barron M: A disposable corneal trephine, Ophthalmic Surg 11:730, 1980.

Hesse RJ, Smith AD, Roberts AD, and Mosteller C: The effect of carbachol combined with intraoperative viscoelastic substances on postoperative IOP response, Ophthalmic Surg 19:224, 1988.

Hu BV, Shin DH, Gibbs KA, and Hong YJ: Implantation of posterior chamber lens in the absence of capsular and zonular support, Arch Ophthalmol 106:416, 1988.

Kasner D: Vitrectomy: a new approach to the management of vitreous, Highlights of Ophthalmology 11:304, 1968.

Katz HR and Forster RK: Intraocular lens calculation in combined penetrating keratoplasty, cataract extraction and intraocular lens implantation, Ophthalmology 92:1203, 1985.

Kaufman HE: The correction of aphakia, Am J Ophthalmol 89:1, 1980.

Kaufman HE: Astigmatism after keratoplasty: possible cause and prevention, Am J Ophthalmol 94:556, 1982.

Kaufman HE and Katz JI: Endothelial damage from intraocular lens insertion, Invest Ophthalmol 15:996, 1976.

Kaufman HE, Varnell ED, and Kaufman S: Chondroitin sulfate in a new cornea preservation medium, Am J Ophthalmol 98:112, 1984.

Kaufman HE and Werblin TP: Epikeratophakia for the treatment of keratoconus, Am J Ophthalmol 93:342, 1982.

Kelley CG: Surgical management of postkeratoplasty astigmatism. In Kaufman HE, Barron BA, McDonald MB, and Waltman SR, editors: The cornea, New York, 1988, Churchill Livingstone.

enyon KR, Wagoner MD, and Hettinger ME: Conjunctival autograft transplantation for advanced and recurrent pterygium, Ophthalmology 92:1461, 1985.

Klyce SD and Beuerman RW: Structure and function of the cornea. In Kaufman HE, Barron BA, McDonald MB, and Waltman SR, editors: The cornea, New York, 1988, Churchill Livingstone.

Krachmer JH and Ching SST: Relaxing corneal incisions for postkeratoplasty astigmatism, Int Ophthalmol Clin 23:153, 1983.

Krachmer JH, and Fenzl RE: Surgical correction of high postkeratoplasty astigmatism: relaxing incisions vs wedge resection, Arch Ophthalmol 98:1400, 1980.

Lass JH, Stocker EG, Fritz ME, and Collie DM: Epikeratoplasty: the surgical correction of aphakia, myopia, and keratoconus, Ophthalmology 94:912, 1987.

correction of aphakia, myopia, and keratoconus, Ophthalmology 94:912, 1987.

Lavery GW and Linstrom RL: Clinical results of trapezoidal astigmatic keratotomy, J Refract Surg 1:70, 1985.

Lavery GW and Lindstrom RL: Trapezoidal astigmatic keratotomy in human cadaver eyes, J Refract Surg 1:18, 1985.

Lavery GW, Lindstrom RL, Hofer LA, and Doughman DJ: The surgical management of corneal astigmatism after penetrating keratoplasty, Ophthalmic Surg 16:165, 1985.

Laughrea PA and Arentsen JJ: Lamellar keratoplasty in the management of recurrent pterygium, Ophthalmic Surg 17:106, 1986.

Lemp MA, Pfister RR, and Dohlman CH: The effect of intraocular surgery on clear corneal grafts, Am J Ophthalmol 70:719, 1970.

Lindquist TD, Rubenstein JB, Rice SW, Williams PA, and Lindstrom RL: Trapezoidal astigmatic keratotomy: quantification in human cadaver eyes, Arch Ophthalmol 104:1534, 1986.

Machemer R, Parel JM, and Buettner H: A new concept for vitreous surgery. 1. Instrumentation, Am J Ophthalmol 73:1, 1972.

Mackman G and Brightbill FS: Combined penetrating keratoplasty and mechanical anterior vitrectomy, Ophthalmic Surg 11:330, 1980.

Maguire LJ: Corneal topography. In Kaufman HE, Barron BA, McDonald MB, and Waltman SR, editors: The cornea, New York, 1988, Churchill Livingstone.

Maguire LJ, Singer DE, and Klyce SD: Graphic presentation of computer analyzed keratoscope photographs, Arch Ophthalmol 105:223, 1987.

Mandel MR, Shapiro MB, and Krachmer JH: Relaxing incisions with augmentation sutures for the correction of postkeratoplasty astigmatism, Am J Ophthalmol 103:441, 1987.

Maxwell WA and Nordan LT: Trapezoidal relaxing incision for post keratoplasty astigmatism, Ophthalmic Surg 17:88, 1986.

McCarey BE and Kaufman HE: Improved corneal storage, Invest Ophthalmol 13:165, 1974.

McCartney DL, Whitney CE, Stark WJ, Wong SK, and Bernitsky DA: Refractive keratoplasty for disabling astigmatism after penetrating keratoplasty, Arch Ophthalmol 105:954, 1987.

McDonald MB, Kaufman HE, Aquavella JV, Durrie DS, Hiles DA, Hunkeler JD, Keates RH, Morgan KS, and Sanders DR: The nationwide study of epikeratophakia for aphakia in adults, Am J Ophthalmol 103:358, 1987.

McDonald MB, Kaufman HE, Aquavella JV, Durrie DS, Hiles DA, Hunkeler JD, Keates RH, Morgan KS, and Sanders DR: The nationwide study of epikeratophakia for myopia, Am J Ophthalmol 103:375, 1987.

McDonald MB, Kaufman HE, Durrie DS, Keates RH, Sanders DR, and the other medical monitors of the National Epikeratophakia Study: Epikeratophakia for keratoconus: the nationwide study, Arch Ophthalmol 104:1294, 1986.

McDonald MB, Klyce SD, Suarez H, Kandarakis A, Friedlander MH, and Kaufman HE: Epikeratophakia for myopia correction, Ophthalmology 92:1417, 1985.

McDonald MB, Koenig SB, Safir A, Friedlander MH, Morgan KS, Kaufman HE, and Granet N: Epikeratophakia: the surgical correction of aphakia: update, 1982, Ophthalmology 90:668, 1983.

McDonald MB, Koenig SB, Safir A, and Kaufman HE: On-lay lamellar keratoplasty for the treatment of keratoconus, Br J Ophthalmol 67:615, 1983.

McDonald MB, Safir A, Waring GO, Schlichtemeier WR, Kissling GE, and Kaufman HE: A preliminary comparative study of epikeratophakia or penetrating keratoplasty for keratoconus, Am J Ophthalmol 103:467, 1987.

McNeill JI, Goldman KN, and Kaufman HE: Combined scleral ring and blepharostat, Am J Ophthalmol 83:592, 1977.

McNeill JI and Kaufman H: Early visual rehabilitation after keratoplasty: a double running suture technique, Ann Ophthalmol 10:652, 1978.

Merck MP, Williams PA, and Lindstrom RL: Trapezoidal keratotomy: a vector analysis, Ophthalmology 93:719, 1986.

Morgon KS, Arffa RC, Marvelli TL, and Verity SM: Five year followup of epikeratophakia in children, Ophthalmology 93:423, 1986.

Morgan KS, McDonald MB, Hiles DA, Aquavella JV, Durrie DS, Hunkeler JD, Kaufman HE, Keates RH, and Sanders DR: The nationwide study of epikeratophakia for aphakia in children, Am J Ophthalmol 103:366, 1987.

Morgan KS, Stephenson GS, McDonald MB, and Kaufman HE: Epikeratophakia in children, Ophthalmology 91:780, 1984.

Morgan KS, Werblin TP, Asbell PA, Loupe DN, Friedlander MH, and Kaufman HE: The use of epikeratophakia grafts in pediatric monocular aphakia, J Pediatr Ophthalmol Strabismus 18:23, 1981.

Mosteller MW, Goosey JD, and Kaufman HE: Accidental heat destruction of corneal graft tissue, Am J Ophthalmol 98:380, 1984.

Olson RJ: Variation in corneal graft size related to trephine technique, Arch Ophthalmol 97:1323, 1979.

Olson RJ: The effect of scleral fixation ring placement and trephine tilting on keratoplasty wound size and donor shape, Ophthalmic Surg 12:23, 1981.

Olson RJ and Kaufman HE: A mathematical description of causative factors and prevention of elevated intraocular pressure after keratoplasty, Invest Ophthalmol Vis Sci 16:1085, 1977.

Pape LG: Intracapsular and extracapsular technique of lens implantation with Healon, Am Intraocul Implant Soc J 6:342, 1980.

Pearlman G, Susal AL, Hushaw J, and Bartlett RE: Recurrent pterygium and treatment with lamellar keratoplasty with presentation of a technique to limit recurrences, Ann Ophthalmol 2:763, 1970.

Phillips RL: Vacuum trephination of the hypotonous eye, Ophthalmic Surg 14:513, 1983.

Pievse D and Casey TA: Lamellar keratoplasty, Br J Ophthalmol 43:733, 1959.

Poirier RH and Fish JR: Lamellar keratoplasty for recurrent pterygium, Ophthalmic Surg 7:38, 1976.

Refojo MF, Dohlman CH, and Koliopoulos J: Adhesives in ophthalmology: a review, Surv Ophthalmol 15:217, 1971.

Richard JM, Paton D, and Gassett AR: A comparison of penetrating keratoplasty and lamellar keratoplasty in the surgical management of keratoconus, Am J Ophthalmol 86:807, 1978.

Robin JB, Gindi JJ, Koh K, Schanzlin DJ, Rao NA, York KK, and Smith RE: An update of the indications for penetrating keratoplasty: 1979 through 1983, Arch Ophthalmol 104:87, 1986.

Rowsey JJ: Curent concepts in astigmatism surgery, J Refract Surg 2:85, 1986.

Salz JJ, Rowsey JJ, Caroline P, Azen SP, Suter M, and Monlux R: A study of optical zone size and incision redeepening in experimental radial keratotomy, Arch Ophthalmol 103:590, 1985.

Sanders N: New treatment for bullous keratopathy: penetrating grafts and radical anterior vitrectomy, Highlights of Ophthalmology 11:296, 1968.

Sanders N: Penetrating corneal transplants for aphakic bullous keratopathy, South Med J 61:869, 1968.

Sanders N: Wedge resection in host cornea to correct post-keratoplasty astigmatism, Ophthalmic Surg 10:53, 1979.

Sanitato JJ, Kelley CG, and Kaufman HE: Surgical management of peripheral fungal keratitis (keratomycosis), Arch Ophthalmol 102:1506, 1984.

Sato T, Akiyama K, and Shibata H: A new surgical approach to myopia, Am J Ophthalmol 36:823, 1953.

Smith PW, Wong SK, Stark WJ, Gottsch JD, Terry AC, and Bonham RD: Complications of semiflexible closed-loop anterior chamber intraocular lenses, Arch Ophthalmol 105:52, 1987.

Smith RE, Beatty RF, and Clifford WS: Pseudophakic keratoplasty: posterior chamber lens implantation in the presence of ruptured capsule, Ophthalmic Surg 18:344, 1987.

Smith RE, McDonald HR, Nesburn AB, and Minckler DS: Penetrating keratoplasty: changing indications, 1947 to 1978, Arch Ophthalmol 98:1226, 1980.

Stainer GA, Perl T, and Binder PS: Controlled reduction of postkeratoplasty astigmatism, Ophthalmology 89:668, 1982.

Stark WJ, Goodman G, Goodman D, and Gottsch J: Posterior chamber intraocular lens implantation in the absence of posterior capsular support, Ophthalmic Surg 19:240, 1988.

Steinert RF and Wagoner MD: Long-term comparison of epikeratoplasty and penetrating keratoplasty for keratoconus, Arch Ophthalmol 106:493, 1988.

Sugar J and Kirk AK: Relaxing keratotomy for post-keratoplasty high astigmatism, Ophthalmic Surg 14:156, 1983.

Swinger CA: Keratomileusis for myopia. In Sanders DR, Hofmann RF, and Salz JJ, editors: Refractive corneal surgery, Thorofare, NJ, 1985, Charles B Slack, Inc.

Swinger CA: Keratophakia and keratomileusis for hyperopia. In Sanders DR, Hofmann RF, and Salz JJ, editors: Refractive corneal surgery, Thorofare, NJ, 1985, Charles B Slack, Inc.

Swinger CA: Postoperative astigmatism, Surv Ophthalmol 31:219, 1987.

Tanne E: Corneal trephines and cutting blocks. In Brightbill FS, editor: Corneal surgery: theory, technique, and tissue, St Louis, 1986, The CV Mosby Co.

Taylor DM, Stern AL, and McDonald PL: Combined procedures: long-term observations. In Brightbill FS, editor: Corneal surgery: theory, technique, and tissue, St Louis, 1986, The CV Mosby Co.

Terry AC and Stark WJ: Removal of closed-loop anterior chamber lens implants, Ophthalmic Surg 15:575, 1984.

Terry MA and Rowsey JJ: Dynamic shifts in corneal topography during the modified Ruiz procedure for astigmatism, Arch Ophthalmol 104:1611, 1986.

Thoft RA, Gordon JM, and Dohlman CH: Glaucoma following keratoplasty, Trans Am Acad Ophthalmol Otolaryngol 78:OP352, 1974.

Thornton SP: A guide to pachymeters, Ophthalmic Surg 15:993, 1984.

Thornton SP and Sanders DR: Graded nonintersecting transverse incisions for correction of idiopathic astigmatism, J Cataract Refract Surg 13:27, 1987.

Tragakis MP and Brown SI: The significance of anterior synechiae after corneal transplantation, Am J Ophthalmol 74:532, 1972.

Troutman RC: Microsurgical control of corneal astigmatism in cataract and keratoplasty, Trans Am Acad Ophthalmol Otolaryngol 27:563, 1973.

Troutman RC: Microsurgery of the anterior segment of the eye, vol 2, The cornea: optics and surgery, St Louis, 1977, The CV Mosby Co.

Troutman RC: Improved techniques in refractive surgery for astigmatism, Cornea 1:57, 1982.

Troutman RC: Corneal wedge resections and relaxing incisions for postkeratoplasty astigmatism, Int Ophthalmol Clin 23:161, 1983.

Troutman RC and Swinger C: Relaxing incision for control of postoperative astigmatism following keratoplasty, Ophthalmic Surg 11:117, 1980.

Uozato H and Guyton DL: Centering corneal surgical procedures, Am J Ophthalmol 103:264, 1987.

Urrets-Zavalia A: Fixed, dilated pupil, iris atrophy, and secondary glaucoma: a distinct clinical entity following penetrating keratoplasty in keratoconus, Am J Ophthalmol 56:257, 1963.

van Rij G, Cornell FM, Waring GO, Wilson LA, and Beekhuis WH: Postoperative astigmatism after central vs eccentric penetrating keratoplasties, Am J Ophthalmol 99:317, 1985.

van Rij G and Vijfvinkel G: Correction of postkeratoplasty astigmatism by razor blade and V-shaped knife wedge resection, Ophthalmic Surg 14:406, 1983.

Villaseñor RA: The history of radial keratotomy. In Sanders DR and Hofmann RF, editors: Refractive surgery: a text of radial keratotomy, Thorofare, NJ, 1985, Charles B Slack, Inc.

Villaseñor RA: Homoplastic keratomileusis for myopia. In Sanders DR, Hofmann RF, and Salz JJ, editors: Refractive corneal surgery, Thorofare, NJ, 1985, Charles B Slack, Inc.

Villaseñor RA, Salz J, Steel D, and Krasnow MA: Changes in corneal thickness during radial keratotomy, Ophthalmic Surg 12:341, 1981.

Waring GO: The changing status of radial keratotomy for myopia. Parts I and II, J Refract Surg 1:81, 119, 1985.

Waring GO: Management of pseudophakic corneal edema with reconstruction of the anterior ocular segment, Arch Ophthalmol 105:709, 1987.

Waring GO: Radial keratotomy. In Kaufman HE, Barron BA, McDonald MB, and Waltman SR, editors: The cornea, New York, 1988, Churchill Livingstone.

Waring GO, Moffitt SD, Gelender H, Laibson PR, Lindstrom RL, Myers WD, Obstbaum SA, Rowsey JJ, Safir A, Schanzlin DJ, Bourque LB, and the PERK Study Group: Rationale for and design of the National Eye Institute Prospective Evaluation of Radial Keratotomy (PERK) study, Ophthalmology 90:40, 1983.

Werblin TP, Kaufman HE, Friedlander MH, and Granet N: Epikeratophakia: the surgical correction of aphakia. III. Preliminary results of a prospective clinical trial, Arch Ophthalmol 99:1957, 1981.

Werblin TP, Kaufman HE, Friedlander MH, McDonald MB, and Sehon K: Epikeratophakia: the surgical correction of aphakia: update, 1981, Ophthalmology 89:916, 1982.

Werblin TP, Kaufman HE, Friedlander MH, Sehon K, McDonald MB, and Granet N: A prospective study of the use of hyperopic epikeratophakia grafts for the correction of aphakia in adults, Ophthalmology 88:1137, 1981.

Wiener M and Alvis BY: Transplantation of cornea by means of a mechanically obtained beveled-edge segment, Am J Ophthalmol 23:877, 1940.

Wong SK, Stark WJ, Gottsch JD, Bernitsky DA, and McCartney DL: Use of posterior chamber lenses in pseudophakic bullous keratopathy, Arch Ophthalmol 105:856, 1987.

Wood TO: Lamellar transplants in keratoconus, Am J Ophthalmol 83:543, 1977.

Yamaguchi T, Kanai A, Tanaka M, Ishii R, and Nakajima A: Bullous keratopathy after anterior-posterior radial keratotomy for myopia and myopic astigmatism, Am J Ophthalmol 93:600, 1982.

Zimmerman TJ, Krupin T, Grodzki W, Waltman SR, and Kaufman HE: Size of donor corneal button and outflow facility in aphakic eyes, Ann Ophthalmol 11:809, 1979.

Zimmerman T, Olson R, Waltman S, and Kaufman H: Transplant size and elevated intraocular pressure postkeratoplasty, Arch Ophthalmol 96:2231, 1978.

Zirm E: Eine erfolgreiche totale Keratoplastik, Arch Ophthalmol 64:580, 1906.

Chapter 6

Allansmith MR, Kerb DR, Greiner JV, et al: Giant papillary conjunctivitis in contact lens wearers, Am J Opthalmol 83:697, 1977.

Aquavella JV: Clinical experience with the Cardona keratoprosthesis, Cornea 2:177, 1983.

Aquavella JV, Rao GN, Brown AC, and Harris JK: Keratoprosthesis: results, complications, and management, Ophthalmology 89:655, 1982.

Bath PE: Keratoprosthesis: an alternative in anterior segment reconstruction, Am Intraocular Implant Soc J 6:126, 1980.

Bath PE, Fridge DL, Robinson K, and McCord RC: Photometric evaluation of YAG-induced polymethylmethacrylate damage in a keratoprosthesis, Am Intra-ocular Implant Soc J 11:253, 1985.

Bath PE, McCord RL, and Cox KC: Nd:YAG laser discission of retroprosthetic membrane: a preliminary report, Cornea 2:225, 1983.

Bath PE and Prendiville K: Keratoprosthesis in a clinically phthisical eye, Cornea 2:203, 1983.

Blencke A, Hagen P, Bromer H, and Deutscher K: Study of the use of glass ceramics in osteo-odontokeratoplasty, Ophthalmologica 176:105, 1978.

Cardona H: Keratoprosthesis, Am J Opthalmol 54:284, 1962.

Cardona H: Plastic keratoprostheses—human application. The Cornea World Congress, Washington, DC, 1965, Butterworth & Co.

Cardona H: Keratoprosthesis: elimination of light reflection from the walls of the optical cylinder, Int Ophthalmol Clin 6:111, Boston, 1966, Little, Brown & Co.

Cardona H: Prosthokeratoplasty: techniques and results, Corneoplastic Surgery, Proc Second International Corneo-Plastic Conference, Oxford and New York, 1969, Pergamon.

Cardona H: Prosthokeratoplasty, Cornea 2:179, 1983.

Cardona H, Castroviejo R, and DeVoe AG: The Cardona keratoprosthesis: first clinical evaluation, Acta XIX Cong. Ophthalmol 2:1211, 1962.

Cardona H and DeVoe, AG: Prosthokeratoplasty, Trans Am Acad Ophthalmol Otolaryngol 83:271, 1977.

Carroll CP and Keates RH: Bone formation in a periosteal graft, Arch Ophthalmol 97:916, 1983.

Choyce DP: Perforating keratoprosthesis, Trans Ophthalmol Soc UK 92:727, 1972.

Choyce DP: The Choyce 2-piece performing keratoprosthesis: 101 cases—1967-1976, Ophthalmol Surg 8:117, 1977.

DeVoe AG: Symposium keratoprosthesis: history, technique, and indications, Trans Am Acad Ophthalmol Otolaryngol 83:249, 1977.

Girard LJ: Keratoprosthesis, Cornea 2:207, 1983.

Girard LJ, Hawkins RS, Nieves R, et al: Keratoprosthesis: a 12 year follow-up, Trans Am Acad Ophthalmol Otolaryngol 83:252, 1977.

Greiner JV, Covington HI, and Allansmith MR: Surface morphology of giant papillary conjunctivitis in contact lens wearers, Am J Ophthalmol 85:242, 1978.

Harris JK, Rao GN, Aquavella JV, and Lottman LE: Keratoprosthesis: technique and instrumentation, Ann Ophthalmol 16:481, 1984.

Heimke G and Polack FM: Ceramic keratoprosthesis: biomechanics of extrusion in through the lid implantation, Cornea 2:197, 1983.

Kozarsky AL, Knight SH, and Waring GO: Clinical results with a ceramic keratoprosthesis placed through the eyelid, Ophthalmology 94:904, 1987.

Mazhdrakova I: Implantation of ungual particles in the eye tissue of rabbit, Bul Oftalmologiya (Sofia) 25:125, 1977.

Mondino BJ, Bath PE, Foos Y, et al: Absent meibomian glands in the ectrodactyly, ectodermal dysplasia, cleft lip-palate syndrome, Am J Ophthalmol 97:497, 1984.

Nussbaum, JN: Cornea artificialis, Munich, 1853, Carl Robert Schurich Press.

Olson RJ and Kaufman HE: An abscess associated with a through-the-lid keratoprosthesis one year after intraocular lens insertion, Ophthalmic Surg 11:203-205, 1980.

Polack F: Keratoprosthesis, Invest Ophthalmol 15:593, 1976.

Polack FM: Clinical results with a ceramic keratoprosthesis, Cornea 2:185, 1983.

Polack FM, editor: Keratoprosthesis conference, Cornea 2:229, 1983.

Polack FM and Heimke G: Ceramic keratoprosthesis, Ophthalmology 87:693, 1980.

Schimmelpfennig B: Study on the tissue compatibility of intracorneal horn lenses in experimental animals, Klin Monatsbl Augenheilkd 172:464, 1978.

Srinivasan BD, Jakobiec FA, Iwamoto T, and DeVoe AG: Giant papillary conjunctivitis with ocular prostheses, Arch Ophthalmol 87:892, 1979.

Stone W and Siderman M: The plastic artificial cornea (an 18 year study): basic principles. In Rycroft PV, editor: Corneo-plastic surgery, Oxford, 1967, Pergamon Press.

Stone W, Yasuda H, and Refojo MD: A 15 year study of the plastic artificial cornea: basic principles. In King JH and McTigue JW, editors: The Cornea World Congress, Washington, DC, 1965, Butterworth & Co.

Strampelli B: Osteo-odontoceratoprostesi, Ann Ottal 89:1039, 1963.

PART TWO

Allarakhia L, Knoll RL, and Lindstrom RL: Soft intraocular lenses, J Cataract Refract Surg 13:607, 1987.

Alpar JJ: A study of the anterior chamber before and after implantation of the Choyce Mark VIII lens, Am Intraocular Implant Soc J 6:363, 1980.

Apple DJ and Olson RJ: Closed-loop anterior chamber lenses, Arch Ophthalmol 105:19, 1987.

Beckman H: Bending of excessively long intra-ocular suture material by argon laser, Am J Ophthalmol 91:401, 1981.

Binkhorst CD, Kats A, Tijan TT, and Loones LH: Retinal accidents in pseudophakia: intraocular versus extracapsular surgery, Trans Am Acad Ophthalmol Otolaryngol 81:120, 1976.

Bloomberg LB: Administration of periocular anesthesia, J Cataract Refract Surg 12:677, 1986.

Bourne WM, Waller R, Liesegang T, and Brubaker R: Corneal trauma in intracapsular and extracapsular cataract extraction with lens implantation, Arch Ophthalmol 99:1375, 1981.

Bresnick GH: Eyes containing anterior chamber acrylic implants: pathological complications, Arch Ophthalmol 82:726, 1969.

Choyce DP: Intraocular lenses and implants, London, 1964, Lewis & Co, Ltd.

Choyce DP: The evolution of the anterior chamber implant up to, and including the Choyce Mark IX, Ophthalmology 86:177, 1979.

Choyce DP: The first 1000 Mark IX implants in the practice of the Regional Eye Centre, Southend General Hospital, Essex, England: 1978-1983, Contact Lens Assoc Ophthalmol J 10:218, 1984.

Clayman HM: Technique for insertion of the superior loop of the Shearing-style posterior chamber lens, Am Intra-Ocular Implant Soc J 4:383, 1980.

Clayman HM, Jaffe NS, Light DS, Jaffe MS, Cassady JC: Intraocular lenses, axial length and retinal detachment, Am J Ophthalmol 92:778, 1981.

Cohan BE: The broken nylon iris fixation suture, Am J Ophthalmol 93:507, 1982.

Cohan BE, Pearch AC, and Schwartz S: Broken nylon iris fixation sutures, Am J Ophthalmol 88:982, 1979.

Colvard DM, Mazzocco TR, Davidson B, Kratz RP, and Johnson SH: Technique for implanting secondary posterior chamber lenses, Am Intraocular Implant Soc J 9:463, 1983.

Cozean CH: A longer view of secondary intraocular lens implantation with special emphasis on the role of the vitreous, Am Intraocular Implant Soc J 6:361, 1980.

Cozean CH and Waltman SR: The effects of posterior chamber phacoemulsification and secondary Kelman anterior chamber implantation on the corneal endothelium, Am Intraocular Implant Soc J 7:237, 1981.

Curtin VT: Retinal detachment surgery following intraocular lens implantation, Trans Ophthalmol Soc NZ 30:45, 1978.

Davidson JA: Analysis of capsular bag defects and intraocular lens positions for consistent centration, J Cataract Refract Surg 12:124, 1986.

Davis DB II and Mandel MR: Posterior peribulbar anaesthesia: an alternative to retrobulbar anaesthesia, J Cataract Refract Surg 12:182, 1986.

Davis JL, Tsiligianni AK, Pflugfelder SC, Miller D, Flynn HW, and Forster RK: Coagulase negative staphylococcal endophthalmitis increase in antimicrobial resistance, Ophthalmology 95:1404, 1988.

Drews RC: Intermittent touch syndrome, Arch Ophthalmol 100:1440, 1982.

Drews RC: Polypropylene in the human eye, Am J Ophthalmol 93:507, 1982.

Eichenbaum DM, Jaffe NS, Clayman HM, and Light DS: Pars plana vitrectomy as a primary treatment for acute bacterial endophthalmitis, Am J Ophthalmol 86:167, 1978.

Elk JR, Wood J, and Holladay JT: Pulmonary edema following retrobulbar block, J Cataract Refract Surg 14:216, 1988.

Emery JM and Little JH: Phacoemulsification and aspiration of cataracts: surgical techniques, complications and results, St Louis, 1979, The CV Mosby Co.

Emery JM and McIntyre DJ: Extracapsular cataract surgery, St Louis, 1983, The CV Mosby Co.

Faulkner GD: Folding and inserting silicone intraocular lens implants, J Cataract Refract Surg 13:678-681, 1987.

Fechner PU: Laser-coagulation of ruptured fixation suture after lens-implantation, Am Intraocular Implant Soc J 4:54, 1978.

Feldman F and Stein H: Delayed glaucoma after implantation of a Choyce intraocular lens, Can J Ophthalmol 14:190, 1980.

Forster RK: Endophthalmitis: diagnostic cultures and visual results, Arch Ophthalmol 92:387, 1974.

Forster RK, Zachary IG, Cottingham AJ Jr, and Norton EWD: Further observations on the diagnosis, cause and treatment of endophthalmitis, Am J Ophthalmol 81:52, 1976.

Forster RK, Abbott RL, and Gelender H: Management of infectious endophthalmitis, Ophthalmology 87:313, 1980.

Friedberg HL and Kline OR Jr: Contralateral amaurosis after retrobulbar injection, Am J Ophthalmol 101:688, 1986.

Galin MA, Goldstein JM, Tuberville A, Perez HD, and Kaplan H: Intraocular lenses generate chemotactic activity in human serum: Binkhorst lecture, part III, Arch Ophthalmol 99:1434, 1981.

Galin MA, Poole TA and Obstbaum SA: Retinal detachment in pseudophakia, Am J Ophthalmol 88:49, 1979.

Gerding DN, Poley B, Hall WH, LeWin DP, and Clark MD: Treatment of pseudomonas endophthalmitis associated with prosthetic intraocular lens implantation, Am J Ophthalmol 88:902, 1979.

Girard LJ, Madero R, and Monasterio R: Complications of the Simcoe flexible loop phacoprostheses in the anterior chamber, Ophthalmic Surg 14:332, 1983.

Graether JM: A new method of inserting the J-loop posterior chamber lens to achieve capsular fixation and consistent centering, Am Intraocular Implant Soc J 7:70, 1981.

Hagan JC III: Complications while removing the IOLAB 91Z lens for the UGH-UGH$^+$ syndrome, Am Intraocular Implant Soc J 10:209, 1984.

Hales RH: Dislocation of the Kelman II anterior chamber intraocular lens, Am Intraocular Implant Soc J 8:376, 1982.

Handa J, Henry C, Krupin T, and Keates E: Extracapsular cataract extraction with posterior chamber lens implantation in patients with glaucoma, Arch Ophthalmol 105:765, 1987.

Heslin KB and Guerriero PN: Extracapsular cataract extraction and primary posterior chamber lens implantation, J Cataract Refract Surg 12:44, 1986.

Jaffe NS: Cataract surgery and its complications, ed 3, St Louis, 1981, The CV Mosby Co.

Jaffe NS and Clayman HM: Pathophysiology of corneal astigmatism after cataract extraction, Trans Am Acad Ophthalmol Otolaryngol 79:615, 1975.

Jaffe NS and Clayman HM: Cataract extraction in eyes with congenital colobomata, J Cataract Refract Surg 13:54, 1987.

Jaffe NS, Clayman HM, and Jaffe MS: Cystoid macular edema after intracapsular and extracapsular cataract extraction with and without an intraocular lens, Ophthalmology 89:25, 1981.

Jaffe NS, Clayman HM, and Jaffe MS: Retinal detachment in myopic eyes after intracapsular and extracapsular cataract extraction, Am J Ophthalmol 97:48, 1984.

Johnson SJ and Kratz RP: Improved technique for secondary anterior lens insertion, Am Intraocular Implant Soc J 8:267, 1982.

Jungschaffer OH: Retinal detachments after intraocular lens implants, Arch Ophthalmol 95:1203, 1977.

Kaufman HE and Katz JI: Endothelial damage from intraocular lens insertion, Invest Ophthalmol 15:996, 1976.

Kaufman HE and Katz JI: Effects of intraocular lens on the corneal endothelium, Trans Ophthalmol Soc UK 97:265, 1977.

Keates RH and Lichtenstein RB: Surgical complications of Choyce type implants, Ophthalmology 86:625, 1979.

Keates RH and Lichenstein RB: The Kelman and other anterior chamber lenses, Ophthalmic Surg 11:708, 1980.

Kelman CD: Phacoemulsification and aspiration: the Kelman technique of cataract removal, New York, 1975, Aesculapius Publishers Inc.

Klein RM, Katzin HM, and Yannuzi LA: The effect of indomethacin pretreatment of aphakic cystoid macular edema, Am J Ophthalmol 87:847, 1979.

Koenig SB, Snyder RW, and Kay J: Respiratory distress after a Nadbath block, Ophthalmology 95:1285, 1988.

Kokoris N and Macy JI: Laser iridectomy treatment of acute pseudophakic pupillary block glaucoma, Am Intraocular Implant Soc J 8:33, 1982.

Kraff MC, Sanders DR, and Lieberman HL: Specular microscopy in cataract and intraocular lens implantation, Arch Ophthalmol 98:1782, 1980.

Kraff MC, Sanders DR, and Lieberman HL: Monitoring for continuing endothelial cell loss with cataract extraction and intraocular lens implantation, Ophthalmology 89:30, 1982.

Kraff MC, Sanders DR, Peyman GA, Lieberman HL, and Tarabishy S: Slit-lamp fluorophotometry in intraocular lens patients, Ophthalmology 87:877, 1980.

Kraff MC, Sanders DR, and Raanan MG: A survey of intraocular lens explantations, J Cataract Refract Surg 12:644, 1986.

Kratz RP, Mazzocco TR, Davidson B, and Colvard DM: The Shearing intraocular lens: a report of 1,000 cases, Am Intraocular Implant Soc J 7:55, 1981.

Leibowitz HM, Laing RA, Chang R, Theodore JA, and Oak SS: Corneal edema secondary to vitreocorneal contact, Arch Ophthalmol 99:417, 1981.

Levy JH and Pisacano A: Initial clinical studies with silicone intraocular implants, J Cataract Refract Surg 14:294, 1988.

Lichter PR: Avoiding complications from local anesthesia, Ophthalmology 95:565, 1988.

Liesegang TJ, Bourne WM, and Ilstrup DM: Short and long term endothelial cell loss associated with cataract extraction and intraocular lens implantation, Am J Ophthalmol 97:32, 1984.

Lindstrom RL, Harris WS, and Lyle A: Secondary and exchange posterior chamber lens implantation, Am Intraocular Implant Soc J 8:355, 1982.

Lindstrom RL and Herman WK: Pupil capture: prevention and management, Am Intraocular Implant Soc J 9:201, 1983.

Lindstrom RL and Nelson JD: Anterior chamber lens subluxation through a basal peripheral iridectomy, Am Intraocular Implant Soc J 9:53, 1983.

Lindstrom RL, Nelson JD, and Neist RL: Anterior chamber lens subluxation through a basal peripheral iridectomy, Am Intraocular Implant Soc J 9:53, 1983.

Lippmann JI: Pupillary abnormalities associated with posterior chamber lens implantation, Ophthalmic Surg 13:197, 1982.

Mackool RJ: Closed vitrectomy and the intraocular implant, Ophthalmology 88:414, 1981.

Mackool RJ: Simultaneous closed vitrectomy and secondary intraocular lens implantation, Am Intraocular Implant Soc J 7:233, 1981.

Mackool RJ and Holtz J: Descemet membrane detachment, Arch Ophthalmol 95:459, 1977.

Mamalis N, Apple DJ, Brady SE, Notz RG, and Olson RJ: Pathological and scanning electron microscopic evaluation of the 91Z intraocular lens, Am Intraocular Implant Soc J 10:191, 1984.

Maynor RC Jr: Five cases of severe anterior chamber lens implant complications, Am Intraocular Implant Soc J 10:223, 1984.

Mazzocco TR, Kratz RP, Davidson B, and Colvard DM: Secondary posterior chamber intraocular lens implants, Am Intraocular Implant Soc J 7:341, 1981.

McCannel MA: A retrievable suture idea for anterior uveal problems, Ophthalmic Surg 7:98, 1976.

The Miami Study Group: Cystoid macular edema in aphakic and pseudophakic eyes, Am J Ophthalmol 88:45, 1979.

Mondino FJ and Rao H: Effect of intraocular lens on complement levels in human serum, Acta Ophthalmol 61:76, 1983.

Morgan CM, Schatz H, Vine AK, Cantrill HL, Davidorf FH, Gitter, KA, and Rudich R: Ocular complications associated with retrobulbar injections, Ophthalmology 95:660, 1988.

McGalliard JN: Respiratory arrest after two retrobulbar injections, Am J Ophthalmol 105:90, 1988.

McGuigan LJB, Gottsch J, Stark WJ, Maumenee AE, and Quigley HA: Extracapsular cataract extraction and posterior chamber lens implanation in eyes with preexisting glaucoma, Arch Ophthalmol 104:1301, 1986.

Neumann AC, Molyet E, Teal C, and McCarty G: Phacoemulsification devices: a consumer's update, J Cataract Refract Surg 13:669, 1987.

Obstbaum SA: Glaucoma and intraocular lens implantation, J Cataract Refract Surg 12:257, 1986.

Ostbaum SA and Galin MA: Cystoid macular and ocular inflammation: the corneoretinal inflammatory syndrome, Trans Ophthalmol Soc UK 99:187, 1979.

Olson RJ and Kolodner H: The position of the posterior chamber intraocular lens, Arch Ophthalmol 97:715, 1979.

Olson RJ, Sevel D, and Stevenson D: A histopathological study of the Choyce VIII intraocular lens, Am J Ophthalmol 92:781, 1981.

Pallin SL and Walman GB: Vitreous management during secondary implantation, Am Intraocular Implant Soc J 7:271, 1981.

Pallin SL and Waldman GB: Posterior chamber intraocular lens implant centration: in or out of "the bag," Am Intraocular Implant Soc J 8:254, 1982.

Pape LG: Intracapsular and extracapsular technique of lens implantation with Healon, Am Intraocular Implant Soc J 6:342, 1980.

Passo MS, Ernest JT, and Goldstick TK: Hyaluronate increases intraocular pressure when used in cataract extraction, Br J Ophthalmol 69:572, 1985.

Pearce JL: Sixteen months' experience with 140 posterior chamber intraocular lens implants, Br J Ophthalmol 61:310, 1977.

Percival SPB and Das SK: UGH syndrome after posterior chamber lens implantation, Am Intraocular Implant Soc J 9:200, 1983.

Percival SPB and Gillam AF: Central cornea guttata, age and specular microscopy, Am Intraocular Implant Soc J 6:347, 1980.

Pettitt TH, Olson RJ, Foos RY, and Martin WJ: Fungal endophthalmitis following intraocular lens implantation: a surgical epidemic, Arch Ophthalmol 98:1025, 1980.

Ramsay RC and Knobloch WH: Ocular perforation following retrobulbar anesthesia for retinal detachment surgery, Am J Ophthalmol 86:61, 1978.

Rao GN, Stevens RE, Harris JK, and Aquavella JV: Long-term changes in corneal endothelium following intraocular lens implantation, Ophthalmology 88:386, 1981.

Richburg FA: Anterior chamber lenses and severe segmental uveal ectropion, Am Intraocular Implant Soc J 7:328, 1981.

Rock RL and Rylander HG: Spontaneous iris retraction occurring after extracapsular cataract extraction and posterior lens implantation in patients with glaucoma, Am Intraocular Implant Soc J 9:45, 1983.

Sanders DR, Kraff MC, Lieberman HL, Peyman GA, and Tarabishy S: Breakdown and reestablishment of blood-aqueous barrier with implant surgery, Arch Ophthalmol 100:588, 1982.

Schneider ME, Milstein DE, Oyakawa RT, Ober RR, and Campo R: Ocular perforation from a retrobulbar injection, Am J Ophthalmol 106:35, 1988.

Shammas HJF and Milke CF: Cystoid macular edema following secondary lens implantation, Am Intraocular Implant Soc J 7:40, 1981.

Shearing SP: Evolution of the posterior chamber intraocular lens, Am Intraocular Implant Soc J 10:343, 1984.

Sheets JH and Maida JW: Lens glide in implant surgery, Arch Ophthalmol 96:145, 1978.

Shepard DD: Consultation selection, Am Intraocular Implant Soc J 9:60, 1983. (Editorial.)

Shields MB, Campbell DG, and Simmons RJ: The essential iris atrophies, Am J Ophthalmol 85:749, 1978.

Siepser SB and Kline OR Jr: Aborted posterior chamber intraocular lens insertions: a "second Choyce," Am Intraocular Implant Soc J 10:51, 1984.

Simcoe CW: Simcoe posterior chamber lens: theory, techniques and results, Am Intraocular Implant Soc J 7:155, 1981.

Simel PJ: Posterior chamber implants without iridectomy, Am Intraocular Implant Soc J 8:141, 1982.

Sinskey RM and Patel J: Posterior chamber intraocular lens implants in children: report of a series, Am Intraocular Implant Soc J 9:157, 1983.

Skorpik C, Menapace R, Gnad HD, Grasl M, and Scheidel W: Evaluation of 50 silicone posterior chamber lens implantations, J Cataract Refract Surg 13:640, 1987.

Skuta GL, Parrish RK, Hodapp E, Forster RK, and Rockwood EJ: Zonular dialysis during extracapsular cataract extraction in pseudoexfoliation syndrome, Arch Ophthalmol 105:632, 1987.

Stanley JA, Shearing SP, Anderson RR, Avallone AN: Endothelial cell density after posterior chamber lens implantation, Ophthalmology 87:381, 1980.

Taylor DM, Atlas BF, Romanchuk KG, and Stern A: Pseudophakic bullous keratopathy, Ophthalmology 90:19, 1983.

Terry AC and Stark WJ: Removal of closed-loop anterior chamber lens implants, Ophthalmic Surg 15:575, 1984.

Van Buskirk EM: Pupillary block after intraocular lens implantation, Am J Ophthalmol 95:55, 1983.

Vastine DW, Weinberg RS, Sugar J, and Binder PS: Stripping of Descemet's membrane associated with intraocular lens implantation, Arch Ophthalmol 101:1042, 1983.

Waltman SR: Penetrating keratoplasty for pseudophakic bullous keratopathy, Arch Ophthalmol 99:415, 1981.

Wang HS: Management of a posterior capsule rupture in planned extracapsular cataract extraction and posterior chamber lens implantation, J Cataract Refract Surg 12:73, 1986.

Wang HS: Peribulbar anesthesia for ophthalmic procedures, J Cataract Refract Surg 14:441, 1988.

Wiley RG, Neville RG, and Martin WG: Late postoperative hemorrhage following intracapsular cataract extraction with the IOLAB 91Z anterior chamber lens, Am Intraocular Implant Soc J 9:466, 1983.

Woodhams JT, Maddox R, Hunkeler JD, Bruhl D, Lester JC, Key C, Knolle G Jr, and Sheets J: A review of 1,147 cases of Sheets lens implantations, Am Intraocular Implant Soc J 10:185, 1984.

Worst JGF: Iris sutures for artificial lens fixation: Perlon vs. stainless steel, Trans Am Acad Ophthalmol Otolaryngol 81: OP 102, 1976.

PART THREE

Abraham RK and Miller GL: Outpatient argon laser iridectomy for angle-closure glaucoma: a two-year study, Trans Am Acad Ophthalmol Otolaryngol 79:529, 1975.

Barkan O: Operation for congenital glaucoma, Am J Ophthalmol 25:552, 1942.

Barkan O: Goniotomy for the relief of congenital glaucoma, Br J Ophthalmol 32:701, 1948.

Barkan O: Surgery of congenital glaucoma, Am J Ophthalmol 37:1523, 1953.

Cairns JE: Trabeculectomy: preliminary report of a new method, Am J Ophthalmol 66:673, 1968.

Coleman DJ, Lizzi FL, Driller J, et al: Therapeutic ultrasound in the treatment of glaucoma. II. Clinical applications, Ophthalmology 92:347, 1985.

Curran EJ: A new operation for glaucoma involving a new principle of aetiology and treatment of chronic primary glaucoma, Arch Ophthalmol 49:131, 1920.

David R, Livingston DG, and Luntz MH: Ocular hypertension—a long-term follow-up of treated and untreated patients, Br J Ophthalmol 61: 668, 1977.

Duke-Elder S: System of ophthalmology, London, 1969, Henry Kimpton, vol. XI.

Fankhauser F: The Q-switched laser: principles and clinical results. In Trokel SL, editor: YAG laser ophthalmic microsurgery, Norwalk, CT, 1983, Appleton-Century-Crofts.

François J: Combined operation for cataract and glaucoma, Ophthalmologica 177:158, 1978.

Gregersen E and Kessing SV: Congenital glaucoma before and after the introduction of microsurgery, Acta Ophthalmol 55:422, 1977.

Harrison R: Glaucoma in the aphakic eye. In Jakobiec F and Sigelman J: Advanced techniques in ocular surgery, Philadelphia, 1984, WB Saunders Co.

Hoskins HD, Shaffer RN, and Hetherington J: Anatomical classification of the developmental glaucomas, Arch Ophthalmol 102(9):1331, 1984.

Jerndal T: Dominant goniodysgenesis with late congenital glaucoma, Am J Ophthalmol 74:28, 1972.

Jerndal T and Lundstrom M: Trabeculectomy combined with cataract extraction, Am J Ophthalmol 81:227, 1976.

Klapper RM: The role of neodymium:YAG laser in microsurgery of the glaucomas, Int Ophthalmol Clin 25(3):101, 1985.

Krejci L, Harrison R, and Wichterle O: Hydroxyethyl methacrylate capillary strip: animal trials with a new glaucoma drainage device, Arch Ophthalmol 84:76, 1970.

Krupin T, Kaufman P, Mandell A, et al: Filtering valve implant surgery for eyes with neovascular glaucoma, Am J Ophthalmol 89:338, 1980.

Lowe RF: Primary angle-closure glaucoma, Br J Ophthalmol 51:727, 1967.

Luntz MH: Angle-closure glaucoma. In Turtz AI: Ophthalmology, St. Louis, 1969, The CV Mosby Co, vol 1.

Luntz MH: Congenital, infantile and juvenile glaucoma, Trans Am Acad Ophthalmol Otolaryngol 86:793, 1979.

Luntz MH: Surgical management of aphakic glaucoma, Doc Ophthalmol Proc Ser 21:793, 1979.

Luntz MH: Congenital, infantile, and juvenile glaucoma, Ophthalmology (Rochester) 86:793, 1979.

Luntz MH: Advances in glaucoma: surgical techniques. In Boyd BF: Highlights of ophthalmology, 1981, vol 2; Box 1189, Panama 1, Republic of Panama.

Luntz MH and Berlin MS: Combined trabeculectomy and cataract extraction, Trans Ophthalmol Soc UK 100:533, 1980.

Luntz MH, Harrison R, and Schenker HI: Glaucoma surgery, Baltimore, 1984, The Williams & Wilkins Co.

Luntz MH and Livingston DG: Trabeculectomy ab externo and trabeculotomy in congenital and adult-onset glaucoma, Am J Ophthalmol 83:174, 1977.

Luntz MH and Schenker HI: Retinal vascular accidents in glaucoma and ocular hypertension, Surv Ophthalmol 25:163, 1980.

McGuigan LJB, Luntz MH, Freedman J, and Harrison R: The role of subscleral Scheie procedure in glaucoma surgery, Ophthalmic Surg 17(12):802, 1986.

McPherson SD: Result of external trabeculotomy, Am J Ophthalmol 76:918, 1973.

Molteno ACB: New implant for drainage in glaucoma: animal trial, Br J Ophthalmol 53:161, 1969.

Molteno ACB, Van Biljon G, and Ancker E: Two-stage insertion of glaucoma drainage implants, Trans Ophthalmol Soc NZ 31:17, 1979.

Molteno ACB and Luntz MH: The use of plastic in glaucoma surgery, Proc First Int S Afr Ophthalmolog Symp, p 125, Durban, 1969, Butterworth Pubs.

Nauman GOH: Direct pars plicata diathermy. In Heilmann K and Paton D, editors: Atlas of ophthalmic surgery, Stuttgart and New York, 1987, Georg Thieme Verlag, vol 2.

Pollack IP: Use of argon laser energy to produce iridotomies, Trans Am Ophthalmol Soc 77:674, 1979.

Ritch R: A new lens for argon laser trabeculoplasty, Ophthalmic Surg 16(5):331, 1985.

Schwartz AL, Whitten ME, Bleiman B, et al: Argon laser trabecular surgery in uncontrolled phakic open-angle glaucoma, Ophthalmology (Rochester) 88:203, 1981.

Shields MB and Simmons RJ: Combined cyclodialysis and cataract extraction, Ophthalmic Surg 7:62, 1976.

Smith RJ: A new technique for opening the canal of Schlemm, Br J Ophthalmol 44:370, 1960.

Smith RJ: Medical versus surgical therapy in glaucoma simplex, Br J Ophthalmol 56:277, 1972.

Sugar HS: Experimental trabeculectomy in glaucoma, Am J Ophthalmol 51:623, 1961.

Sugar HS: The filtering operations—past, present, and future, Int Ophthalmol Clin 21:1, 1981.

Ticho U and Zauberman H: Argon laser application to the angle structures in the glaucomas, Arch Ophthalmol 94:61, 1976.

Wilensky JT and Jampol LM: Laser therapy for open-angle glaucoma, Ophthalmology (Rochester) 88:213, 1981.

Wise JB: Glaucoma treatment by trabecular tightening with the argon laser, Int Ophthalmol Clin 21:69, 1981.

Wise JB and Witter LS: Argon laser therapy for open-angle glaucoma: a pilot study, Arch Ophthalmol 97:319, 1979.

Yablonski ME, Masonson HN, el-Sayyad F, Dennis PH, Hargrave S, and Coleman DJ: Use of therapeutic ultrasound to restore failed trabeculectomies, Am J Ophthalmol 103(4):492, 1987.

PART FOUR

Chapter 18

Harada M and Ito Y: Surgical correction of cyclotropia, Jpn J Ophthalmol 8:88, 1964.

Helveston EM and Birchler C: Class VII superior oblique palsy: subclassification and treatment suggestions, Am Orthoptic J 32:104, 1982.

PART SIX

Benson WE: Retinal detachment, Hagerstown, Md, 1980, Harper & Row, Publishers.

Delaney WV Jr, Torrisi PF, Hampton GR, Hay PB, and Hart K: Complications of scleral buckling procedures, Arch Ophthalmol 105:702, 1987.

Gass JDM: Stereoscopic atlas of macular diseases, St Louis, 1987, The CV Mosby Co.

Kaplan HJ: Immunology of retinal and choroidal disease. In Tso MOM, editor: Retinal diseases, Philadelphia, 1988, JB Lippincott Co.

Michels RG: Vitreous surgery, St Louis, 1981, The CV Mosby Co.

Michels RJ: Vitrectomy, St Louis, 1985, The CV Mosby Co.

Schepens CL: Retinal detachment, Philadelphia, 1984, WB Saunders Co.

Sigelman J: Advanced management and photocoagulation of peripheral retinal diseases. In Jakobiec F and Sigelman J: Advanced techniques in ocular surgery, Philadelphia, 1984, WB Saunders Co.

Sigelman J: Retinal diseases: pathogenesis, laser therapy, and surgery, Boston, 1984, Little, Brown & Co.

Tso MOM, editor: Retinal diseases, Philadelphia, 1988, JB Lippincott Co.

Index

Page numbers in *italics* indicate illustrations.

U

V